AF341982

RETINA
Medical and Surgical Management

RETINA
Medical and Surgical Management

Editor-in-Chief

Atul Kumar MD FAMS FRCS (Ed)
Professor and Chief
Dr Rajendra Prasad Centre for Ophthalmic Sciences
All India Institute of Medical Sciences
New Delhi, India

Assistant Editor

Raghav Ravani MD FICO
Dr Rajendra Prasad Centre for Ophthalmic Sciences
All India Institute of Medical Sciences
New Delhi, India

Foreword

Shunji Kusaka MD

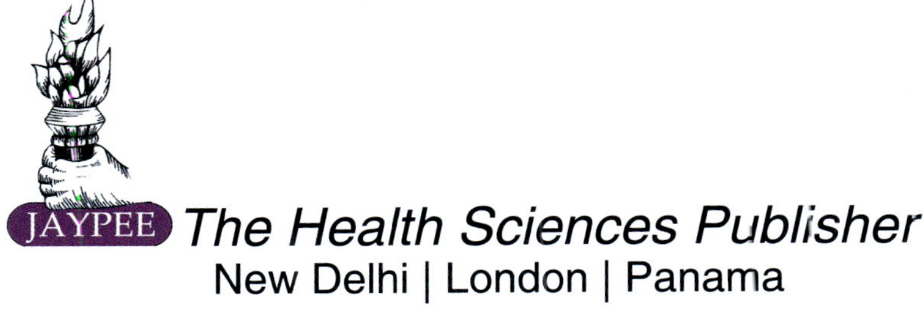

JAYPEE *The Health Sciences Publisher*
New Delhi | London | Panama

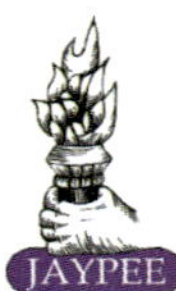 **Jaypee Brothers Medical Publishers (P) Ltd**

Headquarters
Jaypee Brothers Medical Publishers (P) Ltd.
4838/24, Ansari Road, Daryaganj
New Delhi 110 002, India
Phone: +91-11-43574357
Fax: +91-11-43574314
E-mail: jaypee@jaypeebrothers.com

Overseas Offices

JP Medical Ltd.
83 Victoria Street, London
SW1H 0HW (UK)
Phone: +44-20 3170 8910
Fax: +44(0)20 3008 6180
E-mail: info@jpmedpub.com

Jaypee-Highlights Medical Publishers Inc.
City of Knowledge, Bld. 235, 2nd Floor, Clayton
Panama City, Panama
Phone: +1 507-301-0496
Fax: +1 507-301-0499
E-mail: cservice@jphmedical.com

Jaypee Brothers Medical Publishers (P) Ltd.
17/1-B, Babar Road, Block-B, Shyamoli
Mohammadpur, Dhaka-1207
Bangladesh
Mobile: +08801912003485
E-mail: jaypeedhaka@gmail.com

Jaypee Brothers Medical Publishers (P) Ltd.
Bhotahity, Kathmandu, Nepal
Phone: +977-9741283608
E-mail: kathmandu@jaypeebrothers.com

Website: www.jaypeebrothers.com
Website: www.jaypeedigital.com

Inquiries for bulk sales may be solicited at: jaypee@jaypeebrothers.com

Retina: Medical and Surgical Management

First Edition: **2018**

ISBN: 978-93-5270-294-7

Printed at: Sanat Printers

Dedication

Dedicated to my late loving parents whose blessings helped me continue my work with dedication and passion to its conclusion, and to my wonderful family Parul, Aman and Aarshi whose positive attitude and encouragement was always there with me through these tough over 2 years that it took to write this useful textbook on 'RETINA'.

Contributors

Divya Agarwal MBBS
Dr Rajendra Prasad Centre for
Ophthalmic Sciences
All India Institute of Medical Sciences
New Delhi, India

Sumeet Agarwal MS FVRS
Narayana Nethralaya
Bengaluru, Karnataka, India

Sahil Agrawal MD
Dr Rajendra Prasad Centre for
Ophthalmic Sciences
All India Institute of Medical Sciences
New Delhi, India

Rajendra S Apte MD PhD
Translational Research and
Jeffrey Fort Innovation Fund
Washington University School of Medicine
St Louis, Missouri, USA

Yamini Attiku MD
Dr Rajendra Prasad Centre for
Ophthalmic Sciences
All India Institute of Medical Sciences
New Delhi, India

Mayank Bansal MD
Dr Rajendra Prasad Centre for
Ophthalmic Sciences
All India Institute of Medical Sciences
New Delhi, India

Reema Bansal MS
Advanced Eye Center
Department of Ophthalmology
Postgraduate Institute of Medical
Education and Research
Chandigarh, India

Aswini Behera MD
Dr Rajendra Prasad Centre for
Ophthalmic Sciences
All India Institute of Medical Sciences
New Delhi, India

Shashwat Behera MD
Dr Rajendra Prasad Centre for
Ophthalmic Sciences
All India Institute of Medical Sciences
New Delhi, India

Pramod S Bhende MS
Sankara Nethralaya
Shri Bhagwan Mahavir
Vitreoretinal Services
Chennai, Tamil Nadu, India

Anand S Brar MBBS
Dr Rajendra Prasad Centre for
Ophthalmic Sciences
All India Institute of Medical Sciences
New Delhi, India

Parijat Chandra MD
Dr Rajendra Prasad Centre for
Ophthalmic Sciences
All India Institute of Medical Sciences
New Delhi, India

Rohan Chawla MD FRCS (Glasg)
Dr Rajendra Prasad Centre for
Ophthalmic Sciences
All India Institute of Medical Sciences
New Delhi, India

Annu Chohan MSc
Dr Rajendra Prasad Centre for
Ophthalmic Sciences
All India Institute of Medical Sciences
New Delhi, India

Nagesha CK MS
Sankara Nethralaya
Shri Bhagwan Mahavir
Vitreoretinal Services
Chennai, Tamil Nadu, India

Kaustubh Deshmukh MS
Sankara Nethralaya
Shri Bhagwan Mahavir
Vitreoretinal Services
Chennai, Tamil Nadu, India

Chirakshi Dhull MD
Dr Rajendra Prasad Centre for
Ophthalmic Sciences
All India Institute of Medical Sciences
New Delhi, India

Mangat R Dogra MS
Advanced Eye Center
Department of Ophthalmology
Postgraduate Institute of Medical
Education and Research
Chandigarh, India

Mohit Dogra MS
Advanced Eye Center
Department of Ophthalmology
Postgraduate Institute of Medical
Education and Research
Chandigarh, India

Kavitha Duraipandi MD
Dr Rajendra Prasad Centre for
Ophthalmic Sciences
All India Institute of Medical Sciences
New Delhi, India

Amit Gadkar MD
Dr Rajendra Prasad Centre for
Ophthalmic Sciences
All India Institute of Medical Sciences
New Delhi, India

Meghal Gagrani MBBS
Dr Rajendra Prasad Centre for
Ophthalmic Sciences
All India Institute of Medical Sciences
New Delhi, India

Itika Garg MD
Dr Rajendra Prasad Centre for
Ophthalmic Sciences
All India Institute of Medical Sciences
New Delhi, India

Neha Goel MS
ICARE Eye Hospital and
Postgraduate Institute
Noida, Uttar Pradesh, India

Siddhi Goel MD
Dr Rajendra Prasad Centre for
Ophthalmic Sciences
All India Institute of Medical Sciences
New Delhi, India

Amod Gupta MS
Advanced Eye Center
Department of Ophthalmology
Postgraduate Institute of Medical
Education and Research
Chandigarh, India

Vishali Gupta MS
Advanced Eye Center
Department of Ophthalmology
Postgraduate Institute of Medical
Education and Research
Chandigarh, India

Yogita Gupta MD
Dr Rajendra Prasad Centre for
Ophthalmic Sciences
All India Institute of Medical Sciences
New Delhi, India

Nasiq Hasan MD
Dr Rajendra Prasad Centre for
Ophthalmic Sciences
All India Institute of Medical Sciences
New Delhi, India

Astha Jain MS
Narayana Nethralaya
Bengaluru, Karnataka, India

Shreyans Jain MD
Dr Rajendra Prasad Centre for
Ophthalmic Sciences
All India Institute of Medical Sciences
New Delhi, India

Chaitra Jayadev MS
Narayana Nethralaya
Bengalure, Karnataka, India

Hemant K Joshi MOptom
Dr Rajendra Prasad Centre for
Ophthalmic Sciences
All India Institute of Medical Sciences
New Delhi, India

Prateek Kakkar MD
Dr Rajendra Prasad Centre for
Ophthalmic Sciences
All India Institute of Medical Sciences
New Delhi, India

Deeksha Katoch MS
Advanced Eye Center
Department of Ophthalmology
Postgraduate Institute of Medical
Education and Research
Chandigarh, India

Alisha Kishore MD
Dr Rajendra Prasad Centre for
Ophthalmic Sciences
All India Institute of Medical Sciences
New Delhi, India

Aman Kumar MBBS
Advanced Eye Center
Department of Ophthalmology
Postgraduate Institute of Medical
Education and Research
Chandigarh, India

Atul Kumar MD FAMS FRCS (Ed)
Professor and Chief
Dr Rajendra Prasad Centre for
Ophthalmic Sciences
All India Institute of Medical Sciences
New Delhi, India

Naveen Kumar BCom
Dr Rajendra Prasad Centre for
Ophthalmic Sciences
All India Institute of Medical Sciences
New Delhi, India

Pradeep Kumar MS
Dr Rajendra Prasad Centre for
Ophthalmic Sciences
All India Institute of Medical Sciences
New Delhi, India

Vinod Kumar MD
Dr Rajendra Prasad Centre for
Ophthalmic Sciences
All India Institute of Medical Sciences
New Delhi, India

Devesh Kumawat MD
Dr Rajendra Prasad Centre for
Ophthalmic Sciences
All India Institute of Medical Sciences
New Delhi, India

Suman Lata MBBS
Dr Rajendra Prasad Centre for
Ophthalmic Sciences
All India Institute of Medical Sciences
New Delhi, India

Ashish Markan MD
Dr Rajendra Prasad Centre for
Ophthalmic Sciences
All India Institute of Medical Sciences
New Delhi, India

Thirumalesh MB MD
Narayana Nethralaya
Bengaluru, Karnataka, India

Aditi Mehta MD
Dr Rajendra Prasad Centre for
Ophthalmic Sciences
All India Institute of Medical Sciences
New Delhi, India

Aditya Modi DNB FVRS
Narayana Nethralaya
Bengaluru, Karnataka, India

Kabiruddin Molla BOptom
Dr Rajendra Prasad Centre for
Ophthalmic Sciences
All India Institute of Medical Sciences
New Delhi, India

Cynthia Montana MD PhD
Translational Research and
Jeffrey Fort Innovation Fund
Washington University School of Medicine
St Louis, Missouri, USA

Vineet Mutha MD
Dr Rajendra Prasad Centre for
Ophthalmic Sciences
All India Institute of Medical Sciences
New Delhi, India

Ajay Panwar DOpt
Dr Rajendra Prasad Centre for
Ophthalmic Sciences
All India Institute of Medical Sciences
New Delhi, India

Karthikeya R MD
Dr Rajendra Prasad Centre for
Ophthalmic Sciences
All India Institute of Medical Sciences
New Delhi, India

Priyanka Ramesh MD
Dr Rajendra Prasad Centre for
Ophthalmic Sciences
All India Institute of Medical Sciences
New Delhi, India

Raghav Ravani MD FICO
Dr Rajendra Prasad Centre for
Ophthalmic Sciences
All India Institute of Medical Sciences
New Delhi, India

Manasa S MD
Dr Rajendra Prasad Centre for
Ophthalmic Sciences
All India Institute of Medical Sciences
New Delhi, India

Pranita Sahay MD
Dr Rajendra Prasad Centre for
Ophthalmic Sciences
All India Institute of Medical Sciences
New Delhi, India

Nitesh Salunkhe MD
Dr Rajendra Prasad Centre for
Ophthalmic Sciences
All India Institute of Medical Sciences
New Delhi, India

Parveen Sen MS
Sankara Nethralaya
Shri Bhagwan Mahavir
Vitreoretinal Services
Chennai, Tamil Nadu, India

Sagnik Sen MBBS
Dr Rajendra Prasad Centre for
Ophthalmic Sciences
All India Institute of Medical Sciences
New Delhi, India

Anin Sethi MD
Dr Rajendra Prasad Centre for
Ophthalmic Sciences
All India Institute of Medical Sciences
New Delhi, India

Manthan Shah MD PhD
Translational Research and
Jeffrey Fort Innovation Fund
Washington University School of Medicine
St Louis, Missouri, USA

Pooja Shah MD
Dr Rajendra Prasad Centre for
Ophthalmic Sciences
All India Institute of Medical Sciences
New Delhi, India

Farin Shaikh MD
Dr Rajendra Prasad Centre for
Ophthalmic Sciences
All India Institute of Medical Sciences
New Delhi, India

Nawazish Shaikh MBBS
Dr Rajendra Prasad Centre for
Ophthalmic Sciences
All India Institute of Medical Sciences
New Delhi, India

Sufiyan Shaikh MS
Sankara Nethralaya
Shri Bhagwan Mahavir
Vitreoretinal Services
Chennai, Tamil Nadu, India

Anu Sharma MOptom
Dr Rajendra Prasad Centre for
Ophthalmic Sciences
All India Institute of Medical Sciences
New Delhi, India

Abhishek Sheemar MD
Dr Rajendra Prasad Centre for
Ophthalmic Sciences
All India Institute of Medical Sciences
New Delhi, India

Sharan Shetty MS
Sankara Nethralaya
Shri Bhagwan Mahavir
Vitreoretinal Services
Chennai, Tamil Nadu, India

Sriram Simakurthy MD
Dr Rajendra Prasad Centre for
Ophthalmic Sciences
All India Institute of Medical Sciences
New Delhi, India

Shilky Singh MOptom
Dr Rajendra Prasad Centre for
Ophthalmic Sciences
All India Institute of Medical Sciences
New Delhi, India

Ankita Srivastava MOptom
Dr Rajendra Prasad Centre for
Ophthalmic Sciences
All India Institute of Medical Sciences
New Delhi, India

Neha Pareka Sudhakar MS
Narayana Nethralaya
Bengaluru, Karnataka, India

Dheepak Sundar MD
Dr Rajendra Prasad Centre for
Ophthalmic Sciences
All India Institute of Medical Sciences
New Delhi, India

Abhidnya Surve MD
Dr Rajendra Prasad Centre for
Ophthalmic Sciences
All India Institute of Medical Sciences
New Delhi, India

Akshay Tayade MD
Dr Rajendra Prasad Centre for
Ophthalmic Sciences
All India Institute of Medical Sciences
New Delhi, India

Stanford C Taylor MD PhD
Translational Research and
Jeffrey Fort Innovation Fund
Washington University School of Medicine
St Louis, Missouri, USA

Ruchir Tewari MD
Dr Rajendra Prasad Centre for
Ophthalmic Sciences
All India Institute of Medical Sciences
New Delhi, India

Jaya Prakash V MD
Sankara Nethralaya
Shri Bhagwan Mahavir
Vitreoretinal Services
Chennai, Tamil Nadu, India

Foreword

It is a great honor and pleasure for me to be invited to write the foreword for book '*Retina: Medical and Surgical Management*' by Prof Atul Kumar. Professor Kumar is currently the Chief and Professor of Ophthalmology at Dr Rajendra Prasad Centre for Ophthalmic Sciences (RPC-AIIMS), the national apex ophthalmic center at All India Institute of Medical Sciences in New Delhi, India. He is a renowned retina specialist, particularly in vitreoretinal surgery for various diseases such as macular holes, retinal detachment, myopic traction maculopathy and so forth. In 2007, he was awarded the Padma Shri, the fourth highest civilian award in India for his contribution to the field of medicine. In 2016, he was appointed Honorary Advisor Ophthalmology to the Government of India. To date, he has published more than 260 articles, 16 book chapters and 5 books. Fortunately, I had an opportunity to become acquainted with him recently, and I soon realized how sincerely dedicated he is to ophthalmology practice, research and education. I believe that this book has been accomplished through his extraordinary passion for education, particularly of young physicians who wish to acquire the cutting-edge knowledge of the retina. Needless to say, this book also represents the efforts of many distinguished contributing authors.

After reading through the manuscript, I am convinced that this is the ideal textbook for ophthalmology residents, retina fellows and even for senior retina specialists, who want to update their knowledge of retinal diseases and treatment within a relatively short time. The content is condensed, yet core information is never omitted.

In Section 1, essential information related to the basics of science and clinical knowledge, such as the imaging findings and electrophysiology of the retina are described. From Sections 2 to 9, the pathophysiology and medical and surgical treatments of various retinal disorders are discussed in detail. Readers will appreciate the presence of many high-quality images and illustrations throughout this book, which will facilitate greater reader comprehension. This is certainly a 'must-have' textbook for clinicians to improve their understanding of retinal diseases.

Shunji Kusaka MD
Professor
Kindai University Sakai Hospital
Osaka, Japan

Preface

It was about 2 years ago that I conceived the idea of a comprehensive textbook on retina for residents and vitreoretinal fellows, and also a reference book to flip through, lying on the desk of the practicing Ophthalmologist and so decided to put down my thoughts and ideas of all what I see and do daily since the last 30 years into a book-form.

I have always been passionate about Retina as a sub-specialty since my residency days at RP Centre and this amazing field of vitreoretinal disease where rapid changes in technology meets newer techniques and continues to evolve rapidly expanding itself into a complex practice of ophthalmic medicine and surgery that utilizes a wide range of diagnostic and therapeutic modalities to treat ocular diseases. From case reports to phase 3 multicenter clinical trials, published data continues to accumulate in exponential fashion. As a result it is increasingly difficult for the clinician dealing with vitreoretinal disease, both general and specialist alike to apply the amassed information to patient care.

This textbook is primarily intended to provide the ophthalmology resident and practicing comprehensive ophthalmologist with an up-to-date, clinically oriented source that covers the full spectrum of medical and surgical vitreoretinal disease. Subspecialists in the field should also find it useful as a review and selected reference.

Although this text is meant to be comprehensive, we have tried to highlight the essential, clinically important aspects of vitreoretinal medical and surgical practice. Chapter dealing with disease state emphasize clinical feature, diagnosis, and management. Entire chapters are devoted to the most commonly encountered problems.

The text is divided into 9 sections, each section having many chapters in a systematic fashion devoted to the various retinal diseases and their signs, symptoms and management. The latest imaging platforms with illustrations and surgical techniques have been described in this new textbook of Retinal diseases. Assembling a textbook that attempts to have the chapters both current and detailed in content along with uniform layout requires a special effort from all the contributors to adhere to strict guidelines and I am grateful to all those invited to participate in the writing of this textbook for their applaudable efforts.

About the Book: An Introduction

This book is intended to serve as an in-depth textbook and guide for understanding the subject of retina and vitreous and the diseases related to it with well-illustrated colored images and all the recent updates. It is broadly divided into 9 sections with relevant chapters in each section. Section I is dedicated to Basic sciences and Diagnostics and covers useful anatomy and physiology of the eye, the all important retinal imaging with the latest imaging platforms and crisp pictures of retinal diseases imaged with the latest high technology hardware. Ocular Electrophysiology and ophthalmic USG which provides information of retinochoroidal disorders completes this section.

Section 2 is devoted to retinal degenerations and fundal dystrophies. This includes pathological myopia and its lesions with pictorial representation, Retinitis Pigmentosa and related syndromes, Hereditary Retinal and Choroidal Vitreoretinopathy and Dystrophies.

Section 3 is totally devoted to Macular diseases including central serous chorioretinopathy (CSR), AMD and etiologies leading to secondary CNV membranes. Vitreomacular interface diseases and VMT are explained next, closely followed by a chapter each devoted to ERM's and Macular holes each.

Myopic Traction Maculopathy is now imaged more commonly in Myopic eyes especially with the SS-OCT device and is next described, followed by Optic disc pit maculopathy and its management with ILM stuffing. Submacular bleeding is now seen often especially in Polypoidal Choroidal Vasculopathy eyes and RAM eyes requiring an effective management with submacular tPA injection and is described in detail. Low vision aids still plays an important role in eyes with end-stage AMD lesions and scar formation and a detailed explanation of the available aids and their usage provides a place in this book.

The next section is devoted to vascular occlusions including Ocular ischemic syndrome (OIS). The all important Diabetic retinopathy is explained in great detail including its epidemiology, pathogenesis, classification and trials till date. DME being the prime cause for visual disturbance is discussed with its management in a separate chapter. PDR and its laser, anti-VEGF and surgical treatment comes next and then Macular Telangiectasia followed by miscellaneous vascular retinopathies in one chapter.

Section 5 of this compendium is devoted to Pediatric retinal disease including ROP, FEVR, Coats disease and Iridofundal coloboma.

Section 6 is devoted to Uveal diseases including both Infectious and Noninfectious uveitis with illustrations to support the text.

Section 7 details with 'Surgical Retina including management of RD, Retinal lasers, Scleral Buckling procedures including Pneumatic retinopexy, Vitreous substitutes, techniques for pars plana vitrectomy, GRT management, Vitrectomy for diabetic TRD, Dislocated nucleus and IOL followed by complications of VR surgery including Endophthalmitis. This section ends with newer innovations and techniques in Vitreo-Retina.

The last 2 sections covers the useful topic of Ocular trauma as Section 9 and comprehensively covers classification, Globe injury, Disc avulsion, RIOFB, post-traumatic endophthalmitis and shaken baby syndrome. The last section of retinal diseases covers the newly described entities of Cancer-associated and autoimmune retinopathies, Toxic and Photic retinopathies and lastly Phacomatosis.

This book will provide the specific academic requirements for postgraduate students as well as ophthalmic fellows pursuing retina. It shall also be useful for all the ophthalmic practitioners and researchers as it contains extensive and easily accessible material with special focus on medical and surgical management of various diseases in retina and vitreous from basics to the current concept in a comprehensive and easy to understand manner. I hope the book proves useful to provide a better understanding of various vitreoretinal conditions and its medical and surgical management.

Atul Kumar MD FAMS FRCS (Ed)

Acknowledgments

I wish to acknowledge the support of the staff and my co-authors from India and abroad, colleagues at RP Centre, Senior and Junior Residents in particular for all their hard work and dedication without whom I would have found it tough to complete the writing/editing on time with special reference to Vineet Mutha, Raghav Ravani, Yogita Gupta, Alisha Kishore and Abidnye Surve for taking time-out at odd hours to help the proof-reading which they managed admirably. Thank you all so much. Patients at our institutions always deserve credit as they are continued sources of inspiration for such academic endeavours.

I also wish to thank Mr Jitendar P Vij (Group Chairman), Mr Ankit Vij (Group President) and the editorial team at Jaypee Brothers Medical Publishers (P) Ltd for their dedicated guidance and expertise with special mention of Ms Chetna Malhotra Vohra (Associate Director—Content Strategy), Ms Kritika Dua (Development Editor) and Vipin Kaushik (Team Leader—Typesetting Department) who nearly pushed me of the cliff, to help me complete the chapters. It was a pleasure working with all the publishing team at Jaypee Brothers Medical Publishers (P) Ltd, New Delhi, India for the book proofs and editing, etc. Finally, I wish to thank my family for their unwavering enthusiastic support and encouragement.

Contents

Section 4: Retinal Vascular Disorders

Section 8: Ocular Trauma

Section 9: Miscellaneous Retinal Conditions

List of Videos

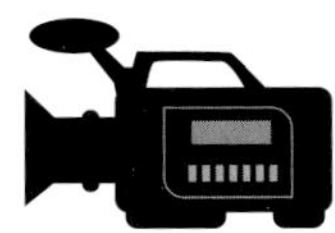

Basic Sciences and Diagnostics

Chapter 1

Clinical Anatomy and Physiology of Vitreous and Retina

Raghav Ravani, Aman Kumar, Yogita Gupta, Rohan Chawla, Atul Kumar

THE VITREOUS

The word *vitreous* literally means like a glass (in appearance or properties). The vitreous is a transparent, hydrophilic, optically clear media that constitutes about 80% of the eye volume. Anteriorly, it is limited by the ciliary body, the zonules, and the lens while posteriorly, it is limited by the retina and forms the vitreoretinal interface. Topographically, vitreous may be classified into: The central or *core vitreous* and the peripheral or *cortical vitreous*.

The anterior cortex, consists of condensation of collagenous fibers that attach to the posterior surface of capsule of lens forming the *Wieger's ligament* or hyaloideocapsular ligament (Fig. 1.1). The presence of crystalline lens leads to a concave, retrolental indentation of the anterior cortex called as the patellar fossa. The potential space between lens and anterior vitreous (anterior hyaloid) which is bordered by Wieger's ligament is called the *Berger's space* (Fig. 1.1). The preequatorial and postequatorial lens zonules enclose a space called the *Canal of Hannover*. *Vitreous base* is an area that extends about 2 mm anterior and 3 mm posterior to the ora serrata where the collagen fibers are especially dense and insert firmly (Fig. 1.2). The vitreous cortex is firmly adherent to the internal limiting membrane (ILM) in certain areas: at the region of the vitreous base,[1] around the optic disc, at the retinal vessels and around foveola.[2,3]

Embryology and Development of Vitreous

Embryologically, the vitreous can be divided into primary (primitive), secondary (definitive) and tertiary vitreous, which represent different phases of development of vitreous from various layers of the developing embryo (Table 1.1).

Structural development: In the first month of gestation, at 5–13 mm fetus stage, a fibrillar vascular structure, the *primary vitreous,* forms from the mesenchymal layer and fills the space formed as the optic cup grows with its lens vesicle. Later the cells of the hyaloid arterial wall presumably secrete the

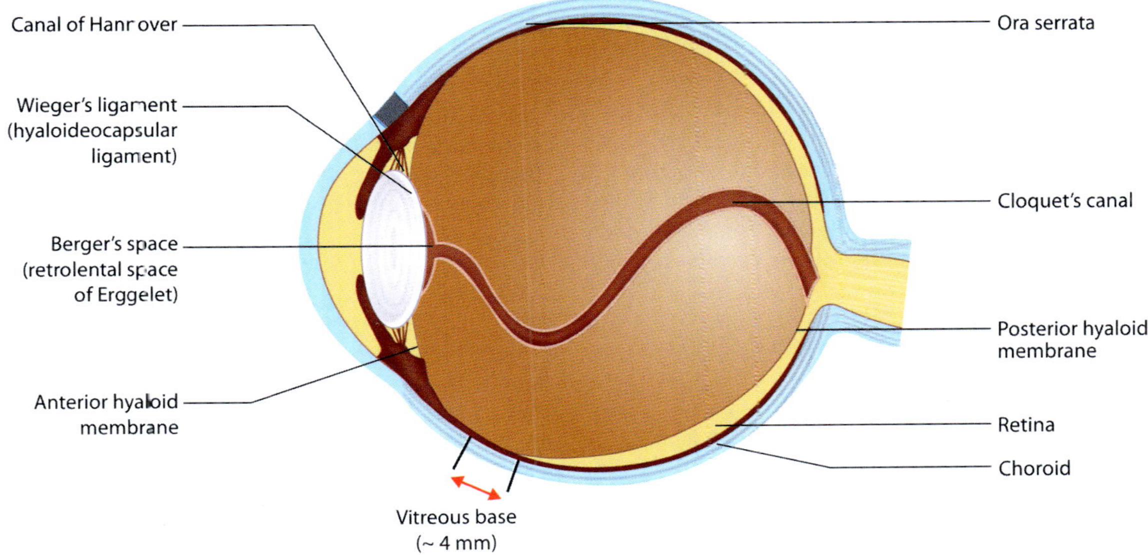

Fig. 1.1: Gross anatomy of vitreous.

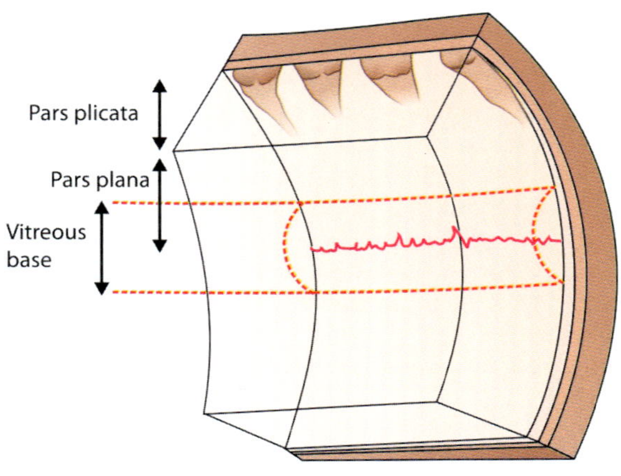
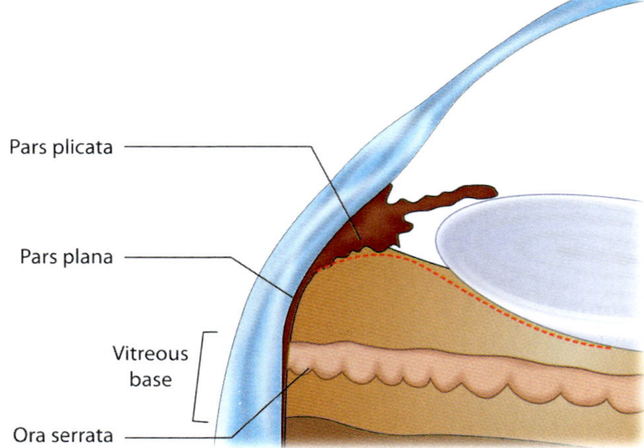

Fig. 1.2: Anatomy of vitreous base.

Table 1.1: Embryological phases of vitreous development.	
Developmental vitreous	*Origin*
Primary (primitive) vitreous	Mesenchymal (secreted by embryonic retinal cells and later from cells of penetrating hyaloid artery).[4-8]
Secondary (definitive) vitreous	Neuroectodermal (Neuroectoderm of optic cup)
Tertiary vitreous	Neuroectodermal (neuroectoderm of the ciliary region)

fibrillar material forming the primary vitreous.[4-8] It has a dense vascular plexus (anterior and posterior tunica vasculosa lentis) that mainly provides nourishment to the developing lens.

In the second month of gestation at 14–70 mm fetus stage, primary vitreous with its vasculature is seen to regress and *secondary vitreous* forms which is an avascular and compact network of type II collagen fibrils secreted from the neuroectoderm of the optic cup by the 6th week. The primary vitreous is thus eventually replaced by secondary vitreous and the main hyaloid artery disappears and leaves a residual tube of primary vitreous, called *Cloquet's canal* (*see* Fig. 1.1), surrounded by the secondary vitreous, which extends from the retrolental space to the optic nerve (area of Martegiani). If the regression of primary vitreous fails to occur, it leads to a condition known as persistent fetal vasculature (PFV) (formerly known as persistent hyperplastic primary vitreous or PHPV).

The *tertiary vitreous* develops from neuroectoderm in the third month of gestation at stage of 71–110 mm fetal length, which develops as the suspensory fibrils, contains no vessels or nerves and has two main parts: collagen fibers and hyaluronic acid (HA) with high (~98%) water content.

Molecular and cellular development: The two main components of vitreous, i.e. the collagen and HA, are produced in the primary and secondary vitreous. The cells in the primary vitreous differentiate as hyalocytes and fibroblasts in secondary vitreous. The hyalocytes supposedly produces glycosaminoglycans (GAGs), especially HA.[9] The collagen may be synthesized from fibroblast or from retina.[10,11] The hyalocytes are mononuclear cells found in the posterior vitreous cortex, approximately 30 microns (20–50 microns) from the ILM, with highest density near the vitreous base and posterior pole, and lowest near the equator.[12,13]

Biochemical Properties of the Vitreous

Clinical implication: Hyalocytes play an important role in macular pucker when there occurs anomalous posterior vitreous detachment (APVD) and vitreoschisis, wherein hyalocyte proliferate on the surface of the retina, resulting in hypercellular membrane and also cause tangential traction by recruitment of cells from circulation and retina and inducing collagen gel contraction in response to platelet-derived growth factor (PDGF) and other cytokines.[14]

Vitreous consists of three major structural components: water, collagen fibers, and GAGs. The vitreous contains more than 99% of water. The vitreous exists as a gel-like structure due to the arrangement of long, nonbranching, collagen fibrils which are suspended in a network of HA.[15-17] The most common type of collagen fibrils are collagen type II, which are composed of helices made of three α-chains, stabilized by hydrogen bonds between opposing residues in different chains.[8] Collagen type IX functions as a link between type II collagen fibrils.[16,18,19]

Posterior Vitreous Detachment and Anomalous Posterior Vitreous Detachment

The vitreoretinal interface is a complex formed by the posterior vitreous cortex, the ILM and an intervening extracellular matrix, consisting of fibronectin, laminin, etc. The vitreous at this interface is believed to be adhered to ILM by an extracellular matrix, causing the adhesion to be fascial.[20,21] Chondroitin sulfate exists at sites of strong vitreoretinal adhesions like vitreous base and optic disc, and hence the rationale for pharmacologic vitreolysis using chondroitinase derivatives for disorders of vitreoretinal interface. Posterior vitreous detachment (PVD) means separation of posterior vitreous cortex from ILM. PVD begins in the perifoveal region. This is due to vitreous degeneration which may be age-related or due to other secondary causes. The mechanism of age-related vitreous degeneration and hence PVD is briefly discussed in following sections.

Synchysis (Liquefaction)[22,23]

There is age-related increase in central liquid volume of vitreous and decrease in the gel volume leading to formation of vitreous pockets (lacunae) which coalesce to form larger posterior lacuna or bursa or precortical pocket.[24] A study observed 20% of the total volume as liquid vitreous as the human eye reaches adult size.[22] Changes in collagen or conformational change in HA with subsequent cross-linking of fibrils is postulated mechanism for liquefaction of vitreous.[19,25] Changes in minor GAGs and chondroitin sulfate may also play a role in vitreous liquefaction.[26] Biochemically, vitreous HA concentration is steady after the age of 20 years[22] and liquid vitreous increases with age. With age, an increase in HA content of the liquid vitreous and a concomitant decrease in HA content of the gel vitreous is seen. Thus, a reduction of vitreous HA concentration results in decreased viscosity of vitreous gel, which may be accelerated by cataract surgery or a breach in the posterior capsule of the lens.

Syneresis

Along with age-related liquefaction, there occurs thickening and tortuosity of vitreous fibers and resulting collapse of the vitreous. This collapse of vitreous body is called as *syneresis*. This is an age-related process, but may occur earlier in some cases like high myopia,[27] posttrauma to ocular structures, ocular inflammation and congenital vitreoretinopathies (arthro-ophthalmopathies).[28,29]

A clean separation between the cortical vitreous and retinal internal limiting lamina (ILL) is called an innocuous PVD.[30] In most cases, this may be asymptomatic leading to total separation of cortical vitreous from ILL, resulting in a ring of tissue composed of fibrous astrocytes and collagen at its attachment to the optic disc, called as Weiss ring. This may lead to symptom of a floater. Incidence of PVD is 66% between the ages of 66 years and 86 years,[31] and 53% after 50 years.[32]

Anomalous Posterior Vitreous Detachment

This results from liquefaction of vitreous without concurrent weakening of vitreoretinal adherence, leading to various manifestation depending on the level of separation, site of firm adherence and liquefaction. This may lead to either partial thickness detachment called as vitreoschisis,[14,33] wherein there is splitting of the posterior vitreous cortex with anterior displacement of a part of cortex, with posterior layer still attached to the retina. Note, this is not to be confused with partial PVD, which means full thickness but incomplete separation of cortical vitreous.

RETINA

> *Clinical implication:* A PVD may lead to consequences like macular hole, macular pucker, vitreomacular traction syndrome (VMTS), exudative age-related macular degeneration (exudative AMD), vitreo-papillary traction or retinal tears and detachment.[14] Further details have been described in the "Chapter 13: Vitreomacular Interface and Anomalous Posterior Vitreous Detachment".

The retina (Latin: *rete* = net) is the innermost layer and the most comprehensive sensory structure of the eye. It is derived from the optic vesicle and grossly is a thin, transparent membrane with two main components: (1) a pigmented layer (called as retinal pigment epithelium or RPE), and (2) a sensory layer (the neurosensory retina). Embryologically, both are derived from outer and inner layers of the optic vesicle, respectively (Fig. 1.3).

The two layers are attached loosely to each other by various mechanisms, failure of which leads to separation of neurosensory retina from the RPE with accumulation of subretinal fluid, a clinical entity called as retinal detachment.

Forces that keep the retina attached can be divided into:
- Mechanical forces
- Subretinal fluid transport
- Metabolic factors

Mechanical Forces

- Fluid pressure and resistance to flow:
  - Hydrostatic pressure: Contributed by intraocular pressure (IOP)
  - Osmotic pressure: Contributed by extracellular fluid in the choroid
    - Both of the above mentioned forces enhance absorption of fluid out of subretinal space which in turn enhance the binding properties of interphotoreceptor matrix (IPM).
  - Retinal flow resistance because of retina and RPE:[34,35] Acts to push neurosensory retina against RPE.
- *Vitreous support:* Does not directly contribute to attachment of retina, but intact gel form vitreous has a role in preventing pathologic fluid access to subretinal space.[36-41]

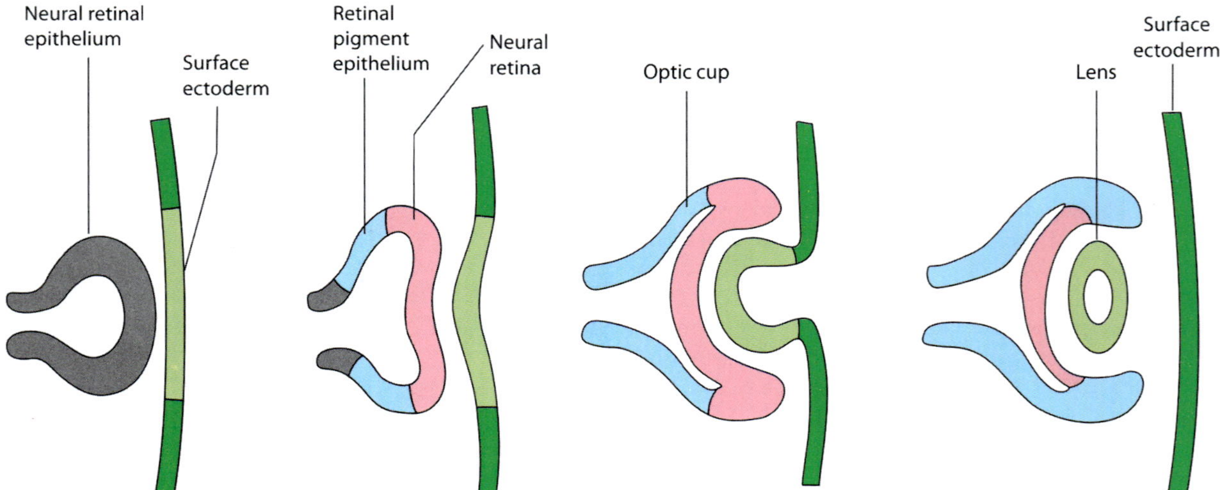

Fig. 1.3: Formation of lens vesicle and optic cup. The thin outer wall of optic cup forms the pigmented layer of retina. The thick inner wall forms the neurosensory retina.

- *Mechanical interdigitation:* RPE microvilli wrap closely around the tips of outer segments, thus acting as mechanical interdigitation between the RPE and neurosensory retina. Exact mechanism is unknown, but close ensheathment might provide frictional resistance to separation of neurosensory retina and RPE. Electrostatic forces that oppose separation of the membranes may also play a role.[42]
- *Interphotoreceptor matrix properties:* Various properties of IPM like the presence of the viscous material,[43] largely due to proteins and glycoproteins and the presence of GAGs[44] helps in attachment of the two layers. The presence of cone matrix sheath that remains attached to both RPE and photoreceptors cells may also play a role in attachment of retina.[45-47]

Subretinal Fluid Transport

Retinal pigment epithelium actively transports water from the subretinal space to the choroid.[37,48,49] Conditions that keep the subretinal space dehydrated and thereby keeping the matrix viscous, contribute to keep the retina closely apposed, e.g. raising systemic osmolality with mannitol passively increases subretinal fluid absorption[50] and thus increases adhesiveness of retina.[51-53]

Metabolic Factors

Metabolic factors like oxygenation, pH, calcium concentration which affect RPE activity and bonding of IPM influence attachment of RPE and neurosensory retina.

Topography of the Retina

The retina proper has a surface area of about 266 mm². The major landmarks of the retina are: the optic disc, area centralis (macula lutea), and the peripheral retina.

The retina is thickest near the optic disc, where it measures approximately 0.56 mm. The retina becomes thinner in the periphery (approximately 0.18 mm at equator to 0.3 mm at the ora serrata).[54-57]

The Optic Disc

It is a circular to oval well-defined pale pink structure of about 1.5 mm in diameter. All the retinal layers terminate at the optic disc, except the nerve fiber layer (NFL), which pass through the lamina cribrosa and form the optic nerve. The depression within the optic disc is called as the physiological cup. Increase in the size of the cup and/or difference in the size of cup of two eyes should arouse suspicion of glaucomatous damage to nerve fibers and should be evaluated.

Area Centralis[55]

This region of the retina, located in the posterior fundus temporal to the optic disc, is divided into the fovea and foveola with parafoveal and a perifoveal ring around the fovea. The area is a horizontally elliptical area demarcated approximately by the upper and lower arcuate and temporal retinal vessels with an average diameter of about 5.5 mm. This area corresponds to approximately 15° of the visual field. Histologically, it is the area that contains two or more ganglion cell layers.

Fovea Centralis (Figs. 1.4 and 1.5)

It is the central depressed part of the macula around 1.85 mm in diameter and 0.25 mm in thickness and is approximately 3–4 mm temporal (approximately 2 disc diameter) and 0.8 mm below the center of the optic disc. It corresponds to visual field of 5°.[55]

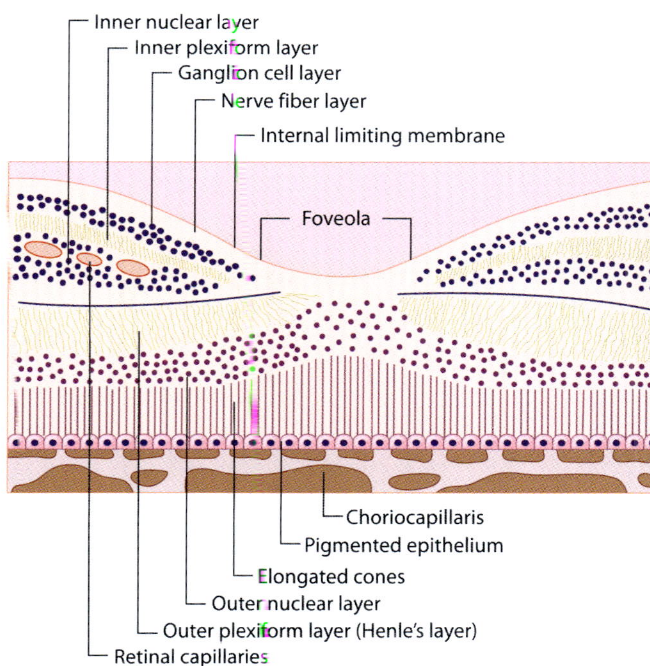

Fig. 1.4: Schematic diagram of microscopic structure of fovea centralis.

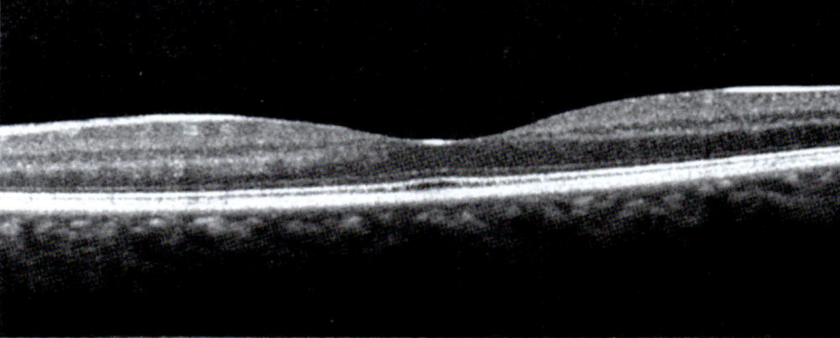

Fig. 1.5: Optical coherence tomography picture of the macula depicting all the layers.

Foveola

It measures 0.35 mm in diameter, 0.13 mm in thickness, and corresponds to the 1° of visual field. It represents area of the highest visual acuity in the retina, consists solely of cone photoreceptors and is avascular.

Parafoveal and Perifoveal Zone

These are areas around the fovea about 0.5 mm and 1.5 mm in diameter, respectively.

Peripheral Retina

It can be divided into following regions:[54,55]
- Near periphery--is a circumscribed region of 1.5 mm around the area centralis.
- Mid periphery--is a 3 mm wide zone around the near periphery.
- Far periphery is a region that extends from the optic disc, 9–10 mm on the temporal side and 16 mm on the nasal side in the horizontal meridian.

Ora Serrata

It is the anterior most region of the retina, where the retina ends and ciliary body starts.
- Dentate processes: These are jetties of retinal tissue extending anteriorly into the pars plana. These are more prominent nasally.
- Ora bays: These are posterior extension of the pars plana towards the retinal side.
- Enclosed ora bay: Dentate processes may wrap around a portion of ora bay to form an enclosed ora bay.
- Meridional fold: It is prominent thickening of retinal tissue extending into the pars plana.
- Meridional complex: Meridional fold when aligned with a ciliary process is known as meridional complex.

Microscopic Architecture of the Retina

As seen by light microscopy, the cross-section of the retina consists of different cell types and their synapses, arranged in 10 layers from without inwards as follows (Figs. 1.6 to 1.8):
- Retinal pigment epithelium (RPE)
- Photoreceptor layer of rods and cones
- External limiting membrane (ELM)
- Outer nuclear layer
- Outer plexiform layer (OPL)
- Inner nuclear layer
- Inner plexiform layer
- Ganglion cell layer
- Nerve fiber layer
- Internal limiting membrane

Retinal Pigment Epithelium

It is the outermost layer of retina consisting of a monolayer of hexagonal pigmented cells derived from the outer layer of the optic cup. The RPE cells in the macula are taller and denser than in the periphery. It maintains apex-to-apex arrangement with Mullerian glia. RPE layer is continuous with the pigment epithelium of the ciliary body and iris.

Electron microscopy shows that each RPE cell has an apical portion with microvilli which envelope the photoreceptor outer segments. Its basal portion shows plasma membrane infolding and is firmly adherent to the underlying basal lamina of the choroid (Bruch's membrane). These cells are connected with each other by tight junctions (zonula occludens and zonula adherens) near the apices, and thus forming the *outer blood-retinal barrier.*

Function of RPE with clinical implications:
- Fundus on examination has a granular appearance due to unequal pigmentation of the RPE cells giving mottled appearance.

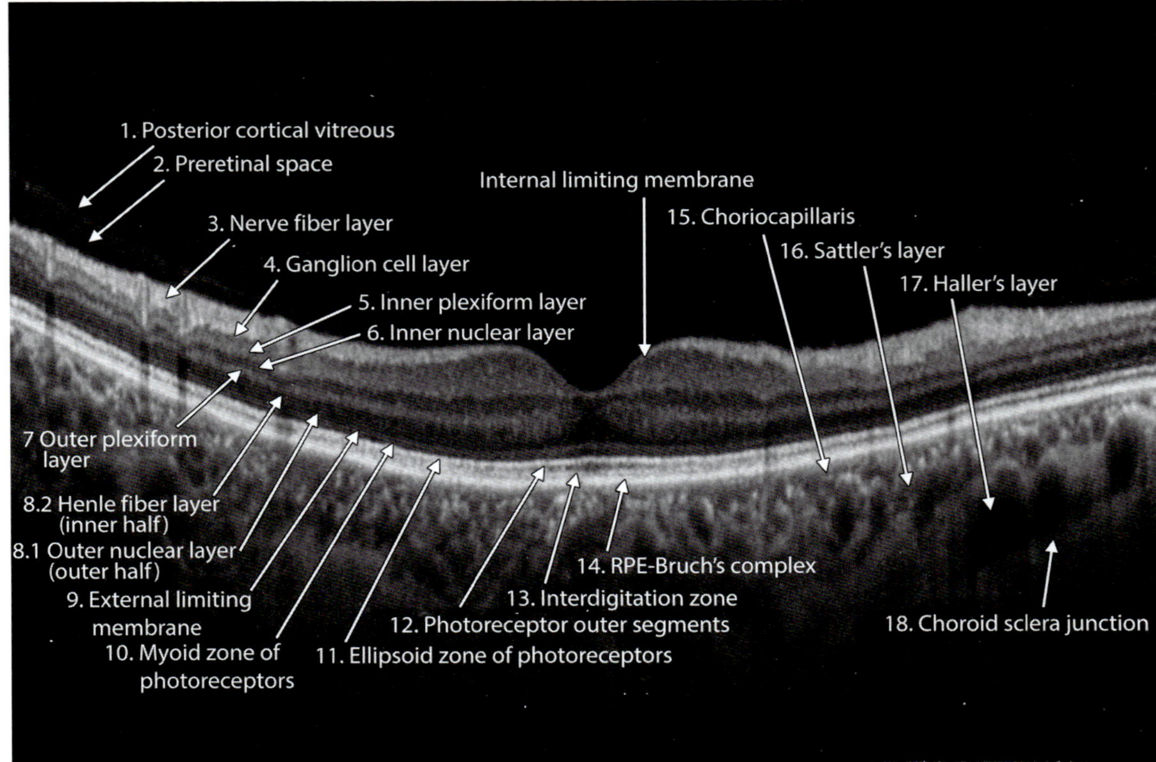

Fig. 1.6: Optical coherence tomography image depicting various layers of the retina.

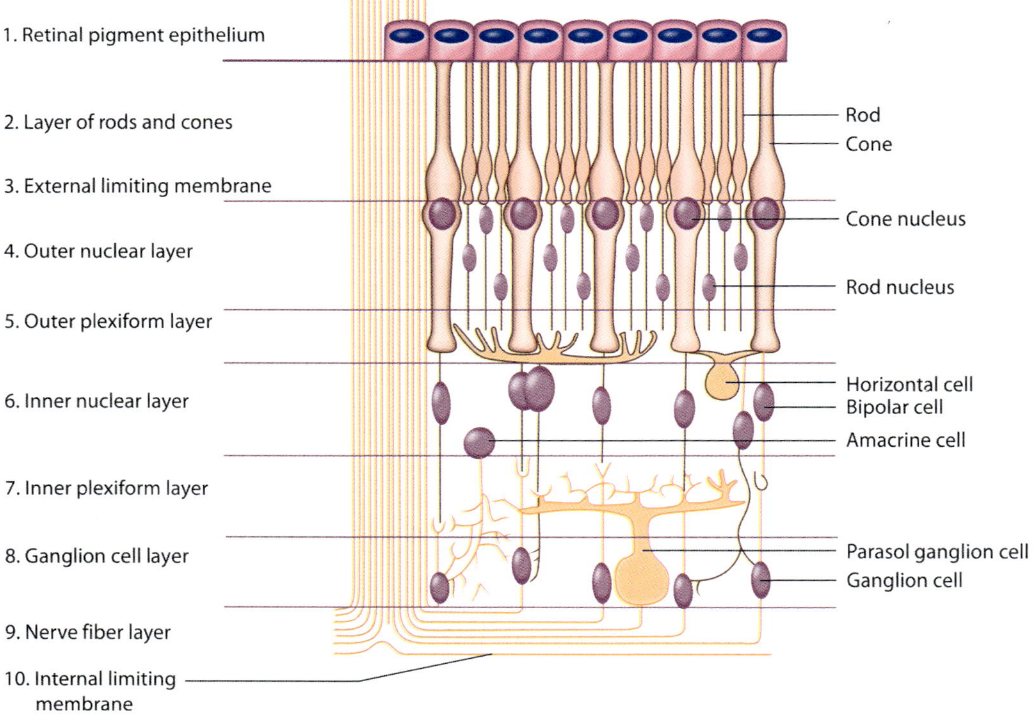

Fig. 1.7: Schematic diagram of microscopic structure of the retina.
Source: Modified with permission from textbook on 'Anatomy and Physiology of eye, 2nd edition, CBS, 2011' by Dr AK Khurana

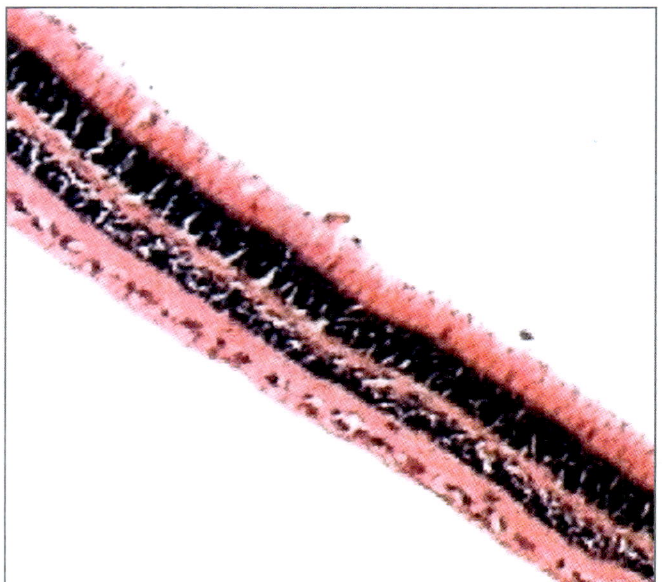

Fig. 1.8: Photograph of histological specimen of human retina. *Courtesy:* Dr Seema Kashyap, Department of Ocular Pharmacology, Dr RP Centre for Ophthalmic Sciences, AIIMS, New Delhi.

- The pigment granules of RPE has melanin pigment that absorbs photons of light and minimizes light scatter within the retina.[58]
- As explained above, the potential space between RPE and sensory retina is called as subretinal space, and fluid collection in this layer is called as subretinal fluid which leads to retinal detachment. RPE pumps this fluid from the subretinal space at a rate of about 0.3 µL/h/mm^2 of RPE (measured in microliters per hour per millimeter square area).[59-63] Resorption rate of detachment in human eyes has been measured as 0.11 µL/h/mm^2 of RPE[64] which is about 3.5 mL of fluid per day.
- The tight junctions between the RPE cells forms the outer blood-retinal barrier. Thus, the selective transport properties of the RPE regulating transepithelial diffusion through paracellular spaces helps maintain environment of the photoreceptors.[65]
- RPE is responsible for transport of metabolites through the blood-retinal barrier and for elaboration of the extracellular matrix.[66]
- It phagocytoses outer segments of photoreceptors being shed according to their circadian rhythm.[67,68] (Rods shed discs at dawn and cones shed at dusk).
- It helps in polyunsaturated fatty acid metabolism.
- Majority of the regeneration process of 11-cis retinaldehyde (the chromophore found in rhodopsin) occurs in the RPE. This helps in perpetuation of the Wald's visual cycle. Defect in *RPE65* (retinal pigment epithelium-specific 65-kDa) gene on chromosome 17 leads to a condition called as Leber's congenital amaurosis (LCA type 2) and retinitis pigmentosa. Recently, gene therapy for LCA with subretinal injection of recombinant adeno-associated virus gene vector carrying altered human *RPE65* is being tried and trials are on.[69]

Photoreceptor Layer (of Rods and Cones)

The photoreceptor layer of the retina consists of the rods and cones. These are the end organs of the visual pathway that transform light energy into visual impulse. On an average, there are about 120 million rods and 6.5 million cones in the human eye. As seen on electron microscopy, these photoreceptors are arranged as mosaic, composition of which varies in different regions of the retina depending on the density variation of both rods and cones in different regions of the retina (Figs. 1.9 and 1.10).

Rod photoreceptor: These are about 40–60 microns long. The highest density of rods are below the optic disc and their number gradually reduces towards the periphery. Rods are absent at the fovea in an area of 0.35 mm, which corresponds to 1.25° of the visual field. It consists of the following:

- *Outer segment:* It is cylindrical, refractile, transversely serrated and contains a photosensitive substance—rhodopsin. The Rod photoreceptor outer segment is composed of numerous lamellar lipo-protein discs (around 6,000–10,000/rod, each about 22.5–24.5 nm thick) stacked together and surrounded by a cell membrane.
- *Inner segment:* Is thicker than the outer segment consisting of two regions, ellipsoid and myoid.
  - *Ellipsoid* (the outer portion) contains abundant mitochondria.
  - *Myoid* (the inner portion) contains glycogen and other organelles.
- *Cell body and nucleus:* lies in the outer nuclear layer. It arises from the inner end of the rod, passes through the ELM and swells into a densely staining nucleus called the rod granule. This terminates into a bulbous structure called the spherule.

Cone photoreceptor: It has following parts:

- *Outer segment:* Cone outer segment is conical in shape, shorter than that of the rod. It contains pigment––iodopsin. The outer segment is composed of lamellar discs (around 1,000–1,200 discs/cone) which are in continuity with the surface plasma membrane.
- *Inner segment:* It is similar in structure to rod inner segment, consisting of ellipsoid and myoid. Ellipsoid is larger than that of rod and has more numerous mitochondria.
- *Cell body and nucleus:* Cone inner segment becomes directly continuous with its nucleus and lies in the outer nuclear layer. A stout cone inner fiber runs from the nucleus which ends in lateral processes called cone pedicle.

Interphotoreceptor matrix: The IPM occupies the space between the photoreceptor outer segments and the RPE. It is a

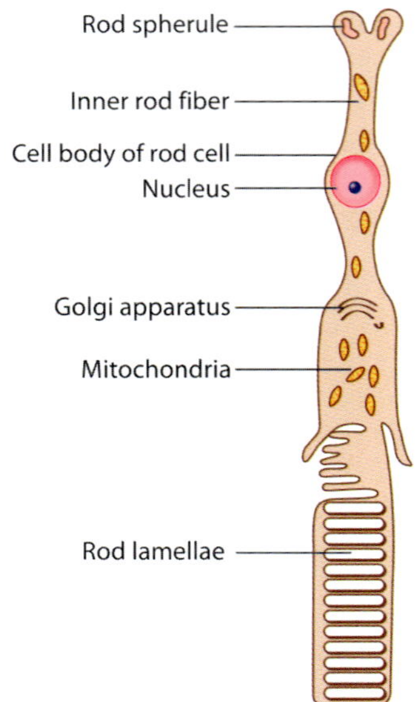

Fig. 1.9: Microscopic (schematic) structure of rod cell.

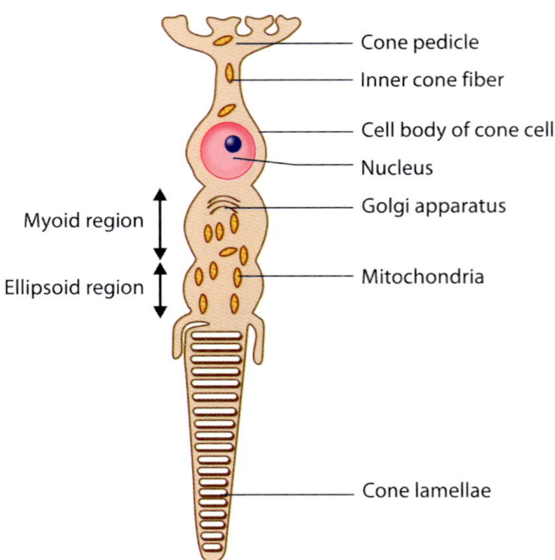

Fig. 1.10: Microscopic (schematic) structure of cone cell.

viscous structure consisting of proteins, glycoproteins, GAGs and proteoglycans. Functionally, IPM plays a role in physiological attachment of retina, facilitation of phagocytosis and probably in alignment of photoreceptor outer segment. The interphotoreceptor retinoid binding protein (IRBP) accounts for 70% of the soluble proteins in the IPM. Its primary function is transport of retinoids between the photoreceptors and the RPE. Thus, minimizes the fluctuations in retinoid availability and protects the plasma membranes from the toxic effects of high retinoid concentration.

External Limiting Membrane

It is a fenestrated membrane through which the processes of the photoreceptors pass. It is not a true basement membrane and electron microscopy studies show that the ELM is formed by the zonula adherens between the Muller cells and the plasma membrane of photoreceptors.

Outer Nuclear Layer

This multilayered outer nuclear layer is formed by the nuclei of rods and cones. Rod nuclei forms the major bulk of this layer except in the foveal region which is dominated by cone nuclei.

> *Clinical implication:* Recently, a study showed that the postoperative integrity of the ELM layer appears to be a critical factor for the restoration of the photoreceptor layer and for predicting a successful visual outcome following macular hole repair.[70]

Outer Plexiform Layer

This layer consists of synapses between photoreceptors with bipolar cells and processes of the horizontal cells. Thus, it represents junction of the end organs of visual pathway and its

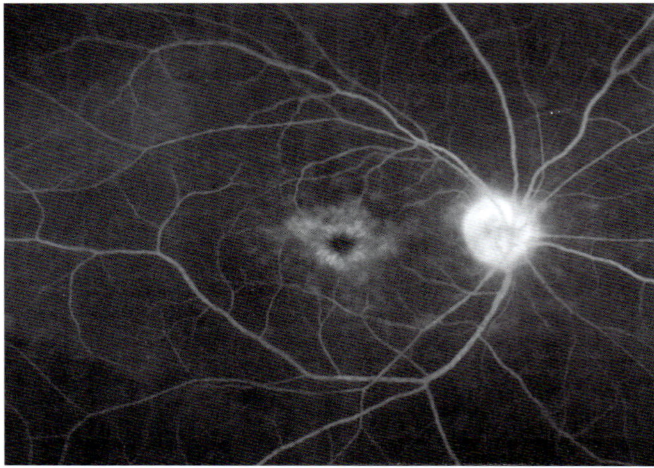

Fig. 1.11: Fundus fluorescein angiography showing typical petalloid leak in cystoid macular edema (CME).

first-order neurons in the retina.[55] This layer is thickest at the macula and consists predominantly of oblique fibers from the fovea known as Henle's layer.

> *Clinical implication:* The arrangement of oblique fibers over macula (Henle's layer) gives typical appearance on fundus fluorescein angiography of petalloid leak in cases of cystoid macular edema (Fig. 1.11).

- Consists of intercellular junctions and synapses, which may act as a functional barrier to diffusion of fluids and metabolites. This functional barrier may retard or prevent the spread of exudates, hemorrhages, and cysts from spreading through the entire retinal thickness.

- It is in a watershed zone of vascular supply of the retina and is sensitive to variations in the circulatory supply from either of the vascular sources, i.e. choroidal or retinal. Thus it is vulnerable to metabolic insult due to senile choriocapillary atrophy or age related thickening of Bruch's membrane.
- The OPL is established site of formation of retinal cysts during aging, advanced stage of which is represented by senile retinoschisis.
- OPL is the most frequent site of exudate and hemorrhage accumulation in patients with retinal vasculopathy.

Inner Nuclear Layer

The inner nuclear layer consists of 8–12 rows of closely packed nuclei of the bipolar cells, horizontal cells, amacrine cells, interplexiform cells and supportive Muller cells.[55]

Horizontal cells: The flat horizontal cells serve to modulate and transform visual information received from the photoreceptors. The concentration of horizontal cells is highest at the fovea and decreases towards the periphery. Horizontal cells are seen by light microscopy to have short processes and long processes that stem from the base of a short process or directly from the perikaryon. A characteristic feature of horizontal cells is the presence of an intracytoplasmic inclusion, the Kolmer crystalloid or body.

Bipolar cells: The bipolar cells are the second-order neurons in the visual pathway and are radially oriented in the retina. Nine main type of bipolar cells have been distinguished[71] based on morphology and synaptic relationships.
- Rod or mop
- Invaginating midget
- Flat midget
- Flat diffuse or brush
- Invaginating diffuse
- On-center blue cone
- Off-center blue cone
- Giant bistratified
- Giant diffuse invaginating.

Rod bipolar cells constitute 20% of the total population and are present 1 mm from the fovea. The invaginating midget cells are the smallest of the bipolar cells. There is a one-to-one ratio (1:1) of midget bipolar cells and the cones at the fovea.[71] All types of bipolar cells have a similar ultrastructure. Most of the midget and diffuse bipolar cells are glutamatergic. A subpopulation of bipolar exhibits strong immunolabeling for glycine. The bipolar cells transmit signals from the photoreceptors and pass it on to the ganglion cells either directly or indirectly via amacrine cells.

Muller cells: Muller cells are the largest of all cells in the retina, and extend from the external to the ILMs. The cell bodies of Muller cells occupy most of the inner intermediate layer of the inner nuclear layer. Embryonically, Muller cells are derived from the inner layer of the optic vesicle. During development of the retina, these cells have an important role in the orientation, displacement and positioning of the developing neurons. They are the principal glial cells of the retina and conserve the structural alignment of its neuronal elements.

Amacrine cells: The cell body of the amacrine cells lie internal to the nuclei of the Muller cells. Each amacrine cell has a single process with extensive branching. The amacrine processes thus extends over a wide area in the inner plexiform layer. The neurotransmitter substances associated with amacrine cell function include both neuroactive substances [acetylcholine, gamma aminobutyric acid (GABA), glycine, dopamine, serotonin] and neuropeptides (cholecystokinin, enkephalin, glucagon, neurotensin, somatostatin, substance P, neuropeptide Y and vasoactive intestinal peptide). Two or more of these neuromodulating chemicals may be present in one cell. Most amacrine cells contain γ-aminobutyric acid and glycine, which have an inhibitory action on the ganglion cells.[72,73]

Inner Plexiform Layer

It is the junction of the bipolar cells (the second-order neurons) with ganglion cells (the third-order neurons). The bipolar cells act as afferent and the ganglion cell acts as efferent to this layer. The amacrine cells mediate interactions within the layer which in turn provides input to the interplexiform cells. Thus, bipolar cells synapse with process of amacrine cells and the dendrites of ganglion cells. In addition to synapses between various cell types, this layer contains processes of the Muller cells and an abundant microvasculature. This layer is absent from the foveola. The dendrites of all bipolar cells have receptors for GABA-A suggesting that inhibition feedback from amacrine cells is mediated by GABA-A.

Ganglion Cell Layer

This layer is composed of the cell bodies of ganglion cells (the third-order neurons). Processes of Muller cells and branches of retinal vessels are also present. It forms two layers at the temporal side of the optic disc, about 6–8 layers at the edge of the foveola and is single layered in the peripheral retina. Ganglion cell layer is absent at foveola and at optic nerve head. Ganglion cells are packed closely together except at the periphery. There are about 1.2 million ganglion cells in the retina with overall cone: ganglion cell ratio of 2.9:1–7.5:1. The axons of these cells form the optic nerve. The ganglion cells can be divided into two major types—M cells and P cells. The *M cells* project to the magnocellular layer of the lateral geniculate body and exhibit nonopponent responses. The *P cells* project to the parvocellular layers of the lateral geniculate body. The P cells are further divided into P1 cells or midget and P2 or small bistratified.

Nerve Fiber Layer

The nerve fiber layer contains the axons of the ganglion cells (also called as the *centripetal* fibers), a rich capillary bed and centrifugal (efferent) fibers along with glial cells. The axons remain unmyelinated until they reach the lamina cribrosa of the optic nerve. The nerve fiber layer is thickest at the nasal edge of the disc, (about 20–30 μm). The thickness decreases

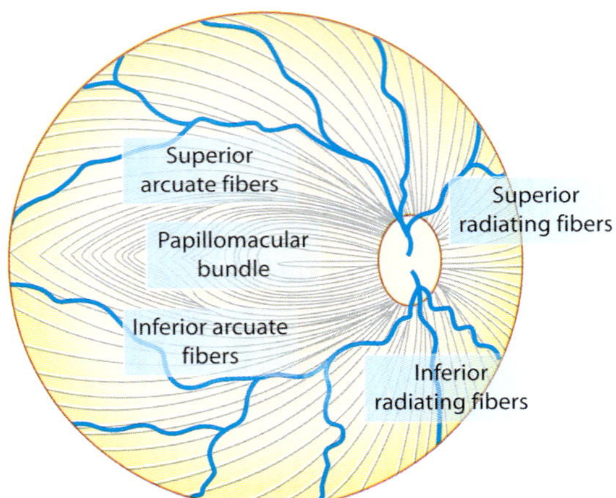

Fig. 1.12: Arrangement of nerve fibers in the retina.

from the optic disc to the ora serrata. The papillomacular bundle represents the thinnest portion of the nerve fiber layer around the optic disc.

Arrangement of nerve fibers in the retina (Fig. 1.12):
- The fibers within the nerve fiber layer course parallel to the surface of the retina, compared to the rest of the fibers of the sensory retina which are perpendicular to it.
- Nasal retina: Fibers of the nasal half of the retina reach to the optic nerve as superior and inferior radiating fibers.
- Temporal retina: Fibers from the macular region pass straight in the temporal part of the optic disc as papillomacular bundle.
- Fibers from rest of the temporal retina arch above and below the macular and papillomacular bundle as superior and inferior arcuate fibers.

Nerve fiber layer thickness at the disc (From thinnest to thickest): In eyes with normal optic nerves, the RNFL at the optic disc border shows a double hump configuration with the mean highest mean thickness in the inferior quadrant (mean ± S.D: 266 ± 64 micron), followed by the superior quadrant (240 ± 57 micron), the nasal quadrant (220 ± 70 micron), and finally the temporal quadrant (170 ± 58 micron).

Clinical implication:
- *Glaucoma:* One of the earliest indication for glaucoma (preperimetric glaucoma) is retinal nerve fiber layer (RNFL) thinning. Arcuate nerve fibers (temporal) are most sensitive to glaucomatous damage and lead to corresponding visual field loss documented on perimetry. Macular fibers occupying the lateral quadrant are most resistant to glaucomatous damage and thus cause a preservation of the central vision even in most advanced stages of glaucoma.
- *Papilledema:* Papillomacular fibers being the thinnest fibers form the last affected portion of the optic disc in papilledema. Papilledema appears first of all in the thickest quadrant of the optic disc, i.e. upper nasal and lower nasal quadrants.

Internal limiting membrane: It forms the innermost layer of the retina. The ILM along with posterior vitreous cortex form the vitreoretinal interface. The fibrils of the vitreous merge with the internal lamellae of the ILM. This layer mainly consists of a periodic acid-Schiff (PAS) positive true basement membrane, unlike ELM. The ILM consists mainly of four elements:
1. Collagen fibrils
2. Proteoglycans of the vitreous (especially HA)
3. The basement membrane
4. The plasma membrane of the Muller cells and other glial cells of the retina

Clinical implication: Recently, ILM peeling has been considered to be one of the important steps to remove the tangential traction in macular hole surgery. Michalewska Z et al. have proposed the role of inverted ILM flap in surgery for large macular hole.[74] For details, refer to the Chapter on Macular Hole.

In posterior retina, the ILM attains a thickness of 0.5–2.0 µm. It is thickest at the fovea, but is absent at the edge of the optic disc. The ILM generally thickens with ageing and is interrupted at the ora serrata.

Blood Supply of the Retina (Fig. 1.13)

- *Outer four layers of retina:* Receive nutrition from the choriocapillaris.
- *Inner six layers of the retina:* Receive blood supply from the central retinal artery.
- Capillary network exists in most of the extramacular fundus, which can be divided into superficial and deep.
  - Superficial capillary network lies at the level of the nerve fiber layer.
  - Deep capillary network lies between inner nuclear layer and outer plexiform layer.
- Fovea is an avascular zone and receives its nutrition from choriocapillaris.
- Macula receives its blood supply by branches from superior and inferior temporal branches of the central retinal artery. In approximately 10% cases, cilioretinal artery (from the ciliary system) is seen to supply the macula.
- *Foveal avascular zone* is a capillary-free zone in the fovea of about 500 µm in diameter.
- Parafoveal zone has a three-layered capillary network, which becomes four-layered in the peripapillary region to support the extremely thick nerve fiber layer.

Choroidal circulation: The nutrition to retina is from two different circulatory systems—the retinal circulation and the choroidal or uveal circulation. Both the circulatory systems are derived from the ophthalmic artery, the first branch of the internal carotid artery.

The major branches of the ophthalmic artery are the central retinal artery, the posterior ciliary arteries, and the muscular branches. Typically, two posterior ciliary arteries

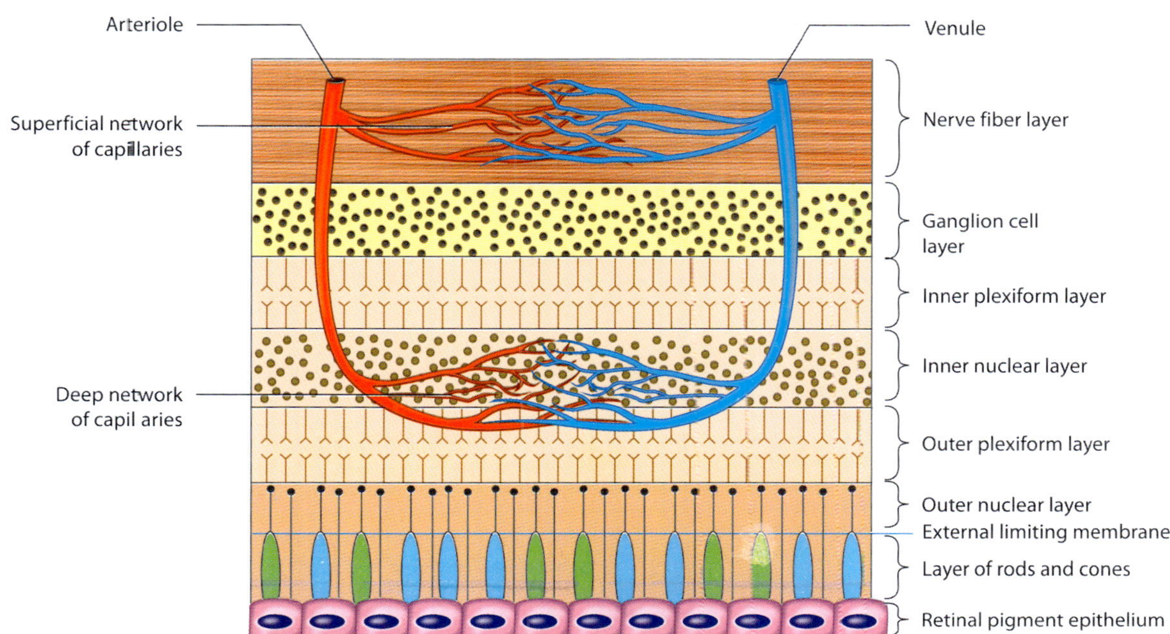

Fig. 1.13: Schematic diagram showing arrangement of retinal capillaries.

exist—a medial and a lateral—but occasionally a third superior posterior ciliary artery is seen.

The posterior ciliary arteries further divide into two long posterior ciliary arteries and numerous short posterior ciliary arteries. The outer layer of choroidal vessels, known as the *Haller's layer* merges with smaller vessels in middle *Sattler's layer.* The posterior choriocapillaris is supplied by these short posterior ciliary arteries, which enter the choroid in the peripapillary and submacular region. The anterior choriocapillaris is supplied by recurrent branches from the long ciliary arteries and anterior ciliary arteries. The watershed zone of the anterior and posterior choroidal circulatory systems is at the equator.

The choroid is by far the most vascular portion of the eye with following functions:

- It is responsible for the nourishment of the photoreceptor–RPE complex.
- Acts as a heat sink and removes the large amount of heat that develops as a result of the metabolic processes initiated when photons strike the photopigments and the melanin of the RPE and choroid.
- It probably also serves as a mechanical cushion for the internal structures of the eye.

PHYSIOLOGY OF THE VISION

The term visual cycle was given by George Wald (1906–1997; who received the Nobel prize in 1967 for this cycle named after him). It is a chain of biochemical reactions following exposure to light so that a steady state equilibrium is maintained between the rate of photo decompensation and photo regeneration. The processing of visual information begins with the detection of light by photoreceptor cells. In the photoreceptors, there occurs a cycle of rhodopsin bleaching and regeneration.

Rhodopsin is a photosensitive visual pigment in the rod outer segments. It has protein opsin and a carotenoid called retinal. The first step in the visual cycle is the absorption of photon's energy by 11-cis retinal inducing it to convert into a more stable all-trans retinal. This process is called *bleaching.* Then a series of conformational changes in rhodopsin leads to the formation of photoexcited metarhodopsin II (Fig. 1.14). Rhodopsin (500 nm)→Bathorhodopsin (543 nm) →Lumirhodopsin (497 nm)→Metarhodopsin-I (480 nm) →Metarhodopsin-II (380 nm).

After release from opsin, the fate of all-trans retinal differs in rods and cones. In cones, re-isomerization can occur in neural retina regenerating 11-cis retinal that recombines with the bleached rhodopsin. In rods all-trans retinal is converted to all-trans retinol by retinol dehydrogenase and transported to interphotoreceptor retinoid binding protein to the RPE. In the RPE, all-trans retinol is esterified to all-trans retinyl ester which is re-isomerized to 11-cis-retinol. It is then stored in RPE as 11-cis-retinyl palmitate or converted back to 11-cis-retinal and transported to rod outer segments.

Transduction

The process of translation of the information in light stimulus into electrical signals is known as visual transduction.

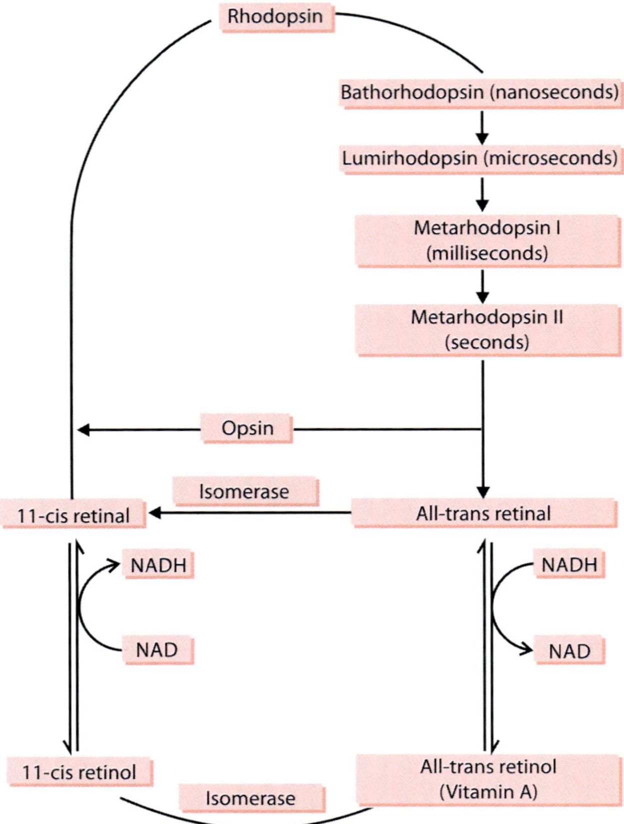

Fig. 1.14: Wald's visual cycle
(NAD: Nicotinamide adenine dinucleotide; NADH: Nicotinamide adenine dinucleotide reduced)

Metarhodopsin-II activates the heterotrimeric G-protein–transducins. Transducin is a G protein that consists of alpha, beta and gamma subunits. It binds to opsin after a conformational change at metarhodopsin II. Guanosine diphosphate (GDP) is bound to the T alpha subunit and during transduction, it is displaced by guanosine-5'-triphosphate (GTP)-causing transducing molecule to separate into a T-alpha GTP and a beta-gamma complex. Activated phosphodiesterase (PDE) catalyzes conversion of cyclic adenosine monophosphate (cAMP) to 5' guanosine monophosphate (GMP) (Fig. 1.15).

This leads to the hyperpolarization of these cells, which changes the transmission of *glutamate*-mediated neuronal signals. This initiates a downstream action potential by ganglion cells that convey signals to the brain. The cells return to its resting state (depolarized) by production of cyclic GMP by guanylate cyclase (GC) activated by Ca^{+2} entering the cells.

Recoverin Cycle

Inhibition of the photocascade can occur at several stages. Activated rhodopsin may be switched off by phosphorylation or by binding of arrestin to its phosphorylation sites. Activated PDE will continue to hydrolyze cyclic GMP until it recombines with the PDE gamma subunits. Tα-GTP is then inactivated by hydrolysis to Tα-GDP which recombines with Tβγ complex. During light stimulation calcium influx through cGMP controlled channels is inhibited. This stimulates the activity of recoverin which in turn activates GC. This enzyme increases cyclic GMP production leading to reopening of ion channels and membrane depolarization.

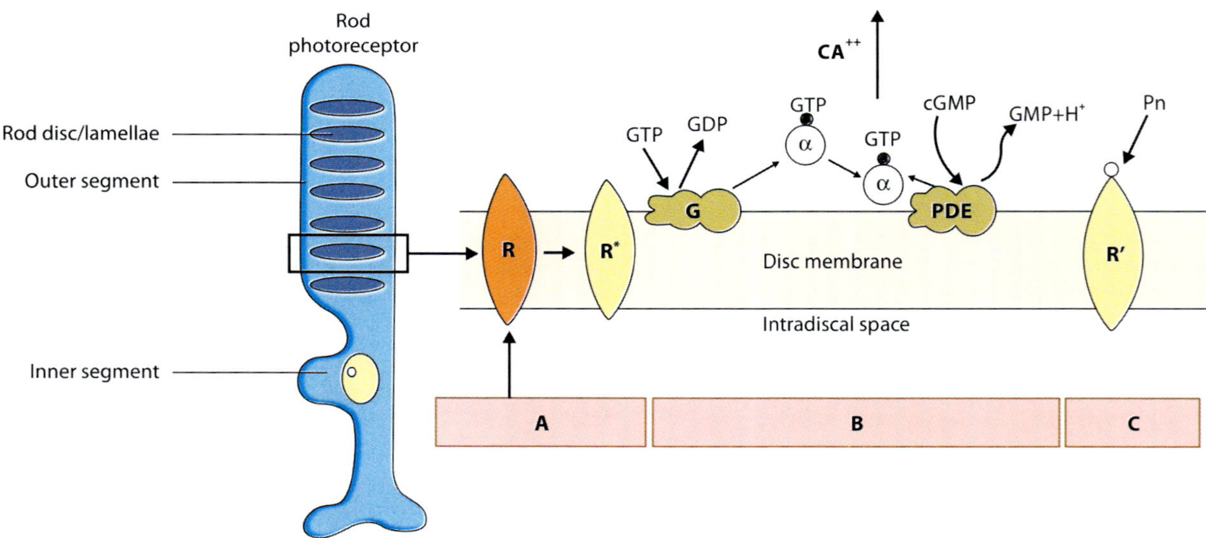

Fig. 1.15: Schematic diagram depicting the process of transduction
(GDP: Guanosine diphosphate; GTP: Guanosine-5'-triphosphate; GMP: Guanosine monophosphate; cAMP: cyclic adenosine monophosphate; PDE: Phosphodiesterase)

REFERENCES

1. Fine BS, Tousimus AJ. The structure of the vitreous body and the suspensory ligaments of the lens. Arch Ophthalmology. 1961;65:95-110.

2. Hogan M, Alvarado J, Weddell J. Histology of the Human Eye. Philadelphia: WB Saunders; 1971.

3. Schubert H. Cystoid macular edema: The apparent role of mechanical factors. Prog Clin Biol Res. 1989;312:299.

4. Davson D. Physiology of the Eye, 3rd edition. New York: Churchill Livingstone; 1972.

5. Duke-Elder F. Textbook of Ophthalmology. London: Henry Kimpton; 1938.

6. Gloor BP. The vitreous. In: Moses RA, Hart WM. (Eds.): Adlers's Physiology of the Eye, 7th Edition. St. Louis: Mosby; 1981. pp. 255-76.

7. Sebag J. Surgical anatomy of the vitreous and the vitreoretinal interface. In: Tasman W. (Ed.). Duane's Clinical Ophthalmology. Philadelphia: Lippincott; 1994. pp. 1-36.

8. Swann D. Chemistry and biology of the vitreous body. Int Rev Exp Pathol. 1989;22:2.

9. Sebag J. Macromolecular structure of the corpus vitreum. Prog Polym Sci. 1998;23:415.

10. Newsome D, Linsenmayer T, Trelstad R. Vitreous body collagen. J Cell Biol. 1976;71:59.

11. Sebag J. Age-related differences in the vitreoretinal interface. Arch Ophthalmology. 1991;109:966.

12. Balazs EA, Toth LZ, Eckl EA. Studies on the structure of the vitreous body: XII. Cytological and histochemical studies on the cortical tissue layer. Exp Eye Res. 1964;3:57.

13. Gloor BP. Cellular proliferation on the vitreous surface after photocoagulation. Graefes Arch Clin Exp Ophthalmology. 1969;178:99.

14. Sebag J. Anomalous PVD—a unifying concept in vitreoretinal diseases. Graefes Arch Clin Exp Ophthalmology. 2004;242:690-8.

15. Balazs EA, Denlinger JL. The vitreous. In: Davson H. (Ed.) The Eye, Volume 1A. New York: Academic Press; 1972.

16. Berman E. Biochemistry of the eye. New York: Plenum Press, 1991.

17. Sebag J. The vitreous. In: Hart W. (Ed.): Adler's Physiology of the Eye, 9th Edition. St. Louis: Mosby; 1985.

18. Funderburgh J, Funderburgh ML, Mann MM, et al. Physical and biological properties of keratan sulphate proteoglycan. Biochem Soc Trans. 1991;19:871-6.

19. Snowden J. The stabilization of in vivo assembled collagen fibrils by proteoglycans/glycosaminoglycans. Biochim Biophys Acta. 1982;703:21.

20. Nishitsuka K, Kashiwagi Y, Tojo N, et al. Hyaluronan production regulation from porcine hyalocyte cell line by cytokines. Exp Eye Res. 2007;85:539-45.

21. Kita T, Hata Y, Kano K, et al. Transforming growth factor-beta2 and connective tissue growth factor in proliferative vitreoretinal diseases: Possible involvement of hyalocytes and therapeutic potential of Rho kinase inhibitor. Diabetes. 2007;56:231-8.

22. Balazs EA, Denlinger JL. Aging changes in the vitreous. In: Dismukes K, Sekular R. (Eds.): Aging and Human Visual Function. New York: Alan R Liss Inc; 1982. pp. 45-57.

23. O'Malley P. The pattern of vitreous syneresis: a study of 800 autopsy eyes. In: Irvine AR, O'Malley C (Eds.): Advances in Vitreous Surgery. Springfield, III: Charles C Thomas; 1976. pp. 17-33.

24. Kishi S, Shimizu K. Posterior precortical vitreous pocket. Arch Ophthalmology. 1990;108:979-82.

25. Aguayo J, Glaser B, Mildvan A, et al. Study of vitreous liquefaction by NMR spectroscopy and imaging. Invest Ophthalmology Vis Sci. 1985;26:692.

26. Kamei A, Totani A. Isolation and characterization of minor glycosaminoglycans in the rabbit vitreous body. Biochem Biophys Res Commun. 1982;109:881-7.

27. Goldmann H. Senile changes of the lens and the vitreous. Am J Ophthalmology. 1964;57:1-13.

28. Maumenee IH. Vitreoretinal degeneration as a sign of generalized connective tissue diseases. Am J Ophthalmology. 1979;88:432-49.

29. Takahashi M, Jalkh A, Hoskins J, et al. Biomicroscopic evaluation and photography of liquefied vitreous in some vitreoretinal disorders. Arch Ophthalmology. 1981;99:1555-9.

30. Foos RY. Ultrastructural features of posterior vitreous detachment. Graefes Arch Clin Exp Ophthalmology. 1975;196:103-11.

31. Favre M, Goldmann H. Zur Genese der hinteren Glaskorperabhebung. Ophthalmologica. 1956;132:86-97.

32. Pischel DK. Detachment of the vitreous as seen with slit-lamp examination. Trans Am Ophthalmology Soc. 1952;50:329-46.

33. Streeten BA. Disorders of the vitreous. In: Garner A, Klintworth GK. (Eds.): Pathobiology of Ocular Disease—A Dynamic Approach. New York: Marcel Dekker; 1982. p. 1381-419.

34. Fatt I, Shantinath K. Flow conductivity of retina and its role in retinal adhesion. Exp Eye Res. 1971;12:218-26.

35. Tsuboi S. Measurement of the volume flow and hydraulic conductivity across the isolated dog retinal pigment epithelium. Invest Ophthalmology Vis Sci. 1987;28:1776-82.

36. Foulds WS. The vitreous in retinal detachment. Trans Ophthalmology Soc UK. 1975;95:412-6.

37. Osterlin S. On the molecular biology of the vitreous in the aphakic eye. Acta Ophthalmology. 1977;55:353-61.

38. Marmor MF. Retinal detachment from hyperosmotic intravitreal injection. Invest Ophthalmology Vis Sci. 1979;18:1237-44.

39. Foulds WS. Experimental retinal detachment. Trans Ophthalmology Soc UK. 1963;83:153-70.

40. Negi A, Kawano S, Marmor MF. Effects of intraocular pressure and other factors on subretinal fluid resorption. Invest Ophthalmology Vis Sci. 1987;28:2099-102.

41. Marmor MF, Maack T. Local environmental factors and retinal adhesion in the rabbit. Exp Eye Res. 1982;34:727-33.

42. Gingell D, Fornes JA. Demonstration of intermolecular forces in cell adhesion using a new electrochemical technique. Nature. 1975;256:210-11.

43. Porello K, LaVail MM. Histochemical demonstration of spatial heterogeneity in the interphotoreceptor matrix of the rat retina. Invest Ophthalmology Vis Sci. 1986;27:1577-86.

44. Berman ER. Mucopolysaccharides (glycosaminoglycans) of the retina: identification, distribution, and possible biological role. Mod Prob Ophthalmology. 1969;8:5-31.

45. Hageman GS, Kirchoff MA, Anderson DH. Biochemical characterization and distribution of retinal interphotoreceptor matrix glycoconjugates. Glycoconj J. 1990;7:512.

46. Hollyfield JG, Varner H, Rayborn ME, et al. Retinal attachment to the pigment epithelium. Retina. 1989;9:59-68.

47. Hageman GS, Marmor MF, Yao XY, et al. The interphotoreceptor matrix mediates primate retinal adhesion. Arch Ophthalmology. 1995;113:655-60.

48. Hughes BA, Miller SS, Machen TE. Effects of cyclic AMP on fluid absorption and ion transport across frog retinal pigment epithelium: measurements in the open-circuit state. J Gen Physiol. 1984;83:875-99.

49. Frambach DA, Weiter JJ, Adler AJ. A photogrammetric method to measure fluid movement across isolated frog retinal pigment epithelium. Biophys J. 1985;47:547-52.

50. Negi A, Marmor MF. Effects of subretinal and systemic osmolality on the rate of subretinal fluid resorption. Invest Ophthalmology Vis Sci. 1984;25:616-20.

51. Kita M, Marmor MF. Retinal adhesive force in living rabbit, cat, and monkey eyes: normative data and enhancement by mannitol

and acetazolamide. Invest Ophthalmology Vis Sci. 1992;33:1879-82.

52. Kita M, Marmor MF. Systemic mannitol increases the retinal adhesive force in vivo. Arch Ophthalmology. 1991;109:1449-50.

53. Yao XY, Moore KT, Marmor MF. Systemic mannitol increases retinal adhesiveness measured in vitro. Arch Ophthalmology. 1991;109:275-7.

54. Singelman J, Ozanics V. Retina. In: Jakobiec (Ed.): Ocular Anatomy, Embryology and Teratology. Philadelphia: Harper and Row; 1982. p. 441.

55. Tripathi RC, Tripathi BJ. Anatomy of the human eye, orbit and adnexa. In: Davson H (Ed.): The Eye, 3rd Edition. London: Academic Press; 1984. pp. 40,145.

56. Ryan SJ, Ogde T (Eds). Retina, 5th Edition. St. Louis: Mosby CV; 1989.

57. Ogden T. Topography of the retina. In: Ryan SJ, Ogde (Eds): Retina, 5th Edition. St. Louis: Mosby CV; 1989. p. 32.

58. Schmidt SY, Peisch RD. Melanin concentration in normal human retinal pigment epithelium: Regional variation and age-related reduction. Invest Ophthalmology Vis Sci. 1986;27:1063-7.

59. Cantrill HL, Pederson JE. Experimental retinal detachment. VI. The permeability of the blood–retinal barrier. Arch Ophthalmology. 1984;102:747-51.

60. Frambach DA, Marmor MF. The rate and route of fluid resorption from the subretinal space of the rabbit. Invest Ophthalmology Vis Sci. 1982;22:292-302.

61. Negi A, Marmor MF. Quantitative estimation of metabolic transport of subretinal fluid. Invest Ophthalmology Vis Sci. 1986;27:1564-8.

62. Pederson JE, Cantrill HL. Experimental retinal detachment. V. Fluid movement through the retinal hole. Arch Ophthalmology. 1984;102:136-9.

63. Hamann S, Kiilgaard JF, La Cour M, et al. Cotransport of H+, lactate, and H2O in porcine retinal pigment epithelial cells. Exp Eye Res. 2003;76:493-504.

64. Chihara E, Nao IN. Resorption of subretinal fluid by trans-epithelial flow of the retinal pigment epithelium. Graefes Arch Ophthalmology. 1985;223:202-4.

65. Fine BS. Limiting membranes of the sensory retina and pigment epithelium. An electron microscopic study. Arch Ophthalmology. 1961;66:847-60.

66. Zinn KM, Benjamin-Henkind J. Retinal pigment epithelium. In: Jakobiec F (Ed.): Ocular Anatomy, Embryology and Teratology. Philadelphia: Harper and Row; 1982. p. 553.

67. Tamai M, Chader GJ. The early appearance of disk shedding in the rat retina. Invest Ophthalmology Vis Sci. 1979;18:913-7.

68. Tamai M, Teirstein P, Goldman A, et al. The pineal gland does not control rod outer segment shedding and phagocytosis in the rat retina and pigment epithelium. Invest Ophthalmology Vis Sci. 1978;17:558-62.

69. Hauswirth WW, Aleman TS, Kaushal S, et al. Treatment of leber congenital amaurosis due to RPE65 mutations by ocular subretinal injection of adeno-associated virus gene vector: short-term results of a phase I trial. Hum Gene Ther. 2008;19(10):979-90.

70. Landa G, Gentile RC, Garcia PM, et al. External limiting membrane and visual outcome in macular hole repair: spectral domain OCT analysis. Eye (Lond). 2012;26(1):61-9.

71. Kolb H, Linberg KA, Fisher SK. Neurons of the human retina: a Golgi study. J Comp Neurol. 1992;318(2):147-87.

72. Davanger S, Ottersen OP, Storm-Mathisen J. Glutamate, GABA, and glycine in the human retina: An immunocytochemical investigation. J Comp Neurol. 1991;311:483-94.

73. Crooks J, Kolb H. Localization of GABA, glycine, glutamate and tyrosine hydroxylase in the human retina. J Comp Neurol. 1992;315:287-302.

74. Michalewska Z, Michalewski J, Adelman RA, et al. Inverted internal limiting membrane flap technique for large macular holes. Ophthalmology. 2010;117(10):2018-25.

Chapter 2

Retinal Imaging

Atul Kumar, Devesh Kumawat, Raghav Ravani, Kavitha Duraipandi, Anu Sharma

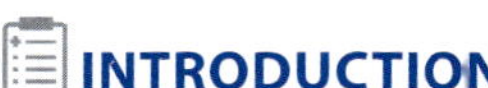

INTRODUCTION

The past decade has witnessed a huge leap from the traditional ophthalmic equipment to the radical cutting-edge technologies for retinal imaging. Diseases involving the eye and other systems of the body can manifest themselves in the retina. With continuing advancement, we can image the retina layer by layer which aids in early diagnosis of otherwise unseen pathologies. While many structures of the eyeball contribute to vision, this chapter highlights the basics of retinal imaging, equipment, techniques involved, image analysis methods and their clinical implications, focusing on the prevalent causes of retinal blindness.

FUNDUS FLUORESCEIN ANGIOGRAPHY

History and Evolution

Fundus angiography has long played an important role in the understanding, diagnosis, and management of retinal vascular disorders. A standard fundus angiogram is a good baseline tool for fine-tuning the diagnosis of choroidal and retinal disorders. As early as in 1954, Edward Maumenee, one of the greatest scholars in retinal vascular diseases, while at Stanford University, used intravenously injected fluorescein with Goldmann slit lamp, contact lens and cobalt blue filter to study choroidal hemangiomas. Subsequently, Milton Flocks and Peter Chao did substantial work to study circulation time in cats using fluorescent dyes. Later, an outstanding contribution toward modern fundus fluorescein angiography (FFA) came from *Harold Novotny*, a junior medical student at Indiana University along with *David Alvis*, a medical intern, who have determined the absorption and emission wavelengths of fluorescein dye and subsequently attached a fundus camera with a blue filter in the path of the activating light and also a green filter for transmission of the dye fluorescence while absorbing most of the background fluorescence. This was photographed on black and white paper to produce an image. Novotny and Alvis, in their 1961 publication in "*Circulation*" had so clearly described the camera and

filter details and the fluorescein technique that it has largely remained unchanged.[1] A new standard for the use of stereoscopic fluorescein angiography was later set by Dr J Donald Gass in 1967 in his book "*Atlas of Macular Diseases*" for diagnosis of retinal diseases.[2]

Basic Principle

To understand the principle of FFA, process like luminescence, fluorescence and phosphorescence should be known.

Luminescence is the emission of light from any source not resulting due to high temperature. Free electrons are excited into higher energy states when light energy is absorbed by a luminescent material. As the excited electrons decay into their lower energy states, an equivalent amount of energy is re-emitted, which when present in the visible spectrum, is called *luminescence*. Fluorophores absorb electromagnetic energy, temporarily exciting them to a higher energy state. As the molecules return to their original energy level, they emit light of a different, usually longer wavelength. *Fluorescence* is *luminescence* that is maintained only by continuous excitation whereas phosphorescence continues to emit light even after the excitation is stopped. In FFA, sodium fluorescein, which is 80% protein bound is injected intravenously. The remaining 20% which freely circulates in the bloodstream fluoresces on excitation at a particular wavelength. In a fundus camera, a blue excitation filter permits only the blue light from a white source to enter the retina and absorbs all other light. This blue light excites the fluorescein in the bloodstream which starts emitting green-yellow light at 520–530 nm. A barrier filter keeps out the blue excitation light (all wavelengths <520 nm) and allows only green-yellow light (all wavelengths >520 nm) to be captured electronically as a digital image.

Pseudofluorescence is a phenomenon that occurs when nonfluorescent light cannot be filtered by the entire filter system as seen in case of old worn-out filters. It causes nonfluorescent structures to fluoresce leading to difficulty in interpretation. It decreases the contrast and resolution of the fundus image. *Pseudofluorescence* must be avoided by careful and regular replacement of filters.

Materials and Equipments

Solution: Fluorescein sodium ($C_{20}H_{10}Na_2O_5$) is water-soluble orange-red crystalline hydrocarbon, also known as "resorcinol phthalein sodium", or uranine ($C_{20}H_{12}O_5Na$), having a low molecular weight (376.27 Da). Fluorescein emits wavelength of ~520–530 nm when it is excited by blue light of ~465–490 nm. 80% of the dye is protein-bound and this fraction does not fluoresce, only the unbound 20% fluoresces. The dye was first synthesized in 1871 by Adolf Von Baeyer, who later received the Nobel Prize in Chemistry (in 1905) for his work on organic dyes. 10 mL of 5% fluorescein, 5 mL of 10% fluorescein and 3 mL of 25% fluorescein solution are available commercially in vials of which 3 mL of 25% and 5 mL of 10% solution are preferred to obtain good contrast images. The fluorescein diffuses through most of the body fluids and through the choriocapillaris, but cannot diffuse through the tight junctions between the retinal vascular endothelial cells (inner blood-retinal barrier) or the zona occludentes between the retinal pigment epithelium (RPE) cells (outer blood-retinal barrier). It is usually eliminated by the liver and kidneys within 1 day, although traces can be found in the body for few weeks.

Various side effects and complications have been described with fluorescein injection.

- *Local side effects:*
  - Extravasation of dye during the injection procedure can be extremely painful and can lead to overlying skin necrosis. Cold compresses and subcutaneous 2% xylocaine injection can be helpful in reducing pain.
  - Inadvertent arterial injection
  - Thrombophlebitis
  - Peripheral nerve palsy
- *Systemic side effects:*
  - Nausea is the most common systemic side effect of fluorescein injection, vomiting occurs infrequently. Oral promethazine hydrochloride (*Phenergan*) 25–50 mg can be used to premedicate patients who previously have had an episode of nausea or vomiting during the procedure.
  - Vasovagal attack can occur in some anxious patients wherein the angiogram needs to be abandoned.
  - Although rare, more severe adverse reactions include anaphylaxis, laryngeal edema, bronchospasm, tonic-clonic seizures, myocardial infarction and cardiac arrest and even death.[3,4]

Contraindications: A known allergy or history of severe adverse reaction during previous fluorescein dye injection is an absolute contraindication. Heart disease or cardiac pacemakers are not a contraindication to fluorescein injection. While there have been no reports of fetal complications from fluorescein injection during pregnancy, the current practice is to avoid angiography in women who are pregnant, especially those in the first trimester.

Film-based versus Digital Fluorescence

The accessibility of digital-based fluorescein angiography has gained wider acceptance over film-based imaging. Despite higher resolution and better viewing of stereo images in film-based imaging, images are comparatively difficult to manipulate, and training and effort are required to process and duplicate film. Film-based images are also difficult to transmit or share as the process is time-consuming compared with digital images.

A digital imaging unit is classically used for FFA. Its advantages include software to improve image quality, storage and reproducibility, exporting images for telemedicine, and measurements and analysis. Main limitations with digital fundus camera include absorption effects of the lens, nonconfocality, light scattering and weak autofluorescence signal.[5] More recently, digital fundus-camera-based systems have been developed which use high-sensitivity monochrome sensors with shifting of excitation filter (580 nm) and barrier filter (695 nm) toward longer wavelength to avoid confounding autofluorescence from the lens.

Alternatively one can use a *confocal scanning laser ophthalmoscope (cSLO)* which instead of a flash-bulb technology in digital cameras, uses near-infrared laser beam (NIR) that quickly scans the retina, captured by a confocal detector and creates a high-resolution, high-contrast image, however of smaller field (30°) (Table 2.1). Webb et al. developed confocal scanning laser ophthalmoscope (cSLO) which scans the retina in two directions: X and Y using a low-energy laser source.[6] The crystalline lens is highly fluorescent in the short-wavelength range (excitation between 400 nm and 600 nm results in peak emission at 520 nm) forming the principal barrier for capturing fundus images. The principle of confocality ensures that the reflectance and fluorescence correspond to the same focal plane, suppressing the defocused light. The original technique used a confocal SLO with the excitation wavelength set at 488 nm and a wide band-pass filter with short wavelength cut-off at 521 nm. Digital fundus photography and confocal scanning laser ophthalmoscopy (cSLO) are the two methods used for capturing fundus photographs. A digital camera captures a single image of the retina, whereas cSLO captures point-by-point image of the retina using laser light projected through a pinhole aperture to produce light of a single wavelength. Different depths and scans are captured in a raster pattern by adjusting the distance of the pinhole aperture. cSLO adds false color to the fundus image by using lasers of different wavelength; whereas, digital fundus photography captures a true color image. cSLO makes it quite strenuous for patients to stay motionless while capturing image as the intensity of laser light is low, but fast acquisition speeds and after-image processing help correct movement artifacts. cSLO can also use longer wavelengths to capture images, making them an ideal tool for fundus autofluorescence (FAF) and indocyanine green (ICG) angiograms.

Table 2.1: Differences between digital fundus camera and confocal scanning laser ophthalmoscope (cSLO).

Modified fundus camera	Confocal scanning laser ophthalmoscope (cSLO)
One single flash at maximum intensity, hence a single image of the fundus is captured.	Continuous scanning at low light intensities. So, scans are obtained in raster fashion through a pinhole aperture.
Entire cone of light	Confocal system
True color image	Pseudo color image
Bandwidth filters for excitation and emission	One excitation wavelength (laser source) Large emission spectrum (cut off filter)
Slower image acquisition capability	Faster acquisition speed, faster after-image processing and thus decreased motion artifacts
Uses shorter wavelengths for FAF and ICG images	cSLO uses longer wavelengths, hence captures higher resolution images for FAF and ICG
Difficult to use in media opacity and poor dilation.	Penetrates media opacity and possible in eyes with poor dilation

Stereoscopic imaging during angiography enhances diagnostic information. Stereoscopic photography helps the ophthalmologist to appreciate different depths and view retinal and choroidal circulation independently. It is obtained by laterally shifting the fundus camera a few millimeters between subsequent photographs, photographing from one side to opposite side of pupil, which are later combined with stereo-viewers. This shift causes the light beam of the fundus camera to project on opposite slopes of the cornea. A hyperstereoscopic effect is created from the resulting cornea-induced parallax which is evident when the sequential pair of photographs is viewed together.

Camera and Ancillary Equipments

Digital fundus cameras range from 30° to 50° field of view and are routinely employed for FFA (Fig. 2.1). Wide-field angiography cameras range from 35° to 200° ultra-wide field systems exist at present, like the Optos system. Wide-angle angiography has the advantage of capturing a single high-resolution image of the retina well beyond the equator and help image the retinal periphery at the same time.

Filters: The exciter filter transmits blue light at 465–490 nm which is the absorption peak of fluorescein excitation and the barrier filter transmits light at 525–530 nm which is the fluorescent or emitted peak of fluorescein. In order to achieve a good image, the filters must allow maximal transmission of light in the appropriate spectral range without the use of an excessively bright flash unit. One should request the transmission curves of the filter combination while choosing the camera to be sure that no significant overlap exists; an overlap usually results in pseudofluorescence.

Technique of Fundus Fluorescein Angiography

Patient positioning: Inform patient about the procedure of fluorescein angiography. A written informed consent from

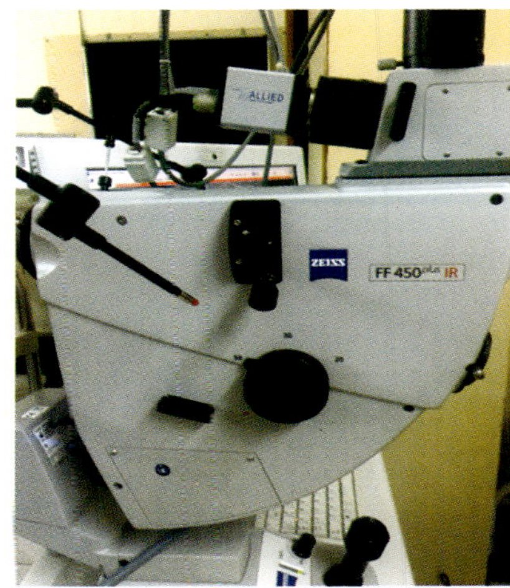

Fig. 2.1: Digital fundus camera used for performing fundus autofluorescence (FAF), flucrescein and indocyanine green (FA and ICG) angiography.

the patient or parents (if minor) should be obtained. Maximum pupil dilatation is required for capturing peripheral areas of retina. Patient sits comfortably with a loose neck collar in front of camera. Patient should ideally be fasting for 3 to 4 hours while performing FFA given the high likelihood of nausea and vomiting during the procedure. Patient should be identified and the demographic data are entered into the database. Patient should be positioned for proper alignment, focus and comfort.

Dye injection: Color fundus photographs and black-and-white monochromatic red-free filter images are routinely taken as baseline pictures before administration of the dye. The early transit phase, which usually lasts less than a minute, is the most critical part of the angiogram. Before injecting the dye, the illuminating beam of the fundus camera is centered

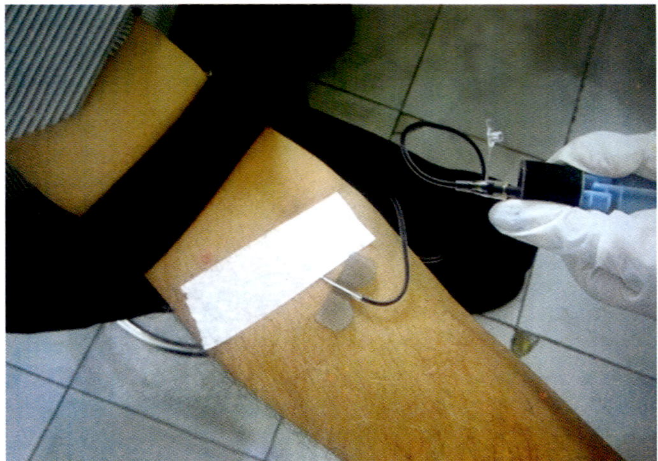

Fig. 2.2: Intravenous injection of 20% fluorescein dye being injected via the antecubital vein using a 24-G scalp vein attached to the 10 cc syringe.

Table 2.2: The approximate timing of normal circulatory dye filling in the eye.

Phase of angiogram	Timing from the start of injection (approximate)
Injection of dye	0 sec
Posterior ciliary arteries	9.5 sec
Choroidal flush (or prearterial phase)	10 sec
Retinal arterial phase	10–12 sec
Arteriovenous phase (laminar stage or early venous stage)	14–15 sec
Venous phase	16–17 sec
Late phase	5 min

within the dilated pupil. The area of interest on the retina is prefocused by the angiographer and then a bolus injection of the dye is administered using a small gauge scalp vein needle (24–25 G) into an antecubital vein (Fig. 2.2).

Fluorescein photography: The timer is started as soon as the dye is injected and the angiographer starts capturing images. The arm-to-retina circulation time usually takes 10–12 seconds in normal individuals. Images are usually taken at a speed of one frame per second until maximum fluorescence occurs. During this early phase only the images of one eye can be captured. Photographs of the other eye or other areas of retina in the primary eye can be captured as soon as the early phase is complete.

The appearance of the dye stabilizes and starts to fade slowly over the next few minutes. Unlike during the early phase, now the angiographer can capture appropriate images as needed. Late phase fundus images are captured as the dye dissipates, anywhere between 7 minutes and 15 minutes after injection. Post angiography, the patient should be informed of dyschromatopsia and yellowish discoloration of urine and skin for a day or so.

Interpretation of a Normal Fundus Angiogram

Dynamic interaction of fluorescein with both normal and abnormal anatomical structures is recorded by fluorescein angiography. Fluorescein dye flows through the internal carotid artery to the ophthalmic artery and then enters the ocular circulation through the short posterior ciliary arteries which supplies the choroid and central retinal artery which supplies the retina. There is a short delay between the "choroid flush" and retinal filling since the route to the choroid is typically less tortuous than the route to the retina. In a normal fluorescein angiogram, the fluorescence starts to be evident in the choriocapillaris approximately 10–12 seconds after injection in younger patients and it may be prolonged up to 12–15 seconds in older patients. Table 2.2 demonstrates the normal phases of an angiogram in human eye.

The choriocapillaris are arranged in a lobular fashion in the posterior fundus, which gives a patchy choroidal fluorescence in the early phase of the angiogram. The foveal avascular zone is relatively hypofluorescent due to the presence of more pigmented and taller RPE cells along with the presence of xanthophyll pigment and absence of retinal capillaries in the center of the fovea.

Phases of Angiography

Choroidal flush: The choroid occasionally begins to fluoresce 1 or 2 seconds before the initial filling of the central retinal artery. This early phase is referred to as the choroidal flush. In presence of a cilioretinal artery, it usually fluoresces along with the choroidal flush. Choroidal fluorescence is less visible in areas where the RPE is darker and vice versa.

Arterial phase: It starts at approximately 1–2 seconds after the choroidal flush as the central retinal artery fills and the dye flows into the retinal arterioles; therefore, the normal "arm-to-retina" circulation time is around 12 seconds (Fig. 2.3). Any delay in the arm-to-retina time may reveal a problem with the injection of fluorescein dye or circulatory disorders including internal carotid artery stenosis.

Arteriovenous phase: Arterial phase is followed by filling of the retinal capillary bed and the retinal veins. Thin column of fluorescein is seen along the walls of the larger veins in this phase as dye from the venules enters the veins (known as *laminar flow*) (Fig. 2.4).

Venous phase: The arteriovenous phase is followed by venous phase where the venous columns become broader as the dye fills up the venous lumen. Over the next 10 seconds the vein gets completely filled with the dye causing maximum vessel fluorescence occurring ~30s after injection, called the "peak

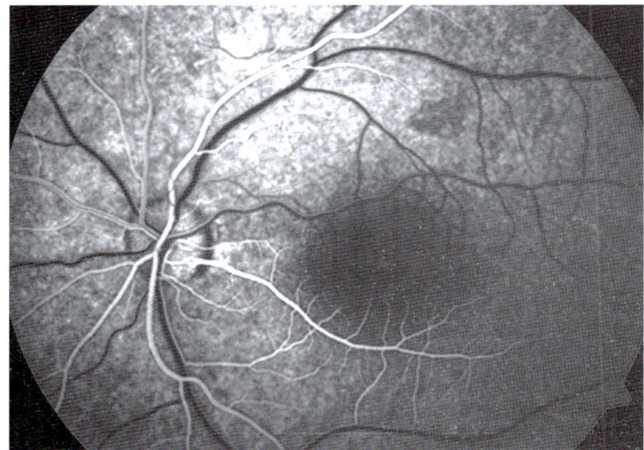

Fig. 2.3: Arterial phase of fluorescein angiogram.

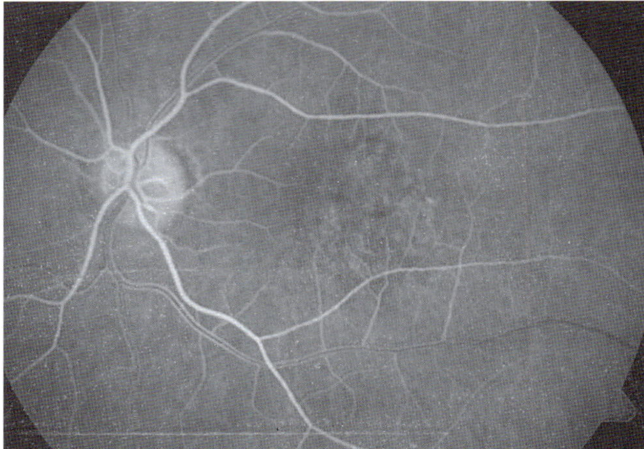

Fig. 2.4: Arteriovenous phase showing laminar flow in the veins.

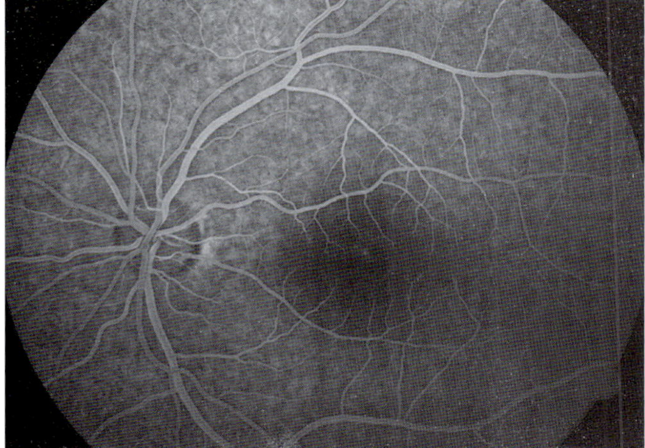

Fig. 2.5: Venous phase showing the complete filling of the arterial and venous systems.

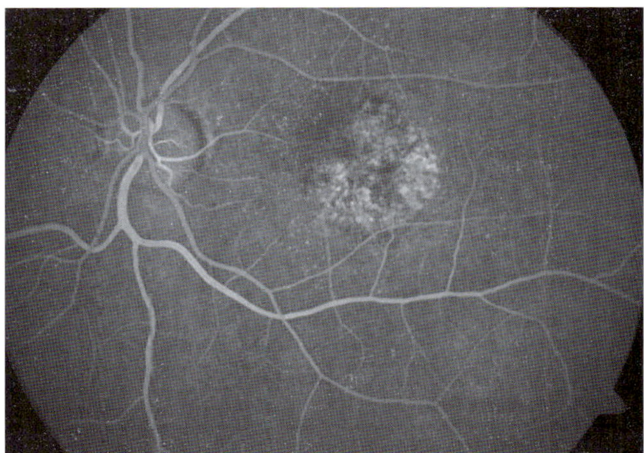

Fig. 2.6: Mid phase of the fluorescein angiogram showing equal filling of arteries and veins with macula showing mottled fluorescence.

phase" of angiogram (Fig. 2.5). This phase is best to visualize the perifoveal capillary network.

Mid phase: Also known as the recirculation phase, this occurs at 2–4 minutes after injection. The veins and arteries remain roughly equal in brightness (Fig. 2.6).

Late phase: The late or elimination phase demonstrates the gradual elimination of dye from the retinal and choroidal vasculature and is visible at ~5 minutes post injection. Late staining of the optic disc is a normal finding. Central area of late hyperfluorescence suggests staining from a choroidal neovascularization (CNV) lesion (Fig. 2.7).

Abnormal Fluorescein Angiogram

Various patterns of abnormal fluorescence may be seen and one must first determine, if they are hypofluorescent or hyperfluorescent in nature.

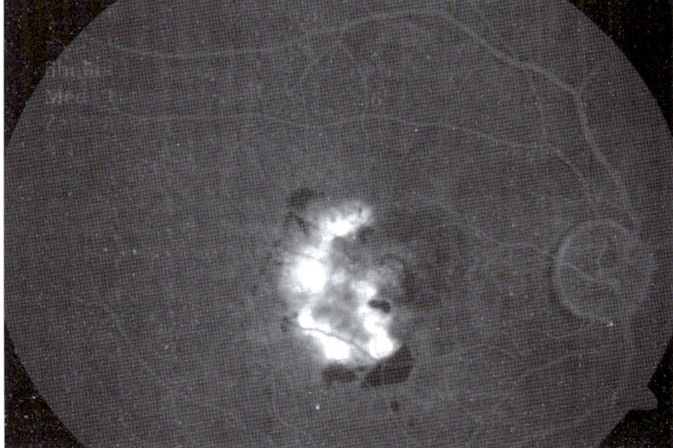

Fig. 2.7: Late phase of the fluorescein angiogram showing the disappearance of dye and associated hyperfluorescent leaking CNV with surrounding edge hypofluorescence secondary to the hemorrhage.

Hypofluorescence

Hypofluorescence is reduced or absent normal fluorescence, which can be categorized into "blocked fluorescence" (masking of fluorescence) or "vascular filling defects". Flame-shaped hemorrhages are superficial and block all retinal vascular fluorescence, while deeper dot or blot hemorrhages block capillary fluorescence but do not block larger superficial vessels (*see* Fig. 2.7). Pathologies located anterior to the choroid and in the subretinal space such as hemorrhage, melanin, lipofuscin (LF), lipid, fibrin, and inflammatory materials can block choroidal fluorescence.

Vascular filling defects result from vascular obstruction (Figs. 2.8A and B), absence of vessels. Conditions involving retinal vasculature include central or branch artery occlusion, capillary nonperfusion secondary to diabetes, vein occlusion, radiation, etc. Conditions involving choroidal vasculature include occlusion of large choroidal vessels or choriocapillaris, malignant hypertension, toxemia, lupus choroidopathy also cause hypofluorescence.

Hyperfluorescence

Hyperfluorescence can be secondary to dye leakage, pooling, staining, pseudofluorescence, autofluorescence, and transmitted fluorescence.

Leakage: Leakage of fluorescein dye is defined as hyperfluorescence due to fluorescein in the extravascular space. The area of fluorescence increases in both size and intensity with time. Retinal neovascularization, other retinal vascular abnormalities, such as vasculitis or inflammatory lesions or macular edema due to breakdown of blood-retinal barrier, can cause leakage of fluorescein because of the increased permeability of blood vessels (Figs. 2.9A and B).

Optic nerve pathology, such as papilledema and ischemic optic neuropathy, produces leakage of the optic nerve head during the late phase of the angiogram.

Pooling: Accumulation of dye into a confined anatomical space with resulting increasing fluorescence although no increase in area of leakage. Pooling is seen in the detachments of neurosensory retina and RPE (Figs. 2.10A and B).

Staining: Staining refers to a pattern of hyperfluorescence where the fluorescence gradually increases in intensity through transit views and more so in late frames. There occurs deposition of fluorescein dye within the involved tissues like fibrous tissue or scar (Fig. 2.11). It is seen in staphyloma, disc, sclera and chorioretinal scar. Normal structures, such as the optic disc and sclera demonstrate staining physiologically. Scleral staining is seen more easily in high myopes and patients who have lightly pigmented fundi.

Transmitted fluorescence: Increased fluorescence from the underlying choroidal vasculature due to absence of overlying RPE is termed as transmitted fluorescence. The major cause of pigment epithelial window defect is atrophy of the pigment epithelium, as in dry AMD. Transmitted fluorescence appears early in study, along with choroidal filling and increases in intensity as dye concentration increases in the choroid which remain uniform in size and gradually declines in fluorescence in the later phases of angiography (Fig. 2.12). It may appear similar to hyperfluorescence, hence it is important to differentiate between the two.

Autofluorescence: It is the continuous emission of fluorescent light from ocular structures in the absence of fluorescein dye. Optic nerve head drusen and astrocytic hamartoma on the disc can cause autofluorescence (Figs. 2.13 to 2.15).

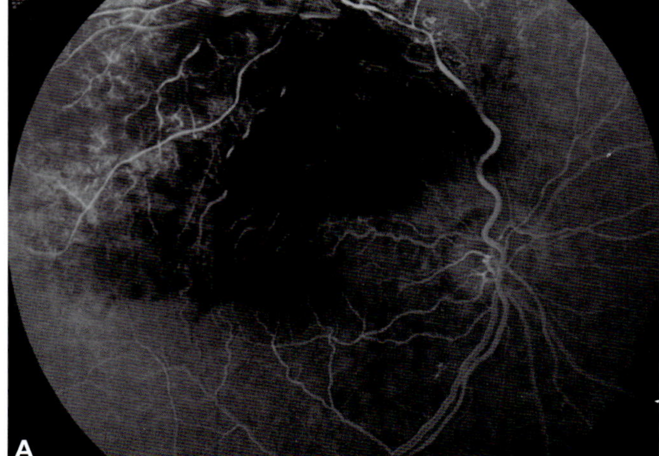
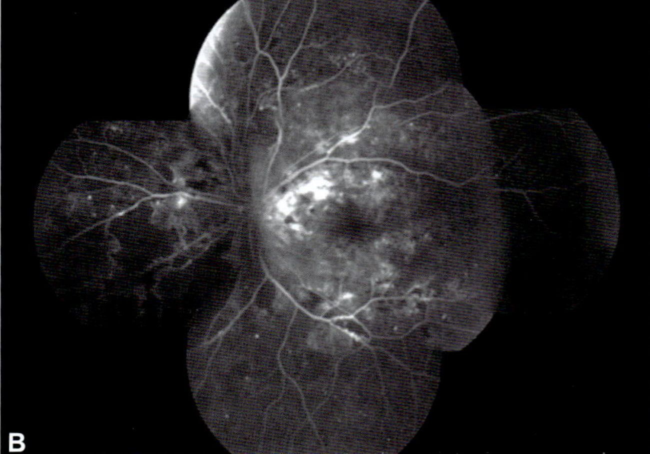

Figs. 2.8A and B: Blocked fluorescence secondary to preretinal hemorrhages in an eye with branch vein occlusion (BVO). (B) Nasal quadrant hypofluorescence due to capillary nonperfusion in an eye with BVO.

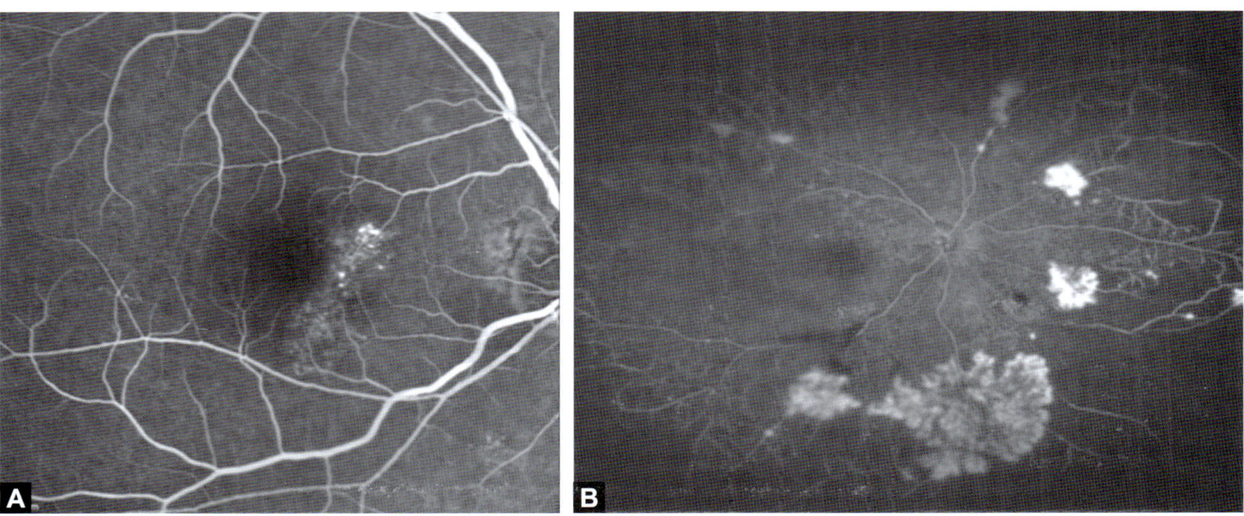

Figs. 2.9A and B: (A) Dye leakage in the macular area in an eye with polypoidal choroidal vasculopathy (PCV) with leaking polyps. (B) Dye leak from multiple NVEs in an eye with PDR.

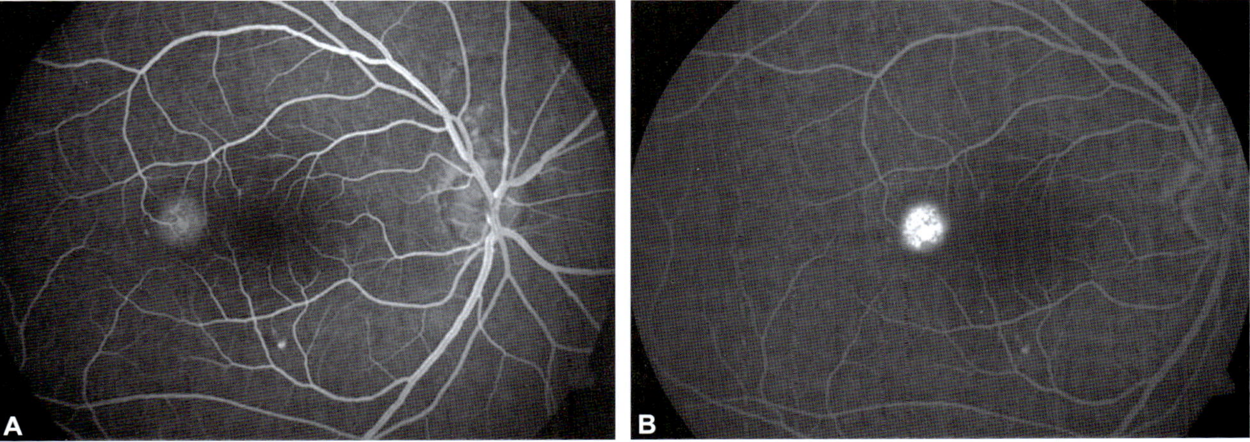

Figs. 2.10A and B: Pooling as seen in the early (A) and late (B) frames where the dye intensity increases within confined boundaries.

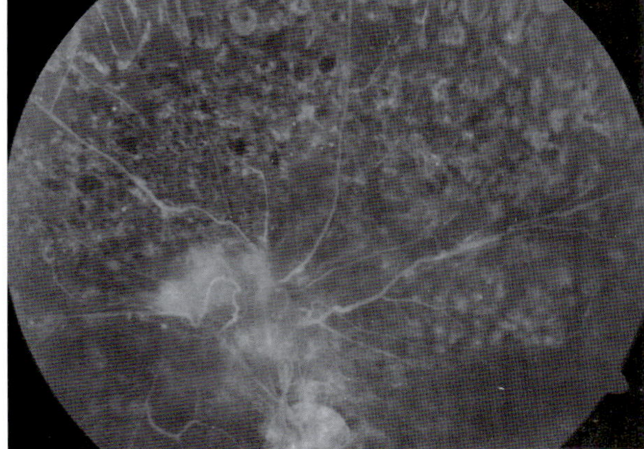

Fig. 2.11: Lasered diabetic retinopathy eye showing hyperfluorescence and late phase staining of fibrous tissue over and around the optic disc.

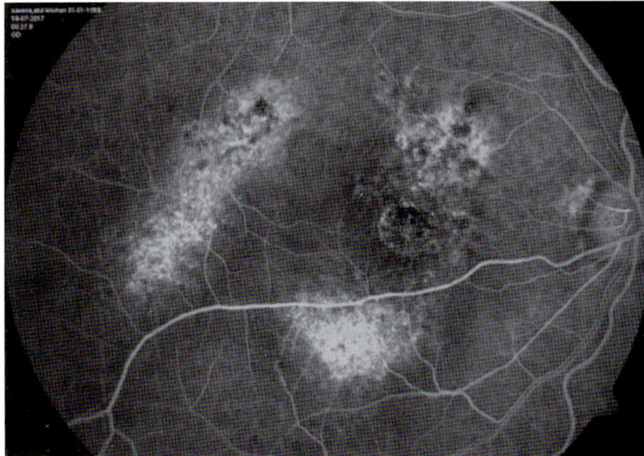

Fig. 2.12: Late phase of fluorescein angiogram showing transmitted fluorescence (window defect) due to retinal pigment epithelium (RPE) disturbance (gravitational tracks) in an eye with chronic central serous chorioretinopathy (CSC).

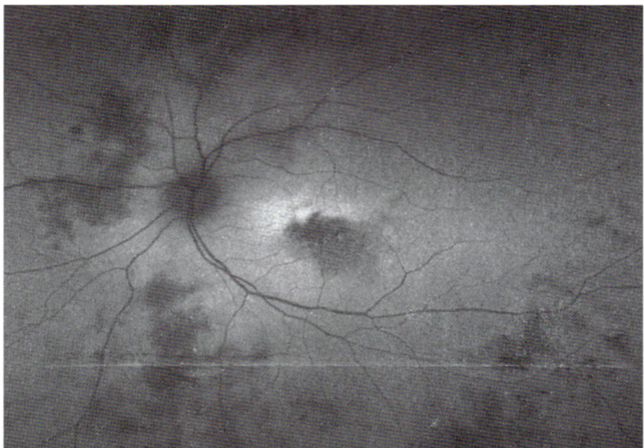

Fig. 2.13: Retinal pigment epithelium (RPE) hypoautofluorescence in an eye with retinitis pigmentosa.

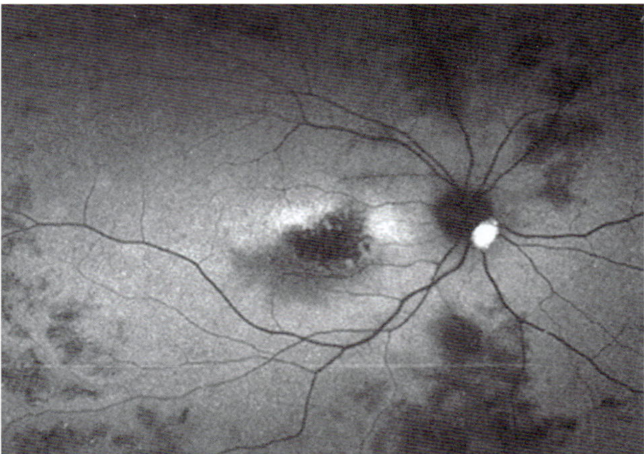

Fig. 2.14: Retinitis pigmentosa (RP) in the fellow eye showing hypoautofluorescence with increased autofluorescence (AF) from disc drusen.

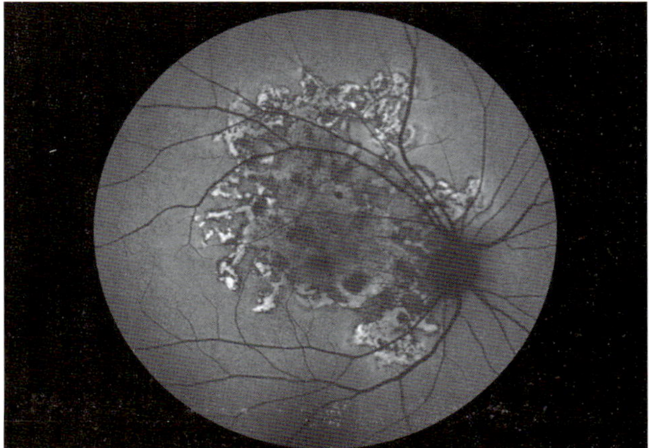

Fig. 2.15: Active serpiginous choroiditis with hyperautofluorescent lesions and hypoautofluorescent borders.

Advances in Fundus Fluorescein Angiography

The first fundus camera was developed by Carl Zeiss and J W Nordenson in 1926 which provided a 20° fundoscopic image which increased to 30° field over the years. Recently, imaging of the ocular fundus has been made possible through the use of scanning laser ophthalmoscopy (SLO), which uses laser light and the principle of confocal laser scanning. The prototype Heidelberg HRA can be used to create widefield images, if used in conjunction with wide-angle lenses.

Confocal scanning laser ophthalmoscopy (cSLO) was used initially by von Rückmann and coworkers in a clinical imaging system.[7] A low-power laser beam on the retina which is swept across the fundus in a raster pattern.[6] The detector then records the intensity of the reflected light at each point, after passing through the confocal pinhole, and a two-dimensional image is subsequently created. Image contrast is enhanced as out-of-focus reflected light is omitted by confocal optics (Figs. 2.16A and B). The standard image field of the typical cSLO encompasses a retinal field of 30° × 30°.

The present day cSLO platform is a modular design including real-time infra-red reflectance imaging, blue reflectance, autofluorescent imaging, FA and ICG simultaneous imaging with video angiography facility and wide-field imaging using non-contact 55 degree, 102 degree and a contact 155 degree lens option. This proves to a very versatile imaging option with high resolution images.

Ultra-wide-field (UWF) imaging has opened areas of study previously unknown in the vitreoretinal subspecialty. FAF can now be acquired in less than 2 seconds by using green light excitation (532 nm) which has been recently introduced in widefield scanning laser ophthalmoscope (P200Tx, Optos) (Figs. 2.17A and B). It uses ellipsoid mirror and two focal points to obtain images from the retinal periphery even in a nonmydriatic eye. The Optos camera also employs scanning laser ophthalmoscopy technology and is capable of producing widefield images with 200° field of view, which equates to 82.5% of total retinal surface area.[8] It employs multiple wavelength imaging using different lasers. The first commercially available Optos camera was built with 532 nm and 633 nm for red and green laser acquired two-color images. With the addition of 488 nm blue laser, it is capable of producing high-resolution fluorescein angiogram images of the retinal periphery and autofluorescence images, which are valuable in disorders that affect the retinal pigment epithelium (Figs. 2.18A and B). The latest addition is an 805 nm infrared laser which has been incorporated to acquire ICG angiography images.

Ultra-wide-field imaging helps us to image the retina anterior to the equator and helps to identify areas of capillary nonperfusion, peripheral vascular changes and neovascularization which is helpful in cases with diabetic retinopathy, retinal vasculitis and vascular occlusions etc.

Ultra-wide-field fluorescein angiography helps in accurate delineation of retinal capillary nonperfusion and precise application of photocoagulation—so called targeted retinal

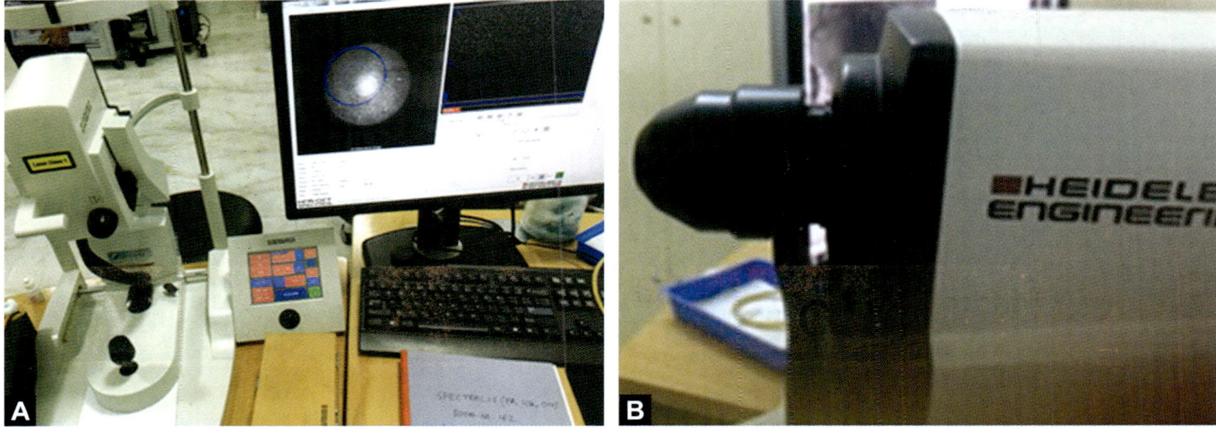

Figs. 2.16A and B: (A) Confocal scanning laser ophthalmoscope with multimodal imaging platform having autofluorescence imaging, infrared fluorescence imaging, real-time fluorescein angiography (FA), indocyanine green (CG), spectral-domain optical coherence tomography (SD-OCT) and optical coherence tomography angiography (OCTA). (B) Heidelberg scanning laser ophthalmoscope (SLO) has options of a noncontact 55° lens seen above, and wide-field 105° lens besides a contact 155° lens.

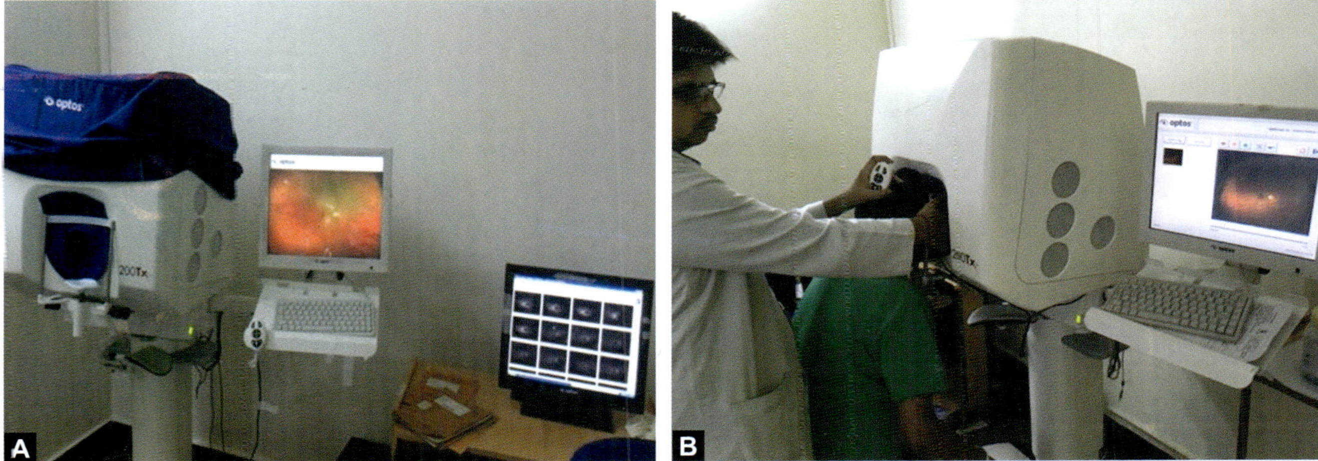

Figs. 2.17A and B: The ultrawide-field Optos 200Tx device offers multiple wavelength imaging, including options for colour, fluorescein angiography and autofluorescence.

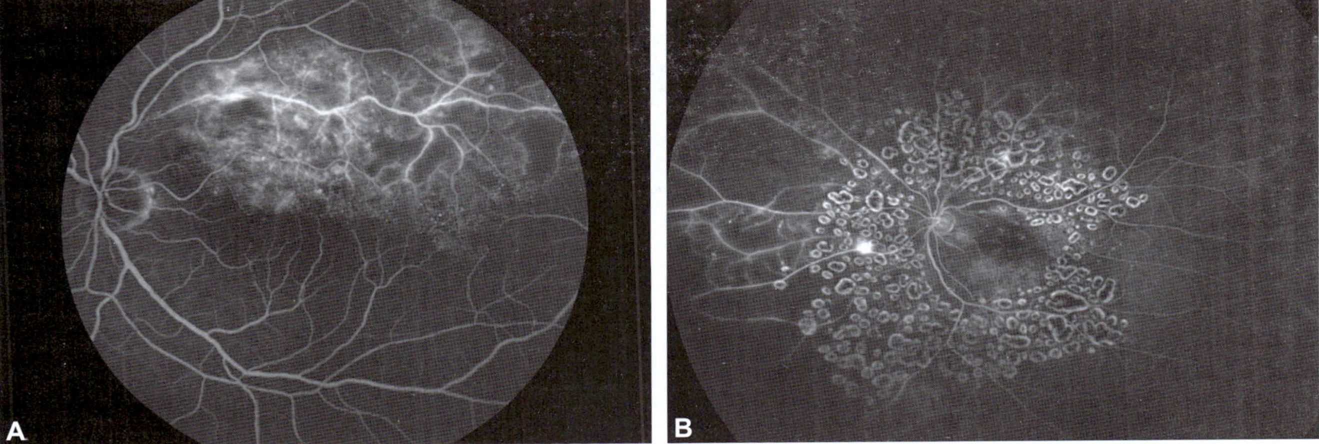

Figs. 2.18A and B: (A) A fundus image of a ST BRVO eye, with the noncontact 55° lens using the SLO. (B) UWF fundus imaging using Optos in a diabetic retina with 200° field of view showing nasal NVE and nonperfusion areas.

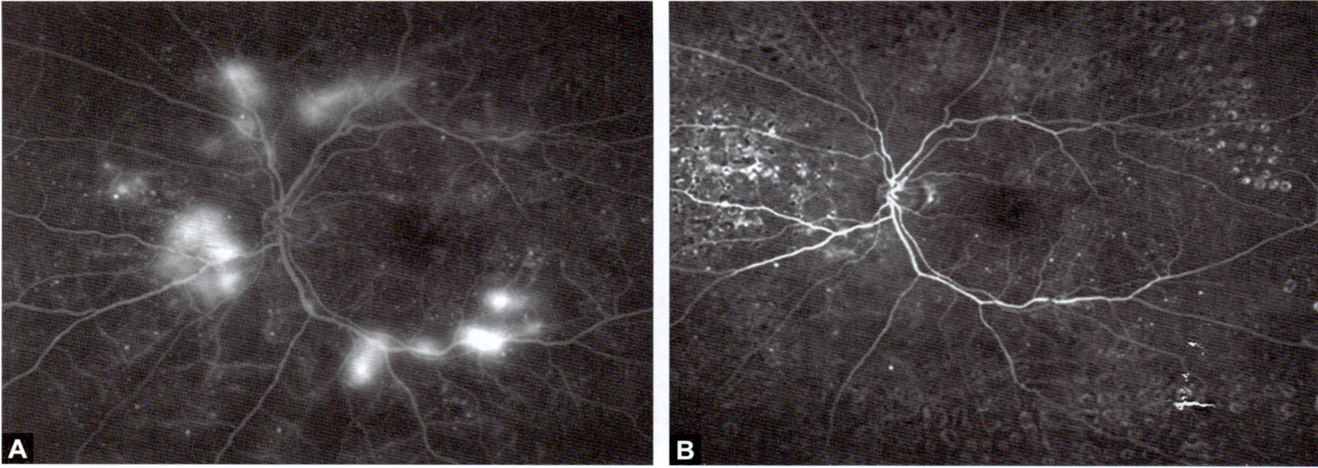

Figs. 2.19A and B: (A) UWF fundus imaging of prelaser PDR eye reveals peripheral CNP areas and multiple NVE. (B) Postlaser regression of NVE on UWFA.

photocoagulation (TRP).[9] Better targeting of laser therapy could reduce the risk of reduced contrast ,delayed dark adaption, visual field disturbance and accommodation loss more associated with a full laser PRP and possibly enhance the efficacy of anti-VEGF injections (Figs. 2.19A and B).

Recent imaging modalities provide ICG angiography along with FFA, FAF and infrared imaging. They permit interweaved angiography which allows parallel acquisition of FFA and ICG without the need for manually switching modes between imaging modalities. Compact versions of UWF devices, are scaled down in size to accommodate smaller work space while providing similar ultra-wide-field and high-resolution images similar to present day UWF equipment.

FUNDUS AUTOFLUORESCENCE

Basic Principle

Fundus autofluorescence imaging is a noninvasive imaging tool for in vivo detection of naturally or pathologically occurring fluorophores of the ocular fundus. Lipofuschin (LF) granules in the retinal pigment epithelium (RPE) and collagen and elastin occurring in choroidal blood vessel wall are the major source of fluorophores.[10] There is gradual accumulation of LF granules which is a by-product of the constant phagocytosis of shed photoreceptor outer-segment discs in RPE cells. Studies have shown that various LF components like A2E (*N*-retinylidene-*N*-retinyl ethanolamine) produce autofluorescence. LF granules emit a green-yellow fluorescence when stimulated with light blue light.[11] As the RPE cells die either due to senescence or apoptosis due to a genetic defect, the fundus AF disappears. We can obtain fundus AF with fundus digital camera using a green 550 nm excitation filter, or a SLO using blue laser excitation at 488 nm with a 500 nm barrier filter.

It is helpful for diagnosis and follow-up of hereditary retinal disorders (Figs. 2.20 and 2.21). Besides it also marks out

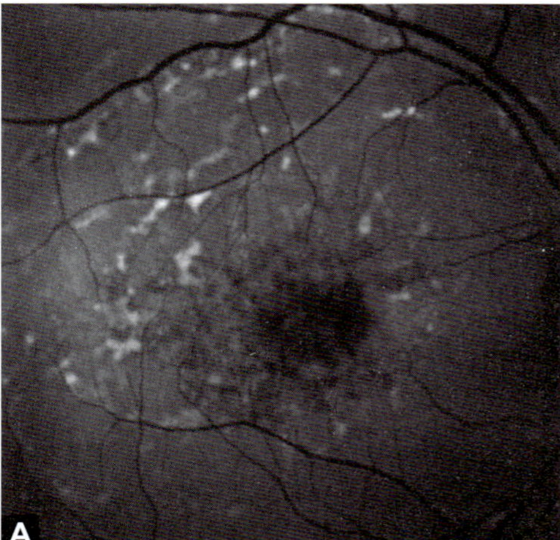

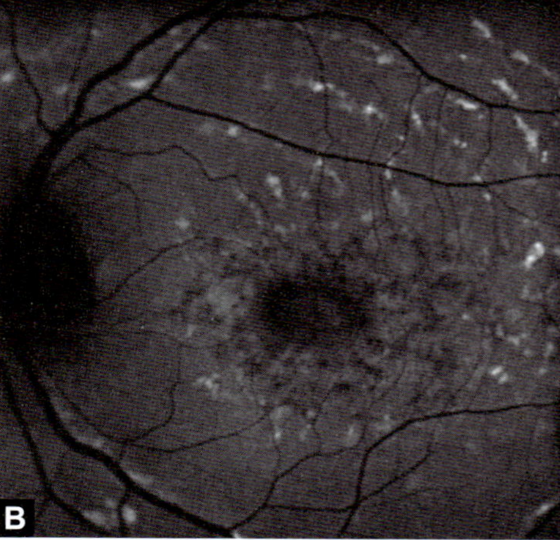

Figs. 2.20A and B: Fundus autofluorescence on the cSLO, in Stargardt's disease reveals hypoautofluorescence in the center due to the degenerated RPE, while the surrounding paramacular area has hyperautofluorescence due to degenerating RPE containing lipofuscin.

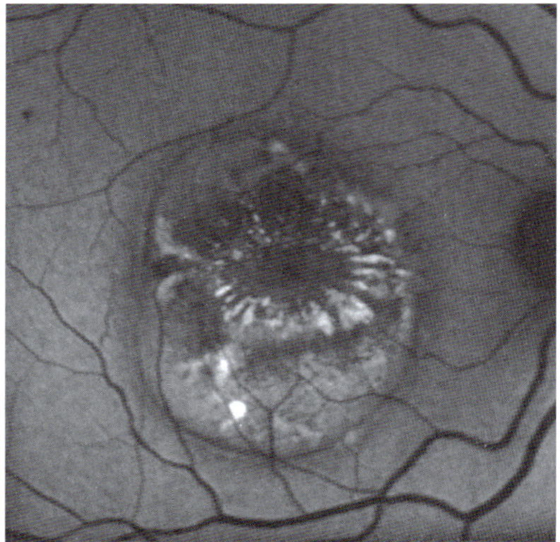

Fig. 2.21: Fundus autofluorescence (blue light) reveals spoke-like distribution of hyperautofluorescence in a case of Best disease.

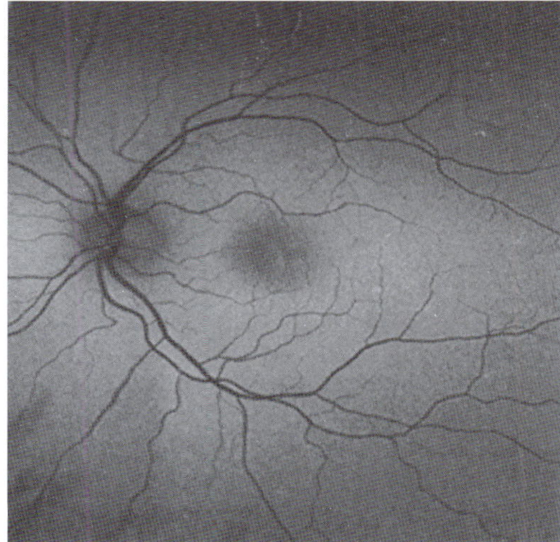

Fig. 2.22: Fundus autofluorescence of a normal retina (200° wide-field image) where the disc and blood vessels appear dark.

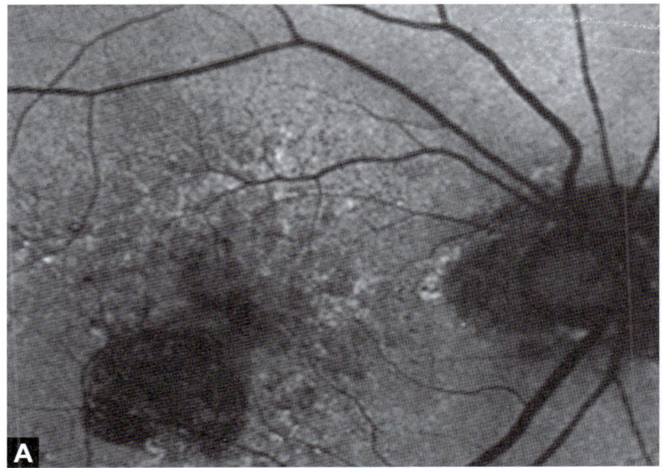

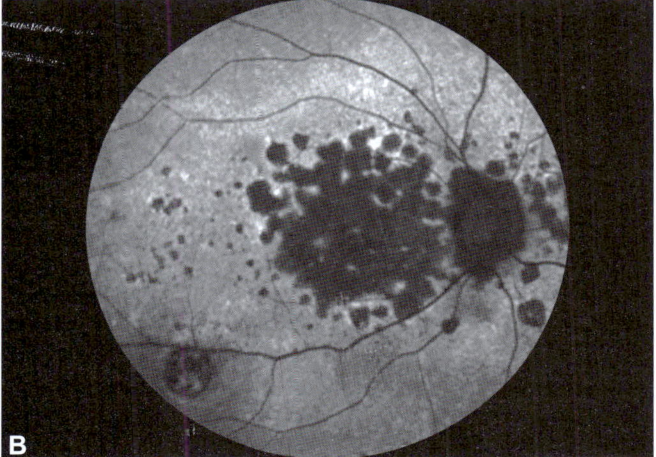

Figs. 2.23A and B: Fundus autofluorescence in a case of dry ARMD as captured on SLO imaging and on UWF-AF imaging.

RPE alterations due to fluid movement in CSC and helps in delineating pigment epithelium detachments (PEDs). Another useful role is in dry AMD lesions when it helps to monitor the size of the lesion and progression (Figs. 2.23A and B).

Technique of Fundus Autofluorescence Imaging

Autofluorescent imaging is noninvasive and requires relatively little time.

Fundus Spectrophotometry

Delori and coworkers using a fundus spectrometer performed pioneering work on the spectral analysis of the origin of the autofluorescence signal.[10] It was designed to determine the spectrum of excitation and fluorescence emission from small areas of the retina. Presently, two systems are available to examine the autofluorescence of the human eye in vivo: confocal scanning laser ophthalmoscope and digital camera.

Interpretation and Clinical Utility of Fundus Autofluorescence Images

The topographical distribution of LF granules and melanin in normal eyes demonstrates a higher FAF signal in the parafoveal area which tends to increase as we move away from it, peaking at the most peripheral retinal areas. In normal eyes, a diffuse FAF signal over the posterior pole can be seen, while the retinal vessels, fovea and the optic nerve head appear dark (Fig. 2.22). The absence of RPE in the optic nerve head region makes it appear dark. The retinal vessels are associated with a markedly reduced FAF signal because of the blocked fluorescence.

Autofluorescence imaging maps the retina metabolically with regard to the health of the retina. Hyperautofluorescence is a sign of increased LF accumulation, whereas areas of hypoautofluorescence indicate missing or dead RPE cells. This imaging technique has potential applications in a variety of retinal diseases including: age-related macular degeneration, retinitis pigmentosa, central serous chorioretinopathy, macular dystrophies, and pseudoxanthoma elasticum.

Age-related Macular Degeneration

Early Age-related Macular Degeneration

Large drusen are often associated with marked FAF abnormalities compared to small drusen, with the exception of basal laminar drusen. Delori and coworkers elaborated a pattern of FAF distribution associated with drusen which consists of decreased FAF in the middle of the druse with a surrounding ring of increased FAF.[12]

Geographic Atrophy

These are associated with death of the RPE cell along with attenuation of the outer neurosensory retina and the choriocapillaris resulting in a corresponding marked decrease in FAF intensity causing hypoautofluorescence. The presence of areas of hyperautofluorescence at the junction around the area of atrophy suggests viable RPE (Fig. 2.24).[13]

Pigment Epithelium Detachment

Fundus autofluorescence imaging in eyes with PED secondary to AMD shows varied features like marked, evenly distributed increase of the FAF signal over the lesion (Figs. 2.25A and B) surrounded by a well-defined hypoautofluorescent halo or an intermediate or a decreased FAF signal over the lesion. Rarely, a cartwheel pattern of increased autofluorescence due to hyperpigmented radial lines can also be seen.

Choroidal Neovascularization

Fundus autofluorescence imaging may be helpful to assess the integrity of the RPE thus leading to the better understanding of the development and behavior of new vessels as well as monitoring the therapeutic success (Figs. 2.26A and B).

Macular Telangiectasia (Mac Tel)

There are two types of macular telangiectasia (MT) as described by Gass and Blodi. The type 1 variety is called macular aneurysmal telangiectasia (MAT) and type 2 which is named as macular perifoveal telangiectasia (MPT). Reduced macular pigment density in MacTel type 2 reduces the normal masking of the foveal 488 nm blue-light FAF leading to abnormally increased FAF in the macular area to a variable degree, with blue-light FAF imaging.

Central Serous Chorioretinopathy

Central serous chorioretinopathy (CSC) is a condition characterized by serous pigment epithelial and neurosensory retinal detachments due to the hyperpermeability in the choroidal vasculature.

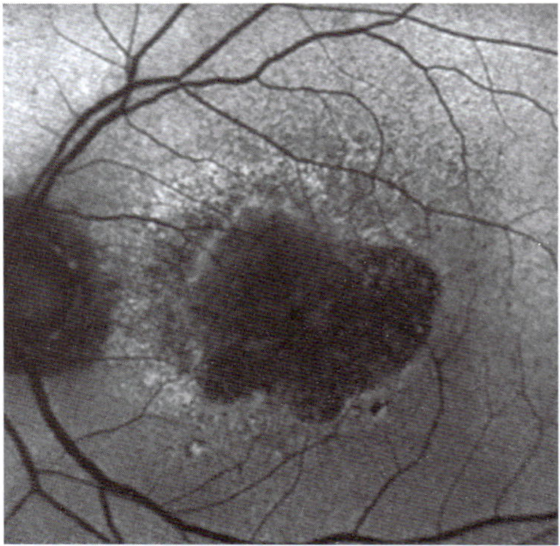

Fig. 2.24: Presence of areas of hyperautofluorescence surrounding areas of atrophy suggests viable RPE around an area of GA.

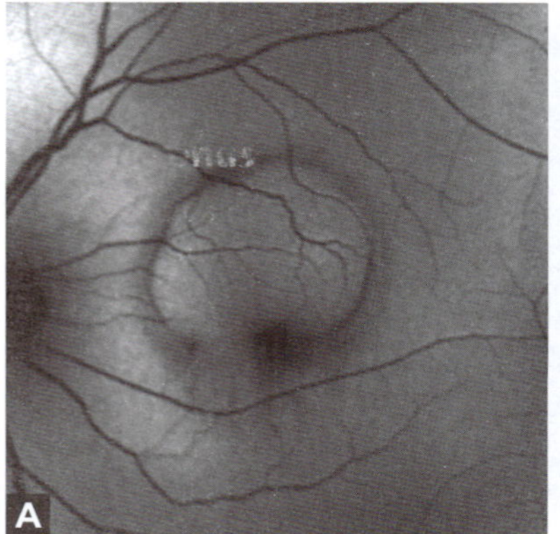

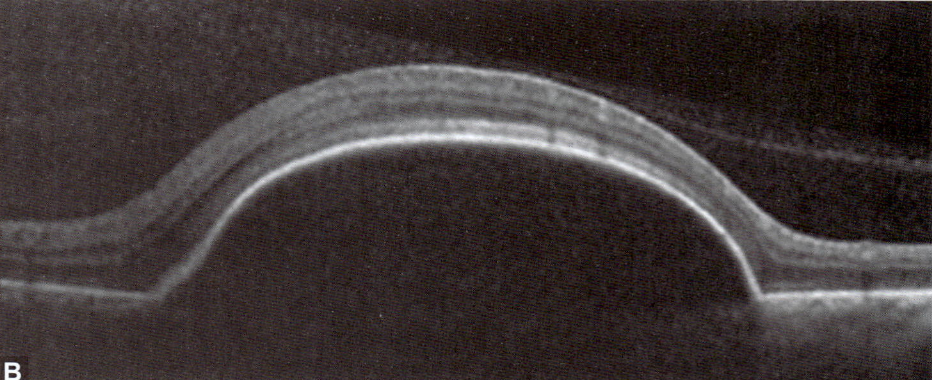

Figs. 2.25A and B: (A) Fundus autofluorescence (FAF) imaging in an eye with PED secondary to AMD shows varied features like evenly distributed increase of the FAF signal over the lesion; (B) Optical Coherence Tomogrpahy (OCT) showing large pigment epithelium detachment (PED)

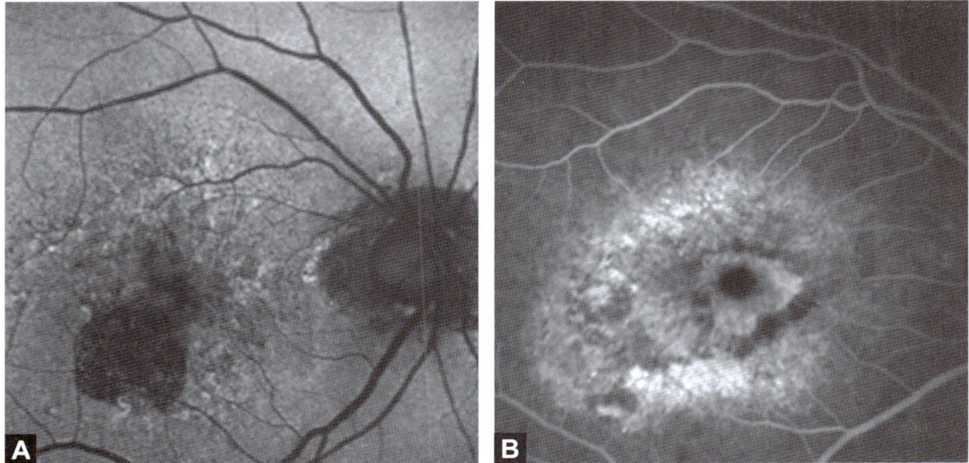

Figs. 2.26A and B: The CNVM lesions show irregular FAF intensities (A) with alternating areas of increased, normal and decreased signal intensity; (B) Fundus angiography showing window defects corresonding to RPE abnormalities.

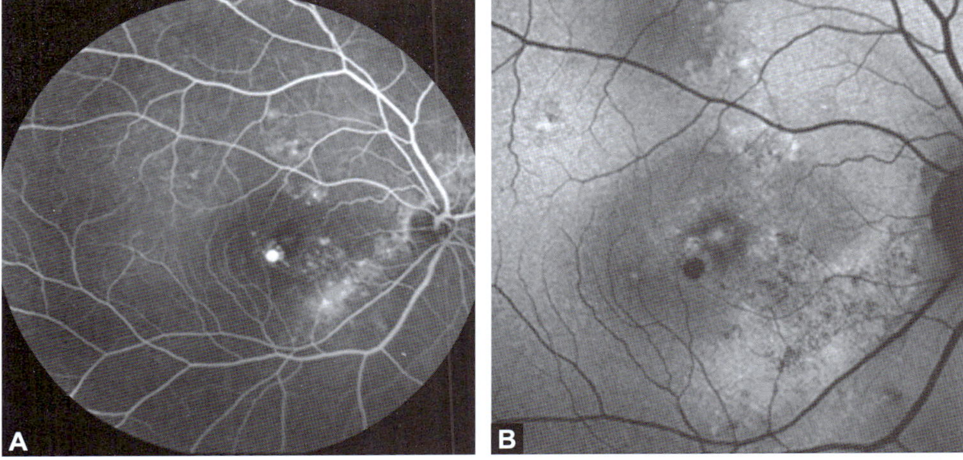

Figs. 2.27A and B: Fundus Fluorescein Angiography of a patient with chronic CSC showing 'Ink Blot' leak with surrounding window defects corresponding to RPE abonormalities. (B) Eye with Chronic CSC showing RPE disturbances on FAF.

Chronic CSC is associated with degenerative changes of the retina and RPE showing irregular levels of autofluorescence with decreased intensity over areas of atrophy called as diffuse retinal pigment epitheliopathy (DRPE). Some patients may have gravitational descending tracts in inferior retina (Figs. 2.27A and B).

Ultra-wide-field Fundus Autofluorescence

Ultra-wide-field FAF (UWFAF) imaging portrays a "metabolic map" of the RPE with peculiar macular abnormalities described in numerous diseases, including inherited retinal dystrophies (Fig. 2.28), central serous retinopathy and age-related macular degeneration.[14] Recently, peripheral pigmentary changes have been reported on UWFAF in patients with AMD.[12] The prognostic implications of these peripheral changes are currently unknown.

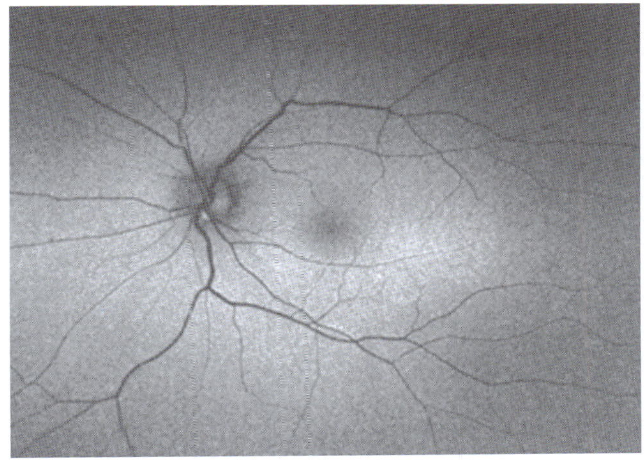

Fig. 2.28: Fundus AF in an eye with "salt and pepper retinopathy".

INDOCYANINE GREEN ANGIOGRAPHY

Indocyanine green is a water soluble, tricarbocyanine anionic dye with a molecular weight of 774.96 Da, which has the maximum absorption at 790 nm and maximum emission at approximately 835 nm in the near infrared wavelength, which allows penetration through macular pigment, blood, melanin and pigment.[15] About 98% of ICG is bound to serum proteins compared to only 80% of fluorescein. The advantage of being more protein bound is that the amount of leakage through the choriocapillaris is less, resulting in enhanced definition of larger choroidal vascular channels, the normal choroidal circulation, and associated pathologies. In this infra-red based, dye imaging technique in the early phase of the angiogram at about 1 minute after injection large choroidal arteries and veins are seen along with the retinal vessels. During the intermediate phase, 5–15 minutes postinjection; a diffuse choroidal fluorescence is seen. In the late phase after 15 minutes, no vascular details are visible.

Elimination of the dye takes place into the bile unchanged, hence has been used by transplant surgeons to assess the function of the transplanted organ. Side effects rate of indocyanine green are lower as compared to fluorescein dye. The dye is however contraindicated in patients with shellfish intolerance or iodine allergies, liver disease, and end-stage renal disease. No studies in animal models have been made regarding use of the dye in pregnancy; however it is best avoided in pregnancy.

The two technologies used for imaging ICG are the standard digital camera based systems and SLO based systems. The SLO systems can produce high-speed frames with 30 images/second in a continuous recording, thus even highlighting feeder vessels, which appear for a very short time. Choroidal neovascularization appears on ICG angiography as a focal hot spot and occult CNV usually form plaques. ICG is extremely useful in eyes with polypoidal choroidal vasculopathy (Figs. 2.29 and 2.30), central serous chorioretinopathy, retinal angiomatous proliferans when the intraretinal vascular network becomes visible, intraocular tumors (choroidal hemangioma, choroidal melanoma) which delineates the neovascular vessels, vascular patterns in choroidal inflammatory conditions such as serpiginous choroidopathy, acute multifocal placoid pigment epitheliopathy (AMPPE), and multifocal choroiditis.

Indocyanine green angiography (ICGA) helps in classifying choroidal neovascularization into the following morphologic types: focal spot or "hot spot", plaques and mixed (i.e. a combination of the previous two). The most common type being plaques (61% of the cases) which carried poor visual prognosis, compared to focal spots or "hot spots" (29%) which had a relatively better prognosis, and they were considered to be potentially treatable by ICG-guided laser photocoagulation.

In conclusion, ICGA remains necessary when the diagnosis proves uncertain despite FA and OCT; in certain cases of

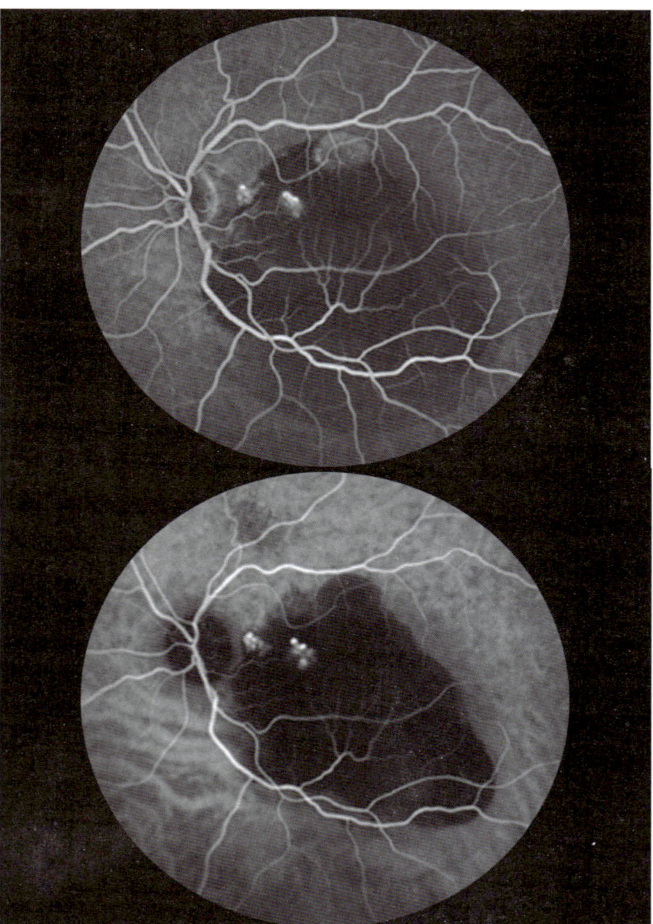

Fig. 2.29: Combined FA-ICG imaging on the cSLO device reveals multiple hyperfluorescent polyps in an eye with polypoidal choroidal vasculopathy, besides blocked fluorescence secondary to subretinal hemorrhage.

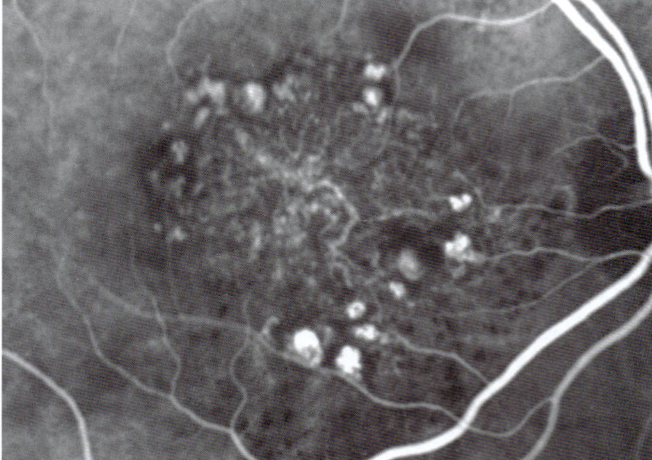

Fig. 2.30: Indocyanine green frame reveals multiple polyps with branching vascular network (BVN) in an eye with polypoidal choroidal vasculopathy.

OCNV with PEDs (particularly in cases of suspected PCV and RAP) or conditions such as central serous chorioretinopathy (CSC), which may require a different therapeutic approach from that used in neovascular AMD; and in the re-evaluation of nonresponding patients. Recently there has been a resurgence of interest in ICGA and multimodality imaging facilitates combined FA-ICG angiography along with OCT for a better diagnosis.

RETCAM

Retcam is an indispensible retinal-imaging tool for widefield pediatric retinal imaging. Retcam 3 and Retcam shuttle are the two models available in the market. The Retcam 3 features an integrated body with monitor, inbuilt keyboard, FA module and a printer (Fig. 2.31). Shuttle is more portable as the major components are integrated into a laptop, so it can be easily transported for use in the OT, NICU and screening in peripheral centers.

Lenses

Multiple lenses with different magnifications are available. The lenses provided are the retinopathy of prematurity (ROP) Lens - 130° field-of-view for premature infants, children's lens - 120° field for pediatric to young adult patients, high magnification lens - 30° field-of-view for details (optional), portrait lens—for adnexal and maxilofacial image acquisition. The most commonly used lens has a field of view of 130°.

Benefits

Photographic records of ROP screening can be saved across the entire period of follow-up and images can be compared to decide the progression or regression of the disease (Figs. 2.32 and 2.33). Indirect ophthalmoscopy requires good skill, and more expertise is needed when coupled with scleral indenta-

tion. The Retcam makes the task much easier for the examiner. Documentation of fundus images has become essential in this era of increase in the number of medicolegal cases. Inter-observer variability is prevented with Retcam which is useful for telemedicine purposes and consultation with experts. A Karnataka Internet Assisted Diagnosis of Retinopathy of Prematurity (KIDROP) program for ROP screening in underserved rural areas using an indigenously developed tele-ROP model has been in place since 2014.[16] KIDROP currently provides ROP screening and treatment services in three zones and 81 neonatal units in Karnataka, India. Technicians are trained to use a portable Retcam Shuttle (Clarity, USA) and validated against ROP experts performing indirect ophthalmoscopy. An indigenously developed 20-point score (STAT score) grades their ability (Level I to III) to image and decide follow-up based on a three-way algorithm. Images are also uploaded on a secure tele-ROP platform and accessed and reported by remote experts on their smart phones (iPhone,

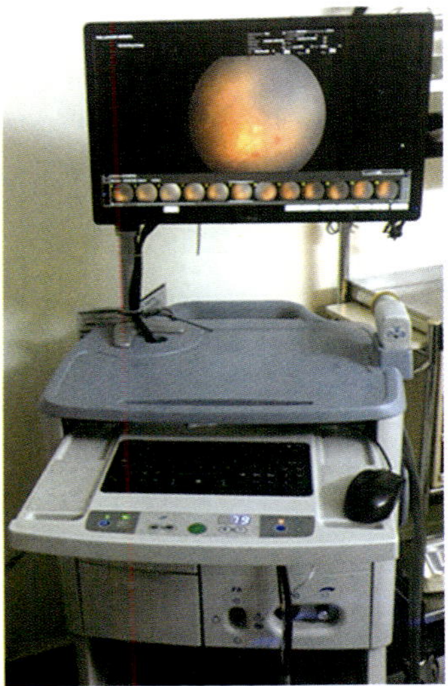

Fig. 2.31: The Retcam 3 machine.

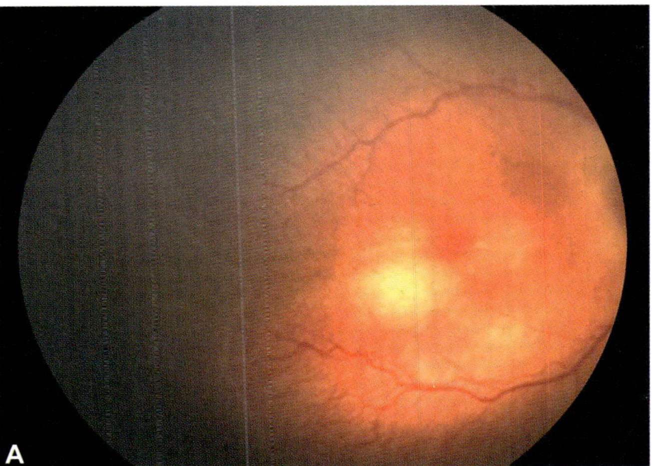

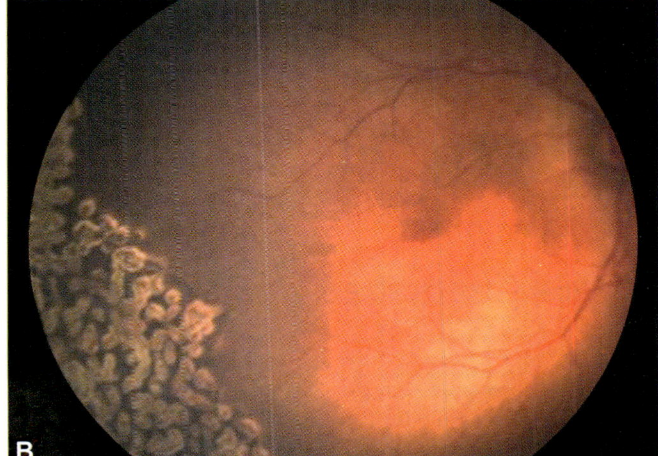

Figs. 2.32A and B: A case of ROP regressed with laser. (A) Pre laser; (B) Post laser RetCam images of a patient with retinopathy of prematurity (ROP)

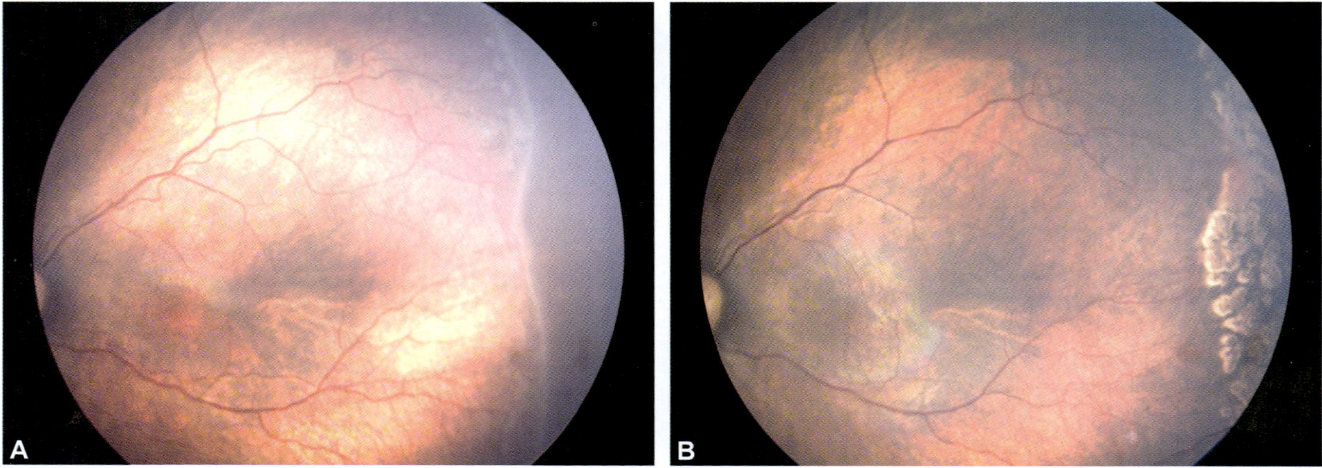

Figs. 2.33A and B: (A) Prelaser picture showing extraretinal ridge in an eye with ROP and regression postlaser (B).

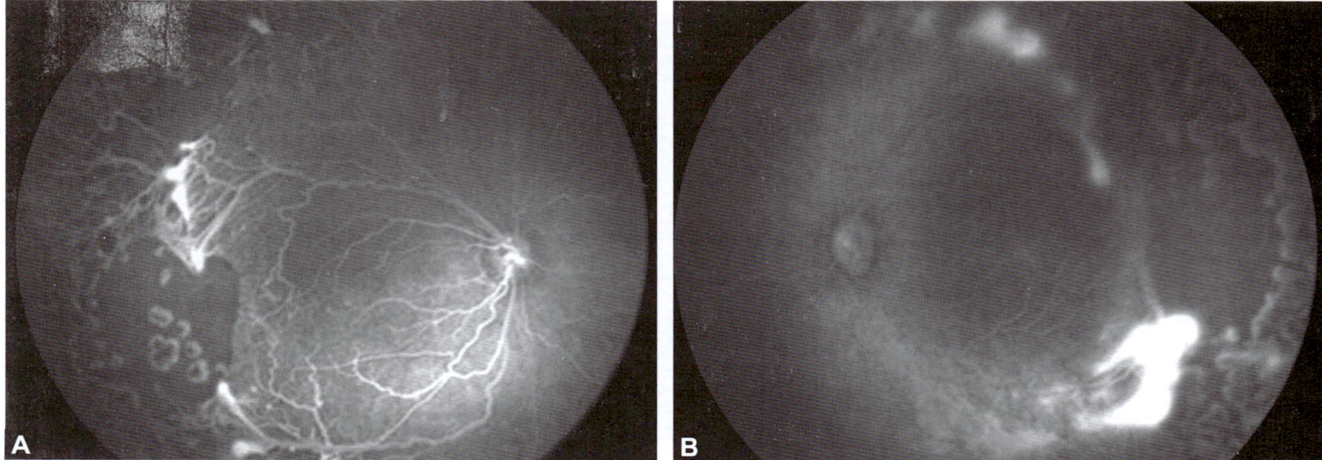

Figs. 2.34A and B: Fluorescein angiography of a case of ROP showing incompletely lasered periphery with neovascular ridge.

Apple). A level III technician agrees with 94.3% of all expert decisions. The sensitivity, specificity, positive predictive value and negative predictive value for treatment grade disease are 95.7%, 93.2%, 81.5% and 98.6%, respectively. This model demonstrates that ROP services can be delivered to the outreach despite lack of specialists.

Retcam-assisted Fluorescein Angiography

Retcam-assisted FA can be performed in Retcam 3. Blue light is emitted and a yellow filter in inserted inside the camera handpiece (Figs. 2.34A and B). Sodium fluorescein 20% dye is injected intravenously (0.04 mL/kg) via a preplaced cannula. It allows clear visualization of the avascular retina and flat neovascularization, which may not be visible to the naked eye. Missed areas of disease and skip areas of treatment can be detected easily, especially in aggressive posterior ROP. While its indications are selective, it does provide useful information for a new ROP trainee.

OPTICAL COHERENCE TOMOGRAPHY

It is a noninvasive diagnostic technique that provides an in vivo cross-sectional view of the retina (Fig. 2.35). OCT was first introduced in 1991 and has many applications beyond ophthalmology, where it has been used to image certain nontransparent tissues. Due to the transparency of the eye (i.e. the retina can be viewed through the pupil), OCT has gained wide recognition as an ophthalmic diagnostic tool. OCT has now become a mainstay tool for retinal imaging in the field of ophthalmology. It is based on the principle of interferometry. It is similar to ultrasound except that it uses near-infrared light (810 nm) in place of sound as the medium to create an image from the backscatter which is reflected.

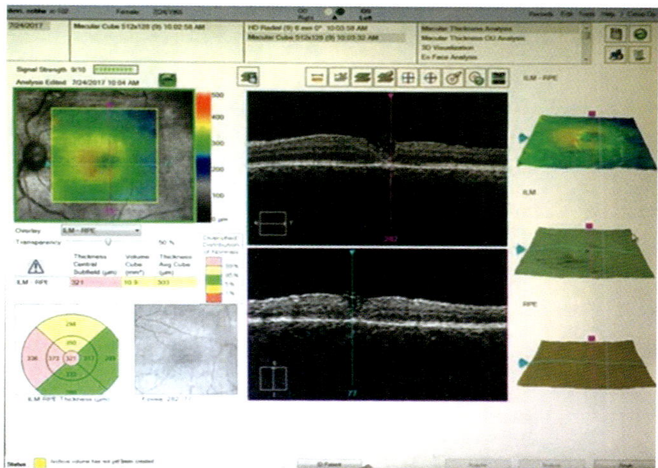

Fig. 2.35: Compact spectral domain OCT device with the screen containing the overlay map, ETDRS grid for thickness measurement, horizontal and vertical scans and 3D cube scan image.

Principle

Optical coherence tomography is based on the principle of low-coherence interferometry, where a low-coherence light beam is directed on the target and the back-reflected light is combined with a reference beam. The interference patterns between the reference beam and reflected beam is reconstructed to form an axial A-scan. A compilation of A-scans is created by moving the beam of light along the tissue line with each A-scan having a different incidence point which creates a two-dimensional cross-sectional image of the tissue known as a B-scan. If these B-scans are repeated at multiple adjacent positions using a raster scan pattern, then a three-dimensional volume can be obtained.

Physical Parameters

Typically, OCT instruments use a light source with wavelength of about 840 nm (infrared spectrum). Keeping the same wavelength, axial resolution depends on the bandwidth of source of light. Newer instruments have an axial resolution of approximately 2–5 μm. The lateral resolution is limited by the diffraction caused by the pupil (20 μm). Patient's ability to avoid eye movements increases the image acquisition time. The availability of scanning techniques to adjust for movements, the availability of tracking software and the instrument's scanning speed (number of A-scans acquired per second) are essential for obtaining quick data.

Generations

From the beginning, OCT images were captured in a time domain fashion (TD-OCT). Single photon detector was used to detect A-scan by moving a mirror to change the optical path of the reference beam in order to match different axial depths in the target tissue. 400 A-scans per second can be acquired by time domain systems using six radial slices at 30° apart. Care was required to prevent missing lesions between the slices as the slices were 30° apart.[17]

Spectral Domain Optical Coherence Tomography

Spectral domain OCT (SD-OCT) or Fourier domain OCT (FD-OCT), or high-definition OCT (HD-OCT), on the other hand, uses an array of detectors to acquire an entire A-scan. They offer high axial resolution (3–5 um) with scan velocity from 20,000–70,000 scans per second (Fig. 2.35). This increase in scan rate reduces the tendency of motion artifact, increases the resolution and lowers the chance of missing any pathology.[8] Time-domain OCTs (TD-OCT) have been largely replaced by spectral-domain devices (SD-OCT) as they provide better resolution of retinal layers and quicker image-capture, and has increased use in clinical practice. The advent of the novel frequency-domain OCT (FD-OCT) devices by recent research has shown to provide better improvement in resolution and speed.

Spectral domain-OCT differs from TD-OCT as it uses the Fourier mathematical transformation, which sums a single periodic function into a series of sinusoidal functions. This allows simultaneous measurement of light reflection when applied to the OCT, compared to the sequential measurement in TD-OCT which results in improvement in resolution of images from 10 μm to 1 μm, which has further allowed to appreciate small cystic changes like those seen in early stages of wet AMD.[9] The FD-OCT, though not yet available for widespread use, may have the broadest application in clinical practice of the three OCT systems. SD-OCT uses a broadband light source and a spectrometer whereas the FD-OCT utilizes a wavelength-swept laser source. This change allows an improvement from the 40 kHz readout rates of the SD-OCTs to repetition rates as high as 370 kHz in the FD-OCTs. Clinically, the potential of the FD-OCTs is vast because of their wide field of view, and they have found such far-reaching uses as imaging of coronary arteries.

The axial resolution of time domain OCTs is 10–15 microns whereas the spectral domain OCT has around 3 micron axial resolution. TD-OCTs capture six radial slices whereas spectral domain machines continuously image an area of 6 mm (infinite tomography). Hence, the chance of inadvertently missing any pathology is minimal.[18] Comparative evaluation between TD-OCT and SD-OCT has been shown in Table 2.3.

Normal Macular Optical Coherence Tomography

Internal limiting membrane (ILM) is the first layer to be detected in most OCT scans. It is seen as a hyperreflective layer at the vitreoretinal interface. In some patients, the posterior hyaloid can be visualized above the ILM as a hyperreflective layer. Within the inner retina, the hyperreflective layers are the retinal nerve fiber layer and the plexiform layers (both inner and outer) whereas the hyporeflective layers are the ganglion cell layer and the nuclear layers (both inner and outer) (Fig. 2.36).

Table 2.3: Comparative evaluation between time-domain-OCT and spectral-domain OCT.

Parameter	Time-domain OCT (TD-OCT)	Spectral-domain OCT (SD-OCT)	Advantage of SD-OCT
Light source	820 nm	840 nm, broader band width	Better axial resolution
Detector	Single movable detector	Spectrometer	Faster scans, no moving parts
Axial resolution	10–20 µm	5–7 µm	Better visualization of retinal layers
Transverse resolution	20 µm	10 µm	Better visualization of retinal layers
Max A-scans per B-scan	512	8,000	Higher tissue resolution.
Scanning speed	400 A-scans/sec	About 28,000–70,000 A-scans/sec or more	3D scanning, faster image acquisition, larger dataset, scan possible in uveitic eye and in hazy media.

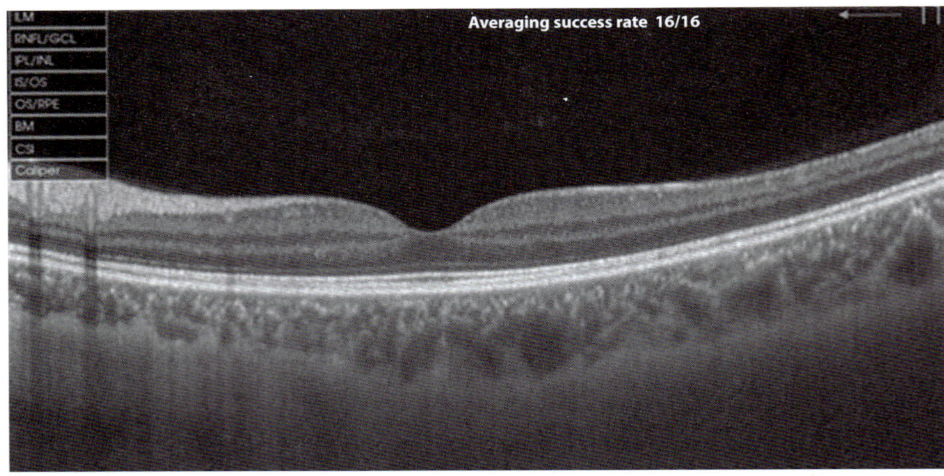

Fig. 2.36: Normal SD-OCT scan image showing a normal VR interface, foveal dip and layers of the retina. The outer ELM, ellipsoid bands and RPE zone is clearly visible. The choroidal layers lie beyond and are seen on the image.

Outside the central fovea, commercially available SD-OCT instruments typically resolve four bands in the outer retina. The innermost band has been attributed to external limiting membrane (ELM). The second band is the boundary between the IS/OS of the photoreceptors and the third band is described as either the OS tips or as Verhoeff's membrane. It was suggested in recent studies that the second band is the ellipsoid section of the photoreceptors (inner segment) instead of the IS/OS junction and that the third band corresponds to the contact cylinder between the external portion of the cone outer segment and the RPE apical processes. Merging of this band occurs with the fourth band in the central fovea, possibly due to greater height of the contact cylinder of the cones and retinal pigment epithelium outside the fovea. The RPE contributes to the fourth hyperreflective outer retinal band, with potential contribution from Bruch's membrane and choriocapillaris. Volumetric assessment can be done by detecting thickness and volume changes, monitoring the efficacy of treatment. A new lexicon for normal anatomical landmarks has been proposed in which lines on OCT have been replaced by the terminology bands as lines represent a one-dimensional image, so they would be replaced by the terminology bands and anatomic regions as zones.[19]

Choroidal Imaging (Enhanced Depth Imaging-Optical Coherence Tomography)

The standard technique of SD-OCT is modified by enhanced depth imaging-optical coherence tomography (EDI-OCT), by positioning the instrument closer to eye to image deeper layers. In this process, the retinal image is inverted (the inner retina faces down and the choroid faces up). The zero delay line is moved posteriorly, which is the point of maximal focus in the interference signal, and is focused on the choroid.[21] Several machines are used for EDI-OCT like the Heidelberg Spectralis OCT (Heidelberg Engineering, Heidelberg, Germany) and the

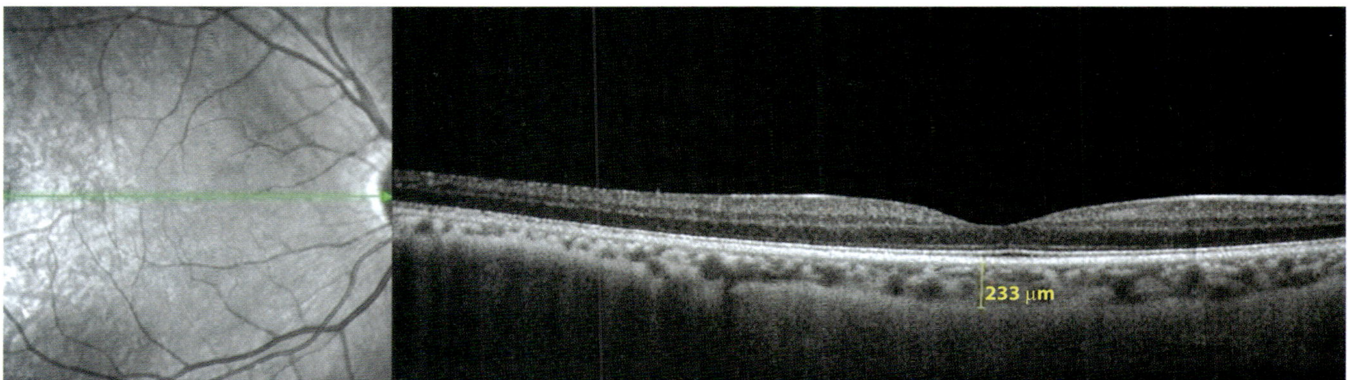

Fig. 2.37: Choroidal th ckness measured on the SLO in a normal eye using EDI.

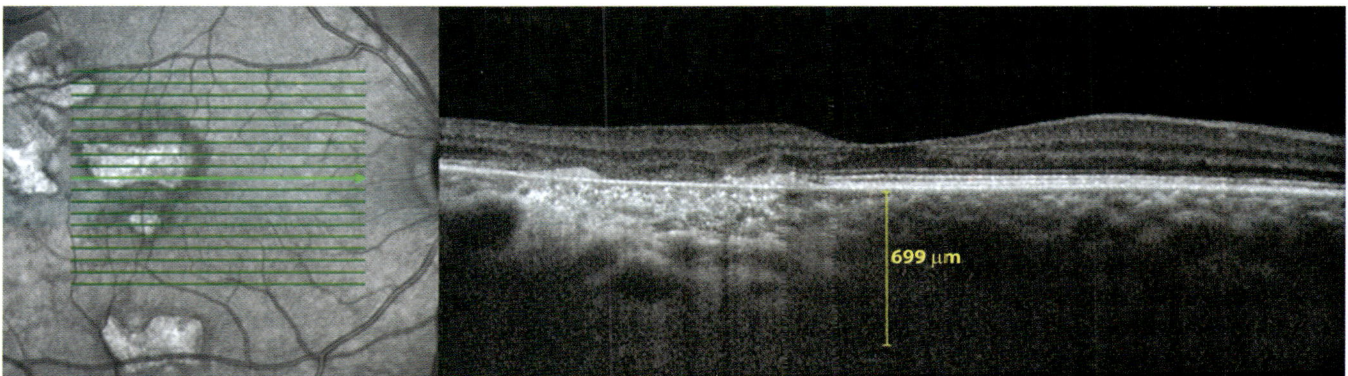

Fig. 2.38: Active serpiginous choroiditis shows increased thickness of choroid on EDI-OCT imaging.

Cirrus HD-OCT (Carl Zeiss Meditec Inc., Dublin, CA). Thus, EDI-OCT has enabled us to obtain a "virtual biopsy", of the ocular structures in a noninvasive, noncontact office-based imaging procedure (Figs. 2.37 and 2.38). Choroidal thickness is described as the distance between the outer border of the retinal pigment epithelium and the inner border of sclera.

Swept-Source Optical Coherence Tomography

The latest development in retinal and choroidal imaging is the Swept-source OCT (SS-OCT; DRI-OCT, Topcon Japan) (Fig. 2.39). The modifications include adoption of longer wavelength for this machine (1,050 nm vs 840 nm in SD-OCT), overcoming scattering by the RPE, which causes poor visualization of deeper lying structures. Use of photodetectors instead of CCD cameras adds to a further increase in resolution (1 μm). The scan speed in SS-OCT is twice that of SD-OCT devices (100,000 A-scans/sec compared with 50,000 A-scans/sec), enabling quicker acquisition of B-scans. This allows us to obtain wide-field B-scans (12 mm vs 6–9 mm with conventional SD-OCT) leading to more accurate 3D imaging of the vitreous, retina, and choroid. Wide scans help to present the optic nerve and macula on the same scan. SS-OCT gives simultaneous high-quality resolution of the vitreous, retina,

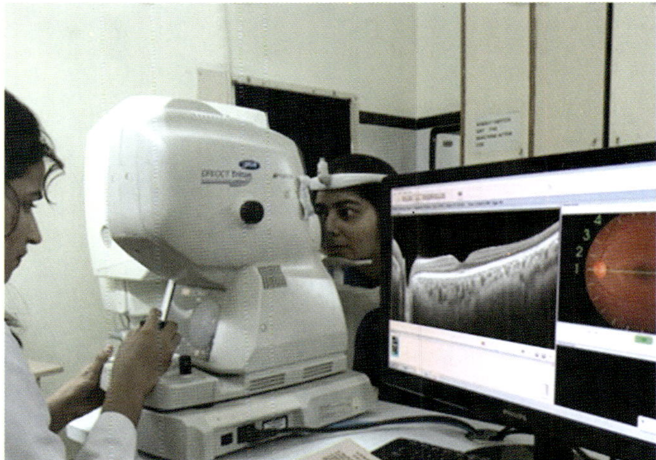

Fig. 2.39: Swept-source OCT (SS-OCT; DRI-OCT, Topcon Japan).

and choroid. Choroidal layers become clearly visible on SS-OCT imaging.

The structure of the choroid has been confirmed by SS-OCT consisting of multiple layers starting from innermost

Box 2.1: Choroidal structure.

Choroidal structure can be precisely visualized with swept-source OCT. Choroidal thickness, unlike retinal thickness, can change during the course of the day. Hence choroidal thickness should be measured around the same time of the day at all follow-ups. The choroid is thickest in the early morning hours and at night compare to other time. Age, refractive error and axial length are other factors responsible for changes of choroidal thickness. Younger and emmetropic patients, therefore, have thicker choroids than older and myopic patients.

Bruch membrane, choriocapillaris, Sattler layer (layer of medium diameter blood vessels), Haller layer (outermost layer of the choroid consisting of larger diameter blood vessels), and lamina suprachoroidea. A hyperreflective line indicating the choroidoscleral boundary—sclera of diminishing reflectivity can be seen, usually behind the lamina suprachoroidea. Scleral vessels can also be visualized. In some eyes, a hyperreflective linear structure between the lamina suprachoroidea and sclera has been attributed to the suprachoroidal space. Using a longer wavelength overcomes cataractous lens opacities and allows visualization of the macula in eyes with disabled fundus view. This may enhance the ability to identify patients who will need additional vitreoretinal treatment in such eyes (Box 2.1).

En-face Optical Coherence Tomography Imaging

En-face imaging is another modification which allows the clinician to visualize three-dimensional data in a fundus projection wherein the retinal and/or choroidal layers at a given depth are projected onto an en-face view (Figs. 2.40A and B). This provides numerous advantages, most notably the ability to precisely localize lesions within specific subretinal layers, using their axial location on OCT cross-sections, as well as the ability to register projected OCT images to other fundus imaging modalities, using retinal vessels as landmarks. This is expected to improve as en-face imaging provides further detail about the subtle pathological features in the retina and choroid in diseased states.[22]

Optical Coherence Tomography—Clinical Applications

Many retinal conditions can be diagnosed with the help of OCT, especially when the media is clear. In general, it is easier to capture lesions in the macula than lesions in the mid- and far-periphery. OCT can be particularly helpful in diagnosing: macular hole, macular pucker, vitreomacular traction, macular edema, detachments of the neurosensory retina and retinal pigment epithelium (e.g. central serous chorioretinopathy or age-related macular degeneration). OCT is gaining increasing popularity when evaluating optic nerve disorders such as glaucoma. OCT can accurately and reproducibly evaluate the nerve fiber layer thickness.

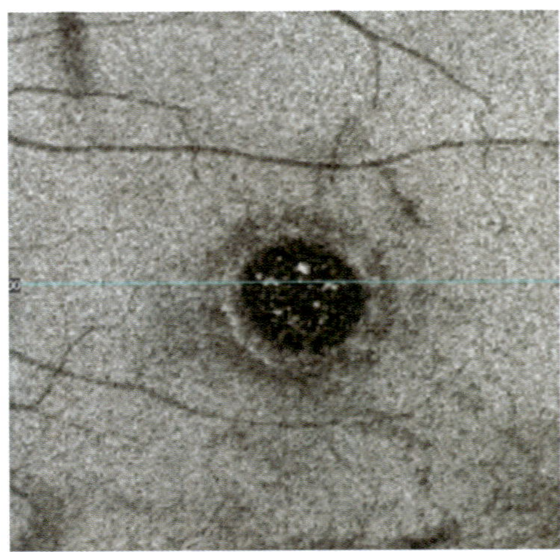

Fig. 2.40A: En-face analysis: Macular cube 200 x 200 μm (Macular Hole). IS/OS-Ellipsoid: Offset = −39 μm, thickness = 20 μm.

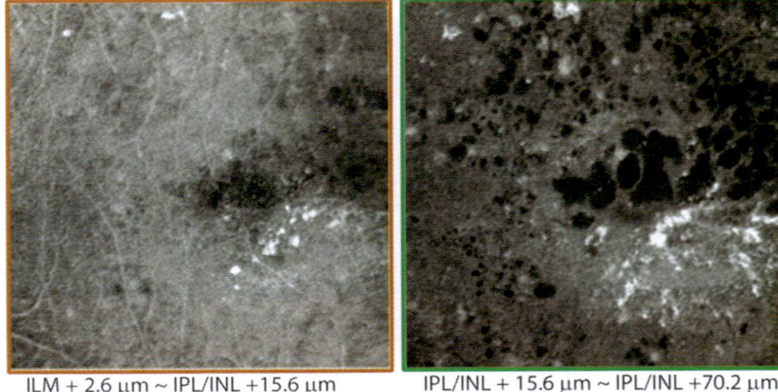

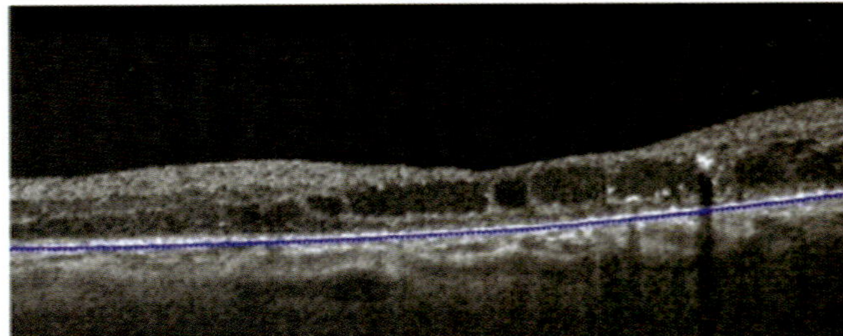

Fig. 2.40B: SS-OCT of a patient with DME showing en-face images at different segmentation levels.

Spectral-domain Optical Coherence Tomography and Vitreomacular Interface Disorders

Natural progression of posterior vitreous detachment, vitreomacular adhesion (VMA) and vitreomacular traction (VMT) have been demonstrated using OCT.[23] Diagnosis of a broad VMA/VMT by biomicroscopy may be difficult. OCT better delineates the VMA/VMT and also visualizes associated ERM and macular edema. According to the International Vitreomacular Traction Study Group,[24] VMA is defined on OCT as "perifoveal vitreous separation with remaining vitreomacular

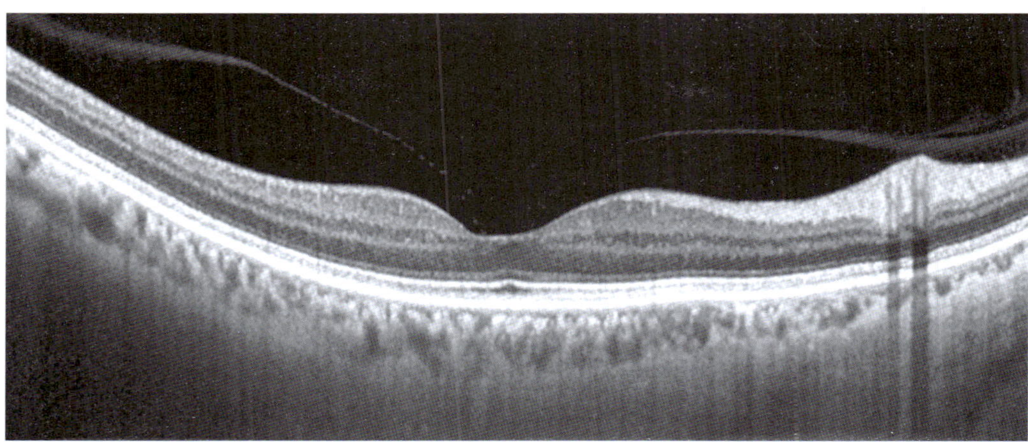

Fig. 2.41: OCT of VMA described as "perifoveal vitreous separation with remaining vitreomacular attachment and unperturbed foveal morphologic features".

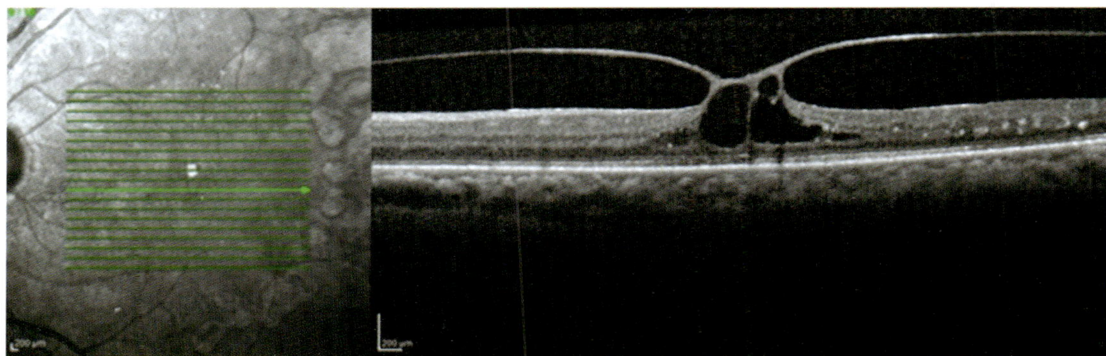

Fig. 2.42: Vitreomacular traction: Anomalous posterior vitreous detachment accompanied by anatomic distortion of the fovea.

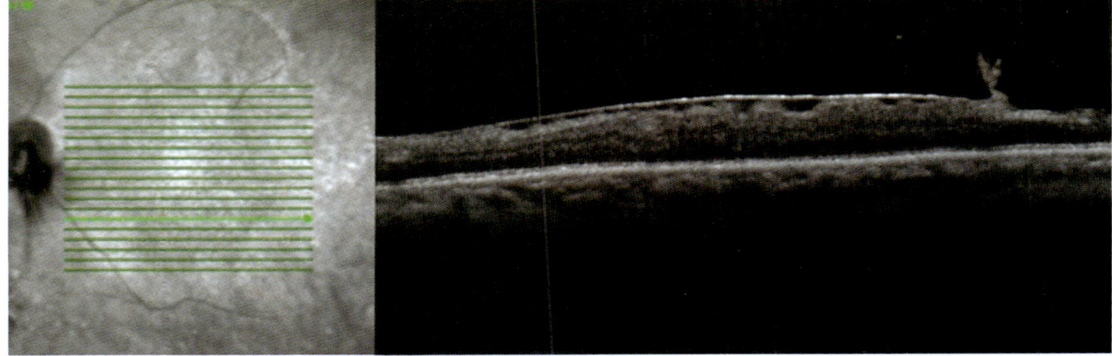

Fig. 2.43: OCT provides qualitative and quantitative information about the retinal anatomy in patients with epiretinal membrane.

attachment and unperturbed foveal morphologic features" (Fig. 2.41).

Vitreomacular traction, on the other hand, is defined by "anomalous posterior vitreous detachment *accompanied by anatomic distortion of the fovea*" (Fig. 2.42).

Both VMA and VMT can be further subclassified as having focal (1,500 µm or less) or broad (more than 1,500 µm) attachment. OCT also allows assessment of structural changes associated with VMA/VMT, such as integrity of the photoreceptor layer, specifically the inner/outer photoreceptor cell junction/ellipsoid zone, as well as the integrity of the external limiting membrane. OCT provides qualitative and quantitative information about the retinal anatomy in patients with epiretinal membrane (Fig. 2.43).[25]

Spectral-domain Optical Coherence Tomography and Macular Holes

Optical coherence tomography can distinguish a full thickness macular hole from a pseudohole or lamellar macular hole (Figs. 2.44A to C). Pseudoholes are present as a central defect within a dense sheet of ERM.[25] Also thickness of the macular hole can be ascertained (partial vs full thickness). The International Vitreomacular Traction Study Group classification divides macular holes based on size of the hole, and the presence or absence of vitreomacular adhesion.[24] Based on the minimum horizontal aperture size (hole width), macular holes are divided as: small holes measure 250 μm or less; medium size holes are between 250 μm and 400 μm, and large holes are larger than 400 μm. Holes are also further subclassified by presence or absence of vitreomacular adhesion. This classification is of clinical importance because it determines the management and prognosis of macular holes.

Optical coherence tomography has increased our perception of the healing process after surgery, and has assisted in determining the pre- and postoperative features that are associated with visual outcome. Macular hole indices are easily calculated from OCT transverse images of the macular area and are predictive of postoperative hole closure.[26] Macular hole closure and restoration of the normal foveal contour can be confirmed with the help of OCT.[27,28] The anatomical and functional recovery of the photoreceptors is relfected by restoration of the ELM and junction of the inner and outer segment of photoreceptors in surgically closed macular holes.[28,29]

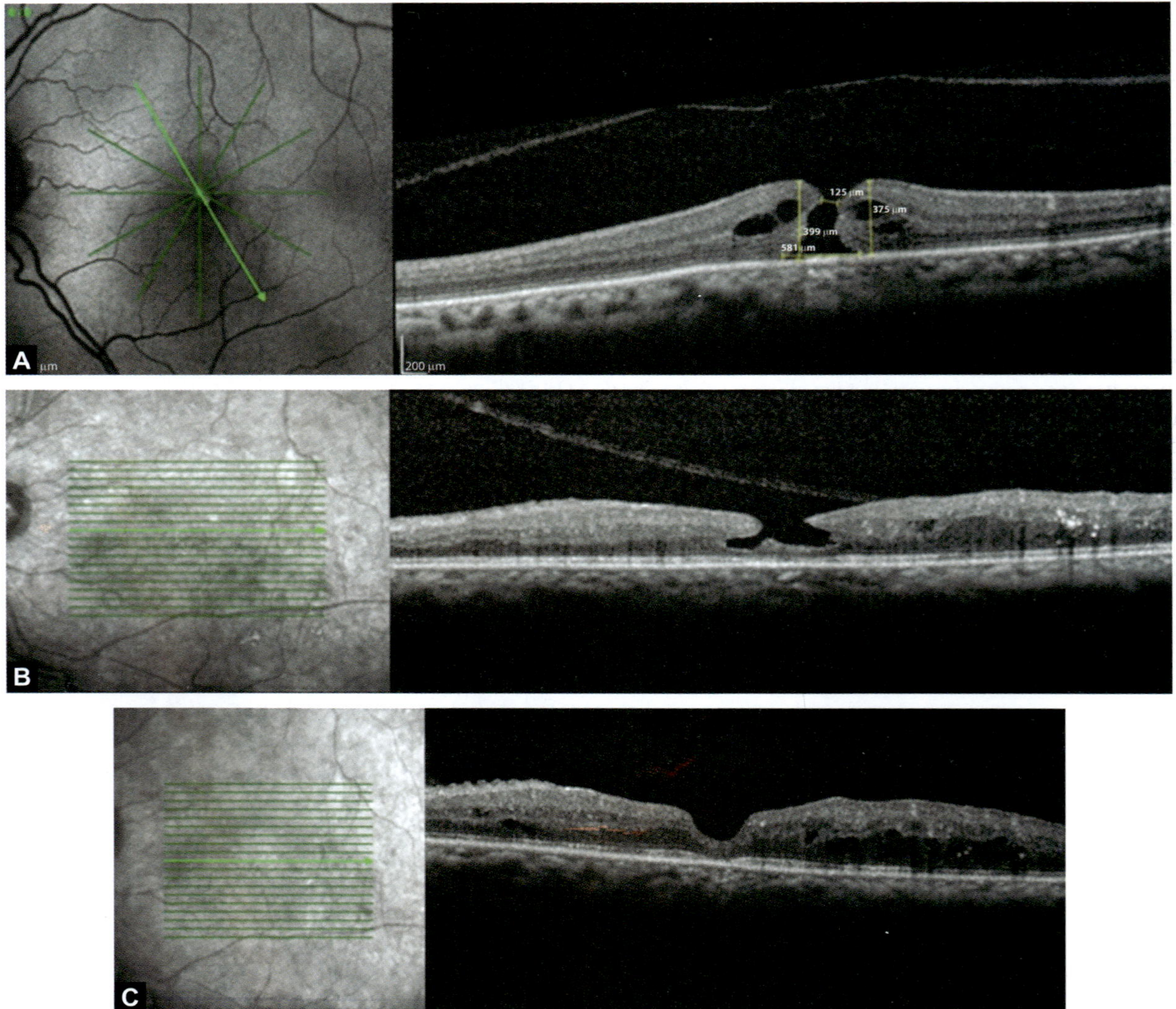

Figs. 2.44A to C: Optical coherence tomography can distinguish a full thickness macular hole (A) from a lamellar hole (B) and a pseudohole (C).

Spectral-domain Optical Coherence Tomography and Age-related Macular Degeneration

Non-neovascular Age-related Macular Degeneration

On SD-OCT, drusen are visualized as areas of RPE elevation with underlying variable reflectivity (Fig. 2.45).[30] OCT can provide a three-dimensional, geometric assessment of drusen. With SD-OCT, one can evaluate the thinning of retinal layers overlying drusen.[31] OCT imaging is also useful for the evaluation of different types of drusen. Typical drusen in AMD are seen as deposits between the RPE and the inner collagenous layer of Bruch's membrane. Subretinal drusenoid deposits are seen as granular hyperreflective material between the RPE and the IS/OS junction.[32] Cuticular drusen appear on OCT imaging as RPE elevation with occasional disruption of the overlying IS/OS junction and ELM.[30]

The RPE pigmentary abnormality can be seen as small discrete hyperreflective material usually within the outer nuclear layer.[33]

GA can now be quantified and evaluated by using SD-OCT. It can present as outer nuclear layer loss or thinning, loss of ELM, IS/OS junctions or choriocapillaris loss.[34] The photoreceptors are lost, often extending beyond the margins of GA.[35] GA appears as a bright area on en-face OCT imaging. This is due to the increased light penetration into the choroid where atrophy has occurred in the macula.[36]

Neovascular Age-related Macular Degeneration

Optical coherence tomography is helpful in detection of intraretinal, subretinal, or sub-RPE fluid. These may be visualized as homogeneous hyporeflective spaces, if the fluid exudation is serous, or may be demarcated by fibrinous membranes in case of profuse proteinaceous exudation. OCT can be used for characterization of retinal PED.[37,38] A serous PED can be seen as a dome-shaped elevation of the RPE with underlying homogeneously hyporeflective space. Bruch's membrane is seen as a thin hyperreflective band underneath the PED. A fibrovascular PED can be seen as they are filled with solid material of medium reflectivity. They are separated by hyporeflective clefts. Hemorrhagic PED can be visualized as a dome-shaped lesion, similar to serous PED. The slope of the elevation in hemorrhagic PED is more acute and appearance of hyperreflective signals, attenuating the signal from deeper structures due to presence of blood. Loss of choroidal detail is also present (Figs. 2.46A and B).

Retinal pigment epithelium tears can be seen as a site of discontinuity in a large PED with the curling of the free edge of the RPE under the PED. Increased reflectivity is noted just adjacent to the tear, where the choroid vessels can be seen due to the absence of the RPE.[39] On OCT imaging, the disciform scar is a highly reflective outer retinal or subretinal lesion. Loss of the overlying photoreceptor layer as disruption of the IS/OS junction and ELM can be associated with scar formation.[40] Subretinal fluid or intraretinal cysts associated with the neovascular lesion can be appreciated in OCT.

Polypoidal Choroidal Vasculopathy

Spectral-domain optical coherence tomography can also show polypoidal lesions underneath the RPE and associated intraretinal, subretinal, and sub-RPE fluid. Tomographic findings highly suggestive of PCV include sharp PED peak, PED notch, and hyporeflective lumen within hyperreflective lesions adherent to RPE (Figs. 2.47A and B).[41]

Central Serous Chorioretinopathy

Optical coherence tomography imaging can demonstrate subretinal fluid and PEDs and can also measure the height and width of the detachments. OCT imaging is also useful for evaluating response as the subretinal fluid resolves and the

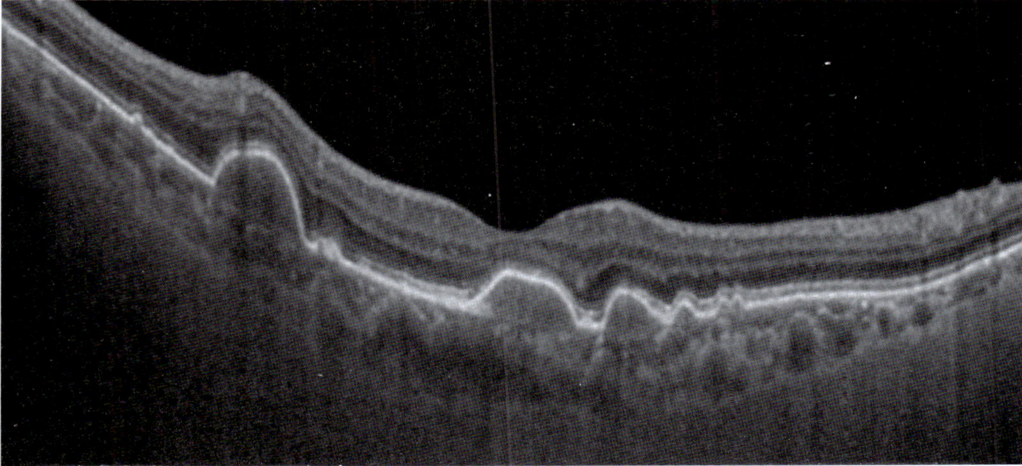

Fig. 2.45: Spectral-domain optical coherence tomography and age-related macular degeneration.

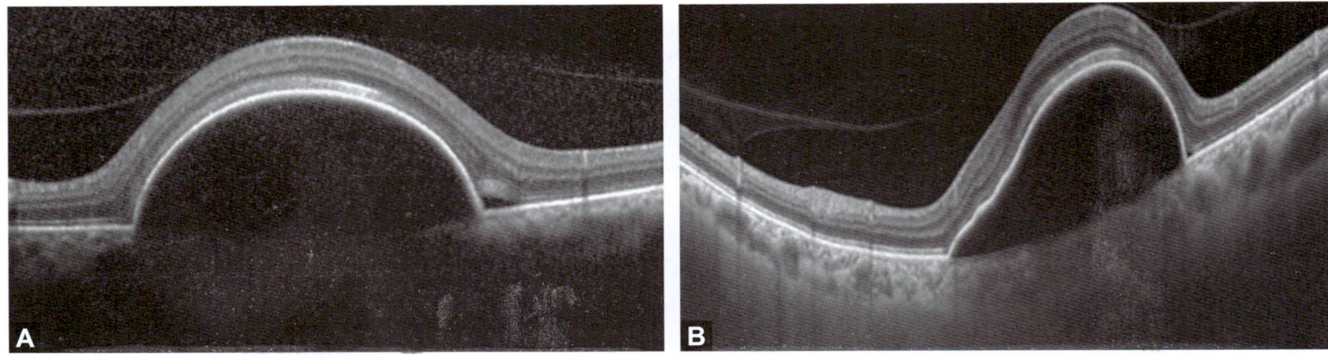

Figs. 2.46A and B: (A) Hemorrhagic PED, showing an optically empty PED with absence of reflectivity from the choroid; (B) Serous PED reveals optically empty space within PED however the choroid is easily visible.

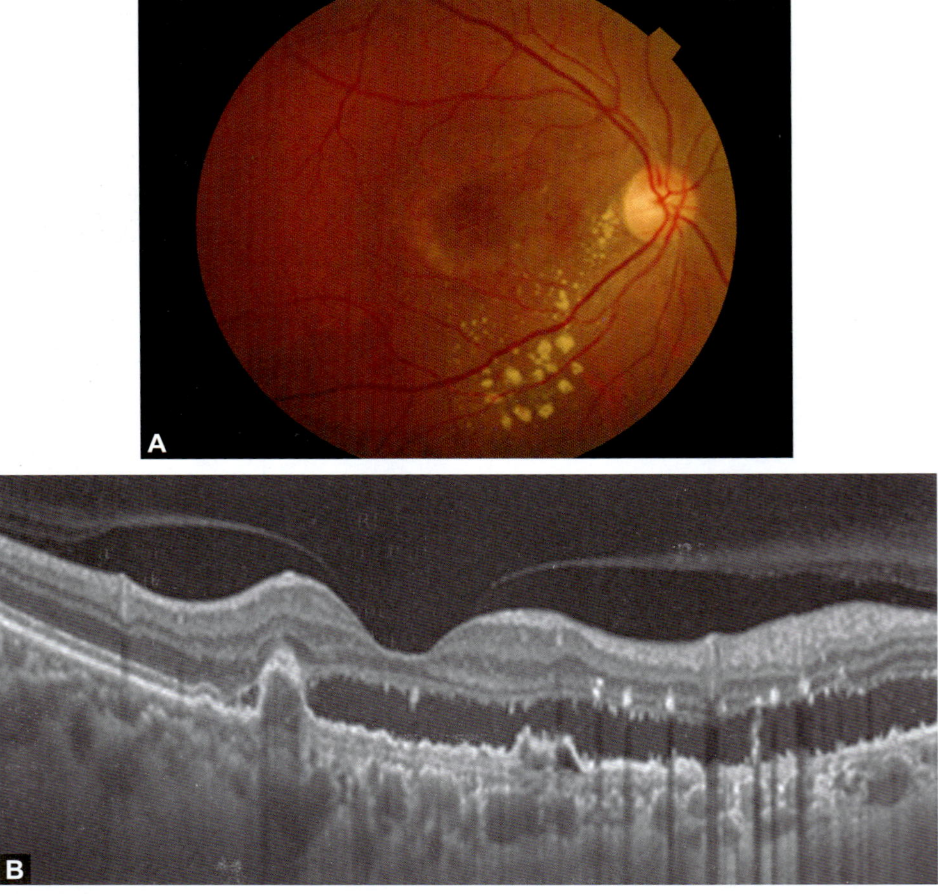

Figs. 2.47A and B: Swept -source OCT image of PCV showing the "thumblike PED" and double layer sign indicative of a branching vascular network beneath the RPE. There is neurosensory RD too.

progression of retinal morphology in chronic cases. Acute CSC shows features of neurosensory retinal thickening within the area of retinal detachment, PED, fibrinous exudates in the subretinal space, and the presence of shaggy outer segments of the neurosensory retina above the leakage site (Figs. 2.48A and B).

Chronic CSC shows foveal atrophy, retinal thinning, and cystoid degenerative changes on OCT (Figs. 2.49A and B).

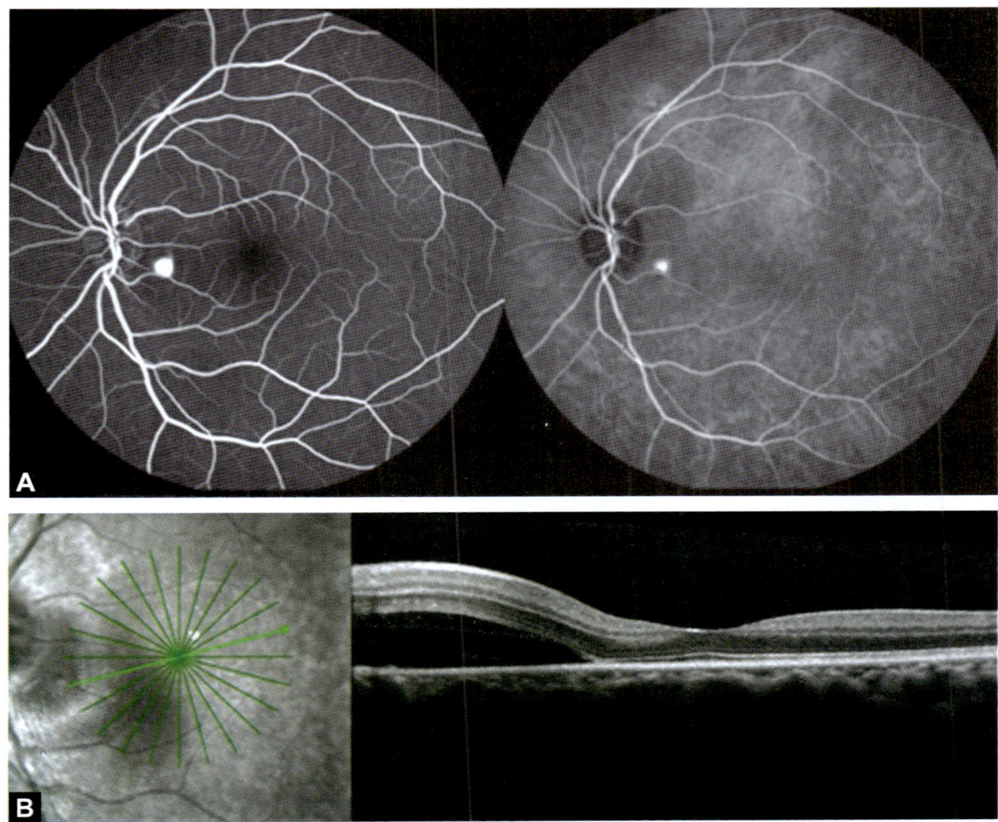

Figs. 2.48A and B: (A) FFA and ICG showing ink blot leak in a case of CSC; (B) OCT of a patient showing NSD sparing fovea in CSC.

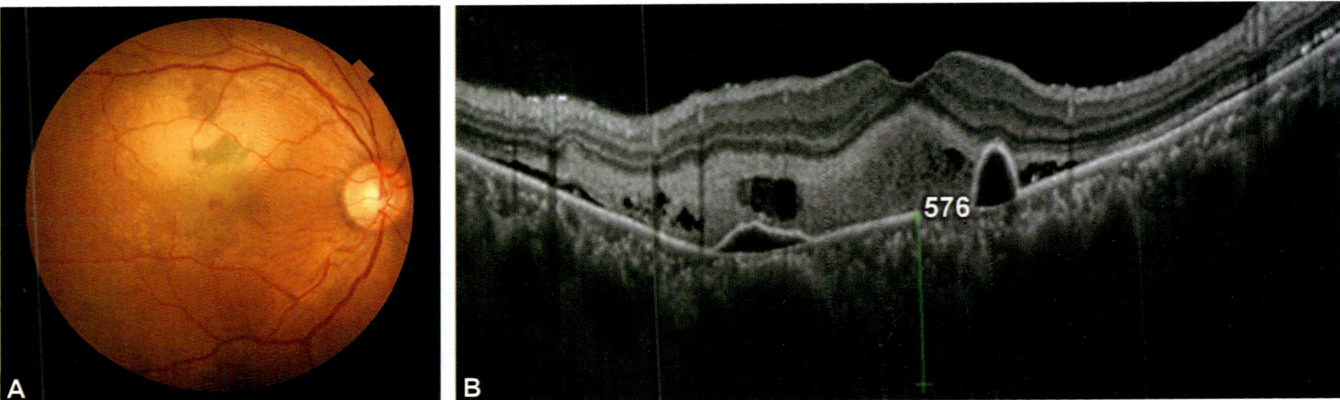

Figs. 2.49A and B: Eye shows chronic CSC with subretinal fibrin on both color picture and SS-OCT. The thumb-like PED is visible with thickened choroid suggesting a pachychoroid clinical spectrum.

Elongation of outer segments of photoreceptors and decreased thickness of the outer nuclear layer are some of the photoreceptor morphological changes seen on OCT.

On EDI-OCT/SS-OCT, eyes with CSC have been found to have much thicker choroid compared with normal.[42,43] Fellow eyes of patients with CSC were also found to have thicker choroids compared with age-matched normal eyes.[44] The changes occurring in the choroid after photodynamic therapy (decrease in choroidal thickening) may reflect a more normalized choroidal permeability.[45]

Cystoid Macular Edema

Cystoid macular edema (CME) is seen as retinal thickening with intraretinal cysts of hyporeflectivity on OCT (Fig. 2.50). CME is characterized by the presence of intraretinal cystoid

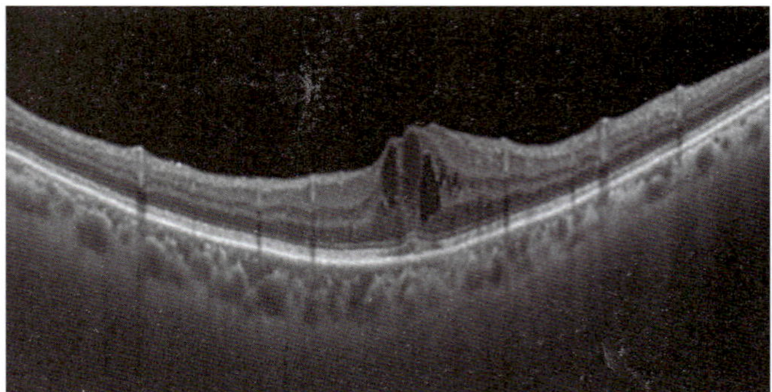

Fig. 2.50: Vertically oriented foveal cystic spaces in an eye with CME.

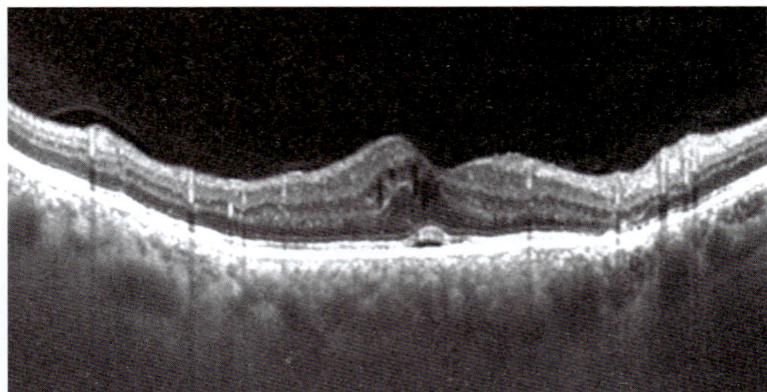

Fig. 2.51: Center-involving DME with cystic spaces on OCT.

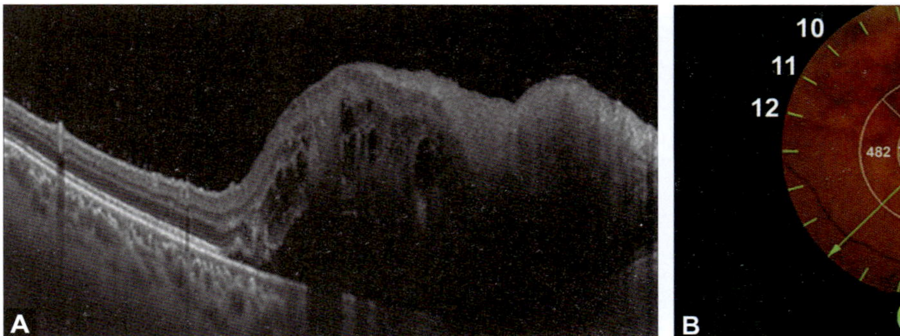

Figs. 2.52A and B: Severe macular edema seen on OCT (A) in an eye with fresh superotemporal branch retinal vein occlusion ; (B) OCT grid showing central macular thickness as 777 micrometres.

areas of low reflectivity, which are typically separated by highly reflective septa (Fig. 2.50).

Diabetic Retinopathy

Optical coherence tomography can be used to classify diabetic macular edema (DME) into several categories: diffuse retinal thickening, CME, serous retinal detachment or subretinal fluid, and vitreomacular interface abnormality.[46] Diffuse retinal thickening is usually defined as a sponge-like swelling of the retina with a generalized, heterogeneous, mild hyporeflectivity (Fig. 2.51).

Optical coherence tomography has become widely accepted in monitoring progression and treatment response in patients with DME.[47,48] OCT imaging is valuable in determining the extent of the tractional component as well as the presence of foveal involvement, assisting in the decision to intervene surgically.[49]

Vascular Occlusion

Both in CRVO and branch retinal vein occlusion eyes, OCT helps in grading the degree of edema and helps as only imaging modality in serial follow-up of such eyes and also deciding the intravitreal anti-VEGF or steroid therapy requirement in such eyes (Figs. 2.52A and B).

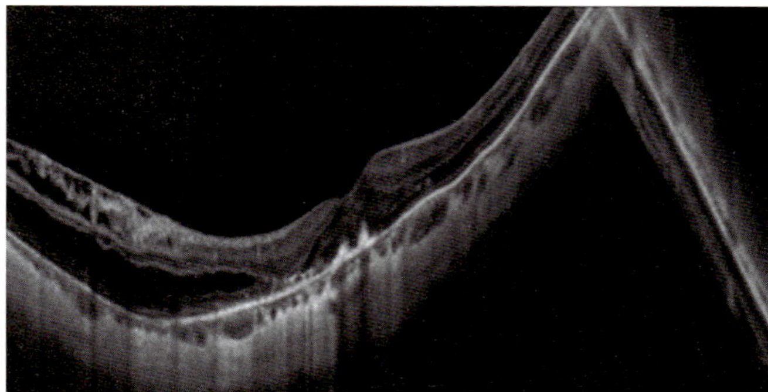

Fig. 2.53: Pathological myopia showing myopic foveoschisis.

Optical Coherence Tomography in High Myopia

Swept-source OCT devices help in scanning details in eyes with pathological myopia due to their longer wavelength and high resolution from vitreoretinal interface to the outer choroid and even sclera. Changes such as myopic foveoschisis, macular CNV and myopic macular holes with and without RD are easily visible and this helps in planning the management of such eyes (Fig. 2.53).

Limitations

Media opacities can hinder imaging as light waves are used instead of sound waves. As a result, the use of OCT will be limited in the setting of vitreous hemorrhage, dense cataract or corneal opacities. Patient cooperation is mandatory as patient movement can decrease the quality of the image. Imaging time is shorter in new machines, which can result in fewer motion-related artifacts. Earlier machines were operator dependent for good quality of image but newer machines like the spectral domain OCT have eye tracking facility which decreases motion related artefacts by limiting acquisition error.

OPTICAL COHERENCE TOMOGRAPHY ANGIOGRAPHY

Principle

Optical coherence tomography angiography (OCTA) involves the principle of high-speed OCT scanning in detection of blood flow by analyzing decorrelation of signals between scans. It is an advanced imaging modality that employs decorrelation angiography technology and high frequency and dense volumetric scanning to detect erythrocyte movement allowing direct visualization of blood vessels in vivo, without the use of exogenous dyes.[50,51] OCTA visualizes the movement of red blood cells by analyzing the changes in the intensity and/or phase signal that arises from repeated B-scans performed in the same location. The motion contrast images produced noninvasively by OCTA are high-resolution (~10 µm), depth-resolved images of the retinal vasculature. Various software algorithms for producing OCTA images exist and include, optical microangiography (OMAG) or split-spectrum amplitude decorrelation angiography (SSADA).

Optical coherence tomography angiography employs the principle of motion contrast imaging to high-resolution volumetric blood flow information. It is based on the fact that in a static tissue, the only moving structures are the erythrocytes. Multiple B-scans of the same cross-section are taken. A computer software generates a decorrelation signal (differences in the backscattered OCT signal intensity or amplitude) between these sequential B-scans. Hence, OCTA requires higher imaging speed than the currently available OCT systems. Since

OCTA images are processed from multiple OCT, flow data is intrinsically linked with the structural data. The flow data is represented as angiographic scans and the structural data is depicted as en-face OCT scans.[1]

The angioplex OCT-A can additionally quantify microvascular changes. It can provide information on the vessel density, perfusion density and the foveal avascular zone (area, perimeter and circularity of FAZ).[2]

Various optical coherence tomography angiography systems and specifications[1,2] are discussed in Table 2.4. OCTA of normal fundus is shown in Figures 2.54A and B.

Artifacts in Optical Coherence Tomography Angiography[3]

Stretch artifact: A defect related to software correction of eye motion in which part of the image seems to have been stretched, as if the images were printed on a rubber sheet, which is then stretched in a nonuniform way.

White-line artifact: A descriptive term for the white line seen in OCTA images associated with an eye movement. The sequential B-scans around the time of a microsaccade vary substantially and, therefore, generate large decorrelation values, which in turn are manifested as white lines in en-face OCTA.

Projection artifact: One of the most important artifacts affecting OCTA. Light incident on a blood vessel may be reflected back toward the observer, as well as scattered elsewhere or refracted. Light which passes through the vessel will fluctuate over time and anything posterior to the vessel will be illuminated by this fluctuating light. Motion contrast techniques detect fluctuations with time, so artifactual images of vessels may be seen at deeper locations in the eye than they actual inhabit (Figs. 2.55A to D).

Image artifact: Anomaly in the visual representation of information derived from an object. In a practical sense, image artifacts generally add unwanted information or subtract necessary information from the representation of the object.

Physical Parameters

Volumetric maps are generated using high-density raster scanning of a two-dimensional area of the retina. Blood flow

Table 2.4: Optical coherence tomography angiography (OCTA) systems and specifications.

OCT-A system	Algorithm	OCT type	Resolution	A scans per second	Scan size
Angiovue, RTVue XR Avanti	SSADA	Spectral domain	304 x 304 pixel density	70,000	2 x 2 mm, 3 x 3 mm, 6 x 6 mm, 8 x 8 mm
Topcon DRI OCT Triton	OCTARA	Swept source	320 x 320 pixel density	100,000	3 x 3, 4.5 x 4.5, 6 x 6
ZEISS, Angioplex™	OMAG	Spectral domain	350 x 350 pixel density	68,000	3 x 3, 6 x 6

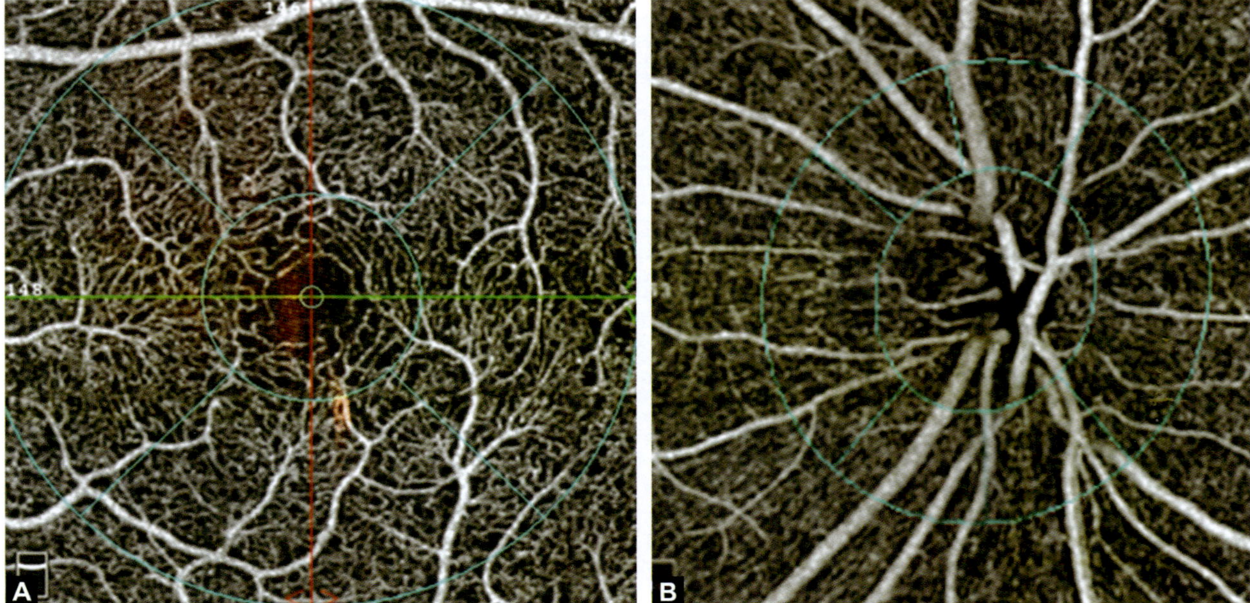

Figs. 2.54A and B: Optical coherence tomography angiography scan of a normal eye through (A) macula (B) optic disc.

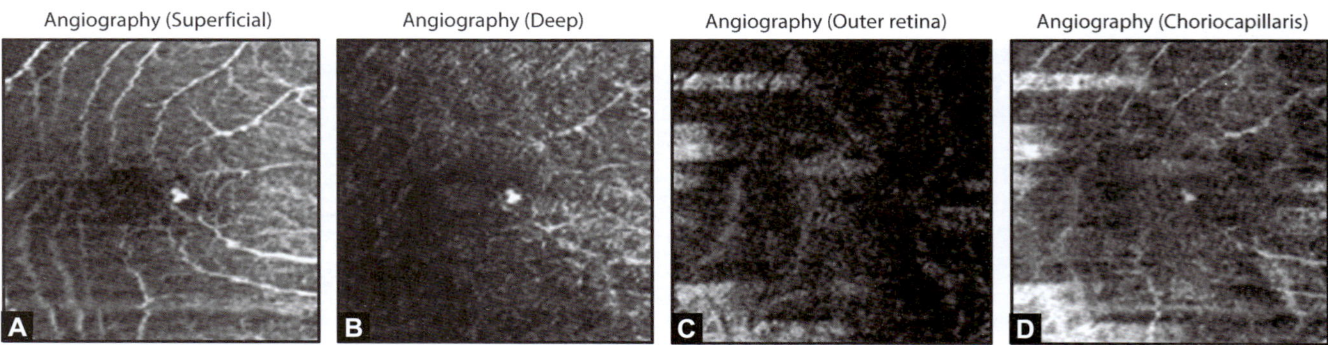

Figs. 2.55A to D: Projection artifact visible as a hyperreflective lesion on all frames from superficial retina to RPE-choriocapillaris layer.

from ILM to the choroid is rendered allowing direct visualization of normal and abnormal blood vasculature. The 70 kHz A-scan rate acquires 3 × 3 mm OCT angiography volume in 3 seconds. The lateral and axial resolutions are both 15 μm.[51]

Optical Coherence Tomography Angiography versus Fundus Fluorescein Angiography

The OCT-A differs from traditional angiography (fluorescein angiography, FA) in numerous domains.

Fluorescein angiography provides two-dimensional images with dynamic visualization of blood flow with a wide-field of view; therefore, patterns of dye leakage, pooling, and staining can be appreciated very well.[52] FA has the disadvantage of being an invasive test that mandates intravenous administration of fluorescein dye and prolonged acquisition imaging for at least 10–15 minutes. Visualization of the intraretinal structures of major capillary networks, superficial and deep networks is not possible on FA.[53] FA does not image the deeper capillary plexus well.[54] Radial peripapillary vascular network cannot be imaged by FA.[55] FA cannot be used on a regular basis in busy settings. Although considered safe, the dye poses risks ranging from nausea to allergic reactions, including anaphylaxis in rare instances and its use is contraindicated in patients with chronic kidney disease.

Optical coherence tomography angiography is a noninvasive technique in comparison to FA. Volumetric angiographic information can be acquired without the use of dye. Each three-dimensional scan set takes very less time of approximately 6 seconds. The vascular plexuses can be studied in details by scrolling the set of en-face images. Segmentation of the inner retina, outer retina, choriocapillaris, or other areas of interest is possible on OCTA. OCT angiography can image all layers of the retinal vasculature very well. Limitations include inability to appreciate leakage, misinterpretation of areas of slow blood flow, such as in microaneurysms or fibrotic CNV and residual motion artifacts which can present as hazy or discontinuous images (Box 2.2).[56]

Optical coherence tomography angiography intrinsically generates data on vascular flow and allows segmentation of retinal layers. This unique feature helps in study of tissue perfusion even in the absence of obvious morphological changes (Figs. 2.56A and B). Disc perfusion can be assessed using flow index of the optic nerve head. For example, optic discs in glaucoma and optic neuritis patients have significantly diminished flow indices compared with normal discs. OCT angiographic measurements are sensitive and remarkably less than that for structural OCT (5 μm) due to signal averaging. Swept-source laser can also be employed on this device, it is centered at 1,040 nm and causes augmented signal penetration depth.[20] Future OCTA devices may be based on approaches, such as phase contrast or intensity variance.

Published studies confirm the clinical efficacy of OCTA in the evaluation of common ophthalmologic diseases, such as diabetic retinopathy, age-related macular degeneration (AMD), CNV, retinal vascular occlusions, macular telangiectasia and sickle-cell disease. Intraretinal (e.g. intraretinal microvascular anomalies) and extraretinal (e.g. neovascularization of the disc or elsewhere) neovascularization can be detected with excellent reliability. The pathology should be within the field of view. Limited field of view is one of the major limitations of OCTA which is improving with advancements (Box 2.3 and Figs. 2.57A and B).

ADAPTIVE OPTICS

Principle

The quality of images acquired for the diagnosis of retinal diseases are limited by both lower-order monochromatic aberrations such as defocus and astigmatism and higher-order monochromatic aberrations, such as coma, trefoil, and spherical aberration in the cornea and lens. These aberrations can be detected by wave-front sensors based on the Hartmann-Shack principle.[57,58] The whole wavelength of incident light are approximated by these sensors which contains an array of lenses. The aberrations which are detected are eliminated using one or more deformable mirrors. These mirrors have small electronically controlled actuators that can move the mirror within a range of ±2 μm, allowing it to adopt desired configuration. With this corrected wavefront, it is then possible to acquire images of the retina with high resolution.[57,58]

Imaging Systems

Initially conventional fundus cameras were modified to incorporate wavefront sensing and correction. Newer "flood-illuminated" fundus cameras are now available for use in clinical settings. These use a light source with a wavelength of 840 nm to provide a near-infrared reflectance image for deep retinal structures with improved transverse resolution. However, their field of view is still limited to 4° × 4°.

Box 2.2: When is optical coherence tomography angiography indicated?

The utility and potential of OCTA has been harnessed for resolution of capillary level details in retina. It can approach the resolution similar to histological studies in human cadaver eyes. Spaide et al. first demonstrated distinct superficial and deep capillary networks using the SSADA technique.[55] OCTA is helpful in elucidating ischemic processes involving different layers of the retinal vasculature, such as superficial plexus ischemia presenting as cotton-wool spots, deep plexus ischemia causing paracentral acute middle maculopathy and macular telangiectasia type 2.

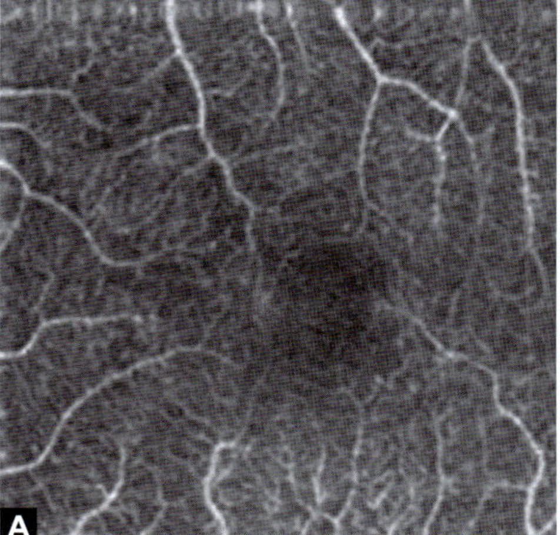
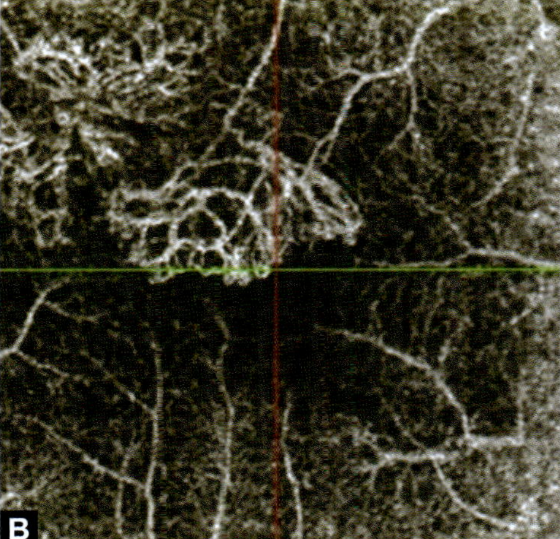

Figs. 2.56A and B: (A) Normal vascular channels and blood flow on OCTA; (B) OCTA reveals an abnormal vascular net.

Box 2.3: Limited field of view is one of the major limitations of OCTA.

Current field-of-view options include 3 x 3 mm, 6 x 6 mm, 8 x 8 mm and 12 x 12 mm scan. Larger fields will be available in the near future. Ophthalmologists still need to perform FA to detect extramacular lesions of any sort, including neovascularization and peripheral nonperfusion in DR. Follow-up examinations for assessment of macular ischemia can be documented with OCTA. OCTA will be most helpful in detection of clinically relevant changes in milder stages of DR, where FA is not indicated. The noninvasive nature of OCTA makes it possible to perform this test causing no significant risk to patients. E.g. those suffering from CKD who are unable to undergo FFA procedure.

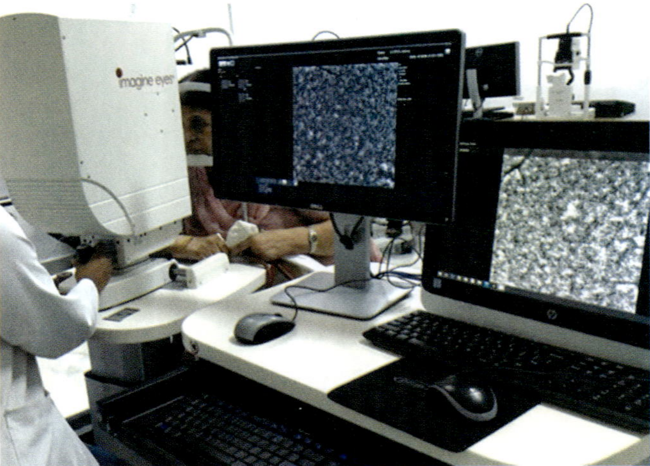

Fig. 2.58: Cone mosaic being captured on a flood illuminated adaptive optics system. Confocal SLO and OCT has also been incorporated in adaptive optics (AO) technology.

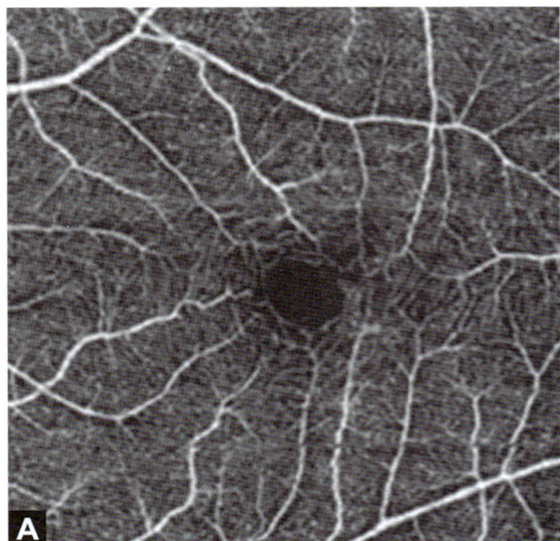

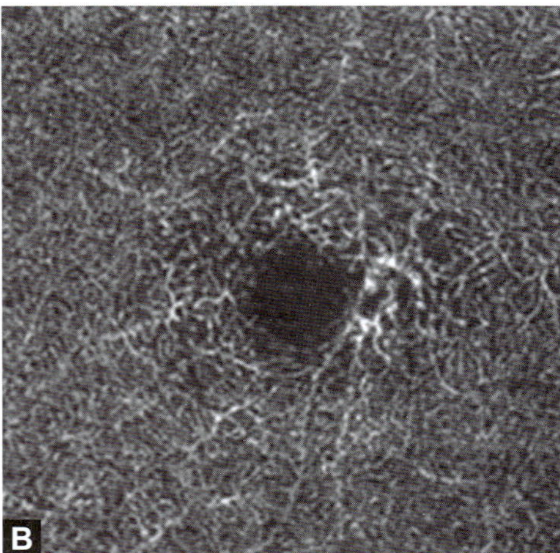

Figs. 2.57A and B: Structural affection of the parafoveal capillaries in an eye with macular telangiectasia. OCTA stays as the most sensitive imaging tool for diagnosis of macular telangiectasia (MacTel).

Confocal SLO systems and OCT systems have also been incorporated with adaptive optics.[59,60] With the adaptive optics, we can acquire images of better contrast, cross-sectional imaging, higher axial resolutions and the measurement of dynamic changes such as blood flow. With the addition of adaptive optics correction to an SLO, the transverse resolution may be increased from approximately 15 µm to less than 3 µm while the axial resolution may be improved from 300 µm to 40 µm (Fig. 2.58).

Ultrastructural Imaging

With adaptive optics, one can now assess photoreceptor cells, retinal pigment epithelium, retinal nerve fiber layer, retinal vessel wall and lamina cribrosa.

Cone photoreceptors are the dominant feature seen with adaptive optics (Figs. 2.59A to C).[61] Cones appear as hyperreflective dots, a manifestation of optical Stiles-Crawford effect.[62] Light from the instrument is reflected back by RPE cells. This reflected light is guided back straight toward the pupil by cone inner segments (acting as optical fibers) and thereby they appear hyperreflective. Other than cone density, arrangement of each cone and regional variabilities in cone topography can also be explored.[63] Rods are difficult to image due to their smaller size (approximately 2 µm in diameter), and their broad angular tuning, which reflects less light back through the pupil.[58,58a-b]

Visualization of single RPE cells also remain challenging due to poor intrinsic contrast of RPE cells and masking of light scatter from RPE cells by overlying photoreceptors, which are also highly scattering.[64] Recently "dark-field" imaging technique has been introduced, where small confocal aperture is replaced by a larger aperture with a central filament. The central filament attenuates the direct signal from photoreceptors, while the larger aperture collects light scattered by the RPE cells (the indirect or so-called dark-field signal).[65]

Density, direction and width of retinal nerve fibers can be identified with adaptive optics.[66] Adaptive optics OCT has

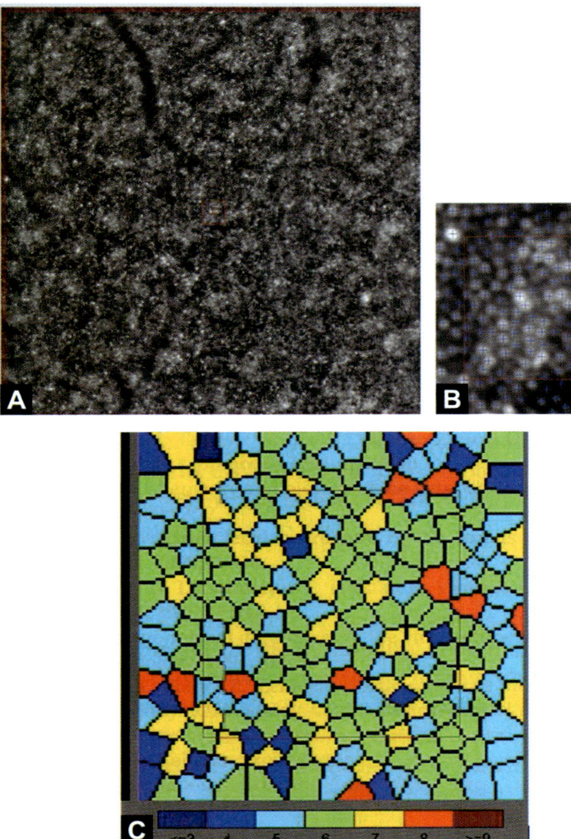

Figs. 2.59A to C: Normal cone mosaic and voronoi diagrams showing each normal cone surrounded by 5–7 adjacent cones.

been used to investigate the micro-architecture of the lamina cribrosa.[67] It also allows high-resolution visualization of the retinal vascular parenchyma and the assessment of retinal blood constituents and flow.[68]

Clinical Implications

Adaptive optics retinal imaging allows measurement of photoreceptor density and diameter and is an important examination for inherited retinal degenerations (cone dystrophy, achromatopsia) and acquired retinal disorders (white dot syndromes, macular telangiectasia type 2, and hydroxychloroquine toxicity).[69-73] Diseased cones do not show the same reflectance pattern as healthy photoreceptors, resulting in dark gaps or areas of "drop-out" within the cone photoreceptor mosaic.[74] With gene therapy trials ongoing, or about to start, adaptive optics imaging of patients with inherited retinal disorders are of particular interest. Adaptive optics has reported evidence of structural changes in cases of glaucoma and other optic neuropathies, where both the peripapillary RNFL bundles and their associated cone photoreceptors have been found to be affected (Figs. 2.60A and B).[75]

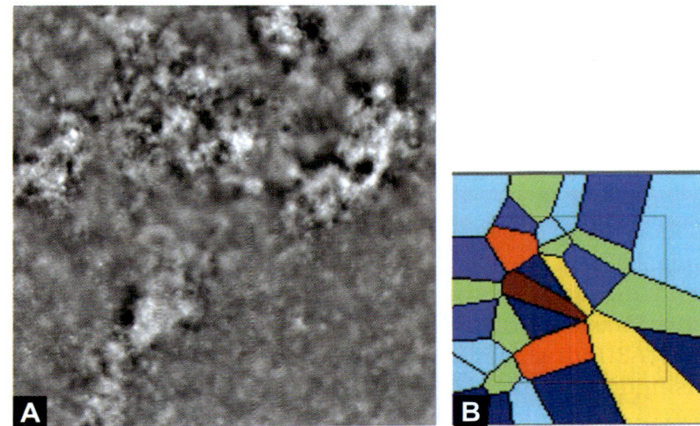

Figs. 2.60A and B: CSC eye with affected cone mosaic and deranged voronoi diagram.

Limitations

The current limitations are imaging eyes with hazy media, formation of normative databases for acquired images, such as cone mosaics, and the cost of the technology. Adaptive optics devices also provide a limited field of view and difficulties in acquiring good quality images in patients with poor fixation, poor compliance, or with significant disruption of their retinal anatomy.

REFERENCES

1. Novotny HR, Alvis DL. A method of photographing fluorescence in circulating blood in the human retina. Circulation. 1961;24:82-6.
2. JD Gass. Atlas of macular diseases: diagnosis and treatment. St. Louis: Mosby; 1970.
3. Pacurariu RI. Low incidence of side effects following intravenous fluorescein angiography. Ann Ophthalmology. 1982;14(1):32-6.
4. Lipson BK, Yannuzzi LA. Complications of intravenous fluorescein injections. Int Ophthalmology Clin. 1989;29(3):200-5.
5. Spaide RF. Fundus autofluorescence and age-related macular degeneration. Ophthalmology. 2003;110(2):392-9.
6. Webb RH, Hughes GW, Delori FC. Confocal scanning laser ophthalmoscope. Appl Opt. 1987;26(8):1492-9.
7. Von Rückmann A, Fitzke FW, Bird AC. Distribution of fundus autofluorescence with a scanning laser ophthalmoscope. Br J Ophthalmology. 1995;79:407-12.
8. Atkinson A, Mazo C. Imaged area of the retina. Data on file, Optos. 2015..
9. Reddy S, Hu A, Schwartz SD. Ultra Wide Field Fluorescein Angiography Guided Targeted Retinal Photocoagulation (TRP). Semin Ophthalmology. 2009;24(1):9-14.
10. Delori FC, Dorey CK, Staurenghi G, et al. In vivo fluorescence of the ocular fundus exhibits retinal pigment epithelium lipofuscin characteristics. Invest Ophthalmology Vis Sci. 1995;36(3):718-29.
11. Lamb LE, Simon JD. A2E: a component of ocular lipofuscin. Photochem Photobiol. 2004;79(2):127-36.
12. Delori FC, Fleckner MR, Goger DG, et al. Autofluorescence distribution associated with drusen in age-related macular degeneration. Invest Ophthalmology Vis Sci. 2000;41(2):496-504.
13. Holz FG, Bellman C, Staudt S, et al. Fundus autofluorescence and development of geographic atrophy in age-related macular degeneration. Invest Ophthalmology Vis Sci. 2001;42(5):1051-6.

14. Spaide RF, Klancnik JM. Fundus autofluorescence and central serous chorioretinopathy. Ophthalmology. 2005;112(5):825-33.

15. Flower RW, Hochheimer BF. Indocyanine green dye fluorescence and infrared absorption choroidal angiography performed simultaneously with fluorescein angiography. Johns Hopkins Med J. 1976;138(2):33-42.

16. Vinekar A, Gilbert C, Dogra M, et al. The KIDROP model of combining strategies for providing retinopathy of prematurity screening in underserved areas in India using widefield imaging, tele-medicine, non-physician graders and smart phone reporting. Indian J Ophthalmology. 2014;62(1):41-9.

17. Huang D, Swanson EA, Lin CP, et al. Optical coherence tomography. Science. 1991;254(5035):1178-81.

18. Wojtkowski M, Bajraszewski T, Gorczyǹska I, et al. Ophthalmic imaging by spectral optical coherence tomography. Am J Ophthalmology. 2004;138(3):412-9.

19. Staurenghi G, Sadda S, Chakravarthy U, et al. Proposed lexicon for anatomic landmarks in normal posterior segment spectral-domain optical coherence tomography: the IN•OCT consensus. Ophthalmology. 2014;121(8):1572-8.

20. Moult E, Choi W, Waheed NK, et al. Ultrahigh-speed swept-source OCT angiography in exudative AMD. Ophthalmic Surg Lasers Imaging Retina. 2014;45(6):496-505.

21. Spaide RF, Koizumi H, Pozzoni MC, et al. Enhanced depth imaging spectral-domain optical coherence tomography. Am J Ophthalmology. 2008;146(4):496-500.

22. Srinivasan VJ, Adler DC, Chen Y, et al. Ultrahigh-speed optical coherence tomography for three-dimensional and en face imaging of the retina and optic nerve head. Invest Ophthalmology Vis Sci. 2008;49(11):5103-10.

23. Uchino E, Uemura A, Ohba N. Initial stages of posterior vitreous detachment in healthy eyes of older persons evaluated by optical coherence tomography. Arch Ophthalmology Chic Ill 1960. 2001;119(10):1475-9.

24. Duker JS, Kaiser PK, Binder S, et al. The International Vitreomacular Traction Study Group classification of vitreomacular adhesion, traction, and macular hole. Ophthalmology. 2013;120(12):2611-9.

25. Wilkins JR, Puliafito CA, Hee MR, et al. Characterization of epiretinal membranes using optical coherence tomography. Ophthalmology. 1996;103(12):2142-51.

26. Kusuhara S, Teraoka Escaño MF, Fujii S, et al. Prediction of postoperative visual outcome based on hole configuration by optical coherence tomography in eyes with idiopathic macular holes. Am J Ophthalmology. 2004;138(5):709-16.

27. Ko TH, Witkin AJ, Fujimoto JG, et al. Ultrahigh-resolution optical coherence tomography of surgically closed macular holes. Arch Ophthalmology Chic Ill 1960. 2006;124(6):827-36.

28. Oh J, Smiddy WE, Flynn HW, et al. Photoreceptor inner/outer segment defect imaging by spectral domain OCT and visual prognosis after macular hole surgery. Invest Ophthalmology Vis Sci. 2010;51(3):1651-8.

29. Sano M, Shimoda Y, Hashimoto H, et al. Restored photoreceptor outer segment and visual recovery after macular hole closure. Am J Ophthalmology. 2009;147(2):313-8.e1.

30. Spaide RF, Curcio CA. Drusen characterization with multimodal imaging. Retina Phila Pa. 2010;30(9):1441-54.

31. Schuman SG, Koreishi AF, Farsiu S, et al. Photoreceptor layer thinning over drusen in eyes with age-related macular degeneration imaged in vivo with spectral-domain optical coherence tomography. Ophthalmology. 2009;116(3):488-96.e2.

32. Zweifel SA, Imamura Y, Spaide TC, et al. Prevalence and significance of subretinal drusenoid deposits (reticular pseudodrusen) in age-related macular degeneration. Ophthalmology. 2010;117(9):1775-81.

33. Ho J, Witkin AJ, Liu J, et al. Documentation of intraretinal retinal pigment epithelium migration via high-speed ultrahigh-resolution optical coherence tomography. Ophthalmology. 2011;118(4):687-93.

34. Schmitz-Valckenberg S, Fleckenstein M, Göbel AP, et al. Optical coherence tomography and autofluorescence findings in areas with geographic atrophy due to age-related macular degeneration. Invest Ophthalmology Vis Sci. 2011;52(1):1-6.

35. Bearelly S, Chau FY, Koreishi A, et al. Spectral domain optical coherence tomography imaging of geographic atrophy margins. Ophthalmology. 2009;116(9):1762-9.

36. Lujan BJ, Rosenfeld PJ, Gregori G, et al. Spectral domain optical coherence tomographic imaging of geographic atrophy. Ophthalmic Surg Lasers Imaging Off J Int Soc Imaging Eye. 2009;40(2):96-101.

37. Zayit-Soudry S, Moroz I, Loewenstein A. Retinal pigment epithelial detachment. Surv Ophthalmology. 2007;52(3):227-43.

38. Lee SY, Stetson PF, Ruiz-Garcia H, et al. Automated characterization of pigment epithelial detachment by optical coherence tomography. Invest Ophthalmology Vis Sci. 2012;53(1):164-70.

39. Chang LK, Sarraf D. Tears of the retinal pigment epithelium: an old problem in a new era. Retina Phila Pa. 2007;27(5):523-34.

40. Landa G, Su E, Garcia PMT, et al. Inner segment-outer segment junctional layer integrity and corresponding retinal sensitivity in dry and wet forms of age-related macular degeneration. Retina Phila Pa. 2011;31(2):364-70.

41. De Salvo G, Vaz-Pereira S, Keane PA, et al. Sensitivity and specificity of spectral-domain optical coherence tomography in detecting idiopathic polypoidal choroidal vasculopathy. Am J Ophthalmology. 2014;158(6):1228-38.e1.

42. Imamura Y, Fujiwara T, Margolis R, et al. Enhanced depth imaging optical coherence tomography of the choroid in central serous chorioretinopathy. Retina Phila Pa. 2009;29(10):1469-73.

43. Hamzah F, Shinojima A, Mori R, et al. Choroidal thickness measurement by enhanced depth imaging and swept-source optical coherence tomography in central serous chorioretinopathy. BMC Ophthalmology. 2014;14:145.

44. Maruko I, Iida T, Sugano Y, et al. Subfoveal choroidal thickness in fellow eyes of patients with central serous chorioretinopathy. Retina Phila Pa. 2011;31(8):1603-8.

45. Maruko I, Iida T, Sugano Y, et al. One-year choroidal thickness results after photodynamic therapy for central serous chorioretinopathy. Retina Phila Pa. 2011;31(9):1921-7.

46. Kim BY, Smith SD, Kaiser PK. Optical coherence tomographic patterns of diabetic macular edema. Am J Ophthalmology. 2006;142(3):405-12.

47. Elman MJ, Bressler NM, Qin H, et al. Expanded 2-year follow-up of ranibizumab plus prompt or deferred laser or triamcinolone plus prompt laser for diabetic macular edema. Ophthalmology. 2011;118(4):609-14.

48. Michaelides M, Kaines A, Hamilton RD, et al. A prospective randomized trial of intravitreal bevacizumab or laser therapy in the management of diabetic macular edema (BOLT study) 12-month data: report 2. Ophthalmology. 2010;117(6):1078-86.e2.

49. Kaiser PK, Riemann CD, Sears JE, et al. Macular traction detachment and diabetic macular edema associated with posterior hyaloidal traction. Am J Ophthalmology. 2001;131(1):44-9.

50. Jia Y, Tan O, Tokayer J, et al. Split-spectrum amplitude-decorrelation angiography with optical coherence tomography. Opt Express. 2012;20(4):4710-25.

51. Makita S, Hong Y, Yamanari M, et al. Optical coherence angiography. Opt Express. 2006;14(17):7821-40.

52. Witmer MT, Parlitsis G, Patel S, et al. Comparison of ultra-widefield fluorescein angiography with the Heidelberg Spectralis®

noncontact ultra-widefield module versus the Optos® Optomap®. Clin Ophthalmology Auckl NZ. 2013;7:389-94.

53. Jia Y, Wei E, Wang X, et al. Optical coherence tomography angiography of optic disc perfusion in glaucoma. Ophthalmology. 2014;121(7):1322-32.

54. Weinhaus RS, Burke JM, Delori FC, et al. Comparison of fluorescein angiography with microvascular anatomy of macaque retinas. Exp Eye Res. 1995;61(1):1-16.

55. Spaide RF, Klancnik JM, Cooney MJ. Retinal vascular layers imaged by fluorescein angiography and optical coherence tomography angiography. JAMA Ophthalmology. 2015;133(1):45-50.

56. De Carlo TE, Romano A, Waheed NK, et al. A review of optical coherence tomography angiography (OCTA). Inter J Retina Vitreous. 2015;1(1):5.

57. Rosenfeld PJ, Durbin MK, Roisman L, et al. ZEISS Angioplex™ spectral domain optical coherence tomography angiography: technical aspects. In: Bandello F, Souied EH, Querques G (Eds). OCT Angiography in Retinal and Macular Diseases 2016 (Vol. 56, pp. 18-29). Basel: Karger Publishers; 2016. pp. I-XI.

58. Spaide RF, Fujimoto JG, Waheed NK. Image artifacts in optical coherence tomography angiography. Retina (Philadelphia, Pa.). 2015;35(11):2163-80.

58a. Roorda A. Adaptive optics ophthalmoscopy. J Refract Surg Thorofare NJ 1995. 2000;16(5):S602-7.

58b. Williams DR. Imaging Single Cells in the Living Retina. Vision Res. 2011;51(13):1379-96.

59. Roorda A, Romero-Borja F, Donnelly Iii W, et al. Adaptive optics scanning laser ophthalmoscopy. Opt Express. 2002;10(9):405-12.

60. Miller DT, Kocaoglu OP, Wang Q, et al. Adaptive optics and the eye (super resolution OCT). Eye Lond Engl. 2011;25(3):321-30.

61. Miller DT, Williams DR, Morris GM, et al. Images of cone photoreceptors in the living human eye. Vision Res. 1996;36(8):1067-79.

62. Miloudi C, Rossant F, Bloch I, et al. The Negative Cone Mosaic: A New Manifestation of the Optical Stiles-Crawford Effect in Normal Eyes. Invest Ophthalmology Vis Sci. 2015;56(12):7043-50.

63. Zhang T, Godara P, Blanco ER, et al. Variability in human cone topography assessed by adaptive optics scanning laser ophthalmoscopy. Am J Ophthalmology. 2015;160(2):290-300.e1.

64. Roorda A, Zhang Y, Duncan JL. High-resolution in vivo imaging of the RPE mosaic in eyes with retinal disease. Invest Ophthalmology Vis Sci. 2007;48(5):2297-303.

65. Scoles D, Sulai YN, Dubra A. In vivo dark-field imaging of the retinal pigment epithelium cell mosaic. Biomed Opt Express. 2013;4(9):1710-23.

66. Takayama K, Ooto S, Hangai M, et al. High-resolution imaging of the retinal nerve fiber layer in normal eyes using adaptive optics scanning laser ophthalmoscopy. PloS One. 2012;7(3):e33158.

67. Nadler Z, Wang B, Schuman JS, et al. In vivo three-dimensional characterization of the healthy human lamina cribrosa with adaptive optics spectral-domain optical coherence tomography. Invest Ophthalmology Vis Sci. 2014;55(10):6459-66.

68. Chui TYP, Gast TJ, Burns SA. Imaging of Vascular Wall Fine Structure in the Human Retina Using Adaptive Optics Scanning Laser Ophthalmoscopy. Invest Ophthalmology Vis Sci. 2013;54(10):7115-24.

69. Morgan JW, Han G, Klinman E, et al. High-resolution adaptive optics retinal imaging of cellular structure in choroideremia. Invest Ophthalmology Vis Sci. 2014;55(10):6381-97.

70. Abozaid MA, Langlo CS, Dubis AM, et al. Reliability and Repeatability of Cone Density Measurements in Patients with Congenital Achromatopsia. Adv Exp Med Biol. 2016;854:277-83.

71. Agarwal A, Soliman MK, Hanout M, et al. Adaptive Optics Imaging of Retinal Photoreceptors Overlying Lesions in White Dot Syndrome and its Functional Correlation. Am J Ophthalmology. 2015;160(4):806-16.e2.

72. Jacob J, Krivosic V, Paques M, et al. Cone density loss on adaptive optics in early macular telangiectasia Type 2. Retina Phila Pa. 2016;36(3):545-51.

73. Debellemanière G, Flores M, Tumahai P, et al. Assessment of parafoveal cone density in patients taking hydroxychloroquine in the absence of clinically documented retinal toxicity. Acta Ophthalmology (Copenh). 2015;93(7):e534-40.

74. Wolfing JI, Chung M, Carroll J, et al. High-resolution retinal imaging of cone-rod dystrophy. Ophthalmology. 2006;113(6):1019.e1.

75. Choi SS, Zawadzki RJ, Keltner JL, et al. Changes in cellular structures revealed by ultra-high resolution retinal imaging in optic neuropathies. Invest Ophthalmology Vis Sci. 2008;49(5):2103-19.

Chapter 3

Electrophysiology

Raghav Ravani, Devesh Kumawat, Priyanka Ramesh, Atul Kumar

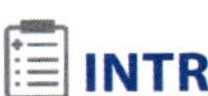 INTRODUCTION

Visual electrophysiological tests are objective tests that help to assess the functional integrity of visual pathway, starting from photoreceptor and retinal pigment epithelial layer in retina to the occipital cortex.

Visual electrophysiological tests include:

- Electroretinography (ERG) (full field): Measures functional integrity of photoreceptors and inner retinal layers of entire retina.
- Multifocal ERG (mfERG): Measures spatial distribution of central retinal cone function.
- Electrooculography (EOG): Measures functional integrity of retinal pigment epithelium (RPE) and its interaction with photoreceptors.
- Visual evoked potential (VEP): Measures functional integrity of optic nerve and occipital cortex.
- Pattern VEP: Objectively assesses the macula and the central retinal ganglion cells.

ELECTRORETINOGRAM

The electroretinogram (ERG) measures the electrical activity generated by the retina in response to light. This is measured at the level of the cornea as there exists a potential difference between the cornea and retina known as corneoretinal potential (range 0.4– 1 mV).[1]

The ERG is a graphical tracing of the summated action potentials generated in retina in response to light stimulus and changes in retinal illumination. Of the electrophysiological test, ERG is the most widely used. Depending upon the stimulus and recording conditions, the ERG provides information regarding the functional state of rods and/or cones and thus, can be used in a diagnosis and prognosis of many inherited or acquired diseases of the retina as a whole.[2]

Full Field Electroretinogram Waveform

It is the summated electrical activity across the entire retina. It represents electrical activity of the photoreceptors, Muller cells and RPE giving rise to multiple wave components of the ERG (Fig. 3.1).[3]

The various wave components are:

"a"-wave: The initial negative deflection is called the "a"-wave (sometimes referred as PIII). The origin of the "a"-wave is taken to be from the photoreceptors. It is due to the local membrane hyperpolarization of the photoreceptors upon stimulation by light resulting in a negative potential at inner photoreceptor segment as compared to the outer photoreceptor segment.

"b"-wave: The large cornea-positive deflection is called the "b"-wave (PII). The origin of the "b"-wave is hypothesized to be from muller cells of the retina and represents the activity of the bipolar cells. The light incident on the photoreceptors leads to local membrane hyperpolarization by release of potassium in the extracellular space. In response, there is a change in membrane potential of muller cells proportionate to the amount of extracellular potassium thus, imparting a relative positive charge and hence, the positive deflection in

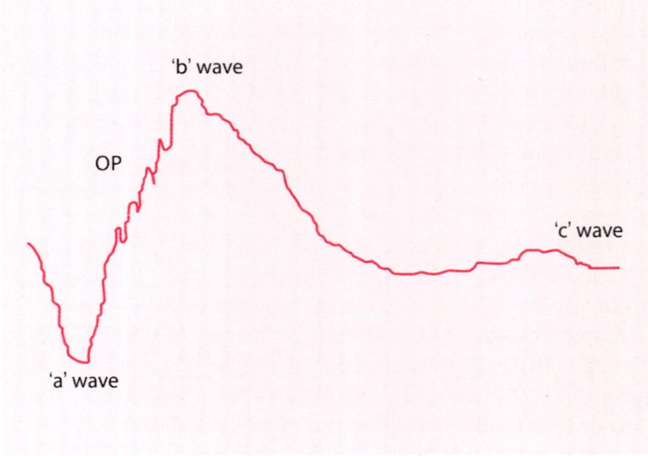

Fig. 3.1: Schematic diagram of waveforms of electroretinography (ERG) (OP: Oscillatory potential).

ERG. As the genesis of both "a"-wave and "b"-wave depends on the intact photoreceptors and the stimulus of light on photoreceptors, the factors affecting generation of "a"-wave also affect "b"-wave. Also it is important to note that since "b"-wave depends on photoreceptors, the "b"-wave recording can be from either cone or rod.

Oscillatory Potential

High frequency, low amplitude wavelets superimposed on the ascending limb of b-wave are known as oscillatory potentials (OP). The origin of OPs is not completely understood but OPs are believed to represent a complex feedback circuit involving the bipolar cells, amacrine cells and interplexiform cells.[4]

"c"-wave: A slow cornea-positive potential is called a "c"-wave (PI). It is generated from the retinal pigment epithelial cells in response to rod photoreceptor stimulation, which are in direct contact with the apex of the RPE cells unlike the cones.[5]

Measurement of Electroretinogram

The amplitude and implicit time of "a"- wave and "b"- wave are measured as follows:

Amplitude: The amplitude of "a"-wave is measured from the baseline to the trough of the negative deflection. The amplitude of "b"-wave is measured from the trough of the "a"-wave to the peak of the "b"-wave.

Time sequences—

Latency: It is the interval between the onset of stimulus and beginning of the "a" -wave response.

Implicit time: The implicit time of "a"-wave is measured from stimulus onset to its trough. Implicit time of "b"-wave is measured from stimulus onset to peak of "b"-wave.

Electroretinogram Records

The International Society for Clinical Electrophysiology of Vision (ISCEV) has published Standards and Guidelines for full field ERG (ffERG). ISCEV specifies six responses based on the adaptation state of the eye and the flash strength:[6,7] (1) Dark-adapted 0.01 ERG (rod ERG); (2) Dark-adapted 3 ERG (combined rod-cone standard flash ERG); (3) Dark-adapted 3 oscillatory potentials; (4) Dark-adapted 10 ERG (strong flash ERG); (5) Light-adapted 3 ERG (standard flash "cone" ERG); and (6) Light-adapted 30 Hz flicker ERG.

Dark-adapted 0.01 ERG (rod ERG)/scotopic rod response: It gives the electrophysiological response of the rod system of the retina. The ERG is recorded under scotopic conditions after at least 20 minutes of dark adaptation using low-intensity white or blue flash. The stimulus is a weak white flash of 0.010 photopic $cd \cdot s \cdot m^{-2}$ with a scotopic strength of 0.025 scotopic $cd \cdot s \cdot m^{-2}$. This stimuli being below the cone threshold, only the rod system responds. This gives a slow positive response with only 'b'-wave being recordable. Clinically, scotopic rod response amplitude is diminished in diseases affecting the rod system like retinitis pigmentosa (RP), choroideremia and congenital stationary night blindness (CSNB).

Dark-adapted 3 ERG (combined rod-cone standard flash ERG)/scotopic maximal combined response: It is a combined response of rods and cones, predominantly rod-dominated. The ERG is recorded under scotopic conditions after dark adaptation using brighter flash stimulus. The strength of the standard flash is 3.0 photopic $cd \cdot s \cdot m^{-2}$ with a scotopic strength of 7.5 scotopic $cd \cdot s \cdot m^{-2}$. It has a larger amplitude and longer implicit time as compared to the photopic response. Since it records the response from both rods and cones, it is affected in diseases that affect either or both the photoreceptors. For example RP and cone dystrophy.

Dark-adapted 3 oscillatory potentials/OPs: These high-frequency wavelets on the ascending limb of 'b'-wave are seen predominantly in the scotopic bright-flash ERG recordings. The response primarily arises from amacrine cells. ERG for OPs can be obtained by using specific filters, which filter out the low frequency 'b'-wave response and allow the higher frequencies to pass. Standard dark-adapted oscillatory potentials are recorded from dark-adapted eyes, using the 3.0 $cd \cdot s \cdot m^{-2}$ standard flash stimulus. These are sensitive to effects of ischemia and commonly used as early indicators of diabetic retinopathy or even progression of severe nonproliferative diabetic retinopathy to proliferative diabetic retinopathy.

Dark-adapted 10 ERG (strong flash ERG): It is a combined response ERG with enhanced "a"-waves which reflect photoreceptor function. The standard strong flash is 10 photopic $cd \cdot s \cdot m^{-2}$, with a scotopic strength of 25 scotopic $cd \cdot s \cdot m^{-2}$.

Light-adapted 3 ERG (standard flash "cone" ERG)/photopic single-flash cone response: It is the measure of the electrophysiological response of the cone system of the retina. The ERG is recorded in photopic conditions after about 10 minutes of adaptation. The background light bleaches the rod system and thereby, suppressing it. The response thus, obtained represents cone system response, which contains both "a"-wave and "b"-wave with a shorter amplitude and shorter implicit time. This is grossly diminished or abnormal in conditions that primarily affect the cone photoreceptors like congenital achromatopsia and acquired cone degeneration. The response is reduced in amplitude and variable in RP depending on the relative involvement of the cone system.[8]

Light-adapted 30 Hz flicker ERG/photopic 30 Hz flicker response: It is a measure of cone activity of the retina using a high frequency repetitive stimulus (30 Hz flicker). The repetitive stimulus at such high frequency generates response from cone system alone since rods cannot respond to rapid stimulation rates. The implicit time of the photopic flicker response is extremely sensitive to changes in the cone system and thus, detects early damage of cone photoreceptors, e.g. RP and progressive cone dystrophy.[9]

Technique and Instrument

Background: For full field ERG response, the background luminance of around 17–34 cd s/m² is provided using Ganzfeld bowl (Fig. 3.2).

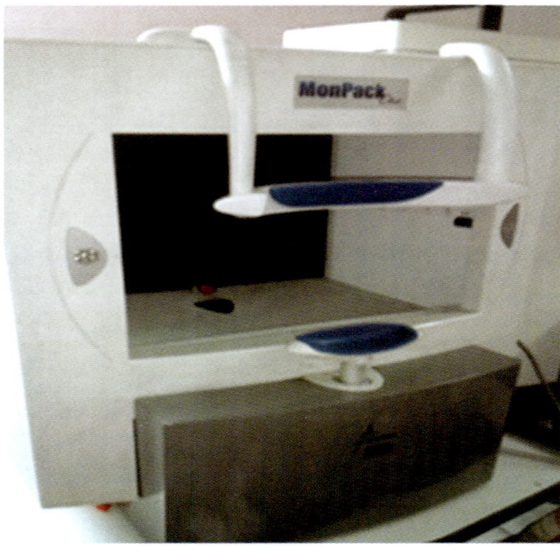

Fig. 3.2: The machine for recording electroretinography (ERG).

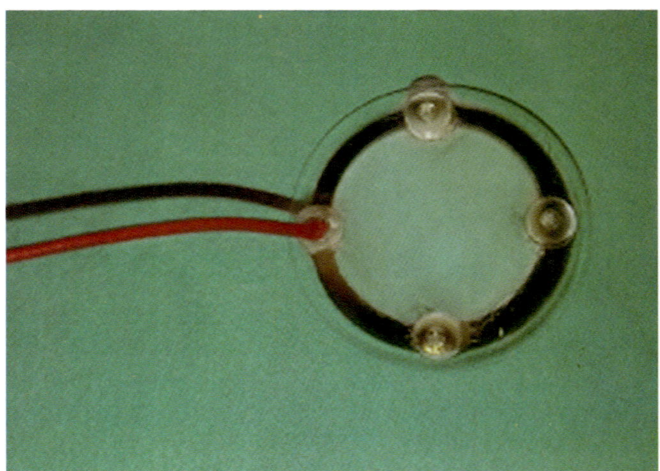

Fig. 3.3: Contact electrode for ERG.

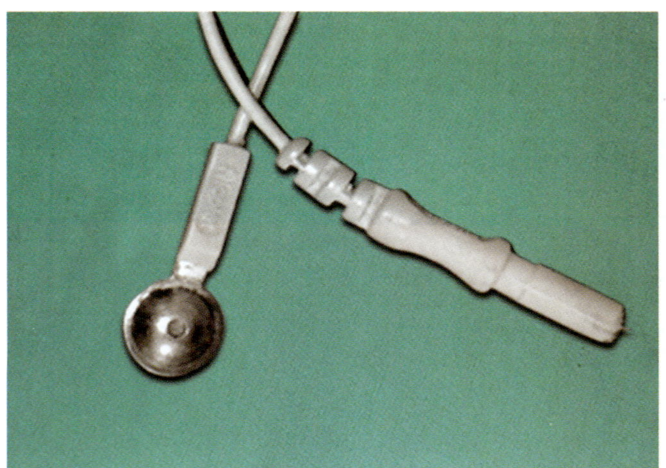

Fig. 3.4: Surface conductive electrode for ERG.

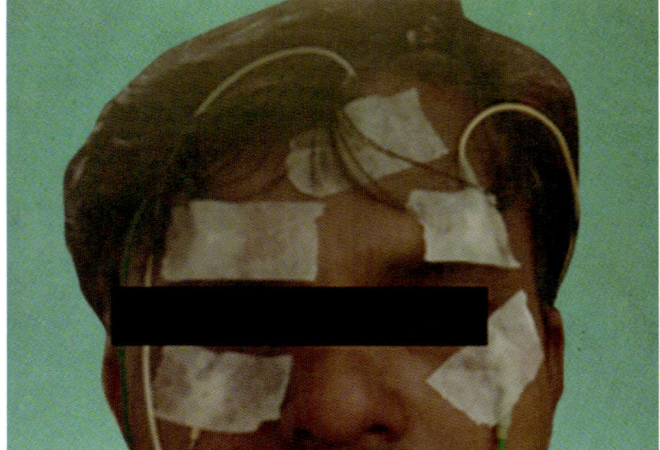

Fig. 3.5: Placement of electrodes during recording an ERG (Note: consent of the patient has been obtained for reproducing the photograph).

Stimulus: A stroboscope flash or cathode ray tube or light emitting diode provides the stimulus flash. The duration of each flash stimulus should not exceed 5 milliseconds, so that duration of each is less than the integration time of any photoreceptors. The ISCEV standard flash produces 1.5–3 cd s/m² of luminous energy at surface of Ganzfeld bowl. Suggested brighter flash by ISCEV standard is of 11–12 cd/m².

Electrodes

Active electrode: These include corneal electrode or surface conductive/skin electrode. Corneal electrodes are contact electrodes, which are optically clear lenses placed in contact with cornea like Jet electrode (unipolar), Dorian Gold lens (bipolar) and Burian-Allen electrode (unipolar or bipolar) (Fig. 3.3).[10]

Surface conductive or skin electrodes are used with conductive paste or gel to achieve good contact with low impedance. In general, the impedance of surface electrode should be less than or equal to 5 kΩ, e.g. gold-foil electrodes,[11] H-K loop[12] and DTL fiber (Fig. 3.4).

Skin electrodes are placed over the upper and lower lid (Fig. 3.5).

Reference electrode: Can be invasive or noninvasive. The latter in turn, can be a unipolar or bipolar electrode. The reference electrode is placed at the outer canthus for unipolar electrodes.

Ground electrode: It is placed either over the forehead or earlobe.

Abnormal Electroretinogram Responses

1. *Negative response*: Is characterized by large "a"-wave and absence of "b"-wave (b/a less than 1.0). This can be seen in severe retinal circulatory disorders like central retinal artery occlusion (CRAO). Negative ERG is also seen in conditions like CSNB,[13] X-linked retinoschisis,[14] Goldmann-Favre syndrome,[15] melanoma associated retinopathy (MAR).
2. *Accentuated response*: It is characterized by a potential with amplitude more than two standard deviations above the mean for both "a"-wave and "b"-wave. Such response is seen in early stages of siderosis bulbi as described by Karpe et al.[16] It is also seen in conditions with subtotal circulatory disturbances of retina and albinism.
3. *Subnormal response*: It is characterized by a potential with amplitude less than two standard deviations below the mean for both "a"-wave and "b"-wave. A subnormal response indicates subnormal functioning of a wider area of retina, e.g. retinal detachment, early RP, chloroquine toxicity.[17]
4. *Extinguished response*: Is characterized by complete absence of response, e.g. advanced RP, Leber's congenital amaurosis, total old retinal detachment, advanced siderosis bulbi.

Pattern Electroretinogram

Contrast-reversing pattern (i.e. a black and white checkerboard) at a rate of about 4.0 ± 0.8 reversals per second (rps)[18] is used to elicit a response known as pattern electroretinogram (pattern ERG or PERG). The mean of the width and the height of the stimulus field should be 15° (±3°). A photopic luminance of greater than 80 cd/m² is required for the white areas. The normal PERG waveform consists of an initial negative wave (N35), followed by a positive component (P50). This is followed by a large negative component at 90–100 ms (N95).[19]

The PERG arises largely in the ganglion cells, driven by the photoreceptors and corresponding retinal cells. Since the PERG (in contrast to the flash ERG) is a local response from the area covered by the retinal stimulus image, it can be used as a sensitive indicator of dysfunction within the macular region. PERGs can be used in patients with abnormal pattern VEPs to differentiate between retinal and optic nerve dysfunction as a cause for the VEP abnormality. It can also be used to monitor other conditions associated with retinal ganglion cell dysfunction, such as glaucoma, optic neuropathies and primary ganglion cell diseases.[20]

MULTIFOCAL ELECTRORETINOGRAPHY

Multifocal electroretinography (mfERG) as the name suggests, is a method of recording local electrophysiological responses from different regions of the retina. The mfERG was developed by Eric Sutter and his colleagues in 1992[21] and introduced as a clinical test in 1995 to provide a topographic measure of retinal electrophysiological activity as opposed to full field ERG, which reflects the summed electrical activity of the retina reflecting global retinal function. Localized lesions of the macula may not alter full field substantially and similarly, a macula sparing retinal disease with normal visual acuity may have abnormal ERG. Herein, lays the utility of multifocal ERG. It is a visual electrophysiological test of local retinal function that measures the spatial distribution of the central retinal cone function. Thus, mfERG responses are recorded from cone-driven retina under light-adapted conditions.[22]

Technique

Patient Preparation

- *Pupils*: Pupils are to be fully dilated.
- *Light adaptation*: It should be done for at least 15 minutes in ordinary room light.
- *Fixation monitoring*: Good, central and steady fixation is essential. Moving the fixation target can compensate for eccentric fixation.
- *Optical correction*: Appropriate optical correction for viewing distance need to be used.
- *Electrodes*: Recording electrodes (active electrodes), reference electrodes and ground electrodes (Fig. 3.6).
  - *Recording electrodes*: These may be contact or noncontact type of electrodes.
    - *Contact electrode*: These can again be unipolar or bipolar. Bipolar corneal contact electrodes yield recordings with highest signal-to-noise ratio (SNR). Thus, the responses have fewer artifacts. Few examples of contact electrodes include: Jet Electrode (unipolar), Dorian Gold lens (Bipolar) and Burian-Allen Electrode (unipolar or bipolar).
    - *Noncontact electrode*: Need longer recording times, repeat measurements are required to obtain comparable SNRs when using noncontact electrodes like gold-foil electrodes, H-K loop and DTL fiber.

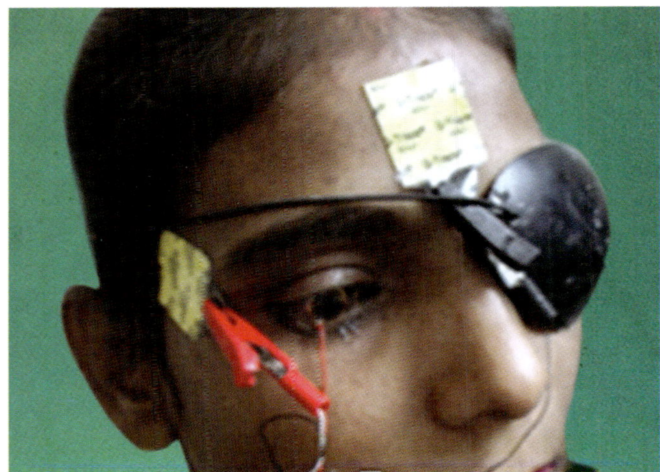

Fig. 3.6: Placement of electrodes for recording multifocal electroretinography (mfERG).

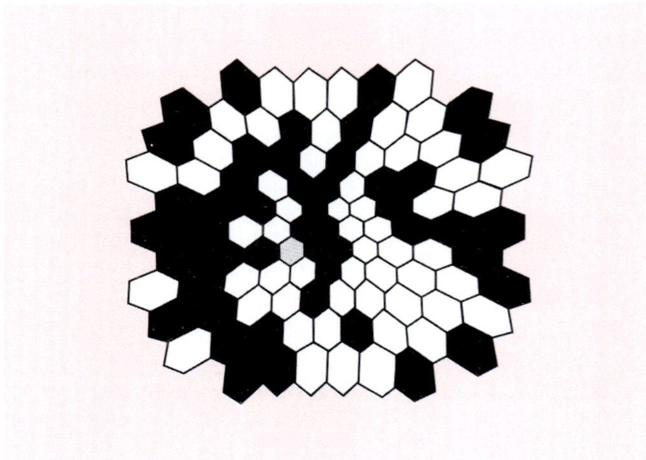

Fig. 3.7: Array of rapidly changing sequence of hexagons as stimulus for multifocal electroretinography (mfERG) recording.

- *Active electrode*: May be placed either in contact with the cornea or in inferior fornix.
- *Reference electrode*: Is placed lateral to the lateral canthus.
- *Ground electrode*: Is placed at center of the forehead or earlobe

Stimulation

Stimulus source: Depending upon the individual equipment, stimulus source may be any one of cathode ray tube (CRT) (earlier versions), light emitting diode (LED), liquid crystal display (LCD) screen or scanning laser ophthalmoscopy (SLO).

Stimulus: Consists of array of hexagons which can be 61, 103 or 241 in number, which are scaled (increased in size with retinal eccentricity from the fovea to periphery to elicit equal amplitude response from all locations since the concentration of cones decreases with increasing distance from the fovea). Thus, the central hexagons are smaller than the peripheral ones (Fig. 3.7).

The stimulus follows a predetermined pseudorandom binary flicker sequence ('m sequence') wherein, each stimulus element has a 50% chance of being illuminated every time the frame changes (Fig. 3.7). Increasing the number of stimulus elements/hexagons improves the spatial resolution but also increases the test duration.

Stimulus size and viewing distance: The overall stimulus pattern should subtend a visual angle of 20–30° on either side of fixation. The Metro Vision System (Vision monitor, Mon Pack 3, Metrovision, France) subtends a field of ± 30° horizontally and ± 24° vertically centered on the fovea at a viewing distance of 30 cm.

Frame frequency: Most widely used CRT frame frequency is 75 Hz. It should never be in line with current frequency (50 or 60 Hz), which may cause interference artifacts.

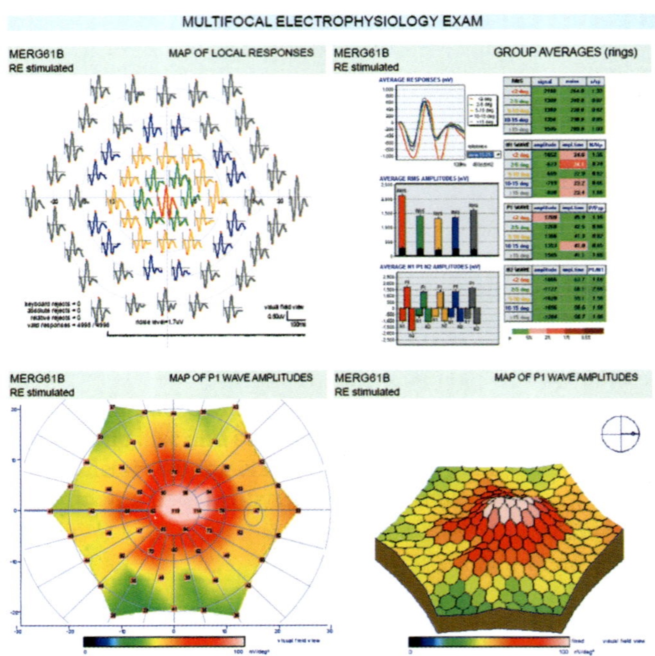

Fig. 3.8: Screenshot of trace array of multifocal electroretinography (mfERG) with 61 elements (upper left image) and 3D-response density plot representation (lower right image).

Fixation target: A red fixation target is presented within the central hexagon. This can be modified in cases with eccentric fixation to test the desired anatomical location.

Luminance: The luminance for the stimulus is 100–200 cd/m² in lighted state and less than1 cd/m² in the dark state. Thus, the mean screen luminance during the test will be 50–100 cd/m².

Contrast and background: The contrast between the lighted and darkened stimulus should be 90% or greater. The background region should have a luminance equal to the mean luminance of the stimulus array to eliminate the rod response.

Test duration: Total time is typically about 4 min for 61 elements or 8 min for 103 elements. The overall recording time is divided into shorter segments of 15–30 sec so that subjects can rest in between and also a poor record due to noise, movement or artifacts can be discarded and run again without losing prior data.

Response and interpretation: Interpretation of mfERG involves interpreting the waveforms in the trace array to look for the variations in amplitude and latency and to detect spatial variations in it. Next is to interpret the numeric data that show amplitudes relative to norms within averaged groups of responses.

Multifocal ERG Interpretation

Trace array: It is the basic mfERG display and is displayed as an array of the mfERG traces using trace lengths of 100 ms or more (Fig. 3.8).

These arrays show topographic variations and demonstrate the quality of records. It is important to specify *field view* or *retinal view* on the array along with notation of width in degrees of the trace array.

Topographic color map/Topographic (3D) response density plots: Shows the 3D topography of overall signal strength per unit area of retina by plotting the amplitude of waveform per unit area of retina (*see* Fig. 3.8). The center of the field being derived from smaller hexagons, show large response and is expressed as nanovolts/deg^2 (area of retina). Normal surface plot gives a *foveal peak* at the center of the retina. Topographic map also helps to monitor fixation by monitoring the location and depth of blind spot. But 3D plots should not be used without simultaneous display of trace array as abnormal or delayed responses can produce normal plots and it also depends on how the local amplitude is measured.

Group averages: Group of responses from the trace arrays can be averaged to compare quadrants, hemiretinal areas, normal versus abnormal regions of two eyes (*see* Fig. 3.8). Comparing successive rings from center to periphery is especially helpful in patients with diseases that produce dysfunction with radial symmetry.

Kernels: The typical waveforms of the mfERG response are technically known as kernels. The most commonly analyzed responses are the first-order and the second-order kernel components.[23]

First-order kernel: The waveform is biphasic with an initial negative deflection (N1) followed by a positive peak (P1) (Fig. 3.9).

First-order kernels are obtained by adding all the records following the presentation of a flash in that hexagon and subtracting all the records following a dark frame.

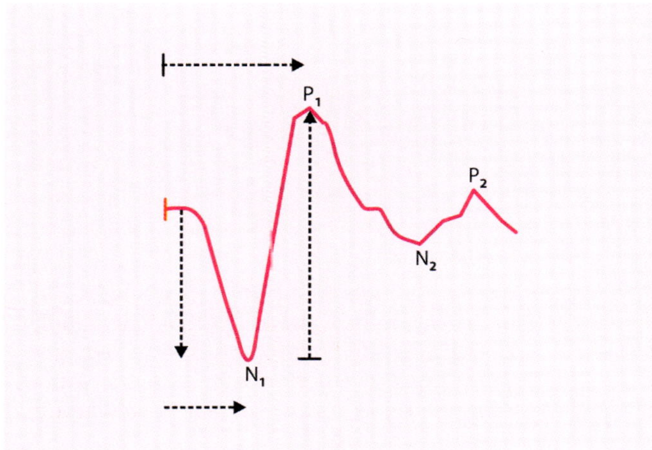

Fig. 3.9: Schematic diagram showing a typical waveform of multifocal electroretinography (mfERG). Second vertical arrow showing the trough-to-peak amplitude and horizontal arrow showing the implicit time.

Second-order kernel: Is a measure of mfERG responses to adaptation by successive flash. This represents the temporal nonlinearity of the local responses and is claimed by many authors to arise from the inner retina. This has especially been useful in retinal vascular occlusions.

Advantages

- As mfERG gives a spatial distribution of retinal function and a topographic representation, it helps in identifying the site of retinal pathology.[24]
- The mfERG distinguishes between the outer and inner retinal diseases.
- It helps in monitoring the progression of the disease.

Indications

- To differentiate diseases that affects the outer retina from those that affect the ganglion cells or optic nerve[25]
- Outer retinal disease: The spatial mfERG responses seem to correlate and match with visual field defects in retinal diseases like multiple evanescent white dot syndrome (MEWDS),[26] retinal detachment, focal cone dystrophy, choroidal neovascularization and commotio retinae.
- Inner retinal disease: The area of field defect correlates and matches with topographic plots of mfERG in retinal artery occlusions. Especially useful in differentiating the inner retinal disease from the optic nerve disease is the second-order kernel.
- Toxic retinopathies: Various studies have demonstrated the role of mfERG in detecting early drug-induced toxic retinopathies.[27]
- Diabetic retinopathy: The implicit time measures are more sensitive in detecting retinal dysfunction in early diabetic retinopathy.[28] The foveal thickness measurement on optical coherence tomography (OCT) has been found to correlate significantly with mfERG recordings.
- Stargardt's disease: Patients have decreased amplitude with normal or minimal delay in implicit time.[29]
- Any retinal fluid [retinal detachment, optic pits, central serous retinopathy and cystoid macular edema (CME)] seems to either diminish the amplitude of the waveform or completely flatten it.
- Retinitis pigmentosa: Both implicit time delay and decreased amplitudes are seen in mfERG waveform in this condition. Delay in implicit time being more important as it has been found at times in patients with normal amplitude responses.[30]
- The mfERG can be used to serially follow-up and monitor response after intervention in patients with retained intraocular foreign body/early siderosis, after photodynamic therapy (PDT), after macular hole surgery, follow-up of CSR or macular edema and after stem cell therapy in retinitis pigmentosa.

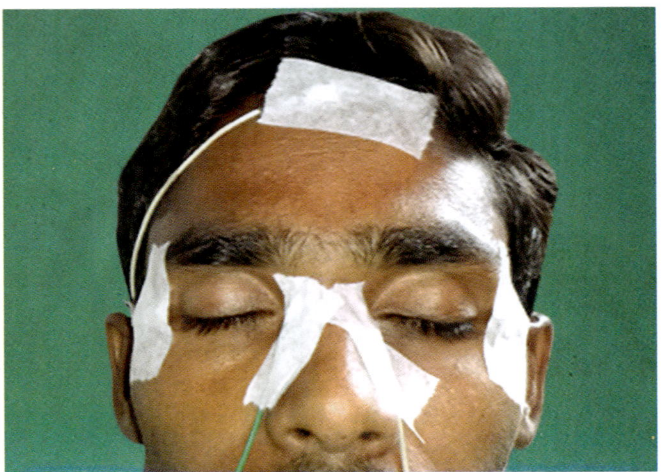

Fig. 3.10: Electrode placement for electrooculography (EOG).

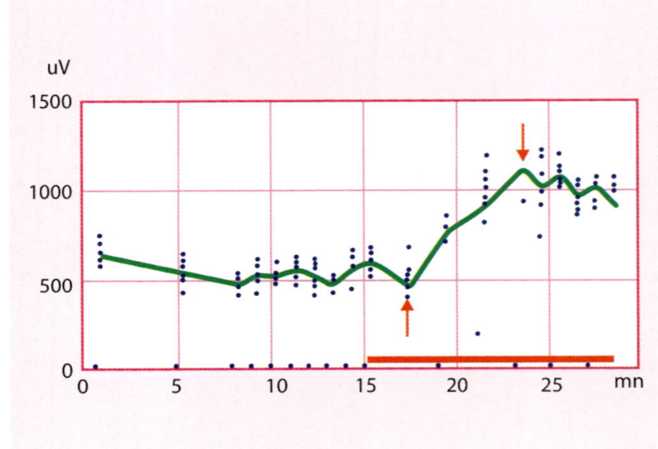

Fig. 3.11: Electrooculography (EOG) waveform showing light peak (LP;upper right red arrow) and dark trough (DT;lower left red arrow). The ratio LP/DT called as Arden ratio.

ELECTROOCULOGRAPHY

Electrooculography (EOG) is the measure of the integrity of the RPE layer of the retina. It is based on the principle of non-invasive measurement of the resting potential difference of the eye that results from the change in polarity from the apical to the basilar end of the RPE in dark versus light-adapted conditions.

Electrodes for EOG are placed on the lateral canthus, medial canthi and one on the forehead (Fig. 3.10).[31] The baseline potential under light adapted state and dark adapted state is recorded.[32]

During the test, a series of lights is linked sequentially and the patient follows the light with saccadic movements during dark and light adapted states. The amplitude of standing potential is recorded over the course of dark adaptation, which decreases with time and reaches a dark trough in about 10 minutes. The amplitude rises with the light adaptation and reaches peak in about 5–10 minutes. The smallest peak-to-trough amplitude in the dark divides the largest Peak-to-trough amplitude in light (Fig. 3.11). This ratio of light peak-to-dark trough amplitude is considered as the measure of RPE integrity and is called the Arden ratio.

A value between 1.65 and 1.85 is normal response; while values more than 1.85 are supernormal and less than 1.65 are subnormal responses.

Like ERG, EOG is a mass response and is not affected by localized disorders. Thus, EOG confirms information provided by ERG and is complementary to ERG. The only exception in which EOG provides unique information is Best vitelliform macular dystrophy (also called Best disease). In Best disease, EOG Arden ratio is abnormal in both the patient and the carrier parent irrespective of signs and symptoms, while the full field ERG is usually normal.

VISUAL EVOKED POTENTIAL

The visual evoked potential (VEP) is the measure of cortically evoked electrical activity and is in fact an electroencephalogram recording of the occipital lobe and is a measure of the integrity of the visual pathway. Thus, it helps to assess the functional state of the visual pathway beyond the ganglion cells. VEP response is primarily driven by macular area due to large macular representation at the cerebral cortex.[33]

The VEP can be measured using either a single midline channel or as a multiple channel recording. However, chiasmal and retrochiasmal disease can be missed using a single midline channel. For placing the electrodes, the distance between the inion and nasion is measured. The active electrode in VEP is placed at 10% distance above the inion. The reference electrode is placed at 30% of the distance from the nasion toward inion. A ground electrode can be placed on the forehead or on an earlobe. The types of VEP differ in the mode of stimulus presentation. The flash VEP is the cortically evoked response to a brief white flash, while the pattern VEP is a response to patterned stimuli like a black-and-white checkerboard or gratings, the mean luminance being constant (Fig. 3.12).

This pattern VEP can in turn be recorded in different ways depending upon the presentation of patterned stimuli, i.e. Pattern appearance-disappearance VEP or pattern reversal VEP. The pattern VEP yields a prominent positive component P100, which is the most consistent measure (Fig. 3.13).

The implicit time of P100 is a sensitive measure of delay in optic nerve transmission caused by demyelination. The P100 is preceded by a negative component at 75 milliseconds called as N75.

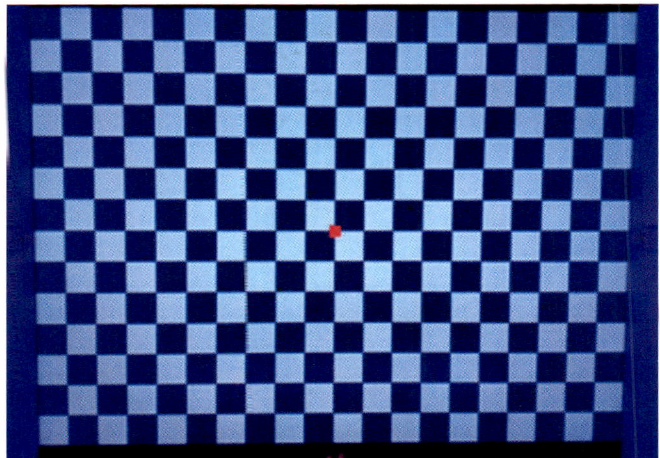

Fig. 3.12: Black-and-white checkerboard stimulus for pattern visual evoked potential (VEP).

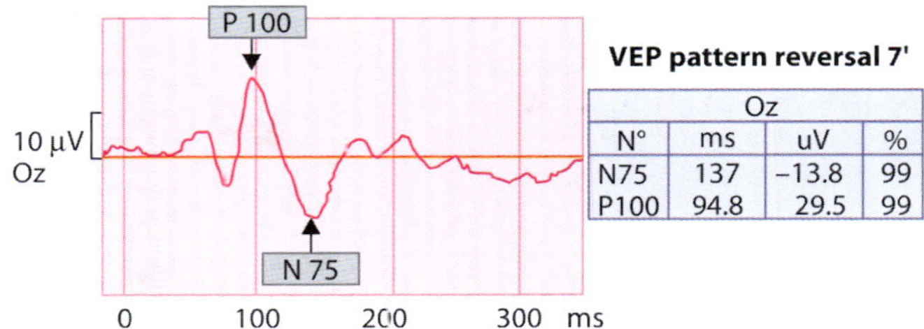

	Oz		
N°	ms	uV	%
N75	137	−13.8	99
P100	94.8	29.5	99

Fig. 3.13: Pattern visual evoked potential (VEP) showing a prominent positive wave P100 (top black arrow).

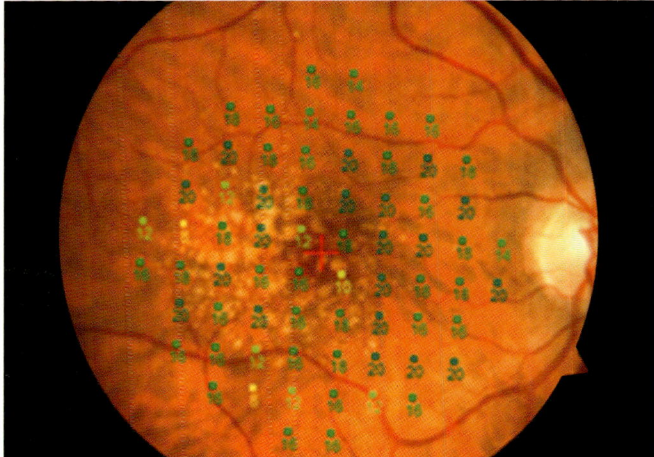

Fig. 3.14: Microperimetry in early age-related macular degeneration (AMD) with patchy loss of macular sensitivity corresponding to drusen deposits.

Advances in Visual Evoked Potential

Sweep VEP (sVEP): Introduced by Regan for objectively measuring refractive errors, sVEP is a steady state pattern VEP to a pattern of elements that varies in some aspect over time. sVEP can measure resolution (grating) acuity and vernier acuity (hyperacuity).

The sVEP usually uses a grating pattern to measure the resolution acuity. An estimation of visual acuity is obtained by sweeping spatial frequency from low to high in about 10s and determining the highest spatial frequency to which a response occurs. To measure contrast sensitivity, contrast is swept with a fixed spatial frequency to determine the lowest contrast to which a response occurs.[34]

Step VEP: An alternative method using a brief staircase for determining the acuity threshold using a steady state VEP.[35]

Motion-onset VEP: Motion-onset VEP has properties that give information not obtainable by standard pattern VEP, e.g. the ability to record up to 50° of eccentricity and the amplitudes being significantly larger to extra-macular stimulation compared to macular, it helps in testing peripheral parts of the retina. Also motion-onset VEPs are being independent of the size of stimulus elements are helpful to record VEPs in patients with low vision and amblyopia.[36]

MICROPERIMETRY

Microperimetry, wherein, a fundus image can be simultaneously observed and monitored for fixation throughout the examination, may be a more accurate tool than visual field examination with conventional perimetry in patients unstable or extrafoveal fixation due to macular pathology.[37-42] It also helps to measure sensitivity at a predetermined location. Hence, fundus-driven perimetry or fundus-controlled perimetry are also other terms considered by some authors.[43-46]

Clinical Application

Age-related Macular Degeneration

Patchy distribution of localized reduction or loss of macular sensitivity associated with drusen is a characteristic microperimetric feature of age-related macular degeneration (AMD).[47,48] Microperimetry parameters when analyzed along with OCT findings show a reduction in sensitivity to correspond with drusen seen as hyper-reflective foci,[49] elevation of RPE and outer retinal thinning[50] on OCT (Fig. 3.14).

In late-stage AMD, choroidal neovascularization, hemorrhage, subretinal tissue and retinal pigment epithelium elevation[51] and disruption of the photoreceptor inner segment to outer segment border (also known as the inner segment ellipsoid zone) is associated with reduced sensitivity.[52] Neovascular complex are seen as absolute defects on field testing with loss of photoreceptor integrity on OCT.[53] When monitoring is done over a period of 2 years, a loss of 1.26 dB per year in mean sensitivity (MP-1) occurs in individuals with geographic atrophy.[54] Similarly, in atrophic macular disease, a loss of 0.88 dB over 1 year occurs in the visual field extending to an eccentricity of 5° with the MP-1.[55] Microperimetry has also been used in various clinical trials as an outcome measure to study various interventions.[56-60]

Retinitis Pigmentosa

Photoreceptor and retinal pigment epithelium cell death leads to progressive visual loss in retinitis pigmentosa (RP).[61] It is typically characterized by concentric, arcuate or mid-peripheral ring visual field loss.[62] With short-wavelength fundus autofluorescence, rings of hyperautofluorescence appear around the fovea in approximately 60% of individuals.[63] Sensitivity in RP is near normal in parafoveal regions.[46] Specifically, in the central 4° around the fovea, sensitivity is normal in individuals who have no evidence of macular change with OCT.[64] A typical relationship is seen between microperimetry findings and the retinal morphology on short-wavelength fundus autofluorescence.[65-67] The sensitivity is relatively preserved inside the hyperautofluorescent ring.[75] Moderately reduced sensitivity is seen across the region of hyperautofluorescence, along with a marked decrease in sensitivity outside the outer border of the ring.[65,66]

Stargardt's disease is a recessively inherited macular dystrophy with loss of central vision. It is characterized by atrophic macular lesions and yellow flecks at the posterior pole and/or mid-periphery.[68] Microperimetry can be used as a measure of macular function in individuals with Stargardt's disease.[46,69-71] Sensitivity is significantly reduced,[46,71] and declines progressively over time at a rate of 1.19 dB/year, using the MP-1 microperimeter.[71] When using red stimuli upon a red background, the sensitivity in the parafoveal area (6–10° eccentricity) is reduced but relatively high in the peripapillary area.[46] This corresponds with photoreceptor layer thickness abnormalities present in the macular area, which are absent in the peripapillary area.[69]

Diabetic Retinopathy

There is a considerable role of microperimetry in diabetic retinopathy, especially diabetic macular edema (DME).[72-80] These individuals have a marked loss of sensitivity in the macular region.[73] A positive correlation has been seen between visual acuity, sensitivity at the fovea[72] and mean sensitivity in the macular area.[75,77] Even diabetic patients without retinopathy have significantly decreased sensitivity compared to controls.[81]

There is increasing evidence in support of the use of microperimetry as a clinical functional measure, as well as in research. However, it is important to interpret the results on these electophyiological tests in association with thorough clinical evaluation and correlation.

REFERENCES

1. Hanitzsch R. Cornea-Negative and Cornea-Positive Slow Components of the ERG and Light-induced Extracellular Potassium Changes. In: Haschke W, Speckmann EJ, Roitbak AI (Eds). Slow Potential Changes in the Brain. Brain Dynamics. Birkhäuser, Boston, MA: Springer; 1993. pp. 203-18.
2. Karpe G. A routine method of clinical electroretinography. Acta Ophthalmology Suppl. 1962;(Suppl 70):15-31.
3. Brown KT. The electroretinogram: its components and their origins. UCLA Forum Med Sci. 1969;8:319-78.
4. Yonemura D, Tsuzuki K, Aoki T. Clinical Importance of the Oscillatory Potential in the Human ERG. Acta Ophthalmology Suppl. 1962;(Suppl 70):115-23.
5. Pearlman JT. The C-Wave of the Human ERG: Its intensity dependence and pupillociliary origin. Arch Ophthalmology. 1962; 68(6): 823-30.
6. Marmor MF, Zrenner E. Standard for clinical electroretinography (1999 update). International Society for Clinical Electrophysiology of Vision. Doc Ophthalmology. 1998-1999;97(2):143-56.
7. Marmor MF, Holder GE, Seeliger MW, et al. Standard for clinical electroretinography (2004 update). International Society for Clinical Electrophysiology of Vision. Doc Ophthalmology. 2004;108(2):107-14.
8. Bush RA, Sieving PA. A proximal retinal component in the primate photopic ERG a-wave. Invest Ophthalmology Vis Sci. 1994;35(2): 635-45.
9. Bush RA, Sieving PA. Inner retinal contributions to the primate photopic fast flicker electroretinogram. J Opt Soc Am A Opt Image Sci Vis. 1996;13(3):557-65.
10. Mohan Ram LS, Jalali S, Faheemuddin S, et al. Safety and efficacy evaluation of a new ERG electrode (the LVP electrode) part II. Flash ERG pilot study. Doc Ophthalmology. 2003;107(2):179-83.
11. Arden GB, Hogg CR, Holder GE. Gold foil electrodes: a two-center study of electrode reliability. Doc Ophthalmology. 1994;86(3): 275-84.
12. Hawlina M, Kosec B. New noncorneal HK-loop electrode for clinical electroretinography. Doc Ophthalmology. 1992;81(2): 253-9.
13. Al Oreany AA, Al Hadlaq A, Schatz P. Congenital stationary night blindness with hypoplastic discs, negative electroretinogram and thinning of the inner nuclear layer. Graefes Arch Clin Exp Ophthalmology. 2016;254(10):1951-6.
14. Neriyanuri S, Dhandayuthapani S, Arunachalam JP, et al. Phenotypic characterization of X-linked retinoschisis: Clinical, electroretinography, and optical coherence tomography variables. Indian J Ophthalmology. 2016;64(7):513-7.
15. Herrador-Montiel Á, Sánchez-Vicente JL, Arias-Alcalá M. Clinical features of Goldmann-Favre vitreoretinal degeneration. Arch Soc Esp Oftalmol. 2012;87(8):260-2.
16. Karpe G. The electroretinogram in siderosis bulbi. Bibl Ophthalmology. 1957;(48):182-90.
17. Nair AA, Marmor MF. ERG and other discriminators between advanced hydroxychloroquine retinopathy and retinitis pigmentosa. Doc Ophthalmology. 2017;134(3):175-83.
18. Holder GE, Brigell MG, Hawlina M, et al. ISCEV standard for clinical pattern electroretinography—2007 update. Doc Ophthalmology. 2007;114(3):111-6.
19. Berninger TA, Arden GB. The pattern electroretinogram. Eye (Lond) 1988;(2 Suppl):S257-83.
20. Cvenkel B, Sustar M, Perovšek D. Ganglion cell loss in early glaucoma, as assessed by photopic negative response, pattern electroretinogram, and spectral-domain optical coherence tomography. Doc Ophthalmology. 2017;135(1):17-28.
21. Sutter EE, Tran D. The field topography of ERG components in man--I. The photopic luminance response. Vision Res. 1992;32(3): 433-46.

22. Hood DC, Bach M, Brigell M, et al. ISCEV standard for clinical multifocal electroretinography (mfERG) (2011 edition). Doc Ophthalmology. 2012;124(1):1-13.

23. Sutter E. The interpretation of multifocal binary kernels. Doc Ophthalmology. 2000;100(2-3):49-75.

24. Rodrigues AR, Filho Mda S, Silveira LC, et al. Spatial distributions of on- and off-responses determined with the multifocal ERG. Doc Ophthalmology. 2010;120(2):145-58.

25. Chan HH, Ng YF, Chu PH. Applications of the multifocal electro-retinogram in the detection of glaucoma. Clin Exp Optom. 2011; 94(3):247-58.

26. Cheng JYC, Luu CD, Yeo IY, et al. The outer and inner retinal function in patients with multiple evanescent white dot syndrome. Clin Experiment Ophthalmology. 2009;37(5):478-84.

27. Adam MK, Covert DJ, Stepien KE, et al. Quantitative assessment of the 103-hexagon multifocal electroretinogram in detection of hydroxychloroquine retinal toxicity. Br J Ophthalmology. 2012;96(5):723-9.

28. Lung JC, Swann PG, Chan HH. The Multifocal On- and Off-Responses in the Human Diabetic Retina. PloS One. 2016;11(5):e0155071.

29. Maia-Lopes S, Silva ED, Silva MF, et al. Evidence of widespread retinal dysfunction in patients with stargardt disease and morphologically unaffected carrier relatives. Invest Ophthalmology Vis Sci. 2008;49(3):1191-9.

30. Todorova MG, Türksever C, Schötzau A, et al. Metabolic and functional changes in retinitis pigmentosa: comparing retinal vessel oximetry to full-field electroretinography, electrooculography and multifocal electroretinography. Acta Ophthalmology. 2016;94(3): e231-41.

31. Constable PA, Bach M, Frishman LJ, et al. International Society for Clinical Electrophysiology of Vision. ISCEV Standard for clinical electro-oculography (2017 update). Doc Ophthalmology. 2017;134(1):1-9.

32. Arden GB, Constable PA. The electro-oculogram. Prog Retin Eye Res. 2006;25(2):207-48.

33. Odom JV, Bach M, Brigell M, et al. ISCEV standard for clinical visual evoked potentials: (2016 update). Doc Ophthalmology. 2016;133(1):1-9.

34. Ridder WH. Methods of visual acuity determination with the spatial frequency sweep visual evoked potential. Doc Ophthalmology. 2004;109(3):239-47.

35. Hamilton R, Bradnam MS, Dutton GN, et al. Sensitivity and specificity of the step VEP in suspected functional visual acuity loss. Doc Ophthalmology. 2013;126(2):99-104.

36. Kreegipuu K, Allik J. Detection of motion onset and offset: reaction time and visual evoked potential analysis. Psychol Res. 2007;71(6):703-8.

37. Inatomi A. A simple fundus perimetry with fundus camera. Doc Ophthalmology Proc Ser. 1979;19:359-62.

38. Kani K, Eno N, Abe K, et al. Perimetry under television ophthalmoscopy. Doc Ophthalmology Proc Ser. 1977;14:231-6.

39. Kani K, Ogita Y. Fundus controlled perimetry. Doc Ophthalmology Proc Ser. 1979;19:341-50.

40. Timberlake GT, Mainster MA, Webb RH, et al. Retinal localization of scotomata by scanning laser ophthalmoscopy. Invest Ophthalmology Vis Sci. 1982;22(1):91-7.

41. Sunness JS, Schuchard RA, Shen NM, et al. Landmark-driven fundus perimetry using the scanning laser ophthalmoscope. Invest Ophthalmology Vis Sci. 1995;36(9):1863-74.

42. Rohrschneider K, Fendrich T, Becker M, et al. Static fundus perimetry using the scanning laser ophthalmoscope with an automated threshold strategy. Graefes Arch Clin Exp Ophthalmology. 1995;233(12):743-9.

43. Acton JH, Smith RT, Greenberg JP, et al. Comparison between MP-1 and Humphrey visual field defects in glaucoma and retinitis pigmentosa. Optom Vis Sci. 2012;89(7):1050-8.

44. Acton JH, Bartlett NS, Greenstein VC. Comparing the Nidek MP-1 and Humphrey Field Analyzer in normal subjects. Optom Vis Sci. 2011;88(11):1288-97.

45. Seiple W, Lima VC, Rosen RB, et al. The physics and psychophysics of microperimetry. Optom Vis Sci. 2012;89(8):1182-91.

46. Cideciyan AV, Swider M, Aleman TS, et al. Macular function in macular degenerations: repeatability of microperimetry as a potential outcome measure for ABCA4-associated retinopathy trials. Invest Ophthalmology Vis Sci. 2012;53(2):841-52.

47. Midena E, Vujosevic S, Convento E, et al. Microperimetry and fundus autofluorescence in patients with early age related macular degeneration. Br J Ophthalmology. 2007;91(11):1499-503.

48. Parisi V, Perillo L, Tedeschi M, et al. Macular function in eyes with early age-related macular degeneration with or without contralateral late age related macular degeneration. Retina. 2007;27(7):879-90.

49. Wu Z, Ayton LN, Luu CD, et al. Relationship between retinal microstructures on optical coherence tomography and microperimetry in age related macular degeneration. Ophthalmology. 2014;121(7):1445-52.

50. Acton JH, Smith RT, Hood DC, et al. The relationship between retinal layer thickness and the visual field in early age-related macular degeneration Invest Ophthalmology Vis Sci. 2012;53(12):7618-24.

51. Hautamaki A, Oikkonen J, Onkamo P, et al. Correlation between components of newly diagnosed exudative age-related macular degeneration lesion and focal retinal sensitivity. Acta Ophthalmology. 2014;92(1):51-8.

52. Landa G, Su E, Garcia PM, et al. Inner segment outer segment junctional layer integrity and corresponding retinal sensitivity in dry and wet forms of age-related macular degeneration. Retina. 2011;31(2):364-70.

53. Sulzbacher F, Kiss C, Kaider A, et al. Correlation of SD-OCT features and retinal sensitivity in neovascular age-related macular degeneration. Invest Ophthalmology Vis Sci. 2012;53(10):6448-55.

54. Meleth AD, Mettu P, Agron E, et al. Changes in retinal sensitivity in geographic atrophy progression as measured by microperimetry. Invest Ophthalmology Vis Sci. 2011;52(2):1119-26.

55. Chen FK, Patel PJ, Webster AR, et al. Nidek MP1 is able to detect subtle decline in function in inherited and age-related atrophic macular disease with stable visual acuity. Retina. 2011;3192: 371-9.

56. Parravano M, Oddone F, Tedeschi M, et al. Retinal functional changes measured by microperimetry in neovascular age-related macular degeneration treated with ranibizumab: 24-month results. Retina. 2010;30(7):1017-24.

57. Parravano M, Parisi V, Ziccardi L, et al. Single-session photodynamic therapy combined with intravitreal ranibizumab for neovascular age-related macular degeneration: a comprehensive functional retinal assessment. Doc Ophthalmology. 2013;127(3):217-25.

58. Cho HJ, Kim CG. Yoo SJ. Retinal functional changes measured by microperimetry in neovascular age-related macular degeneration treated with ranibizumab. Am J Ophthalmology. 2013;155(1):118-26.

59. Ozdemir H, Karacorlu M, Senturk F, et al. Microperimetric changes after intravitreal bevacizumab injection for exudative age-related macular degeneration. Acta Ophthalmology. 2012;90(1):71-5.

60. Munk MR, Kiss C, Huf W, et al. One year follow-up of functional recovery in neovascular AMD during monthly anti-VEGF treatment. Am J Ophthalmology. 2013;156(4):633-43.

61. Kolb H, Gouras P. Electron microscopic observations of human retinitis pigmentosa, dominantly inherited. Invest Ophthalmology. 1974;13(7):487-98.
62. Grover S, Fishman GA, Brown J. Patterns of visual field progression in patients with retinitis pigmentosa. Ophthalmology. 1998;105(6):1069-75.
63. Murakami T, Akimoto M, Ooto S, et al. Association between abnormal autofluorescence and photoreceptor disorganization in retinitis pigmentosa. Am J Ophthalmology. 2008;145(4):687-94.
64. Lupo S, Grenga PL, Vingolo EM. Fourier-domain optical coherence tomography and microperimetry findings in retinitis pigmentosa. Am J Ophthalmology. 2011;151(1):106-11.
65. Greenstein VC, Duncker T, Holopigian K, et al. Structural and functional changes associated with normal and abnormal fundus autofluorescence in patients with retinitis pigmentosa. Retina. 2012;32(2):349-57.
66. Popovic P, Jarc-Vidmar M, Hawlina M. Abnormal fundus auto-fluorescence in relation to retinal function in patients with retinitis pigmentosa. Graefes Arch Clin Exp Ophthalmology. 2005;243(10):1018-27.
67. Wakabayashi T, Sawa M, Gomi F, et al. Correlation of fundus autofluorescence with photoreceptor morphology and functional changes in eyes with retinitis pigmentosa. Acta Ophthalmology. 2010;88(5):e177-183.
68. Walia S, Fishman GA. Natural history of phenotypic changes in Stargardt macular dystrophy. Ophthalmic Genet. 2009;30(2):63-8.
69. Burke TR, Rhee DW, Smith RT, et al. Quantification of peripapillary sparing and macular involvement in Stargardt disease (STGD1). Invest Ophthalmology Vis Sci. 2011;52(11):8006-15.
70. Testa F, Rossi S, Sodi A, et al. Correlation between photoreceptor layer integrity and visual function in patients with Stargardt disease: implications for gene therapy. Invest Ophthalmology Vis Sci. 2012;53(8):4409-15.
71. Testa F, Melillo P, Di Iorio V, et al. Macular function and morphologic features in juvenile stargardt disease: longitudinal study. Ophthalmology. 2014;121(12):2399-405.
72. Soliman W, Hasler P, Sander B, et al. Local retinal sensitivity in relation to specific retinopathy lesions in diabetic macular oedema. Acta Ophthalmology. 2010;90(3):248-53.
73. Deak GG, Bolz M, Ritter M, et al. A systematic correlation between morphology and functional alterations in diabetic macular edema. Invest Ophthalmology Vis Sci. 2010;51(12):6710-4.
74. Vujosevic S, Casciano M, Pilotto E, et al. Diabetic macular edema: fundus autofluorescence and functional correlations. Invest Ophthalmology Vis Sci. 2011;52(1):442-8.
75. Vujosevic S, Midena E, Pilotto E, et al. Diabetic macular edema: correlation between microperimetry and optical coherence tomography findings. Invest Ophthalmology Vis Sci. 2006;47(7):3044-51.
76. Vujosevic S, Pilotto E, Bottega E, et al. Retinal fixation impairment in diabetic macular edema. Retina. 2008;28(10):1443-50.
77. Okada K, Yamamoto S, Mizunoya S, et al. Correlation of retinal sensitivity measured with fundus-related microperimetry to visual acuity and retinal thickness in eyes with diabetic macular edema. Eye (Lond). 2006;20(7):805-9.
78. Carpineto P, Ciancaglini M, Di Antonio L, et al. Fundus microperimetry patterns of fixation in type 2 diabetic patients with diffuse macular edema. Retina. 2007;27(1):21-9.
79. Pearce E, Sivaprasad S, Chong NV. Factors affecting reading speed in patients with diabetic macular edema treated with laser photocoagulation. PLoS One. 2014;9(9):e105696.
80. Vujosevic S, Pucci P, Daniele AR, et al. Extent of diabetic macular edema by scanning laser ophthalmoscope in the retromode and its functional correlations. Retina. 2014;34(12):2416-22.
81. Verma A, Rani PK, Raman R, et al. Is neuronal dysfunction an early sign of diabetic retinopathy? Microperimetry and spectral domain optical coherence tomography (SD-OCT) study in individuals with diabetes, but no diabetic retinopathy. Eye (Lond). 2009;23:1824-30.

Chapter 4

Diagnostic Ophthalmic Ultrasonography

Raghav Ravani, Yogita Gupta, Meghal Gagrani, Atul Kumar

INTRODUCTION AND HISTORY

Ultrasonography (USG) as a noninvasive imaging tool to obtain images has applications in medical science to aid in diagnosis and management of various pathologies. USG is based on the piezoelectric effect to produce acoustic waves more than 20 kHz. It is based on pulse-echo technique. Rapidly repeating bursts of ultrasonic energy are beamed into the ocular and orbital tissues, which are reflected back, depending upon the tissue reflectivity and are then detected, amplified, and converted to electronic display with the help of transducer.

Mundt and Hughes first used the USG as a diagnostic tool in the field of ophthalmology in 1956.[1] First cross-sectional (2D) scan was developed by Baum and Greenwood.[2] Bronson introduced contact B scan and the standardization of A scan[3] and combination of A scan instrument with contact B scan leading to modern day standardized echography was carried out by Ossoinig.[4,5] Coleman developed first ophthalmic 3D scan.[6] Recently, real-time digital 2D B-scan video recording and Doppler USG have become a part of the present day's standardized echography.[7-10]

Ophthalmic USG includes ocular USG and orbital sonography. This chapter deals with ocular USG in reference to retina.

PHYSICS OF THE EQUIPMENT

The ultrasonic transducer is the heart of the USG apparatus. It produces and transmits the sound waves to the ocular tissues. The reflected waves are collected, and converted into electric signal by the transducer depending upon the reflectivity of the tissue. It is the frequency of the transducer that determines the depth of penetrance and resolution of the image. As the frequency increases the resolution of image and thus of the small defects or details in the eye increases, but the penetration decreases. Thus only limited frequencies can be used clinically. The posterior segment scan uses 8–10 MHz frequency while the anterior segment ultrasound biomicroscopy (UBM) with improved resolution uses frequency of 50–100 MHz.[11]

ULTRASOUND IMAGING

Examination Modes

Various examination modes in ophthalmic USG are:
- A scan: Amplitude modulation scan
- B scan: Brightness modulation scan
- Vector A scan
- Doppler USG
- UBM.

A scan: Biometry for axial length and corneal thickness measurement can be done using A scan. It is called as Time-Amplitude scan. The probe used in A scan has probe frequency of around 8 MHz, which emits parallel and nonfocused ultrasound beam with beam width of 5 mm at highest dB and 0.5 mm width at lowest dB. The machine uses mathematical and physics formulae to calculate the speed of sound as it passes through different ocular tissues. This can then be used to measure distance within ocular structures and thus axial length (Fig. 4.1).

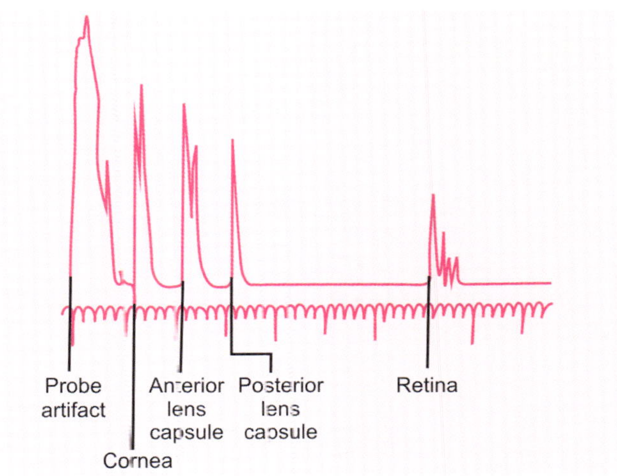

Fig. 4.1: An ophthalmic USG image in A-scan mode showing different tissue spikes.

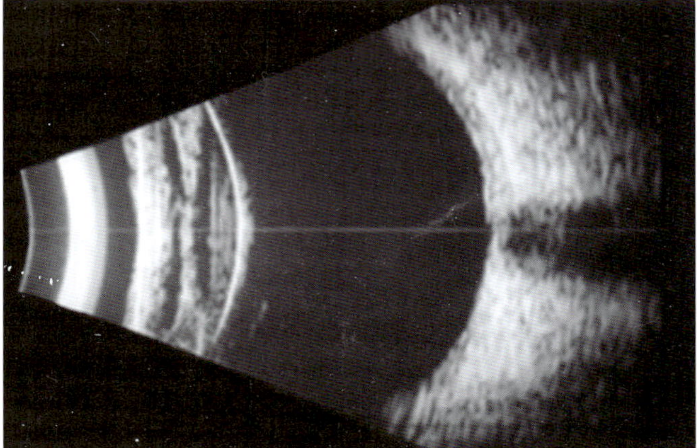

Fig. 4.2: Representative image of a normal B scan of eye.

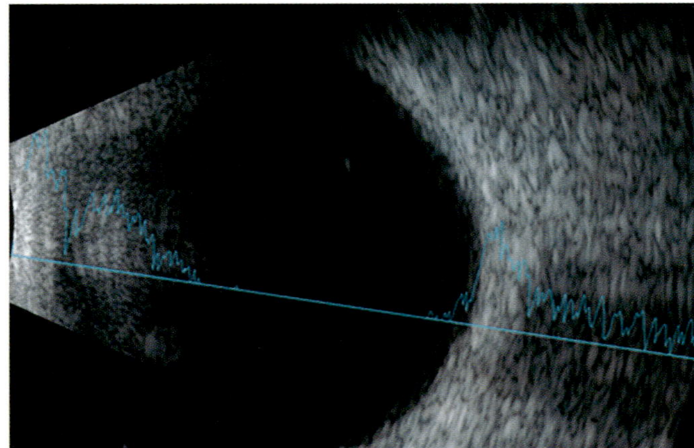

Fig. 4.3: Representative image of vector A scan.

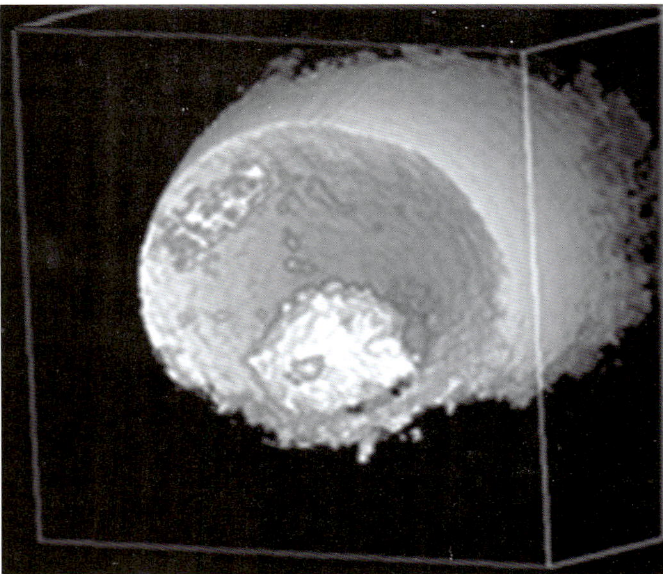

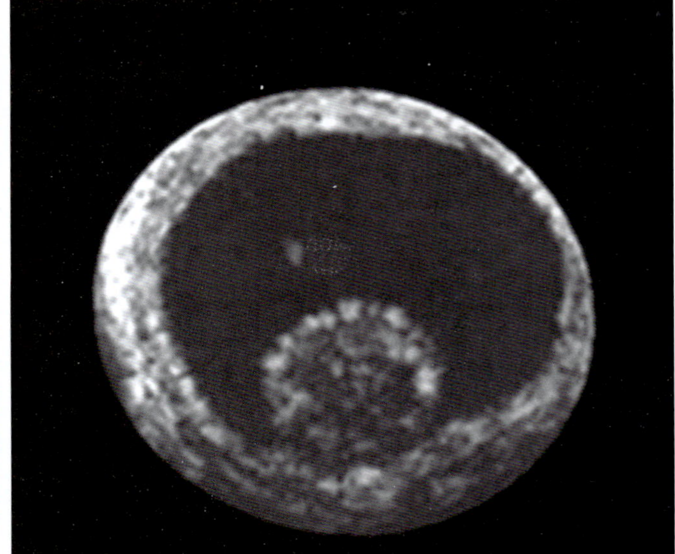

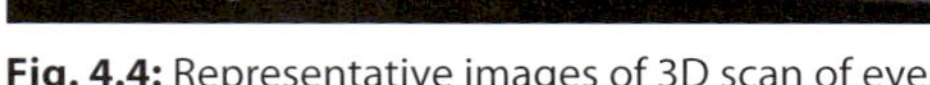

Fig. 4.4: Representative images of 3D scan of eye.

B scan: It is used for diagnostic purpose and for echo structure assessment. It is called as brightness mode 2D scan (Fig. 4.2).

The probe used in B scan is thicker with a marker on the sleeve close to the transducer tip which serves as a guide for imaging orientation purposes such that the marker on the probe corresponds to the top of the scan plane. The transducer uses probe frequency of around 10 MHz, which emits focused sound waves.

Vector A scan: It is a combination of both A and B scans (Fig. 4.3).

Doppler USG: It is important in vascular lesions and is obtained by using frequency shifts from acoustic reflections to measure movement within a tissue and flow within vessels. High flow and low flow states can be differentiated by desig-nating false color codes to the images based on ultrasonic fre-quency of each.

Ultrasound biomicroscopy (UBM): This modality uses high-frequency echograms thus providing better resolution of anterior structures of the eye, especially the cornea, lens, iris and ciliary body. The probe used in UBM has an exposed transducer that is dipped in the cup of coupling fluid placed on the cornea for procuring high-resolution images. The probe is thicker than the B-scan probe with exposed tip with a marker for imaging orientation purposes such that marker on the probe always corresponds to the left side of a UBM scan.

Three-dimensional scan: Unlike some subspecialties, the use of 3D ultrasound in ophthalmology is limited. 3D ultrasonic images of the eye can be reconstructed from a series of scan planes[7-10] (Fig. 4.4).

Examination Technique

The detailed imaging of the eye involves three views as per the probe positioning: axial, transverse, and longitudinal.

Axial View

- *Horizontal axial view*: By placing the probe at the center of the cornea with marker positioned toward the nasal side (Fig. 4.5), this view allows simultaneous imaging of the lens, optic nerve and the macula with nasal side oriented at top of the scan.
- *Vertical axial view*: By placing the probe at the center of the cornea and marker toward the superior aspect (Fig. 4.5), this view allows simultaneous imaging of lens and the optic nerve.

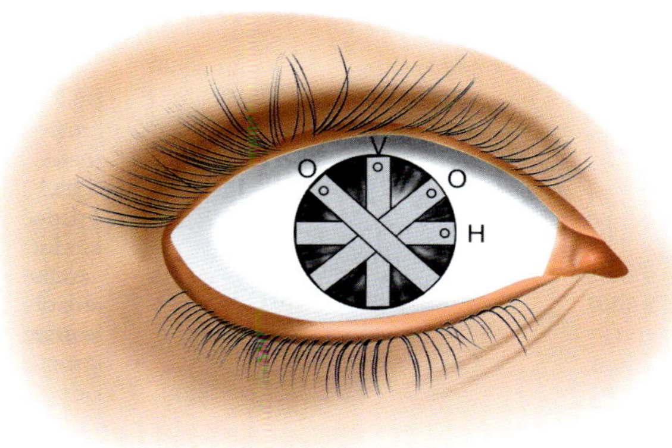

Fig. 4.5: Schematic diagram showing the technique for axial scan.

- *Oblique axial view*: This scan is obtained by placing the probe at center of cornea and marker toward the superior aspect and rotating the probe 45° to the right or the left (Fig. 4.5).

Transverse View

Transverse view provides lateral sweep of one quadrant of the fundus (Fig. 4.6A).

- *Horizontal transverse view*: The tip of the probe is placed on the limbus pointing either superiorly or inferiorly with marker positioned at the nasal side of the eye to image the superior or inferior fundus, respectively such that the nasal side is oriented at the top (Fig. 4.6B).
- *Vertical transverse view*: The tip of the probe is placed on the nasal limbus with probe pointing toward the opposite side and marker positioned on the superior side to view the temporal fundus such that the superior side is oriented at top of the scan (Fig. 4.6B). Similarly changing the position of the probe to the temporal limbus can image the nasal fundus.

Longitudinal View

Longitudinal view provides an anteroposterior scan of a specific meridian of the fundus (Fig. 4.7A).

The longitudinal scans are described as clock hours according to the placement of the probe (Fig. 4.7B). The probe is place on the limbus pointing to the opposite direction with marker directed toward the limbus such that the top of the scan is the anterior peripheral side, while the bottom is the posterior side (close to the optic nerve). To obtain a more peripheral view of a particular meridian, the probe can be shifted away from the limbus.

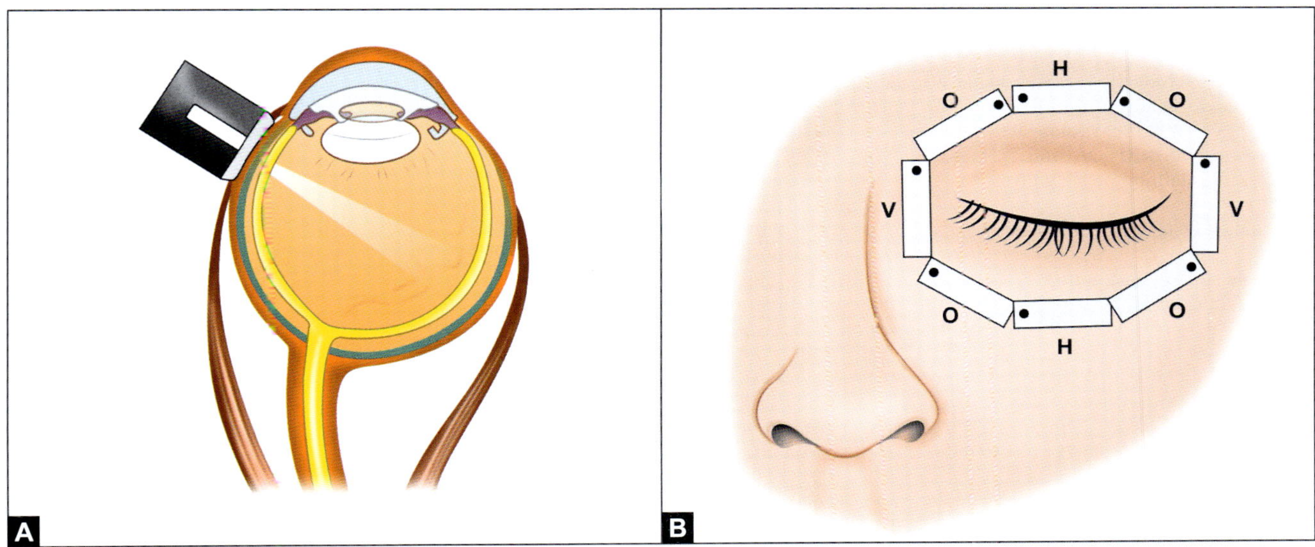

Figs. 4.6 A and B: (A) Schematic diagram showing the lateral sweep on one quadrant of fundus in transverse scan; (B) Schematic diagram showing technique of probe placement for acquiring transverse scan.

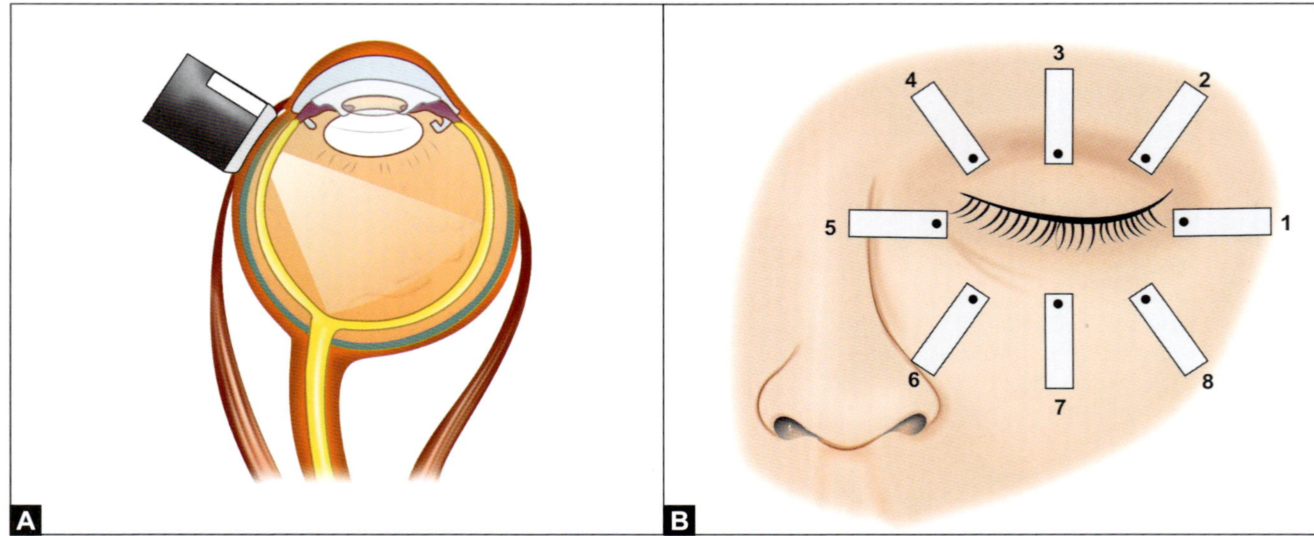

Figs. 4.7A and B: (A) Schematic diagram of longitudinal scan; (B) Schematic diagram showing technique of probe placement for acquiring longitudinal scan.

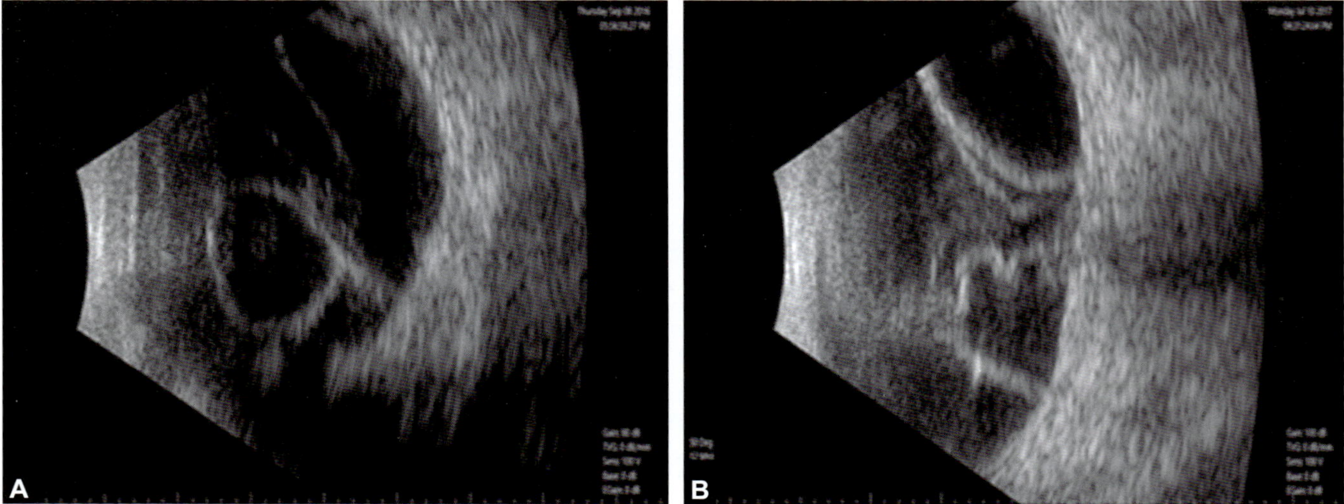

Figs. 4.8A and B: (A) Old retinal detachment (RD) with intraretinal cyst on B-scan; (B) RD with large choroidal detachment.

Ultrasound in Ocular Conditions

Retinal Detachment

Rhegmatogenous retinal detachment on B scan appears as membrane like echogenicity which is continuous, can be traced till the periphery associated with high amplitude reflectivity (80–100%) on vector A scan. The membrane is attached to the disc with a U or V configuration and has limited after-movements on dynamic B scan with clear space underneath suggestive of clear sub-retinal fluid.

Long-standing retinal detachment may show intraretinal cysts and echo dots underneath the membrane suggestive of thick SRF (Figs. 4.8A and B).

Tractional retinal detachment on B scan shows adherence of posterior vitreous at the apex of the tent-like configuration of the localized retinal detachment with limited or no after-movements that does not extend to the ora serrata (Figs. 4.9 and 4.10).

Retinopathy of Prematurity

Ultrasonography proves to be helpful tool in patients with retinopathy of prematurity (ROP), especially in patients with media haze, advanced stages of ROP with tractional retinal detachments from extensive fibrovascular tissue, e.g. stage 5 ROP. The ultrasound helps to define the configuration of the detachment and may show peripheral retinal loops, ridge or cholesterol debris in the subretinal space.

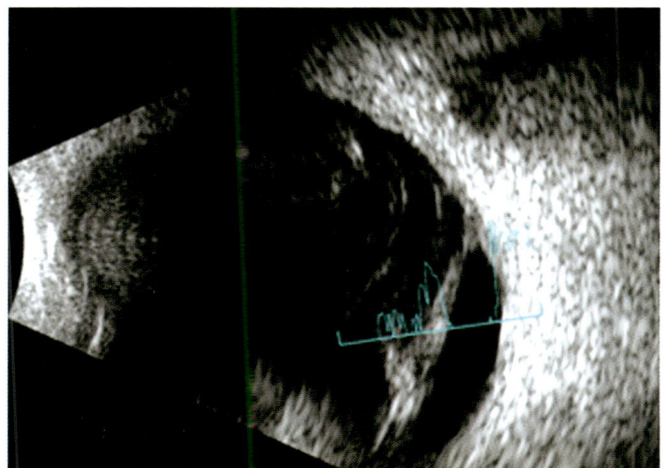

Fig. 4.9: Tractional retinal detachment with tent-like configuration and showing high reflectivity.

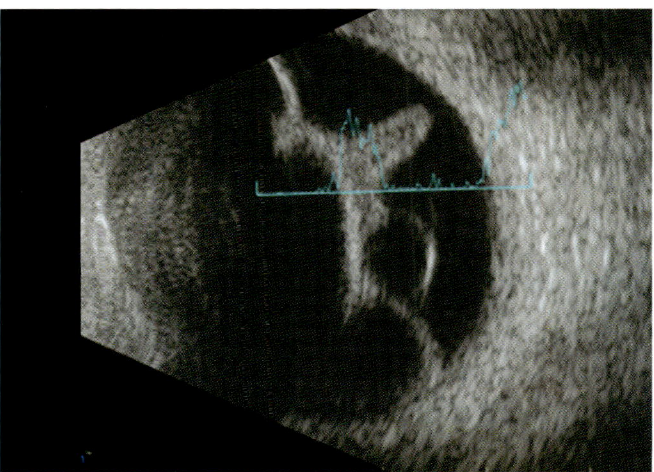

Fig. 4.10: B scan showing a classical diabetic table-top tractional retinal detachment with vector A scan showing high reflectivity spike from the detached retina.

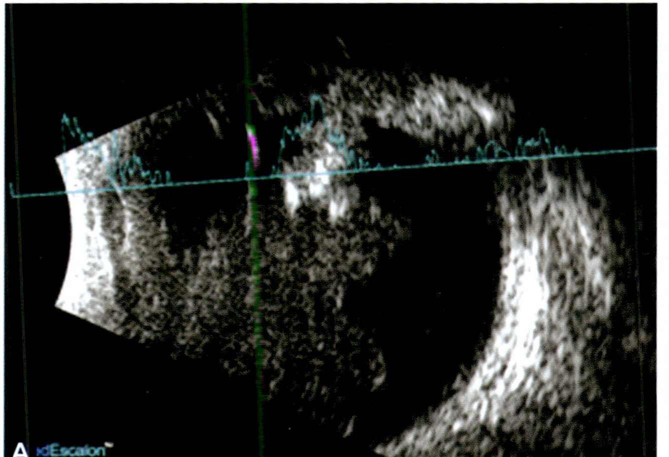

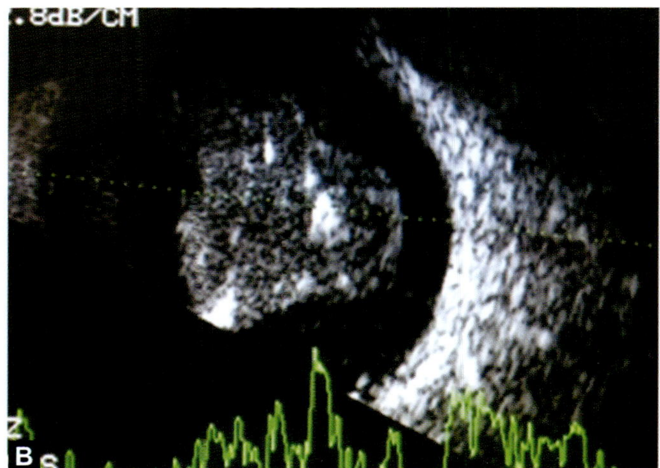

Figs. 4.11A and B: B scans showing presence of mass lesion with irregular configuration with intralesional calcification in both scans. There are classically high-reflectivity spikes producing the *"VW pattern"*, in the latter scan.

Retinoblastoma

It is the most common intraocular tumor of childhood and forms an important differential diagnosis in a child with leukocoria. Echographically, retinoblastoma (RB) is characterized by presence of mass lesion with irregular configuration with presence of areas of high reflectivity with 100% amplitude spike on A scan which persists till low gain with acoustic shadowing suggestive of intralesional calcification (Figs. 4.11A and B).

Usually the A scan shows moderate internal reflectivity, but presence of necrosis and calcification gives highly reflective irregular spikes with moderate to high sound attenuation. The globe may be normal to enlarged in size. Echography may show presence of concomitant retinal detachment in the exophytic variety of RB. Occasionally, echography may show extraocular extension of the tumor, which is of great prognostic and therapeutic importance. Table 4.1 shows the list of ocular conditions with intraocular calcification.

Vitreous Hemorrhage or Exudates

Vitreous cavity may be filled with numerous dot-like echoes with mild-to-moderate amplitude spike on standardized echography (vector scan) suggestive of vitreous hemorrhage or exudates (Fig. 4.12A).

Breakthrough Vitreous Hemorrhage

Subretinal hemorrhage commonly occurs with choroidal neovascular membranes in age-related macular degeneration. Subretinal bleed may dissect through the macula and causes dense premacular hemorrhage (Fig. 4.12B).

Table 4.1: Ocular conditions with intraocular calcification.

Retinal lesions	• Retinoblastoma • Astrocytic hamartoma • Tuberous sclerosis • Coats disease • PHPV/PFV • RPE metaplasia • Toxoplasmosis (chorioretinitis)
Choroidal lesions	• Choroidal osteoma • Choroidal hemangiomas (calcify occasionally)
Miscellaneous	• Optic nerve head drusen • Metastatic calcification, e.g. hyperparathyroidism, pseudo-hypoparathyroidism, and renal tubular acidosis • Dystrophic calcification, e.g. phthisis bulbi

PHPV: Persistent hyperplastic primary vitreous; PFV: Persistent fetal vasculature; RPE: Retinal pigment epithelium

Subhyaloid Hemorrhage

It is seen as either organized mass-like echoes under membrane-like vitreous reflection or as diffuse point-like echoes under mild amplitude membrane-like echo with good after-movements of posterior hyaloid membrane (Fig. 4.13).

Asteroid Hyalosis

It is degenerative vitreous condition, usually asymptomatic in which calcium-pyrophosphate globules collect within the vitreous gel. These acts as reflectors and provide distinctive high amplitude echoes floating in the vitreous that are mobile and follow the dynamic vitreous movements. There is usually a clear space visible between particles and posterior globe wall (Fig. 4.14).

Posterior Vitreous Detachment

It is a degenerative process of the vitreous resulting in separation of posterior hyaloid layer from the internal limiting membrane of the retina. Ultrasonographically, posterior vitreous

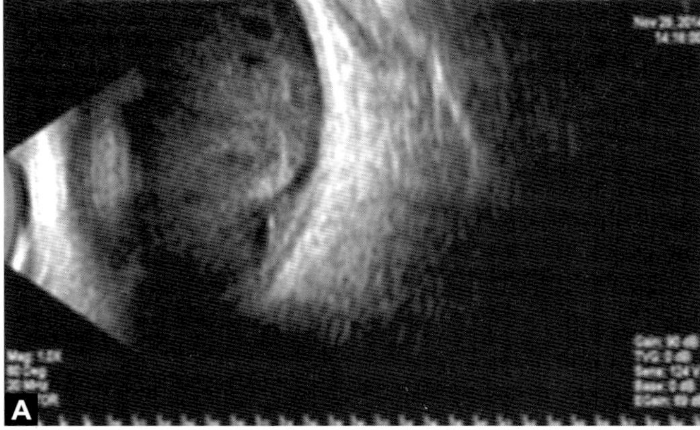
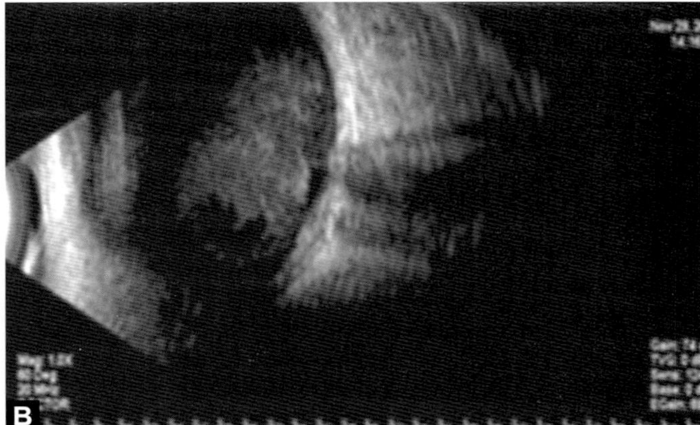

Figs. 4.12A and B: (A) B-scan ultrasonography showing numerous subretinal dot-like echoes suggestive of subretinal blood with breakthrough vitreous hemorrhage; (B) B-scan ultrasonography showing dense premacular hemorrhage.

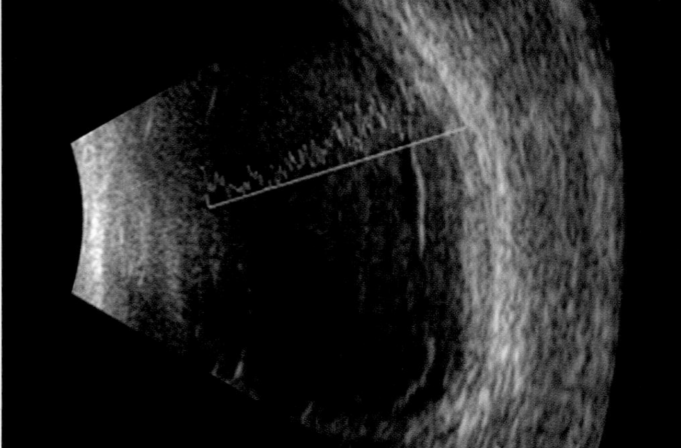

Fig. 4.13: Vector scanning shows retrohyaloid bleed with associated vitreous hemorrhage.

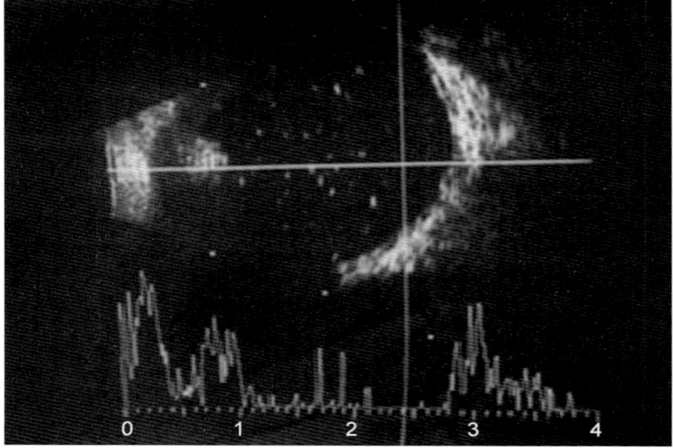

Fig. 4.14: B-scan of a patient with asteroid hyalosis.

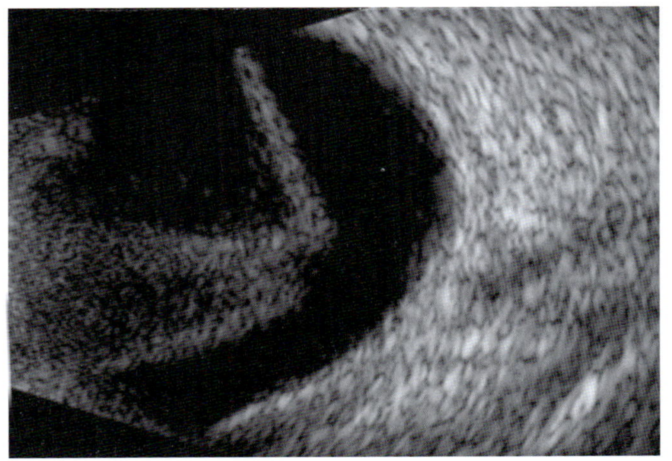

Fig. 4.15: Vitreous hemorrhage with complete posterior vitreous detachment.

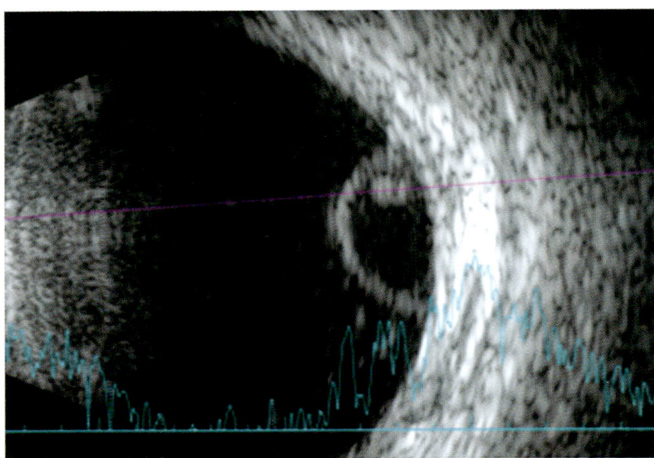

Fig. 4.16: B-scan ultrasound of a patient with intraocular cysticercosis.

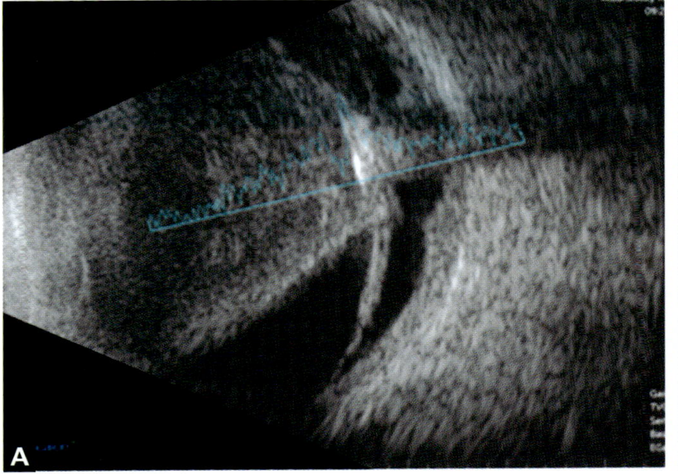

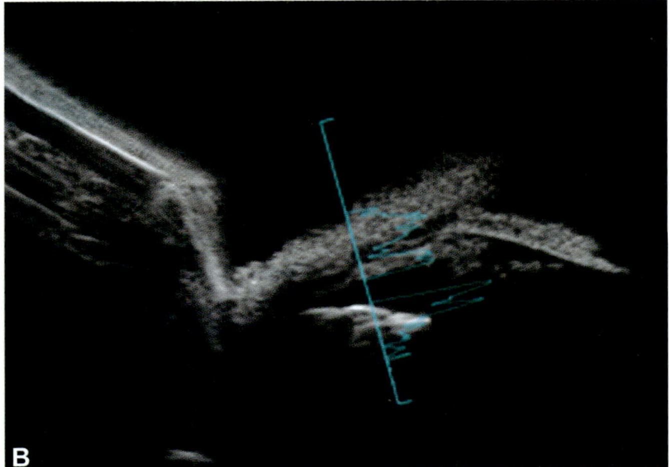

Figs. 4.17A and B: (A) An impacted high-echo foreign body in the region of the optic nerve; (B) Vector scan shows an anteriorly placed foreign body showing high-reflectivity spike (overloaded spike, over 100% reflectivity).

detachment appears as a thin, smooth membrane-like echogenicity with variable attachment to retina and optic disc with clear subvitreal space. It may be small, interrupted, peripheral or continuous with mild-to-moderate amplitude reflectivity on vector A scan with good after-movements on dynamic B scan and variable or nonpersistence till low gain (Fig. 4.15).

Intraocular Cysticercosis

Cysticercosis can present with intraocular cysts. On USG, it is seen as a sharply outlined oval cyst in vitreous cavity or subretinal space with highly reflective echo dense nodule adjacent to the cyst wall—scolex with suckers and hooklets (Fig. 4.16).

Intraocular Foreign Body

Retained intraocular foreign body (RIOFB) is commonly seen as a result of penetrating injury with projectile object.

On USG, RIOFB may be seen as hyper-reflective echogenicity with high amplitude reflectivity (100%) with acoustic shadowing and reverberation echoes behind it and A-scan spike persisting even at low gain (Figs. 4.17A and B).

Ultrasonography helps in localizing the foreign body and approximate sizing of the foreign body. Foreign bodies less than 0.2 mm in size and those in the orbit which are obscured by hemorrhages are best picked up by orbital CT scan.

Posteriorly Dislocated Intraocular Lens

This may appear as point-like echogenicity in the vitreous cavity with high amplitude spike with posterior reverberations with or without orbital shadowing (Fig. 4.18). The intraocular lens (IOL) shows gravity dependent movement and moves against the direction of eye movement.

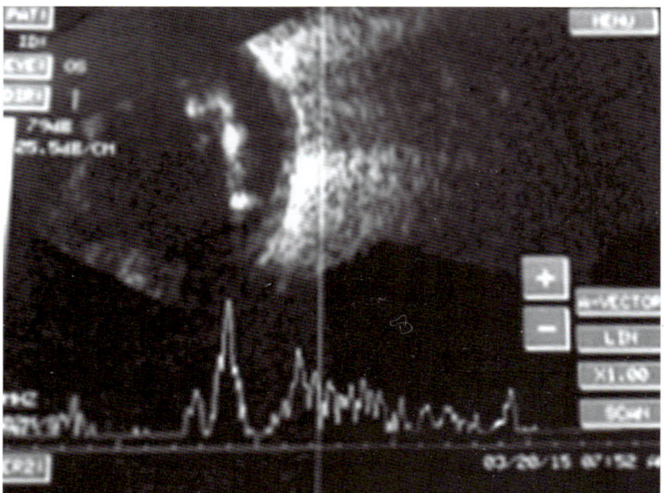

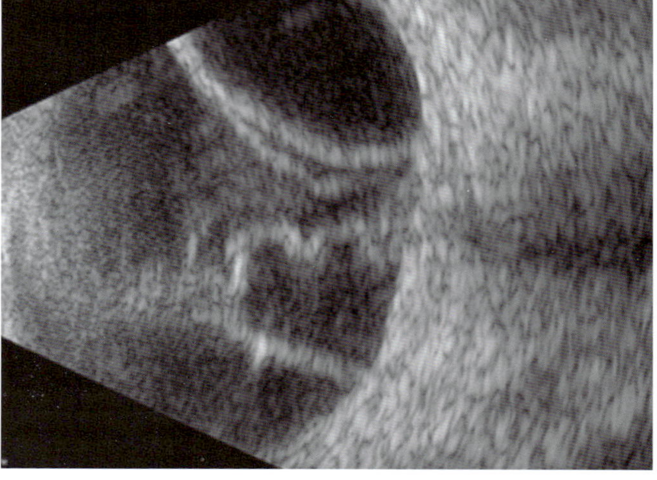

Fig. 4.18: B-scan ultrasonography of a patient with posteriorly dislocated intraocular lens showing acoustic reverberations.

Fig. 4.19: B-scan ultrasonography showing choroidal detachment with retinal detachment.

Choroidal Detachment

Choroidal detachment (CD) may be either serous or hemorrhagic. It is usually seen in the periphery and is usually localized, but may be total. Echographically, CD is characterized by smooth, thick, convex, dome-shaped and immobile elevation with limited after-movement on dynamic B scan. A scan shows steep, high amplitude (100%) spike with characteristic double-peaked spike (Fig. 4.19). Serous CD shows echolucent areas with no reflectivity beneath the choroid. In contrast, the hemorrhagic CD shows dense opacities with variable reflectivity beneath the choroid.

Choroidal Melanoma

B-scan echography shows a pathognomonic collar-button or mushroom-shaped lesion. This appearance is indicative of break in Bruch's membrane and invasion of tumor (Figs. 4.20A to C). A choroidal excavation may be seen on B scan but is not pathognomonic of malignant melanoma. This may be associated with concomitant serous retinal detachment usually extending from margins of the tumor. Scleral thickening with dilation of Tenon's space is suggestive of scleritis associated with tumor necrosis. Occasionally, calcification and extrascleral echolucent nodule behind the sclera suggestive of extrascleral spread may be noted.[12] A large angle kappa (sloping internal signals from higher to lower as the sound beam passes through the lesion) is seen on A scan (Fig. 4.20B).

Metastatic Carcinoma

Metastatic malignancies especially from the lung and breast are seen in eyes, and present with exudative retinal detachment and choroidal metastasis on USG (Fig. 4.21).

Posterior Uveitis

Echography shows diffuse vitreous echogenic opacities with mild-to-moderate amplitude spike with good after-movements. It is to be differentiated clinically from vitreous hemorrhage, which has similar echographic characteristics.

Posterior Scleritis

The characteristic of B scan echographic finding is presence of the classic T-sign, which represents thickened posterior sclera with underlying fluid collection in the Tenon's space (Fig. 4.22).

Infectious Endophthalmitis

The vitreous opacities and exudates along with anterior chamber exudates and corneal edema or opacities preclude detailed posterior segment evaluation in patients with endophthalmitis. Thus B-scan echography plays a key role in evaluation of such patients for diagnosis and follow-up of patients on medical treatment. Echography shows vitreous cavity filled with low-to-moderate intensity spikes with point-like or membrane-like echogenicity with good after-movements and not persisting at low gain (Fig. 4.23).

Ultrasound Biomicroscope

Ultrasound biomicroscope is an instrument for in vivo imaging of anterior segment in noninvasive fashion, with the help of high-frequency ultrasound transducer producing cross-sections of the living eye at microscopic resolution.

Ultrasound biomicroscope was first conceptualized at the Princess Margaret Hospital at Toronto, Canada in 1989 by Dr Charles Pavlin, Professor Stuart and Professor Foster. Initially they developed three probes—50, 80, and 100 MHz for clini-

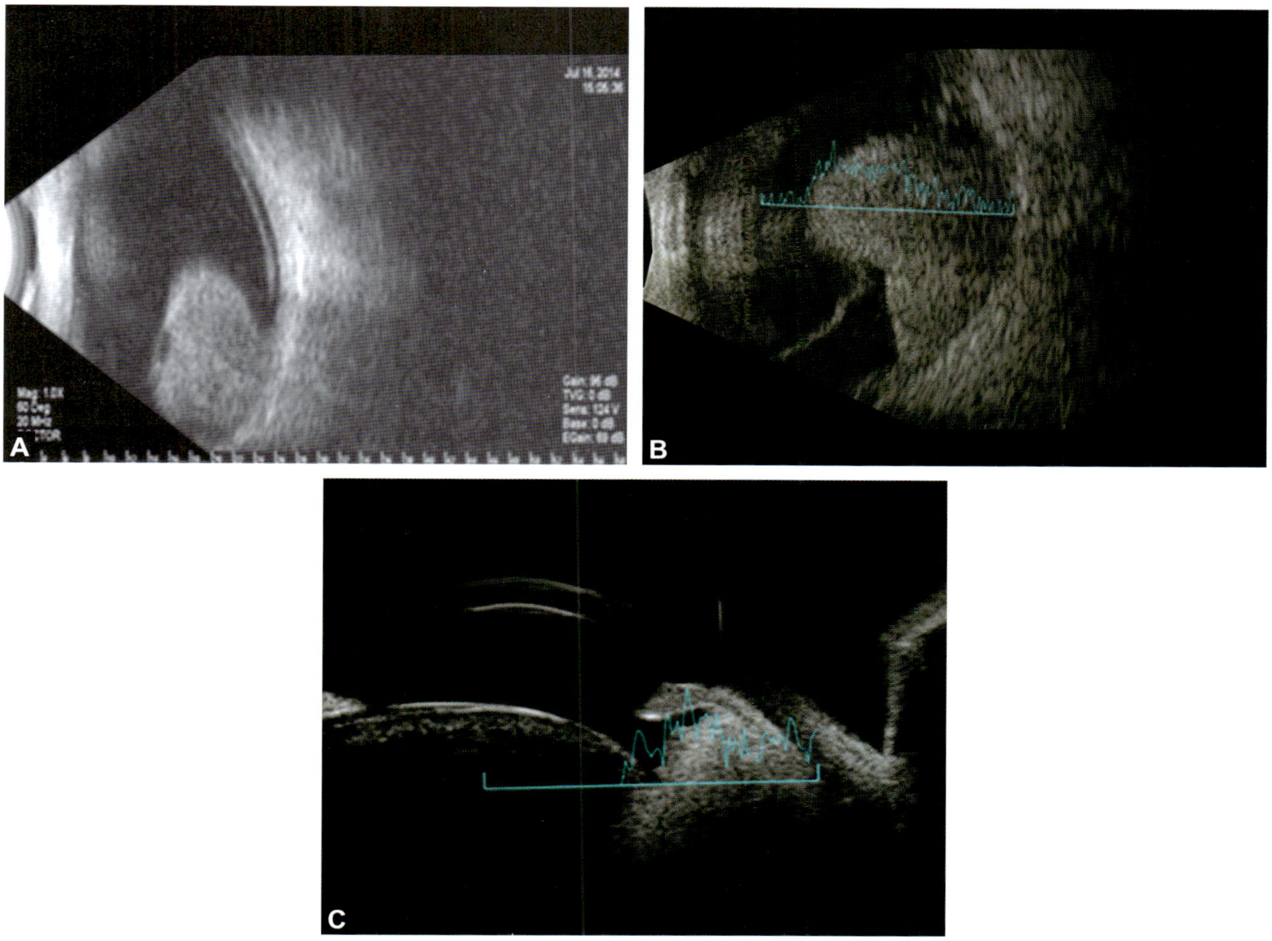

Figs. 4.20A to C: (A and B) B-Scan ultrasonography showing characteristic collar-button or mushroom-shaped lesion of choroidal melanoma in both USG pictures. A large angle kappa on A scan is seen in Figure B. (C) A ciliary body melanoma is visible on ultrasound biomicroscopy in the lowermost scan, again with large angle kappa.

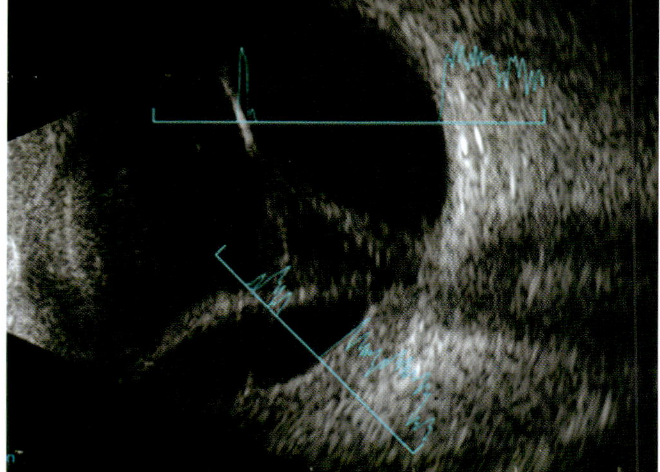

Fig. 4.21: B scan with vector A scan showing high reflectivity spikes from the choroidal metastatic deposits in a patient of metastatic breast cancer, along with retinal detachment

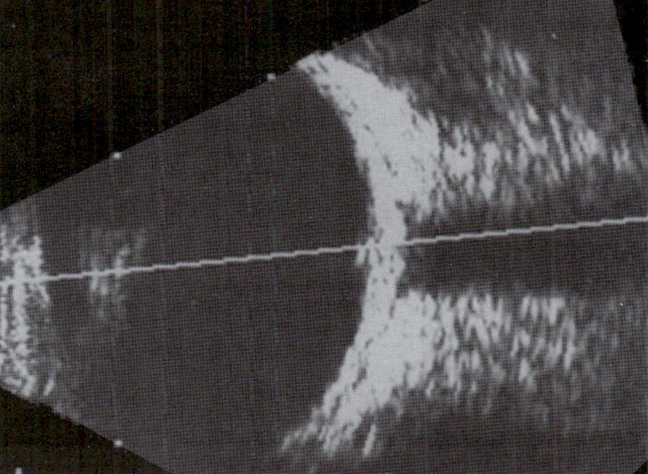

Fig. 4.22: Classical T sign seen in an eye with thickened sclera and sub-tenon's fluid collection.

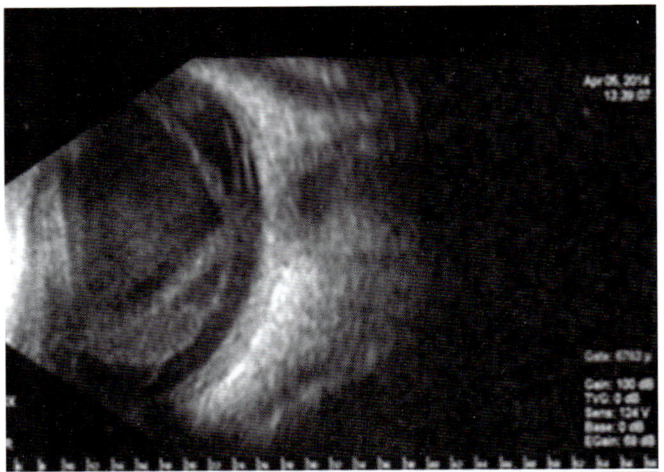

Fig. 4.23: B-scan ultrasonography of a patient with endophthalmitis.

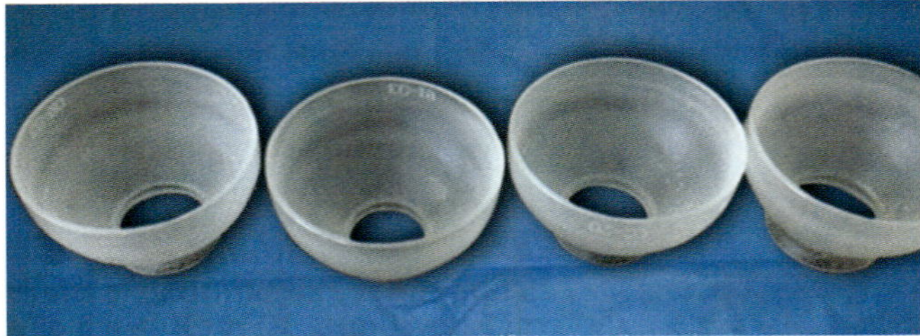

Fig. 4.24: Series of cups to create a water bath for ultrasound biomicroscopy.

cal trials. 80 and 100 MHz probes were used to see the cornea and the anterior chamber as the depth of penetration is only 2 mm. They found that 50 MHz is an ideal compromise between depth and resolution to visualize the entire anterior segment.

Instrument of UBM

Ultrasound biomicroscope mainly consists of a probe, hard disc, video monitor, mouse, foot switch, and printer. There are three main components of the hard disc of the UBM machine—transducer, high-frequency signal processor, and precise motion control device.

The transducer is made up of a piezoelectric crystal produces 50 MHz radiofrequency pulse that travels the body tissue and reflected back to the transducer, which is processed by the signal processing unit. UBM is specially designed to handle high-frequency signals. Special motion control device is used to enable subtle movements to scan adjacent areas in the anterior segment. Series of eye cups are provided with the machine to create a water bath for the coupling agent (Fig. 4.24).

It produces cross-sectional images of anterior segment structures providing a lateral resolution of 50 μm and an axial resolution of 25 μm with a depth of penetration of approximately 4–5 mm. The field of view is 4 mm × 4 mm and the scan rate is 5 frames/sec.

P60 machine: The next generation of ultrasonic biomicroscope provides unprecedented image accuracy and flexibility with 12.5 MHz, 20 MHz, 35 MHz, and 50 MHz probes.

Method

After anesthetizing the eye by instilling 4% lignocaine in the eye, a plastic eye cap is used to gently part the lids and of 2% methylcellulose or saline is used as the coupling agent. The patient is asked to fix at with the fellow eye on a ceiling target to maintain a steady fixation. The probe is kept approximately 2 mm from the eye surface to prevent injury to the cornea. The probe is manually moved perpendicular to the structure to be scanned in each clock hour from the center of the cornea to the ora serrata. Table 4.2 summarizes the key differences between USG and UBM.

Indications for UBM in Retinal and Uveal Diseases

Misplaced IOL Position

Displaced haptics can be imaged and their position in relationship to the ciliary body can be ascertained.[13] Dislocated lenses frequently have a haptic over the pars plana. Any tissue attachment to the ciliary body can be assessed (Fig. 4.25).

Table 4.2: Key differences between USG B scan and UBM scan.	
USG B scan	*UBM*
Structures imaged in the posterior segment have a thickness of more than a millimeter	The anterior segment has a depth of 4–5 mm and the structures are close to each other so we require a higher frequency probe
Frequency of the probe used is 10 MHz	Frequency of the probe used is 50 MHz
10 MHz frequency probe has a depth of 4 cm	The depth of penetration is 4 mm
It has an axial resolution of 940 microns	It has an axial resolution of 30–40 microns

USG: Ultrasonography; UBM: Ultrasound biomicroscopy

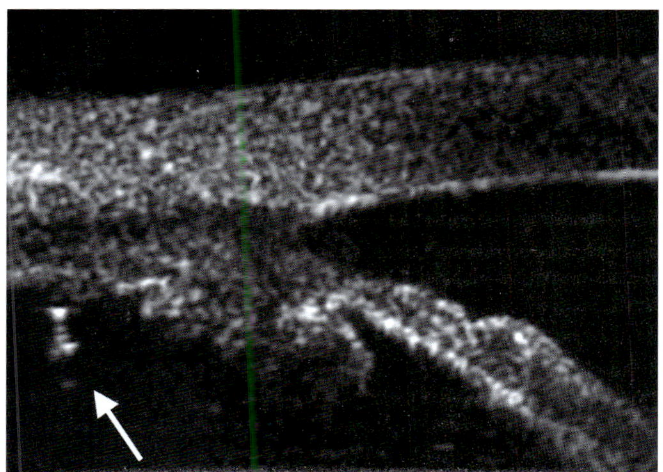

Fig. 4.25: Ultrasound biomicroscopy of a patient with malpositioned intraocular lens showing acoustic reverberation (arrow).

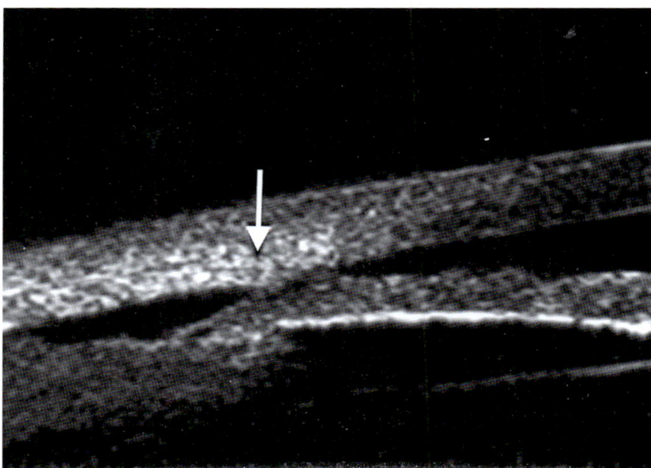

Fig. 4.26: Ultrasound biomicroscopy of a patient showing cyclodialysis cleft (arrow).

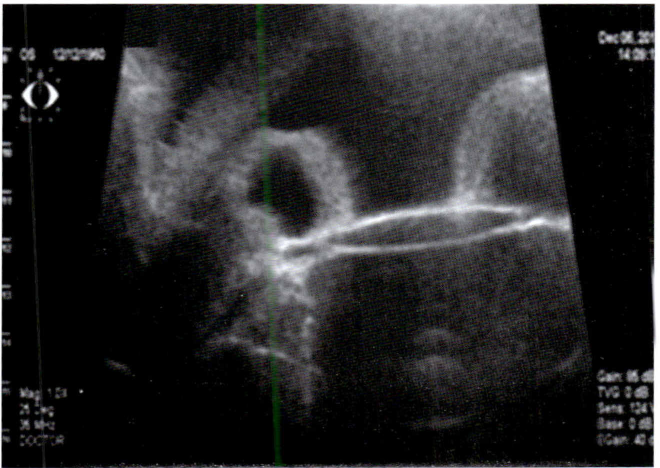

Fig. 4.27: Ultrasound biomicroscopy of a patient with anterior proliferative vitreoretinopathy and iris bombe formation.

Fig. 4.28: Glued intraocular lens with haptic track in sclera visible on ultrasound biomicroscopy.

Trauma

Cyclodialysis is complete disinsertion of the ciliary body from the scleral spur and may be accompanied by a supracillary effusion. UBM is very useful to detect cyclodialysis clefts (Fig. 4.26).[14]

Anterior Proliferative Vitreoretinopathy

Typical features of anterior PVR on UBM may be used to help guide surgery and estimate anatomical prognosis. Circumferential contraction or anterior displacement around the ora serrata can be seen on UBM (Fig. 4.27).

The anterior displacement could be further classified based on UBM images into C-shaped anterior displacement, ciliary body adhesion, and pupil adhesion.

Retained Intraocular Foreign Body

Ultrasound biomicroscope plays an important role in the localization and management of an anteriorly situated intraocular foreign body in ciliary body or pars plana region.[15]

Miscellaneous Conditions

Glued IOL: Figure 4.28 shows a glued IOL with haptic track visible on UBM.

Even caterpillar hairs stuck onto the ciliary body have rarely been detected on UBM.[15,16]

Limitations

The most important limitation of UBM is poor depth of penetration. UBM cannot visualize structures deeper more than 4 mm from the surface. UBM cannot be performed in presence of an open corneal or scleral wound. Being a contact procedure, it cannot be performed in the immediate postoperative period due to the risk of infection.

REFERENCES

1. Mundt GH, Hughes WF. Ultrasonics in ocular diagnosis. Am J Ophthalmology. 1956;41:488.
2. Baum G, Greenwood J. The application of ultrasonic locating techniques to Ophthalmology, part 1. Am J Ophthalmology. 1958;46:319.
3. Bronson N, Fisher Y, Pickering N. Ophthalmic contact B-scan ultrasonography. Westport, CT: Intercontinental; 1976.
4. Ossoinig K. Clinical echo-Ophthalmology. In: Current Concepts of Ophthalmology. Vol III. St Louis, MO: CV Mosby Co; 1972. pp. 101-30.
5. Ossoinig KC. The evaluation of kinetic properties of echo signals. In: Oksala A, Gernet H (Eds). Ultrasonics in Ophthalmology. Basel, Switzerland: Karger; 1967. pp. 88-96.
6. Coleman DJ, Silverman RH, Rondeau MJ, et al. New perspectives: 3-D volume rendering of ocular tumors. Acta Ophthalmology Suppl. 1992;(204):22.
7. Lezzi R, Rosen R, Tello C. Personal computer-based 3-dimensional ultrasound biomicroscopy of the anterior segment. Arch Ophthalmology. 1996;114:520-4.
8. Cusumano A, Coleman D, Silverman R. Three dimensional ultrasound imaging - clinical applications. Ophthalmology. 1998; 105:300-6.
9. Coleman D, Silverman R, Daly S. Advances in ophthalmic ultrasound. Radiol Clin North Am. 1998;36:1073-82.
10. Reinstein D, Raevsky T, Coleman D. Improved system for ultrasonic imaging and biometry. J Ultrasound Med. 1997;16:117-24.
11. Sherer MD, Starkoski BG, Taylor WB, et al. A 100 MHz B-scan ultrasound backscatter microscope. Ultrasound Imaging. 1989; 11:95-105.
12. Barash D, Joan M. Brien O. The role of ultrasound in the management of ocular tumors ophthalmology. Clinics of north America. 1999;12:205-11.
13. Irène MEL, Carl-Gustaf L. Ultrasound biomicroscopy examination of intraocular lens haptic position after phacoemulsification with continuous curvilinear capsulorhexis and extracapsular cataract extraction with linear capsulotomy. Acta Ophthalmologica Scandinavica. 2013;77:45-9.
14. Park M, Kondo T. Ultrasound biomicroscopic findings in a case of cyclodialysis. Ophthalmologica. 1998;212:194-97.
15. Guha S, Bhende M, Baskaran M, et al. Role of ultrasound biomicroscopy (UBM) in the detection and localisation of anterior segment foreign bodies. Ann Acad Med Singapore. 2006;35(8): 536-45.
16. Bhende M, Biswas J, Sharma T, et al. Ultrasound biomicroscopy in the diagnosis and management of pars planitis caused by caterpillar hairs. Am J Ophthalmology. 2000;130:125-6.

Retinal Degenerations and Fundal Dystrophies

Chapter 5

Degenerative Myopia and Retina

Atul Kumar, Rohan Chawla, Devesh Kumawat, Raghav Ravani

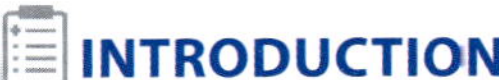

INTRODUCTION

Myopia is a major cause of legal blindness and low vision throughout the world. It is a refractive state of eye in which parallel rays of light coming from infinity are focused in front of the neurosensory retina with the accommodation being at rest. The term myopia is derived from Greek words "mycin" which means "to close" and "ops" meaning "eye". It was first described by Kepler in 1611 in individuals who used to bring their eyelids close to form a stenopaic slit to see better.

"High myopia" (HM) is defined as myopia with spherical equivalent exceeding–6 diopters (D) and/or the axial length longer than 26.5 mm.[1,2] "Pathological myopia" (PM) also known as degenerative myopia, is a type of high axial myopia with characteristic progressive pathological changes in fundus.[3-5] The progressive axial elongation of the eyeball leads to degenerative changes of the sclera, choroid, Bruch's membrane, retinal pigment epithelium (RPE) and neurosensory retina (Fig. 5.1).[6,7] These pathologic changes, especially chorioretinal atrophy and choroidal neovascularization (CNV), are the major causes of progressive loss of vision in PM.[8] CNV secondary to PM is the leading cause of loss of vision in patients younger than 50 years.

EPIDEMIOLOGY AND ETIOLOGICAL FACTORS

Epidemiology of PM and its complications is not consistent throughout the general population. The prevalence of PM varies from 1% to 4%.[5,9,10] PM is more prevalent in Asians than among Africans and Whites. Prevalence is estimated to be 3.1% in China,[9] 1.74% in Japan,[11] and 1.2% in Australia.[10] There are no population studies in India assessing the prevalence of HM. In a study conducted on school-going children in north India, prevalence of HM has been found to be 1.5%.[12] PM is more prevalent in women than in men. In Blue Mountains Eye study, prevalence of PM was 0.4% in women while in men this was 0.06%.[10]

Pathological myopia is the leading cause of unavoidable blindness in Japan, and is second most common cause

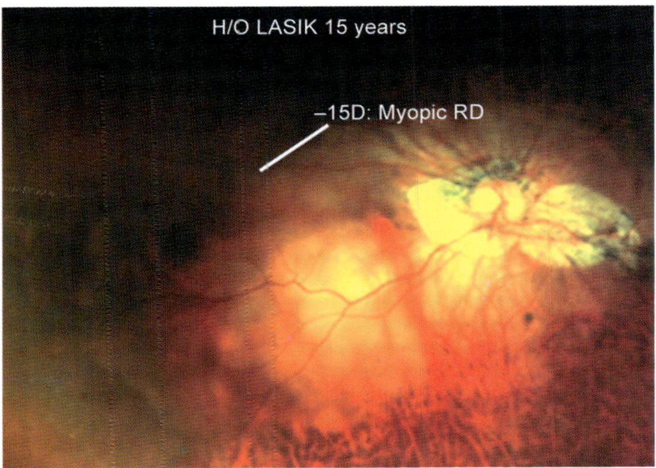

Fig. 5.1: Wide-field pseudocolor image of a patient with pathological myopia showing rhegmatogenous retinal detachment involving posterior pole. Patient had history of refractive surgery (LASIK) 15 years ago.

in Denmark[13] and China.[14] In the west as well, pathological myopia is amongst the leading cause of legal blindness.[15]

Etiological mechanisms are not fully known but a complex interplay of environmental and genetic factors leads to PM.[16,17] Based on studies in families with pathologic myopia, numerous inheritance patterns for pathologic myopia have been identified, including autosomal dominant, autosomal recessive and X-linked forms. The high-myopia genetic loci are heterogeneous[18,19] and these may contribute to varying degrees of myopia.[20,21] Moreover, degenerative myopia is commonly associated with Marfan syndrome, Ehlers-Danlos syndrome, Stickler syndrome, Knobloch syndrome, Noonan and Down syndrome. Refractive status of the parents plays an important role in inheritance of disease.[22,23] High concordance rates of up to 90% have been reported in twin studies.[24]

Possible environmental factors associated with PM include amount of time spent outdoors, water hardness, and use of fluorinated water.[25,26] Time spent indoors has currently been the most studied parameter and thought to be causative for the development of myopia.[27,28]

PATHOPHYSIOLOGY

Pathological changes start occurring in childhood and become prominent in adulthood.[29] To start with, there occurs excessive axial elongation.[30] Axial elongation results in chorioretinal stretching and thinning.

The mechanisms behind pathological axial elongation include emmetropization process and structural alteration of collagen proteins.[31,32] Axial length and corneal curvature are the main factors involved in the process of emmetropization. Anterior chamber depth and lens curvature play a minor role. A defective interplay between these factors leads to ammetropia. Abnormal collagen proteins may lead to degenerative changes in the retina, choroid, and sclera.[32]

Pathological changes like posterior staphyloma and chorioretinal atrophy increase proportionally with increase in axial length.[4] Thinned out chorioretinal tissue (Fig. 5.2B) is associated with poor blood circulation and may lead to CNV development by inducing vascular endothelial growth factor (VEGF) expression.[29,33] Also, scleral thinning may cause deformation of the posterior pole leading to staphyloma formation with a shorter radius of curvature.

Role of Choroid in Axial Elongation

The role of choroid in ocular elongation in response to retinal defocus is recently been talked about.[34-36] With defocus, choroidal thickness varies moving the retina towards the plane of focus.[35] Also, choroid affects the molecular signals arising from retina that modulate scleral growth.[36] Thus, choroid also plays an active role in development of PM.

FEATURES OF PATHOLOGICAL MYOPIA

The typical features of PM include myopic conus, tigroid fundus, posterior staphyloma, diffuse or patchy chorioretinal atrophy, lacquer cracks, Forster–Fuchs' spots, choroidal neovascular membrane and foveoschisis. The clinical features seen in early phase are myopic conus, super traction and tessellation of fundus.

Myopic Conus or Crescent

Myopic conus or crescent is formed by the differential scleral expansion in the peripapillary area. It is a sharply defined concentric area of depigmentation present adjacent to the optic disc, where the inner surface of sclera is visible (Fig. 5.2A). It occurs due to premature termination of the choriocapillaris complex before the optic disc edge. It can be either a scleral crescent alone or choroidal crescent or both.[37] Based on the extent of involvement, it can be temporal conus, nasal conus, inferior conus, or annular conus. Temporal conus are reported to be the most common variant.[4]

Super Traction

It is caused by expansion of the posterior pole leading to retinochoroidal tissue drag over the nasal edge of optic disc.

Posterior Staphyloma

Outward protrusion of all coats of the eye at the posterior pole is called posterior staphyloma and is considered pathognomonic of PM. It is also known as Scarpa's staphyloma. Spaide defined it as an "out-pouching of the wall of the eye that has a radius of curvature less than the surrounding radii of curvature".[38] It is seen as an area with bending of vessels at the margin and a dark crescentic nasal reflex (Figs. 5.2 and 5.3). Curtin has described 10 different types of staphyloma.[39] Its incidence increases with age, and is most commonly seen in the 5th decade.[40] Posterior staphyloma is now known to be the cause of development of myopic maculopathy.[3] The eyes with shallow staphyloma have a higher incidence of CNV and

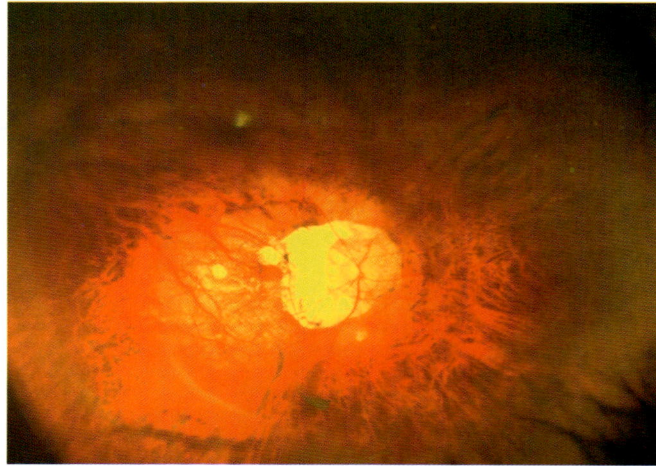

Fig. 5.2A: Ultra-wide-field pseudocolor image of a patient with high myopia showing chorioretinal atrophy, posterior staphyloma and temporal scleral crescent.

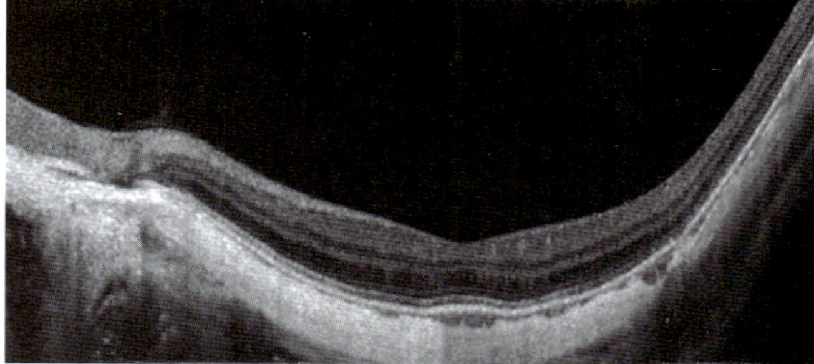

Fig. 5.2B: The optic disc is also tilted. OCT shows evidence of posterior staphyloma and marked choroidal thinning, as sclera is literally in apposition with the RPE
(OCT: Optical coherence tomography; RPE: Retinal pigment epithelium)

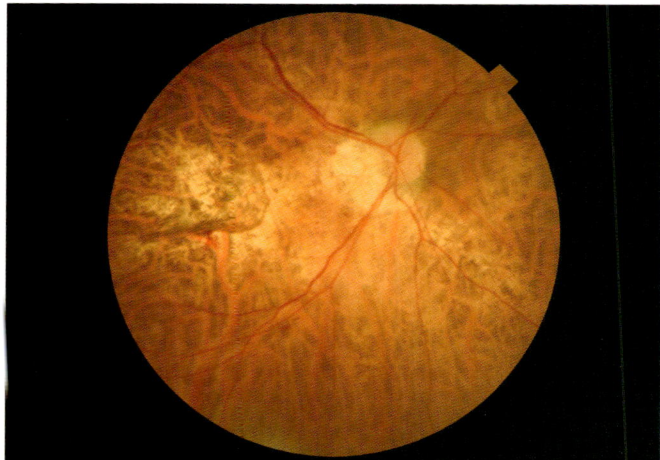

Fig. 5.3: Color image of a patient with pathological myopia showing posterior staphyloma.

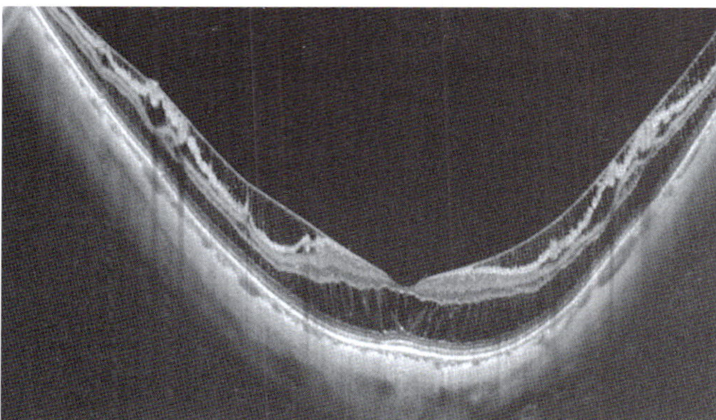

Fig. 5.4: Swept-source optical coherence tomography (OCT) of a patient with pathological myopia with myopic traction maculopathy with foveoschisis. Note the presence of highly thinned out choroid in this enhanced-depth OCT image.

macular hemorrhage.[41] A large number of patients with posterior staphyloma do not have the normal choroidal flush, suggesting the possibility of ischemia and thereby increasing the future risk for development of CNV in these eyes.[42]

Convex elevation of macula within the concavity of a posterior staphyloma has been described as dome-shaped macula on optical coherence tomography (OCT) and ultrasonography in pathologically myopic eyes. Probable pathological causes include tangential vitreomacular traction, localized choroidal or scleral thickening, hypotony and retinal resistance to scleral deformation.[43] It may be a cause of unexplained visual loss in such eyes.

Macular Changes

Myopic maculopathy usually progresses from tessellated fundus to the development of diffuse atrophy and lacquer cracks. This further progresses to patchy atrophy and CNV usually develops adjacent to these areas. Avilla et al.[44] gave a grading of myopic maculopathy with severity from 0 to 5 as follows:

- M0, normal-appearing posterior pole
- M1, choroidal pallor and tessellation
- M2, choroidal pallor and tessellation with posterior staphyloma
- M3, choroidal pallor and tessellation with posterior staphyloma and lacquer cracks
- M4, choroidal pallor and tessellation with lacquer cracks, posterior staphyloma, and focal areas of deep choroidal atrophy
- M5, posterior pole with large geographic areas of deep chorioretinal atrophy and "bare" sclera.

Hayashi et al. also proposed a progression pattern of myopic maculopathy from a tessellated fundus to macular atrophy.[3]

Macular Chorioretinal Atrophy

Chorioretinal atrophy occurs due to progressive thinning of the choroid, loss of choroidal vessels, RPE and photoreceptors.[29] The cause of atrophy is probably choroidal vascular occlusion and abiotrophic degeneration.

Chorioretinal atrophy is of two types: (1) diffuse atrophy, and (2) patchy atrophy.[7] Diffuse atrophy usually appears as yellowish-white areas of atrophy with ill-defined borders, while patchy atrophy has a grayish-white, well-defined area of atrophy (*see* Fig. 5.2A) and on visual fields, it appears as an absolute scotoma. CNV development occurs usually adjacent to the areas of patchy atrophy.[45]

Choroidal Imaging

Enhanced depth imaging OCT or swept-source OCT shows a very thin choroid in highly myopic eyes (Figs. 5.2B and 5.4), which progressively gets thinner with increasing degree of myopia and age.[46]

Lacquer Cracks

These are breaks in the Bruch's membrane at the posterior pole in high myopia (Fig. 5.5A). These are usually associated with a posterior staphyloma. These appear as multiple yellowish-white irregular lines, usually horizontally oriented and coursing the posterior pole. Lacquer cracks can be linear or stellate, and sometimes show branching or crisscrossing or both. These are seen more commonly in males and decreases with increasing age. On fluorescein angiography, these appear as hyperfluorescent tracks due to window defect without any leakage (Fig. 5.5B).[47] On fundus autofluorescence imaging, these appear hypo-autofluorescent. Similarly, they appear hypofluorescent on indocyanine green angiography.[48]

Subretinal bleeding may occur in the absence of CNV in cases of fresh lacquer cracks.[49] Lacquer cracks are also fre-

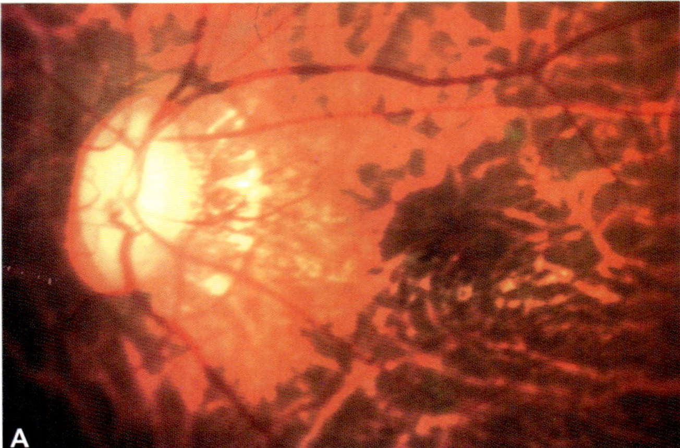

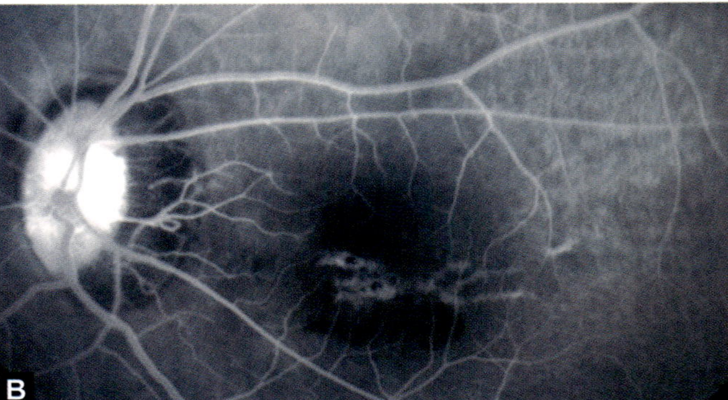

Figs. 5.5A and B: (A) Fundus photograph of a myopic patient with lacquer crack; (B) Fundus angiograph of the same patient showing window-defect corresponding to lacquer cracks.

quently associated with formation of a choroidal neovascularization at the margins or in adjacent areas.[45]

Forster–Fuchs' Spot

Forster–Fuchs' spot is a pigmented lesion that is predominantly dark but can have a gray, yellow, red, or green hue. It is usually raised, round or elliptical in shape. It is named after Ernst Fuchs, who described such a pigmented lesion in 1901, and Carl Förster, who described neovascularization of the retina in 1862. It arises due to proliferation of RPE secondary to choroidal hemorrhage.[50] These are primarily small retinal scars which are formed following degeneration and neovascularization related to HM.

Myopic Choroidal Neovascularization

Approximately 10–11% of highly myopic eyes may develop CNV over a period of 11–12 years.[45] Eventually 30% of the fellow eyes also develop CNV. Macular CNV is the most common complication that results in reduced central vision in patients with PM.[51] Myopic CNV may account for up to 62% of CNV occurring in young patients with age less than 50 years.[52]

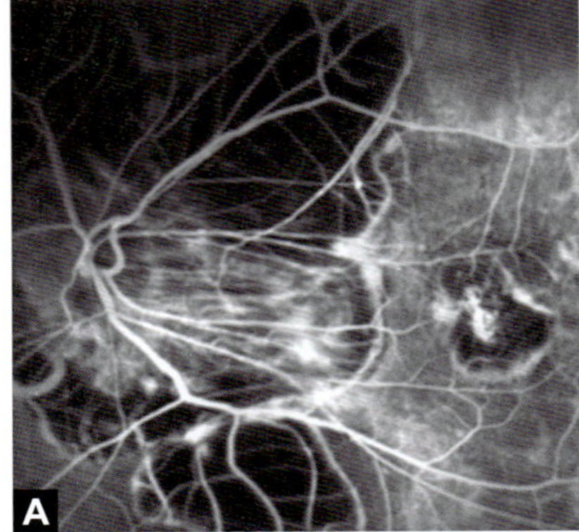

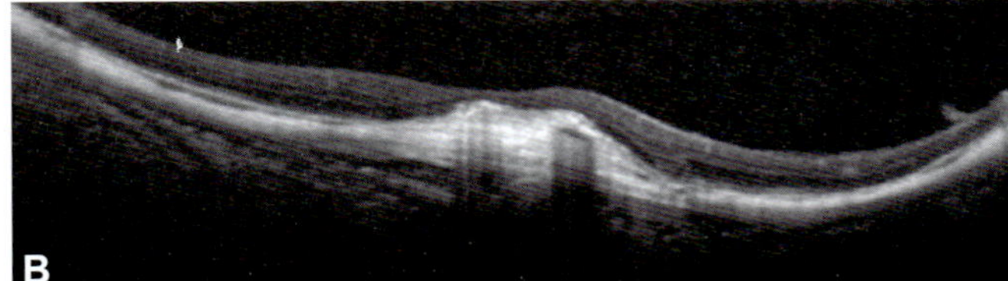

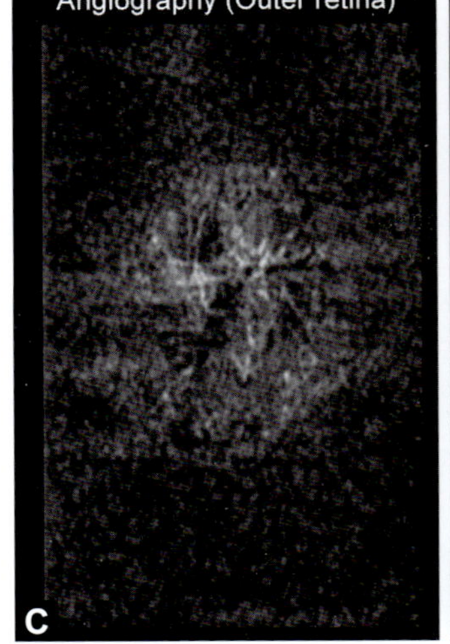

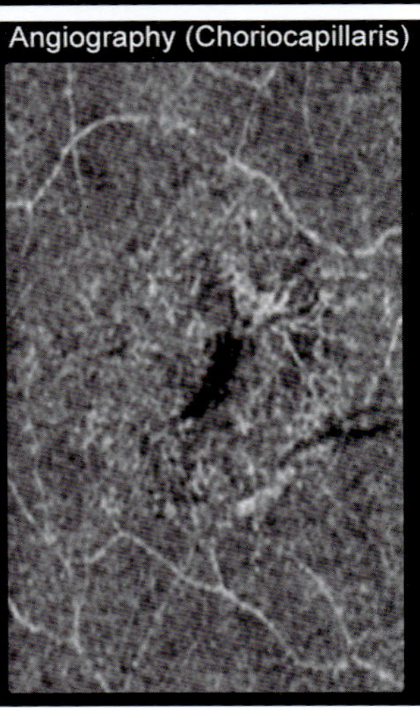

Figs. 5.6A to C: (A) Myopic CNV stains on FA; (B) Showing no leak on OCT due to a tiny membrane and thinned retina; (C) However, OCTA reveals the arborescent new vessels in the sub-RPE and under the neurosensory retina. (CNV: Choroidal neovascularization; FA: Fluorescein angiography; OCT: Optical coherence tomography; OCTA: Optical coherence tomography angiography; RPE: Retinal pigment epithelium)

Myopic CNV is seen as a grayish subretinal membrane with hyperpigmented borders (Figs. 5.6 to 5.8). As the retina is thin, bleeding in these cases usually do not obscure the lesion and is easily observed on clinical examination.

On OCT, a typical type 2 CNV with hyperreflective elevated lesion in the subretinal space, usually without neurosensory detachment or intraretinal edema is seen (Fig. 5.6B). On fundus fluorescein angiography (FFA), myopic CNV is mostly classic with well-defined hyperfluorescence in the

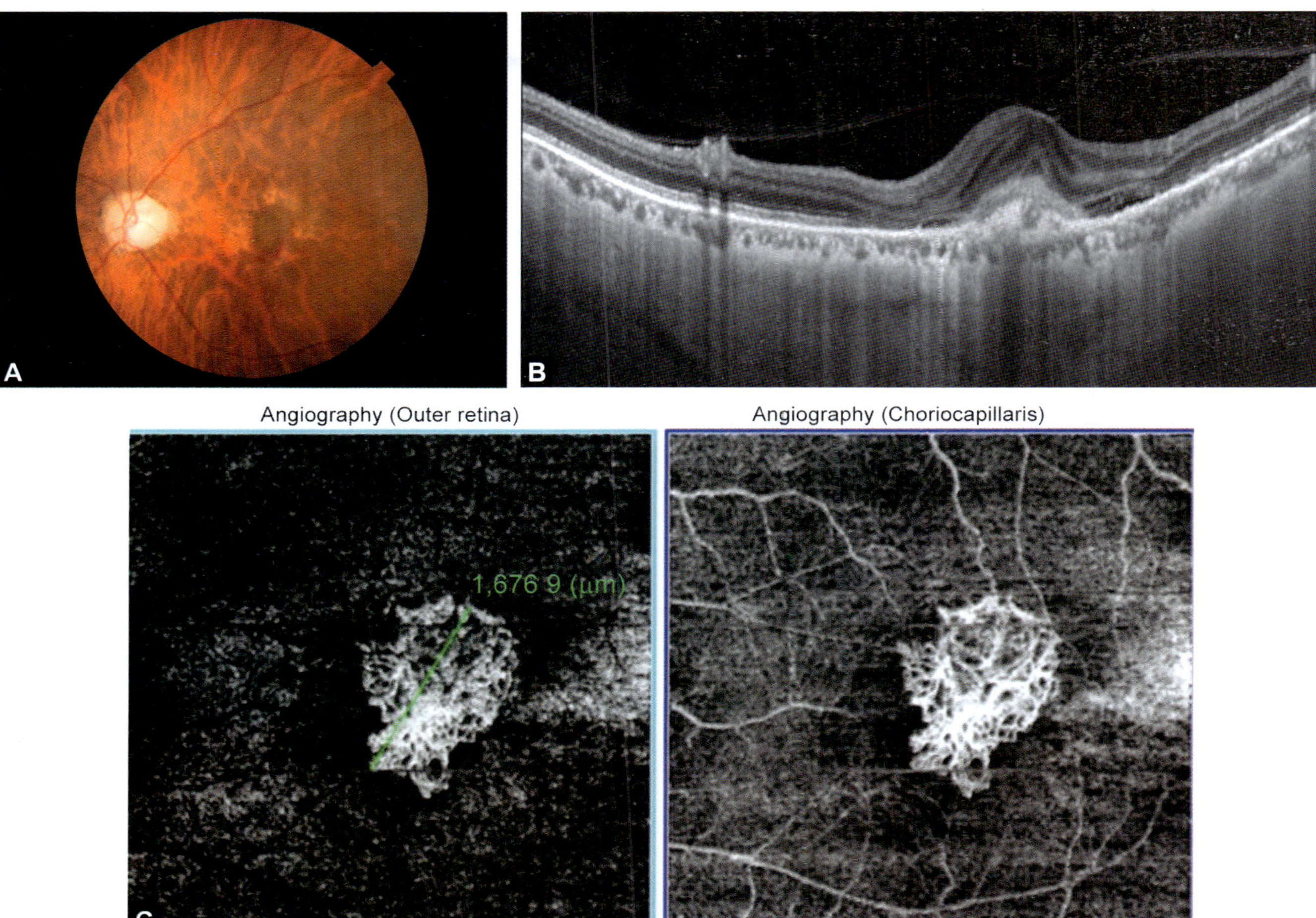

Figs. 5.7A to C: Myopic CNV visible on color photo, OCT and OCTA. A typical lacy network of new vessels is visible on OCTA which originates from the sub-RPE space (Type 1 CNV). (CNV: Choroidal neovascularization; OCT: Optical coherence tomography; OCTA: Optical coherence tomography angiography)

early phases and leakage of fluorescein dye during the late phases (Fig. 5.6A).[53,54]

Unpublished data from our center has revealed type 1 sub-RPE CNV mostly in myopic CNV eyes on OCTA which is in contradistinction to the reported type 2 CNV in literature.

Optical coherence tomography angiography (OCTA) has a definite role in diagnosis of myopic CNV. As subretinal hemorrhage can be caused by both CNV and new lacquer crack formation in eyes with pathologic myopia, OCTA can help identify CNV noninvasively (Fig. 5.6C).

Active CNV is characterized by lacy wheel pattern, widely anatomized network and perilesional hyperintense halo. On the other hand, long filamentous linear large matures vessels, rare anastomosis and dead tree appearance characterize quiescent CNV.[55] OCTA has a higher sensitivity in picking up CNV in myopic patients as compared to FFA and/or OCT. Current limitations of this technique include a relatively small field of view, inability to show leakage, and tendency for image artifacts.

Focal chorioretinal atrophy, steeper posterior staphyloma and lacquer cracks are thought to be the risk factors for development of myopic CNV.[3,51] There are three main stages of myopic CNV. In the initial stage, there is direct damage to photoreceptors causing central visual loss. As the CNV regresses, a pigmented fibrous scar is seen, referred to as Forster–Fuchs' spot. Finally, chorioretinal atrophy develops around the regressed CNV resulting in poor long-term visual outcome.[56]

Photodynamic therapy (PDT), anti-VEGF therapy and a combination of these has been tried for treatment of myopic CNV. Intravitreal anti-VEGF therapy remains the mainstay of treatment. Prior to the use of anti-VEGF, laser photocoagulation, verteporfin PDT and surgical excision or macular translocations were performed to treat CNV.

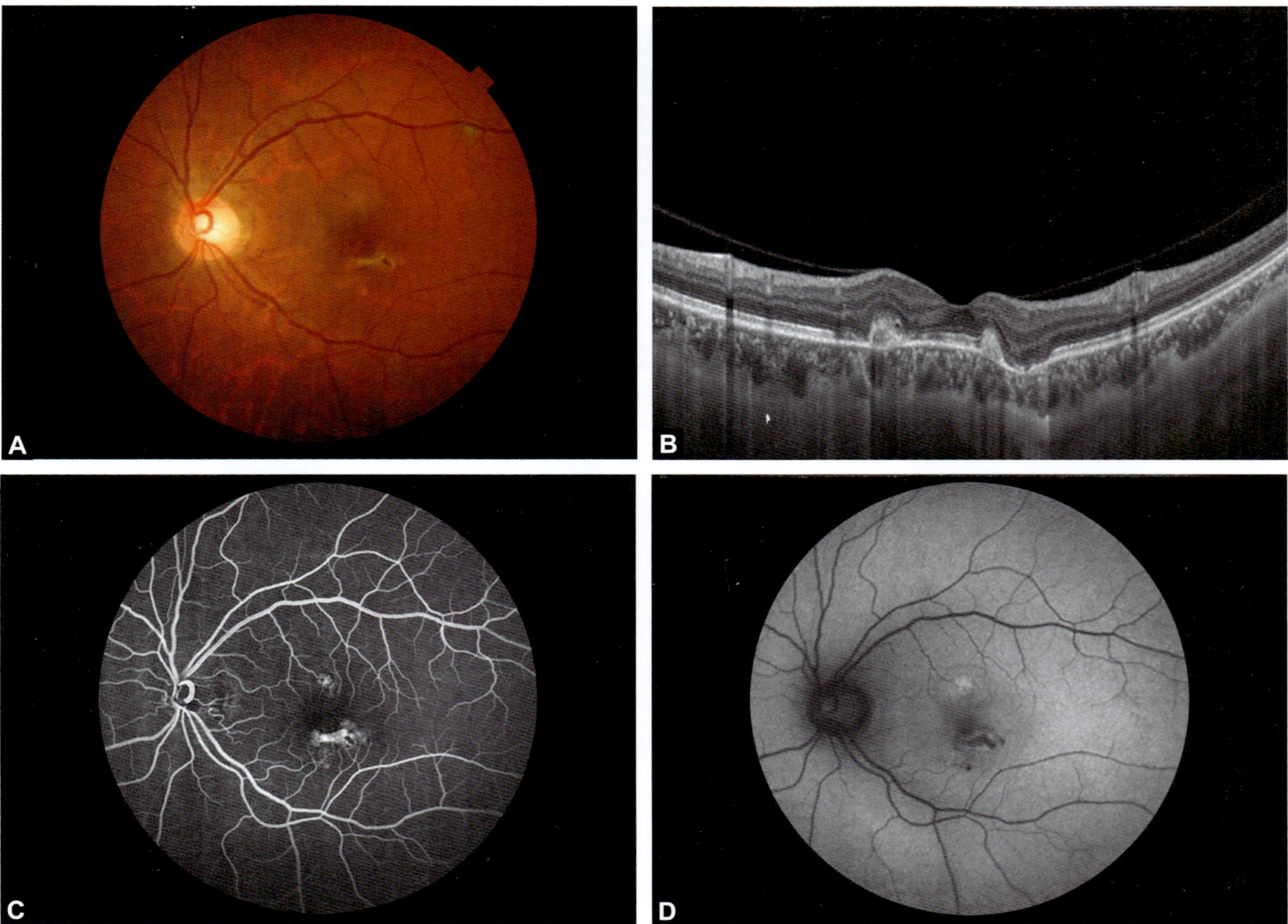

Figs. 5.8A to D: Myopic eye with two separate CNVs visible on (A) Color picture; (B) OCT; (C) FA; and (D) Autofluorescence imaging (Patient had -5.50D myopia). (CNV: Choroidal neovascularization; FA: Fluorescein angiography; OCT: Optical coherence tomography)

REPAIR and RADIANCE study showed efficacy and safety of Ranibizumab in this condition.[57,58] The pro-re-nata (PRN) dosing of ranibizumab was found to be superior to PDT in RADIANCE study.[58] MYRROR study for aflibercept in myopic CNV in Asian population has found it to be safe and effective. Bevacizumab is also used but its intraocular use is not Food and Drug Administration (FDA) approved.

Verteporfin PDT is approved for the treatment of subfoveal myopic CNV. The "Verteporfin in Photodynamic Therapy" (VIP trial) showed that though it generally stabilized but did not improve visual acuity.[59] Although in the long term, some patients may develop vision loss due to chorioretinal atrophy following PDT.

MYOPIC TRACTION MACULOPATHY

Myopic Macular Retinoschisis

Takano and Kishi et al. first described foveal retinoschisis and retinal detachment without retinal holes in severely myopic eyes based on OCT.[60] In 2004, Panozzo and Mercanti et al. coined the term "myopic traction maculopathy" (MTM) to refer to a group of posterior pole pathologies in HM, such as macular retinoschisis, shallow retinal detachment, lamellar macular holes, and macular holes with or without retinal detachment.[61]

Myopic macular retinoschisis has been reported in 9% of highly myopic eyes with posterior staphyloma.[62] Myopic macular retinoschisis or myopic foveoschisis describes a schisis like thickening of neurosensory retina at the macula of highly myopic eyes with posterior staphyloma.[63] MTM always occurs within a posterior staphyloma.

The pathogenesis behind MTM is probably splitting of retina due to relative tautness and noncompliance of inner retina compared with outer retina within the posterior staphyloma (*see* Figs. 5.2 and 5.3) The split occurs at the level of the external limiting membrane.[64] The tractional mechanisms responsible include vitreomacular traction from incomplete posterior vitreous detachment, remnant preretinal cortical

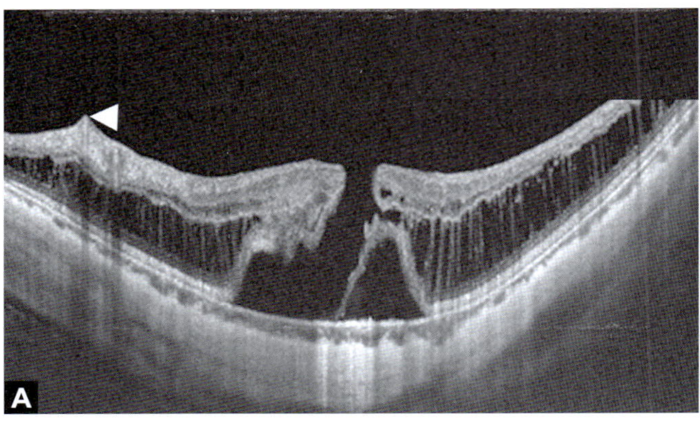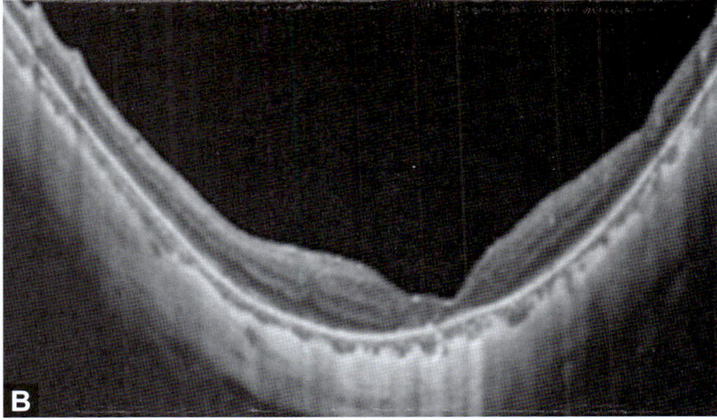

Figs. 5.9A and B: (A) SD-OCT image of a patient with myopic traction maculopathy showing full thickness macular hole traction along retinal vessel with tenting of inner retina (white arrowhead); (B) Postoperatively, the schisis appears settled with hole closure. (SD-OCT: Spectral domain optical coherence tomography)

vitreous layer after posterior vitreous detachment, epiretinal membrane, taut internal limiting membrane (ILM) and shortened and stiff retinal arterioles (Figs. 5.9A and B) (vascular microfolds).[65-72]

Visual complaints are minimal and progress gradually. Patients may complain of blurring of vision or distortion of vision (metamorphopsia).[63] Vision loss occurs with outer lamellar hole formation or foveal detachment. Early stages may be easily underestimated by biomicroscopic examination. The diagnosis is confirmed on OCT, which shows the typical splitting of neurosensory retina, bridging columns and intraretinal cysts.[63,67]

Optical coherence tomography based progression of myopic foveal retinoschisis to retinal detachment has been described in detail by Shimada et al.[73] Stage 1 shows focal irregularity of the thickness of external retinal layer. In stage 2, an outer lamellar hole develops within the thickened area with a small retinal detachment. Vertical enlargement of the outer lamellar hole occurs in stage 3. Lastly in stage 4, elevation of the upper edge of the external retinal layer occurs accompanied by increase in height of the retinal detachment and resolution of schisis.

No definitive literature exists on when to intervene surgically in MTM. Most researchers believe that surgery should be performed in MTM at risk of visual loss. Vitrectomy is widely performed for the treatment of MTM. However, ILM peeling remains a controversial intervention. The ILM is an important factor in the pathogenesis of MTM, and ILM peeling can reduce retinal traction. It can also stimulate the proliferation of the pigment epithelial layer, which is helpful for closing macular holes.

Using intraoperative OCT (iOCT) in such cases may facilitate complete removal of traction and help ensure that no residual membrane leading to continued traction is remaining. The author has described a novel technique of microscope-integrated intraoperative OCT-guided center-sparing ILM peeling for treatment of myoic foveoschisis.[74] The added advantage of center sparing ILM peeling using iOCT is to assist in sparing the ILM over areas of major cystic change and thus avoid surgical complications like deroofing of a large cyst leading to macular hole formation. Macular buckling with or without vitrectomy has also been recommended by few authors for MTM.[75]

Paravascular Microhole-related Retinal Detachment

Retinal detachment from a paravascular microhole associated with posterior major vessels can also develop in highly myopic eyes. The vitreoretinal adhesion is quite strong at the paravascular region, and vitreous traction at this site leads to formation of retinal cysts and breaks.[76]

MYOPIC MACULAR HOLE

Macular hole formation in myopic eyes may be related to the early onset of vitreous degeneration with development of tangential traction at the level of the premacular cortex.[77] Macular holes may also form as an end stage of MTM.

These eyes may further progress to a retinal detachment which may be limited to the posterior pole or could even be a total rhegmatogenous retinal detachment. Additional factors which lead to a retinal detachment in myopic eyes with a macular hole include presence of a posterior staphyloma causing centrifugal traction, chorioretinal atrophy leading to weak adhesion between the neurosensory retina and RPE and anteroposterior tractional forces leading to lifting of hole edge and inelasticity of stretched retinal vessels.[78] Surgery is the mainstay treatment, in which the primary aim is to relieve these tractional forces (Figs. 5.10A to D). Triamcinolone helps us in the complete removal of posterior vitreous cortex by adhering to it. Microscope-integrated intraoperative optical coherence tomography (MI-OCT) has further enabled to us to identify the fine layer of posterior vitreous cortex and complete removal of tractional forces at the edge of the macular hole.[79]

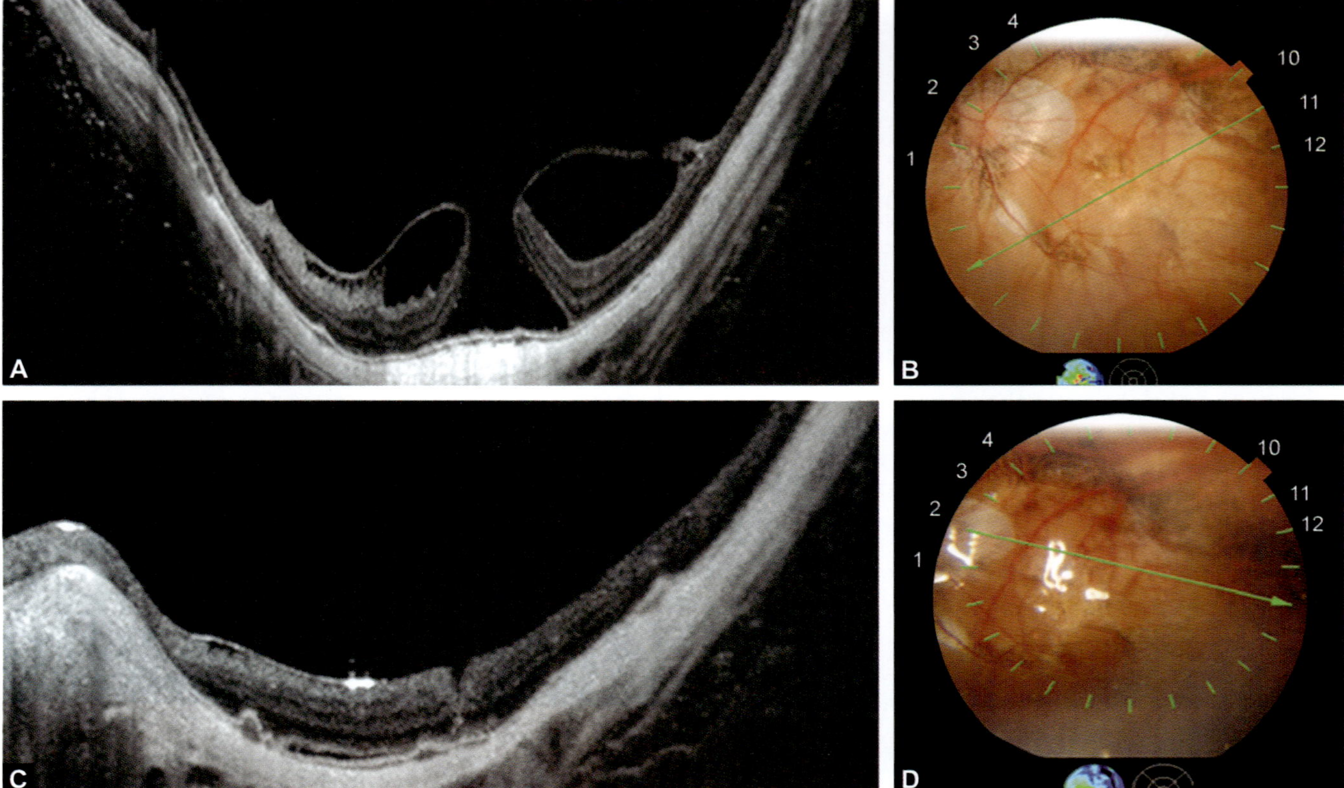

Figs. 5.10A to D: Myopic macular hole shown (A and B) preoperatively; and (C and D) postoperatively, closed using the inverted internal limiting membrane flap technique and C_3F_8 gas injection. Numbers in Figures 5.10B and D denotes the axis in which the scan is taken.

Myopic macular hole formation tends to occur at a younger age as compared to idiopathic age-related macular holes. The degree of myopia and axial length have been shown to have an inverse correlation to the age of onset of the macular hole.[77]

MARFAN SYNDROME

Marfan syndrome (MFS) is a dominantly inherited connective tissue disorder. It primarily involves the ocular, cardiovascular, and skeletal systems. Classic MFS (MFS type 1 or MFS1) is caused by the deficiency of a structural extracellular matrix protein, fibrillin-1. Studies of pathogenic models have shown dysregulation of cytokine-transforming growth factor beta (TGF-β) signaling. MFS1 affects about 1:5,000 to 1:10,000 individuals.[80,81]

Patients who have clinical findings of MFS, and genetic variants in the transforming growth factor-beta receptor-1 gene (TGFβR1) and the transforming growth factor-beta receptor-2 gene (TGFβR2), are designated as having MFS type 2 (MFS2). Marfanoid habitus is also commonly seen as observed at our center, where tall statured individuals, usually males, have a positive arm span to height ratio greater than 1.0, unusually long limbs, pectus excavatum and associated ocular features of moderate to high myopia with lattice degeneration.

Ocular Findings

The "major criterion" for the ocular system is "ectopia lentis" (the dislocation or displacement of the eye's natural crystalline lens) (Figs. 5.11A and B). About 50% of patients have lens dislocation, with the dislocation position described as superior and temporal. Ectopia lentis may be present at birth or develop in childhood or adolescence.

"Minor criteria" for the ocular system are as follows (At least 2 minor criteria must be present):

- Flat cornea (as measured by keratometry)
- Increased axial length of the globe (as measured by ultrasonography)
- Cataract, described as nuclear sclerotic (patients <50 years)
- Hypoplastic iris or hypoplastic ciliary muscle that causes decreased miosis
- Nearsightedness (myopia), regardless of whether or not the lens is properly positioned. Myopia is the most com-

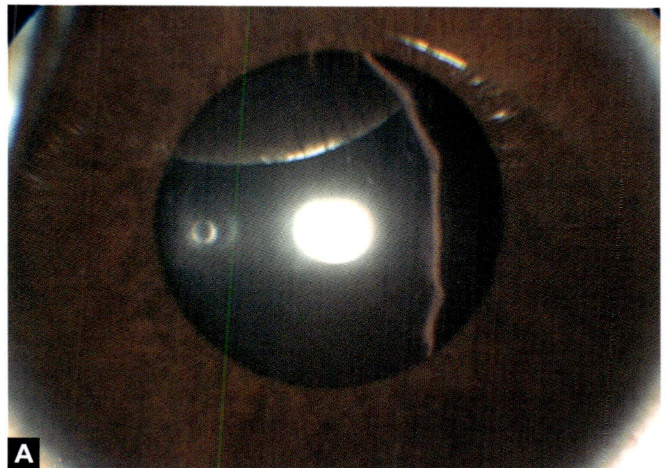 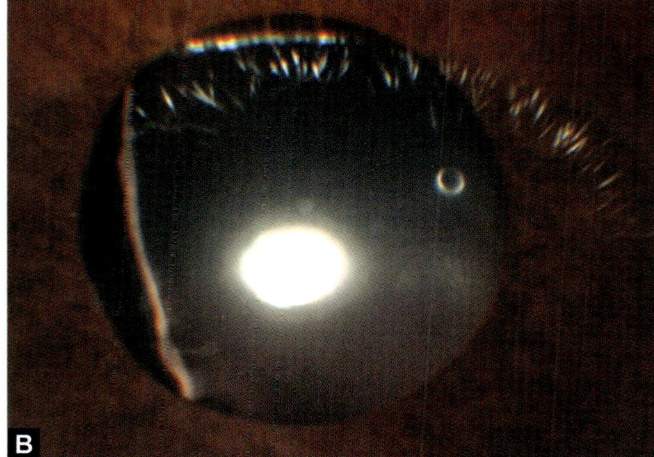

Figs. 5.11A and B: Ectopia lentis OU in a patient of Marfan's syndrome.

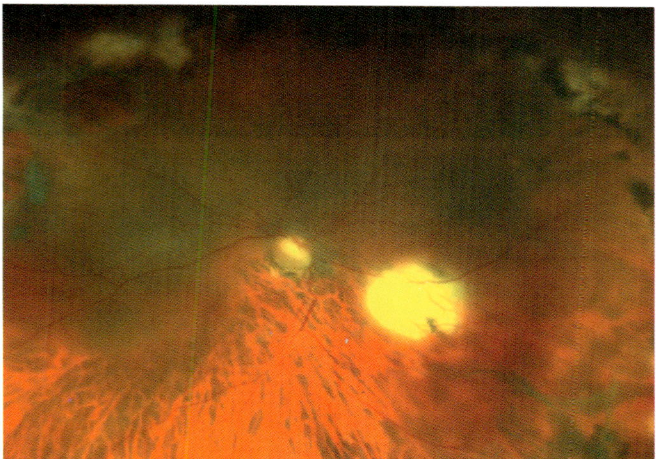

Fig. 5.12: Recurrent retinal detachment (RD) in the superior quadrant in the same patient who has ectopia lentis as in Figure 5.11A and B, post silicon oil removal, 13 years after first surgery for RD.

mon refraction error and is due to an elongated globe and amblyopia ("lazy eye")

- Glaucoma (patients <50 years)
- Retinal detachment (Fig. 5.12).

According to the "revised Ghent nosology (2010) (Ghent-2) criteria", the diagnosis of MFS depends on the following seven rules:[81]

- In the absence of family history:
  - *Aortic root dilatation Z score more than or equal to 2 and ectopia lentis is equal to MFS [Ao (Z ≥2) and EL = MFS]:* The diagnosis of MFS is confirmed when the patient demonstrates aortic root dilatation (Z ≥2 when standardized to age and body size) or dissection and ectopia lentis, irrespective of presence or absence of systemic features.
  - *Aortic root dilatation Z score more than or equal to 2 and FBN1 is equal to MFS [Ao (Z ≥2) and FBN1 = MFS]:* Even in the absence of ectopia lentis, the diagnosis of MFS can be confirmed by aortic root dilatation (Z ≥2) or dissection and the identification of a bona fide *FBN1* mutation.
  - *Aortic root dilatation Z score more than or equal to 2 and systemic score more than or equal to 7 points is equal to MFS [Ao (Z ≥2) and Syst (≥7 points) = MFS]:* Sufficient systemic findings can confirm the diagnosis of MFS when aortic root dilatation (Z ≥2) or dissection is present in the absence of ectopia lentis and the *FBN1* status is either unknown or negative (≥7 points, according to a scoring system).
  - *Ectopia lentis and FBN1 with known aortic root dilatation is equal to MFS (EL and FBN1 with known Ao = MFS):* If ectopia lentis is present with a known aortic root dilatation/dissection, the diagnosis of MFS can be confirmed by the identification of an aortic disease-associated *FBN1* mutation.
- In the presence of family history:
  - Ectopia lentis and family history of MFS = MFS
  - Systemic score ≥7 points and family history of MFS = MFS
  - Aortic root diameter (Z-score ≥2 above 20 years old, ≥3 below 20 years) and family history of MFS (as defined above) = MFS.

Scoring of Systemic Features of Marfan Syndrome

- Wrist and thumb sign–3 points (wrist or thumb sign–1 point)
- Pectus carinatum deformity–2 points (pectus excavatum or chest asymmetry–1 point)
- Hindfoot deformity–2 points (plain pes planus–1 point)
- Protrusio acetabuli–2 points

- Reduced upper segment/lower body segment ratio and increased arm/span height ratio and no severe scoliosis–1 point
- Scoliosis or thoracolumbar kyphosis–1 point
- Reduced elbow extension–1 point
- Facial features (3/5)–1 point (dolichocephaly, enophthalmos, downslanting palpebral fissures, malar hypoplasia, retrognathia)
- Pneumothorax–2 points
- Skin striae–1 point
- Myopia >3 diopters–1 point
- Mitral valve prolapse (all types)–1 point
- Dural ectasia–2 points

(The systemic features number 1–13 are used for the systemic score in the Ghent-2 nosology, where a maximum total score points of 20 points can be obtained. We number the systemic features as 1–8 and address these as "skeletal score", and the systemic features as 9–12 and address these as "non-skeletal score".)

PREVENTION OF MYOPIA AND ITS PROGRESSION

There is no definitive evidence of prevention or delay in progression of myopia by alteration of the pattern of spectacle wear, bifocals, ocular hypotensives, or contact lenses. Undercorrection leads to progression of myopia by enhancing the accommodative effort. So optimal refractive correction is necessary.[82] Progressive or bifocal lenses may also slow the progression by limiting ocular accommodation.[83] Increased time spent outdoors may be effective in preventing and delaying the onset of myopia, although it is not effective in slowing progression in eyes that are already myopic.[84]

The best results so far have been observed with atropine eye drops with a dose-effect relationship.[85,86] In a study by Chia et al, Atropine 0.01% has minimal side effects compared with atropine at 0.1% and 0.5%, and retains comparable efficacy in controlling myopia progression. More selective antimuscarinic agents such as pirenzipine are under investigation. Scleral reinforcement surgeries have also been described as a measure to slow down progression, but are usually reserved for severe progressive myopia.[87]

CONCLUSION

Pathological myopia is a challenge for the ophthalmologist because it requires comprehensive evaluation and management during course of the disease. With better understanding of the pathological progression, safer and effective treatments will develop in future.

REFERENCES

1. Morgan IG, Ohno-Matsui K, Saw SM. Myopia. Lancet. 2012; 379(9827):1739-48.
2. Miller DG, Singerman LJ. Natural history of choroidal neovascularization in high myopia. Curr Opin Ophthalmology. 2001;12(3): 222-4.
3. Hayashi K, Ohno-Matsui K, Shimada N, et al. Long-term pattern of progression of myopic maculopathy: a natural history study. Ophthalmology. 2010;117(8):1595-611,1611.
4. Curtin BJ, Karlin DB. Axial length measurements and fundus changes of the myopic eye. Am J Ophthalmology. 1971;71(1 Pt 1): 42-53.
5. Wong TY, Ferreira A, Hughes R, et al. Epidemiology and disease burden of pathologic myopia and myopic choroidal neovascularization: an evidence-based systematic review. Am J Ophthalmology. 2014;157(1):9-25.
6. Grossniklaus HE, Green WR. Pathologic findings in pathologic myopia. Retina Phila Pa. 1992;12(2):127-33.
7. Ohno-Matsui K, Kawasaki R, Jonas JB, et al. International photographic classification and grading system for myopic maculopathy. Am J Ophthalmology. 2015;159(5):877-83.
8. Saw SM. How blinding is pathological myopia? Br J Ophthalmology. 2006;90(5):525-6.
9. Liu HH, Xu L, Wang YX, et al. Prevalence and progression of myopic retinopathy in Chinese adults: the Beijing Eye Study. Ophthalmology. 2010;117(9):1763-8.
10. Vongphanit J, Mitchell P, Wang JJ. Prevalence and progression of myopic retinopathy in an older population. Ophthalmology. 2002;109(4):704-11.
11. Asakuma T, Yasuda M, Ninomiya T, et al. Prevalence and risk factors for myopic retinopathy in a Japanese population: the Hisayama Study. Ophthalmology. 2012;119(9):1760-5.
12. Saxena R, Vashist P, Tandon R, et al. Prevalence of myopia and its risk factors in urban school children in Delhi: the North India Myopia Study (NIM Study). PloS One. 2015;10(2):e0117349.
13. Buch H, Vinding T, La Cour M, et al. Prevalence and causes of visual impairment and blindness among 9980 Scandinavian adults: the Copenhagen City Eye Study. Ophthalmology. 2004;111(1): 53-61.
14. Xu L, Wang Y, Li Y, et al. Causes of blindness and visual impairment in urban and rural areas in Beijing: the Beijing Eye Study. Ophthalmology. 2006;113(7):1134.
15. Cotter SA, Varma R, Ying-Lai M, et al. Causes of low vision and blindness in adult Latinos: the Los Angeles Latino Eye Study. Ophthalmology. 2006;113(9):1574-82.
16. Jacobsen N, Jensen H, Goldschmidt E. Does the level of physical activity in university students influence development and progression of myopia?--a 2-year prospective cohort study. Invest Ophthalmology Vis Sci. 2008;49(4):1322-7.
17. Lyhne N, Sjolie AK, Kyvik KO, et al. The importance of genes and environment for ocular refraction and its determiners: a population based study among 20-45 year old twins. Br J Ophthalmology [Internet]. 2001;85(12):1470-6.
18. Paluru P, Ronan SM, Heon E, et al. New locus for autosomal dominant high myopia maps to the long arm of chromosome 17. Invest Ophthalmology Vis Sci. 2003;44:1830-6.
19. Young TL, Ronan SM, Alvear AB, et al. A second locus for familial high myopia maps to chromosome 12q. Am J Hum Genet. 1998;63(5):1419-24.
20. Ibay G, Doan B, Reider L, et al. Candidate high myopia loci on chromosomes 18p and 12q do not play a major role in susceptibility to common myopia. BMC Med Genet. 2004;5(1):20.
21. Mutti DO, Semina E, Marazita M, et al. Genetic loci for pathological myopia are not associated with juvenile myopia. Am J Med Genet. 2002;112(4):355-60.
22. Ashton GC. Segregation analysis of ocular refraction and myopia. Hum Hered. 1985;35:232-9.
23. Yap M, Wu M, Liu ZM, et al. Role of heredity in the genesis of myopia. Ophthalmology Physiol Opt. 1993;13:316-9.

24. Dirani M, Chamberlain M, Shekar SN, et al. Heritability of refractive error and ocular biometrics: the Genes in Myopia (GEM) twin study. Invest Ophthalmology Vis Sci. 2006;47(11):4756-61.

25. Daubs J. Environmental factors in the epidemiology of malignant myopia. Am J Optom Physiol Opt. 1982;59(3):271-7.

26. Daubs JG. Some geographic, environmental and nutritive concomitants of malignant myopia. Ophthalmic Physiol Opt J Br Coll Ophthalmic Opt Optom. 1984;4(2):143-9.

27. Jones LA, Sinnott LT, Mutti DO, et al. Parental history of myopia, sports and outdoor activities, and future myopia. Invest Ophthalmology Vis Sci. 2007;48(8):3524-32.

28. Sherwin JC, Reacher MH, Keogh RH, et al. The association between time spent outdoors and myopia in children and adolescents: a systematic review and meta-analysis. Ophthalmology. 2012;119(10):2141-51.

29. Silva R. Myopic maculopathy: a review. Ophthalmology J Int Ophtalmol Int J Ophthalmology Z Augenheilkd. 2012;228(4): 197-213.

30. Curtin BJ. The Myopias: Basic Science and Clinical Management. Philadelphia, PA: Harper & Row; 1985.

31. Siegwart JT, Norton TT. Perspective: how might emmetropization and genetic factors produce myopia in normal eyes? Optom Vis Sci. 2011;88(3):E365-72.

32. Hornbeak DM, Young TL. Myopia genetics: a review of current research and emerging trends. Curr Opin Ophthalmology. 2009;20(5):356-62.

33. Wakabayashi T, Ikuno Y. Choroidal filling delay in choroidal neovascularization due to pathological myopia. Br J Ophthalmology. 2010;94(5):611-5.

34. Wallman J, Turkel J, Trachtman J. Extreme myopia produced by modest change in early visual experience. Science. 1978 29;201(4362):1249-51.

35. Wallman J, Wildsoet C, Xu A, et al. Moving the retina: choroidal modulation of refractive state. Vision Res. 1995;35(1):37-50.

36. Wallman J, Winawer J. Homeostasis of eye growth and the question of myopia. Neuron. 2004 19;43(4):447-68.

37. Kobayashi K, Ohno-Matsui K, Kojima A, et al. Fundus characteristics of high myopia in children. Jpn J Ophthalmology. 2005;49(4):306-11.

38. Spaide RF. Staphyloma: Part 1. In: Spaide RF, Ohno-Matsui K, Yannuzzi LA. (Eds). Pathologic Myopia. New York: Springer; 2014. pp. 167-76.

39. Curtin BJ. The posterior staphyloma of pathologic myopia. Trans Am Ophthalmology Soc. 1977;75:67-86.

40. Hsiang HW, Ohno-Matsui K, Shimada N, et al. Clinical characteristics of posterior staphyloma in eyes with pathologic myopia. Am J Ophthalmology. 2008;146(1):102-10.

41. Steidl SM, Pruett RC. Macular complications associated with posterior staphyloma. Am J Ophthalmology. 1997;123(2):181-7.

42. Moriyama M, Ohno-Matsui K, Futagami S, et al. Morphology and long-term changes of choroidal vascular structure in highly myopic eyes with and without posterior staphyloma. Ophthalmology. 2007;114(9):1755-62.

43. Ellabban AA, Tsujikawa A, Muraoka Y, et al. Dome-shaped macular configuration: longitudinal changes in the sclera and choroid by swept-source optical coherence tomography over two years. Am J Ophthalmology. 2014;158(5):1062-70.

44. Avila MP, Weiter JJ, Jalkh AE, et al. Natural history of choroidal neovascularization in degenerative myopia. Ophthalmology. 1984;91(12):1573-81.

45. Ohno-Matsui K, Yoshida T, Futagami S, et al. Patchy atrophy and lacquer cracks predispose to the development of choroidal neovascularization in pathological myopia. Br J Ophthalmology. 2003;87(5):570-3.

46. Fujiwara T, Imamura Y, Margolis R, et al. Enhanced depth imaging optical coherence tomography of the choroid in highly myopic eyes. Am J Ophthalmology. 2009;148(3):445-50.

47. Ikuno Y, Sayanagi K, Soga K, et al. Lacquer crack formation and choroidal neovascularization in pathologic myopia. Retina Phila Pa. 2008;28(8):1124-31.

48. Ohno-Matsui K, Morishima N, Ito M, et al. Indocyanine green angiographic findings of lacquer cracks in pathologic myopia. Jpn J Ophthalmology. 1998;42(4):293-9.

49. Ohno-Matsui K, Ito M, Tokoro T. Subretinal bleeding without choroidal neovascularization in pathologic myopia. A sign of new lacquer crack formation. Retina Phila Pa. 1996;16(3):196-202.

50. Levy JH, Pollock HM, Curtin BJ. The Fuchs' spot: an ophthalmoscopic and fluorescein angiographic study. Ann Ophthalmology. 1977;9(11):1433-43.

51. Ikuno Y, Jo Y, Hamasaki T, et al. Ocular risk factors for choroidal neovascularization in pathologic myopia. Invest Ophthalmology Vis Sci. 2010;51(7):3721-5.

52. Cohen SY, Laroche A, Leguen Y, et al. Etiology of choroidal neovascularization in young patients. Ophthalmology. 1996;103(8):1241-4.

53. Neelam K, Cheung CMG, Ohno-Matsui K, et al. Choroidal neovascularization in pathological myopia. Prog Retin Eye Res. 2012;31(5):495-525.

54. Chan WM, Ohji M, Lai TYY, et al. Choroidal neovascularization in pathological myopia: an update in management. Br J Ophthalmology. 2005;89(11):1522-8.

55. Miyata M, Ooto S, Hata M, et al. Detection of myopic choroidal neovascularization using optical coherence tomography angiography. Am J Ophthalmology. 2016;165:108-14.

56. Yoshida T, Ohno-Matsui K, Yasuzumi K, et al. Myopic choroidal neovascularization: a 10-year follow-up. Ophthalmology. 2003;110(7):1297-305.

57. Tufail A, Narendran N, Patel PJ, et al. Ranibizumab in myopic choroidal neovascularization: the 12-month results from the REPAIR study. Ophthalmology. 2013;120(9):1944-5.

58. Wolf S, Balciuniene VJ, Laganovska G, et al. RADIANCE: a randomized controlled study of ranibizumab in patients with choroidal neovascularization secondary to pathologic myopia. Ophthalmology. 2014;121(3):682-92.

59. Verteporfin in Photodynamic Therapy Study Group. Photodynamic therapy of subfoveal choroidal neovascularization in pathologic myopia with verteporfin. 1-year results of a randomized clinical trial--VIP report no. 1. Ophthalmology. 2001;108(5):841-52.

60. Takano M, Kishi S. Foveal retinoschisis and retinal detachment in severely myopic eyes with posterior staphyloma. Am J Ophthalmology. 1999;128(4):472-6.

61. Panozzo G, Mercanti A. Vitrectomy for myopic traction maculopathy. Arch Ophthalmology Chic Ill 1960. 2007;125(6):767-72.

62. Baba T, Ohno-Matsui K, Futagami S, et al. Prevalence and characteristics of foveal retinal detachment without macular hole in high myopia. Am J Ophthalmology. 2003;135(3):338-42.

63. Gohil R, Sivaprasad S, Han LT, et al. Myopic foveoschisis: a clinical review. Eye Lond Engl. 2015;29(5):593-601.

64. Sayanagi K, Morimoto Y, Ikuno Y, et al. Spectral-domain optical coherence tomographic findings in myopic foveoschisis. Retina Phila Pa. 2010;30(4):623-8.

65. Panozzo G, Mercanti A. Optical coherence tomography findings in myopic traction maculopathy. Arch Ophthalmology Chic Ill 1960. 2004;122(10):1455-60.

66. Wu PC, Chen YJ, Chen YH, et al. Factors associated with foveoschisis and foveal detachment without macular hole in high myopia. Eye Lond Engl. 2009;23(2):356-61.

67. Fang X, Weng Y, Xu S, et al. Optical coherence tomographic characteristics and surgical outcome of eyes with myopic foveoschisis. Eye. 2008 3;23(6):1336-42.

68. Gaucher D, Haouchine B, Tadayoni R, et al. Long-term follow-up of high myopic foveoschisis: natural course and surgical outcome. Am J Ophthalmology. 2007;143(3):455-62.

69. Benhamou N, Massin P, Haouchine B, et al. Macular retinoschisis in highly myopic eyes. Am J Ophthalmology. 2002;133(6):794-800.

70. Sayanagi K, Ikuno Y, Tano Y. Tractional internal limiting membrane detachment in highly myopic eyes. Am J Ophthalmology. 2006;142(5):850-2.

71. Ikuno Y, Gomi F, Tano Y. Potent retinal arteriolar traction as a possible cause of myopic foveoschisis. Am J Ophthalmology. 2005;139(3):462-7.

72. Sayanagi K, Ikuno Y, Gomi F, et al. Retinal vascular microfolds in highly myopic eyes. Am J Ophthalmology. 2005;139(4):658-63.

73. Shimada N, Ohno-Matsui K, Yoshida T, et al. Progression from macular retinoschisis to retinal detachment in highly myopic eyes is associated with outer lamellar hole formation. Br J Ophthalmology. 2008;92(6):762-4.

74. Kumar A, Ravani R, Mehta A, et al. Outcomes of microscope-integrated intraoperative optical coherence tomography-guided center-sparing internal limiting membrane peeling for myopic traction maculopathy: a novel technique. Int Ophthalmology. 2017 Jul 4.

75. Mateo C, Gómez-Resa MV, Burés-Jelstrup A, et al. Surgical outcomes of macular buckling techniques for macular retinoschisis in highly myopic eyes. Saudi J Ophthalmology. 2013;27(4):235-9.

76. Spencer LM, Foos RY. Paravascular vitreoretinal attachments. Role in retinal tears. Arch Ophthalmology Chic Ill 1960. 1970;84(5):557-64.

77. Kobayashi H, Kobayashi K, Okinami S. Macular hole and myopic refraction. Br J Ophthalmology. 2002;86(11):1269-73.

78. Morita H, Ideta H, Ito K, et al. Tanaka S. Causative factors of retinal detachment in macular holes. Retina Phila Pa. 1991;11(3):281-4.

79. Kumar A, Kakkar P, Ravani R, et al. Utility of microscope integrated optical coherence tomography (MIOCT) in the treatment of myopic macular hole retinal detachment. BMJ case rep. 2017;2017.

80. Bolar N, Van Laer L, Loeys BL. Marfan syndrome: from gene to therapy. Curr Opin Pediatr. 2012;24(4):498-504.

81. Loeys BL, Dietz HC, Braverman AC, et al. The revised Ghent nosology for the Marfan syndrome. J Med Genet. 2010;47(7):476-485.

82. Chung K, Mohidin N, O'Leary DJ. Undercorrection of myopia enhances rather than inhibits myopia progression. Vision Res. 2002;42(22):2555-9.

83. Cheng D, Woo GC, Drobe B, et al. Effect of bifocal and prismatic bifocal spectacles on myopia progression in children: three-year results of a randomized clinical trial. JAMA Ophthalmology. 2014;132(3):258-64.

84. Xiong S, Sankaridurg P, Naduvilath T, et al. Time spent in outdoor activities in relation to myopia prevention and control: a meta-analysis and systematic review. Acta Ophthalmology (Copenh). 2017;95(6):551-66.

85. Chia A, Chua WH, Cheung YB, et al. Atropine for the treatment of childhood myopia: safety and efficacy of 0.5%, 0.1%, and 0.01% doses (Atropine for the Treatment of Myopia 2). Ophthalmology. 2012;119(2):347-54.

86. Li SM, Wu SS, Kang MT, et al. Atropine slows myopia progression more in Asian than white children by meta-analysis. Optom Vis Sci Off Publ Am Acad Optom. 2014;91(3):342-50.

87. Avetisov ES, Tarutta EP, Iomdina EN, et al. Nonsurgical and surgical methods of sclera reinforcement in progressive myopia. Acta Ophthalmology Scand. 1997;75(6):618-23.

Chapter 6

Retinitis Pigmentosa and Allied Disorders

Vinod Kumar, Karthikeya R, Raghav Ravani, Annu Chohan, Atul Kumar

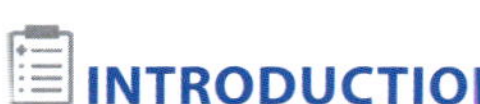 INTRODUCTION

Retinitis pigmentosa (RP) refers to a group of hereditary, clinically, and genetically diverse disorders of progressive retinal dysfunction characterized by photoreceptor, retinal pigment epithelium, and eventually diffuse retinal atrophy. The term RP first used by Donders[1] in 1857. Though RP is not primarily an inflammatory disorder, the terminology is still widely used. Several terms have been used in the past to describe RP such as pigmentary retinopathy, rod cone dystrophy and tapetoretinal degeneration.

CLASSIC RETINITIS PIGMENTOSA

Retinitis pigmentosa is termed typical RP if it occurs in isolation. In the presence of associated systemic disease, the terminology used is syndromic RP. The approximate prevalence of typical RP worldwide is 1 in 5,000.

Genetics

Retinitis pigmentosa can be inherited in autosomal recessive (AR), autosomal dominant (AD) or X-linked (XL) manner though it occurs in isolated sporadic forms as well. The XL pattern is the least common but is the most severe form of RP. Autosomal dominant RP on the other hand is the mildest form and these patients tend to retain useful central vision for long. Approximately, 46 genes associated with RP have been identified, most of them causing AR RP.[2]

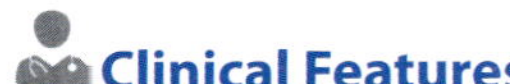 Clinical Features

Night blindness is the most common presenting feature in patients with RP. The age of onset of this symptom depends upon the type of inheritance. While most patients with AR and XL RP present within the first or early second decade, patients with AD RP tend to present in the second half of third decade.[3] Patients, who live in well-lighted urban areas, often present late.

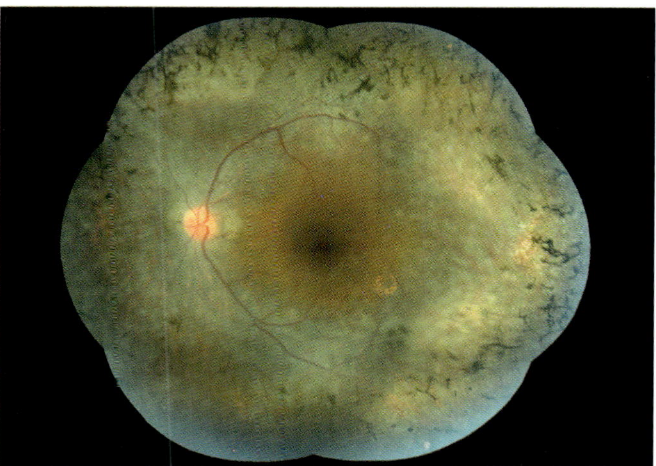

Fig. 6.1: Color montage of left eye of a patient with retinitis pigmentosa showing arterial attenuation, bony spicule pigmentation, and mild optic disc pallor.

Gradual progressive contraction of the visual field (VF) is the second most common symptom of RP. Relatives often complain that the patients bump into objects frequently, especially at night. Superior field is affected first and VF loss tends to be symmetrical between the two eyes.[4] It is important to assess the VFs in RP, as it may lead to visual handicap in spite of good central visual acuity.

The central vision may be affected due to a host of abnormalities seen in the macula, as would be discussed in examination. Color vision gets affected in the later stages of disease especially if central vision is affected. Patients may also complain of photopsia or floaters.

The classical triad of findings in patients with RP includes arterial attenuation, bony spicule pigmentation, and waxy pallor of the disc in that order (Fig. 6.1). The fundus in the initial stages may virtually be normal or show only mild retinal pigment epithelium (RPE) granularity or mottling in the midperiphery. As the disease progresses, photoreceptors and

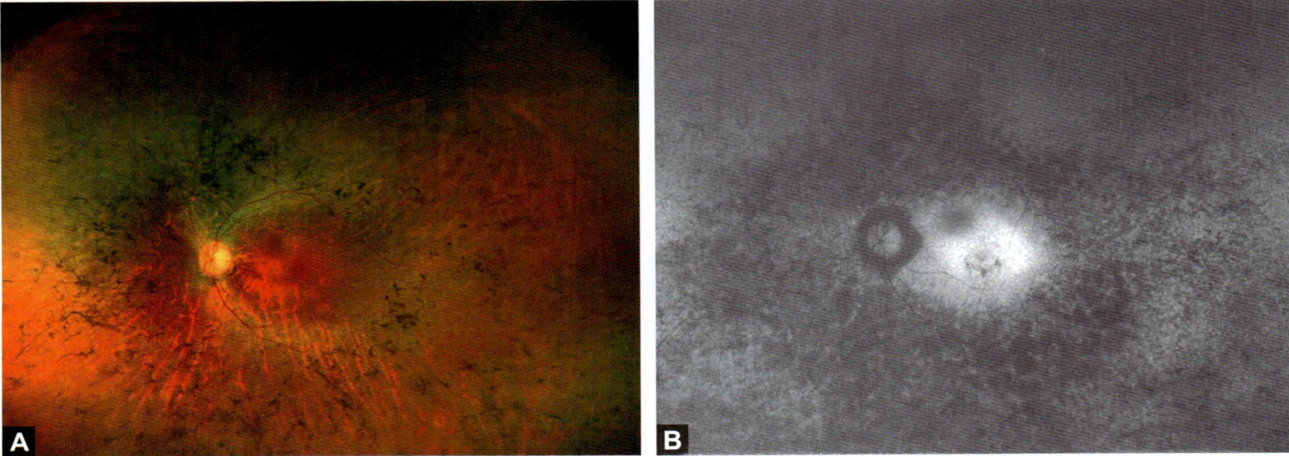

Figs. 6.2A and B: (A) Retinitis pigmentosa showing bony corpuscular pigmentation and (B) lesional hypo-autofluorescence on Fundus autofluorescence imaging.

RPE undergo degeneration leading to pigment release. This pigment migrates into the retina giving characteristic bony spicule pigmentation that has a perivascular distribution. The pigment deposition progresses both centripetally and centrifugally and reaches up to the vascular arcades.

Retinitis pigmentosa without bony spicules was earlier known as "*RP sine pigmento*". Now it is accepted that absence of pigment (Figs. 6.2A and B) is just a stage in the development of typical RP. Virtually all RP would have bony spicule pigmentation sooner or later. The RPE gradually undergoes atrophy and large choroidal vessels become discernable. The optic disc, which may show hyperemia in early stages, becomes pale over a period of time and eventually undergoes atrophy. The surface gliosis provides it a typical waxy pale look.

It was earlier considered that macula is spared in RP. With growing knowledge, several abnormalities have been identified in the macula in patients with RP. These include cystoid macular edema (CME) (Fig. 6.3), epiretinal membrane, and macular atrophy.[5] In addition, macular hole and macular pigment abnormalities may also be encountered.

Other Ocular Features

Associated ocular findings are common in patients with RP. These include:

- *Posterior subcapsular cataract (PSC):*[6] It is seen in 35–50% of RP patients. The age at which cataract occurs is very variable
- High myopia and astigmatism[7]
- Primary open angle glaucoma and keratoconus
- Vitreous cells are common and indicate ensuing rapid photoreceptor degeneration. Fine pigment-like dusting is also common.
- Optic disc drusen (Figs. 6.4A and B) (seen in 10% of RP patients)[8]
- Coats-like response[9] and vasoproliferative tumor have also been reported.

Investigations

Electrophysiology

Electroretinography (ERG) is an important test in the diagnosis and management of patients with RP. Scotopic and

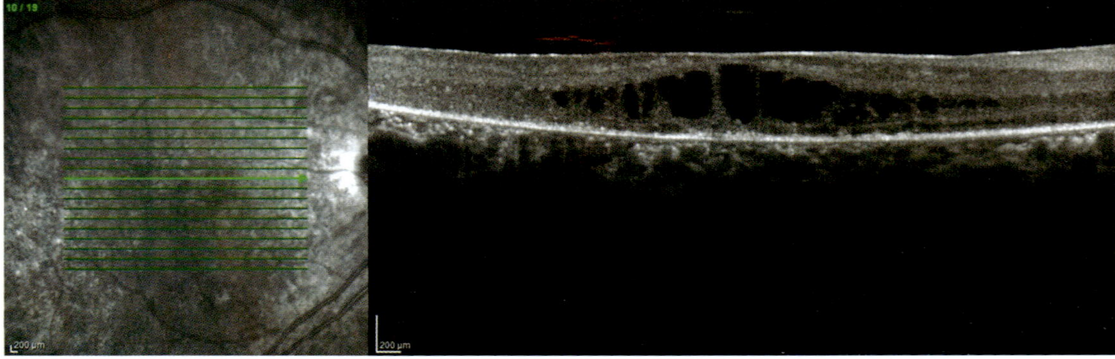

Fig. 6.3: Spectral-domain optical coherence tomography of macula of a patient with retinitis pigmentosa showing cystoid macular edema.

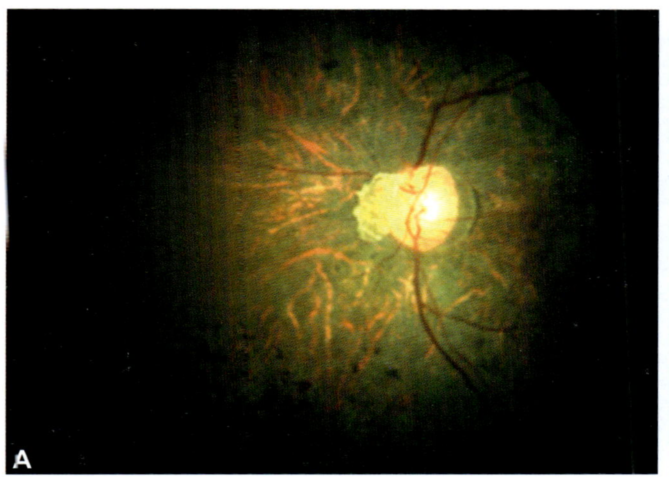 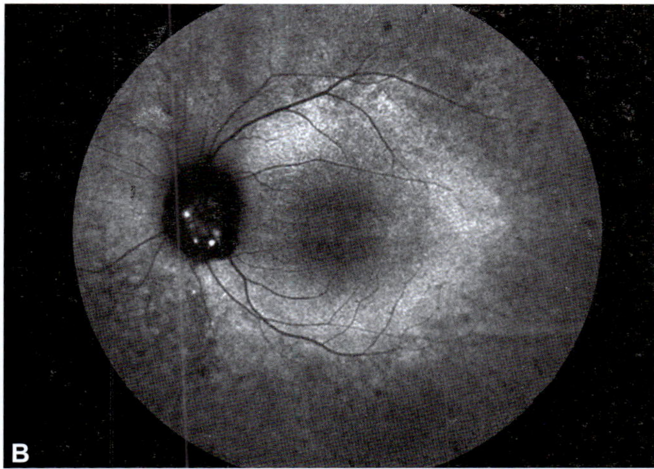

Figs. 6.4A and B: (A) Optic disc drusen in a patient with retinitis pigmentosa; (B) Fundus autofluorescence of another patient of retinitis pigmentosa with optic disc drusen.

combined responses are often severely diminished even when fundus may seem normal. Though the cones are not affected initially, cone responses are also often depressed eventually. Subsequently, both cone and rod responses are undetectable and ERG becomes extinguished. In electrooculogram) (EOG), slow and fast oscillations of resting potential induced by light are diminished in patients with RP.

Visual Fields

Visual fields are an important marker of the disease progression and are also useful to quantitate the visual handicap. The VF changes correlate with the fundus findings. Initially, relative scotoma is seen in mid-periphery. These become denser with disease progression and coalesce to form typical ring scotoma (Fig. 6.5) leaving behind only a central tunnel of vision (tubular or tunnel vision). Central VF may also be affected when macular involvement occurs.

Fluorescein Angiography and Optical Coherence Tomography

Fluorescein angiography (FA) shows areas of RPE atrophy as window defects and may also be useful for detecting macular leakage if any. Optical coherence tomography (OCT) has largely replaced FA to detect macular abnormalities like outer retinal layer abnormalities, macular edema, and epiretinal membrane.[10] OCT is also very useful in monitoring the treatment response and follow-up of patients with macular edema.

Autofluorescence

It is an important tool to assess and monitor RPE damage in patients with RP.

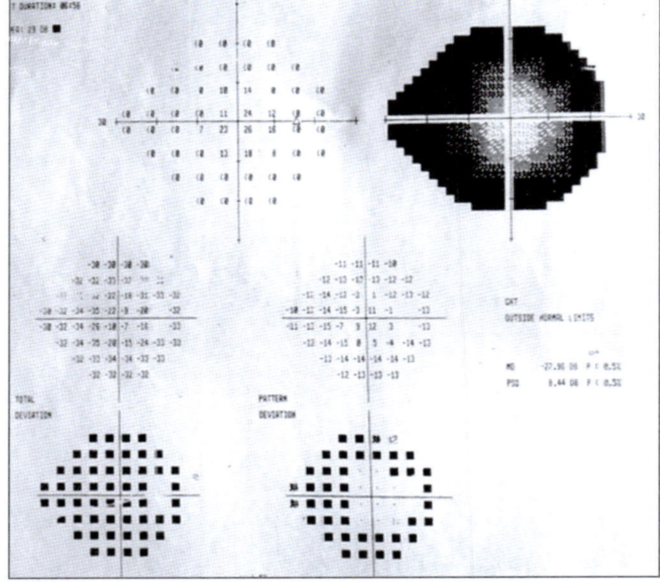

Fig. 6.5: Ring scotoma in a patient with retinitis pigmentosa.

Dark Adaptometry

Prolonged dark adaptation is seen in all types of RP irrespective of the stage of RP.

VARIANTS OF RETINITIS PIGMENTOSA

Sectoral Retinitis Pigmentosa

In this subtype of RP, the pigmentary changes are limited to a sector of retina, either a quadrant or two (Fig. 6.6). The patients are usually asymptomatic. VF changes coincide with the area involved, while ERG is frequently normal. Sectoral RP has been found to be nonprogressive.

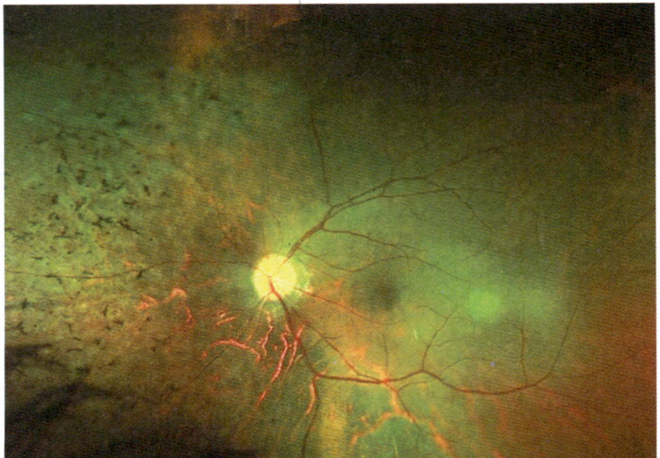

Fig. 6.6: Ultra wide field color photograph of a patient with sectoral retinitis pigmentosa showing only nasal involvement.

Unilateral Retinitis Pigmentosa

True unilateral RP is very rare. Most of these cases tend to be pseudo-RP. Two genetic scenarios may lead to true unilateral RP: carriers of XL RP and somatic mosaicism of a dominant gene for RP.

Pericentral Retinitis Pigmentosa

In this subtype of RP, the involvement is closer to the fixation. The pigmentary changes occur closer to the macula as compared to typical RP. Earlier involvement of macula may occur and hence this subtype of RP has prognostic significance.

Retinitis Punctata Albescens[11]

Retinitis punctata albescens (RPA) is subtype of RP. It is a fleck retinal degeneration (Figs. 6.7A and B) characterized by slowly progressive visual loss along with the macular atrophic degeneration. A similar appearing condition fundus albipunctatus can be differentiated by its stationary nature.

SYNDROMIC RETINITIS PIGMENTOSA

Several systemic disorders are known to occur with RP, most common being Usher syndrome. These are listed below.

Usher Syndrome (Figs. 6.8A and B)

It is an AR condition characterized by congenital deafness and typical RP. It accounts for up to 18% of cases of RP. Three clinical types are known:

- *Type 1* (most common): Severe congenital deafness, speech impairment, vestibular symptoms, and early onset RP.
- *Type 2*: Moderate congenital deafness, absence of speech and vestibular abnormalities, and late onset RP.
- *Type 3* (least common): Progressive hearing and visual loss that starts late.

Deafness in association with RP is not a diagnostic feature of Usher syndrome and is also seen in other disorders like Refsum disease, Bardet-Biedl syndrome, Cockayne syndrome, and Kearns-Sayre syndrome. It is important to distinguish these disorders before labeling the patient as Usher syndrome.

Bardet-Biedl Syndrome

It is also known as Laurence-Moon-Bardet-Biedl syndrome (Figs. 6.9A to D) has recently been named as polydactyly-obesity-kidney-eye syndrome. The disease is characterized by following features:

- Mental retardation
- Polydactyly (postaxial)/syndactyly/brachydactyly

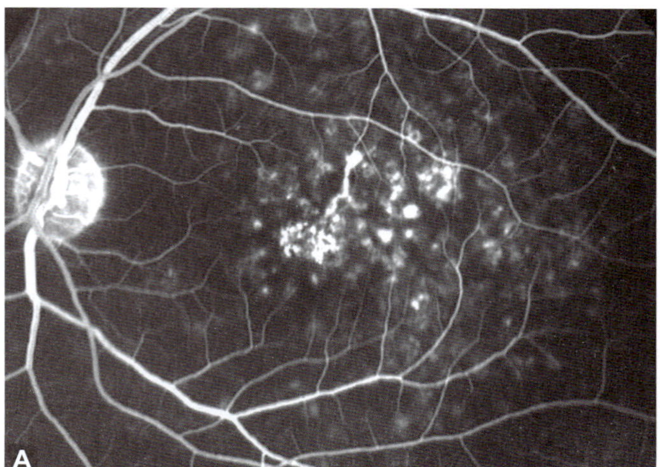
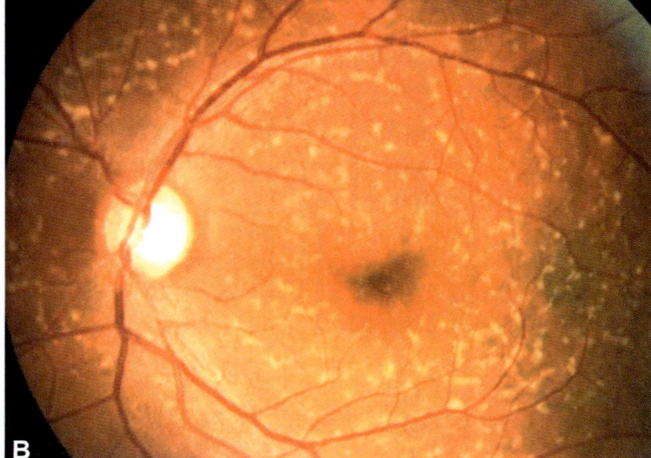

Figs. 6.7A and B: (A) Fundus fluorescence angiography; (B) Fundus photograph of eye with retinitis punctata albescens.

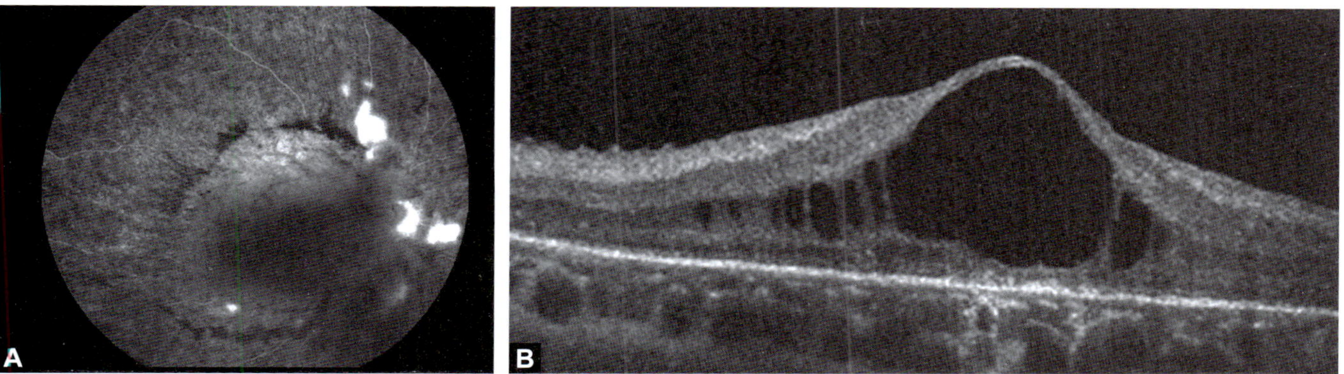

Figs. 6.8A and B: (A) Usher syndrome with retinitis pigmentosa on fluorescein angiography with associated retinal neovascularization elsewhere (NVE) for which scatter laser was done at multiple sittings; (B) Presence of cystoid macular edema on optical coherence tomography.

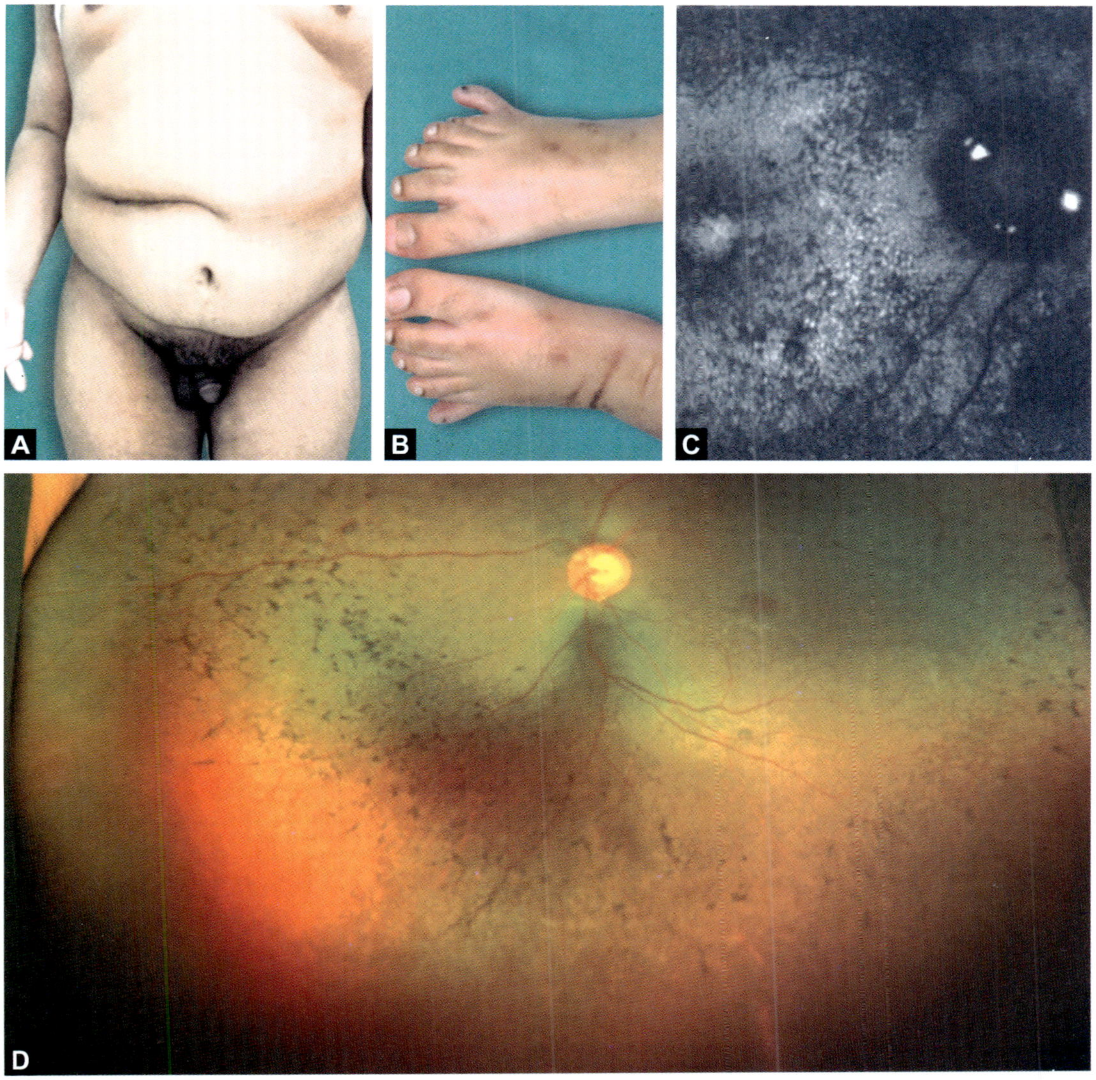

Figs. 6.9A to D: A 17-year-old male patient with Bardet-Biedl syndrome showing (A) truncal obesity and hypogenitalism, (B) polydactyly, (C) Pigment mottling at posterior pole and optic disc drusen on fundus autofluorescence (FAF) imaging and (D) Pigmentary retinopathy on widefield pseudocolor image.

- Truncal obesity
- Hypogenitalism
- Renal abnormalities.

The retinal abnormalities tend to differ from typical RP. The retinal disease is characterized by less pigmentation giving it a "sine pigmento" or RP albescence appearance. The visual loss occurs early leading to blindness by second or third decade.

Refsum Syndrome

Refsum syndrome (RS) consists of two distinct AR abnormalities in peroxisomal phytanic acid alpha-hydrolase resulting in phytanic acid accumulation all over the body. The disease is characterized by progressive neurological deficit, deafness, liver disease, and pigmentary retinopathy. Two forms are recognized:

1. *Infantile form*: Phytanic acid levels are moderately elevated and the patients have craniofacial deformities, generalized hypotony, psychomotor retardation, bleeding episodes, liver dysfunction, and severe deafness.
2. *Adult (classical) form*: It is characterized by highly elevated serum phytanic acid levels. The patients have ataxia, polyneuropathy and muscle wasting, anosmia, deafness, cardiomyopathy, skeletal abnormalities, and ichthyosis.

Both types are associated with night blindness and pigmentary retinopathy similar to RP. The progression of systemic and ocular manifestations can be limited by a diet restricted in phytanic acid content, if the disease is diagnosed early.

Other disorders like Bassen-Kornzweig syndrome (abetalipoproteinemia), Kearns-Sayre syndrome, neuronal ceroid lipofuscinoses, Leber congenital amaurosis (LCA), and progressive cone dystrophy can present with RP.

Differential Diagnosis

A variety of disorders can lead to pigmentary retinopathy (pseudo-retinitis pigmentosa), which can mimic RP. These must be suspected and ruled out in all cases with appropriate clinically relevant laboratory investigations. Common causes of pseudo-RP include:

- Rubella retinopathy
- Syphilis
- Cancer associated retinopathy
- Drug toxicities (thioridazine and chlorpromazine)
- Diffuse unilateral subacute neuroretinitis
- Post trauma, self-settled retinal detachment.

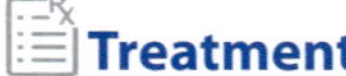 Treatment

While as of now RP is incurable, it is often possible to help patients by providing useful information and support to improve quality of their life. Correction of refractive error, cataract extraction, treatment of macular edema whenever present and low vision aids could be of great help in these patients.

Refractive errors especially myopia is common in RP and can further add to visual disability and nyctalopia. Appropriate refractive correction improves the residual central function in patients with RP.

Cataract is common in patients with RP is of frequent occurrence. PSC is the most common type. The patients with RP often benefit from cataract surgery especially those having PSC[12] and cataract surgery should not be delayed. Cataract surgery does not improve the VF, however, and has no effect on disease progression.

Cystoid macular edema is a common occurrence in RP. This can compromise the residual central vision and worsen the visual handicap. CME is more commonly picked up with the increasing use of OCT in clinical practice. Both topical and systemic carbonic anhydrase inhibitors (CAIs) work well. Initially, dorzolamide drops are used thrice a day.[13] If topical CAIs do not work, systemic acetazolamide works well (Figs. 6.10A and B). Initial dose of 500 mg/day is used followed by 250 mg/day.[14] In refractory cases, intravitreal triamcinolone acetonide,[15] bevacizumab,[16] ranibizumab or dexamethasone implants[17] can be used.

Supplementation of 15,000 IU of vitamin A has been reported to slow down the progression of RP.[18] The patients however should be monitored for hepatotoxicity and osteopenia. The potential teratogenic risks of vitamin A in pregnant women must be kept in mind. Supplementary docosahexaenoic acid (DHA) facilitates and hastens the benefit of high-dose vitamin A in the first 2 years of treatment.[19] Oral valproic acid (VPA) has been shown to improve visual acuity and multifocal electroretinogram (mfERG) amplitudes in patients with RP.[20] This has been postulated to work by mechanisms of preventing photoreceptor cell death, prevention of inflammatory damage to the retina by causing apoptosis of microglial cells and by acting as a pharmacologic chaperone and helping the mutant rhodopsin protein to fold properly.[20]

A study to evaluate the efficacy of VPA in RP was recently carried out at our center. 15 patients with typical RP received 500 mg of oral VPA once a day for 1 year (group 1); 15 patients with typical RP (group 2) were taken as controls and received no treatment.

Patients receiving VPA showed a statistically significant improvement in median best-corrected visual acuity (BCVA) from baseline. A slight deterioration in median BCVA was noted in the control group. mfERG and VER also showed a significant improvement in amplitude and latency/implicit time in patients receiving VPA. This was absent in the control group.[20]

ARTIFICIAL VISION IN RETINITIS PIGMENTOSA

Globally, about 400,000 people are legally blind due to RP and role of artificial retina or electronic prosthesis in RP has been studied widely. Epiretinal implants have shown better results out of all these types. Epiretinal implant Argus II, popularly known as "Bionic Eye", has shown promising results in patients

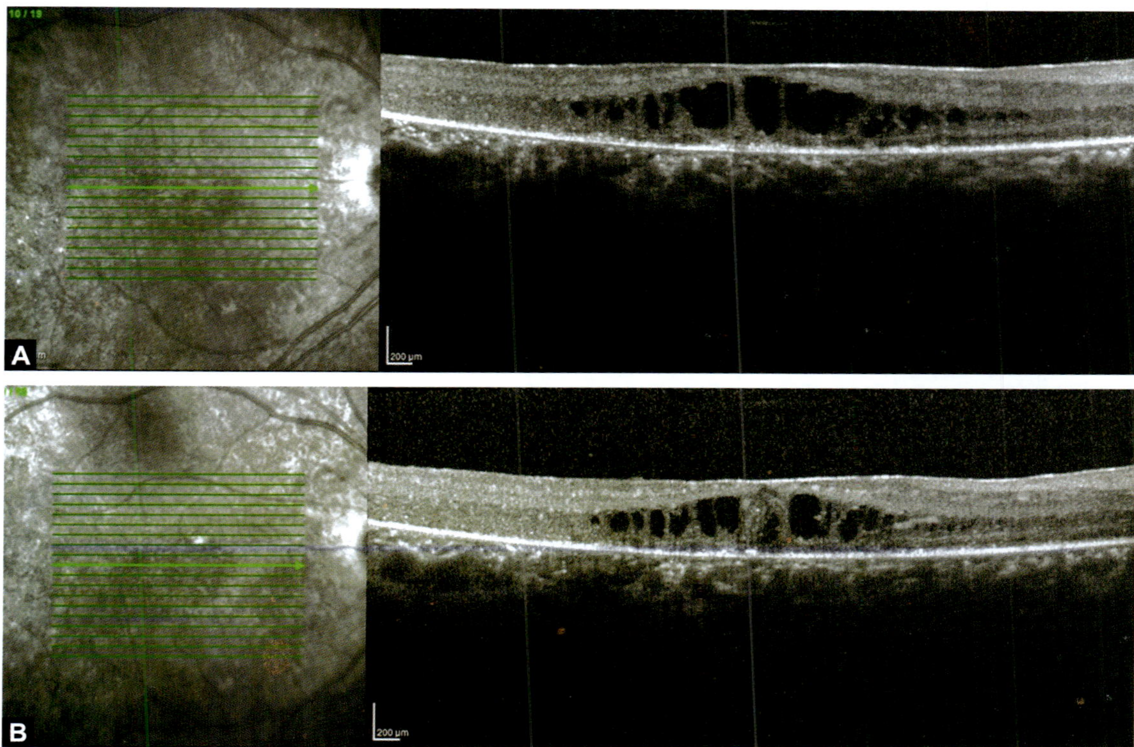

Figs. 6.10A and B: Retinitis pigmentosa with cystoid macular edema (A) before and (B) after treatment with oral acetazolamide.

with RP and has got regulatory approval in both Europe and the USA.[21] The RP patients implanted with Argus II implant were shown to perceive phosphenes when stimulated with lights.

Eligibility for the Argus II: The Argus II is implanted in the worse-seeing eye. It is used in patients with severe RP meeting the following criteria:

- Age 25 or older
- Perception of light without projection of rays or no light perception in both eyes after confirmation of intact functioning of inner retinal layer
- History of some useful form vision in the past
- Aphakic or pseudophakic
- Willing to receive postimplant clinical follow-up and visual rehabilitation.

The Argus II consists of a miniature camera fitted in a pair of glasses that converts video images into electrical impulses. These impulses are wirelessly transmitted to the epiretinal implant (array of electrodes) which in turn stimulates the viable retinal cells which then transmit signals via optic pathway to form an image.

Genome Editing

Clustered Regularly Interspaced Short Palindromic Repeat (CRISPR)/Cas9 is a new gene-editing technology to repair genetic mutation in RP. CRISPR/Cas9 is used to repair the defective gene in the stem cell derived from the skin of the patient with RP.[22] The defective gene is cut and a new gene pasted by specialized proteins. These modified cells when transplanted back into the same patient has the potential of transforming into healthy retinal cell and may help improve vision loss, especially in patients with XL form of RP. The stem cells being autologous have reduced chances of rejection. This technology is yet to be approved for human use.

LEBER CONGENITAL AMAUROSIS

Theodore Leber first described this entity in 1869.[23] LCA is a group of inherited retinal dystrophies, which usually present with severe visual loss in early childhood.[24] LCA is the most common genetic cause of blindness and visual impairment in infants and children.[25]

Genetics

Leber congenital amaurosis is both genetically as well as clinically heterogeneous. It is an AR condition and up to 20 causative mutations have been identified on chromosomes 17, 1, 14, 6, and 7.[26]

 Clinical Features

Leber congenital amaurosis patients typically present with severe visual loss in infancy or early childhood. In addition, the parents may give history of roving eye movements and frequent eye poking by the child. Though night blindness is common, some patients report aversion to light. The visual loss in these patients is severe with visual acuity ranging from 6/60 to light perception.[27] Nystagmus is another common feature in this condition. The pupillary light reflexes are either severely diminished or abolished. High hypermetropia is commonly seen in LCA, though myopia has also been reported.[28] Children with LCA frequently rub or poke their eyes to mechanically stimulate the photoreceptors so as to get sensation of light. This phenomenon is known as Franceschetti's oculo-digital sign and commonly leads to enophthalmos in these children due to atrophy of orbital fat.[29] Though it is considered pathognomonic of LCA, it may be observed in other diseases with poor vision as well.

Fundus findings may vary from near normal or mild retinal involvement to severe pigmentary changes with macular coloboma. Especially in the early stages fundus examination may be normal despite a very poor visual function. Pigment epithelium granularity appears which progresses to pigmentary retinopathy and arteriolar attenuation (Fig. 6.11). In advanced stages, the fundus appearance may be similar to RP. Pigmented macular coloboma may also be seen but these do not represent true macular coloboma (Figs. 6.11 and 6.12). Other fundus findings may include marbled fundus, peripheral nummular pigmentation, disc edema, and retinal vasculitis.

Electrophysiological tests including ERG and visual evoked potential (VEP) are severely depressed or extinguished. Typical ocular features along with extinguished ERG lead to a clinical diagnosis of LCA. The definitive diagnosis however depends on the genetic analysis.

Other ocular associations include squint, keratoconus, keratoglobus, and cataract (Figs. 6.13A and B). Mental retardation (in up to 52% of cases),[30] stereotypic movements and behavior, deafness, renal anomalies, and skeletal and CNS abnormalities are the various systemic associations of LCA.

Common differential diagnoses for LCA are RP, achromatopsia, and congenital stationary night blindness (CSNB).

Extinguished photopic and scotopic ERG, lack of progression, and onset before 1 year of age point more toward the diagnosis of LCA.

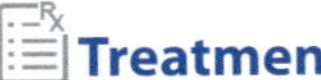

Treatment

Gene therapy trials have shown encouraging result for treatment of LCA. Subretinal injection of human *RPE65* gene along with recombinant adeno-associated virus serotype 2 (rAAV2-RPE65 vector) has shown to be safe and efficacious.[31]

To conclude, LCA is hereditary retinal dystrophy and gene therapy has shown promising result in its treatment.

CONGENITAL STATIONARY NIGHT BLINDNESS

Congenital stationary night blindness refers to a group of retinal disorders that present with a common feature of nonprogressive night blindness or difficulty in dim light. Though most of the patients otherwise have normal visual function, some forms may have myopia, nystagmus, strabismus or decreased vision. Clinical examination, ERG, dark adaptometry, and appropriate genetic testing help in identifying the subtype of CSNB.

Genetics

The wide variety of phenotypes of CSNB results from many mutations, which may be acquired in AR, AD or XL patterns. CSNB is a phenotypically and genetically heterogeneous disease resulting from mutations in 17 genes, identified so far.[32]

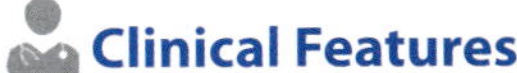

Clinical Features

On the basis of fundus appearance, CSNB is divided into two types:
1. *CSNB with normal fundus*: Patients having CSNB with normal fundus have normal visual and cone function.

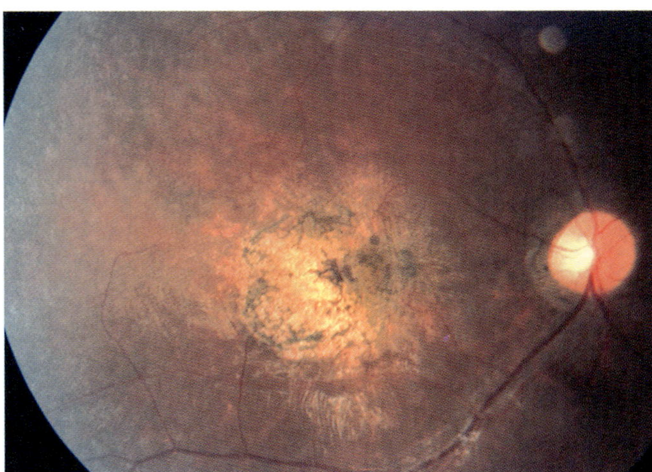

Fig. 6.11: An 18-year-old male with Leber congenital amaurosis showing pigment mottling at the macula and outside the vascular arcades.

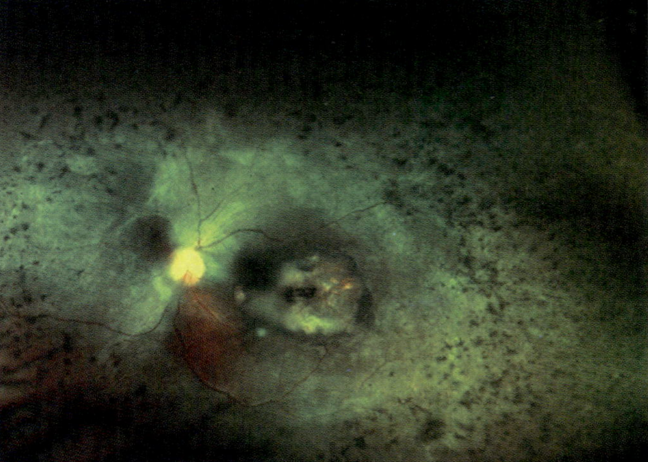

Fig. 6.12: Ultra wide field pseudo color image of left eye of a patient with Leber congenital amaurosis showing macular coloboma and pigmentary retinopathy.

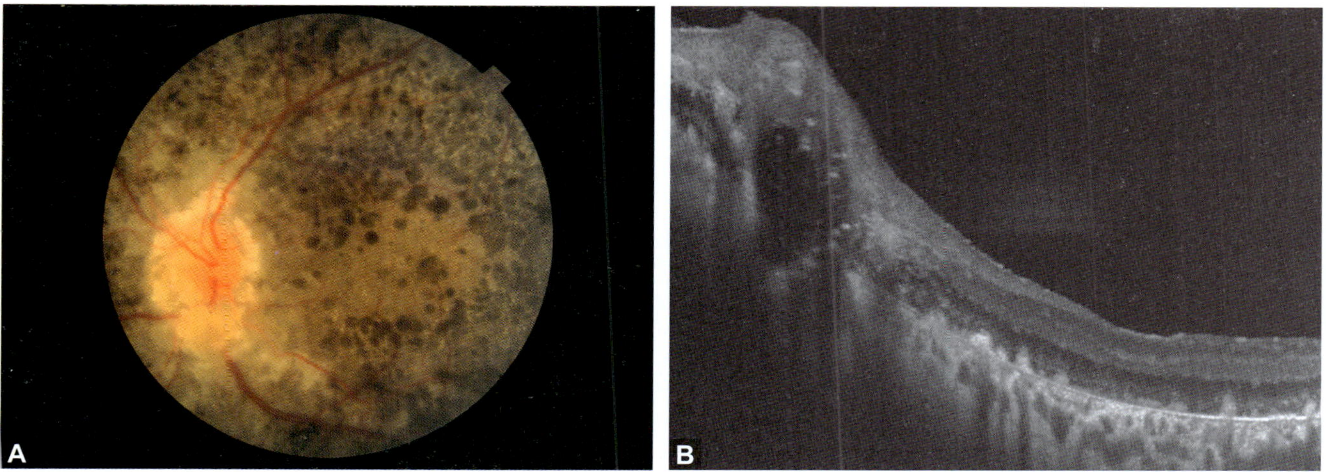

Figs. 6.13A and B: Case of Leber congenital amaurosis with (A) disc drusen, also (B) visible on swept-source optical coherence tomography imaging as hyporeflective well-defined areas.

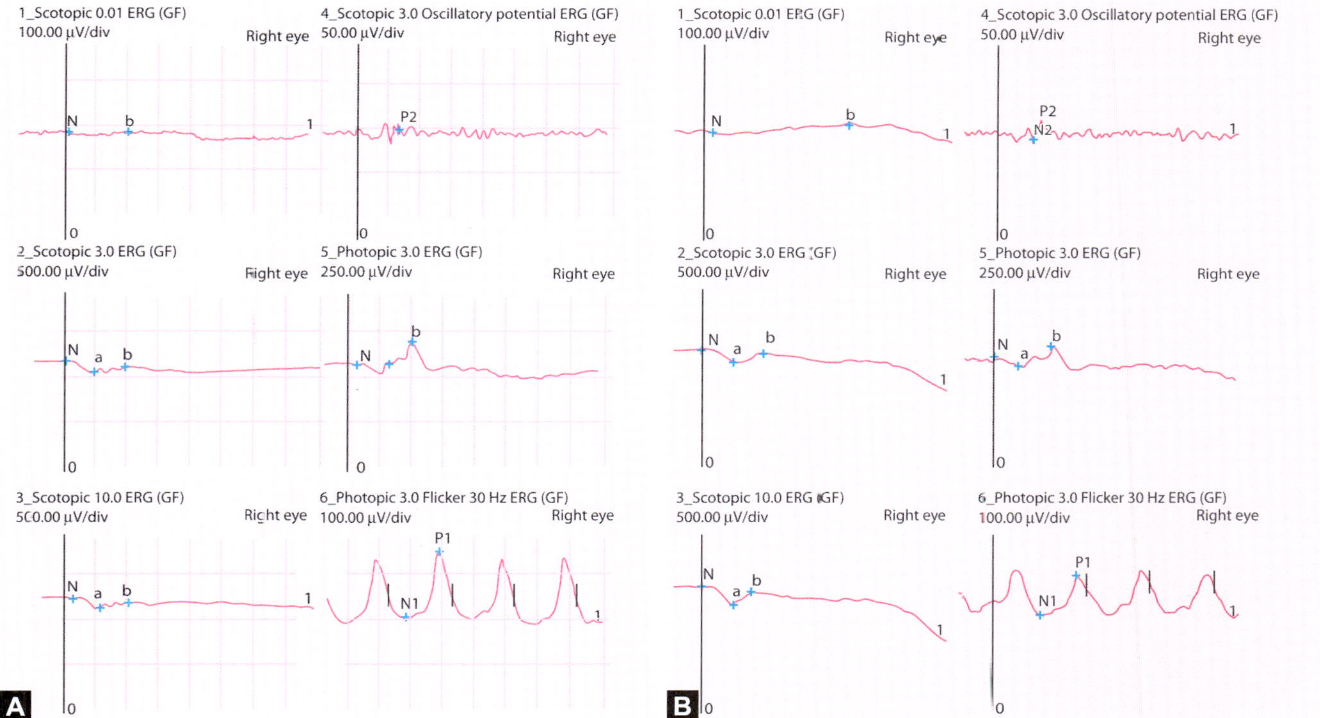

Figs. 6.14A and B: (A) Full field electroretinogram (ERG) showing extinguished scotopic responses and extinguished "a" and "b" waves on maximum bright field stimulation in dark-adapted state indicating congenital stationary night blindness (CSNB) with photoreceptor dysfunction; (B) Full field ERG showing preserved "a" wave but an absent "b" wave on maximum bright field stimulation in dark-adapted state with absent scotopic responses indicating CSNB with bipolar dysfunction.

These are further subdivided into two categories based on ERG findings:

- *Riggs-type (type 1 or CSNB with photoreceptor dysfunction)*: The patients in this type of CSNB have extinguished scotopic responses and also extinguished "a" and "b" waves on maximum bright field stimulation in dark-adapted state (Fig. 6.14A). This points toward primary photoreceptor dysfunction.
- *Schubert-Bornschein (type 2 or CSNB with bipolar cell dysfunction)*: In this type, patients have a preserved

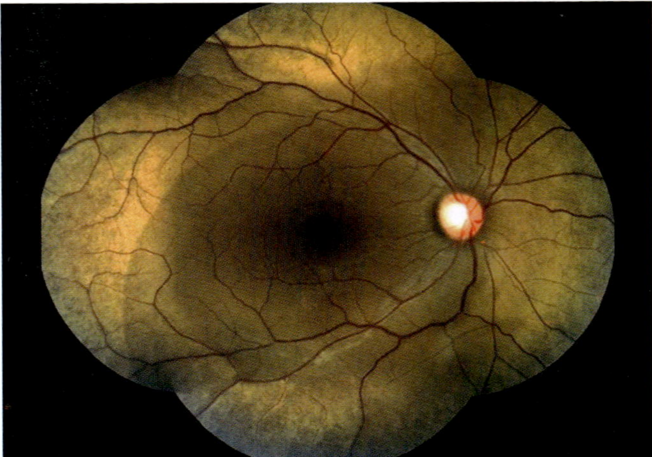

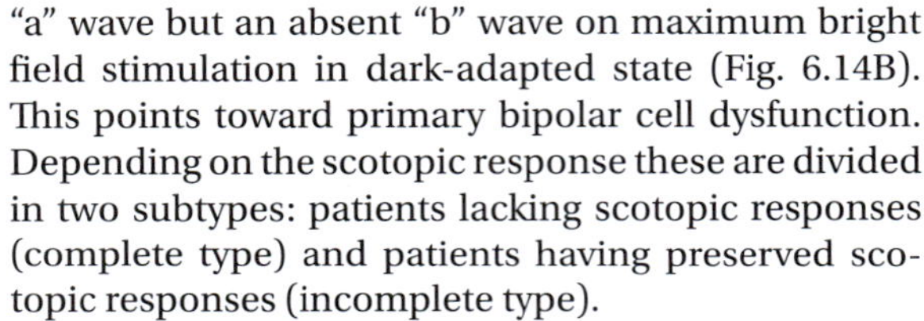

Fig. 6.15: Montage color fundus photograph showing Mizuo-Nakamura phenomenon. The central fundus after prolonged dark adaptation does not show the typical golden sheen. The peripheral fundus however has golden sheen after exposure to light.

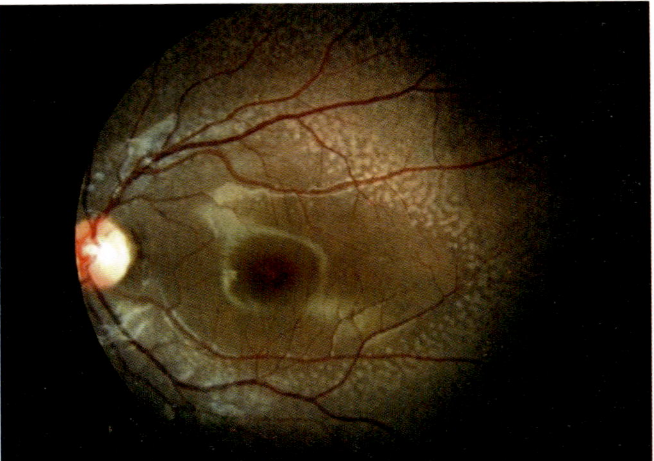

Fig. 6.16: Whitish yellow retinal flecks in a patient with fundus albipunctatus.

"a" wave but an absent "b" wave on maximum bright field stimulation in dark-adapted state (Fig. 6.14B). This points toward primary bipolar cell dysfunction. Depending on the scotopic response these are divided in two subtypes: patients lacking scotopic responses (complete type) and patients having preserved scotopic responses (incomplete type).

2. *CSNB with abnormal fundus*: This includes two distinct entities:
   - *Oguchi disease*: It is an AR form of CSNB, which is characterized by a peculiar fundus feature known as Mizuo-Nakamura phenomenon (Fig. 6.15). Here the fundus has a typical golden sheen, which disappears after prolonged (3–4 hours) dark adaptation. The visual acuity and cone function are normal. The ERG lacks scotopic responses that normalize after prolonged dark adaptation. The exact mechanism of Mizuo–Nakamura phenomenon is not well understood.
   - *Fundus albipunctatus*: Yellow white flecks scattered throughout the fundus characterize this subtype of CSNB (Fig. 6.16), which is inherited in an AR or dominant pattern. These flecks spare the macula and increase in size from the center towards the periphery. There are no optic disc, vascular or pigment abnormalities. While the cone function is normal, the rod responses can be elicited only after prolonged dark adaptation.

REFERENCES

1. Donders FC. Beiträge zur pathologischen Anatomie des Auges. II. Pigmentbildung in der Netzhaut. Graefes Arch Opthalmol. 1857;3:139-50.
2. Uthedu. [online] Available from https://sph.uth.edu/Retnet/ [Accessed on December 2017].
3. Tanino T, Ohba N. Studies on pigmentary retinal dystrophy. II. Recordability of electroretinogram and the mode of inheritance. Jpn J Ophthalmology. 1976;20:482-6.
4. Massof RW, Benzschawel T, Emmel T, et al. The spread of retinal degeneration in retinitis pigmentosa. Invest Ophthalmology Vis Sci. 1984;25(Suppl):196.
5. Fishman GA, Fishman M, Maggiano J. Macular lesions associated with retinitis pigmentosa. Arch Ophthalmology. 1977;95:798-803.
6. Heckenlively J. The frequency of posterior subcapsular cataract in the hereditary retinal degenerations. Am J Ophthalmology. 1982;93:733-8.
7. Sieving PA, Fishman GA. Refractive errors of retinitis pigmentosa patients. Br J Ophthalmology. 1978;62:163-7.
8. Novack RL, Foos RY. Drusen of the optic disc in retinitis pigmentosa. Am J Ophthalmology. 1987;103:44-7.
9. Khan JA, Ide CH, Strickland MP. Coats'-type retinitis pigmentosa. Surv Ophthalmology. 1988;32:317-32.
10. Witkin AJ, Ko TH, Fujimoto JG, et al. Ultra-high resolution optical coherence tomography assessment of photoreceptors in retinitis pigmentosa and related diseases. Am J Ophthalmology. 2006;142:945-52.
11. Franceschetti A, François J, Babel J. Retinitis punctata albescens. In: Franceschetti A, François J, Babel J (Eds). Chorioretinal Heredodegenerations. Springfield, Ill: Charles C Thomas; 1974. pp. 222-31.
12. Bastek JV, Heckenlively JR, Straatsma BR, et al. Cataract surgery in retinitis pigmentosa patients. Ophthalmology. 1982;89:880-4.
13. Genead MA, Fishman GA. Efficacy of sustained topical dorzolamide therapy for cystic macular lesions in patients with retinitis pigmentosa and usher syndrome. Arch Ophthalmology. 2010;128:1146-50.
14. Orzalesi N, Pierrottet C, Porta A, et al. Long-term treatment of retinitis pigmentosa with acetazolamide. A pilot study. Graefes Arch Clin Exp Ophthalmology. 1993;231:254-6.
15. Scorolli L, Morara M, Meduri A, et al. Treatment of cystoid macular edema in retinitis pigmentosa with intravitreal triamcinolone. Arch Ophthalmology. 2007;125:759-64.

16. Yuzbasioglu E, Artunay O, Rasier R, et al. Intravitreal bevacizumab (Avastin) injection in retinitis pigmentosa. Curr Eye Res. 2009;34:231-7.

17. Saatci AO, Selver OB, Seymenoglu G, et al. Bilateral Intravitreal Dexamethasone Implant for Retinitis Pigmentosa-Related Macular Edema. Case Reports in Ophthalmology. 2013;4(1):53-8.

18. Berson EL, Rosner B, Sandberg MA, et al. A randomized trial of vitamin A and vitamin E supplementation for retinitis pigmentosa. Arch Ophthalmology. 1993;111:1465-6.

19. Berson EL, Rosner B, Sandberg MA, et al. A randomized trial of supplemental vitamin A and vitamin E supplementation for retinitis pigmentosa. Arch Ophthalmology. 1993;111:761-72.

20. Kumar A, Midha N, Gogia V, et al. Efficacy of oral valproic acid in patients with retinitis pigmentosa. J Ocul Pharmacol Ther. 2014;30:580-6.

21. Luo YH, da Cruz L. The Argus® II Retinal Prosthesis System. Prog Retin Eye Res. 2016;50:89-107.

22. Bassuk AG, Zheng A, Li Y, et al. Precision Medicine: Genetic Repair of Retinitis Pigmentosa in Patient-Derived Stem Cells. Sci Rep. 2016;6:1996-9.

23. Leber T. Uber retinitis pigmentosa und angeborene amaurose. Graefes Arch Clin Exp Ophthalmology. 1869;15:1-25.

24. Perrault I, Rozet JM, Gerber S, et al. Leber congenital amaurosis. Mol Genet Metab. 1999;68:200-8.

25. Koerekoop RK, Lopez I, den Hollander AI, et al. Genetic testing for retinal dystrophies and dysfunctions: benefits, dilemmas and solutions. Clin Experiment Ophthalmology. 2007;35:473-85.

26. Chacón-Camacho OF, Zenteno JC. Review and update on the molecular basis of Leber congenital amaurosis. World J Clin Cases. 2015;3(2):112-24.

27. den Hollander AI, Roepman R, Koenekoop RK, et al. Leber congenital amaurosis: genes, proteins and disease mechanisms. Prog Retin Eye Res. 2008;27:391-419.

28. Harris EW. Leber's congenital amaurosis and RPE65. Int Ophthalmology Clin. 2001;41:73-82.

29. Fazzi E, Signorini SG, Scelsa B, et al. Leber's congenital amaurosis: an update. Eur J Paediatr Neurol. 2003;7:13-22.

30. Dekaban AS. Mental retardation and neurologic involvement in patients with congenital retinal blindness. Dev Med Child Neurol. 1972;14:436-44.

31. Jacobson SG, Cideciyan AV, Ratnakaram R, et al. Gene therapy for Leber congenital amaurosis caused by RPE65 mutations: safety and efficacy in 15 children and adults followed up to 3 years. Arch Ophthalmology. 2012;130:9-24.

32. Zeitz C, Robson AG, Audo I. Congenital stationary night blindness: an analysis and update of genotype-phenotype correlations and pathogenic mechanisms. Prog Retin Eye Res. 2015;45:58-110.

Chapter 7

Hereditary Vitreoretinopathies

Vinod Kumar, Neha Goel

STICKLER SYNDROME

 ### INTRODUCTION

Stickler syndrome, also known as hereditary arthro-ophthalmopathy, refers to a group of progressive diseases characterized by a distinctive facial appearance, ocular abnormalities, skeletal problems and hearing loss. Stickler syndrome affects one in approximately 7,500–9,000 newborns and is the most common inherited cause of retinal detachment in children. It is also the commonest chondrodysplasia associated with vitreoretinal degeneration; others being Marshall syndrome, Kniest dysplasia, Knobloch syndrome and Weissenbacher–Zweymüller syndrome.

 ### PATHOPHYSIOLOGY

Genetics

Stickler syndrome is an autosomal dominant condition with complete penetrance and variable expression. The disease is a result of defective collagen connective tissue resulting from different mutations. It is now known to have at least five clinically different subgroups. Type I and type II Stickler's syndrome are caused by mutations in *COL2A1* and *COL11A1* genes respectively, which encode for type II and type XI collagen respectively.[1,2] Ocular involvement is seen predominantly in type I and type II of Stickler syndrome which are also the commonest types of Stickler's syndrome constituting more than 90% of total cases.

Clinically, these two types of Stickler syndrome can be differentiated based on the vitreous morphology.[3] While the vitreous is predominantly membranous in type I Stickler syndrome, it is irregular, fibrillary and has a beaded appearance in type II Stickler syndrome. In addition, deafness is usually seen in type II Stickler syndrome.

 ### CLINICAL FEATURES

The diagnosis of Stickler syndrome is based on the clinical features. The ocular features include congenital myopia

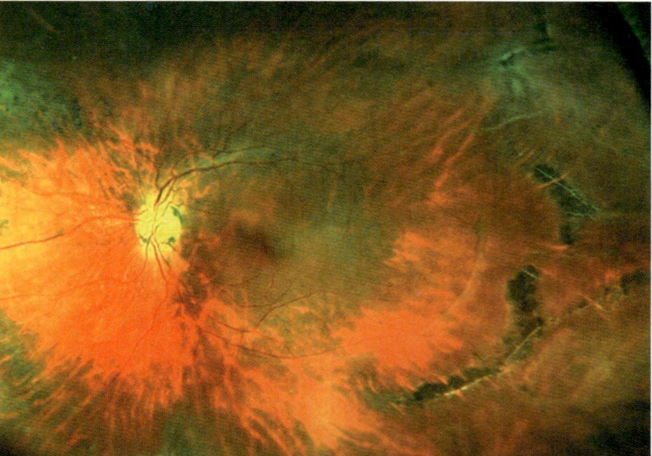

Fig. 7.1: Multiple pigmented radial lattices in a patient with Stickler syndrome and high myopia.

that is usually nonprogressive. Patients frequently present in childhood. The lens is frequently affected leading to early onset cataract or ectopia lentis. Some patients may exhibit a characteristic quadrantic lamellar cortical lenticular opacity, which, if present, is a characteristic sign.[4] Glaucoma can be seen in 5–10% of cases and is a result of angle anomalies. Depending on the type, vitreous can be membranous or fibrillary. Multiple pigmented radial lattices (Fig. 7.1) are the characteristic ocular feature of Stickler syndrome.[5] These patients have a high risk of retinal detachment (50%), which tends to be bilateral and often associated with multiple and giant retinal tears.[6]

Patients with Stickler syndrome exhibit typical facial features consisting of mid-facial hypoplasia, depressed nasal bridge, micrognathia and anteverted nares. Other facial features include cleft lip and palate, bifid uvula and Pierre Robin sequence (opening in the roof of the mouth). Deafness is especially common in type II Stickler syndrome and could be both conductive as well as sensorineural. Skeletal features include mild spondyloepiphyseal dysplasia, joint hypermobility and early onset osteoarthritis.[7]

MANAGEMENT

Management consists of tackling the facial and skeletal anomalies and deafness. Ocular management consists of timely correction of refractive errors, frequent follow-ups to detect retinal breaks and their early treatment to prevent retinal detachment.[8] In case of retinal detachment, vitrectomy with silicone oil or long acting gas is warranted.

WAGNER SYNDROME

INTRODUCTION

Wagner syndrome, also known as erosive vitreoretinopathy, was earlier considered to be a part of Stickler syndrome. However, Wagner syndrome is now known to be a clinically and genetically distinct entity and as opposed to Stickler syndrome does not have systemic manifestations. It forms a component of chromosome 5q retinopathies; other components being erosive vitreoretinopathy and Jansen syndrome.

PATHOPHYSIOLOGY

Genetics

Wagner syndrome is a hereditary disorder transmitted in an autosomal dominant manner. A mutation in the chondroitin sulfate proteoglycan 2 gene (*CSPG2*), now named *VCAN* has been mapped to chromosome 5q12-14.[9,10] *VCAN* encodes for Versican protein and is the causative factor in erosive vitreo-retinopathy as well.

CLINICAL FEATURES

Typically the patients present early in life with night blindness and pseudo-strabismus (because of positive angle kappa) resulting from congenital temporal displacement of the fovea.[11] As opposed to Stickler syndrome, myopia is usually mild to moderate. The crystalline lens frequently develops dot-like cortical cataract. The vitreous is typically optically empty with avascular vitreous veils near the equator, which may also be seen at the posterior pole in certain cases. The retinal blood vessels show sheathing, perivascular pigmentation and may exhibit an abnormal pattern in the form of optic nerve inversion. Retinal and chorioretinal atrophy tends to progress leading to visual loss.[9,12] Retinal traction and retinal detachment are common. FA shows non-perfusion due to gross loss of the choriocapillaris. Electroretinogram (ERG) as well as dark adaptometry are normal early in the life, but tend to progressively deteriorate over a period of time.[13]

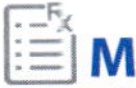

MANAGEMENT

The treatment consists of correction of the refractive error, phacoemulsification for cataracts, frequent screening for early detection of retinal breaks and their treatment with laser photocoagulation. Retinal detachment should be promptly managed with vitreoretinal surgery.[13]

GOLDMANN–FAVRE SYNDROME

INTRODUCTION

Goldmann–Favre syndrome (GFS), also known as Goldmann–Favre vitreo-tapetoretinal degeneration, is an extremely rare inherited vitreoretinal dystrophy. The condition affects the crystalline lens, vitreous, retina and is characterized by clumps of intraretinal pigmentation.[14-16] It is frequently misdiagnosed as retinitis pigmentosa and X-linked retinoschisis (XLRS). Enhanced S cone syndrome (ESCS) is considered to be a milder form of the GFS.

PATHOPHYSIOLOGY

Genetics

Goldmann–Favre syndrome is caused by mutations in *NR2E3* gene, earlier known as PNR (photoreceptor-specific nuclear receptor) located on chromosome 15q23. Its expression is limited to photoreceptors and is essential for proper rod and cone photoreceptor development and maintenance.[17,18] Different mutations in *NR2E3* gene result in ESCS, GFS and clumped pigmentary retinal degeneration (CPRD). All of these are characterized by markedly decreased or absent rod function, night blindness and increased function of S (blue) cones.

CLINICAL FEATURES

The most common presenting feature of patient with GFS is night blindness that has an early onset in the first decade.[16] Patients complain of progressive decrease in vision similar to that in retinitis pigmentosa. This is often caused by development of cataract and macular retinoschisis. Clinically the intraretinal pigments are in the form of clumps and spots (Figs. 7.2 and 7.3) rather than bone spicules as seen in retinitis pigmentosa. These are often concentrated around the vascular arcades and spare the macular area.

Retinoschisis occurs in the macular area and is seen in periphery as well in some cases. These two may be contiguous or separated from each other by normal retina. The macular schisis is similar to that seen in XLRS. This can be confused with cystoid macular edema, but there is absence of leakage on fluorescein angiography in the former. Peripheral dendriform lesions can also be visible in some patients with GFS as seen in patients with XLRS.

The vitreous is usually liquefied leading to an optically empty vitreous cavity on examination. The posterior cortex can become condensed forming a preretinal membrane present through large portions of fundus.

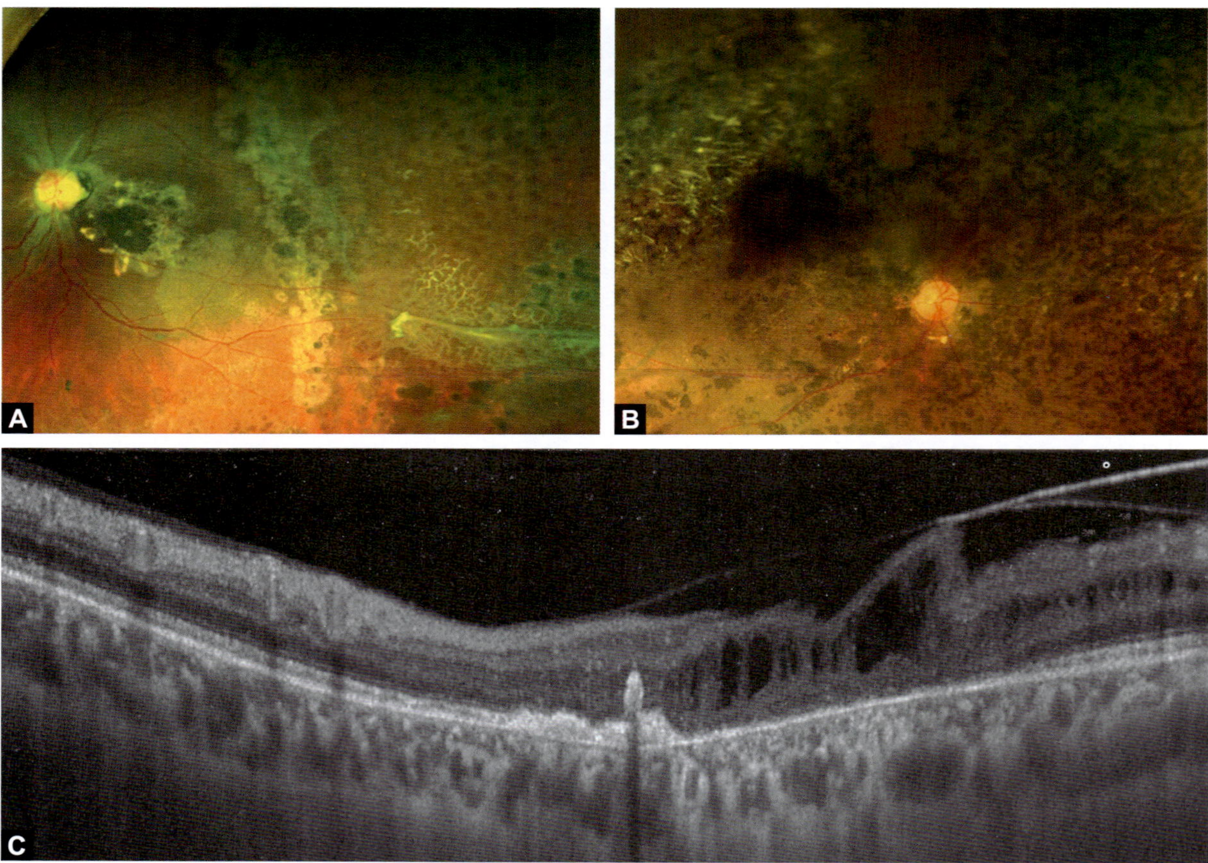

Figs. 7.2A to C: Intraretinal pigment clumps, dendritic patches on color pictures of both eyes and macular foveoschisis in a case with Goldmann–Favre hereditary ocular diseases.

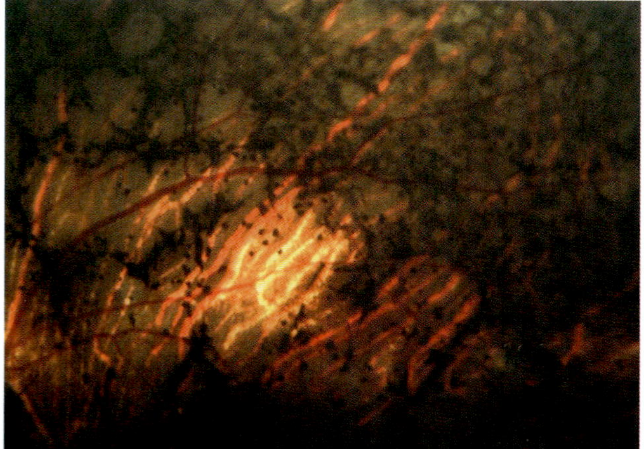

Fig. 7.3: Clumps of pigment and oval areas of retinal atrophy in a patient with Goldmann–Favre syndrome.

Electrophysiology plays an important part in the diagnosis of GFS. Characteristic features on full field ERG include absence of rod responses, presence of similar waveforms in the maximum dark-adapted response and single-flash light-adapted waveform and disproportionately reduced 30-Hz cone flicker to the single-flash cone amplitude. Stimulation of S cones with blue light usually reveals supernormal responses on ERG.[19]

TREATMENT

There is no definite treatment for the GFS. Regular follow-up to look for complications and their early detection is warranted. Macular schisis has been treated with topical dorzolamide (2%) drops in few reports.

REFERENCES

1. Hoornaert KP, Vereecke I, Dewinter C, et al. Stickler syndrome caused by COL2A1 mutations: genotype–phenotype correlation in a series of 100 patients. Eur J Hum Genet. 2010;18:872-80.
2. Majava M, Hoornaert KP, Bartholdi D, et al. A report on 10 new patients with heterozygous mutations in the COL11A1 gene and a review of genotype-phenotype correlations in type XI collagenopathies. Am J Med Genet A. 2007;143:258-64.

3. Ang A, Ung T, Puvanachandra N, et al. Vitreous phenotype: a key diagnostic sign in Stickler syndrome types 1 and 2 complicated by double heterozygosity. Am J Med Genet A. 2007;143:604-7.

4. Snead MP, McNinch AM, Poulson AV, et al. Stickler syndrome, ocular only variants and a key diagnostic role for the ophthalmologist. Eye (Lond). 2011;25:1389-400.

5. Vu CD, Brown Jr J, Korkko J, et al. Posterior chorioretinal atrophy and vitreous phenotype in a family with Stickler syndrome from a mutation in the COL2A1 gene. Ophthalmology. 2003;110:70-7.

6. Watanabe H, Kohzaki K, Kubo H, et al. [Stickler syndrome with rhegmatogenous retinal detachment.] Nippon Ganka Gakkai Zasshi. 2010;114:454-8.

7. Couchouron T, Masson C. Early-onset progressive osteoarthritis with hereditary progressive ophthalmopathy or Stickler syndrome. Joint Bone Spine. 2011;78:45-9.

8. Carroll C, Papaioannou D, Rees A, et al. The clinical effectiveness and safety of prophylactic retinal interventions to reduce the risk of retinal detachment and subsequent vision loss in adults and children with Stickler syndrome: a systematic review. Health Technol Assess. 2011;15:iii-xiv, 1-62.

9. Mukhopadhyay A, Nikopoulos K, Maugeri A, et al. Erosive vitreoretinopathy and Wagner diseases are caused by intronic mutations in CSPG2/Versican that result in an imbalance of splice variants. Invest Ophthalmology Vis Sci. 2006;47:3565-72.

10. Meredith SP, Richards AJ, Flanagan DW, et al. Clinical characterisation and molecular analysis of Wagner syndrome. Br J Ophthalmology. 2007;91:655-9.

11. Maumenee IH, Stoll HU, Mets MB. The Wagner syndrome versus hereditary arthro-ophthalmopathy. Trans Am OphthalmolSoc. 1982;80:349-65.

12. Kloeckener-Gruissem B, Amstutz C. VCAN-related vitreoretinopathy. In: Pagon RA, Bird TD, Dolan CR (Eds). GeneReviews (Internet). Seattle: University of Washington; 2009.

13. Edwards AO. Clinical features of the congenital vitreoretinopathies. Eye (Lond). 2008;22:1233-42.

14. Favre M. [Two cases of hyaloid-retinal degeneration.] Ophthalmologica. 1958;135:604-9.

15. Francois J, de Rouck A, Cambie E. [Goldmann–Favre vitreotapetoretinal degeneration.] Ophthalmologica. 1974;168:81-96.

16. Fishman GA, Jampol LM, Goldberg MF. Diagnostic features of the Favre–Goldmann syndrome. Br J Ophthalmology. 1976;60:345-53.

17. Schorderet DF, Escher P. NR2E3 mutations in enhanced S-cone sensitivity syndrome (ESCS), Goldmann–Favre syndrome (GFS), clumped pigmentary retinal degeneration (CPRD), and retinitis pigmentosa (RP). Hum Mutat. 2009;30:1475-85.

18. Brydak-Godowska J, Makowiec-Tabernacka M. [Goldmann–Favre syndrome—case report.] Klin Oczna. 2009;111:346-7.

19. Jacobson SG, Roman AJ, Roman MI, et al. Relatively enhanced S cone function in the Goldmann–Favre syndrome. Am J Ophthalmology. 1991;111:446-53.

Macular Dystrophies

Vinod Kumar, Neha Goel, Karthikeya R

STARGARDT DISEASE

 ### INTRODUCTION

Stargardt disease is the most common inherited macular dystrophy in both adults and children, with an estimated prevalence of 1 in 10,000.[1] The disease has its usual onset in early teens and carries a great phenotypic and genetic heterogeneity.

GENETICS

Stargardt disease is an autosomal recessive condition caused by sequence variations in *ABCA4* gene that is located on chromosome 1. *ABCA4* is a member of the ATP-binding cassette (ABC) transporter gene family, encoding the retinal specific transmembrane ABCA4 protein, which is involved in the active transport of retinoids from photoreceptor to the retinal pigment epithelium (RPE).[2,3] Abnormalities in this protein leads to deposition of bisretinoids (A2E) in photoreceptors and RPE which degenerate over time. A large number of sequence variations in *ABCA4* gene (more than 600) have been reported till date in cases with Stargardt disease.[4] Stargardt disease is also therefore referred as ABCA4 related retinopathy.

ABCA4 gene has also been associated with cone-rod dystrophy and retinitis pigmentosa.

 ### CLINICAL FEATURES

The age of onset has a wide variation. A later age of onset is usually associated with a better visual prognosis. The common presentation is gradually progressive decline in the visual acuity that may range from mild to severe, dyschromatopsia and central scotoma. The cases with mild visual loss may also be detected on routine examination and are often referred as *abnormal sheen at the macula*. In the early stages

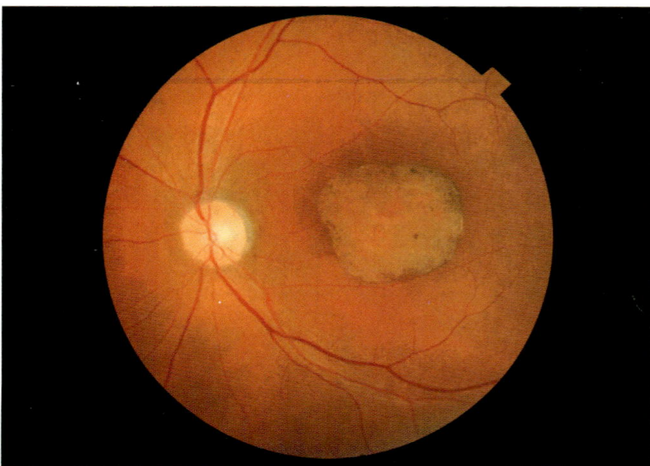

Fig. 8.1: Color photograph showing metallic sheen at the macula in a patient with Stargardt disease.

the macula may be normal or may show mottling of the RPE. A metallic sheen often gives a beaten-bronze appearance to the macula (Fig. 8.1). In the later stages, this leads to outer retinal and geographic atrophy of the RPE. Sometimes lesions may clinically appear as Bull's eye maculopathy.

Accumulation of bisretinoids/lipofuscin in the outer retinal layers leads to an opaque RPE. This causes vermillion fundus and is often appreciated as dark red fundus when compared to a normal eye.

A characteristic feature of Stargardt disease is the presence of multiple yellow flecks at the level of RPE (Fig. 8.2). These may be present just around the central macular lesion or may extend beyond the vascular arcades and typically have a pisciform shape with a branching pattern. The presence of flecks alone was earlier referred to as fundus flavimaculatus. It is now considered within the spectrum of ABCA4 related retinopathy.

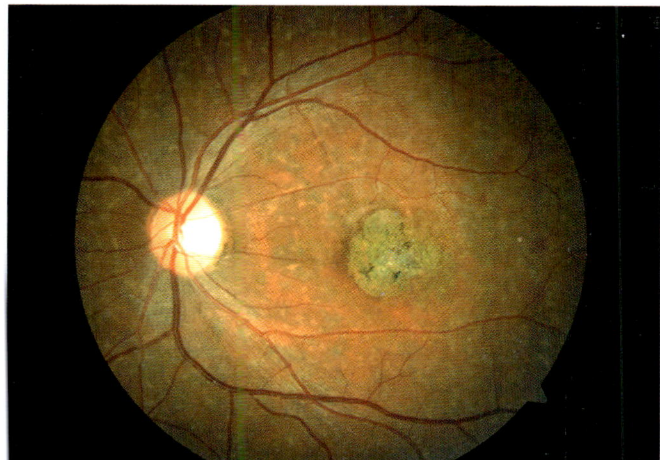

Fig. 8.2: Color photograph showing pisciform flecks along with the central macular lesion in Stargardt disease.

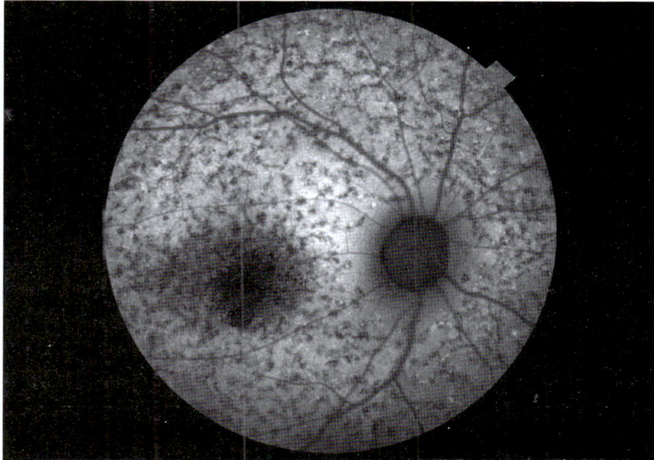

Fig. 8.3: Fundus autofluorescence picture of Stargardt disease showing hypoautofluorescence corresponding to the central area. Flecks are hypoautofluorescent with few being hyperautofluorescent at the periphery. Note the peripapillary sparing seen.

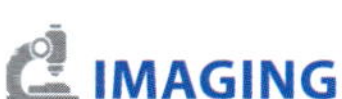

IMAGING

Retinal imaging especially fundus fluorescein angiography (FFA), short wave fundus autofluorescence (FAF) and optical coherence tomography (OCT) play an important role in the diagnosis, management and follow-up of patients with Stargardt disease. Since the basic pathology is of excess deposition of A2E/lipofuscin that makes the RPE opaque on fundus fluorescein angiography (FFA) and prevents the observer from seeing the choroidal blood vessels beneath the retina .This is referred to as the *dark choroid sign*. The sign however is not exclusive for Stargardt disease. As the RPE undergoes degeneration, choroidal hyperfluorescence becomes apparent as window defects.

Fundus autofluorescence is very useful in the assessment of patients with Stargardt disease.[5] The areas with A2E deposition appear as hyperautofluorescent while areas with degenerated RPE appear hypoautofluorescent. The flecks may be hyper- or hypo-autofluorescent but are usually hyperautofluorescent initially. As more peripheral flecks appear, the old ones at the posterior pole become hypoautofluorescent (Fig. 8.3). An area of peripapillary sparing is often considered characteristic of Stargardt disease. FAF is also a useful indicator of advancing central geographic atrophy.[6]

Optical coherence tomography shows the extent of affection of retinal layers at the posterior pole (Fig. 8.4). The outer retinal layers including RPE are often affected and the area usually correlated well with the visual acuity.[7]

Electrophysiology may help in the diagnosis especially when genetic analysis is not available (Fig. 8.5). The full field electroretinogram (ERG) is normal until late stages.[8] The pattern ERG and multifocal ERG show abnormalities even when fundus looks normal. In the late stages however peripheral cone dysfunction followed by combined cone and rod dysfunction may occur. Thus, electrophysiological testing may also aid in prognostication of the disease, depending on

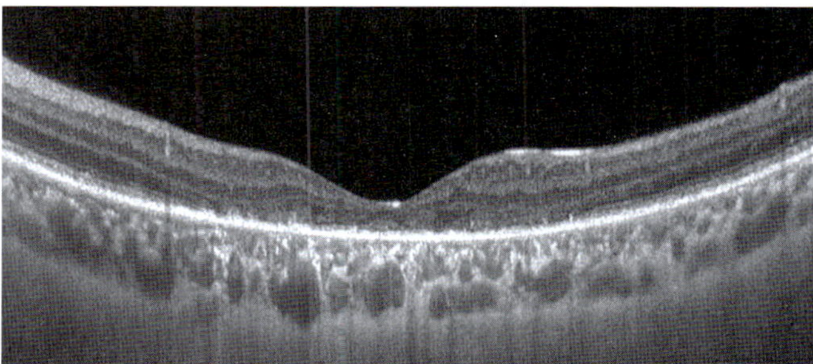

Fig. 8.4: Swept source optical coherence tomography of patient with Stargardt disease showing atrophy of outer retinal layers at the macula.

involvement of the full field ERG. Adaptive Optics testing which increases lateral resolution of retinal images ,reveals affection of of photoreceptors.

TREATMENT

There is no definitive treatment of Stargardt disease. The treatment mainly is supportive in the form of low vision aids whenever required and avoidance of excessive formation of bisretinoids. Vitamin A supplements should thus be avoided in this condition.

There are several active research programs on the treatment of Stargardt disease. These include gene therapy, cell replacement therapy and pharmacotherapy. The major problem with gene therapy in Stargardt disease is the limited carrying capacity of Adeno-associated viruses since *ABCA4* gene is larger than its vector-carrying capacity. Lentivirus vector has been developed recently to deliver *ABCA4* in the subretinal space.[9] Stem cell replacement therapy and pharmacotherapies are still under trials.

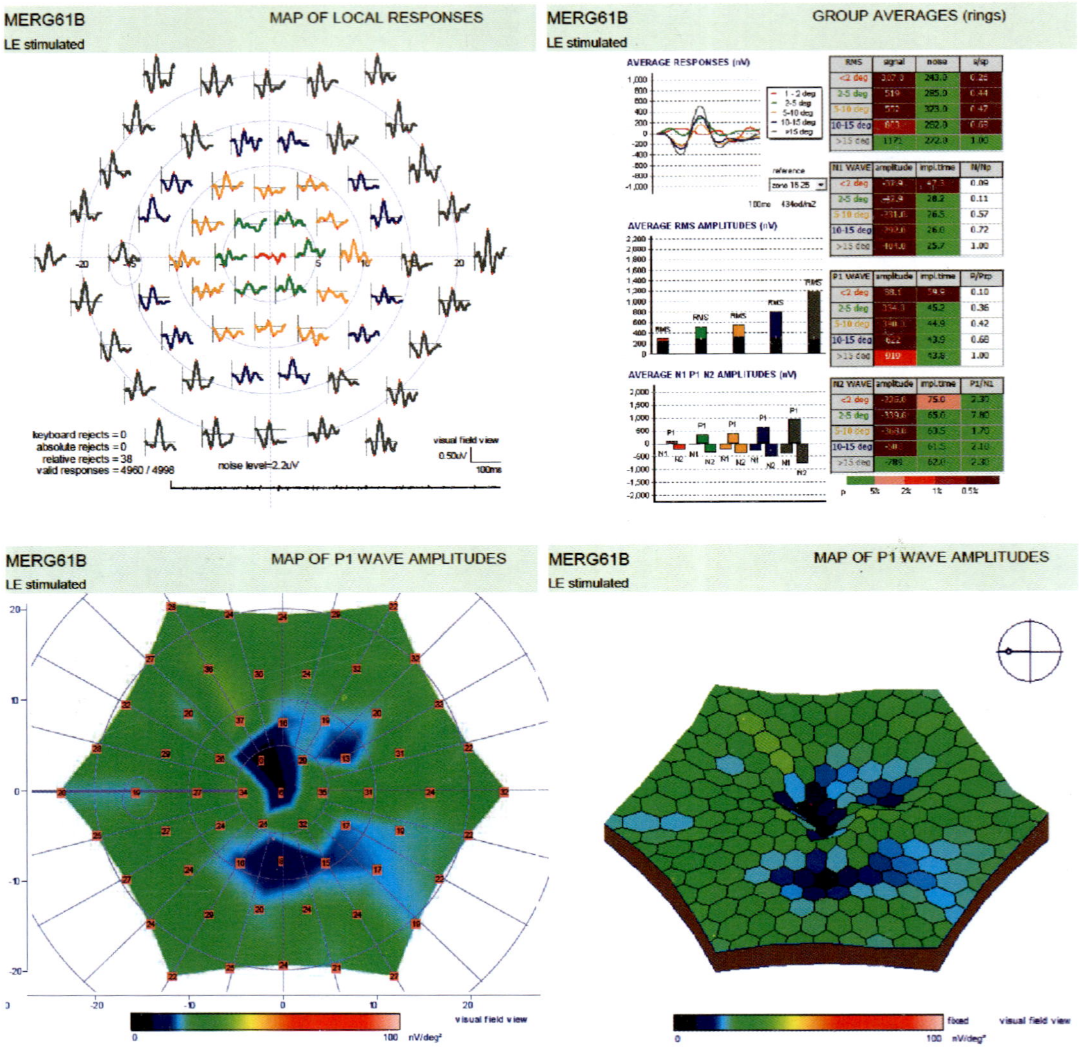

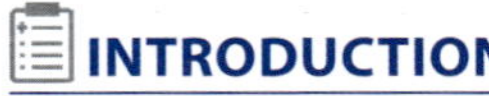

Fig. 8.5: Multifocal ERG of a patient with Stargardt syndrome. Full-field ERG may be within normal limits. Multi-focal ERG shows depressed P1 amplitude.

BEST VITELLIFORM MACULAR DYSTROPHY

INTRODUCTION

Best macular dystrophy also known as Best vitelliform macular dystrophy or Best's disease was first described by Friedrich Best in 1905.[10] It is one of the most common retinal dystrophies with estimated incidence of 1 in 10,000 population. Typically the disease is dominantly inherited with onset in the juvenile age group.

GENETICS

Best macular dystrophy is an autosomal dominant condition caused by mutations in *BEST1* gene that is located on 11q13.[11]

Earlier known as VMD2, the *BEST1* gene encodes a protein, Bestrophin, which is located on the basolateral membrane of the retinal pigment epithelium (RPE). Over a hundred mutations have been identified till date. Apart from the typical presentations, *BEST1* mutations may be associated with other phenotypic presentations including autosomal dominant vitreoretinochoroidopathy, autosomal recessive bestrophinopathy and multifocal Best disease.

CLINICAL FEATURES

The juvenile form of BMD is usually detected on routine examination, as vision is frequently unaffected in the initial stages. The typical fundus lesion is a round to oval, yellow *vitelliform* lesion (called so because of the resemblance to egg yolk) that is centered on the fovea (Fig. 8.6). The lesion

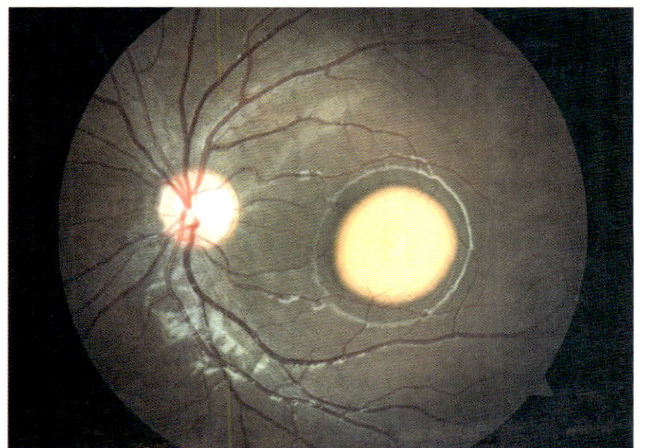

Fig. 8.6: Vitelliform round lesion in a 10-year-old patient with Best macular dystrophy.

size may vary from half to two disc diameters and tends to be smaller as the age of onset increases. This yellow material is composed predominantly of material made of A2E, which is a byproduct of the visual cycle.

Over a period of time the yellow material settles down due to gravity that gives appearance of *pseudohypopyon* (Fig. 8.7A). Later the lesion may develop subretinal fibrosis or RPE pigmentary changes that give appearance of *scrambled egg* (vitelliruptive, Fig. 8.8). A characteristic feature of disease at this stage is fibrotic pillar frequently seen due to sub-RPE fibrosis. This is seen as a yellow dot inside the lesion. Eventually the RPE undergoes atrophy. Choroidal neovascularization is seen in some cases and may significantly worsen the visual acuity.[12] Patients with BMD can develop subretinal hemorrhages with minor head/ocular trauma even in the absence of choroidal neovascularization. Though disease is characteristically symmetric in early stages, the course

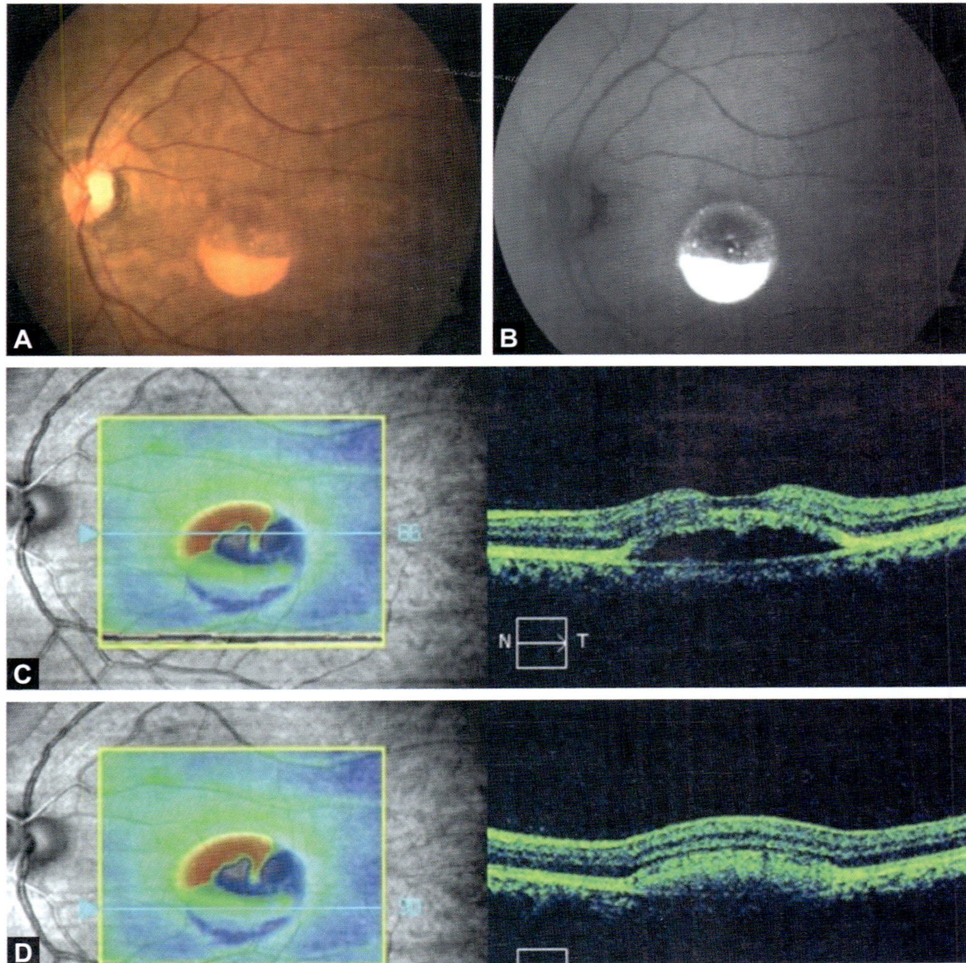

Figs. 8.7A to D: Patient with Best macular dystrophy showing pseudohypopyon (A). Short-wave autofluorescence shows hyperautofluorescence corresponding to yellow material (B) Spectral domain–optical coherence tomography through the upper part of lesion shows hyporeflective subretinal space (C) while spectral domain–optical coherence tomography through the lower part shows subretinal hyperrefective vitelliform material (D).

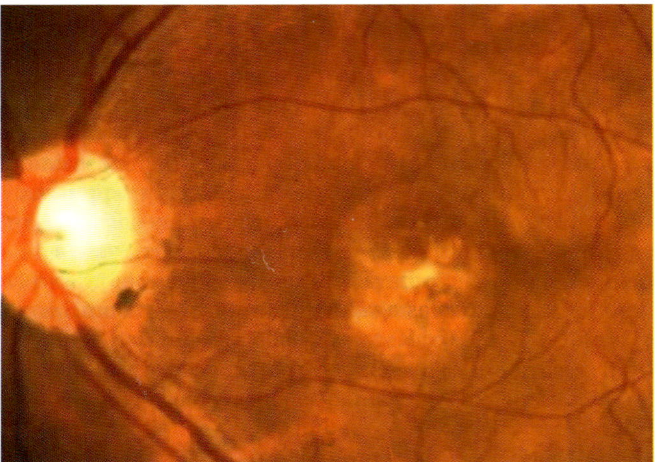

Fig. 8.8: Color fundus photograph of a patient with Best macular dystrophy showing vitelliruptive stage.

may render the disease asymmetric between the two eyes. Visual acuity is usually not affected until the disease reaches vitelliruptive stage.

A minority of patients may have multiple vitelliform lesions scattered over the posterior pole. Multiple lesions are however more common in autosomal recessive forms of disease. Hypermetropia and hence propensity for angle closure is common in patients with BMD.[13]

Imaging plays an important part in the diagnosis and management of BMD. Short wave autofluorescence shows bright hyperautofluorescence in relation to the vitelliform material (Fig. 8.7B). Fluorescein angiography shows hyperfluorescence in the early stages of the disease while it becomes hypofluorescent in the later stages. The main role of the fluorescein angiography is to distinguish or detect the presence of choroidal neovascularization.

Optical coherence tomography[14] shows homogenous hyperreflective material in the subretinal space in the vitelliform lesion. Once the material settles down in the pseudohypopyon stage, the space occupied by the vitelliform material previously is now seen as clear hyporeflective space (black, Fig. 8.7C). The vitelliform material inferiorly is still seen as hyperreflective subretinal material (Fig. 8.7D). The fibrotic pillar is commonly seen corresponding to the yellow spot in the vitelliruptive stage.

Electrooculogram is a useful electrodiagnostic modality for the diagnosis of BMD. The normal value of Arden ratio (ratio of light peak to dark trough of standing positive potential of cornea) ranges from 1.8–2.0. In patients with BMD, Arden ratio typically is decreased below 1.5 (Figs. 8.9A and B). Full-field electroretinogram (ERG) however is normal.

TREATMENT

No definitive treatment of BMD is available and management is mainly supportive. This includes correction of refractive error if any, providing protective glasses and avoiding contact sports. Choroidal neovascularization responds well to anti-vascular endothelial growth factor (VEGF) agents and needs to be treated to prevent further visual loss.[15]

ADULT ONSET FOVEOMACULAR VITELLIFORM DYSTROPHY

INTRODUCTION

Adult onset foveomacular vitelliform dystrophy (AOFVD) is a disease that is often misdiagnosed as age-related macular degeneration or, in rare instances, as Best vitelliform macular dystrophy. It is a condition often seen in asymptomatic adults over 50 years of age.[16] It is a bilateral asymmetric condition in which there is a foveal or parafoveal subretinal yellow dome shaped deposit with a central pigmented spot. It can be inherited as an autosomal dominant condition but is usually sporadic. The clinical presentation can be variable in terms of the size, shape, elevation pigmentation and extent of macular involvement. Occasionally patients are symptomatic and complain of mild blurring of vision or mild metamorphopsia.[17]

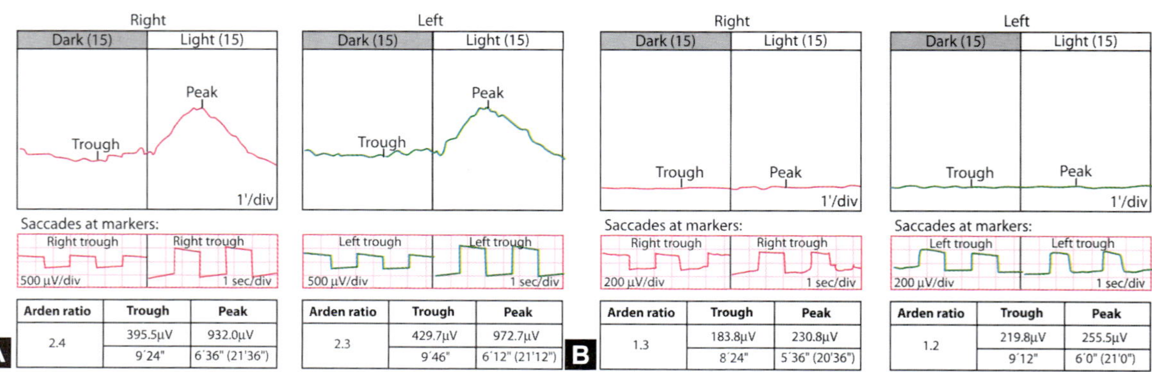

Arden ratio	Trough	Peak
2.4	395.5µV	932.0µV
	9´24"	6´36" (21'36")

Arden ratio	Trough	Peak
2.3	429.7µV	972.7µV
	9´46"	6´12" (21'12")

Arden ratio	Trough	Peak
1.3	183.8µV	230.8µV
	8´24"	5´36" (20'36")

Arden ratio	Trough	Peak
1.2	219.8µV	255.5µV
	9´12"	6´0" (21'0")

Figs. 8.9A and B: (A) Electrooculogram (EOG) of a normal person; (B) Electrooculogram (EOG) of a patient with Best macular dystrophy.

These yellow lesions are hyperautofluorescent, variably stain on fluorescein angiography and distinctly lack a leakage. On OCT, they are seen as hyperreflective material located in the subretinal space between the ellipsoid zone and the RPE-Bruch's membrane complex. The other clues to the diagnosis are absence of subretinal fluid or subretinal blood. Both electrooculography (EOG) and electroretinogram (ERG) are usually with in normal limits in these patients. When confusion persists even after routine work up, an OCT angiography can be used to confirm the absence of a neovascular network within the lesion.

Adult onset foveomacular vitelliform dystrophy is generally slowly progressive and retaining good reading vision in at least one of the eyes is the rule. When there is vision loss, the cause could be RPE degeneration/atrophy, outer retinal atrophy or a secondary choroidal neovascular membrane (CNVM). Secondary CNVM can occur in as many as one third of the patients with AOFVD.

Treatment is not recommended unless the condition is complicated with a secondary CNVM, when the treatment of choice is intravitreal anti-VEGF injections.

CONE DYSTROPHY

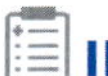

INTRODUCTION

Cone dystrophy is a progressive retinal degeneration primarily affecting cone photoreceptors.[18] This group of varied disorders is characterized by reduced central visual acuity, photophobia and subnormal color vision. Few authors' group achromatopsia and blue cone monochromatism with cone dystrophies,[19] however, the better term for these entities is *cone dysfunction syndrome* as these are clinically stationary.[20] Cone dystrophy is progressive and in advanced stage patients show overlap with cone-rod dystrophies. The diagnosis is based on a strong clinical suspicion, further proven by ERG, OCT and fundus autofluorescence. The advent of adaptive optics has provided new insights into the morphological evaluation of this entity. Conventional treatment options are mainly based on optical vision enhancing devices, however, the decoding of responsible genes in few subtypes have offered a hope for gene therapy in future.

EPIDEMIOLOGY

The disease onset is typically in teenage to early adult life.[21] A case of late onset cone dystrophy at age of 47 years has also been described.[22] It is known to occur in all parts of the world with equal predilection for both the sexes. No racial preference has been described.

GENETICS

All three types of Mendelian inheritance as well as sporadic occurrence have been reported in the literature. Mutations in peripherin/RDS, *CRX 8*, *GUCY2D* and *GUCA1A* gene cause autosomal dominant (AD) cone dystrophy with a better long term prognosis in *GUCA1A* involvement.[23] Mutations in PYK2- binding domain of PITPNM3 protein also cause the AD variant.[24] *ABCR* and *CACNA2D4* gene mutation causes autosomal recessive[25] and *RPGR* gene causes the X-linked recessive variant. Recently *KCNV2* mutation has been linked with cone dystrophy with supernormal rod response (CDSSR).[26] Achromatopsia gene *CNGB3* accounts for the small fraction of late-onset disease and *CNGA3* may have an additive effect.[27] Mutations in the *RDH5* gene of fundus albipunctatus have been reported to cause progressive cone dystrophy as well as night blindness.[28]

PATHOPHYSIOLOGY

The pathological hallmark is widespread degeneration of cone photoreceptors. Histopathological examination of human specimens has revealed loss of photoreceptor cells, both cones and rods, primarily at the macula and periphery with relative sparing of the equatorial area. Lipofuscin like deposits in basal portions of RPE cells with RPE atrophy in the macular area have been seen on electron microscopy.[29]

CLINICAL FEATURES

Classical cone dystrophy patients report an insidious onset of mild decrease in central visual acuity, which usually progresses over a variable period of time to stabilize around 20/200.[19] Central vision loss is usually symmetric.[18] Color discrimination is invariably affected to different degrees in all patients. Formal color vision testing using Farnsworth-Munsell hue test helps in excluding congenital color blindness patients from this subgroup. Patients usually complain of day blindness (hemeralopia) with better vision at dusk. While the presence of photophobia is an important indicator to presence of cone dystrophy (Table 8.1), nystagmus points to congenital diseases like achromatopsia and ocular albinism and reduces the probability of cone dystrophy.[19]

Ophthalmoscopic appearance is essentially normal in early stages as symptoms precede signs and diagnosis at this stage is usually clinched with ERG. With progression of disease, mottling of the RPE in perifoveal area is seen, which is followed by granularity of the RPE. Later stages may have appearance of *bull's eye maculopathy* (Figs. 8.10A and 8.11A and B), an appearance that is shared by multiple diseases. In later stages an area of retinal atrophy develops, centered on the fovea (Figs. 8.10B to D and 8.11C).[18] All cases may not progress to the advanced stage due to their individual genetic basis. Mild temporal optic disc pallor may be present in the later stages. Additional ophthalmoscopic features like appearance of bony spicules and vascular attenuation may signify a rod-cone dystrophy.

Table 8.1: Differential diagnosis for cone dysfunction.

Inheritance	Age-onset	
Hereditary	Nystagmus at birth	Achromatopsia
	Nystagmus at birth	Blue cone achromatism
	Nystagmus at birth	Ocular albinism
	First-second decade	Lebers congenital amaurosis
	Teenage- early adult	Cone dystrophy
	Teenage- early adult	Cone-rod dystrophy
	First-second decade	Rod-cone dystrophy
	Congenital	Protanopia, deuteranopia, tritanopia
Acquired	Variable (Conditions with Bull's eye maculopathy)	Drug toxicity: chloroquine, hydroxychloroquine, clofazimine
		Fundus flavimaculatus, Stargardt, fenestrated sheen dystrophy
	Variable	Chorioretinitis

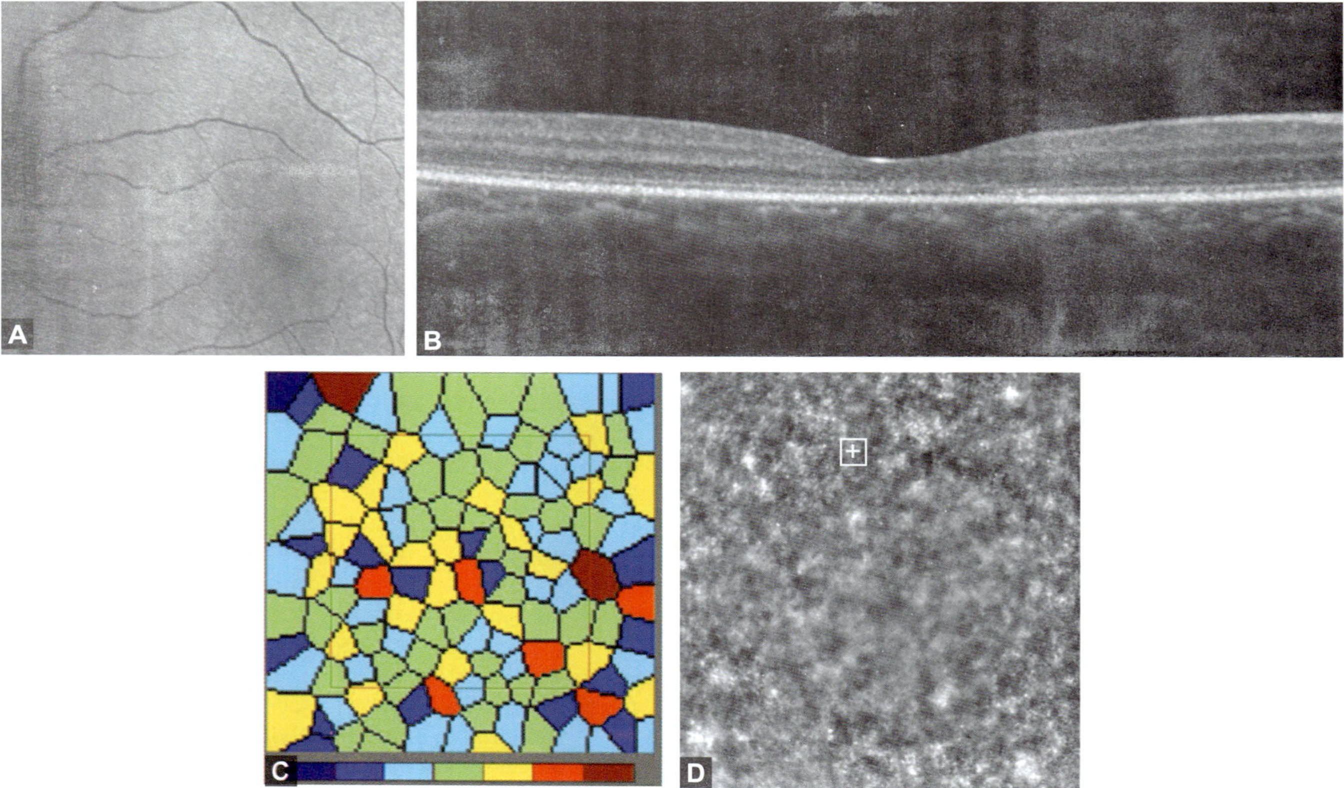

Figs. 8.10A to D: Eye with cone-rod dystrophy, showing (A) bull's-eye maculopathy on fundus autofluorescence imaging; (B) foveal atrophy on optical coherence tomography and (C and D) Adaptive Optics shows affected cone mosaic.

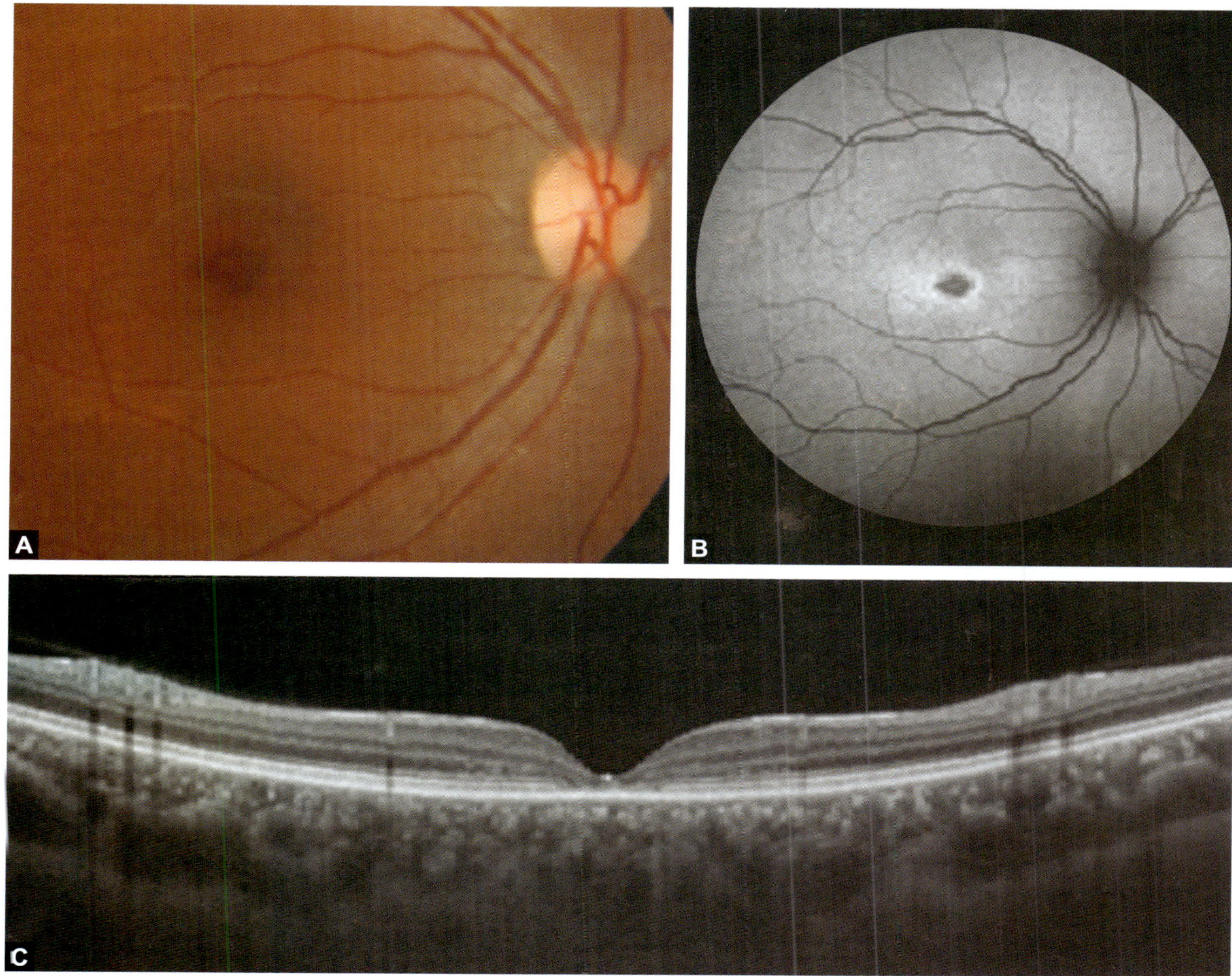

Figs. 8.11A to C: (A) Right eye of a 24-year-old male with BCVA 20/200 showing foveal atrophy; (B) Autofluorescence of the same eye shows a bull's-eye maculopathy pattern with dense focal hypofluorescence at fovea; (C) Optical coherence tomography shows foveal thinning and loss of ellpsoid zone and external limiting membrane.

INVESTIGATIONS

Visual Fields

Visual field testing is an integral part of diagnostic workup. Central field defects are the rule. The importance of visual field charting lies in the detection of peripheral field defects like ring scotomas or field constrictions, which point towards the diagnosis of rod-cone dystrophy. Perimetry also helps in the monitoring of progression of disease and prognostication.

Autofluorescence Imaging

Fundus autofluorescence changes precede ophthalmoscopic changes and classical patterns of RPE alterations help the diagnosis. Initial stages show drusen like dots manifesting hyperautofluorescence.[30] Advanced stage shows ring of hyperautofluorescence around fovea called as *bull's eye maculopathy* (Figs. 8.12 and 8.13). A circumscribed patch of hypoautofluorescence is seen in stage of central foveal atrophy (Figs. 8.12 and 8.13). Recently abnormal wide field autofluorescence has also been used as a predictor of retinal function.[31]

Electroretinography

Full field electroretinography is essential in diagnosis of cone dystrophies (Figs. 8.14A to C). Cone dystrophies are panretinal disorders unlike the macular dystrophies like Stargardt disease, which do not alter the full field ERG. An abnormal photopic ERG in the setting of normal scotopic ERG can either be cone dystrophy or achromatopsia.[32,33]

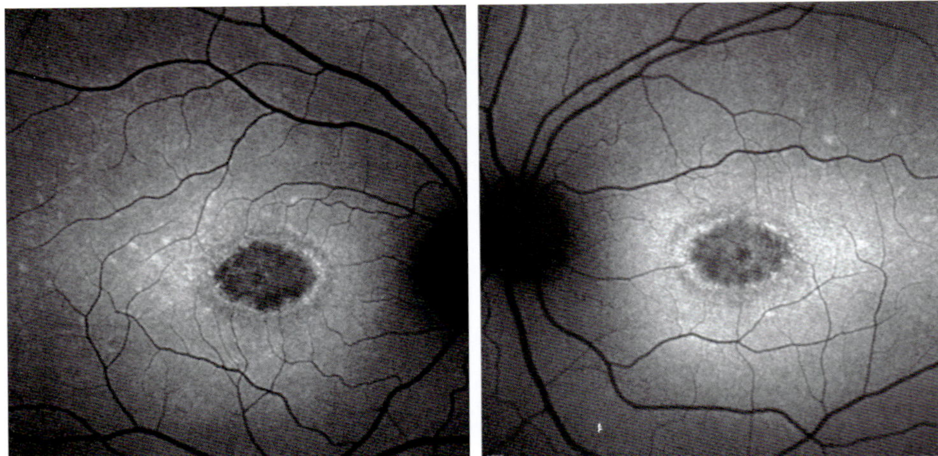

Fig. 8.12: Bull's-eye maculopathy in a case of cone dystrophy.

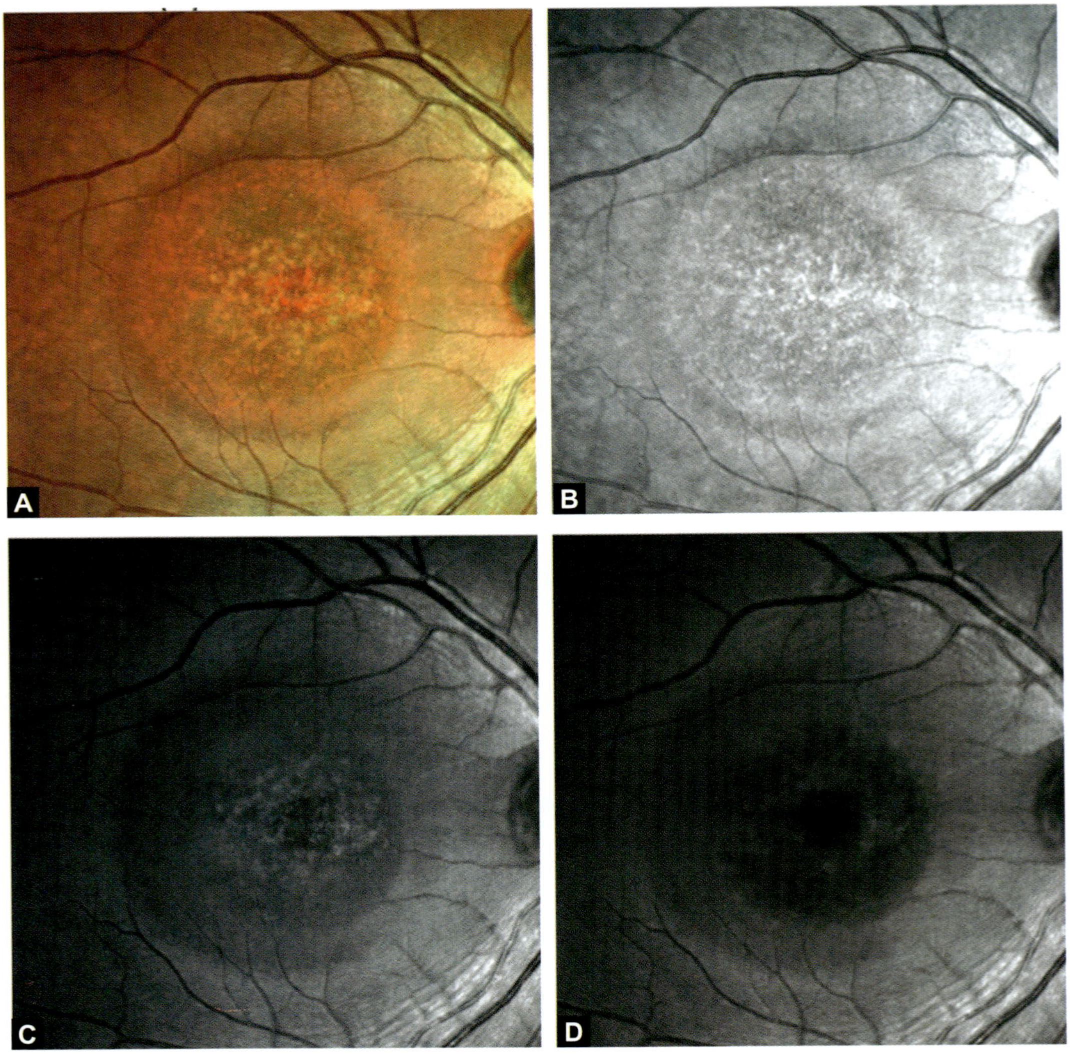

Figs. 8.13A to D: Bull's-eye maculopathy with (A) fundus autofluorescence, (B) infrared, (C) green and (D) blue reflectance images in a case of cone dystrophy.

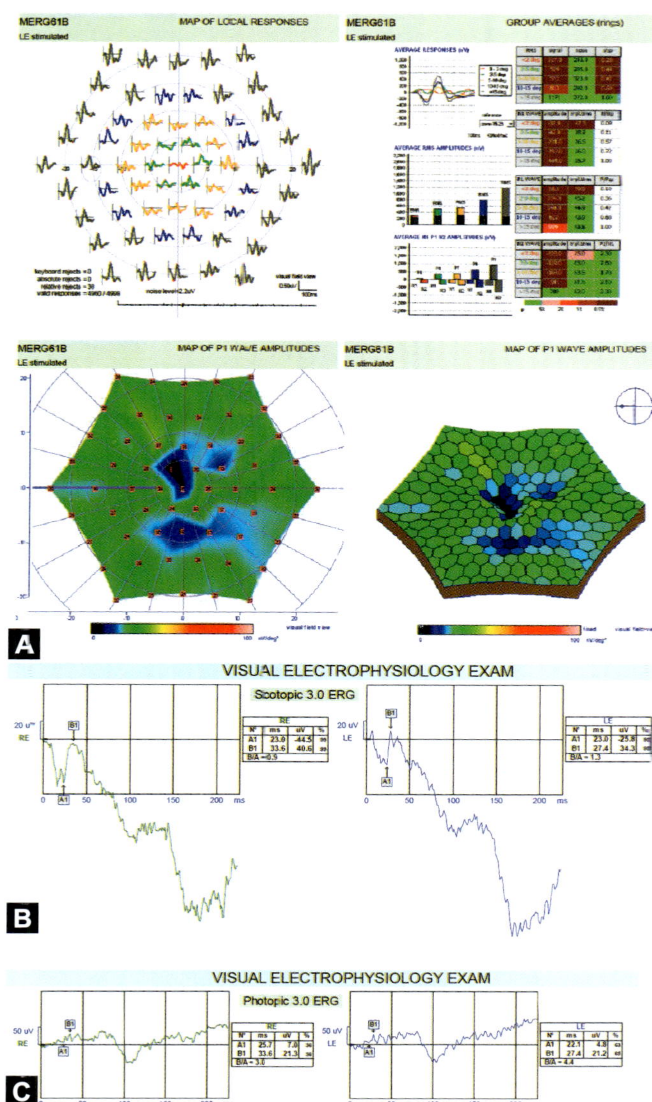

Figs. 8.14A to C: (A) Representative Multifocal ERG of an eye with cone dystrophy showing depressed amplitude in the central 1° region. ERG in these patients show normal scotopic response (B) with markedly depressed photopic response (C).

Optical Coherence Tomography

Optical coherence tomography shows progressive retinal thinning with predominant loss in the ellipsoid zone and outer nuclear layer (Fig. 8.15). RPE attenuation is also apparent.[34]

Other Investigations (Fig. 8.16)

Dark adaptometry is useful to diagnose preclinical cases. Adaptive optics is being applied to determine the clinical correlation of various genetic mutations and its phenotype. Adaptive optics can help in identifying the cone mosaic and in quantifying the cone density (Figs. 8.16D and E).

VARIANTS OF CONE DYSTROPHY

Peripheral Cone Dystrophy

This subset of patients demonstrates a relative paracentral scotoma with central sparing.[35]

Late Onset Cone Dystrophy

Electrophysiological testing is essential in these cases as the symptoms and signs overlap numerous retinal degeneration and inflammation.[22]

MANAGEMENT

The key issue in this group of disorders is formulating a correct diagnosis to allow prognostication of future visual potential and genetic counseling to determine hereditary patterns. Clinical and electrophysiologic testing formulates a diagnosis of cone dystrophy, which must be followed by search for candidate genes to prognosticate the mutation specific clinical course.

The complaints of photophobia can be overcome by use of tinted glasses and contact lenses.[36] They also help in improving daytime vision but lead to loss of depth and color perception in dim lighting. Adequate vocational rehabilitation and low vision aids may be necessary in advanced stages of disease.

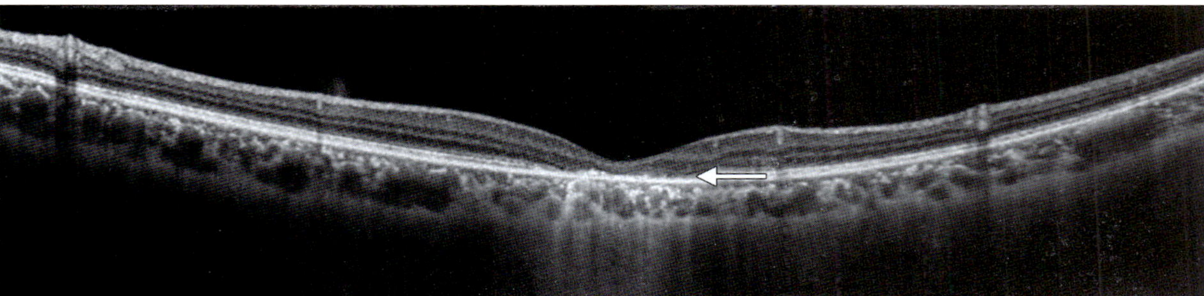

Fig. 8.15: Optical coherence tomography showed foveal thinning with absent ellipsoid zone and attenuated retinal pigment epithelium–Bruch's membrane layer.

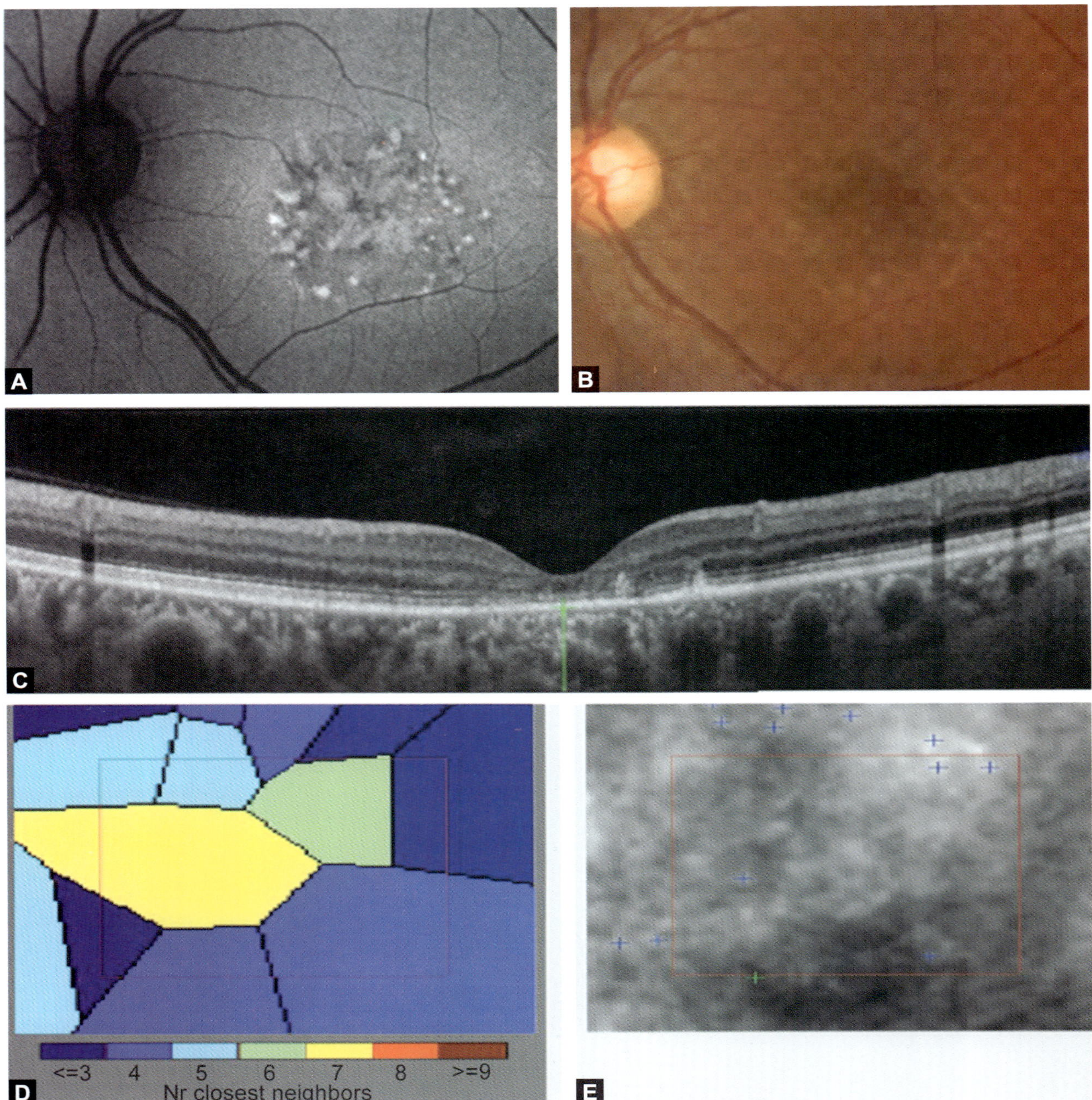

Figs. 8.16A to E: Autofluorescence (A) and color fundus photo (B) reveals a macular degeneration with pigmentary abnormality. Optical coherence tomography shows foveal thinning and outer retinal atrophy (C) adaptive optics reveals reduced cone density (E) and decreased cell adherence ratio on Voronoi diagrams (D)

ACHROMATOPSIA

INTRODUCTION

Achromatopsia (also known as rod monochromatism) is an inherited condition characterized by congenital lack of cone function and is seen in 1 in 30,000 people.[37] While complete Achromatopsia is characterized by total lack of cone function, incomplete Achromatopsia has at least one type of cones, which are functional (blue cone monochromatism being the commonest of these).

GENETICS

Complete Achromatopsia is an autosomal recessive condition. Five genes have been identified so far and all of them are encode components of the cone specific phototransduction cascade.[38,39]

CLINICAL FEATURES

Patients with complete Achromatopsia present in infancy or early childhood with complaints of pendular nystagmus, photophobia, lack of color vision, and poor visual acuity. The visual acuity is usually below 6/60. With aging the visual acuity and photophobia remain stable, but nystagmus becomes better. Stable visual acuity is a useful indicator to distinguish this condition from progressive cone dystrophies. The fundus has normal appearance, subtle pigmentary changes or may even show macular atrophy.

INVESTIGATIONS

Electroretinogram is crucial for establishing the diagnosis of Achromatopsia. While rod responses are well preserved, cone responses and 30 Hz flicker are severely diminished or absent (Fig. 8.17). Multifocal–ERG shows marked depression at macula as well.

Since these patients have congenital color blindness and have learnt various colors as lighter or darker shades of gray, they may be able to identify various colors on routine Ishihara plates despite lacking color vision totally. Visual fields though difficult to obtain because of poor fixation, show central scotoma. Dark adaptation curve shows lack of rod-cone break up, as there is no cone function.

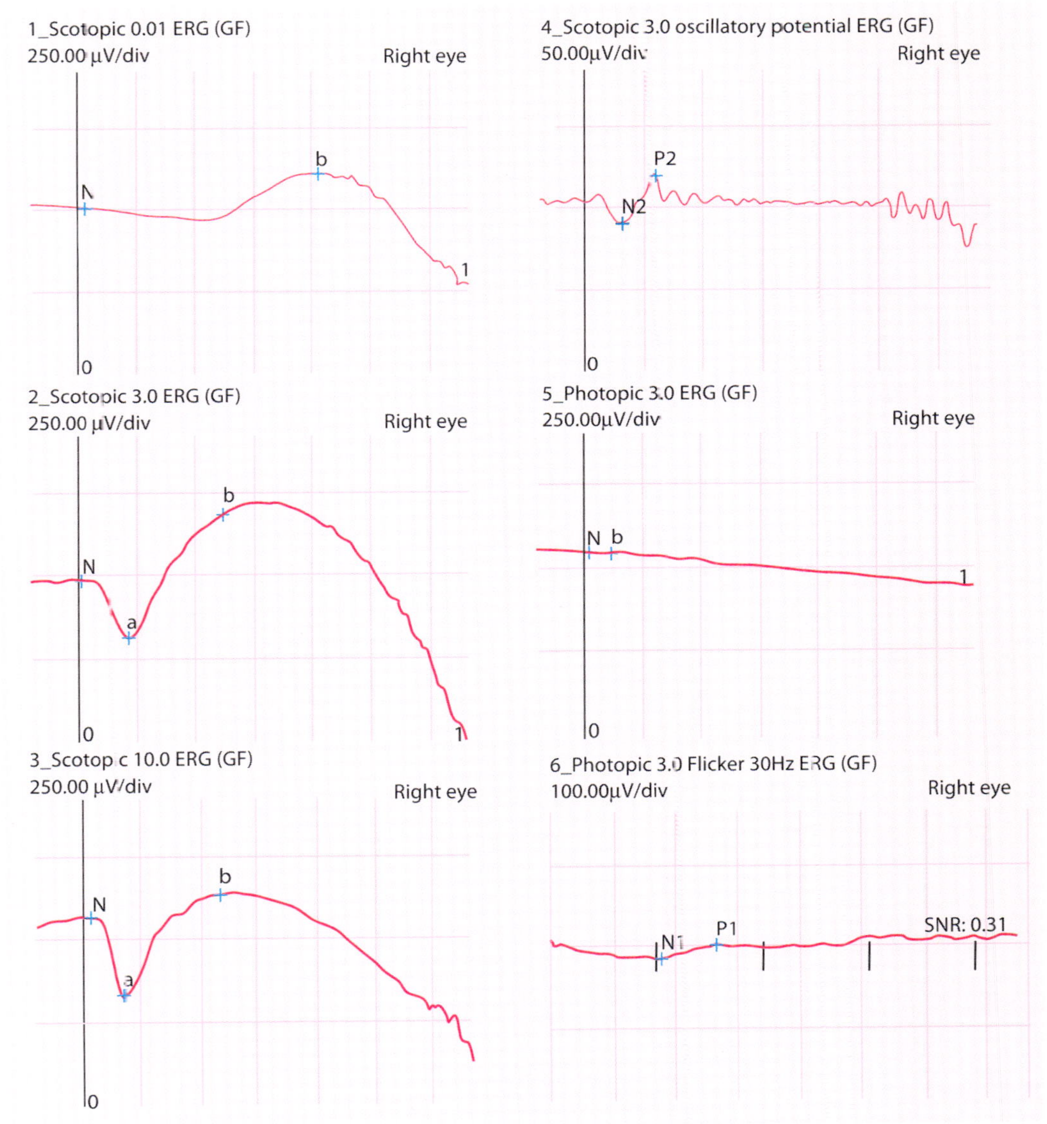

Fig. 8.17: Full-field electroretinogram of a patient with achromatopsia showing normal scotopic responses and extinguished cone and 30 Hz flicker responses.

Recent studies on OCT findings in achromatopsia[40] have revealed varied findings of foveal hypoplasia, defects in ellipsoid layer, and optically empty spaces in cone layer.

TREATMENT

Patients are troubled maximally by photophobia which can be reduced by using tinted glasses or contact lenses. While low vision aids may be prescribed for visual tasks, nystagmus tends to reduce with age.

BLUE CONE MONOCHROMATISM

INTRODUCTION

Incomplete Achromatopsia contains at least one type of functional cones. Blue cone monochromatism (BCM), also known as S cone monochromatism or X-linked incomplete achromatopsia) has preserved S cones (cones sensitive to short wavelengths) and is the commonest. It has X-linked inheritance. The L and M cones (cones sensitive to long and medium wavelengths respectively) are absent. Though L or M cone monochromatism can occur, they are extremely rare and hence not discussed here. BCM has an estimated prevalence of 1 in 100,000. Patients with BCM present with similar features as that of achromatopsia, but have better visual acuity that ranges from 6/24 to 6/60. BCM patients have preserved color vision for blue colors. ERG shows absent cone function. Blue stimulus on a yellow background may elicit S cone function and is a very useful marker of BCM as opposed to achromatopsia.

CONGENITAL RED-GREEN COLOR BLINDNESS

INTRODUCTION

The Young-Helmholtz trichromatic color vision theory basically names red, green and blue as the three primary colours present within the photoreceptors. These colors of varying wavelengths combine and produce the visible spectrum. Deficiences of any ,or a combination of these primary colors leads to color blindness of varying types. Color vision deficiency is an inherited condition affecting males (8%) more that the females (0.5%). This is because of X-linked inheritance pattern of congenital red-green color blindness. The ability of the patient to identify colors may be either defective (anomalous) or totally absent (anopia).

The three primary colors red, green and blue are referred to as prota, deutera and trita respectively. Based on the color defect and its severity the patients can therefore be named. Protanopia, deuteranopia, protanomaly, and deuteranomaly are commonly inherited forms of red-green color blindness that commonly affect human population. Those affected have difficulty with discriminating red and green hues due to the absence or mutation of the red or green retinal photoreceptors.

The Ishihara color plates (Fig. 8.18) typically test for red-green color deficiency. A number is embedded within the pseudo-isochromatic chart in a slightly different color which can be read by a normal person, but not by a color deficient person.

The Eldridge-green lantern test is another color vision test which asks the individual to be tested to see different color shades and apertures sitting at 6 metres distance. Farns-

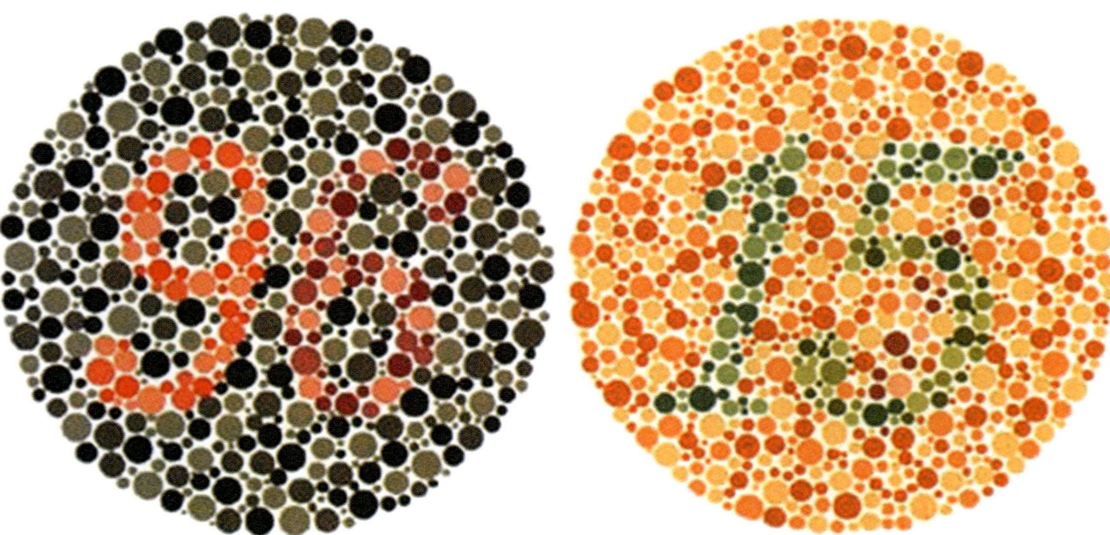

Fig 8.18: Representative pseudoisochromatic plates (Ishihara) showing the embedded digits in a slightly different colour is often difficult to perceive by the congenital red-green colour deficient person, and finds great use for ophthalmic check conducted prior to taking up a profession.

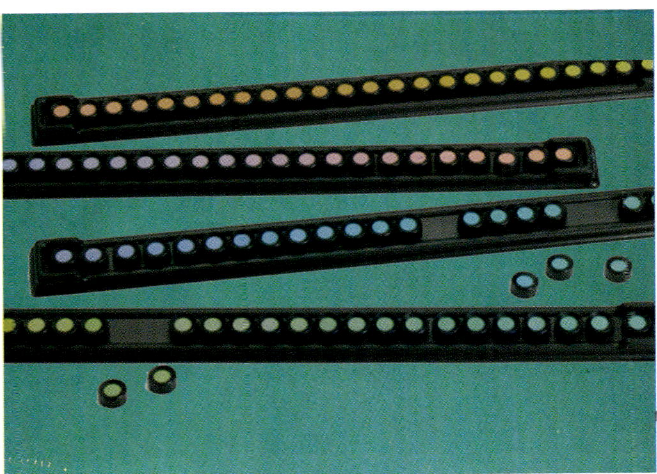

Fig. 8.19: Arrangement tests" require the examinee to arrange the colour caps in a sequence of either their hues (or saturation) or to group greys and colors. The Farnsworth-Munsell 100 Hue discrimination test (FM 100 Hue) is an arrangement test and tests for subtle colour defects.

worth-Munsell 100 Hue is a hue/chromatic discrimination by arranging a set of coloured caps based on their hue (Fig. 8.19).

Finally the Nagels Anomaloscope helps match green and red colour against a predetermined yellow color and is a sensitive test for all the primary colour deficiences.

REFERENCES

1. Fujinami K, Lois N, Davidson AE, et al. A longitudinal study of Stargardt disease: clinical and electrophysiologic assessment, progression, and genotype correlations. Am J Ophthalmology. 2013; 155(6):1075-88.
2. Cideciyan AV, Aleman TS, Swider M, et al. Mutations in ABCA4 result in accumulation of lipofuscin before slowing of the retinoid cycle: a reappraisal of the human disease sequence. Hum Mol Genet. 2004;13(5):525-34.
3. Tsybovsky Y, Molday RS, Palczewski K. The ATP-binding cassette transporter ABCA4: structural and functional properties and role in retinal disease. Adv Exp Med Biol. 2010;703:105-25.
4. Zernant J, Xie YA, Ayuso C, et al. Analysis of the ABCA4 genomic locus in Stargardt disease. Hum Mol Genet. 2014;23:6797-806.
5. Lois N, Halfyard AS, Bird AC, et al. Fundus autofluorescence in Stargardt macular dystrophy-fundus flavimaculatus. Am J Ophthalmology. 2004;138(1):55-63.
6. Gelman R, Smith RT, Tsang SH. Diagnostic accuracy evaluation of visual acuity and fundus autofluorescence macular geographic atrophy area for the discrimination of Stargardt groups. Retina. Philadelphia, PA; 2016.
7. Strauss RW, Munoz B, Wolfson Y, et al. Assessment of estimated retinal atrophy progression in Stargardt macular dystrophy using spectral-domain optical coherence tomography. Br J Ophthalmology 2015;0:1-7.
8. Oh KT, Weleber RG, Stone EM, et al. Electroretinographic findings in patients with Stargardt disease and fundus flavimaculatus. Retina. 2004;24(6):920-8.
9. Tanna P, Strauss RW, Fujinami K, Michaelides M. Stargardt disease: clinical features, molecular genetics, animal models and therapeutic options. Br J Ophthalmology. 2016.
10. Best F. Ueber eine hereditaere Makulaaffection. Zschr Augenheilk. 1905;13:199-212.
11. Stone EM, Nichols BE, Streb LM, et al. Genetic linkage of vitelliform macular degeneration (Best's disease) to chromosome 11q13. Nat Genet. 1992;1(4):246-50.
12. Miller SA, Bresnick GH, Chandra SR. Choroidal neovascular membrane in Best's vitelliform macular dystrophy. Am J Ophthalmology. 1976;82(2):252-5.
13. Wittstrom E, Ponjavic V, Bondeson ML, et al. Anterior Segment abnormalities and angle-closure glaucoma in a family with a mutation in the Best1 gene and Best vitelliform macular dystrophy. Ophthalmic Genet. 2011;32(4):217-27.
14. Querques G, Regenbogen M, Quijano C, et al. High-definition optical coherence tomography features in vitelliform macular dystrophy. Am J Ophthalmology. 2008;146(4):501-7.
15. Querques G, Bocco MC, Soubrane G, et al. Intravitreal ranibizumab (Lucentis) for choroidal neovascularization associated with vitelliform macular dystrophy. Acta Ophthalmology. 2008;86(6): 694-5.
16. Gass JD. A clinicopathologic study of a peculiar foveomacular dystrophy. Trans Am Ophthalmology Soc. 1974;72:139-56.
17. Grob S, Yonekawa Y, Eliott D. Multimodal imaging of adult-onset foveomacular vitelliform dystrophy. Saudi J Ophthalmology. 2014;28(2):104-10.
18. Wu DM, Fawzi AA. Abnormalities of Cone and Rod Function. In: Ryan SJ (Ed). Retina, 5th edition. USA: Elsevier Saunders; 2013. pp. 899.
19. Atmaca-Sonmez P, Khan NW, Heckenlively JR. Hereditary Cone Dystrophies. In: Albert DM, Miller JW (Eds). Albert Jakobiec's Principles and Practice of Ophthalmology, 3rd edition. Philadelphia: Saunders Elsevier; 2008. pp. 2253.
20. Michaelides M, Hardcastle AJ, Hunt DM, Moore AT. Progressive Cone and Cone-Rod Dystrophies: Phenotypes and Underlying Molecular Genetic Basis. Surv Ophthalmology. 2006 May;51(3):232-58.
21. Cone Dystrophies. In: Retina and Vitreous Basic and Clinical Science Course 2015-16. American Academy of Ophthalmology. pp. 236.
22. Langwinska-Wosko E, Szulborski K, Broniek-Kowalik K. Late onset cone dystrophy. Doc Ophthalmology. 2010;120(3):215-8.
23. Miyake Y. Cone Dystrophy. In: Electrodiagnosis of Retinal Diseases. Tokyo: Springer-Verlag; 2006. pp. 126.
24. Köhn L, Kadzhaev K, Burstedt MSI, et al. Mutation in the PYK2-binding domain of PITPNM3 causes autosomal dominant cone dystrophy (CORD5) in two Swedish families. Eur J Hum Genet. 2007;15(6):664-71.
25. Wycisk KA, Zeitz C, Feil S, et al. Mutation in the Auxiliary Calcium-Channel Subunit CACNA2D4 Causes Autosomal Recessive Cone Dystrophy. Am J Hum Genet. 2006;79(5):973-7.
26. Zelinger L, Wissinger B, Eli D, et al. Cone Dystrophy with Supernormal Rod Response: Novel KCNV2 Mutations in an Underdiagnosed Phenotype. Ophthalmology. 2013;120(11):2338-43.
27. Thiadens AA, Roosing S, Collin RWJ, et al. Comprehensive Analysis of the Achromatopsia Genes CNGA3 and CNGB3 in Progressive Cone Dystrophy. Ophthalmology. 2010;117(4):825-30.
28. Nakamura M, Hotta Y, Tanikawa A, et al. A high association with cone dystrophy in fundus albipunctatus caused by mutations of the RDH5 gene. Invest Ophthalmology Vis Sci. 2000;41(12):3925-32.
29. Rabb MF, Tso MO, Fishman GA. Cone-Rod Dystrophy. Ophthalmology. 1986;93(11):1443-51.
30. Wang NK, Chou CL, Lima LH, et al. Fundus autofluorescence in cone dystrophy. Doc Ophthalmology. 2009;119(2):141-4.

31. Oishi M, Oishi A, Ogino K, et al. Wide-Field Fundus Autofluorescence Abnormalities and Visual Function in Patients With Cone and Cone-Rod DystrophiesWide-Field FAF in Cone-Rod Dystrophy. Invest Ophthalmology Vis Sci. 2014;55(6):3572-7.

32. David AQ, Barbara AB. Clinical Retina. 1st edition. AMA Press; 2002.

33. Langwińska-Wośko E, Szulborski K, Zaleska-Żmijewska A, et al. Electrophysiological testing as a method of cone–rod and cone dystrophy diagnoses and prediction of disease progression. Doc Ophthalmology. 2015;130(2):103-9.

34. Ito N, Kameya S, Gocho K, et al. Multimodal imaging of a case of peripheral cone dystrophy. Doc Ophthalmology. 2015;130(3):241-51.

35. Kondo M, Miyake Y, Kondo N, et al. Peripheral cone dystrophy: A variant of cone dystrophy with predominant dysfunction in the peripheral cone system1. Ophthalmology. 2004;111(4):732-9.

36. Rajak SN, Currie AD, Dubois VJ, et al. Tinted Contact Lenses as an Alternative Management for Photophobia in Stationary Cone Dystrophies in Children. J Am Assoc Pediatr Ophthalmology Strabismus. 2006;10(4):336-9.

37. Michaelides M, Hunt DM, Moore AT. The cone dysfunction syndromes. Br J Ophthalmology. 2004;88(2):291-7.

38. Remmer MH, Rastogi N, Ranka MP, et al. Achromatopsia: a review. Curr Opin Ophthalmology. 2015;26(5):333-40.

39. Aboshiha J, Dubis AM, Carroll J, Hardcastle AJ, Michaelides M. The cone dysfunction syndromes. Br J Ophthalmology. Mar 13, 2015.

40. Thiadens AA, Somervuo V, van den Born LI, et al. Progressive loss of cones in achromatopsia: an imaging study using spectral-domain optical coherence tomography. Invest Ophthalmology Vis Sci. 2010;51(11):5952-7.

Chapter 9

Choroidal and Other Fundal Dystrophies

Vinod Kumar, Karthikeya R, Pradeep Kumar

CHOROIDEREMIA

INTRODUCTION

Choroideremia is an X-linked recessive disorder characterized by degeneration of retina, retinal pigment epithelium (RPE) and choroid. It was first described by Mauthner[1] in 1872 and has an estimated prevalence of one in 50,000.[2]

PATHOPHYSIOLOGY

Genetics

Choroideremia occurs because of mutation in the *CHM* gene, localized on the X chromosome (Xq21).[3] The *CHM* gene encodes the 95 kDa protein Rab escort protein 1 (REP1).[4] Mutations in the *CHM* gene cause truncation or deletion of REP1, which is known to play an essential role in the intracellular vesicular transport. Although the X-linked diseases manifest in males, in choroideremia, female carriers may also be affected because of lyonization phenomenon. In this phenomenon, one of the two copies of the X chromosome present in females is inactivated leading to expression of gene even with one copy.

CLINICAL FEATURES

Affected males present in the first or second decade with difficulty in vision in the night or dim light conditions.[4] The visual acuity is frequently normal at this stage. With disease progression, visual acuity as well as the field of vision decrease. The field of vision is affected significantly by the fourth decade but patients often retain useful vision by this time.

In early stages, the fundus may be normal or have subtle RPE changes that may mimic retinitis pigmentosa. With progression mid-peripheral retinal, RPE and choroidal atrophy sets in which progresses both centripetally and centrifugally. The macula is spared till late, i.e. 5th to 6th decade. In the last stages only a small cruciate shaped area of normal retina may persist (Fig. 9.1A). Extensive RPE atrophy results in visible large choroidal vessels initially and bare sclera in late stages. This gives a pale appearance to the fundus.

Carrier females are often asymptomatic. They may show patchy atrophy and pigment mottling in the peripheral retina.

INVESTIGATIONS

Fluorescein angiography shows filling of large choroidal vessels only. It is also helpful in determining the residual capillary bed in the macular area (Fig. 9.1B).

Visual fields show a ring scotoma and defects which commensurate with the chorioretinal degeneration seen in the midperiphery. With disease progression, contraction of visual fields is observed.

Electroretinogram (ERG) shows absent scotopic and severely diminished photopic responses even in early stages. Both photopic and scotopic responses become extinguished eventually in cases with choroideremia.

Optical coherence tomography (OCT) may be a useful tool to document and monitor cystoid macular edema seen frequently in these patients.[5]

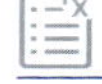

MANAGEMENT

Phase 1-2 clinical trials assessing gene therapy using the AAV2-REP1 vector have been recently published. The therapy was found to be safe and had a positive effect on visual acuity and retinal sensitivity.[6]

GYRATE ATROPHY

INTRODUCTION

It is a rare choroidal disease with low prevalence characterized by progressive chorioretinal atrophy especially in peripheral retina. The first case of this disease was described in 1888 by Jacobsohn[7] as an example of "atypical retinitis pigmentosa". The disease was first recognized as a distinct entity by Cut-

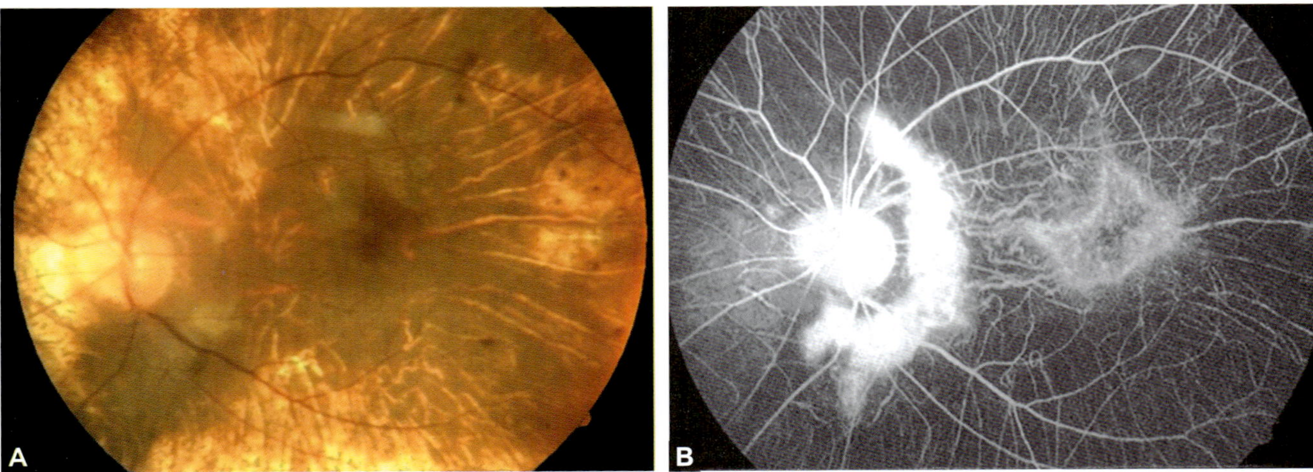

Figs. 9.1A and B: (A) Color fundus photograph of a patient with choroideremia showing chorioretinal atrophy, visible large choroidal vessels, areas of scleral show and preserved macular area; (B) Fluorescein angiogram of same patient showing filling of large choroidal vessels only. Note preserved choriocapillaris in macular and peripapillary area.

ler[8] and Fuchs[9]. Ornithine-δ-aminotransferase (OAT) gene mutation causes gyrate atrophy. The *OAT* gene is essential for the synthesis of enzyme ornithine aminotransferase which helps in breaking down ornithine in the mitochondria of cells.

 **PATHOPHYSIOLOGY**

Genetics

The disease is inherited as an autosomal recessive trait, due to a genetic defect in the mitochondrial encoded enzyme 'OAT'.[10] A number of mutations have been identified in the OAT gene on chromosome 10q26.[11-13] OAT catalyzes interconversion of ornithine, glutamate and proline and has pyridoxal phosphate (vitamin B6) as a cofactor. This leads to hyperornithinemia, and reduced levels of plasma lysine, glutamine, glutamate and creatinine.[14-16]

Mutations in *OAT* gene result in a reduced amount of functional ornithine aminotransferase enzyme which impedes the conversion of ornithine into pyrroline-5-carboxylate (P5C). It is not clear how these changes result in the specific signs and symptoms of gyrate atrophy. Studies have suggested that a deficiency of P5C may interfere with the normal function of the retina and excess ornithine may suppress the production of creatine. Creatine is needed by many tissues in the body to store and use energy.

 **CLINICAL FEATURES**

The symptoms usually begin in the second to third decades of life and include poor night vision and constriction of peripheral field of vision with high myopia. Since the disease is progressive and spreads from periphery to center, macula may be involved in later phases and hence, diminution of

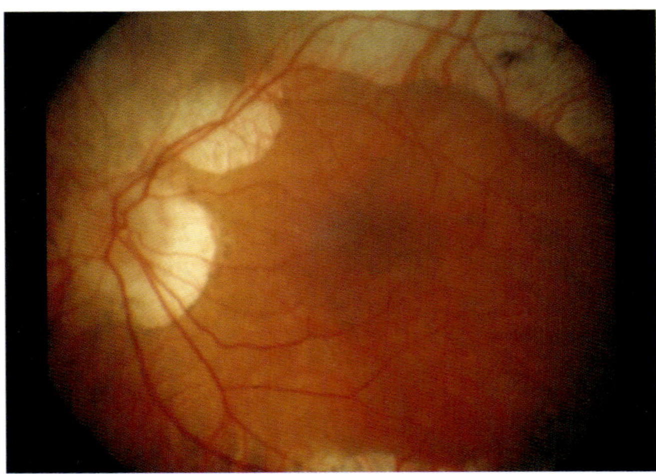

Fig. 9.2: Color fundus picture showing patches of chorioretinal atrophy with scalloped margins.

vision is a late presentation. Frequent association involves myopia, posterior subcapsular cataracts and vitreous opacities.[17]

The fundus changes involves characteristic well circumscribed patches of chorioretinal atrophy with hyperpigmented margins that begin in the mid-peripheral and peripheral retina with thinning and atrophy of RPE with either normal or sclerotic underlying choroidal vessels. The lesions typically have scalloped margin between the affected and unaffected retina and are distinct to begin with, but later become confluent as they progress both centrally and peripherally (Fig. 9.2).

In later stages, the retinal vessels may be attenuated and the optic nerve may appear pale. Cystoid macular edema has been reported in patients with gyrate atrophy.[18-20]

 ## INVESTIGATIONS

Visual field testing most commonly shows a concentric peripheral constriction of the visual field. In later stages, annular ring or paracentral scotomas may be seen. Central scotoma is seen if the fovea is involved.

Full-field ERG in early stages shows only a mild abnormality in rod and cone amplitude which deteriorates and may become undetectable as the disease progresses. In early stages, rods are more affected, but later both cones and rods are severely impaired.[21,22] The electro-oculography (EOG) light peak to dark trough ratio may become markedly reduced at later stages.

Histopathology is remarkable in that there is complete loss of the retina, RPE, and choroid in the affected areas, with an abrupt transition to unaffected retina.[23]

MANAGEMENT

Arginine being a precursor of ornithine, a diet restricted in arginine and low in protein has been advised as a form of therapy in patients with gyrate atrophy of the choroid and retina.[24-26] Since ornithine is produced from other amino acids as well, some investigators advocate a strict low-protein diet with near total elimination of arginine with essential amino acid supplementation.

Some cases of gyrate atrophy may respond to oral pyridoxal phosphate (vitamin B6) with resultant decrease in plasma ornithine levels. Others may be nonresponsive to B6 and are called as nonresponders.[27] Overall, ERG responses are better maintained by B6-responders compared to nonresponders.[23,27] The dietary approach to reducing plasma ornithine levels in patients with gyrate atrophy showed varied effectivity in different studies.[24-27] Intravitreal injection of 4-mg triamcinolone acetonide for macular edema in gyrate atrophy has shown short-term therapeutic effects, with recurrence of edema after drug clearance.[20]

X-LINKED RETINOSCHISIS (XLRS)

 ## INTRODUCTION

Haas[28] first described X-linked retinoschisis (XLRS) in 1898. The currently accepted terminology, XLRS, was first used in 1953.[29] XLRS is one of the most common genetic causes of progressive vitreoretinal degeneration in young male children. The disease is relatively common and prevalence of disease varies from one in 5,000–25,000.[30,31]

 ## PATHOPHYSIOLOGY

Genetics

X-linked retinoschisis (XLRS) is caused by mutations in *RS1* gene on chromosome Xp22.1. Since its first identification

by Sauer et al[32] in 1997, approximately 200 mutations have been identified till date.[33] Though all kinds of mutations may be seen, missense mutations in exons 4–6 are most common. *RS1* is expressed in the photoreceptors and retinal bipolar cells,[34] and encodes a 224-amino-acid highly conserved 23 kDa protein complex—Retinoschisin. Retinoschisin is a cell adhesion protein which helps to maintain structural integrity of the photoreceptor-bipolar synapse and the cellular organization of the retina. Mutations of *RS1* disrupt subunit assembly of protein structure and cause XLRS.

Female carriers of *RS1* mutation do not show any visual dysfunction. However, they act as carriers and transmit the gene to half of their children. Males having the mutation are uniformly affected, and pass their mutation to their daughters only.

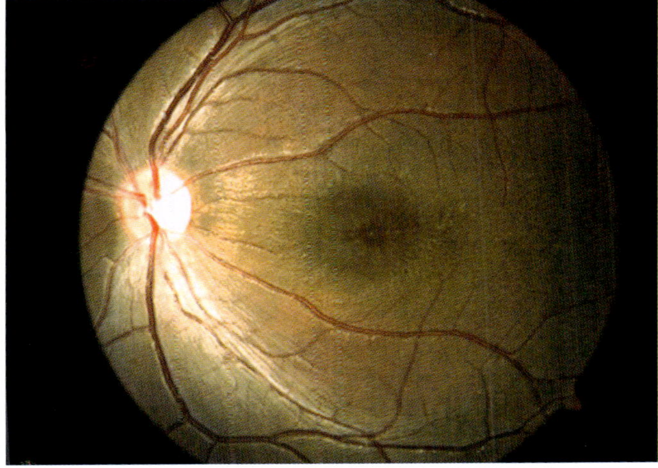 ## CLINICAL FEATURES

The patients typically present in the first or early second decade with complaints of decreased vision. In severe cases, presentation can be earlier with squint or nystagmus.

The characteristic finding is bilateral foveal schisis (Fig. 9.3) seen in 98–100% of the cases in patients with XLRS.[35] The typical pattern of radiating folds like a spoke-wheel pattern in the macula is however seen in 70% of the patients only.[36] Though disease is bilateral, asymmetric involvement may be seen.

Peripheral retinoschisis (Fig. 9.4) is seen in approximately 50% of cases and is predominantly seen in inferotemporal quadrant (Fig. 9.5). Peripheral schisis usually occurs in the inner retinal layers. The retinal blood vessels can be seen in the inner or outer layer of retinoschisis, sometimes crossing from one to another. Breaks develop in the inner and/or outer layers and may range from small holes to total absence of retinal tissue. With progression, only blood vessels or

Fig. 9.3: Color fundus photograph showing foveal schisis and radiating folds in a patient with XLRS ("cart-wheel appearance").

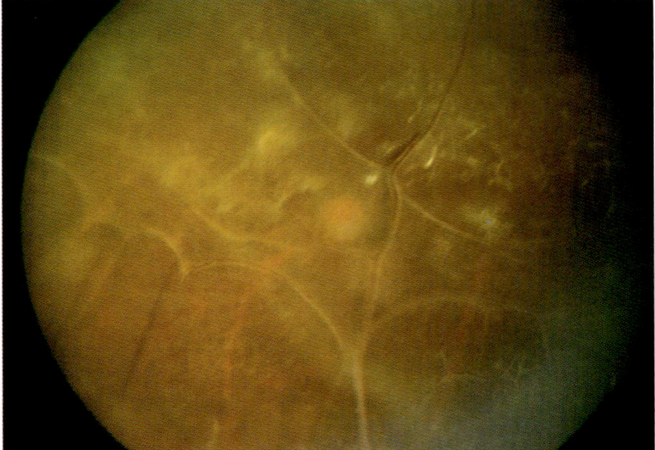

Fig. 9.4: Color fundus photograph of a patient with XLRS showing peripheral retinoschisis, holes in inner layer and vitreous veils. Note the silver dendriform lesions.

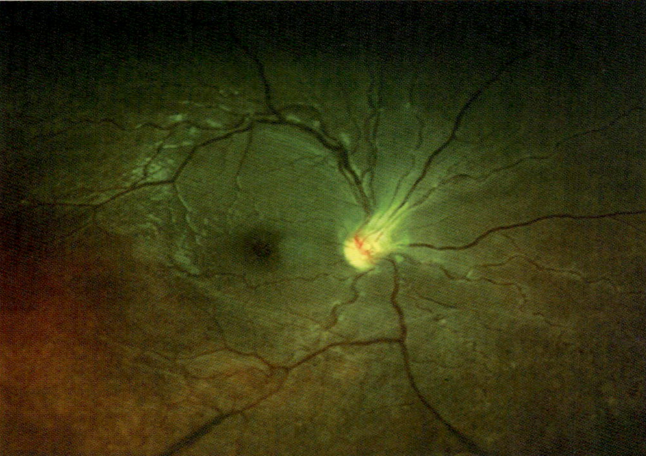

Fig. 9.5: Ultrawide field pseudocolor photograph of right eye showing foveal and peripheral schisis and vitreous veils in the inferior fundus.

small remnants of retinal tissue persist, which are known as "vitreous veils". Other common clinical features include silver dendriform lesions in the periphery, vascular attenuation, sheathing and subretinal fibrosis.

Common causes of vision loss include retinal detachment (5–20%),[36] vitreous hemorrhage (one-third of cases),[37] hemorrhages in the schitic cavities, splitting of the macular layers and macular hole formation.[38] The visual acuity ranges from 6/18 to 6/60 and remains stable up to 5th to 6th decade after which progression frequently leads to legal blindness.

INVESTIGATIONS

Optical coherence tomography is a useful tool to assess the pathology in the macula (Fig. 9.6). The outer retina shows schisis cavities at the macula, whereas in more peripheral regions splitting of the retina typically occurs more superficially. This is in contrast to degenerative retinoschisis, where the peripheral schisis occurs in deeper retinal layers. Also, the schitic cavities at macula in XLRS are seen in multiple layers.[39] The OCT may show additional findings like lamellar or full thickness macular hole. OCT is also helpful in follow-up and monitoring of macular changes in these patients. The OCT picture mimics that of cystoid macular edema (CME) and it is important to distinguish the two.

Electroretinogram is a helpful tool in the diagnosis of XLRS. The selective depression of b-wave amplitude with preservation of a-wave amplitude [negative ERG, (Fig. 9.7)] is a typical feature of XLRS[40] and in combination with clinical findings makes the diagnosis of XLRS highly likely.

Fluorescein angiography, though not usually performed is helpful in differentiating foveal schisis from CME, as no leakage is seen in the former.

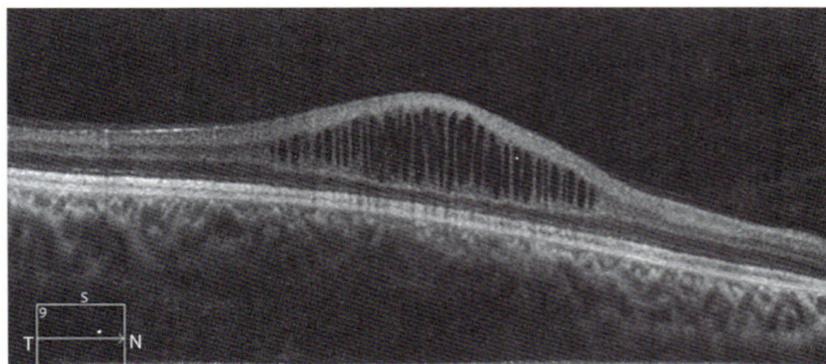

Fig. 9.6: Spectral domain optical coherence tomography (SD-OCT) of macula in a patient with XLRS showing foveal schisis in inner nuclear layer.

DIFFERENTIAL DIAGNOSIS

Goldmann-Favre vitreoretinal degeneration (GFVD) can closely mimic XLRS. However, severely diminished vision, nyctalopia, presence of pigmentation and affection of both a- as well as b-wave on ERG point towards GFVD.

Degenerative retinoschisis is seen in elderly, is unilateral and predominantly peripheral. Macular schisis is not seen in these cases. It is important to distinguish CME from various disorders; fluorescein angiography may be a helpful tool in such cases.

MANAGEMENT

No definitive medical treatment for XLRS exists. The carbonic anhydrase inhibitor Dorzolamide has been used for foveal schisis in patients with XLRS with some positive effect.[41]

Laser photocoagulation may be employed for progressive retinoschisis. However, the role of laser photocoagulation

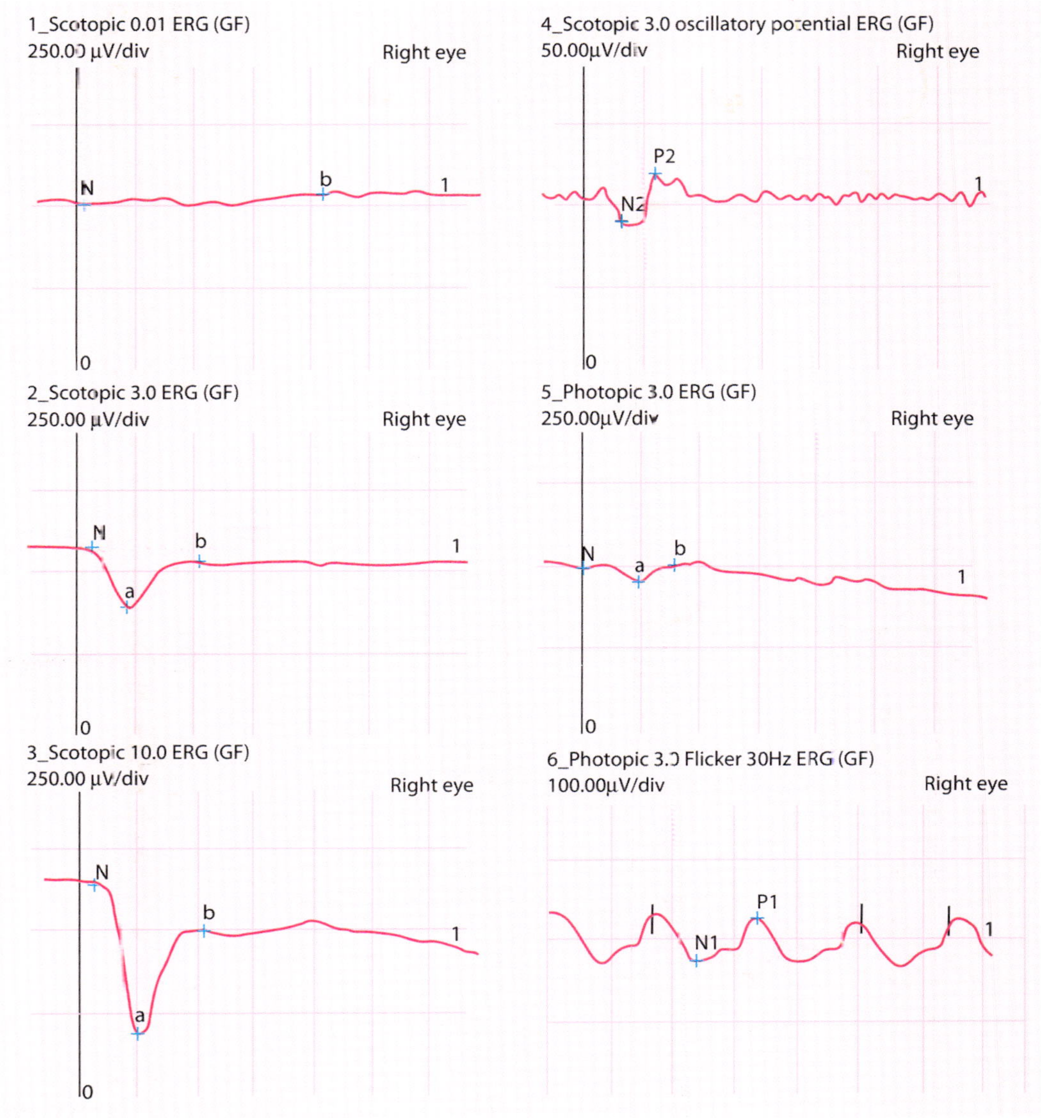

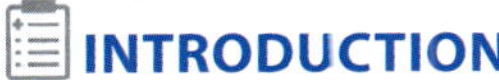

Fig. 9.7: Electroretinogram (ERG) in X-linked retinoschisis showing selective decrease of the b-wave amplitude.

remains controversial, as there are reports of increased incidence of retinal detachment following laser photocoagulation.[42]

Vitreoretinal surgery is reserved for complications of XLRS like retinal detachment and vitreous hemorrhage. Vitreous hemorrhage occurring in the setting of XLRS resolves frequently and vitrectomy is indicated only in cases of dense vitreous hemorrhage. Hemorrhage into the schitic cavities also resolves spontaneously and vitrectomy is done only if the blood filled schitic cavity overhangs the macula. During vitrectomy it is important to relieve the traction on blood vessels to prevent recurrence of bleeding. Removal of the inner wall is often required to relieve traction on the retina in case of retinal detachment in XLRS.

OCULOCUTANEOUS ALBINISM

INTRODUCTION

Oculocutaneous albinism (OCA) is a genetic disorder caused by a complete deficiency or dysfunction in melanin synthesis resulting in the hypomelanosis of skin, hair and eyes. The patients have normal number of melanocytes in the skin and follicles, but the melanin pigment is totally or partially absent.[43] The skin and hair are not affected in ocular albinism, with eye being the only organ affected. Albinism occurs all over the world with a prevalence of 1 in 17,000, and the prevalence is more in sub-Saharan Africa.

 **PATHOPHYSIOLOGY**

Genetics

The disease is predominantly autosomal recessive. Ocular albinism (*OA1* gene) is transmitted in an X-linked manner. Four distinct types of OCA are known depending on the gene involved. The types and genes are as described in Table 9.1.

Oculocutaneous albinism type 1A is the most severe type with complete lack of melanin biosynthesis. Other types have some amount of melanin production, which can be determined by hair bulb incubation test. The test however is reliable only after 5 years of age.

CLINICAL FEATURES

Reduction in melanin makes the skin pale and hair look white in patients with OCA (Fig. 9.8). This also predisposes to increased risk of skin malignancies that are a major cause of mortality in these patients. Deafness may be an associated feature in ocular albinism.

Ocular features overlap in all types of OCA and ocular albinism. Patients are intolerant to ambient light conditions and complain of intense photophobia. They have poor visual acuities that range from 6/18 to 6/120 and horizontal pendular nystagmus, which improves with age. The iris lacks pigment leading to a translucent pink appearance of the eye (Fig. 9.9). In other types of OCA, the iris color may vary depending on the amount of melanin pigment.

Reduced or absent pigment in the RPE makes the fundus appearance pale with visible underlying large choroidal vessels (Fig. 9.10). Foveal hypoplasia is common; it is diagnosed by absent foveal reflex and absence of yellow xanthophyll as well as hyperpigmentation of RPE cells at the macula. Fluorescein angiography shows absence of foveal avascular zone and OCT reveals absence of foveal contour (Fig. 9.11). In addition, patients have high incidence of refractive errors, squint and positive angle kappa. One peculiar feature of OCA is increased crossover of optic nerve fibers at the optic chiasma.

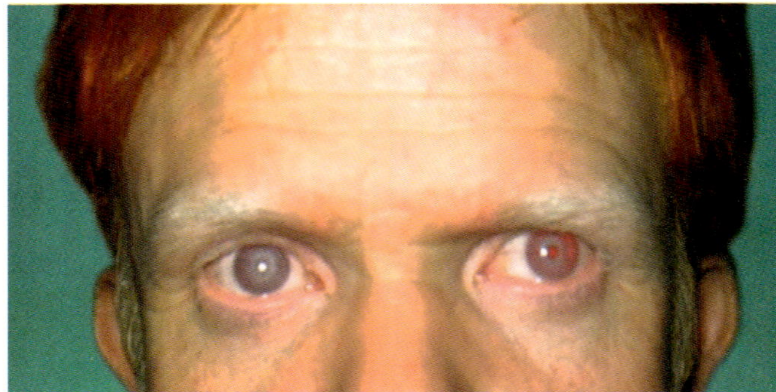

Fig. 9.8: Patient with Oculocutaneous albinism (some pigmentation present) shows red hair, pale skin and iris.

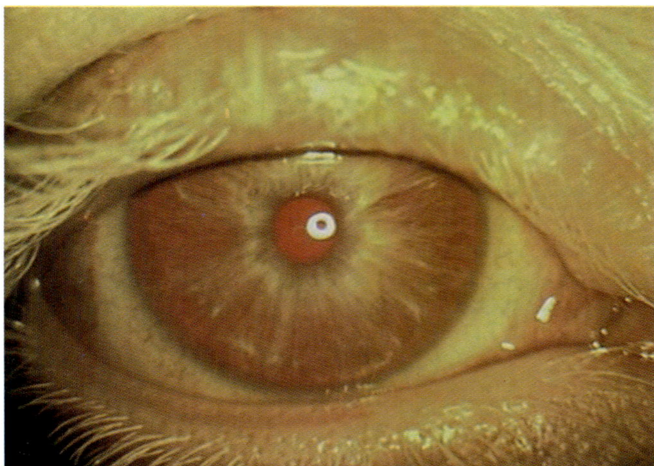

Fig. 9.9: Translucent iris and pink eye appearance in albinism.

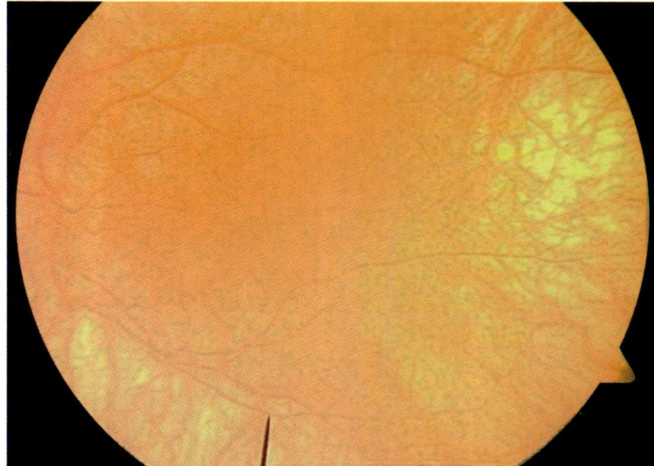

Fig. 9.10: Color fundus photograph of a patient with oculocutaneous albinism showing hypopigmented RPE and visible large choroidal vessels.

Table 9.1: Various types of oculocutaneous albinism (OCA).	
Type	*Gene*
OCA type 1A	TYR
OCA type 1B	TYR
OCA type 2	OCA2
OCA type 3	TYR P1
OCA type 4	SCL45A2

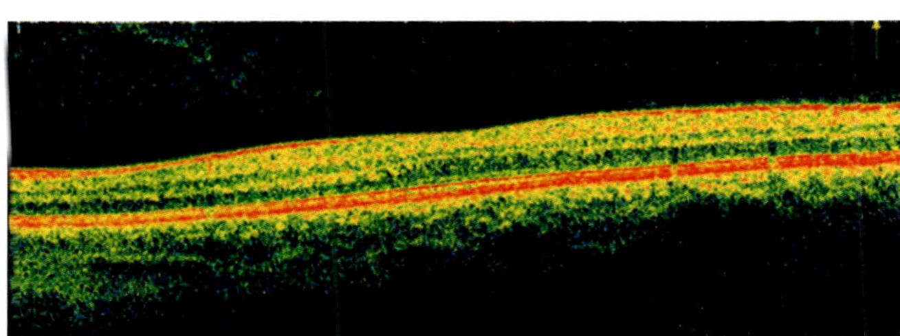

Fig. 9.11: Spectral domain optical coherence tomography (SD-OCT) scan of a patient of a patient with albinism showing flattening of foveal contour suggestive of foveal hypoplasia.

INVESTIGATIONS

Visual-evoked potential (VEP) is a useful tool in the diagnosis of patients with OCA as VEP is often asymmetrical in the two eyes because of faulty crossover at optic chiasma.[44]

Oculocutaneous albinism may be a part of syndromes such as Hermansky-Pudlak syndrome (HPS), Chediak-Higashi syndrome (CHS) and Waardenburg syndrome type II.

The HPS is an autosomal recessive condition characterized by hypopigmentation and accumulation of the ceroid material in tissues throughout the body. These patients have immunologic deficiency. The systemic problems in HPS include interstitial lung fibrosis, granulomatous colitis and bleeding diathesis due to deficiency of granules in the platelets.

The CHS is a rare condition associated with increased susceptibility to bacterial infections, hypopigmentation, prolonged bleeding time, bruisability, and peripheral neuropathy. Appropriate testing is mandatory to rule out syndromes in affected patients.

MANAGEMENT

The most troublesome symptom of OCA patients is photophobia, which can be managed by dark glasses. Dark glasses also help in reducing nystagmus. Refractive errors if any, should be corrected. These patients often benefit from bifocal glasses and low vision aids.

REFERENCES

1. Mauthner L. Ein Fall von Choroideremia. Berl Natur-med Ver Innsbruck. 1872;2:191.
2. MacDonald IM, Sereda C, McTaggart K, et al. Choroideremia gene testing. Expert Rev Mol Diagn. 2004;4:478-84.
3. Lewis RA, Nussbaum RL, Ferrell R. Mapping X-linked ophthalmic diseases. Provisional assignment of the locus for choroideremia to Xq13-q24. Ophthalmology. 1985;92:800-6.
4. Roberts MF, Fishman GA, Roberts DK, et al. Retrospective, longitudinal, and cross sectional study of visual acuity impairment in choroideremia. Br J Ophthalmology. 2002;86: 658-62.
5. Genead MA, Fishman GA. Cystic macular oedema on spectral-domain optical coherence tomography in choroideremia patients without cystic changes on fundus examination. Eye (Lond). 2011; 25:84-90.
6. MacLaren RE, Groppe M, Barnard AR, et al. Retinal gene therapy in patients with choroideremia: initial findings from a phase 1/2 clinical trial. Lancet. 2014;383:1129-37.
7. Jacobsohn E. Ein fall von Retinitis pigmentosa atypica. Klin Monatsbl Augenheilkd. 1888;26:202-6.
8. Cutler C. Dri ungewohnliche Falle von retino-choroideak Degeneration. Arch Augenheilkd. 1895;30:117.
9. Fuchs E. Ueber awei der Retinitis pigmentosa verwandte Krankheiten (retinitis punctata albescens und atrophia gyrata choriodeae et retinae). Arch Augenheilkd. 1896; 32:111.
10. Simell O, Takki K. Raised plasma-ornithine and gyrate atrophy of the choroid and retina. Lancet. 1973;1:1031-3.
11. Valle D, Walser M, Brusilow SW, et al. Gyrate atrophy of the choroid and retina: amino acid metabolism and correction of hyperornithinemia with an arginine-deficient diet. J Clin Invest. 1980;65:371-8.
12. Valle D, Walser M, Brusilow S, et al. Gyrate atrophy of the choroid and retina. Biochemical considerations and experience with an arginine-restricted diet. Ophthalmology. 1981;88:325-30.
13. Kaiser-Kupfer MI, de Monasterio FM, Valle D, et al. Gyrate atrophy of the choroid and retina: improved visual function following reduction of plasma ornithine by diet. Science. 1980;210:1128-31.
14. Inana G. Hotta Y, Zintz C, et al. Expression defect of ornithine aminotransferase gene in gyrate atrophy. Invest Ophthalmology Vis Sci. 1988;7:1001-5.
15. Mitchell GA, Brody LC, Siplia I, et al. At least two mutant alleles of ornithine delta-aminotransferase cause gyrate atrophy of the choroid and retina in Finns. Proc Natl Acad Sci USA. 1989;86: 197-201.
16. McClatchey AI, Kaufman DL, Berson EL, et al. Splicing defect at the ornithine amino-transferase (OAT) locus in gyrate atrophy. Am J Hum Genet. 1990;47:790-4
17. Takki KK, Milton RC. The natural history of gyrate atrophy of the choroid and retina. Ophthalmology. 1981;88:292-301.
18. Feldman RB, Mayo SS, Robertson DM, et al. Epiretinal membranes and cystoid macular edema in gyrate atrophy of the choroid and retina. Retina. 1989;9:139-42.
19. Oliveira TL, Andrade RE, Muccioli C, et al. Cystoid macular edema in gyrate atrophy of the choroid and retina: a fluorescein angiography and optical coherence tomography evaluation. Am J Ophthalmology. 2005;140:147-9.
20. Vasconcelos-Santos DV, Magalhães EP, Nehemy MB. Macular edema associated with gyrate atrophy managed with intravitreal triamcinolone: a case report. Arq Bras Oftalmol. 2007; 70:858-61.
21. Weleber RG, Kennaway NG. Clinical trial of vitamin B6 for gyrate atrophy of the choroid and retina. Ophthalmology. 1981;88: 316-24.
22. Raitta C, Carlson S, Vannas-Sulonen K. Gyrate atrophy of the choroid and retina: ERG of the neural retina and the pigment epithelium. Br J Ophthalmology. 1990;74:363-7.
23. Wilson DJ, Weleber RG, Green WR. Ocular clinicopathologic study of gyrate atrophy. Am J Ophthalmology. 1991: 111:24-33.
24. Berson EL, Hanson 3rd AH. Rosner B, et al. A two year trial of low protein, low arginine diets or vitamin B6 for patients with gyrate atrophy. Birth Defects Orig Artic Ser. 1982;18:209-18.
25. Kaiser-Kupfer MI, Caruso RC, Valle D. Gyrate atrophy of the choroid and retina. Long-term reduction of ornithine slows retinal degeneration. Arch Ophthalmology. 1991;109:1539-48.
26. Vannas-Sulonen K, Simell O. Sipilä I. Gyrate atrophy of the choroid and retina. The ocular disease progresses in juvenile patients despite normal or near normal plasma ornithine concentration. Ophthalmology. 1987;94:1428-33.

27. Weleber RG, Kennaway NG. Clinical trial of vitamin B6 for gyrate atrophy of the choroid and retina. Ophthalmology. 1981;88:316-24.

28. Haas J. Ueber das Zusammenvorkommen von Veranderungen der Retina und Choroidea. Arch Augenheilkd. 1898;37:343-8.

29. Jager G. A hereditary retinal disease. Trans Ophthalmology Soc UK. 1953;73:617-9.

30. Tantri A, Vrabec TR, Cu-Unjieng A, et al. X-linked retinoschisis: Report of a family with a rare deletion in the XLRS1 gene. Am J Ophthalmology. 2003;136:547-9.

31. Functional implications of the spectrum of mutations found in 234 cases with X-linked juvenile retinoschisis. The Retinoschisis Consortium. Hum Mol Genet. 1998;7:1185-92.

32. Sauer CG, Gehrig A, Warneke-Wittstock R, et al. Positional cloning of the gene associated with X-linked juvenile retinoschisis. Nature Genet. 1997;17:164-70.

33. Human and Clinical Genetics. (2008). X-linked Retinoschisis sequence variation database. [Online] Available from http://www.dmd.nl/rs/index.html. [Accessed November, 2017]

34. Molday LL, Hicks D, Sauer CG, et al. Expression of X-linked retinoschisis protein RS1 in photoreceptor and bipolar cells. Invest Ophthalmology Vis Sci. 2001;42:816-25.

35. Falcone PM, Brockhurst RJ. X-chromosome-linked juvenile retinoschisis: Clinical aspects and genetics. Int Ophthalmology Clin. 1993;33:193-202.

36. Kellner U, Brummer S, Foerster MH, et al. X-linked congenital retinoschisis. Graefes Arch Clin Exp Ophthalmology. 1990;228:432-7.

37. George ND, Yates JR, Moore AT. Clinical features in affected males with X-linked retinoschisis. Arch Ophthalmology. 1996; 114:274-80.

38. Gautam M, Muralidhar NS, Murthy H. Bilateral macular holes in X-linked retinoschisis: now the spectrum is wider. Indian J Ophthalmology. 2011;59:507-9.

39. Muscat S, Fahad B, Parks S, et al. Optical coherence tomography and multifocal electroretinography of X-linked juvenile retinoschisis. Eye (Lond). 2001;15:796-9.

40. Tanimoto N, Usui T, Takagi M, et al. Electroretinographic findings in three family members with X-linked juvenile retinoschisis associated with a novel Pro192Thr mutation of the XLRS1 gene. Jpn J Ophthalmology. 2002;46:568-76.

41. Genead MA, Fishman GA, Walia S. Efficacy of sustained topical dorzolamide therapy for cystic macular lesions in patients with X-linked retinoschisis. Arch Ophthalmology. 2010;128:190-7.

42. Tantri A, Vrabec TR, Cu-Unjieng A, et al. X-linked retinoschisis: a clinical and molecular genetic review. Surv Ophthalmology. 2004;49: 214-30.

43. Bolognia JL, Jorizzo JL, Schaffer JV, et al. Dermatology, 3rd edition. Philadelphia, PA: Saunders Elsevier; 2012.

44. Witkop CJ. Albinism: hematologic-storage disease, susceptibility to skin cancer, and optic neuronal defects shared in all types of oculocutaneous and ocular albinism. Ala J Med Sci. 1979;16:327-30.

Macular Disease and Degeneration

Chapter 10

Central Serous Chorioretinopathy

Mayank Bansal, Ashish Markan, Raghav Ravani, Itika Garg, Atul Kumar

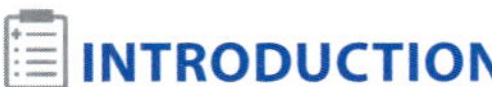 INTRODUCTION

Central serous chorioretinopathy (CSCR) is a chorioretinal disease with multifactorial etiology, and a complex pathogenesis. According to recent literature, CSCR has been identified as a disorder of choroidal vasculature primarily. Increased permeability of the choriocapillaris leads to focal or diffuse dysfunction of the retinal pigment epithelium (RPE)[1] causing neurosensory detachment.

ETIOLOGY AND RISK FACTORS

The exact etiology of CSCR is not fully understood. CSCR has been associated with patients having high levels of endogenous corticosteroids as well as in patients with secondary hypercortisolism. Other associations are "type A" personality, stress, lack of sleep, Cushing's syndrome, sleep apnea, gastroesophageal reflux disease (GERD), exogenous use of steroids (intravenous, cutaneous, or even nasal sprays) (Figs. 10.1A to C). Cases of CSCR associated with the above associations are more commonly bilateral and atypical (Figs. 10.2A and B). Choroidal vascular hyperpermeability plays a major role in the pathogenesis of CSCR.[2]

Psychosomatic Factors

Several psychosocial stressors have been associated with the onset of CSCR. Individuals with Type A personality have a higher risk.[3] Higher levels of circulating catecholamines and corticosteroids have been reported to cause increased risk of CSCR in Type A personalities.[4]

Pregnancy

Increased endogenous corticosteroids during pregnancy may be responsible for increased risk of developing CSCR.[5] Third trimester is the most common time of presentation, and CSCR resolves within 1–2 months after delivery.

Tuberculosis

Tuberculosis had been implicated as potential cause of CSCR (Fig. 10.3) in certain cases probably due to an improvement seen in few cases on antitubercular therapy (ATT). However, presently the response to ATT is attributed to induction of cytochrome *P450* in the liver by rifampicin that leads to an increased metabolism of the endogenous steroids.[6]

Other Factors

Recent meta-analysis indicates that hypertension, *H. pylori* infection, steroid use, disturbed sleep, obstructive sleep apnoea (OSA), autoimmune disorders, psychopharmacologic medication use, gastroesophageal reflux disease, peptic ulcer, antihistaminic drug use, antacids/anti-reflux agents and alcohol consumption were significant risk factors for the occurrence of CSCR.[7]

Another hypothesis is based on activation of the mineralocorticoid pathway. Vasodilation in the choroid could be due to overactivation of mineralocorticoid pathway in ocular tissues. This hypothesis links CSCR to other comorbidities with increased mineralocorticoid activity such as systemic hypertension and psychological stress.

CLINICAL FEATURES

Symptoms

Central scotoma is the most common presenting symptom that may be associated with metamorphopsia. Best corrected visual acuity (BCVA) at presentation generally ranges from 6/6 to 6/60.[8] The detached neurosensory retina causes the eye to become more hyperopic, so the vision improves with the use of a plus correction lens.

Signs

On fundus examination (Figs. 10.4A and B), CSCR typically has a well-demarcated oval area of neurosensory retinal detachment (NSD) in the posterior pole. Serous pigment epithelial detachments (PED) can also occur. Fundus examination with slit lamp biomicroscopy using a +90D lens is the preferred method of examination. In mild cases, the loss of the normal foveal reflex might be the only indicator of CSCR. Yellow dots are frequently observed on the posterior surface of the detached

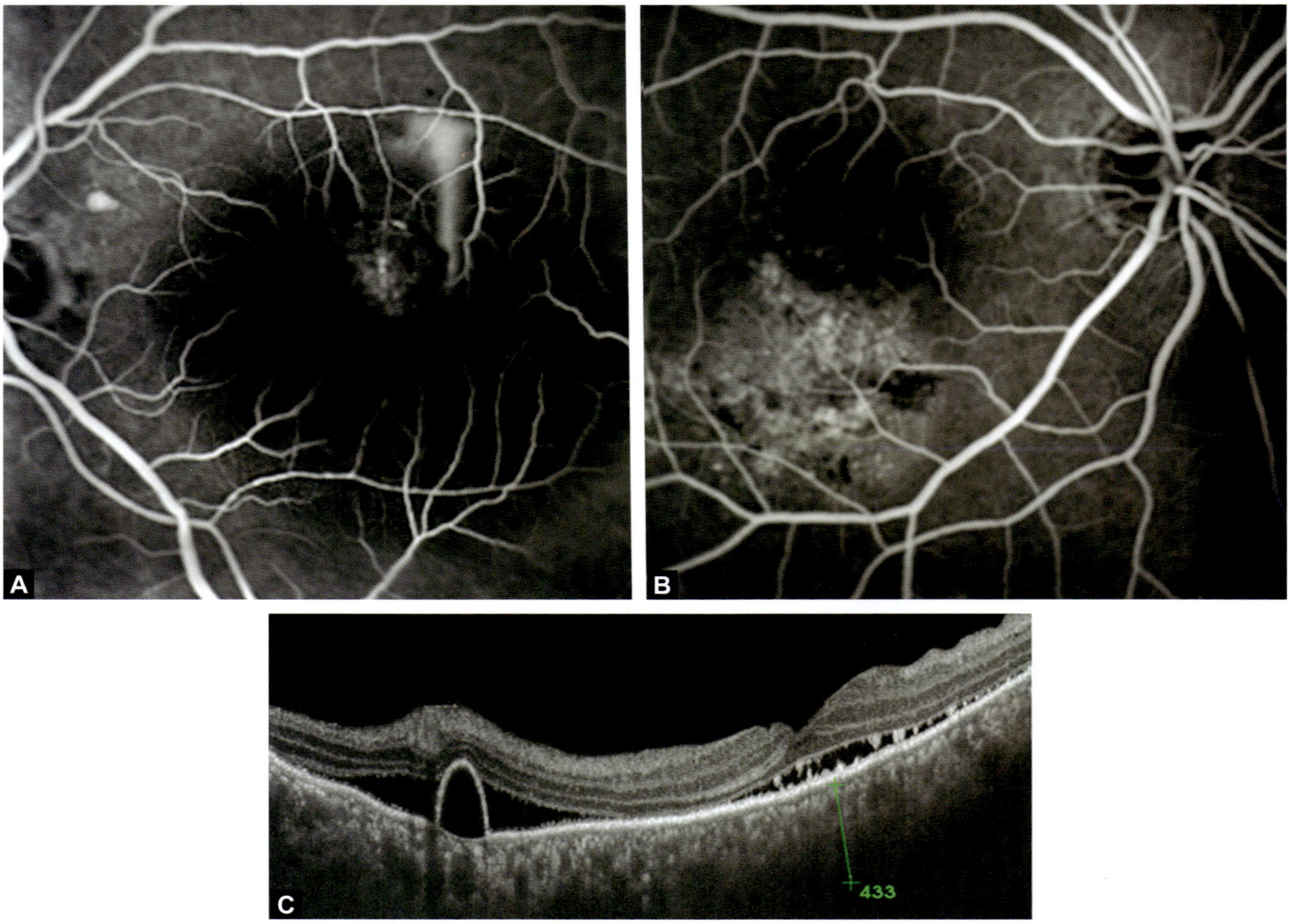

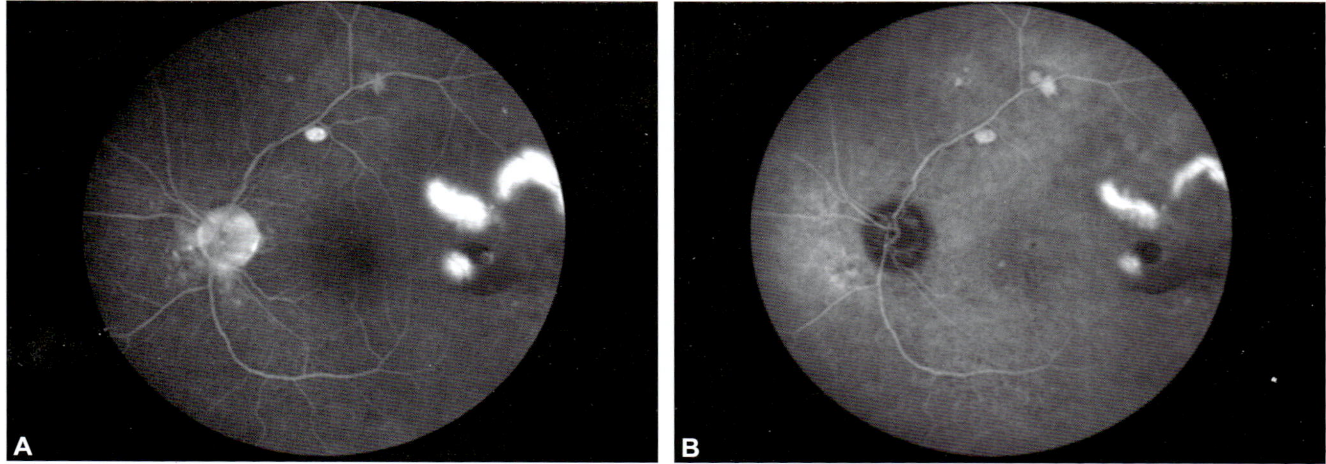

Figs. 10.1A to C: (A) and (B) Fundus fluorescein angiography (C) spectral domain-optical coherence tomography (SD-OCT) image shows serous detachment of the retina with a single pigment epithelial detachment (PED), besides the choroidal thickening. The patient has chronic multifocal CSCR and was on oral methylprednisolone for a systemic disease.

Figs. 10.2A and B: (A) Fundus fluorescein angiography and (B) indocyanine green angiography (ICGA) reveals large multifocal leaks in patient with chronic central serous chorioretinopathy (CSCR).

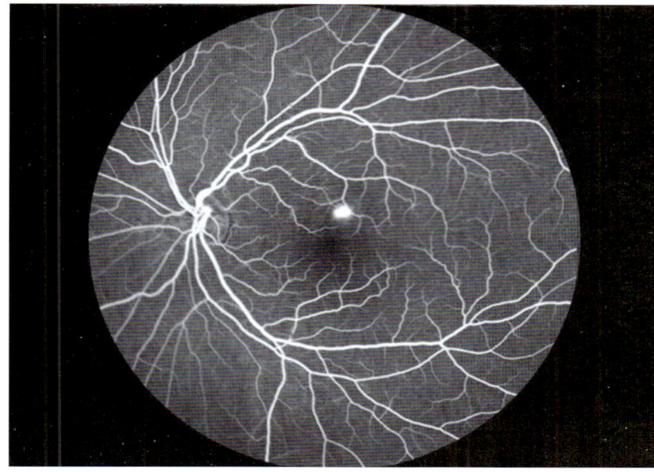

Fig. 10.3: Fluorescein angiography (FA) picture of a 20-year-old female with history of spinal tuberculosis before 4 years for which she received a full course of antitubercular therapy (ATT). A year after completing ATT, she presented with acute ink blot leakage suggestive of central serous chorioretinopathy (CSCR).

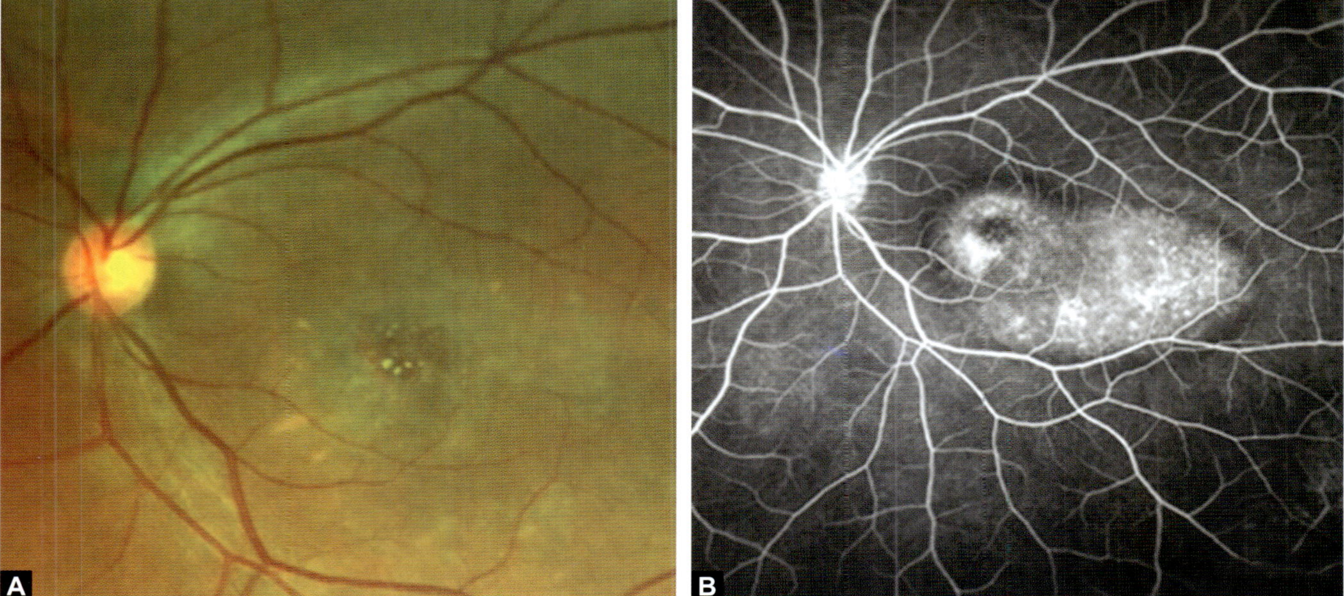

Figs. 10.4A and B: (A) Wide field fundus photograph and (B) Fluorescein angiography image of a patient with chronic central serous chorioretinopathy (CSCR) showing retinal pigment epithelium (RPE) mottling with window defect on fundal fluorescein angiography (FFA).

retina. They are postulated to be due to the phagocytosis of shed photoreceptor outer segments. Cream-colored subretinal deposits with or without a central clearing might be seen due to fibrin deposition.

Natural Course and Sequelae

Although 90% of the acute cases show resolution of subretinal fluid (SRF) over 2–3 months, sequelae may be seen in some cases. These include retinal pigment epithelium (RPE) depigmentation, subretinal fibrinous deposits, geographic atrophy and choroidal neovascularization (CNV). The risk of CNV formation is 0.3% and 2% per patient per year and it may develop at any time after the occurrence of CSCR.[9,10]

Chronic Central Serous Chorioretinopathy

There is no consensus on what constitutes chronic CSCR. It may be defined on the basis of the duration of subretinal fluid being present for more than 4–6 months. According to Yannuzzi, chronic CSCR is defined by the development of a diffuse pigment epitheliopathy and decompensation of the retinal pigment epithelium.[11] In a recent review article on CSCR the following terminology has been proposed.[12]

- *Acute CSCR*—spontaneous resolution of NSD within 4 months.
- *Nonresolving CSCR*—persistence of NSD beyond 4 months.

- *Recurrent CSCR*—recurrence of CSCR after complete resolution of the previous episode.
- *Chronic CSCR*—CSCR with widespread diffuse pigment epitheliopathy.
- *Inactive CSCR*—patients who have had CSCR, but at present do not have NSD.

The prognosis in chronic CSCR is guarded.

DIFFERENTIAL DIAGNOSIS FOR CENTRAL SEROUS CHORIORETINOPATHY

- Choroidal hemangioma
- Neovascular age-related macular degeneration (AMD)
- Exudative retinal detachment
- Macular hole
- Nonexudative (Dry) AMD
- Pseudophakic (Irvine-Gass) macular edema
- Rhegmatogenous retinal detachment
- Choroidal neovascular membranes
- Tuberculous choroiditis
- Vogt-Koyanagi-Harada disease

An optic nerve head pit can mimic a CSCR lesion (Figs. 10.5A and B); however, no leak is visible in the macula as the fluid tracks from the pit to the macula. Neovascular AMD and CNV with a serous detachment can also resemble CSCR; however, the presence of drusen, hemorrhage and/or exudates would point toward AMD or a CNV. An inferior retinal detachment just involving the fovea may also be confused with CSCR. An indirect ophthalmoscopic examination can help in establishing the correct diagnosis in these cases, as retinal detachment would generally extend much into the periphery up to the ora and will not be limited to the posterior pole. There might even be a break or dialysis seen in the peripheral retina.

In some cases, there is presence of fluid at the fovea due to a secondary cause and may mimic CSCR, as seen in Vogt-Koyanagi-Harada disease, posterior scleritis, multifocal choroiditis, uveal effusion, shallow choroidal tumors such as a nevus or hemangioma and dome-shaped maculopathy. The comprehensive clinical picture along with clues from investigations like optical coherence tomography (OCT), fundus fluorescein angiography (FFA), indocyanine green angiography (ICGA) and ultrasound B/A scan helps to establish the correct diagnosis in such cases.

Neovascular AMD with a picture of macular detachment can mimic CSCR too.

 INVESTIGATIONS

Optical Coherence Tomography

Optical coherence tomography can demonstrate the presence of neurosensory detachment (Fig. 10.6) or PED (Figs. 10.7A and B) and helps in differentiating between the two in

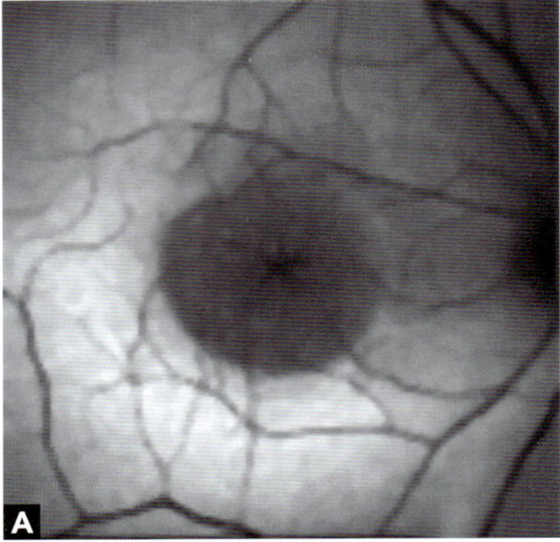

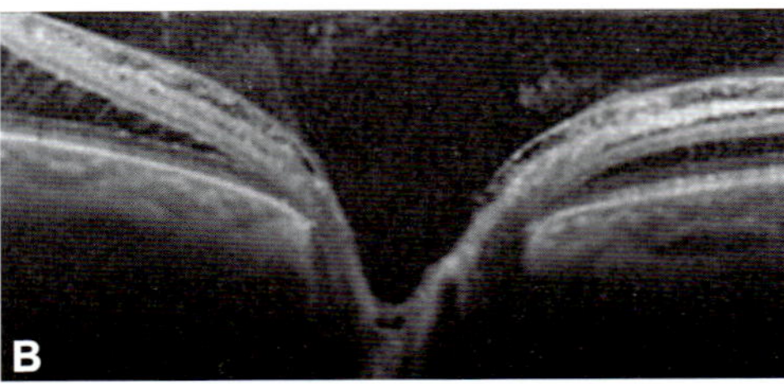

Figs. 10.5A and B: (A) Fundus autofluorescence image in optic disc pit and (B) spectral domain-optical coherence tomography (SD-OCT) image of a patient with optic nerve head pit. An optic nerve head pit with macular detachment mimics a picture akin to central serous chorioretinopathy (CSCR), however there are no point leaks over the fovea.

cases with CSCR. Subretinal yellow dots observed clinically, appear as hyperreflective structures on OCT. On follow-up, serial scans help in assessing treatment response and disease progression. Quantitative measurements can provide further objective documentation.

A hyporeflective area within hyperreflective subretinal fibrin seen on OCT has been shown to correlate with focal leakage on fluorescein angiography.[13]

Enhanced depth imaging (EDI) OCT has enabled the visualization of choroid on OCT. In CSCR, the subfoveal choroidal thickness is typically found to be increased. Specifically, larger hyporeflective lumens of choroidal vessels have been described, denoting vascular engorgement.[14] There is a spectrum of disorders thought to be associated with increased choroidal thickness and dilated outer layer (Haller's layer) choroidal vessels—referred to as "pachychoroid". It is hypothesized that CSCR may also be one such disease as part of the spectrum.[15]

Fluorescein Angiography

Fluorescein angiography (FA) in acute CSCR typically shows two types of leakage patterns: ink blot or smoke stack (Figs. 10.8A to C). In the former, the leakage starts as a pinpoint in the early phase which diffuses out concentrically in the late phase appearing like an ink blot. In the latter, the leak-

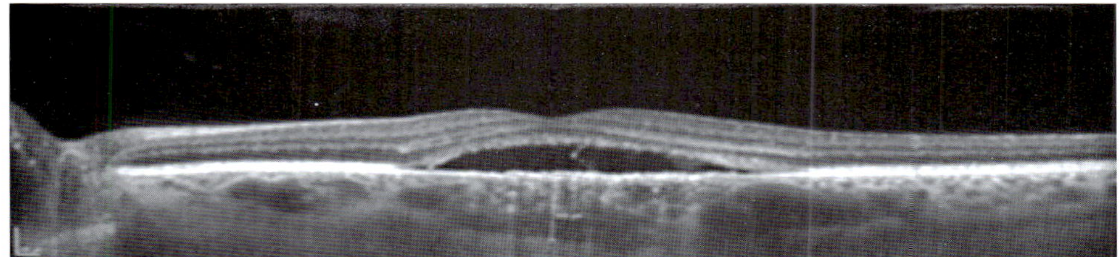

Fig. 10.6: Neurosensory detachment with thickened choroid in an eye with central serous chorioretinopathy (CSCR).

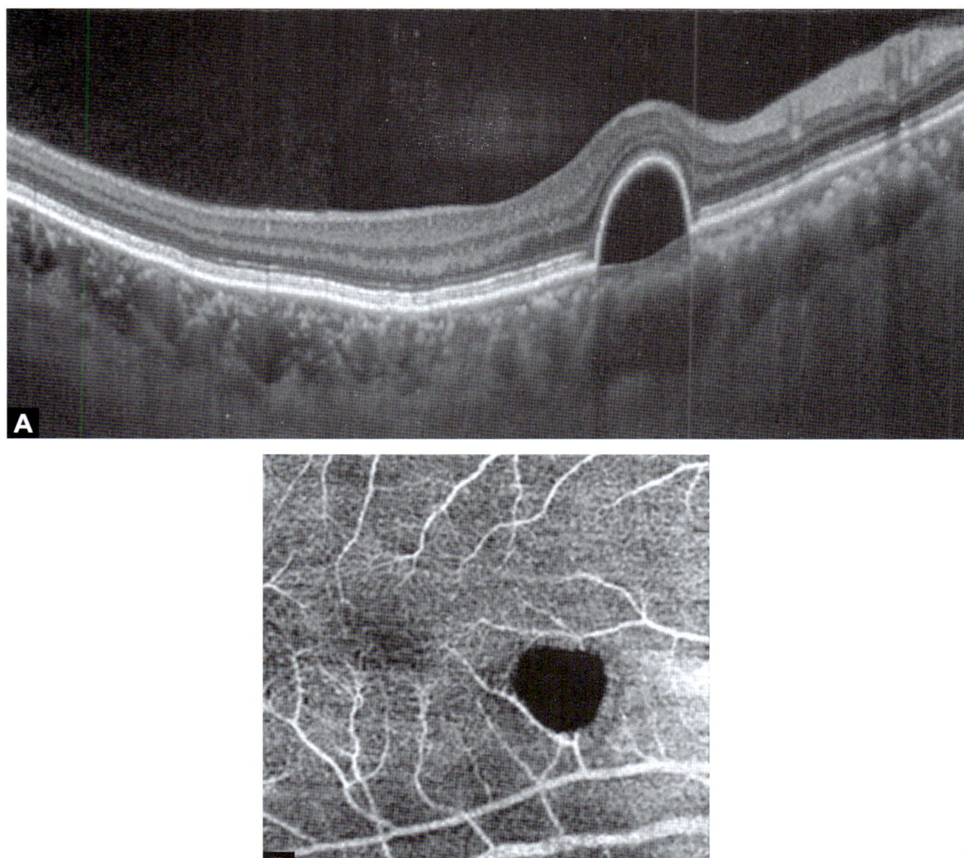

Figs. 10.7A and B: Type II central serous chorioretinopathy (CSCR) w th pigment epithelial detachment (PED) seen on optical coherence tomography (OCT) and optical coherence tomography angiography (OCTA).

age starts as a pinpoint in the early phase tracking upward gradually and expanding further to form a mushroom cloud or umbrella-like appearance. Smoke stack appearance is less common and only appears in about 10–15% of patients with acute CSCR. An increased concentration of protein in the subretinal fluid leads to smokestack pattern.[16]

Fundal fluorescein angiography of chronic CSCR reveals multiple RPE window defect due to RPE atrophy. As the fluid gravitates inferiorly, pigment epithelial tracks also become visible along the course of the fluid movement.

Fundus Autofluorescence

In acute CSCR, within the first 1–2 months, there is a minimal change on fundus autofluorescence (FAF). Hyperautofluorescence outlining the area of serous detachment is subsequently seen.[17]

In chronic CSCR, areas of geographic atrophy appear as hypoautofluorescent. It can be in the form of confluent hypoautofluorescence, or descending gravitational tracts, having a granular hypoautofluorescent appearance (Figs. 10.9A to D).

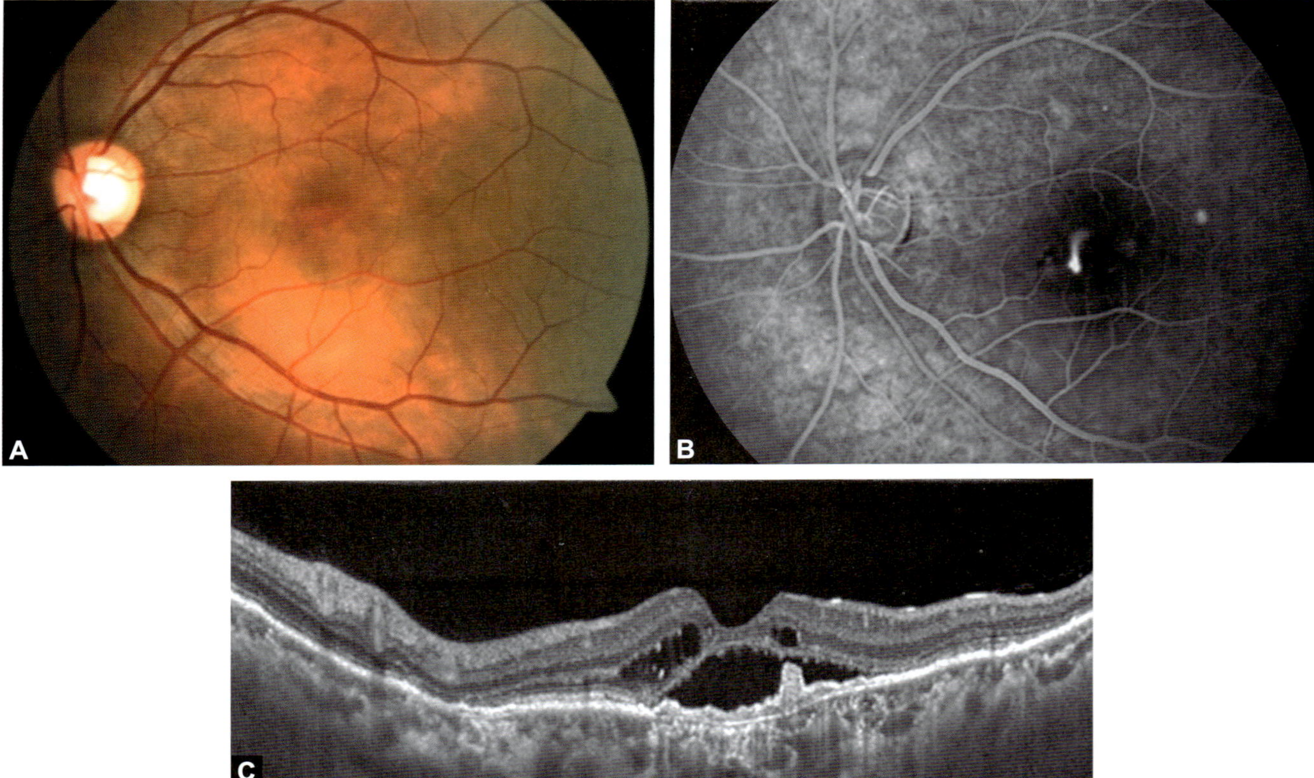

Figs. 10.8A to C: Mixed central serous chorioretinopathy (CSCR) showing serous macular detachment on color picture, classic smokestack leak and serous pigment epithelial detachments (PEDs) on fundus fluorescein angiography (FFA) and neurosensory detachment with thickened (pachy) choroid on swept source optical coherence tomography (SSOCT).

Indocyanine Green Angiography

Indocyanine green angiography is useful for both detecting the abnormalities in choroidal vasculature and also for guiding the treatment, e.g. photodynamic therapy (PDT). Abnormally dilated choroidal vasculature is typically seen in the early phase with choroidal hyperpermeability seen as hyperfluorescent patches in the late phase. We have seen a case in which an ink blot leak was picked up well on ICG whereas it was not visible on FFA (Figs. 10.10A and B).

Choroidal Imaging in Central Serous Chorioretinopathy

Both EDI-OCT and swept source OCT (Fig. 10.11) reveal a thicker choroid (Figs. 10.12A and B) in active CSCR. The abnormally dilated large choroidal vessels of the Haller's layer can also be visualized.

Optical Coherence Tomography Angiography

Costanzo et al. have shown dark areas and abnormal choroidal flow pattern on optical coherence tomography angio-graphy (OCT-A) in cases of CSCR. The authors report that the pathological choroidal vascular pattern observed in many CSCR cases is distinct from CNV.[18] In our experience, OCT-A is very helpful in detecting secondary CNV formation in cases of CSCR.

TREATMENT

Medical Treatment

Majority of acute cases resolve spontaneously (Figs. 10.13A to C). Removal of psychological stressors and discontinuation of exogenous steroids is helpful. Treatment is considered when the serous detachment is persistent for 3–4 months, because beyond this time, irreversible photoreceptor atrophy may occur. Antidepressants and tranquilizers may play a role in stressful Type A personality patients. Avoid corticosteroid use as it may exacerbate the serous detachments which are already present. The safety and efficacy of finasteride, a dihydrotestosterone synthesis inhibitor, was evaluated by Forooghian et al.[19] and they found that in five patients with chronic CSCR, the drug led to decrease in macular thickness

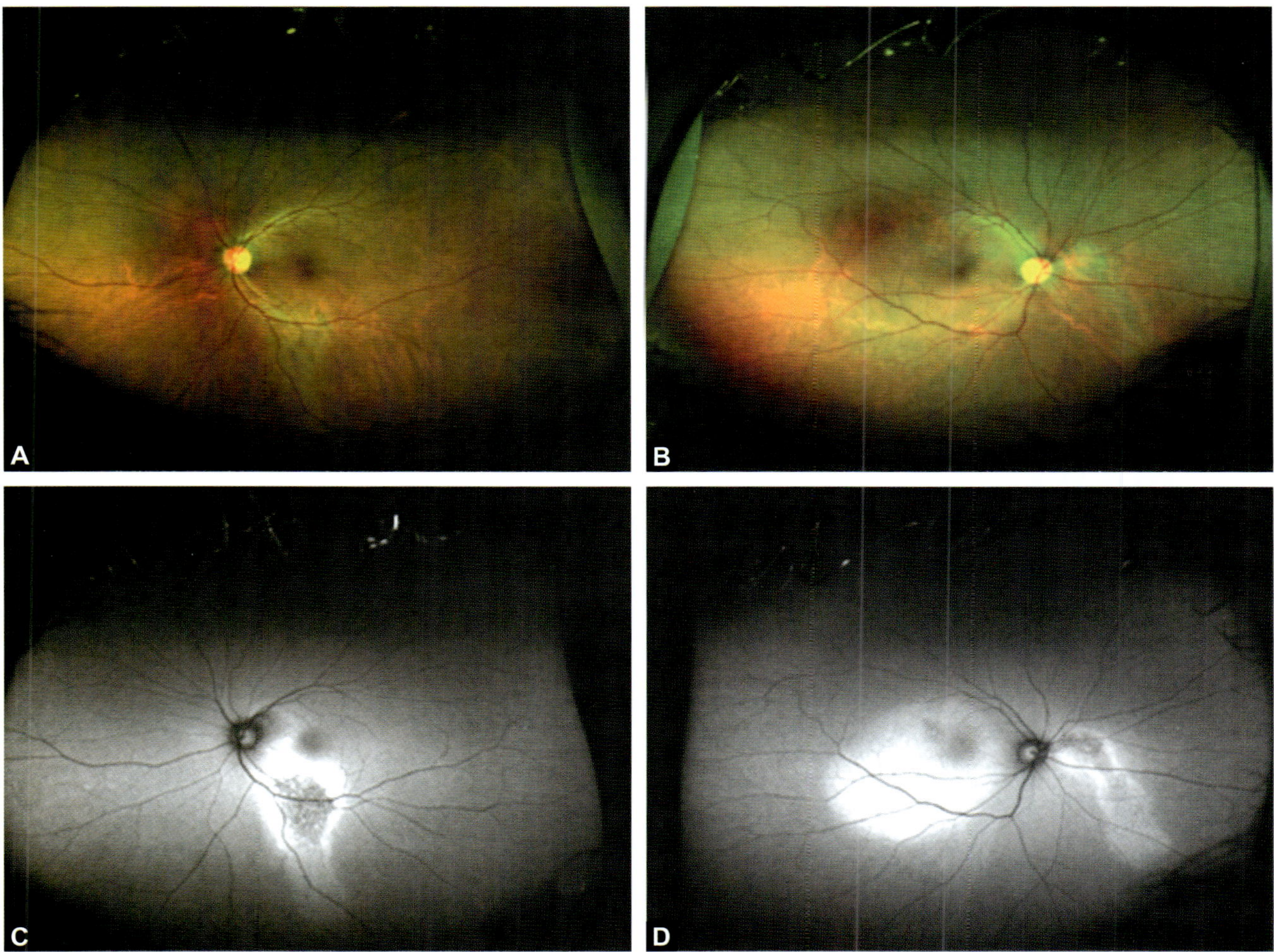

Figs. 10.9A to D: (A) and (B): Wide field pseudocolor image of a patient having chronic central serous chorioretinopathy (CSCR) with retinal pigment epithelium (RPE) atrophy. (C) and (D) shows fundus autofluorescence image of the same patient showing hypoautofluorescence along the gravitational tracts (RPE atrophy) with surrounding hyperautofluorescence.

and subretinal fluid, but it recurred on planned cessation of the medication. A patient with chronic subretinal fluid for over 2 years was reported after 1 month of treatment with rifampicin.[20] A prospective pilot study showed that in long-standing chronic CSCR, oral rifampin may be an option for treatment.[21] Rifampin, and cytochrome P450 inducer, accelerate the metabolism of steroids and hence the benefit of using Rifampin. However, side-effects and potential hepatotoxicity should be kept in mind when treating these patients with oral rifampicin.[22]

Oral Mineralocorticoid Receptor Antagonists for the Treatment of Central Serous Chorioretinopathy

In a rat model of oxygen-induced retinopathy (OIR), Wilkinson-Berka and colleagues characterized the adverse effects of MR overactivation on the retinal microvasculature wherein increased angiogenesis in OIR was noted with aldosterone + salt but was reduced with the MR antagonist spironolactone.[28]

Spironolactone is a nonselective competitive antagonist of the aldosterone receptor. Due to its nonselectivity, it additionally results in coantagonism of the androgen, glucocorticoid, and progesterone receptors.[26]

Eplerenone is the first member in a new class of selective aldosterone antagonists originally approved for the treatment of hypertension and congestive heart failure following myocardial infarction. Derived from spironolactone, eplerenone was designed to enhance selective binding to the MR while minimizing binding to the other steroid receptors.[27] Eplerenone has a 10- to 20-fold lower binding affinity for the MR in vitro, compared to spironolactone.[27]

In a series of 120 patients that showed a response to mineralocorticoid antagonists, eplerenone or spironolactone; a positive effect was found in 50% of the patient with recalcitrant disease.[23] The beneficial role of mineralocorticoid antag-

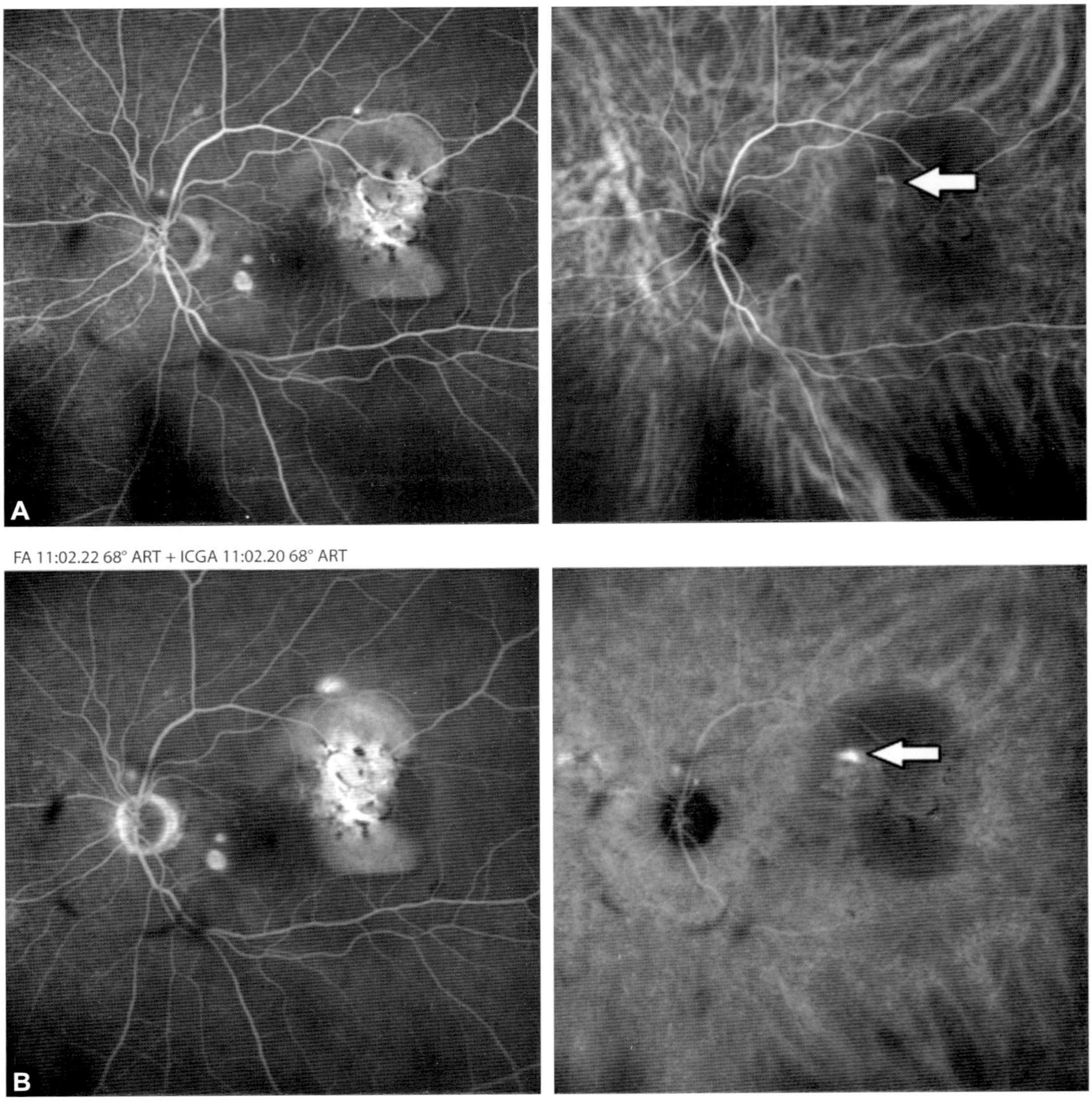

FA 11:02.22 68° ART + ICGA 11:02.20 68° ART

Figs. 10.10A and B: Fundus fluorescein angiography (FFA) and indocyanine green angiography (ICG) of a patient with chronic central serous chorioretinopathy (CSCR). Note the leak noted on ICG (white arrows) without corresponding leak on FFA.

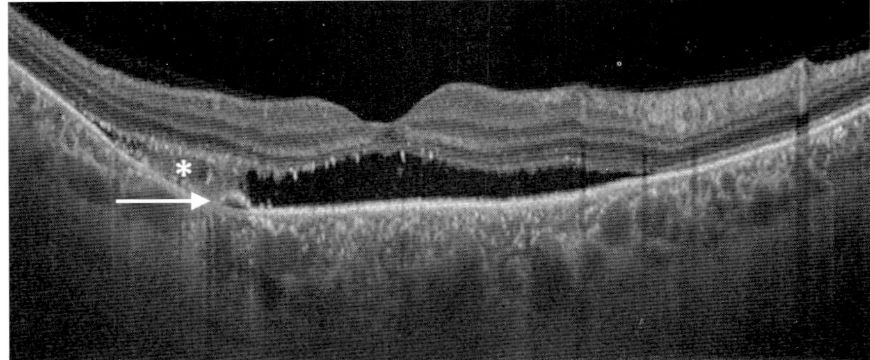

Fig. 10.11: Swept source optical coherence tomography (SS-OCT) image of a patient with central serous chorioretinopathy (CSCR) showing subretinal fibrin (asterisk), serous pigment epithelial detachment (PED) (white arrow), neurosensory detachment and underlying pachychoroid.

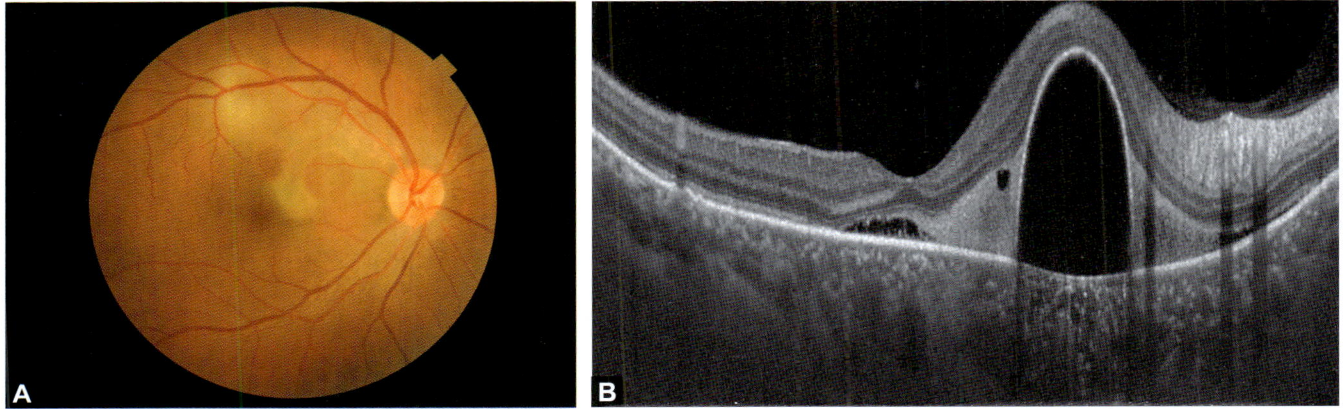

Figs. 10.12A and B: Chronic central serous chorioretinopathy (CSCR) with subretinal fibrin and thumb-like pigment epithelial detachment (PED). There is associated choroidal thickening.

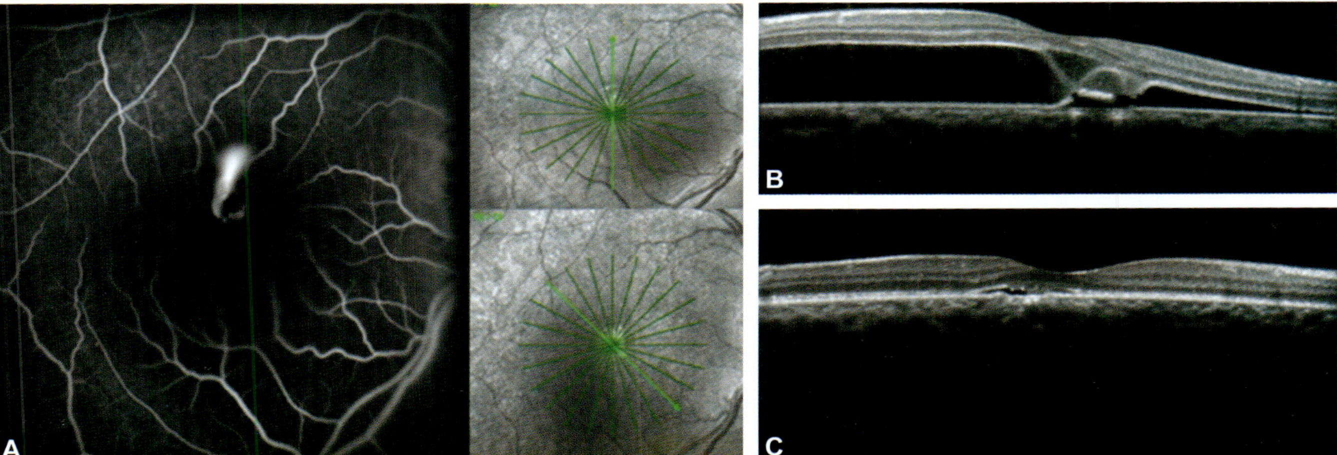

Figs. 10.13A to C: Acute central serous chorioretinopathy (CSCR) (first attack) showing early smokestack leak on (A) fundus fluorescein angiography (FFA) and (B) spectral domain-optical coherence tomography (SD-OCT). (C) After 1 month, on conservative treatment, SD-OCT reveals reduction of subretinal fluid (ellipsoid layer still disrupted).

onists in the treatment of CSCR has also been seen in other studies.[24-27]

There is emerging evidence implicating the mineralocorticoid receptor (MR) pathway in the disease pathogenesis which has sparked interest in the use of MR antagonists as a potentially viable treatment option for CSCR. Eplerenone is a selective aldosterone receptor blocker, and hence has reduced risk of adverse effects such as hyperkalemia and libido disturbances. It is administered as an initial loading dose of tablet 25 mg/day increasing after 2–3 days to 50 mg/day for about 3–4 months. This drug is used in for both acute and chronic cases of CSCR.

Adverse effects of both spironolactone and eplerenone include potentially life-threatening hyperkalemia, which can be potentiated by concurrent renal insufficiency, diabetes mellitus, advanced CHF, older patient age, and interactions with other drugs. While both medications can produce dose-dependent rises in serum potassium concentrations, this effect appears to be greater with spironolactone when both are administered at the recommended dosages.

Additionally, due to its structural similarity to progesterone and its interaction with other steroid receptors, spironolactone is known to inhibit free testosterone from binding to androgen receptors, resulting in undesirable hormonal effects (gynecomastia, decreased libido, menstrual irregularities, and erectile dysfunction).

As a recommendation, avoid MR antagonists if the baseline serum potassium concentration is greater than 5.5 mEq/L, the creatinine clearance is less than 50 mL/min, or the serum creatinine is greater than 2 mg/dL in men.

Response to Eplerenone

The response to oral eplerenone is variable as we feel after treating many patients and is identical with the trials carried out also. Further prospective, controlled studies in a larger population of patients are warranted and currently ongoing to evaluate the most appropriate dose and duration of oral MR-antagonist treatment in nonresolving CSCR.

Laser Treatment

Photodynamic Therapy

Photodynamic therapy has been reported to cause choriocapillaris narrowing, choroidal hypoperfusion, reduction of choroidal exudation. Choroidal vascular remodeling has been proposed as the mechanism by which PDT may cause resolution of CSCR[28] (Figs. 10.14A and B). ICG-guided PDT is highly efficacious in CSCR.

However, it may be accompanied with complications like RPE atrophy and choriocapillaris ischemia with long-term retinal thinning. The incidence may be higher with the conventional verteporfin full-fluence treatment..

Photodynamic therapy with reduced dosage: Considering the above complications, PDT with reduced dosage, i.e. 3 mg/m² instead of the conventional 6 mg/m² has been advocated. This regime has been reported to have same efficacy as conventional PDT (Figs. 10.15A and B) but with lesser complications including risk of long-term choroidal ischemia and resulting drop in vision.[29]

Photodynamic therapy with reduced laser fluence: Standard-fluence PDT (50 J/cm²) has been compared with low-fluence PDT (25 J/cm²). Reduced fluence PDT was found to be comparable to standard fluence PDT, with lesser choroidal hypoperfusion (Figs. 10.16A and B).[30]

Intravitreal ranibizumab has also been tried in cases of CSCR. In terms of anatomical outcomes, fewer eyes achieve resolution of SRF with ranibizumab injections as compared to low-fluence PDT.[31]

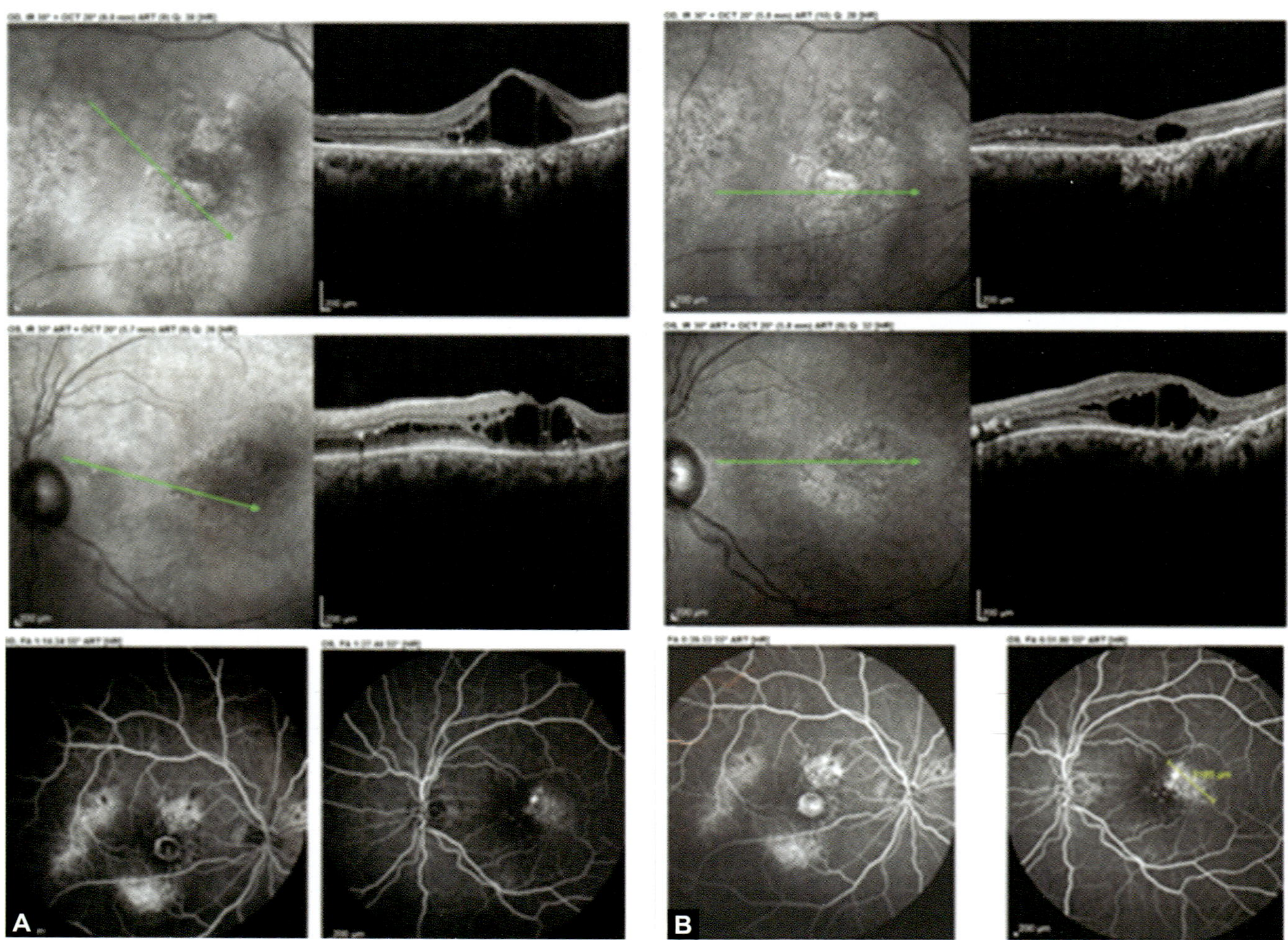

Figs. 10.14A and B: (A) Prephotodynamic therapy (PDT) and (B) post-PDT imaging in a patient with bilateral chronic multifocal central serous chorioretinopathy (CSCR).

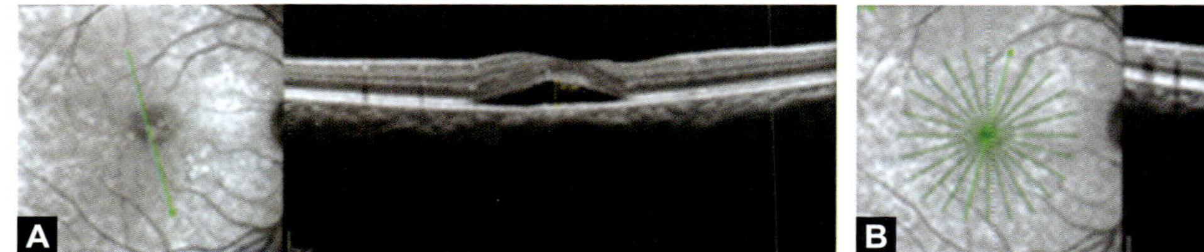

Figs. 10.15A and B: Spectral domain-optical coherence tomography (SD-OCT) showing (A) prereduced laser fluence (rf)-photodynamic therapy (PDT) treatment and (B) post-rf-PDT treatment resulting in subretinal fluid (SRF) absorption.

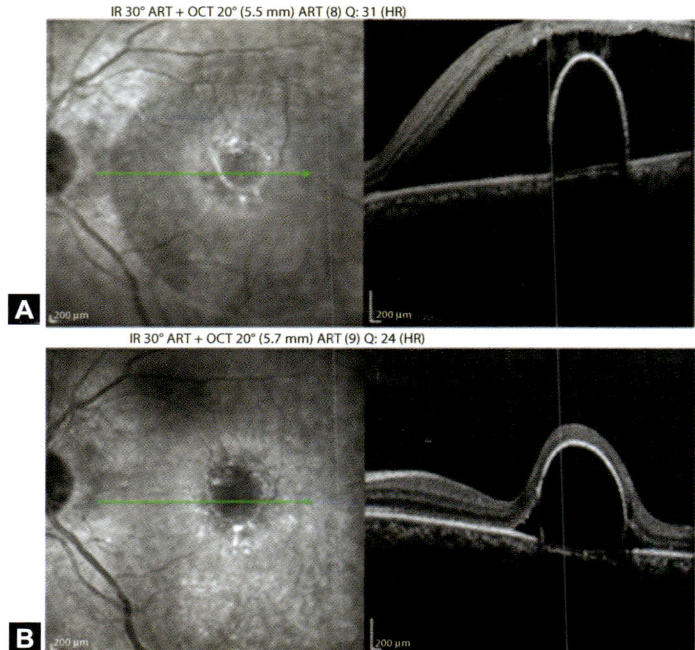

Figs. 10.16A and B: (A) Prereduced fluence photodynamic therapy (PDT) and (B) postreduced fluence PDT in an eye with mixed central serous chorioretinopathy (CSCR) (PED with neurosensory detachment).

Focal Laser

Focal thermal laser photocoagulation can be considered for extrafoveal lesions (Figs. 10.17 and 10.18). However, laser photocoagulation may not alter the recurrence rate but the gain in visual acuity would depend on multiple factors including duration of CSCR and integrity of the photoreceptors. Heavy laser can result in CNV formation. In one study, CNV was seen at the site of laser in less than 10% of treated patients and it was detected only on FFA because it was extrafoveal and asymptomatic.[32]

Subthreshold Micropulse Diode Laser and "Selective" Laser Treatment

In few studies subthreshold micropulse diode laser (810 nm) to the leaking site has been found to be effective.[33-35] In another study, subthreshold diode laser micropulse photocoagulation was enhanced by indocyanine green dye in seven patients with chronic CSCR with no spontaneous resolution 6 months after the onset. At 12 months follow-up, resolution of the neurosensory retinal detachment was seen in all patients without recurrence.[36]

"Selective laser treatment" aimed at the RPE with sparing of photoreceptors has also been attempted. This is performed by using very short duration pulses of laser. In one study, no collateral retinal damage was seen on spectral domain-OCT (SD-OCT) after selective laser treatment (527 nm, 200 nsec pulse duration (30 pulses at 100 Hz); energy 100–200 µJ/pulse; 200 µm retinal spot diameter) at 1 year follow-up unlike in those patients who underwent conventional laser photocoagulation (532 nm; power 100–200 mW; retinal spot diameter 100 µm; pulse duration 100 msec).[37]

Role of Antivascular Endothelial Growth Factor Therapy Agents

Choroidal neovascularization secondary to CSCR may be treated successfully with intravitreal bevacizumab.

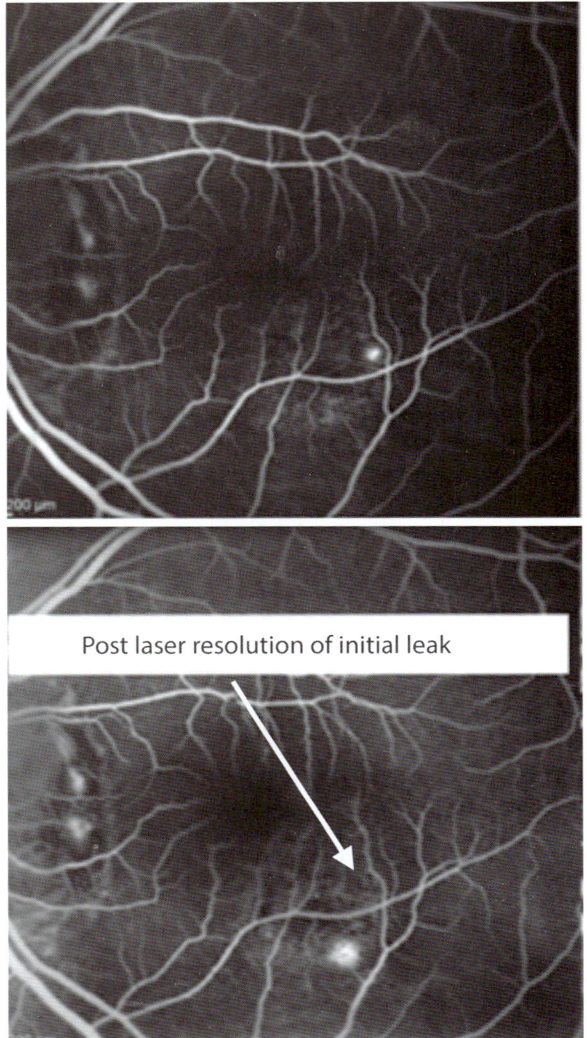

Fig. 10.17: Recurrent leak in central serous chorioretinopathy (CSCR) treated with focal laser. The lower picture shows a fresh leak at a new location suggesting recurrence.

Intravitreal aflibercept (Eylea) and ranibizumab (Lucentis) are being used to treat the neurosensory detachment of CSCR. A prospective randomized study that compared outcomes of intravitreal ranibizumab to low-fluence photodynamic therapy in chronic CSCR showed that the anatomic outcomes in ranibizumab group were "not promising" when compared to low-fluence PDT at follow-up of 6 months.[38] Thus, presently we do not advocate the use of anti-VEGF in CSCR without any neovascularization.[39,40]

Perhaps at present the role of any particular drug or laser treatment often does not alter or cure the disease per se; however, these treatments in the absence of large randomized controlled studies remain the only available modalities of treatment in our armamentarium.

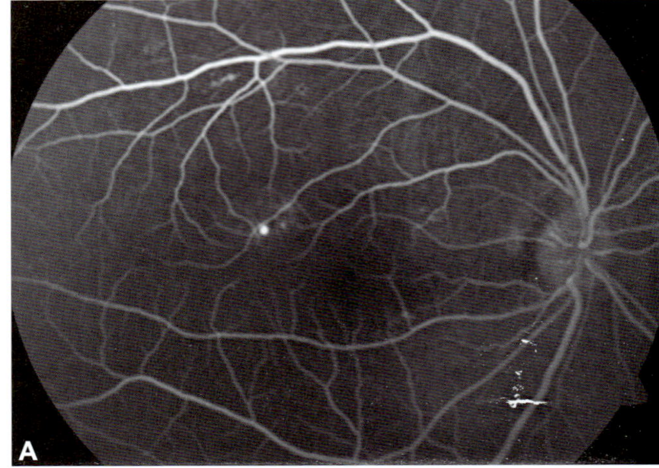

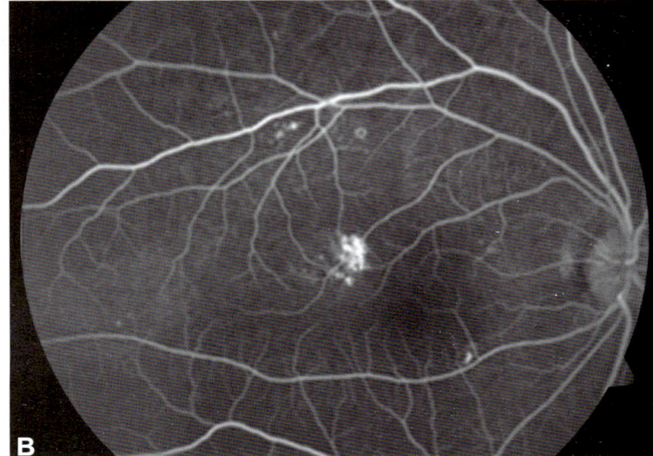

Figs. 10.18A and B: (A) Active paramacular central serous chorioretinopathy (CSCR) with point leak and (B) postlaser treatment.

REFERENCES

1. Nicholson B, Noble J, Forooghian F, et al. Central serous chorioretinopathy: update on pathophysiology and treatment. Surv Ophthalmology. 2013;58(2):103-26.
2. Liew G, Quin G, Gillies M, et al. Central serous chorioretinopathy: a review of epidemiology and pathophysiology. Clin Experiment Ophthalmology. 2013;41(2):201-14.
3. Yannuzzi LA. Type-A behavior and central serous chorioretinopathy. Retina. 1987;7(2):111-31.
4. Yannuzzi LA. Type A behavior and central serous chorioretinopathy. Trans Am Ophthalmology Soc. 1986;84:799-845.
5. Chumbley LC, Frank RN. Central serous retinopathy and pregnancy. Am J Ophthalmology. 1974;77(2):158-60.
6. Ravage ZB, Packo KH, Creticos CM, et al. Chronic central serous chorioretinopathy responsive to rifampin. Retin Cases Brief Rep. 2012;6(1):129-32.
7. Liu B, Deng T, Zhang J. Risk factors for central serous chorioretinopathy: A Systematic Review and Meta-Analysis. Retina.. 2016;36(1):9-19.
8. Wang M, Munch IC, Hasler PW, et al. Central serous chorioretinopathy. Acta Ophthalmology (Copenh). 2008;86(2):126-45.

9. Yannuzzi LA, Shakin JL, Fisher YL, et al. Peripheral retinal detachments and retinal pigment epithelial atrophic tracts secondary to central serous pigment epitheliopathy. Ophthalmology. 1984;91(12):1554-72.

10. Bandello F, Virgili G, Lanzetta P, et al. ICG angiography and retinal pigment epithelial decompensation (CRSC and epitheliopathy). J Fr Ophthalmology. 2001;24(4):448-51.

11. Yannuzzi LA, Slakter JS, Kaufman SR, et al. Laser treatment of diffuse retinal pigment epitheliopathy. Eur J Ophthalmology. 1992;2(3):103-14.

12. Daruich A, Matet A, Dirani A, et al. Central serous chorioretinopathy: Recent findings and new physiopathology hypothesis. Prog Retin Eye Res. 2015;48:82-118.

13. Yannuzzi NA, Mrejen S, Capuano V, et al. A Central Hyporeflective Subretinal Lucency Correlates With a Region of Focal Leakage on Fluorescein Angiography in Eyes With Central Serous Chorioretinopathy. Ophthalmic Surg Lasers Imaging Retina. 2015;46(8):832-6.

14. Yang L, Jonas JB, Wei W. Choroidal vessel diameter in central serous chorioretinopathy. Acta Ophthalmology (Copenh). 2013;91(5):e358-62.

15. Gallego-Pinazo R, Dolz-Marco R, Gómez-Ulla F, et al. Pachychoroid Diseases of the Macula. Med Hypothesis Discov Innov Ophthalmology. 2014;3(4):111-5.

16. Bujarbarua D, Nagpal PN, Deka M. Smokestack leak in central serous chorioretinopathy. Graefes Arch Clin Exp Ophthalmology. 2010;248(3):339-51.

17. Spaide RF, Klancnik JM. Fundus autofluorescence and central serous chorioretinopathy. Ophthalmology. 2005;112(5):825-33.

18. Costanzo E, Cohen SY, Meier A, et al. Optical Coherence Tomography Angiography in Central Serous Chorioretinopathy. J Ophthalmology. 2015;2015:134783.

19. Forooghian F, Meleth AD, Cukras C, et al. Finasteride for chronic central serous chorioretinopathy. Retina. 2011;31(4):766-71.

20. Steinle NC, Gupta N, Yuan A, et al. Oral rifampin utilisation for the treatment of chronic multifocal central serous retinopathy. Br J Ophthalmology. 2012;96(1):10-3.

21. Shulman S, Goldenberg D, Schwartz R, et al. Oral Rifampin treatment for longstanding chronic central serous chorioretinopathy. Graefes Arch Clin Exp Ophthalmology. 2016;254(1):15-22.

22. Nelson J, Saggau DD, Nielsen JS. Rifampin induced hepatotoxicity during treatment for chronic central serous chorioretinopathy. Retin Cases Brief Rep. 2014;8(1):70-2.

23. Chin EK, Almeida DR, Roybal CN, et al. Oral mineralocorticoid antagonists for recalcitrant central serous chorioretinopathy. Clin Ophthalmology. 2015;9:1449-56.

24. Zhao M, Célérier I, Bousquet E, et al. Mineralocorticoid receptor is involved in rat and human ocular chorioretinopathy. J Clin Invest. 2012;122(7):2672-9.

25. Kapoor KG, Wagner AL. Mineralocorticoid Antagonists in the Treatment of Central Serous Chorioretinopathy: A Comparative Analysis. Ophthalmic Res. 2016;56(1):17-22.

26. Ghadiali Q, Jung JJ, Yu S, et al. Central serous chorioretinopathy treated with mineralocorticoid antagonists: a one-year pilot study. Retina. 2016;36(3):611-8.

27. Schwartz R, Habot-Wilner Z, Martinez MR, et al. Eplerenone for chronic central serous chorioretinopathy—a randomized controlled prospective study. Acta Ophthalmology. 2017;95(7):e610-8.

28. Wilkinson-Berka JL, Tan G, Jaworski K, et al. Identification of a retinal aldosterone system and the protective effects of mineralocorticoid receptor antagonism on retinal vascular pathology. Circ Res. 2009;104(1):124-33.

29. Chan WM, Lam DS, Lai TY, et al. Choroidal vascular remodelling in central serous chorioretinopathy after indocyanine green guided photodynamic therapy with verteporfin: a novel treatment at the primary disease level. Br J Ophthalmology. 2003;87(12):1453-8.

30. Chan WM, Lai TY, Lai RY, et al. Safety enhanced photodynamic therapy for chronic central serous chorioretinopathy: one-year results of a prospective study. Retina. 2008;28(1):85-93.

31. Reibaldi M, Cardascia N, Longo A, et al. Standard-fluence versus low-fluence photodynamic therapy in chronic central serous chorioretinopathy: a nonrandomized clinical trial. Am J Ophthalmology. 2010;149(2):307-15.e2.

32. Bae SH, Heo JW, Kim C, et al. A randomized pilot study of low-fluence photodynamic therapy versus intravitreal ranibizumab for chronic central serous chorioretinopathy. Am J Ophthalmology. 2011;152(5):784-92.e2.

33. Ficker L, Vafidis G, While A, et al. Long-term follow-up of a prospective trial of argon laser photocoagulation in the treatment of central serous retinopathy. Br J Ophthalmology. 1988;72(11):829-34.

34. Chen SN, Hwang JF, Tseng LF, et al. Subthreshold diode micropulse photocoagulation for the treatment of chronic central serous chorioretinopathy with juxtafoveal leakage. Ophthalmology. 2008;115(12):2229-34.

35. Lanzetta P, Furlan F, Morgante L, et al. Nonvisible subthreshold micropulse diode laser (810 nm) treatment of central serous chorioretinopathy. A pilot study. Eur J Ophthalmology. 2008;18(6):934-40.

36. Gupta B, Elagouz M, McHugh D, et al. Micropulse diode laser photocoagulation for central serous chorio-retinopathy. Clin Experiment Ophthalmology. 2009;37(8):801-5.

37. Ricci F, Missiroli F, Regine F, et al. Indocyanine green enhanced subthreshold diode-laser micropulse photocoagulation treatment of chronic central serous chorioretinopathy. Graefes Arch Clin Exp Ophthalmology. 2009;247(5):597-607.

38. Framme C, Walter A, Prahs P, et al. Structural changes of the retina after conventional laser photocoagulation and selective retina treatment (SRT) in spectral domain OCT. Curr Eye Res. 2009;34(7):568-79.

39. Semeraro F, Romano MR, Danzi P, et al. Intravitreal bevacizumab versus low-fluence photodynamic therapy for treatment of chronic central serous chorioretinopathy. Jpn J Ophthalmology. 2012;56(6):608-12.

40. Chan WM, Lai TY, Liu DT, et al. Intravitreal bevacizumab (avastin) for choroidal neovascularization secondary to central serous chorioretinopathy, secondary to punctate inner choroidopathy, or of idiopathic origin. Am J Ophthalmology. 2007;143(6):977-83.

Chapter 11

Age-Related Macular Degeneration

Atul Kumar, Mayank Bansal, Raghav Ravani, Annu Chohan

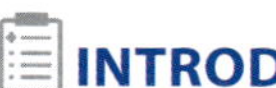 INTRODUCTION

Age-related macular degeneration (AMD) is an acquired disease causing retinal degeneration and significant central visual loss due to both non-neovascular (drusen and retinal pigment epithelium changes), and neovascular etiology [choroidal neovascular membrane (CNVM)]. With progressive disease, localized areas of retinal pigment epithelium (RPE) cell dropouts, subretinal or sub-RPE hemorrhage or serous fluid, and subretinal fibrosis is seen. Genetic as well as non-genetic factors, environmental, nutritional processes and aging have been speculated in the aetiopathogenesis of this disease. Current research has highlighted biochemical pathways, which are now being explored for novel therapeutics. The clinical hallmark of AMD lies in the detection of drusen within the macula. The word *druse* (singular) finds its origin in the German for *potato stone* or geode.

EPIDEMIOLOGY, PATHOPHYSIOLOGY, GENETICS AND RISK FACTORS

Epidemiology

Various studies have reported the incidence of AMD. One of the most significant studies was the Beaver Dam Eye Study, which evaluated individuals between 43 years and 86 years of age and reported the 15-year cumulative incidence of late AMD in people greater than 75 years of age as 8%, which makes it a significant public health problem.[1] The Framingham Eye Study gave us a prevalence of neovascular AMD in subjects aged more than 52 years of age as 1.5%.[2]

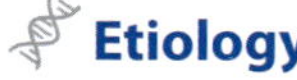 Etiology

A number of risk factors coexist in AMD patients. A study by Klein R et al. showed that early AMD was present in less than 5% in ages less than 34 years and 9.8% in ages greater than 65 years. Multivariate regression analysis revealed age, male sex, cigarette smoking, higher high-density lipoprotein cholesterol level and hearing impairment to be associated with early AMD. There were no associations of blood pressure, body mass index, physical activity, alcohol intake, white blood cell count, hematocrit level, platelet count, serum cholesterol level, or carotid intimal-medial thickness with early AMD.[3] The effect of these risk factors result in geographic atrophy, choroidal neovascularization (CNV) and RPE detachment. Treatment methods variously target the final common pathway of damage (choroidal neovascularization) or may lead to earlier intervention by targeting the *intermediate disease mechanisms*, i.e. the interplay between all the risk factors. Though there is a paucity of such treatments targeting the intermediate disease mechanisms, these are more likely to be successful due to intervention at earlier stages of the disease.

Genetic and Biochemical Pathways in Age-related Macular Degeneration

Biochemical pathways and genetic association studies have found two polymorphisms, Tyr402His at *10q26* (Complement factor H locus), and Ala69Ser (LOC387715) which may be responsible for up to 75% of the genetic risk of AMD.

Complement pathway (complement factor 2, complement factor 3,[4] complement factor B,[5] complement factor H)[6-9] is involved in natural as well as acquired immunity and activation of this system results in cellular damage. This mechanism is evidenced by the presence of many complement system proteins within drusen in patients with AMD.

Pathology

Aging changes in retina and choroid are very similar to those seen in initial stages of AMD.[10] A common pathogenic route in both aging and AMD is cumulative oxidative injury.[11] With age, reduction in the photoreceptor density is seen in the outer retina. Within the RPE, there is a reduction of melanin granules, with the formation of lipofuscin granules. Development of sheet-like deposits called basal laminar deposits is seen between the RPE plasma membrane and basement membrane. Involution of choriocapillaris is also seen with decrease in choroidal blood flow and reduction in lumen diameter. Small amounts of hard drusen alone are not pathognomonic of AMD and as such, focal deposition is a normal finding in aging.[10,12,13]

Age-related drusen are biochemically distinct from drusen associated with AMD.[14] While small hard drusen can be seen as a normal aging process, large, confluent, or soft drusen should be viewed as a marker of AMD.[15]

Nodular drusen appear as eosinophilic dome-shaped structures deposited between Bruch's membrane and RPE and are densely periodic acid-Schiff (PAS) positive. Increasing basophilic nature may indicate an accumulation of calcium (Figs. 11.1A and B). Calcified drusen show calcific granules or stippling on Von Kossa staining. Soft or large drusen appear with associated localized detachments of RPE at locations of basal laminar or basal linear deposits, which represent granular material accumulating between the RPE and its basement membrane or outside the RPE cell basement membrane, respectively.

Fibrous disciform scars result from sub-RPE neovascularization within the Bruch's membrane or between the RPE and retina (Figs. 11.2A to C). Presence of hemosiderin suggests a hemorrhagic antecedent event. RPE hyperplasia is seen along with disciform scarring and may be associated with a lymphocytic infiltrate in the adjacent choroid. There is photoreceptor loss in the overlying retina with cystic changes.[16]

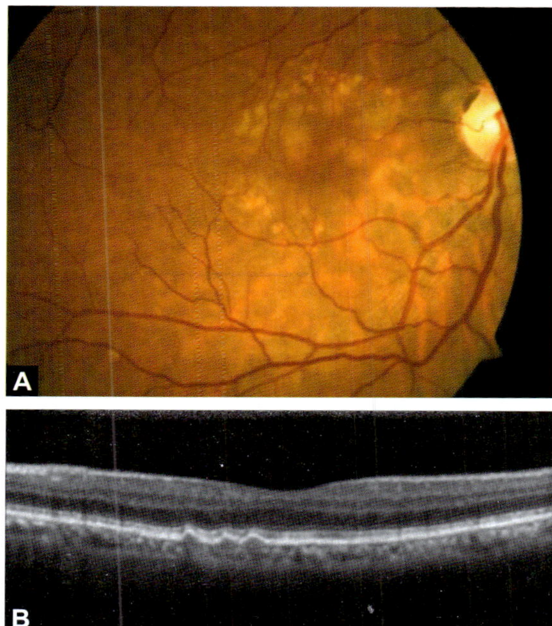

Figs. 11.1A and B: (A) Confluent soft drusen in fundus photography (B) optical coherence tomography (OCT) reveals subretinal pigment epithelium (RPE) humps.

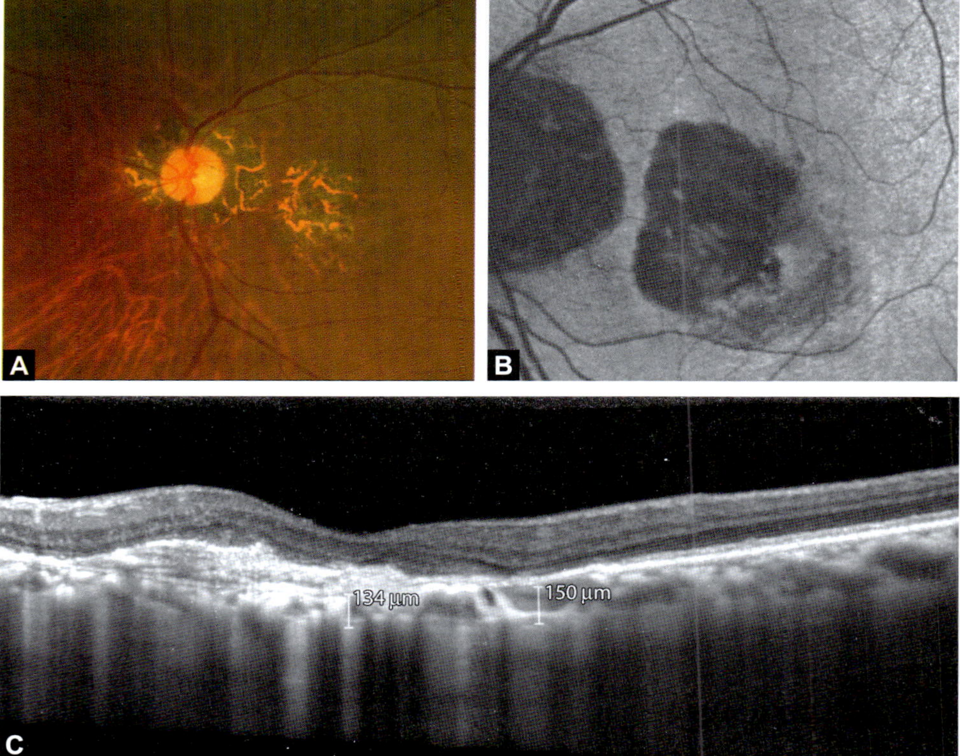

Figs. 11.2 A to C: (A) Fundus color picture, (B) fundus autofluorescence (FAF) image shows dry age-related macular degeneration (AMD) with early scar. (C) spectral domain optical coherence tomography (SD-OCT) reveals atrophic macula with subretinal scar formation. There is associated choroidal thinning.

🏛 Risk Factors

Age

Risk of AMD clearly increases with age. A steep increase (three-fold) is seen in patients of age more than 75 years compared to patients between 65 years and 74 years of age (Beaver Dam Eye Study; Framingham Eye Study).[17,18]

Cigarette Smoking

Significant tobacco smoking history is associated with increased chances of neovascular age-related macular degeneration (NVAMD).[19,20] This increased risk persists even after cessation of smoking (odds ratio 1.13), however, current smokers are at twice the risk of AMD-related vision loss as compared to nonsmokers. After stopping smoking over 20 years earlier patients were not seen to be at higher risk of developing AMD-related vision loss.[21]

Genetic Susceptibility

Genetic factors affect the pathogenesis of AMD and certain genetic loci have been found to be treatment response modifiers, such as seen with intravitreal antivascular endothelial growth factor (VEGF) agents.[22] Further pharmacogenomic studies are required to elucidate the mechanisms, formulate treatment guidelines in future along with proper prognostication indices.

Other Risk factors

Cardiovascular disease, hypertension, female gender, hypercholesterolemia, obesity, hyperopia,[23] family history and light-colored irides.

CLASSIFICATION AND CLINICAL FEATURES

Classification

(A) Non-neovascular or Dry Age-related Macular Degeneration

- *Early AMD*: Characterized by presence of numerous small (<63 microns, "hard") or intermediate (≥63 microns but <125 microns, "soft") drusen. It is worthy to note that small drusen can frequently be seen with aging in patients over 50 years of age, therefore, intermediate drusen are more specific for AMD[24] (Figs. 11.3A and B). Size of drusen can be gauged by comparing with diameter of retinal vein at disc margin which is 125 microns.
- *Intermediate AMD:* Defined by extensive small or intermediate drusen, or any drusen of large size (≥125 microns).[24]
- *Advanced AMD*: May be characterized either by geographic atrophy or choroidal neovascular membrane (Their sequelae-subretinal or sub-RPE hemorrhage or serous fluid, as well as subretinal fibrosis may be seen).[25]

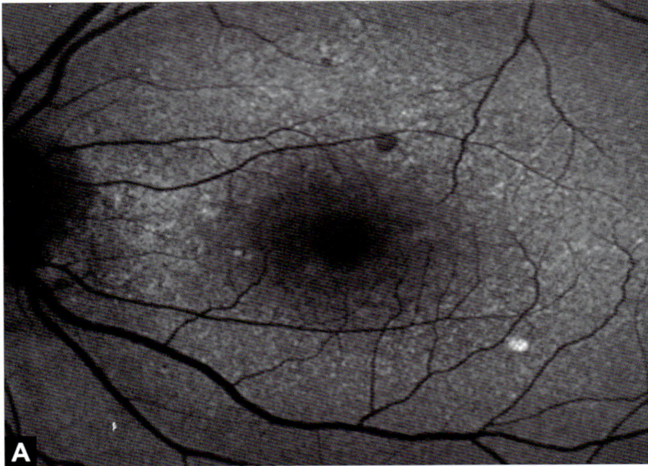

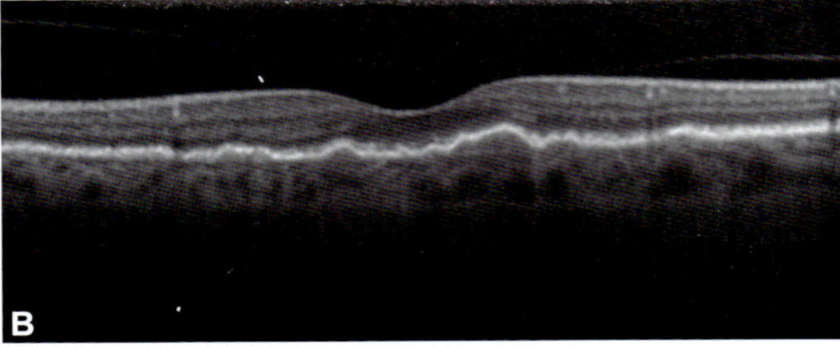

Figs. 11.3A and B: (A) Autofluorescence picture of an eye with pre-age-related macular degeneration (AMD) drusen, visible as (B) subretinal pigment epithelium (RPE) humps on spectral domain optical coherence tomography (SD-OCT).

(B) Neovascular Age-related Macular Degeneration/Wet/Exudative Age-related Macular Degeneration

👤 Clinical Features

Symptoms: Patients with drusen may not complain of visual loss. In non-neovascular AMD, patients with geographic atrophy perceive central scotoma, which is a positive scotoma. Patients with neovascular age-related macular degeneration (nAMD) notice blurred or distorted vision and metamorphopsia. Sudden loss of vision may be a presenting complaint in those with subretinal bleed.[26]

Signs: Patients with non-nAMD show drusen. Hard drusen are yellow in color with discrete margins, clinically seen when the size is more than 30–50 microns. Soft drusen have fuzzy margins and most of them are about 250 microns in size. With progression, RPE degeneration occurs causing loss of adjacent photoreceptors, and juxtaposition of Bruch's membrane to the inner nuclear layer. Geographic atrophy is seen as sharply defined area of hypo- or depigmentation, with loss of RPE.

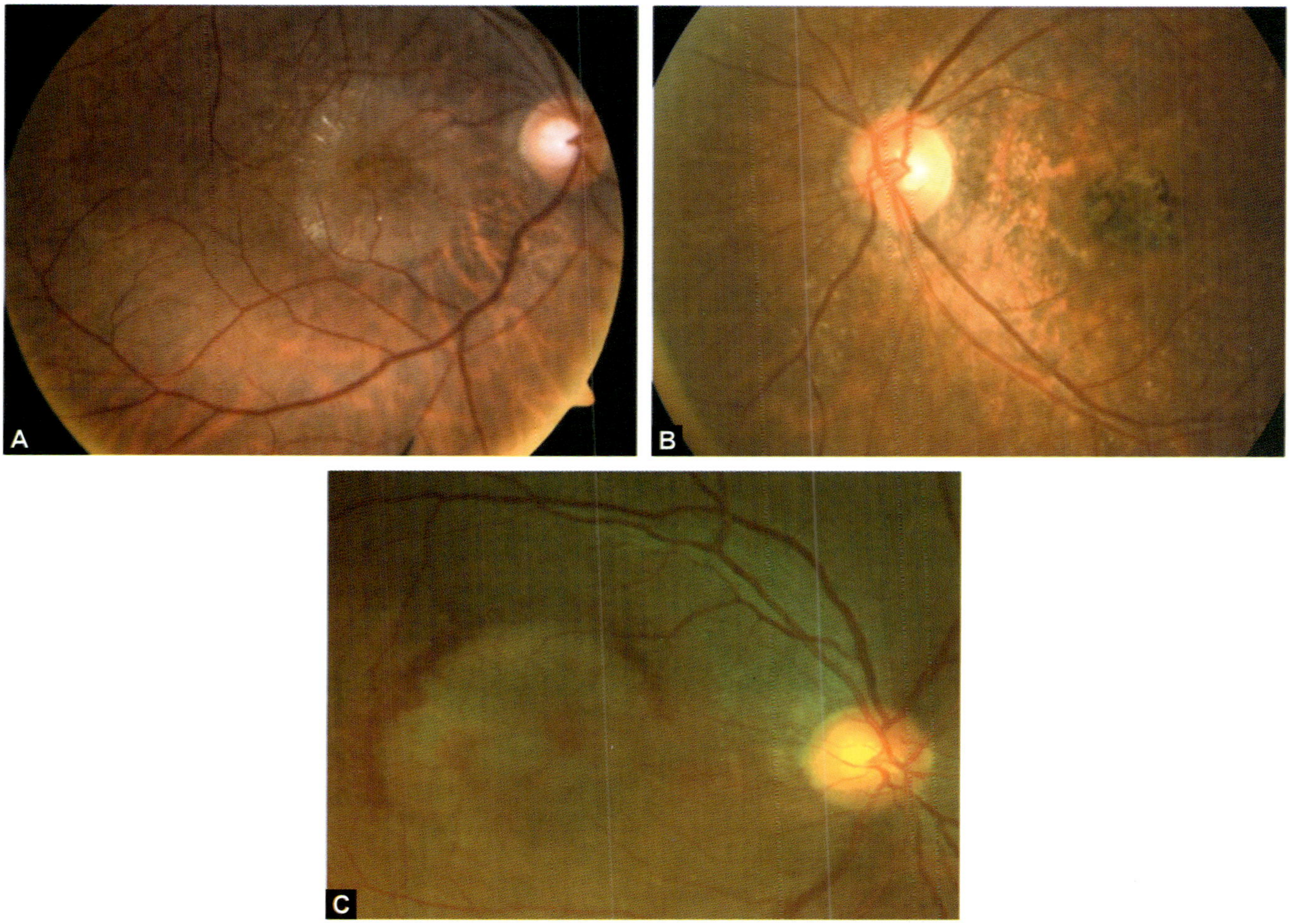

Figs. 11.4A to C: (A) Clinical picture reveals greyish, exudative neovascular membrane (B) Non-neovascular age-related macular degeneration (AMD) (C) Clinical picture reveals greyish, exudative neovascular membrane with advancing edge showing the pathognomonic hemorrhage.

In nAMD, CNV is seen as a green-gray membrane, believed to be due to hyperplasia of RPE (Figs. 11.4 and 11.5). If the CNV bleeds, it may be seen as subretinal hemorrhage, break-through vitreous hemorrhage. The CNVM may eventually undergo fibrosis and form a disciform scar

INVESTIGATIONS

Fluorescein Angiography

Fluorescein angiography (FA) is typically performed with a clinical diagnosis of nAMD. Hypofluorescence (blocked fluorescence) may be caused by hemorrhage, lipid exudation, and pigment hyperplasia. Causes of hyper-fluorescent lesions include drusen (staining in late phase), RPE atrophy (transmission/window defect), choroidal neovascular membranes (leak), serous pigment epithelial detachment (PED) (pooling), and subretinal fibrosis or scar (staining).[27]

Choroidal neovascular membranes are typically classified as *classic* or *occult* on FA. *Classic* CNV is typically seen

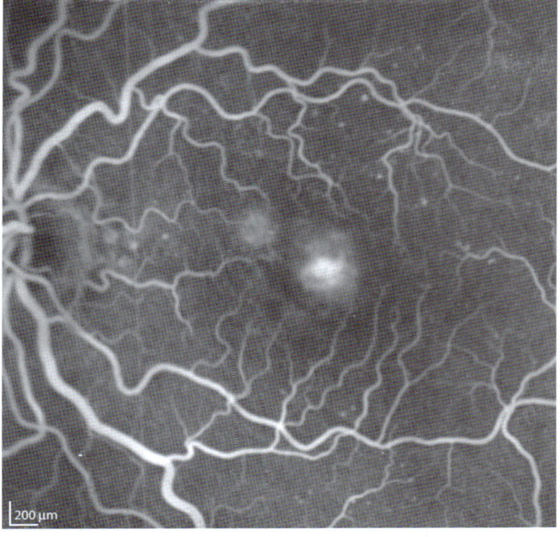

Fig. 11.5: Leaking neovascular membrane AMD (NVAMD) on fluorescein angiography (FA).

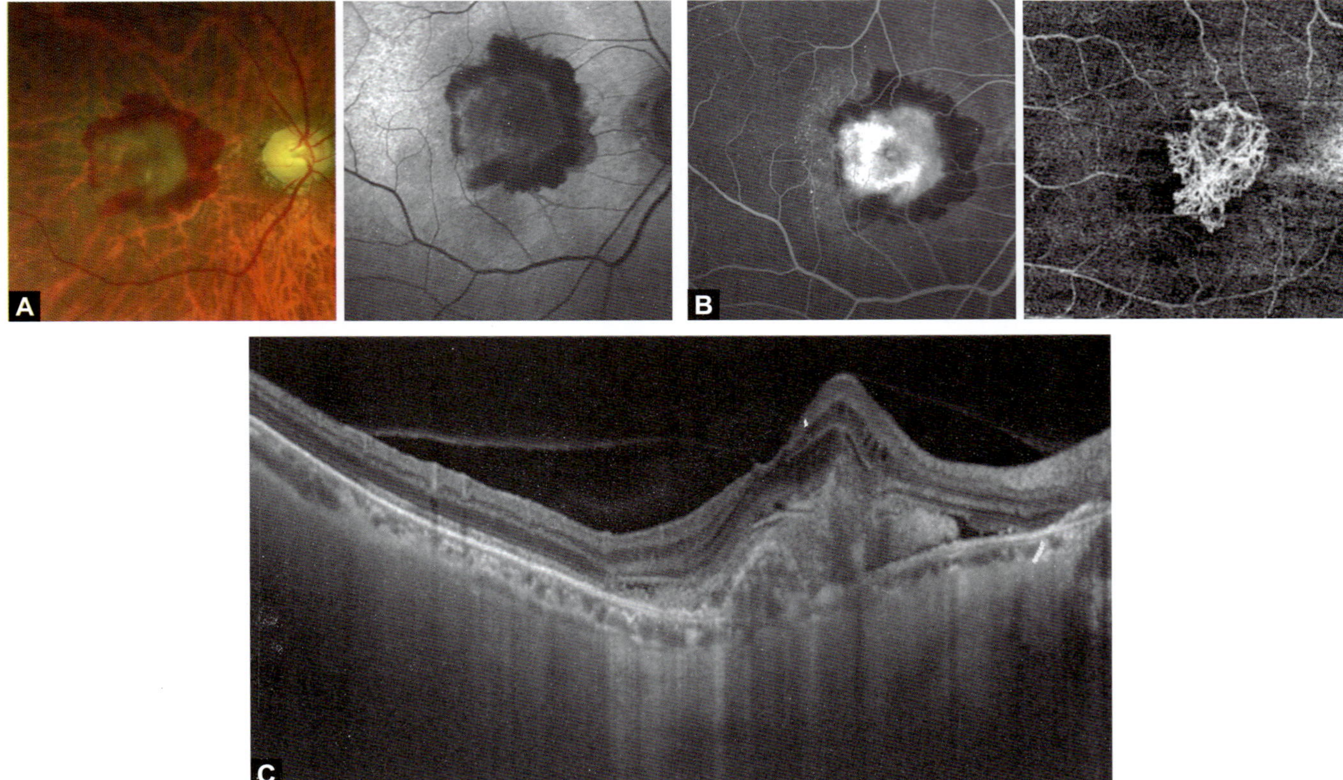

Figs. 11.6A to C: (A and B) Classic choroidal neovascularization (CNV) - color photograph, fluorescein angiography (FA) and fundus autofluorescence (FAF). Optical coherence tomography angiography (OCTA) reveals the neovascular net in the subretinal pigment epithelium (RPE) space. (C) Swept-source OCT (SSOCT) shows the neovascular (NV) membrane with subretinal fluid and hemorrhage.

as a leak, in the early phase, which intensifies throughout the transit phase. It is uniform, with 'lacy' margins (Figs. 11.5 and 11.6). Classic CNV represents subretinal (subneurosensory retina) neovascular tissue, which is also called type 2 CNV.

'Occult' lesions are typically seen in the late phase of FA.[28] It consists of two described forms on FA–a) Fibrovascular PED (FVPED) and b) late leakage of undetermined source (LLUS).

Fibrovascular pigment epithelial detachment is seen as an irregular elevation of the RPE with stippled or granular irregular fluorescence.[29] Late leakage of undetermined source are seen as areas of hyperfluorescence at the level of RPE seen in late phases.

Occult CNV corresponds to sub-RPE CNV or type 1 CNV. As it lies under the RPE, the fluorescent patterns are more appreciable in the late phases.

Optical Coherence Tomography

Optical coherence tomography (OCT) is a noninvasive imaging device, which gives an optical cross-sectional image of the retina. It uses the principle of low-coherence interferometry.[30]

In eyes with non-nAMD, drusen are seen as hyper-reflective structures, at the level of RPE. Drusenoid PEDs, appear as elevation of RPE, with uniform hyper-reflective structure under it whereas serous PEDs are clear and hyporeflective under the RPE (Fig. 11.7).

Eyes with nAMD may also show multiple findings. Of most significance, is the presence of subretinal fluid and intraretinal cystic spaces associated with CNVM, both of which are hypo reflective. The CNVM is hyper-reflective, and OCT is helpful in differentiating the level of the neovascularization, into type 1 and 2 (Fig. 11.8). Scar tissue, typically seen following treatment, is also hyperreflective. While initial exam of a patient with nAMD warrants FA, with OCT patients can be monitored for response following anti-VEGFs.

Optical Coherence Tomography Angiography

Optical coherence tomography angiography (OCTA) is a high-speed OCT scanning device which detects retinal blood flow by analyzing signal decorrelation between scans. Split-spectrum amplitude-decorrelation angiography (SSADA)

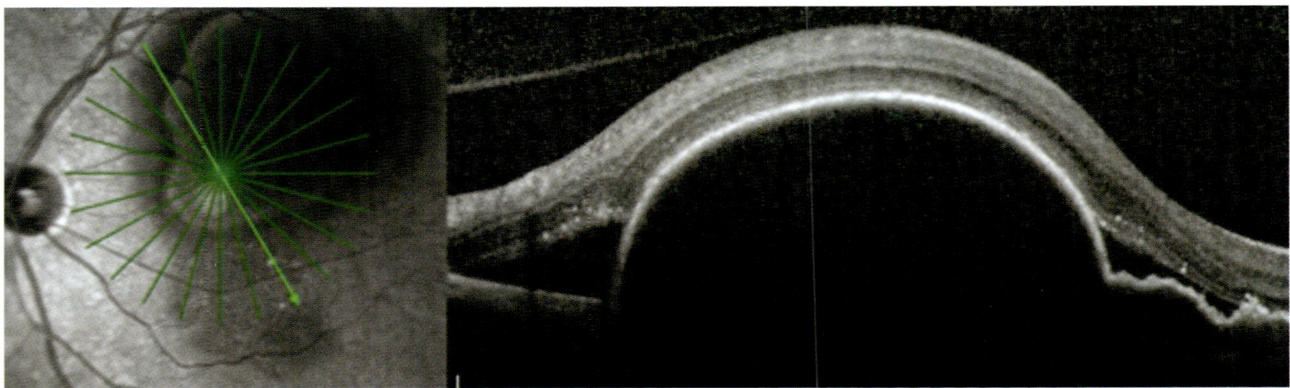

Fig. 11.7: Occult age-related macular degeneration (AMD) with subsensory fluid.

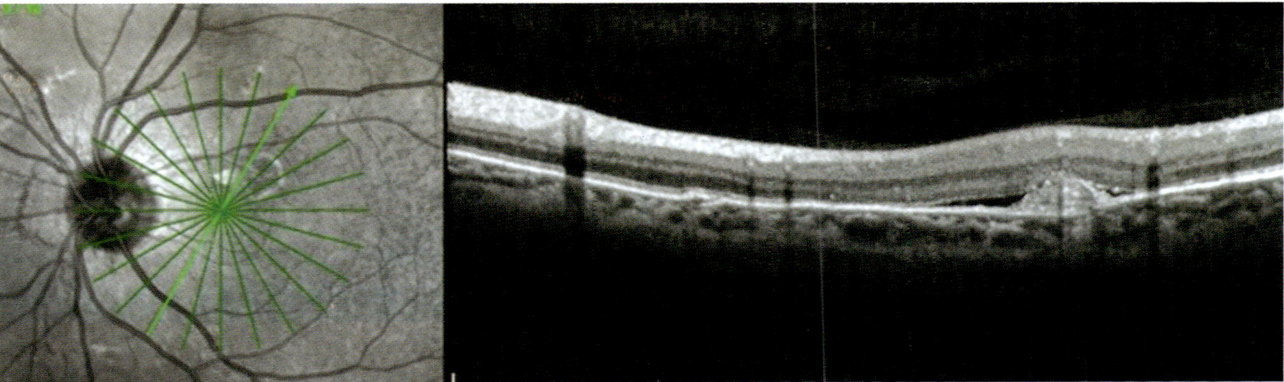

Fig. 11.8: Neovascular age-related macular degeneration (AMD) with subretinal fluid on high resolution optical coherence tomography (HR-OCT).

technology and high frequency dense volumetric scanning detects erythrocyte movement which displays blood vessels in vivo, without using injectable dyes. Further its application in neovascular AMD has been demonstrated in a landmark study where it has helped identify subtypes of choroidal neovascularization and correlate them with the disease course, prognosis, and response to treatment[31] (Figs. 11.9 and 11.10).

Autofluorescence

Autofluorescence is observed due to lipofuscin, and A2E in RPE. Drusen are seen as hyper-autofluorescent lesions and geographic atrophy is seen as hypo-autofluorescent area.

Indocyanine Green Angiography

Indocyanine green angiography (ICGA) is useful to demonstrate choroidal vasculature; hence, its role in CNVM is significant. Areas of active CNVM are seen as hot spots or leaks on ICGA. Only ICGA has the potential to identify CNV hidden by subretinal hemorrhage. It can often reveal occult CNV, not demonstrated on FA.

DIFFERENTIAL DIAGNOSIS

The differential diagnosis of AMD varies greatly depending on the clinical stage of presentation of the patient. So it is useful to organize the differentials by *non-neovascular* and *neovascular* AMD.

Non-neovascular Age-related Macular Degeneration

The differential diagnosis of non-nAMD includes central serous chorioretinopathy (CSCR), Heredomacular dystrophy (HMD), adult onset foveomacular vitelliform dystrophy, cuticular drusen, and drug toxicity (e.g., chloroquine toxicity).

Adult-Onset Foveomacular Vitelliform Dystrophy (Figs. 11.11 and 11.12)

It presents asymptomatically or with mild blurring, after the age of 40 years.[32] Biomicroscopically, it is characterized by a subretinal deposit of oval or round, elevated, yellowish

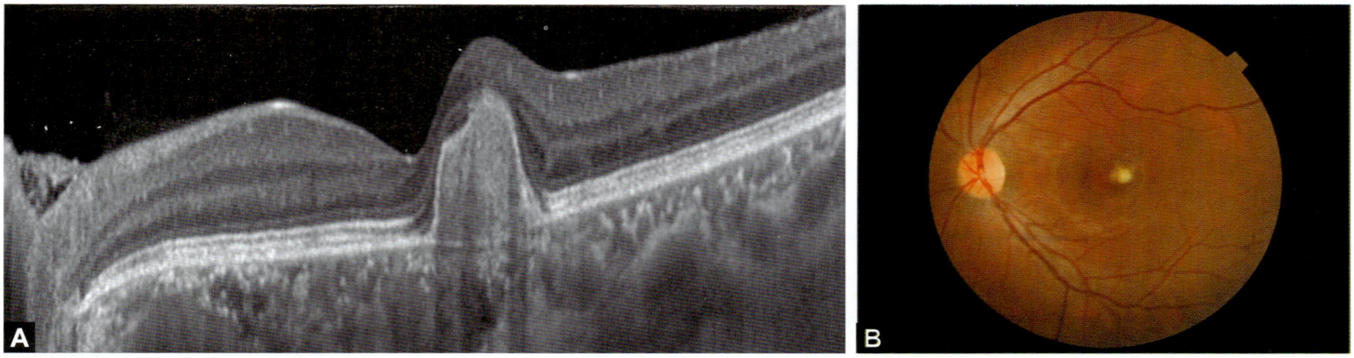

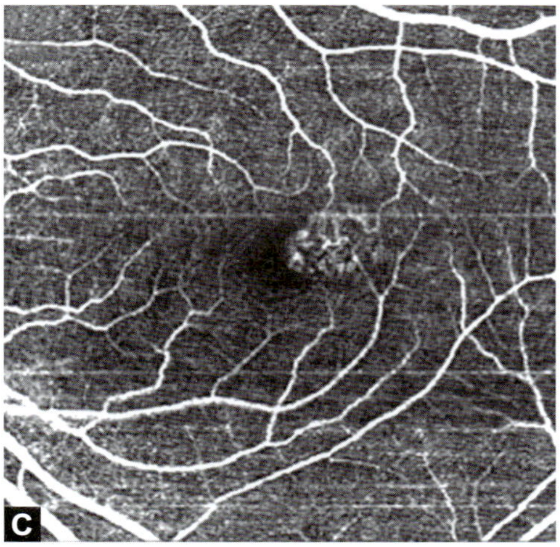

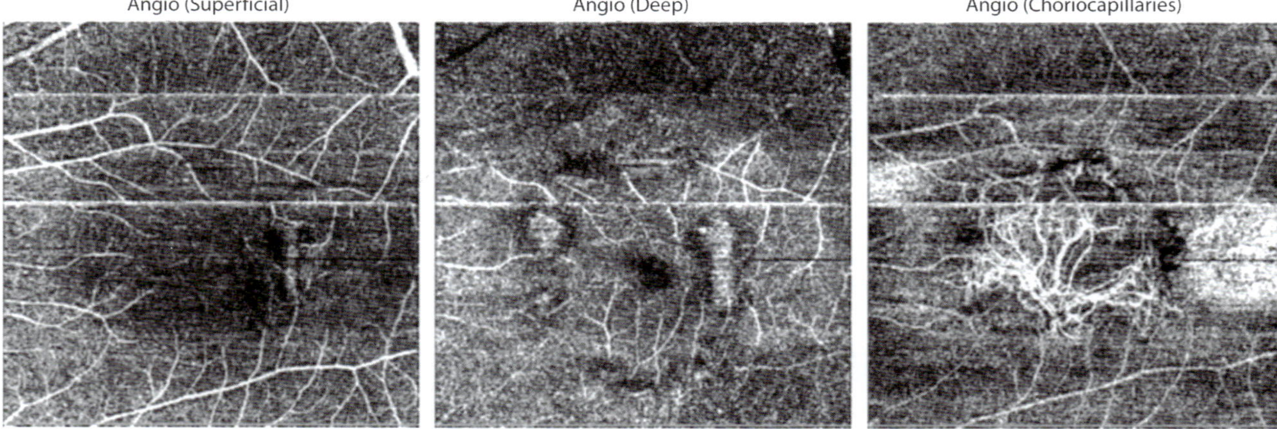

Figs. 11.9A to C: (A and B) Spectral domain optical coherence tomography (SD OCT) shows no subretinal fluid in an eye with idiopathic choroidal neovascularization (CNV) however (C) Angio-OCT reveals minimal neovascular growth. Need to follow-up only.

Angio (Superficial)   Angio (Deep)   Angio (Choriocapillaries)

Fig. 11.10: Angio-optical coherence tomography (OCTA) reveals Type 1 neovascular membrane (sub-RPE location).

material localized in the macular area, and often centered by a pigmented spot.[33] On OCT it is seen as a dome shaped hyperreflective material in the subretinal-space.[34,35]

Multimodal imaging is of great help as it may often be mistaken for neovascular AMD. The subretinal yellowish vitelliform material is seen as a hyper autofluorescent material on AF imaging, while FA reveals a hyperfluorescent center. OCT shows the exact location as bilateral subretinal location. Differentiation from Best's disease is based on electrophysiology which shows normal electrooculogram (EOG) and electroretinogram (ERG) and onset of central scotomas later in life around the 4th decade. Autosomal dominant or

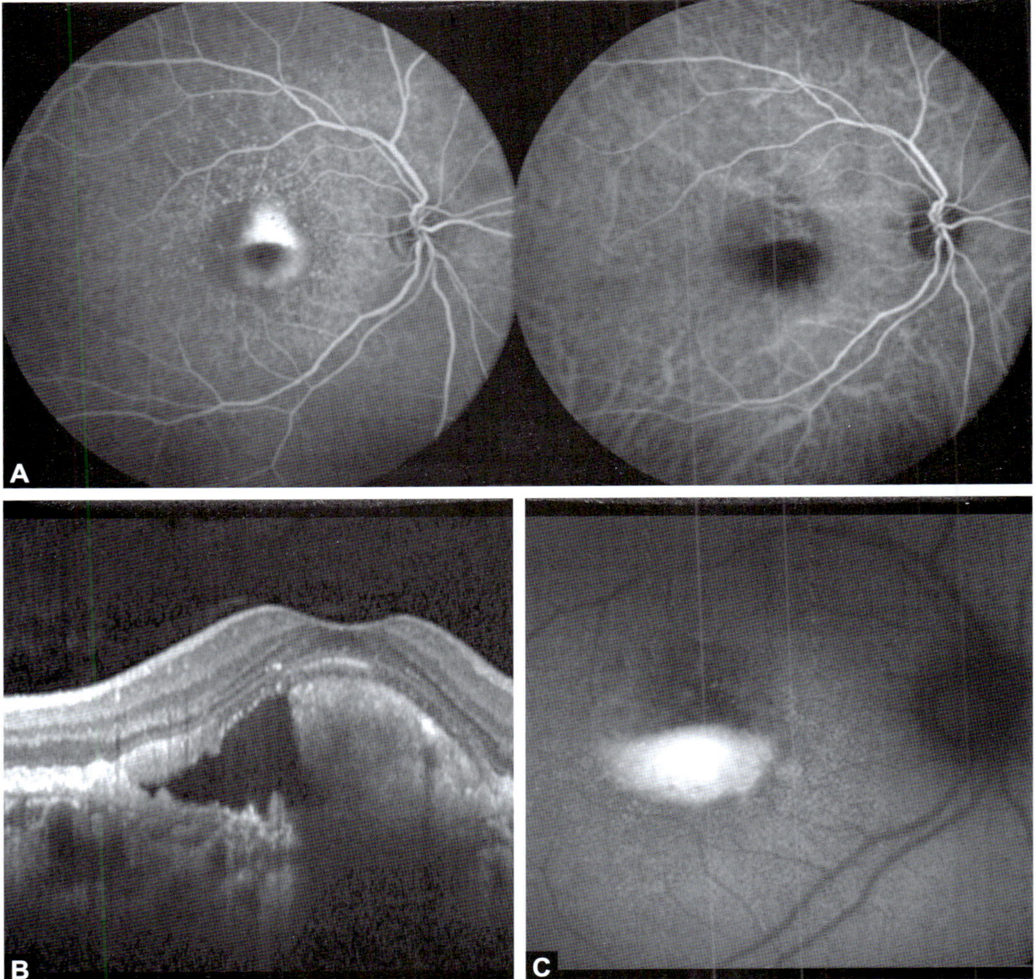

Figs. 11.11A to C: Adult-onset foveomacular vitelliform dystrophy (AOFVD): (A) monthly fluorescein angiography (FA)/indocyanine-green angiography (FA/ICGA): FA shows central hypofluorescence surrounded by an irregular ring of hyperfluorescence, ICGA: central hypofluorescence blocking the choroidal vessels (B) Spectral domain optical coherence tomography (SD-OCT): dome shaped lesion with an inferiorly settled hyper-reflective material and a superior optically empty zone (C) Autofluorescence imaging shows hyperautofluorescent material corresponding to the lipofuscin deposits.

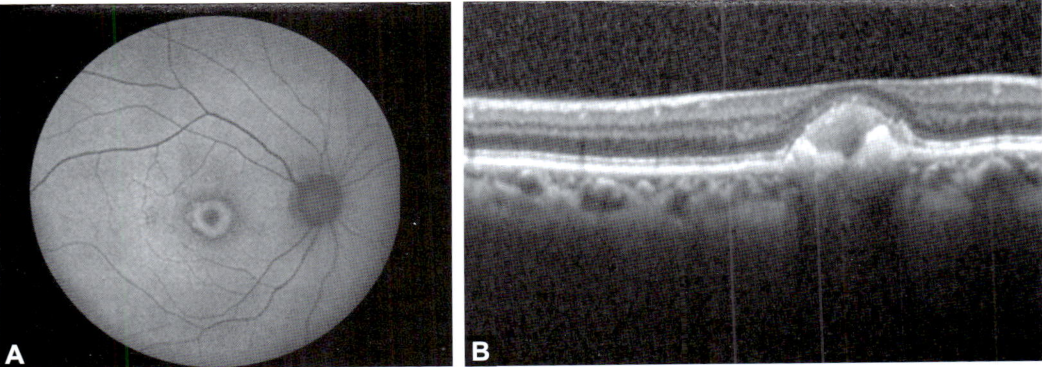

Figs. 11.12A and B: Adult-onset foveomacular vitelliform dystrophy (AOFVD) (A) Autofluorescence imaging showing a ring of hyper-autofluorescence with central hypo-autofluorescence (B) Corresponding spectral domain optical coherence tomography (SD-OCT) image showing accumulation of hyper reflective material.

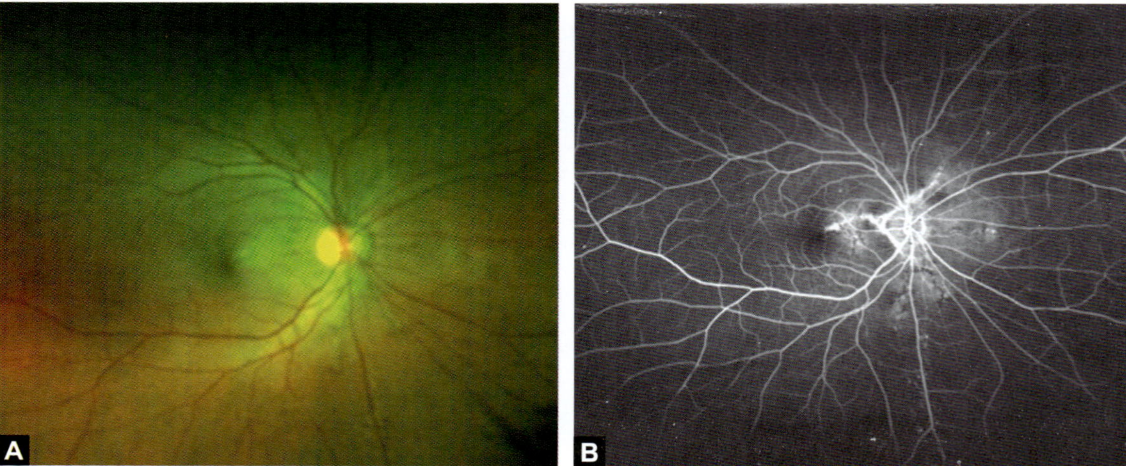

Figs. 11.13A and B: Angioid streaks with secondary choroidal neovascularization (CNV) on spectral domain optical coherence tomography (SD –OCT), color photography (CP) and fluorescein angiography (FA), visible as irregular Bruch's membrane disruptions extending outwards from the disc.

sporadic inheritance has been noted in this disorder. Treatment involves getting best corrected refraction and often the visual disturbance is mild to moderate only. Anti-VEGFs are not indicated.

Neovascular Age-related Macular Degeneration

The differential diagnosis of neovascular AMD includes choroidal neovascularization caused by other conditions like ocular histoplasmosis syndrome, pathologic myopia, Traumatic choroidal rupture and angioid streaks (Figs. 11.13 and 11.14).

TREATMENT

The cornerstone for therapy in non-nAMD is observation with risk factor modification and nutritional supplementation. nAMD is managed more aggressively with close follow up examinations with intravitreal injections of anti-VEGF agents as and when required. Rehabilitation with low vision services is the only alternative in patients with advanced disease in both eyes.

Medical Therapy

Non-Neovascular Age-Related Macular Degeneration Treatment

Antioxidant and nutritional supplementation: Treatment is aimed at reducing the risk of progression. Antioxidant and mineral supplementation have been tried in various studies. The suggested daily regimen by the Age Related Eye Disease Study (AREDS) is:[24]
- 500 milligrams of vitamin C
- 400 International Units of vitamin E

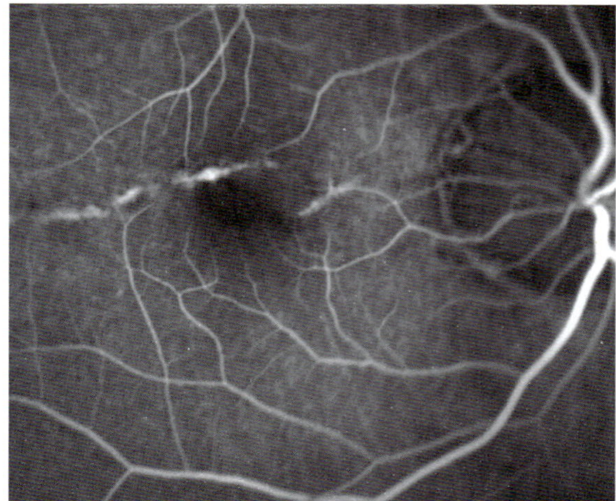

Fig. 11.14: Angioid streaks associated with early choroidal neovascularization (CNV) formation in the juxtafoveal region.

- 15 milligrams of beta-carotene (equivalent of 25,000 International Units of vitamin A)
- 80 milligrams of zinc as zinc oxide
- 2 milligrams of copper as cupric oxide

Copper supplementation was introduced in order to prevent its deficiency, which can be induced by zinc in the AREDS formula. Beta-carotene supplementation at high doses in AREDS formula may possess a potential risk of lung cancer. Non beta-carotene containing supplements may be considered for this subgroup of patients.[36] AREDS reported that in patients with intermediate AMD or those with advanced AMD in one eye, the risk of progression was reduced by about 25% with the above formulation but it failed to prove a similar response in patients with early AMD.

Age Related Eye Disease Study (AREDS2) was a large randomized double control trial designed to test whether adding lutein and zeaxanthin; docosahexaenoic acid (DHA) and eicosapentaenoic acid (EPA); or lutein + zeaxanthin + DHA + EPA; to the AREDS formulation leads to further reduction in the risk of progression to advanced AMD. AREDS2 also explored the effect of elimination of beta-carotene and reduction in the dose of zinc from the original AREDS formulation. Modifications of AREDS2 explored as an alternative included:

- 10 mg lutein and 2 mg zeaxanthin
- 350 mg DHA and 650 mg EPA
- No beta-carotene
- 25 mg zinc

Participants taking AREDS formulation that had lutein/zeaxanthin without beta-carotene had a slight reduction in the risk of advanced AMD, compared to those on formulation with beta-carotene and no lutein/zeaxanthin. This was an important observation for former smokers as such patients who took AREDS with beta-carotene were seen to have a higher incidence of lung cancer. The effect of lowering zinc oxide doses (25 mg) were not significant, however 80 mg of zinc oxide showed more protection from advanced AMD. The final AREDS approved formulation was then recommended which replaces beta-carotene with lutein/zeaxanthin, but does not reduce the dose of zinc oxide.

- *500 milligrams of vitamin C*
- *400 International Units of vitamin E*
- *80 milligrams of zinc as zinc oxide*
- *2 milligrams of copper as cupric oxide*
- *10 mg lutein and 2 mg zeaxanthin*
- *No beta-carotene*

Neovascular Age-related Macular Degeneration Treatments

Macular photocoagulation study (MPS): Initial treatment of nAMD aimed at laser photocoagulation of choroidal neovascular lesions. The MPS was landmark study evaluating laser treatment of extrafoveal, juxtafoveal, and subfoveal neovascular membranes.[37] Extrafoveal or juxtafoveal sites fared better than those receiving direct laser to subfoveal membranes. While laser therapy was found to prevent further deterioration of vision, it did not cause improvement of vision. In current day use of anti-VEGF drugs, use of laser photocoagulation has highly diminished.

Photodynamic Therapy

Verteporfin

Verteporfin is a hydrophobic, lipophilic, synthetic porphyrin, synthesized from blood-derived hematoporphyrin. For intravenous administration, it is dissolved in an organic solvent. Abnormal vessels selectively take up verteporfin. It has an absorption peak at 689 nm, and when activated by laser, 15 minutes after initial infusion, it yields a large quantum of singlet oxygen. It clears rapidly from the body with no significant photo toxicity after 24 hours, which is a major advantage in its clinical applications.

The treatment of AMD with photodynamic therapy (TAP) investigated subfoveal CNV demonstrating a classic component on FA. The study concluded that photodynamic therapy (PDT) could reduce the risk of visual loss in patients with subfoveal CNV compared to sham treatment.

Visudyne in minimally classic (VIM) trial, studied role of PDT in eyes having less than 50% classic CNV on FA. The study concluded, patients with smaller lesions might benefit slightly from verteporfin PDT.

Photodynamic therapy is Food and Drug Administration (FDA) approved for eyes with predominantly classic nAMD. Although PDT is an improvement over subfoveal laser, typically patients maintain, or lose visual acuity with minimal visual gain on monotherapy. Anti-VEGF treatment has gained popularity over PDT as monotherapy for nAMD. Studies have also found the additive benefit of combination therapy of PDT with anti-VEGFs, in cases refractory to anti-VEGFs alone.

Anti-Vascular Endothelial Growth Factor Treatment

Pegaptanib (Macugen: OSI/Eyetech Pharmaceuticals, New York, NY)

RNA oligonucleotide aptamer binding to human VEGF165. The VEGF Inhibition Study in Ocular Neovascularization (VISION) clinical trial studied AMD patients with subfoveal CNV, who received 1 of 3 doses of pegaptanib or sham injection every 6 weeks for 48 weeks. Visual gain of three or more lines was seen in 6% of treated patients as against 2% of control patients after a follow-up of 1 year. Macugen received FDA approval for treating neovascular AMD. However, some patients still lost vision despite treatment, similar to PDT. Therefore, use of pegaptanib has declined in favor of newer anti-VEGF agents.

Ranibizumab (Lucentis; Genentech, South San Francisco, California)

Ranibizumab is a recombinant humanized, antibody (Fab) fragment that binds VEGF. Ranibizumab binds to and inhibits the biologic activity of all active forms of VEGF-A unlike pegaptanib. The minimally classic/occult trial of the anti-VEGF antibody ranibizumab in the treatment of neovascular AMD (MARINA) study was a sham-controlled clinical trial comparing ranibizumab with sham injections. It found that 95% of ranibizumab-treated eyes experienced either visual improvement or maintained vision compared with 62% of sham-treated eyes after 12 months. A striking 40% of ranibizumab treated eyes gained 15 letters or more (Figs 11.15A and B).

Anti-vascular endothelial growth factor antibody for the treatment of predominantly classic choroidal neovascularization in AMD (ANCHOR) study was a sham-controlled clinical trial of eyes with predominantly classic CNV due to nAMD.

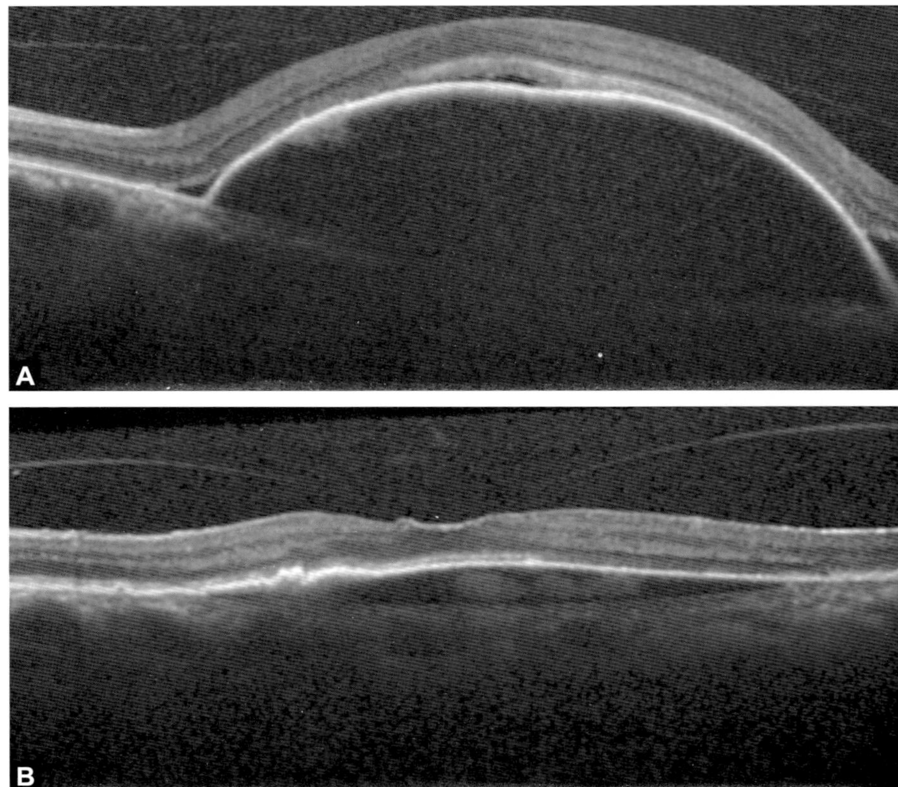

Figs. 11.15A and B: (A) Predominantly occult choroidal neovascularization (CNV) with subretinal fibrosis (SRF) (B) marked flattening of pigment epithelial detachment (PED) with resorption of SRF post antivascular endothelial growth factor (VEGF) injection.

Groups were divided into eyes treated with ranibizumab and sham, verteporfin PDT or sham injection and verteporfin PDT. Ranibizumab-treated eyes maintained or improved vision in 95% of cases compared with 64% of eyes treated with PDT alone.

Prospective optical coherence tomography imaging of patients with nAMD treated with intraocular ranibizumab (PrONTO) study proposed that minimizing the number of reinjections by using an OCT-guided variable dosing regimen gave similar outcomes as those of MARINA and ANCHOR study.

Bevacizumab (Avastin; Genentech, South San Francisco, CA)

Bevacizumab is a full-length monoclonal antibody having both Fab and Fc fragments, binding to VEGF. Bevacizumab has 2 antigen-binding domains, whereas ranibizumab has only one. Avastin (bevacizumab) for choroidal neovascularization (ABC) trial found that 6 weekly injections of intravitreal bevacizumab 1.25 mg showed structural and functional improvement in patients with nAMD. Fabs in general have shorter systemic half-lives than full-length antibodies and intravitreal injections of ranibizumab have a shorter systemic half-life than intravitreal injections of bevacizumab. Comparison of AMD treatment trial (CATT) compared bevacizumab to ranibizumab, and found noninferiority of bevacizumab (Table 11.1).

Recently 5 years CATT results suggest that more frequent anti-VEGF results in increased area of geographic atrophy.

Vascular Endothelial Growth Factor Trap Aflibercept (Regeneron, Tarrytown, NY)

This anti-VEGF is a fusion protein that has both VEGF 1 receptor and VEGF 2 receptor binding site fused to the Fc constant region of IgG. VEGF Trap binds both VEGF and placental-like growth factor (PlGF) and fully penetrates all retinal layers. VEGF Trap is given in dose of 2 mg in 0.05 mL, interval of 2 months. The VIEW 1 and 2 studies have investigated its role in neovascular AMD and have found it to provide visual gain in patients.

The results of the vascular endothelial growth factor trap-eye: Investigation of efficacy and safety in wet AMD studies (VIEW 1 and VIEW 2) support this by demonstrating that aflibercept, dosed every 2 months after a monthly loading dose for 3 months, was noninferior in the proportion of patients who maintained or improved vision at 52 weeks compared with monthly injections of ranibizumab. These results were maintained over the 2 years of the study.

Table 11.1: Comparison of age-related macular degeneration treatment trial (CATT) summary: ranibizumab (R) vs bevacizumab (B) and monthly vs quarterly: multicenter randomized controlled trial in over 1000 patients.

Factor	1 year	2 years
Efficacy	R = B	R = B
Decrease in central retinal thickness	R > B	R > B
Period without fluid	R > B on monthly dosing; R = B on quarterly dosing	R > B on monthly dosing; R = B on quarterly dosing
Decreased visual decline	R = B; Monthly dosing better than quarterly	R = B; Monthly dosing better than quarterly
Adverse effects related to thromboembolic phenomena	B > R but not statistically significant; B 24%, R 19%	B increases the risk of hospitalization

Brolucizumab in Neovascular Age-related Macular Degeneration

The initial 48-week data for its large-scale, phase 3 HAWK and HARRIER clinical trials of its anti-VEGF brolucizumab (RTH258) for wet AMD, demonstrated a durable 12-week retreatment interval for a majority of patients in the 2 studies. The HAWK and HARRIER results at the AAO meeting in New Orleans in 2017, showed impressive efficacy in both eliminating retinal fluid and reducing central subfield thickness in a head-to-head comparison with aflibercept. At week 48, relative to aflibercept, 31% fewer patients on brolucizumab 6 mg had intraretinal fluid and/or subretinal fluid in HAWK, and 41% fewer in HARRIER. Novartis said the absence of fluid for patients in the brolucizumab arm suggests the potential for a long-lasting effect and decreased treatment need.

Additionally, brolucizumab 6 mg demonstrated superior reduction in central subfield thickness. Significantly improved central subfield thickness reduction were evident in both HAWK and HARRIER at week 16 and at week 48. Brolucizumab also met the primary efficacy endpoint of noninferiority to aflibercept in mean change in BCVA from baseline to week 48 in both trials.

Brolucizumab is a single-chain antibody tiny fragment and (Molecular Weight: 26 kD) (Fig. 11.16) offer the advantages of small size, enhanced tissue penetration, rapid clearance from systemic circulation, and versatility in drug delivery.

New Monoclonal Antibody Treatment in Retina

The most common monoclonal antibody-based therapeutics are humanized and fully human antibodies (Table 11.2). Humanized antibodies, like ranibizumab (Lucentis; Genentech) and bevacizumab (Avastin; Genentech), replace only the antigen binding site from the human antibody with that of the specific mouse region.[1] The preparation of fully human antibodies, like adalimumab (Humira; AbbVie, Inc.), is via transgenic mice and phage display technology.[2] Currently, antibodies are produced as monospecific, human, or nearly human molecules. They are modified to produce high affinity target binding.

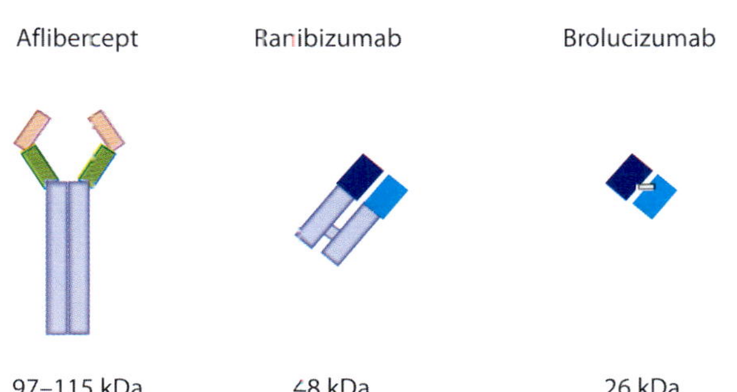

Fig. 11.16: Comparative molecular weights of various antivascular endothelial growth factor (VEGF) drugs.

Radiation Therapy

Radiation can inhibit the cellular proliferation that forms the choroidal neovascular membrane. The CABERNET, MERLOT, and MERITAGE studies have studied the efficacy and safety of epimacular brachytherapy in nAMD. Radiation retinopathy is reported complication in eyes receiving this therapy.[38]

Combination Therapies

The efficacy of ranibizumab and PDT combination compared to PDT alone for treating neovascular AMD was reported by FOCUS trial. PROTECT study had highlighted that the administration of PDT and ranibizumab was safe and more compatible for the patient and the ophthalmologist. TORPEDO trial demonstrated the efficacy of reduced fluence rate PDT in combination with ranibizumab in active neovascular AMD.

Anti-Platelet-Derived Growth Factor

Role of pericytes and endothelial cells have been under study in relation to CNV due to AMD. The angiogenic endothelial cells release platelet-derived growth factor that chemoattracts PDGF receptor-B containing pericytes to which the PDGF binds. The pericytes provides endothelial cells with growth and survival factors, including VEGF, and also plays major role in their survival. Established and mature CNV vessels that have sufficient pericyte coverage may be resistant to anti-VEGF monotherapy.

Table 11.2: Targeted disease process, mechanism of action, manufacturer, and phase of development of new monoclonal antibody-based treatment.

Treatment	Targeted disease	Mechanism of action	Manufacturer	Current status
GSK933776	Geographic atrophy (GA) in age-related macular degeneration (AMD)	Humanized monoclonal antibody against amyloid-beta	GlaxoSmithKline	Phase 2 completed: Drug is safe but did not slow GA growth
Lampalizumab	GA in AMD	Antigen-binding fragment of a humanized monoclonal antibody	Roche	Phase 3 trials under way
THR-317	Diabetic Macular Edema (DME)	Anti-PIGF recombinant monoclonal antibody	Thrombogenics	Phase 2 study under way
RO6867461 (RG7716)	DME, neovascualr AMD (nvAMD)	Bispecific antibody blocking simultaneous Ang-2 and VEGF-A	Hoffman LaRoche	Phase 2 study under way
REGN910 (nesvacumab)	DME, nvAMD	Fully human IgG1 monoclonal antibody that specifically binds and inactivates the Tie2 receptor ligand Ang-2 with high affinity, but shows no binding to Ang-1	Regeneron Pharmaceuticals	Phase 2 study under way
DS7080a	nvAMD	Monoclonal antibody	Daiichi Sankyo, Inc.	Phase 1 study under way
TK001 (sevacizumab)	nvAMD	Recombinant humanized monoclonal antibody	Jiangsu T-Mab Biopharma Co., Ltd.	Phase 1 study under way
Brolucizumab (formerly RTH-258 & ESBA1008)	nvAMD	Humanized, single-chain antibody fragment that is much smaller than commercially available anti-VEGF agents	Alcon	Phase 2 study completed, phase 3 under way
REGN2176-3	nvAMD	Combination antibody to PDGFR-b coformulated with aflibercept	Regeneron Pharmaceuticals	Phase 2 study terminated: no additional efficacy seen with REGN2176-3 over aflibercept alone
iSONEP (LT1009)	nvAMD	Humanized monoclonal antibody against S1P (systemic administration)	Lpath, Inc.	Phase 2a completed: did not meet primary endpoints

Combination therapy with anti-VEGF and anti-PDGF drugs will theoretically "strip" pericytes from endothelium, causing the vasculature of CNV to become more susceptible to anti-VEGF therapy thereby inducing regression, all this while not affecting pericytes on mature normal vasculature.

Fovista

Fovista (Ophthotech, New York, NY) is an anti-PDGF pegylated aptamer, administered via intravitreal injection. It binds with high affinity to PDGF causing stripping of the pericytes from the vessel basement membrane. Intravitreal Fovista, 3 mg with ranibizumab is found to be safe, with a favorable short-term safety profile.[39]

A randomized, multicentric, controlled double-masked study (Multicentric trial OPH-1004) investigated the superiority of combination therapy of Fovista (pegpleranib) (anti-PDGF therapy) and anti-VEGF therapy compared to anti-VEGF monotherapy for treatment of wet-AMD. In phase 3 clinical trial, the combination did not achieve the predetermined primary endpoint of mean change in visual acuity at

12 months. The addition of 1.5 mg of Fovista to an Eylea or Avastin regimen did not result in benefit as measured by the mean change in visual acuity at the 12-month time point.

Surgery

The submacular surgery trials (SST) studied submacular surgery extensively. Macular translocation was not found to yield effective results.[40] Excising choroidal neovascular membranes, did not gain significant usage.

Submacular hemorrhage is a known complication of nAMD causing substantial visual impairment (Figs. 11.17A and B). Mechanisms of vision loss include toxicity of the released iron on the photoreceptors, shearing of photoreceptors by the contraction of fibrin clots, separation of photoreceptors from RPE, progression of the underlying and macular scar formation.

Management of submacular hemorrhage has evolved from invasive procedures like subretinal removal of submacular bleed to lesser invasive procedures like intravitreal or subretinal injection of recombinant tissue plasminogen activator (r-tPA). Surgical removal of submacular bleed and CNVM has been found to result in poor functional outcomes and are therefore not advised. Minimally invasive techniques include vitrectomy with injection of subretinal tPA and aspiration of liquefied blood; intravitreal tPA with pneumatic displacement; subretinal injection of tPA with pneumatic displacement; intravitreal injection of recombinant tPA with evacuation of subretinal bleed followed by gas tamponade; intravitreal injection of anti-VEGF; and subretinal injection of r-tPA during pars plana vitrectomy followed by an intravitreal gas tamponade without evacuation (Figs.11.18A and B).

The technique and efficacy of intravitreal recombinant tPA (r-tPA) with displacement of bleed by gas was described by Heriot, further elucidated by researchers. Haupert et al. demonstrated pars plana vitrectomy with subretinal r-tPA injection with pneumatic displacement with gas along with postoperative propped up positioning.[41]

Kumar A et al. investigated the effectiveness of the modified technique of pars plana vitrectomy with subretinal injection of rtPA (12.5 mg/0.1 mL), bevacizumab (2.5 mg/0.1 mL) along with 0.3 mL of air. The eye was filled with 20% SF6 followed by postoperative propped up positioning. This tech-

nique was found to be extremely effective with only two cases having rebleed.[42]

Breakthrough vitreous hemorrhage in eye with nAMD causes sudden peripheral and central vision loss; as against central vision loss seen in nAMD, and submacular bleed. Additional causes of vitreous hemorrhage need to be kept in mind, considering the age group. It is managed by pars plana vitrectomy, with intravitreal anti-VEGF.

Other complications include RPE dehiscence or tears, which have been associated with CNV, often in an eye with a serous or fibrovascular PED, and secondary to laser photocoagulation. CNV underlying a detached RPE or PCV can contribute to RPE tear formation (Figs. 11.19 and 11.20). Tears occur at the junction of attached and detached RPE, when the PED can no longer resist the stretching forces from the fluid in the sub-RPE space or from the contractile forces of the underlying fibrovascular tissue that may be associated.

POLYPOIDAL CHOROIDAL VASCULOPATHY AND PACHYCHOROID SPECTRUM

Idiopathic polypoidal choroidal vasculopathy (IPCV) was first described by Yannuzzi in 1982 as a pathology consisting of polypoidal, subretinal, vascular lesions with serous and hemorrhagic detachments of the retinal pigment epithelium.[43] Kleiner et al. later identified a series of middle-aged adult African women with recurrent subretinal and sub-RPE bleeding and termed this condition as posterior uveal bleeding syndrome.[44] Subsequently the condition was globally known as PCV.

Though initial reports suggested that PCV was more commonly seen in women, later it was reported to be equally prevalent between both the sexes with the most common age group affected being 50–65.[45-47] Prevalence rates are higher among Asians with presumed AMD (23.9–54.7%) when compared to Caucasians (4–9.8%).[35,48-50]

As per an epidemiological case control study (n = 354; cases = 177; controls = 177) conducted at our center (unpublished data), we found that the mean age of PCV patients was 66 ± 6 years with male predominance (57%). There was no statistically significant difference (p > 0.05) between the two groups with reference to diet, smoking, alcoholism, exercise, diabetes mellitus, ischemic heart disease and plasma

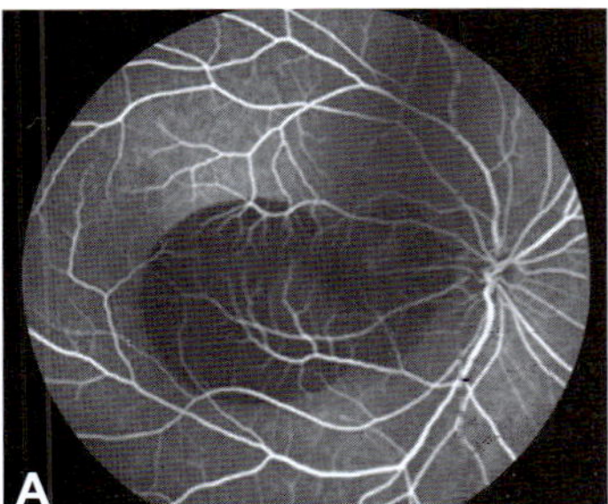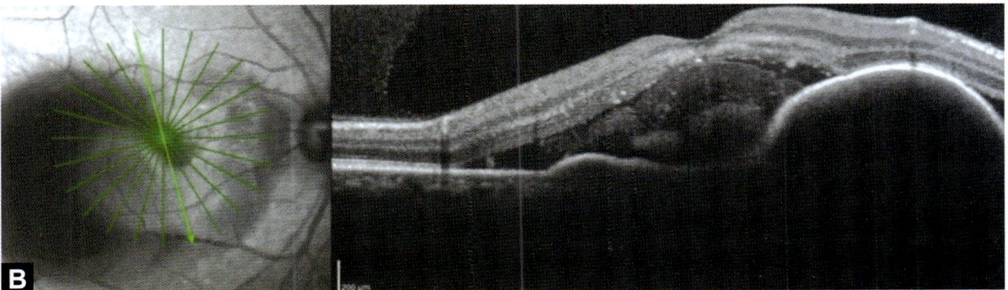

Figs. 11.17A and B: (A) Reveals a submacular bleed on fundus photo; (B) The collected bleed next to the pigment epithelial detachment (PED) in the submacular area.

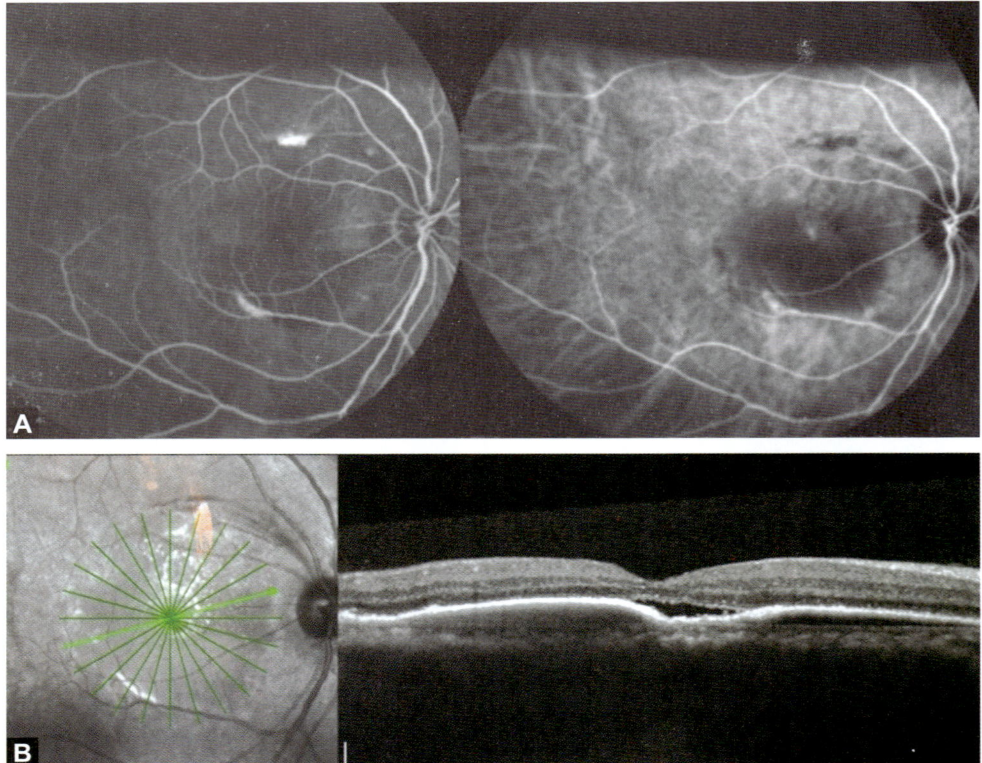

Figs. 11.18A and B: (A) On fluorescein angiography (FA) and indocyanine-green angiography (ICGA) imaging, post recombinant tissue plasminogen activator (r-TPA) submacular injection, the blood has displaced inferiorly. A hot spot is visible on ICGA suggesting a retinal angiomatous proliferation (RAP) lesion (at 2 weeks post injection) (B) Corresponding spectral domain optical coherence tomography (SD-OCT) image showing resolution.

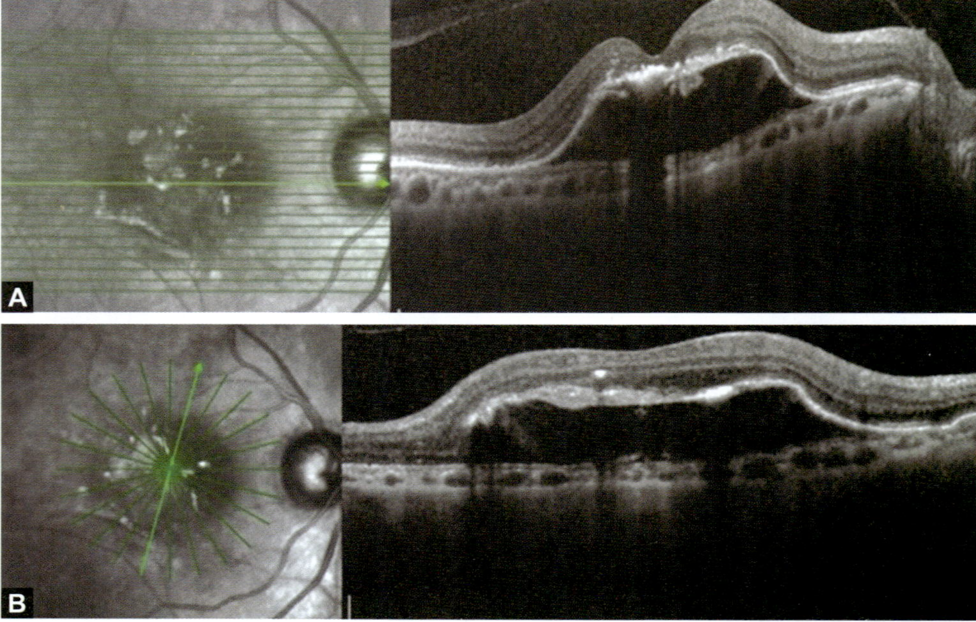

Figs. 11.19A and B: (A) Highly elevated pigment epithelium detachment (PED) on spectral domain optical coherence tomography (SD-OCT); (B) OCT shows ripped retinal pigment epithelium (RPE) from one edge.

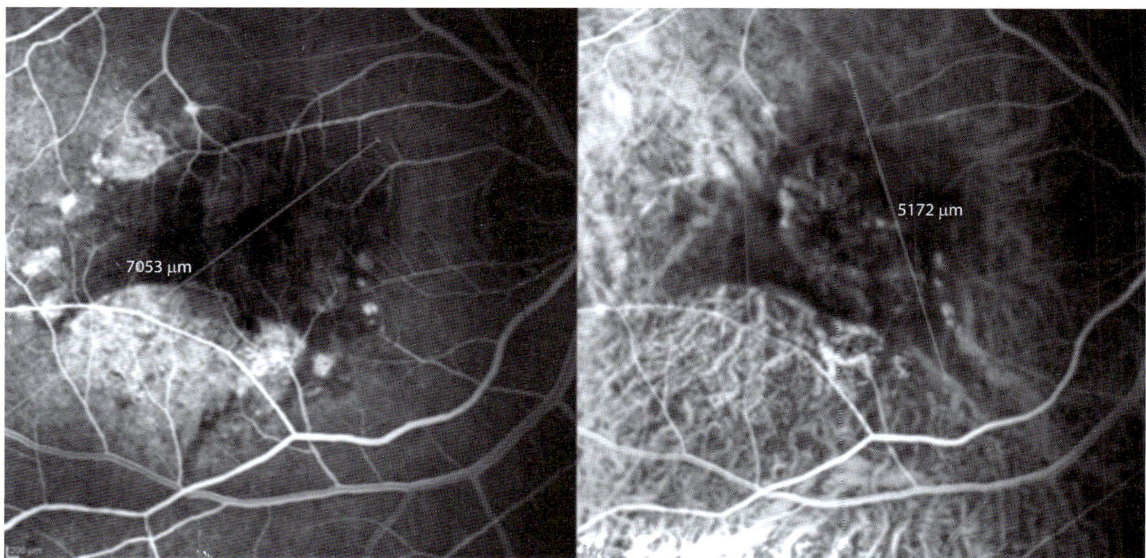

Fig. 11.20: Ripped retinal pigment epithelium (RPE) in an eye with polypoidal choroidal vasculopathy (PCV) on indocyanine-green angiography (ICGA)/fundus fluorescein angiography (FFA) imaging.

homocysteine. Stress, lack of sleep, obesity, hypertension and higher socioeconomic status (p ≤ 0.05) were more commonly seen in PCV cases. Central serous chorioretinopathy (CSC) preceded PCV in 10% cases.

Polypoidal choroidal vasculopathy is characterized by hyalinization and dilatation of inner choroidal vessels. The term hyalinization indicates replacement of smooth muscle component of the vessel wall by amorphous pseudo collagenous tissue with deposition of basement membrane like protein. In contrast, choroidal neovascularization (CNV) consists of granulation tissue proliferation that represents a nonspecific wound healing response. It has also been reported that the aqueous levels of VEGF were significantly lower in PCV when compared to CNV.[51]

Clinical presentation is variable (Figs. 11.21 to 11.23). Indocyanine green angiography (ICGA) is considered to be the gold standard for the diagnosis of PCV. According to evidence-based guidelines, ICGA should be always performed for the diagnosis when routine ophthalmoscopic examination suggests a serosanguineous maculopathy with one of the features as given in Box 11.1.[52]

According to EVEREST study (a multicenter, randomized active controlled study) PCV is defined as the presence of early subretinal focal ICGA hyperfluorescence (Figs. 11.23A and B) appearing within the first 6 minutes after injection of ICGA with at least one of the features as given in Box 11.2.[53]

The Planet study revealed Aflibercept was effective for the eyes with treatment-naive polypoidal choroidal vasculopathy to achieve the resolution of polypoidal lesions. One needs to carefully observe the eyes after confirming complete resolution of polypoidal lesion because of recurrent polyps seen in one-quarter of the study eyes.

Regarding the Laptop study In a recent article, Oishi et al.[1] discussed the 24-month results of the Ranibizumab (Lucentis) and Photodynamic Therapy on Polypoidal choroidal vasculopathy (LAPTOP) study, and reported that patients with polypoidal choroidal vasculopathy (PCV) who were randomized to the ranibizumab arm experienced a gain in visual acuity (VA), while those in the photodynamic therapy (PDT) arm did not show improvement in VA.

The OCT findings include characteristic double layer sign and dome or thumb-shaped elevation of pigment epithelium. (Fig. 11.22B) The double layer sign is a spectral domain OCT finding distinguished by an inner hyper-reflective layer corresponding to RPE and an outer hyper-reflective layer denoting the Bruch's-choriocapillaris complex. It is suspected that the space between the two layers indicates fluid accumulation or the presence of the branching vascular network (BVN). The thumb shaped PED correlates to the polypoidal vascular activity.[54] PEDs may be serous or hemorrhagic with or without an associated notch. The BVN that has infiltrated the Bruchs membrane often terminates as polyps. The polyps correspond to the notch and show moderate hyper-reflectivity.[55]

Optical coherence tomography-angiography helps in identifying and defining BVN better than ICGA. The various patterns of BVN identified using OCT-A include sea-fan, medusa and tangle. The polyp detection rate of OCT-A is however comparatively lesser than ICGA (50–95%). The detection rate depends on the velocity of blood flow in the polyp. According to the principle of SSADA (Split spectrum amplitude decorrelation angiography), the slow velocity in some polyps cannot be picked up in OCT-A due to low decorrelation value[56] (Figs. 11.24A and B).

Classification of Polypoidal Choroidal Vasculopathy[52]

- *Quiescent:* Polyps in the absence of subretinal or intraretinal fluid or hemorrhage;

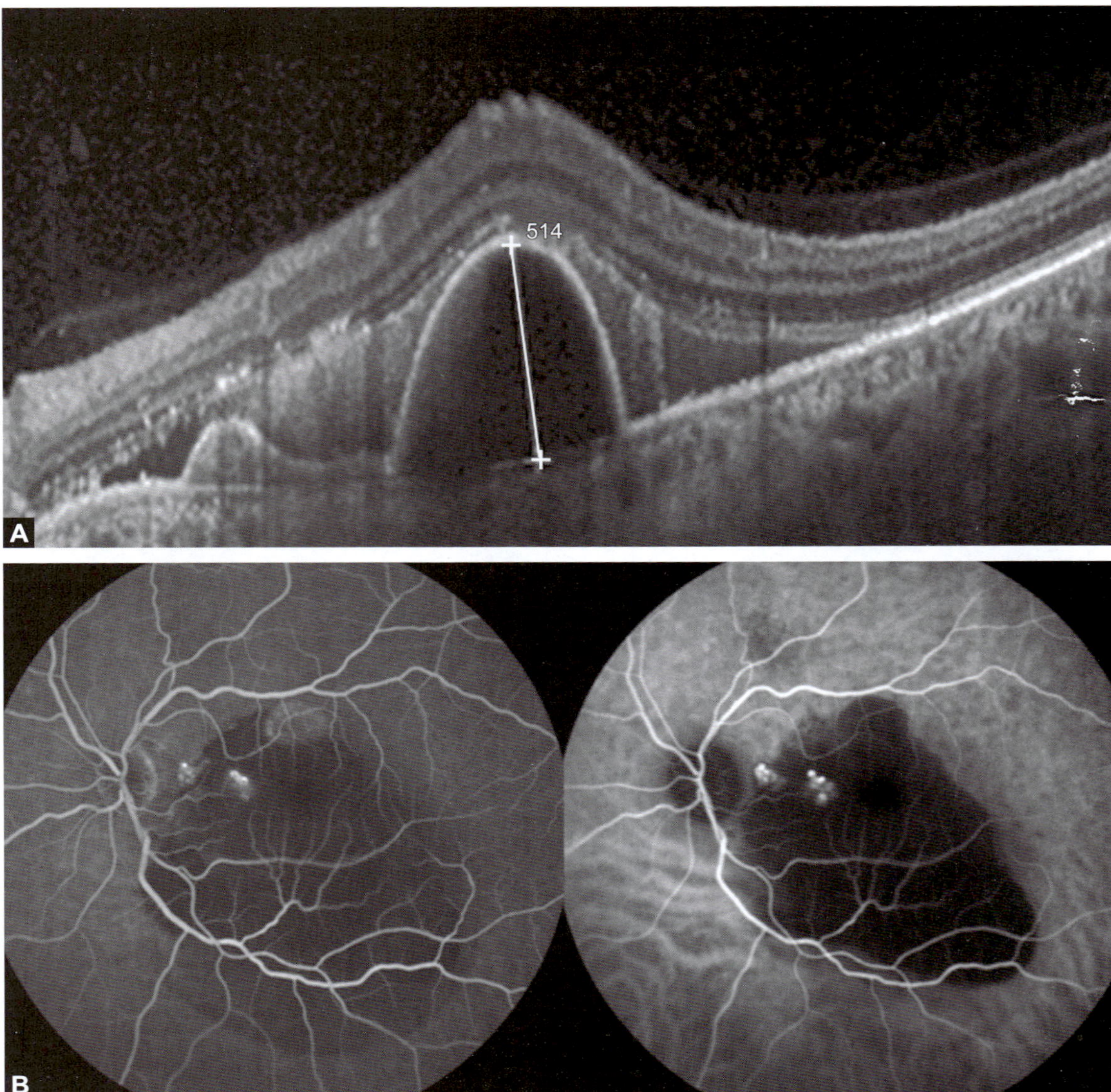

Figs. 11.21A and B: (A) A Case of polypoidal choroidal vasculopathy (PCV) showing serosanguineous pigment epithelial detachments with submacular hemorrhage. (B) Fluorescein angiography (FA) and indocyanine-green angiography (ICGA) of the same patient showing multiple focal hyperfluorescence corresponding to the polyps.

- *Exudative:* Exudation without hemorrhage, which includes sensory retinal thickening, neurosensory detachment, PED, and subretinal lipid exudation;
- *Hemorrhagic:* Any subretinal or sub-RPE hemorrhage with or without other exudative characteristics.

Management

Treatment should be started for active symptomatic PCV. PCV can be considered active, if there is any one of the features as listed in Box 11.3.[52]

Various treatment modalities include thermal laser photocoagulation, verteporfin photodynamic therapy (vPDT) and anti VEGF therapy. Polyp regression is the main goal of treatment. The entire PCV lesion including the BVN as indicated by ICGA needs to be treated by either thermal laser photocoagulation or PDT.

Polyp regression may be better with PDT when compared to anti-VEGF monotherapy. But serious adverse effects of PDT exist and include vision loss, subretinal hemorrhage and choroidal ischemia. Recently, a number of trials have illustrated the superiority of combination therapy of PDT and anti-VEGF over PDT monotherapy (Figs. 11.25A and B). With the advent of intravitreal Aflibercept (VEGF trap), IVA monotherapy (Figs. 11.26 and 11.27) and combination therapy with PDT (Figs. 11.28A and B) have gained recognition

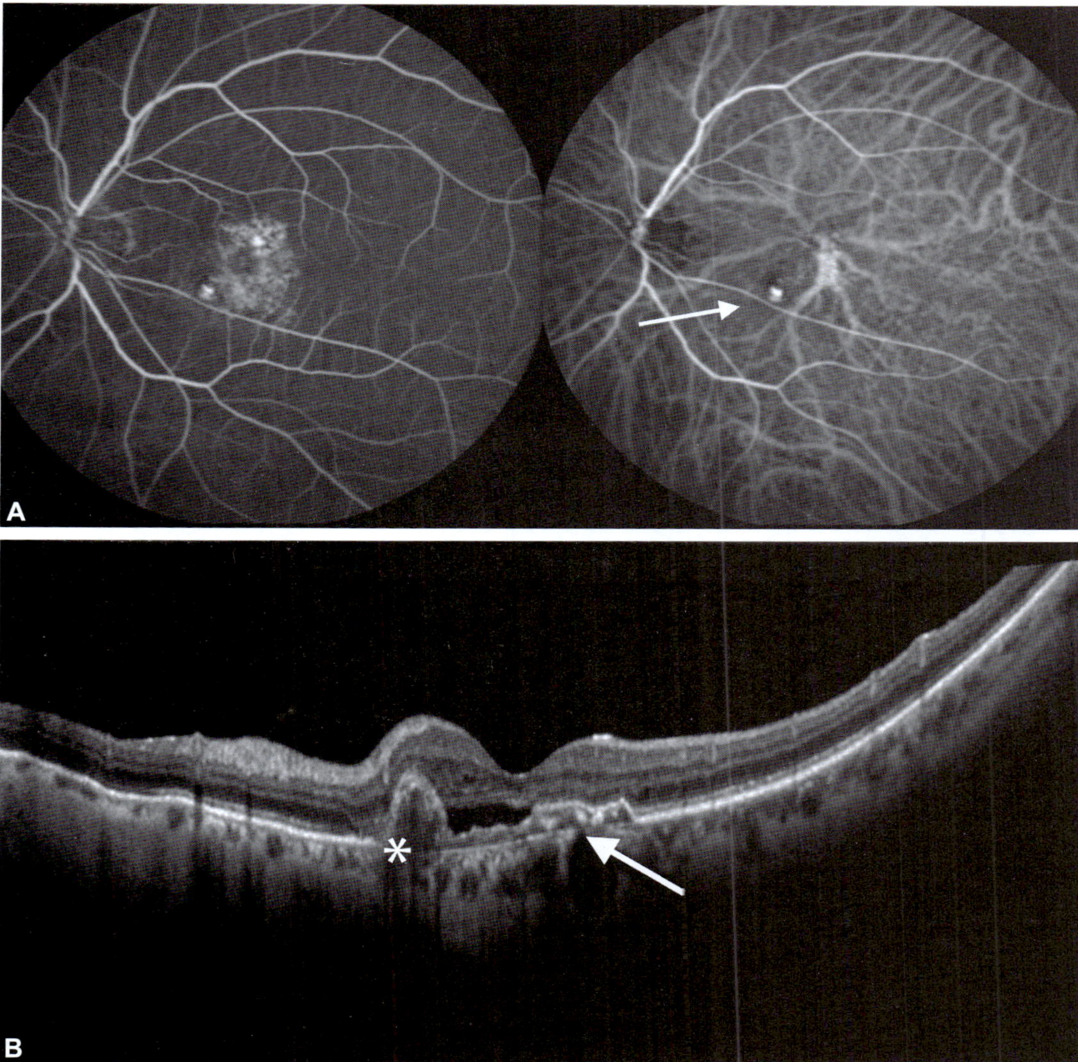

Figs. 11.22A and B: (A) Focal hypofluorescence surrounded by a hyperfluorescent halo in the early phase of ICGA (corresponding to the polyp) (White arrow) (B) Spectral domain optical coherence tomography (SD-OCT) imaging of the same patient showing thumb shaped pigment epithelium detachment (PED) (asterisk) with double layer sign (arrow).

Evidence based treatment; monitoring and re-treatment guidelines with conclusions of some of the prominent trials have been listed (Tables 11.3 to 11.5 and Box 11.4).

Submacular Bleed in Polypoidal Choroidal Vasculopathy

The incidence of sub-RPE or subretinal hemorrhage (Fig. 11.29) is high in PCV patients (30–64%).

Despite combination therapy of intravitreal Aflibercept and rf PDT or Aflibercept monotherapy, sub RPE and sub-retinal bleed has a definite risk in PCV eyes. At our center, we inject a mixture of intravitreal tPA (50 units), Avastin (0.1cc) and air bubble (0.4 cc) using a 41G Translocation needle to displace the clot and maintain propped up position to gravi-

tate the bleed inferiorly (Figs. 11.30A and B). We have an encouraging series of the above mentioned treatment and the results are gratifying.[42]

PACHYCHOROID SPECTRUM

The term pachychoroid (pachy-thick) denotes abnormal and permanent increase in choroidal thickness and is most commonly associated with CSC.[55,59] Dilated large outer choroidal vessels (Haller's layer) compressing the choriocapillaris and the Sattler's layer characterize this entity. The spectrum includes pachychoroid pigment epitheliopathy (PPE), CSC, pachychoroid neovasculopathy (PNV) and PCV.[59]

Pachychoroid pigment epitheliopathy is diagnosed by multimodal imaging and represents a forme fruste form

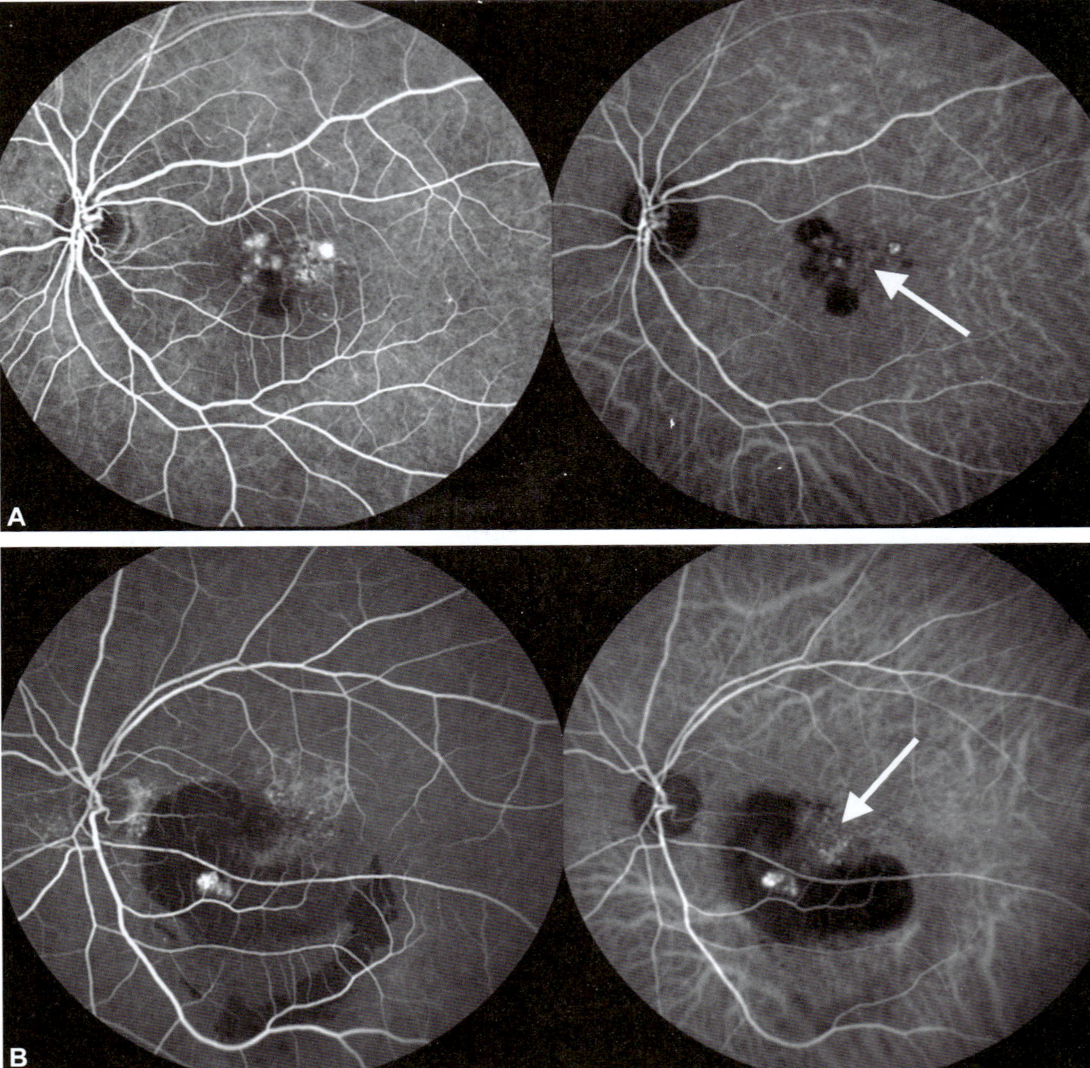

Figs. 11.23A and B: Fluorescein angiography (FA)/indocyanine-green angiography (ICGA) early hyperfluorescence with surrounding hypofluo-rescent halo along with branching vascular network (arrows).

Box 11.1: Clinical features of polypoidal choroidal vasculo-pathy (PCV).

- Clinically visible orange-red subretinal nodules
- Spontaneous massive subretinal hemorrhage
- Notched or hemorrhagic pigment epithelium detachment (PED)
- A lack of response to anti-VEGF therapy

Box 11.2: Clinical features of indocyanine green angio-graphy (ICGA).

- Branching vascular network (BVN) [an interconnected inner choroidal vascular network identified on indocyanine-green angiography (ICGA)] (Figs. 11.3 and 11.4)
- Pulsatile polyp (ICGA video guided)
- Nodular appearance (stereoscopic fundus ophthalmoscopy)
- Hypofluorescent halo around the polyp (ICGA in the first 6 minutes)
- Orange subretinal nodules corresponding to the area of polyp
- Massive submacular hemorrhage (> 4 disc areas)

of CSC manifesting with RPE changes with absence of sub-retinal fluid. Fundus examination shows absence of tessel-lation with orange-red appearance due to the thickened choroid along with RPE alterations. OCT imaging reveals scattered small RPE elevations secondary to RPE hyperpla-sia or sub RPE drusen like deposits. Larger choroidal vessels in outer Haller's layer approximate the Bruch's membrane directly with absence of the underlying Sattler's layer. ICGA reveals mid-phase hyperfluorescence corresponding to choroidal hyperpermeability.[58] PNV may follow PPE or CSC

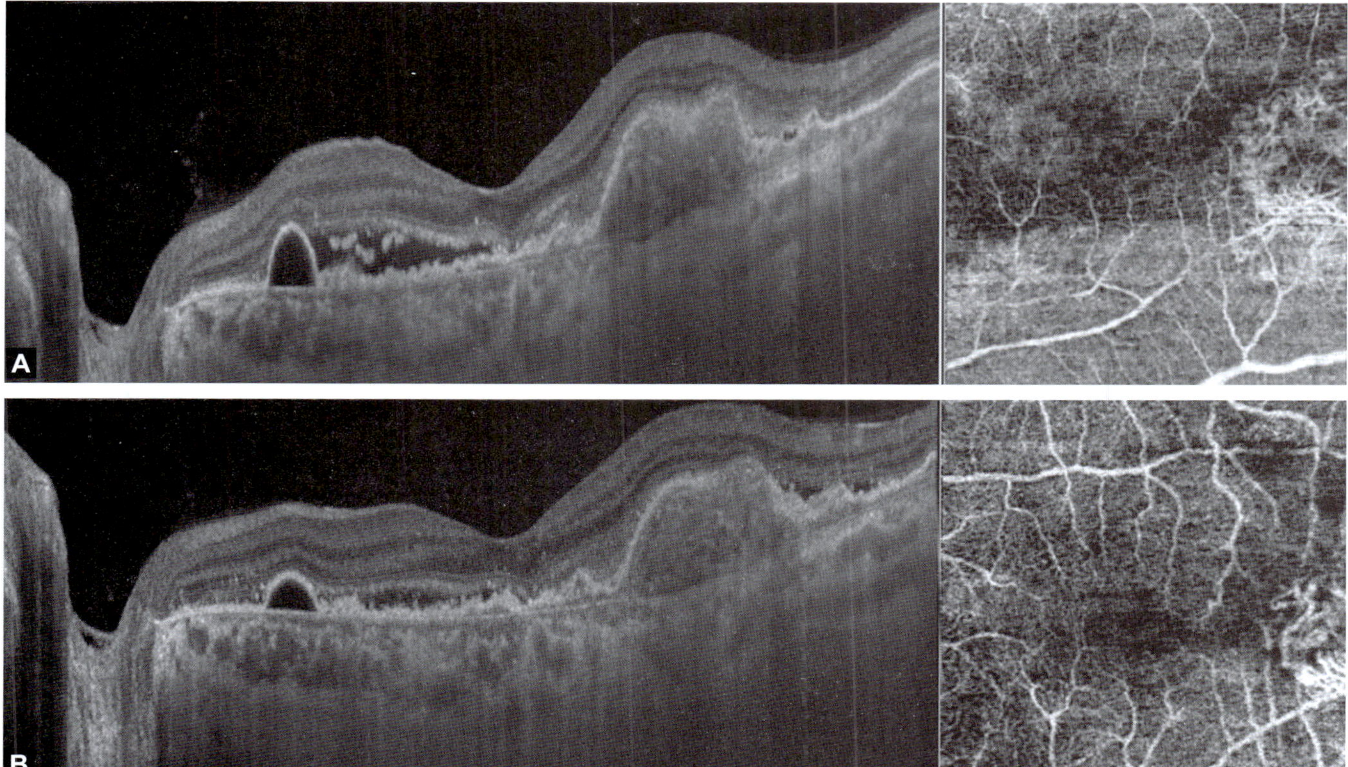

Figs. 11.24A and B: (A) Swept-source optical coherence tomography (OCT) of an eye shows thumb-like polyp with subretinal fluid (SRF) before aflibercept monotherapy and whorl like new subretinal pigment epithelium (RPE) and subretinal new vessels on OCTA; (B) Same eye reveals regression of polyp height with absence of SRF on OCT while OCT-A showing reduction of the neovascular lesion following intravitreal aflibercept monotherapy. Dilated choroidal vessels from Haller's layer appear to be present with associated choroidal thickening.

- Vision loss $\geq$ = 5 letters [Early Treatment Diabetic Retinopathy Study (ETDRS) chart]
- Subretinal or intraretinal fluid on optical coherence tomography (OCT)
- Pigment epithelial detachment on OCT
- Subretinal or sub RPE hemorrhage
- Fluorescein leakage

characterized by similar features along with the presence of type 1 choroidal neovascularization over an area of large choroidal thickening (Figs. 11.31A and B). Eventually PCV may develop within or at the margins of the slow-growing type 1 neovascular tissue.[58,59]

RETINAL ANGIOMATOUS PROLIFERATION (FIGS. 11.32 AND 11.33)

Retinal angiomatous proliferation (RAP) is a common variant of NVAMD characterized by formation of new vessels within the retinal tissue that can invade into the subretinal space or into the choroid, also known as type 3 neovascularization. The vasculogenesis may initiate from the retina, from the choroid, or simultaneously from both. RAP requires ICG angiography for definitive diagnosis. Incidence of the RAP variant among NVAMD cases appears to be approximately 5–10%, and it may be less common in Asians unlike PCV.

The pathophysiology of RAP is unknown but genotyping data shows an association among RAP, PCV and AMD.[13] High-speed ICG angiography best visualizes RAP lesions, particularly the retinal feeding arterioles and draining venules.

Staging of Retinal Angiomatous Proliferation

Clinically, stage 1 RAP lesions present with intraretinal neovascularization with telangiectatic retinal capillaries perfused by the retinal circulation. Stage 2 RAP lesions extend into the subretinal space to form subretinal neovascularization associated with a serous PED. Most stage 2 RAP lesions are perfused by retinal arterioles and drained by retinal venules. In stage 3 RAP, it is presumed that a retinal-choroidal anastomosis (RCA) is formed. Untreated stage 3 RAP lesions lead to formation of large fibrotic scars.

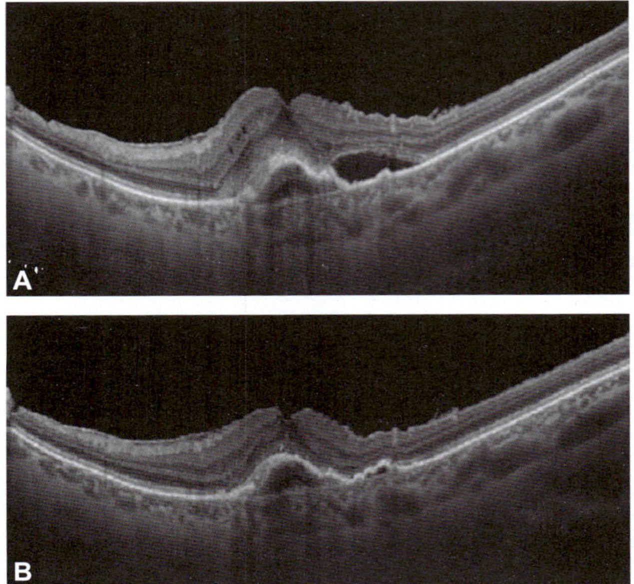

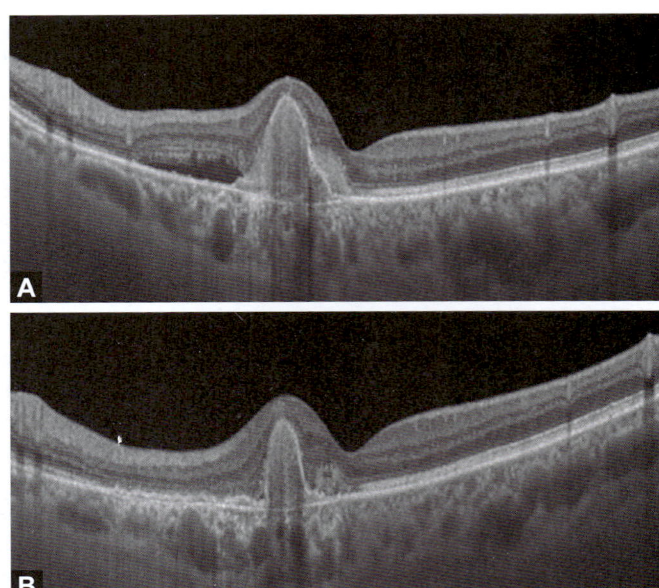

Figs. 11.25A and B: (A) Thumb shaped notched pigment epithelium detachment (PED) with subretinal fluid (SRF) at presentation. (B) The SRF resolved following combination therapy of photodynamic therapy (PDT) and three doses of intravitreal ranibizumab.

Fig. 11.26: Pre and postaflibercept intravitreal injection (2.0 mg) shows resolution of subretinal fluid with persisting thumb like pigment epithelium detachment (PED).

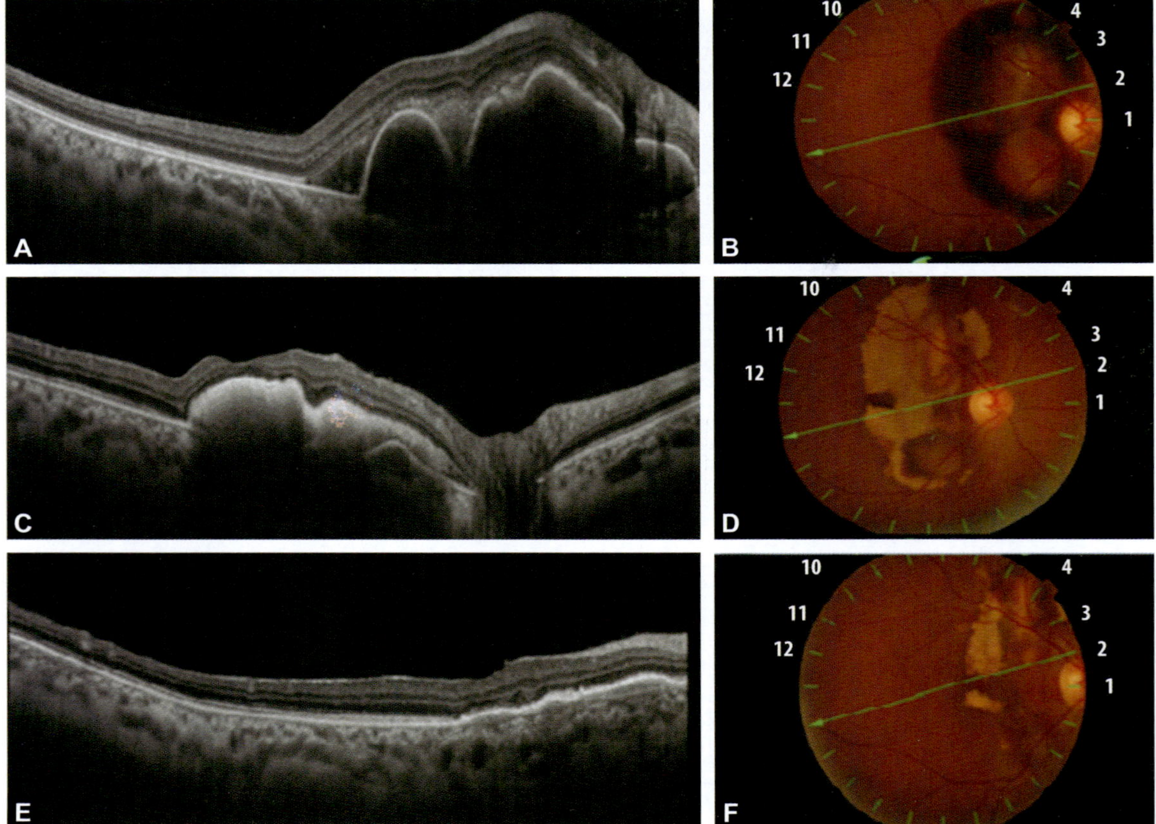

Figs. 11.27A to F: Rapid resolution of hemorrhagic pigment epithelium detachment (PED) and submacular hemorrhage following three doses of intravitreal aflibercept at monthly interval (Loading dose).

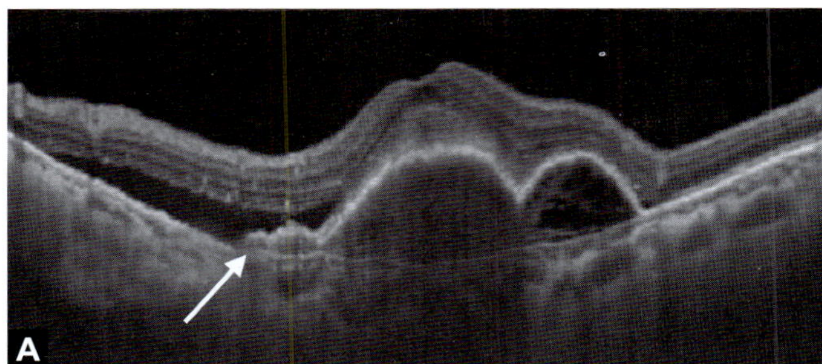

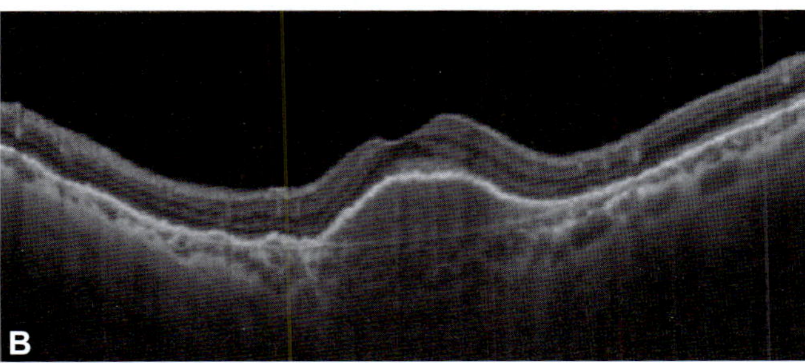

Figs. 11.28A and B: Reduction in serous pigment epithelium detachment (PED), subretinal fluid and double layer sign (arrow) following reduced fluence photodynamic therapy (PDT) and intravitreal aflibercept.

Table 11.3: Initial treatment.

Extrafoveal polypoidal choroidal vasculopathy (PCV)	Photocoagulation, photodynamic therapy (PDT)
Subfoveal, juxtafoveal PCV	Indocyanine-green angiography (ICGA) guided full fluence (FF) or reduced fluence (RF) verteporfin (v) PDT or combination of FF/RF PDT with 3 x 0.5 mg ranibizumab intravitreal injections at monthly intervals.

Table 11.4: Retreatment.

Incomplete regression of polyps [Assessed by indocyanine-green angiography (ICGA)]	Retreat with photodynamic therapy (PDT) monotherapy or combination therapy
Complete regression of polyps but leakage of fluorescein angiography (FA) with clinical or optical coherence tomography (OCT) signs of activity	Retreat with anti-vascular endothelial growth factor (VEGF)

Table 11.5: Conclusions of significant trials.[53,57]

Everest	*Purpose:* To assess the effects of verteporfin photodynamic therapy (vPDT) combined with ranibizumab or alone vs ranibizumab alone in patients with symptomatic macular polypoidal choroidal vasculopathy (PCV)
	 Study: Randomized controlled trial conducted in 61 Asian patients
	 Result:
	 • At month 6:
	   – Polyp regression rate in 3 groups
	     - v-PDT plus Rb: 77.8%
	     - PDT alone: 71.4%
	     - Rb alone: 28.6%
	 Conclusion: v-PDT combined with Ranibizumab or vPDT alone is superior to Ranibizumab monotherapy in achieving complete regression of polyps

Laptop	*Purpose:* To compare the effect of PDT and intravitreal Ranibizumab in patients with PCV *Study:* Randomized multicenter trial conducted in 93 patients *Result:* PDT arm—Improvement in central retinal thickness (CRT) but no change in visual acuity (VA) Ranibizumab arm: Improvement in CRT and VA *Conclusion:* Intravitreal Ranibizumab is more effective than PDT in obtaining better visual outcomes
Planet (ongoing)	*Purpose:* To evaluate the efficacy, safety, and tolerability of intravitreal aflibercept injection (IAI) monotherapy compared with IAI plus PDT in patients with PCV. *Study:* Randomized multicenter trial conducted in 333 patients *Result:* 1 year results have revealed the IAI monotherapy is effective treatment with no need of rescue therapy in more than 85% patients. 80% of patients had no signs of polyp activity at week 52 *Conclusion:* IAI monotherapy was noninferior to IAI plus active PDT

- Monthly examination including visual acuity, fundus biomicroscopy, optical coherence tomography (OCT) and 3-4 monthly fluorescein angiography (FA)/indocyanine green angiography (ICGA) for the first 6 months.

Hence RAP is included as type 3 neovascular AMD in which retinal vessels are responsible to form the CNV. RAP presents similar to other types of nAMD. Multiple hemorrhages are more common and are superficial. OCT helps in differentiating it from other types of neovascular AMD where typically a hyper-reflective area in all layers of retina is seen to

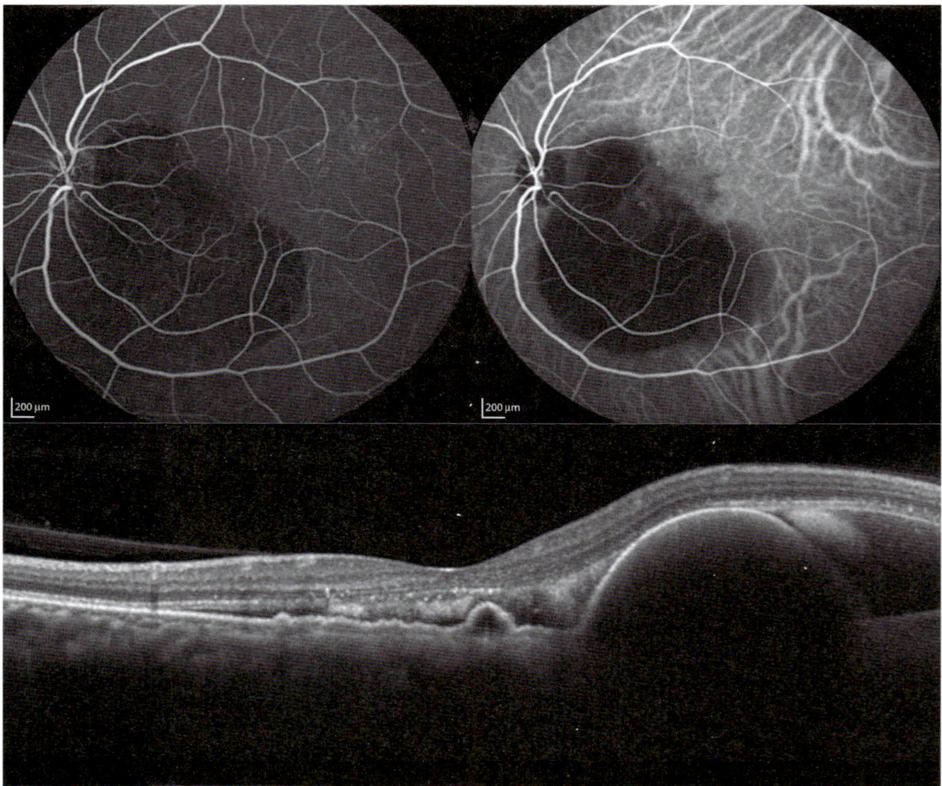

Fig. 11.29: Case of polypoidal choroidal vasculopathy (PCV) with an extensive submacular and retinal pigment epithelial detachment (RPED), bleed and polyps are visible on ICGA frame.

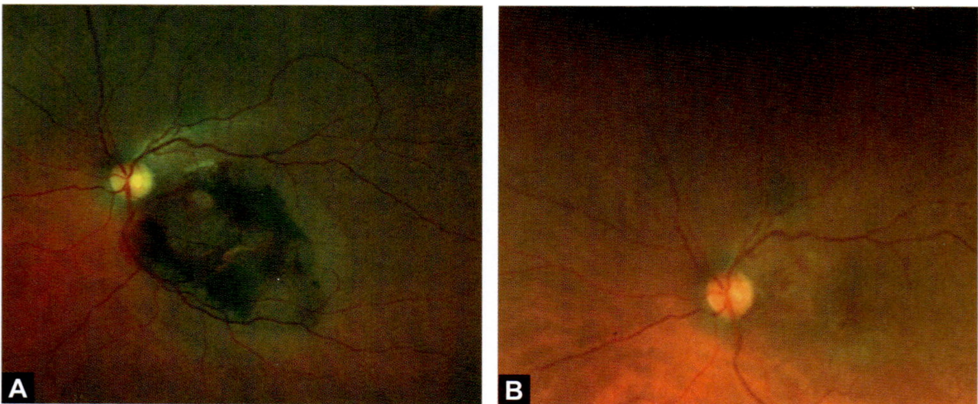

Figs. 11.30A and B: (A) Combined-intraretinal and subretinal pigment epithelium (RPE) blood seen (B) Post subretinal injection of 50 u tissue plasminogen activator (tPA) + 0.1 cc avastin + 0.4 cc air reveals significant displacement of hemorrhage.

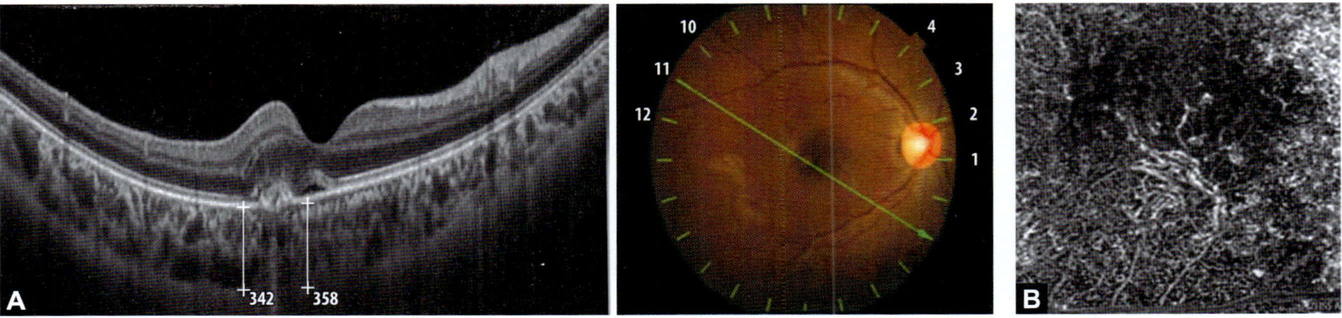

Figs. 11.31A and B: (A) Pachychoroid neovasculopathy with retinal pigment epithelium (RPE) disturbances on clinical picture, choroidal neovascularization (CNV) growing into subretinal space and thickened choroid on swept-source optical coherence tomography (SS-OCT). (B) OCT-A also reveals a type I neovascular membrane.

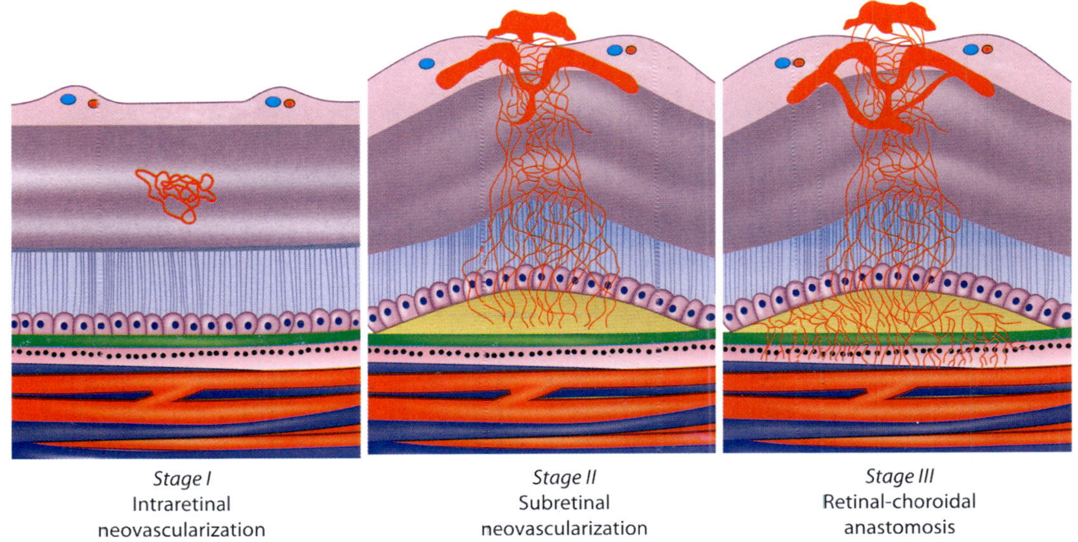

Fig. 11.32: Stages of retinal angiomatous proliferation.

form CNV, in the region of RAP. It is seen as a hyperfluorescent area on ICG. Mainstay of therapy is the anti-VEGFs. Reduced fluence PDT has been tried in nonresponsive cases.[60-63]

Treatment for Retinal Angiomatous Proliferation

Retinal angiomatous proliferation lesions appear exquisitely sensitive to anti-VEGF therapy.[64-67] Since RAP lesions respond well to anti-VEGF therapy, this suggests that the underlying pathophysiology is strongly VEGF-mediated. Identification of the cellular source of VEGF in RAP (i.e. retinal, RPE, or choroid) to explain the origin of new vessel growth in the retina as differentiated from the choroidal origin in typical CNV remains speculative. Focal thermal laser therapy to the afferent arteriole has demonstrated short-term resolution of retinal edema, however with associated combination of PDT or intravitreal triamcinolone acetonide.[68]

It has been observed that unilateral RAP development essentially always predisposes to development of RAP lesions in the fellow eye, hence the importance of retinal screening of the fellow eye. Advanced forms of the disease involving a vascularized RPE detachment and RCA are unlikely to respond well to any form of current treatment.

PERIPHERAL EXUDATIVE HEMORRHAGIC CHORIORETINOPATHY

Peripheral exudative hemorrhagic chorioretinopathy (PEHCR) is a bilateral, degenerative disorder of the peripheral retina and choroid in which there are areas of subretinal pigment epithelial (RPE) hemorrhage and exudation.[64] The underlying disease is considered to be similar to polypoidal choroidal vasculopathy (PCV)[65,66] except that it is occurring at a peripheral location. It is so often confused with choroidal melanoma that it is sometimes called "pseudomelanoma."[65,67] It is seen in elderly caucasian females. Age, hypertension and use of anti-platelet and anticoagulants are considered risk factors for the development of PEHCR.

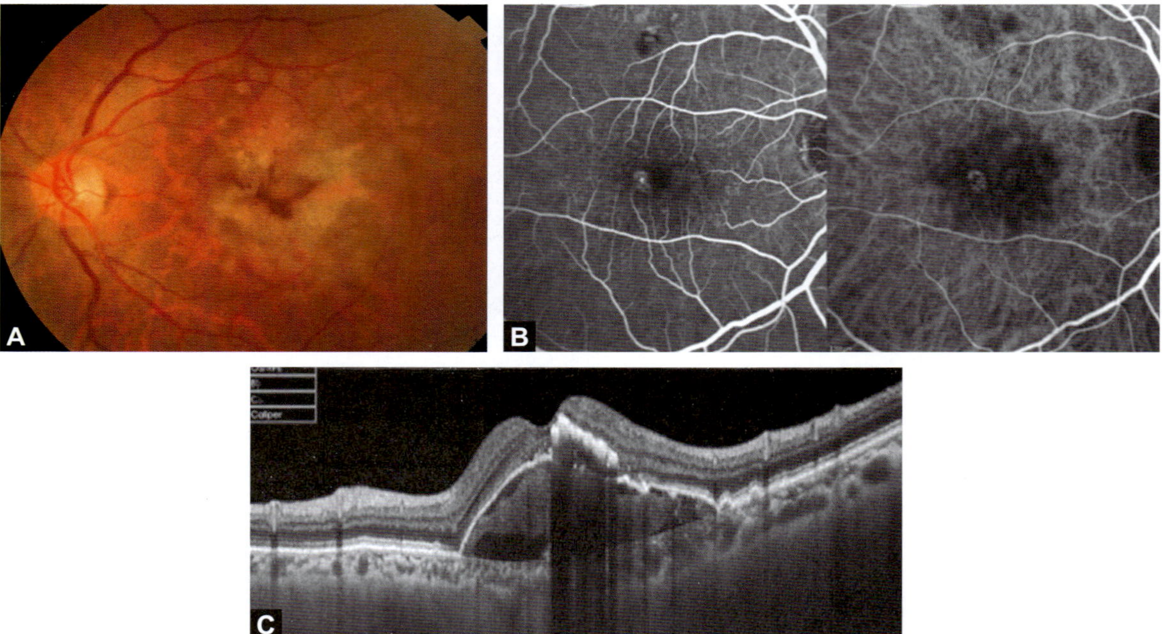

Figs. 11.33A to C: (A) Retinal angiomatous proliferation (RAP) stage IIB with pigment epithelium detachment (PED) showing pre and intraretinal hemorrhages, (B) intraretinal neovascularization on fluorescein angiography (FA)/indocyanine green (ICGA) angiography and (C) Neovascularisation (NV) growing into subretinal pigment epithelium (RPE) space on swept-source optical coherence tomography (SS-OCT).

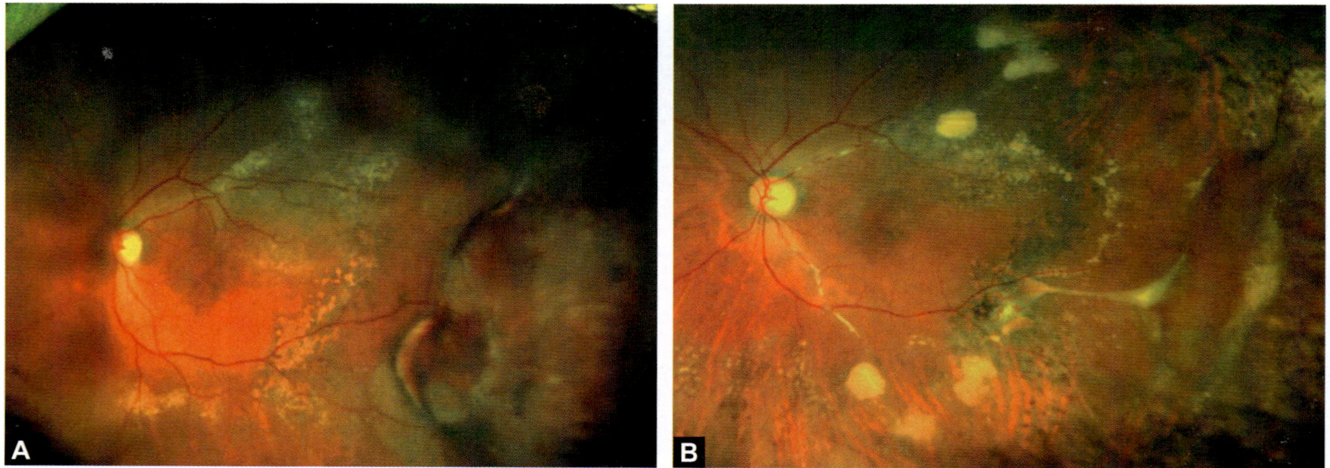

Figs. 11.34A and B: Peripheral exudative hemorrhagic chorioretinopathy (PEHCR) is a peripheral variant of age-related macular degeneration (AMD)/polypoidal choroidal vasculopathy (PCV) and simulates choroidal melanoma. Reticular pseudodrusen are also visible. Post laser and anti-vascular endothelial growth factor (VEGF) injection shows resolution of the lesion.

Often patients are asymptomatic and are only discovered to have this disease on routine fundus screening. But it can lead to visual symptoms and rarely even irreversible blindness. Patients usually present with peripheral subretinal hemorrhage, serous or hemorrhagic RPE detachments, subretinal fluid or lipid exudation and exudative retinal detachment (Figs. 11.34A and B). The large mounds of subretinal and sub-RPE blood can be mistaken for a choroidal melanoma. There are peripheral pigmentary abnormalities, drusen or chorioretinal atrophic patches seen around the lesion. These lesions are mostly located in the temporal periphery and can be variable in size. When there is a breakthrough bleed into the vitreous cavity from these lesions patients present with sudden onset loss of vision. When a lesion in the midperiphery involves the macula either due to exudation or hemorrhage, central visual acuity can be compromised. Not uncommonly, a PEHCR can have a central PCV or an age-related macular degeneration lesion which can cause central vision

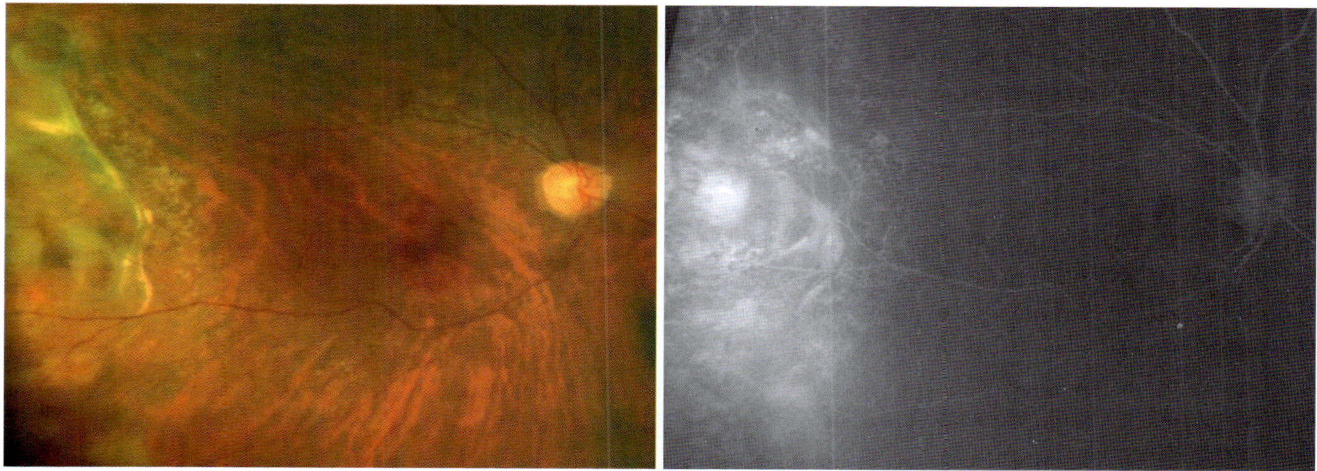

Fig. 11.35: Case of peripheral exudative hemorrhagic chorioretinopathy (PEHCR) with elevated exudative lesion in temporal periphery which reveals dye leakage on FA.

loss and be the primary symptom of patients.[67] Findings in the contralateral eye can range from pigmentary abnormalities or drusen to disciform scarring and is seen in a few series in up to 70% of the patients.[67]

Features that help in differentiating a PEHCR from a choroidal melanoma are surrounding retinal and subretinal exudation, central and peripheral RPE pigmentary changes, blocked fluorescence on fluorescein angiography (Fig. 11.35), lack of intrinsic vascular pulsations and lack of sentinel vessels on slit-lamp biomicroscopy.[67]

Treatment depends on the status of the macular retina. In isolated peripheral lesions without a central PCV or a neo-vascular AMD, observation is a prudent choice. Shields has noted stability or regression of lesion in 89% of the cases.[67] Even in progressive lesions, treatment can be withheld until central vision is threatened. But treatment can be considered in one eyed patients or in patients who have already lost central field due to PCV or AMD. Cryopexy, laser photocoagulation and PDT are the available options

Antivascular endothelial growth factor injections are reported to be effective in reducing subretinal bleeding and exudation in cases of isolated PEHCR without macular exudative lesions or in patients with PEHCR and a concurrent PCV or a neovascular AMD in the macula.[68] We have observed encouraging results with use of anti-VEGFs in our PEHCR patients with flattening of the lesion and marked reduction of exudation.[69-73]

REFERENCES

1. Leibowitz HM, Krueger DE, Maunder LR. The Framingham Eye Study Monograph: An ophthalmological and epidemiological study of cataract, glaucoma, diabetic retinopathy, macular degeneration, and visual acuity in a general population of 2631 adults, 1973-1975. Surv Ophthalmology. 1980; 24(Suppl):335-610.

2. Klein R, Klein BE, Linton KL. Prevalence of age-related maculopathy: The Beaver Dam Eye Study. Ophthalmology. 1992;99(6):933-43

3. Klein R, Cruickshanks KJ, Nash SD, et al. The Prevalence of Age-Related Macular Degeneration and Associated Risk Factors. Arch Ophthalmology. 2010;128(6):750-8.

4. Yates JR, Sepp T, Matharu BK, et al. The Genetic Factors in AMD Study Group. Complement C3 variant and the risk of age-related macular degeneration. N. Engl J Med. 2007;357(6):553-61.

5. Hagman GS, Anderson DH, Johnson LV, et al. A common haplotype in the complement regulatory gene factor H (HF1/CFH) predisposes individuals to age-related macular degeneration. Proc Natl Acad Sci USA. 2005;102(20):7227-32

6. Haines JL, Hauser MA, Schmidt S, et al. Complement factor H variant increases the risk of age-related macular degeneration. Science. 2005;308:419-21.

7. Klein RJ, Zeiss C, Chew EY, et al. Complement factor H polymorphism in age-related macular degeneration. Science. 2005;308:385-9.

8. Edwards AO, Ritter R 3rd, Abel KJ, et al. Complement factor H polymorphism and age-related macular degeneration. Science. 2005;308:421-4.

9. Stone EM, Braun TA, Russell SR, et al. Missense variations in the fibulin 5 gene and age-related macular degeneration. N Engl J Med. 2004;351(4):346-53.

10. Zarbin MA. Current concepts in the pathogenesis of age-related macular degeneration. Arch Ophthalmology. 2004;122(4):598-614.

11. Guymer R, Bird AC. Age Changes in Bruch's Membrane and Related Structures. In: Schahcat AP, Ryan SJ (Eds). Retina, 4th Edition. Elsevier Mosby; 2006.

12. Jager RD, Mieler WF, Miller JW. Age-Related Macular Degeneration. N Engl J Med. 2008;358(24):2606-17.

13. Crabb JW, Miyagi M, Gu X, et al. Drusen proteome analysis: an approach to the etiology of age-related macular degeneration. Proc Natl Acad Sci USA. 2002;99(23):3842-7.

14. Bressler NM, Bressler SB, West SK, et al. The Grading and Prevalence of Macular Degeneration in Chesapeake Bay Waterman. Archives of Ophthalmology. 1989;107(6):847-52.

15. Green WR. Ophthalmic Pathology. Retina. WB Saunders Company; 1996. pp. 982-1047.

16. Zarbin MA, Rosenfeld FJ. Pathway-based therapies for age-related macular degeneration. Retina. 2010;30(9):1350-67.

17. Leibowitz HM, Krueger DE, Maunder LR, et al. The Framingham Eye Study monograph: An ophthalmological and epidemiological study of cataract, glaucoma, diabetic retinopathy, macular degeneration, and visual acuity in a general population of 2631 adults, 1973-1975. Surv Ophthalmology. 1980;24(Suppl):335-610.

18. Clemons TE, Milton RC, Klein R, et al. Risk factors for the incidence of advanced age-related macular degeneration in the Age-Related Eye Disease Study (AREDS): AREDS report no. 19. Ophthalmology. 2005;112(4):533-9.

19. Khan JC, Thurlby DA, Shahid H, et al. Smoking and age-related macular degeneration: the number of pack years of cigarete smoking is a major determinant of risk for both geographic atrophy and choroidal neovascularization. Br J Ophthalmology. 2006; 90(1):75-80.

20. Evans JR, Fletcher AE, Wormald RP. 28,000 Cases of age related macular degeneration causing visual loss in people aged 75 years and above in the United Kingdom may be attributable to smoking. Br J Ophthalmology. 2005;89(5):550-3.

21. Smailhodzic D, Muether PS, Chen J, et al. Cumulative Effect of Risk Alleles in CFH, ARMS2, and VEGFA on the Response to Ranibizumab Treatment in Age-Related Macular Degeneration. Ophthalmology (in press) 2012; p 1-8.

22. Sandberg MA, Tolentino Mj, Miller S, et al. Hyperopia and neovascularization in age-related macular degeneration. Ophthalmology. 1993;100(7):1009-13.

23. Guymer R, Bird AC. Age Changes in Bruch's Membrane and Related Structures. In: Schahcat AP, Ryan SJ (Eds). Retina, 4th Edition. Elsevier, Mosby; 2006.

24. Coleman HR, Chan CC, Ferris FL 3rd, et al. Age-related macular degeneration. 2008. Lancet. 2008;372(9652):1835-45.

25. Gupta OP, Brown GC, Brown MM. Age-related macular degeneration: the costs to society and the patient. Curr Opin Ophthalmology. 2007;18(3):201-5

26. Bressler SB, Do DV, Bressler NM. Age-related macular degeneration: drusen and geographic atrophy. In: Albert DM, Miller JW, Azar DT, et al. (Eds). Albert and Jakobiec's Principles and Practice of Ophthalmology. 3rd edition. Philadelphia: Saunders; 2008.

27. Lim LS, Mitchell P, Seddon JM, et al. Age-related macular degeneration. Lancet. 2012;379(9827):1728-38.

28. Bressler NM, Bressler SB, Fine SL. Neovascular (Neovascular) Age-Related Macular Degeneration. In: Schachat A (Ed). Retina, 4th Edition. Elsevier, Mosby; 2006.

29. Huang D, Swanson EA, Lin CP, et al. Optical coherence tomography. Science. 1991;254(5035):1178-81.

30. Yannuzzi LA, Wong DW, Sforzolini BS, et al. Polypoidal choroidal vasculopathy and neovascularized age-related macular degeneration. Arch Ophthalmology. 1999;117(11):1503-10.

31. Kuehlewein L, Bansal M, Lenis TL, et al. Optical Coherence Tomography Angiography of Type 1 Neovascularization in Age-Related Macular Degeneration. Am J Ophthalmology. 2015; 160(4):739-48.e2.

32. Benhamou N, Souied EH, Zolf R, et al. Adult-onset foveomacular vitelliform dystrophy: a study by opticalcoherence tomography. Am J Ophthalmology. 2003;135(3):362-7.

33. Burgess DB, Olk RJ, Uniat LM. Macular disease resembling adult foveomacular vitelliform dystrophy in older adults. Ophthalmology 1987;94(4):362-6.

34. Puche N, Querques G, Benhamou N, et al. High-resolution spectral domain optical coherence tomographyfeatures in adult onset foveomacular vitelliform dystrophy. Br J Ophthalmology. 2010;94(9):1190-6

35. Bressler NM, Bressler SB, Sarks SH, et al. Age-Related Macular Degeneration: Nonneovascular Early AMD, Intermediate AMD, and Geographic Atrophy. In: Schahcat AP, Ryan SJ (Eds). Retina, 4th edition. Elsevier Mosby;2006.

36. Macular Photocoagulation Study Group. Argon laser photocoagulation for senile macular degeneration. Results of a randomized clinical trial. Arch Ophthalmology. 1982;100(6):912-8.

37. Macular Photocoagulation Study Group. Argon laser photocoagulation for senile macular degeneration. Three-year results from randomized clinical trial. Arch Ophthalmology. 1986; 104(5):694-701.

38. Petrarca R, Dugel PU, Bennett M, et al. Macular epiretinal brachytherapy in treated age-related macular degeneration (MERITAGE): month 24 safety and efficacy results. Retina. 2014; 34(5):874-9.

39. Jaffe GJ, Eliott D, Wells JA, et al. A Phase 1 Study of Intravitreous E10030 in Combination with Ranibizumab in Neovascular Age-Related Macular Degeneration. Ophthalmology. 2016;123(1):78-85.

40. Bressler NM, Bressler SB, Childs AL, et al. Submacular Surgery Trials (SST) Research Group. Surgery for hemorrhagic choroidal neovascular lesions of age-related macular degeneration: ophthalmic findings: SST report. Ophthalmology. 2004;111(11): 1993-2006.

41. Haupert CL, McCuen BW 2nd, Jaffe GJ, et al. Pars plana vitrectomy, subretinal injection of tissue plasminogen activator, and fluid-gas exchange for displacement of thick submacular hemorrhage in age-related macular degeneration. Am J Ophthalmology. 2001;131(2):208-15.

42. Kumar A, Roy S, Bansal M, et al. A Modified Approach in Management of Submacular Hemorrhage Secondary to Wet Age-Related Macular Degeneration Asia-Pacific Journal of Ophthalmology. 2016;5(2):143-6.

43. Yannuzzi LA, Ciardella A, Spaide RF, et al. The expanding clinical spectrum of idiopathic polypoidal choroidal vasculopathy. Arch Ophthalmology. 1997;115(4):478-85.

44. Kleiner RC, Brucker AJ, Johnston RL. The posterior uveal bleeding syndrome. Retina. 1990;10(1):9-17.

45. Yannuzzi LA, Sorenson J, Spaide RF, et al. Idiopathic polypoidal choroidal vasculopathy (IPCV). Retina. 1990;10(1):1-8.

46. Byeon SH, Lee SC, Oh HS, et al. Incidence and clinical patterns of polypoidal choroidal vasculopathy in Korean patients. Jpn J Ophthalmology. 2008;52(1):57-62.

47. Ciardella AP, Donsoff IM, Yannuzzi LA. Polypoidal choroidal vasculopathy. Ophthalmology Clin North Am. 2002;15(4):537-54.

48. Lafaut BA, Leys AM, Snyers B, et al. Polypoidal choroidal vasculopathy in Caucasians. Graefes Arch Clin Exp Ophthalmology. 2000;238(9):752-9.

49. Ladas ID, Rouvas AA, Moschos MM, et al. Polypoidal choroidal vasculopathy and exudative age-related macular degeneration in Greek population. Eye (Lond). 2004;18(5):455-9.

50. Scassellati-Sforzolini B, Mariotti C, Bryan R, et al. Polypoidal choroidal vasculopathy in Italy. Retina. 2001;21:121-5.

51. Nakashizuka H, Mitsumata M, Okisaka S, et al. Clinicopathologic findings in polypoidal choroidal vasculopathy. Invest Ophthalmology Vis Sci. 2008;49(11):4729-37.

52. Koh AH, Chen LJ, Chen SJ, et al. Polypoidal choroidal vasculopathy: evidence-based guidelines for clinical diagnosis and treatment. Retina. 2013;33(4):686-716.

53. Koh A, Lee WK, Chen LJ, et al. EVEREST study: efficacy and safety of verteporfin photodynamic therapy in combination with ranibizumab or alone versus ranibizumab monotherapy in patients with symptomatic macular polypoidal choroidal vasculopathy. Retina. 2012;32(8):1453-64.

54. Sato T, Kishi S, Watanabe G, et al. Tomographic features of branching vascular networks in polypoidal choroidal vasculopathy. Retina. 2007;27(5):589-94.

55. Tsujikawa A, Sasahara M, Otani A, et al. Pigment epithelial detachment in polypoidal choroidal vasculopathy. Am J Ophthalmology. 2007;143(1):102-11.

56. Wang M, Zhou Y, Gao SS, et al. Evaluating Polypoidal Choroidal Vasculopathy With Optical Coherence Tomography Angiography OCT Angiography in Polypoidal Choroidal Vasculopathy. Invest Ophthalmology Vis Sci. 2016;57(9):526-32.

57. Oishi A, Kojima E, Mandai M, et al. Comparison of the effect of ranibizumab and verteporfin for polypoidal choroidal vasculopathy: 12-month LAPTOP study results. Am J Ophthalmology. 2013;156(4):644-51.

58. Lehmann M, Bousquet E, Beydoun T, et al. Pachychoroid: an inherited condition?. Retina. 2015;35(1):10-6.

59. Gallego-Pinazo R, Dolz-Marco R, Gómez-Ulla F, et al. Pachychoroid diseases of the macula. Med Hypothesis Discov Innov Ophthalmology. 2014;3(4):111-5.

60. Freund KB, Ho IV, Barbazetto IA, et al. Type 3 neovascularization: the expanded spectrum of retinal angiomatous proliferation. Retina. 2008;28(2):201-11.

61. Yannuzzi LA, Negrão S, Iida T, et al. Retinal angiomatous proliferation in age-related macular degeneration. Retina. 2001; 21(5):416-34.

62. Rouvas AA, Papakostas TD, Ntouraki A, et al. Angiographic and OCT features of retinal angiomatous proliferation. Eye (Lond). 2010;24(11):1633-43.

63. Scott AW, Bressler SB. Retinal angiomatous proliferation or retinal anastomosis to the lesion. Eye (Lond). 2010;24(3):491-6.

64. Meyerle CB, Freund KB, Iturralde D, et al. Intravitreal bevacizumab (Avastin) for retinal angiomatous proliferation. Retina. 2007;27(4):451-7.

65. Bearelly S, Espinosa-Heidmann DG, Cousins SW. The role of dynamic indocyanine green angiography in the diagnosis and treatment of retinal angiomatous proliferation. Br J Ophthalmology. 2008;92(2):191-6.

66. Engelbert M, Zweifel SA, Freund KB. "Treat and extend" dosing of intravitreal antivascular endothelial growth factor therapy for type 3 neovascularization/retinal angiomatous proliferation. Retina. 2009;29(10):1424-31.

67. Hemeida TS, Keane PA, Dustin L, et al. Long-term visual and anatomical outcomes following anti-VEGF monotherapy for retinal angiomatous proliferation. Br J Ophthalmology. 2010;94(6):701-5.

68. Saito M, Shiragami C, Shiraga F, et al. Comparison of intravitreal triamcinolone acetonide with photodynamic therapy and intravitreal bevacizumab with photodynamic therapy for retinal angiomatous proliferation. Am J Ophthalmology. 2010;149(3):472-81. e1.

69. Reese AB, Jones IS. Hematomas Under the Retinal Pigment Epithelium. Trans Am Ophthalmology Soc. 1961;59:43-79.

70. Goldman DR, Freund KB, McCannel CA, et al. Peripheral polypoidal choroidal vasculopathy as a cause of peripheral exudative hemorrhagic chorioretinopathy: a report of 10 eyes. Retina Phila Pa. 2013;33(1):48-55.

71. Mashayekhi A, Shields CL, Shields JA. Peripheral Exudative Hemorrhagic Chorioretinopathy: A Variant of Polypoidal Choroidal Vasculopathy? J Ophthalmic Vis Res. 2013;8(3):264-7.

72. Shields CL, Salazar PF, Mashayekhi A, et al. Peripheral exudative hemorrhagic chorioretinopathy simulating choroidal melanoma in 173 eyes. Ophthalmology. 2009;116(3):529-35.

73. Takayama K, Enoki T, Kojima T, et al. Treatment of peripheral exudative hemorrhagic chorioretinopathy by intravitreal injections of ranibizumab. Clin Ophthalmology. 2012;6:865-9.

Chapter 12

Choroidal Neovascular Membranes

Pranita Sahay, Shilky Singh, Anand S Brar, Atul Kumar

INTRODUCTION

Choroidal neovascular membrane (CNVM) is character-ized by extension of the choriocapillaris through the Bruch's membrane into subretinal pigment epithelium space (type 1 CNVM) or subretinal space (type 2 CNVM). Recently type 3 CNVM has been recognized as a predominantly intrareti-nal neovascularization which later extend beneath the retina without a preceding type 1 CNVM.[1] The origin of type 3 CNVM has been proposed to be from deep retinal capillary plexus which develops early retinochoroidal anastomosis (RCA) or from the choriocapillaris.[2] CNVM can occur in various disor-ders that compromise the Bruch's membrane and/or retinal pigment epithelium (RPE) function (Table 12.1). CNV in the macular area results in severe vision loss if left untreated.

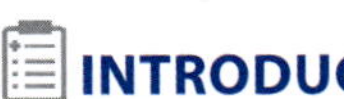

PATHOPHYSIOLOGY

The two basic prerequisites for the formation of CNVM are proliferation of the choriocapillaris and compromised Bruch's membrane and/or RPE function.

Proliferation of the Choriocapillaris

The capillary endothelial cells proliferate from preexisting choriocapillaris due to the imbalance between the angio-genic growth factors [vascular endothelial growth factor[3], (VEGF); platelet-derived growth factor β (PDGF β); trans-forming growth factor α, (TGF α); erythropoietin (EPO); beta fibroblast growth factor (bFGF); and fibroblast growth fac-tor-2 (FGF-2)] and anti-angiogenic growth factors (Pigment epithelium-derived factor (PEDF) and thrombospondin 1).[4-9] Oxidative stress (reactive oxygen species, ROS), complement dysregulation and inflammatory mediators (interleukin IL-1β and tumor necrosis factor, TNF-α) have also been implicated in this process. These proliferating cells align themselves to form new capillary sprouts which later develop into tubes with lumen. Recently hematopoietic stem cells have also been implicated in the development of choroidal neovascu-larization.[10]

Table 12.1: Conditions associated with choroidal neovas-cularization

Degenerative	Age-related macular degenera-tion Myopic degeneration Angioid streaks
Heredodegenerative	Vitelliform macular dystrophy Fundus flavimaculatus Optic nerve head drusen
Inflammatory	Punctate inner choroiditis (PIC) Multifocal choroiditis and panu-veitis (MCP) Serpiginous choroiditis Birdshot chorioretinopathy Vogt-Koyanagi-Harada syndrome Behcet's syndrome Sympathetic ophthalmia
Infectious	Ocular histoplasmosis syndrome (OHS) Toxoplasmosis Toxocariasis Rubella
Tumor	Choroidal nevus Choroidal hemangioma Metastatic choroidal tumors Hamartoma of the retinal pig-ment epithelium
Traumatic	Choroidal rupture Intense photocoagulation
Idiopathic	

Compromised Bruch's Membrane and Retinal Pigment Epithelium Function

Compromise of the Bruch's membrane and RPE is essential for the progression of choroidal neovascularization. Bruch's membrane disruption occurs when the balance between proteolytic enzymes such as matrix metalloproteinases (MMPs) and their inhibitors, the tissue inhibitors of metalloproteinases (TIMPs) tilts towards a proteolytic environment. RPE cells express MMP-1 (collagenase), MMP-3 (stromelysin) MMP-9 (gelatinase) as well as TIMP-1, TIMP-2 and TIMP-3. Macrophages may also produce MMPs causing focal disruption of Bruch's membrane creating passage for entry of activated choroidal endothelial cells to the sub-RPE space. This ultimately leads to destruction of the normal architecture of the photoreceptors and outer retinal layers and results in a disciform scar.

 CLINICAL FEATURES

Symptoms

Patients usually complain of acute/subacute painless blurring of vision with metamorphopsia (especially for near).[11,12] Patient may also complain of scotoma and diminution of vision. Often no symptoms or only vague visual complaints may be present.[13]

Signs

Visual acuity, although frequently decreased, may not always be affected. Stereoscopic slit-lamp biomicroscopy using either plus 90 or 78 D lens or a corneal contact lens is essential to evaluate the subtle clinical findings of CNV. It appears as a gray–green elevation of tissue deep to the retina (due to hypertrophic RPE in response to the CNV). It may be associated with intraretinal and subretinal lipid deposition, subretinal fluid, subretinal and sub-RPE hemorrhage, cystoid macular edema, detachment of neurosensory retina and pigment epithelium detachment (serous, fibrovascular, drusenoid or hemorrhagic pigment epithelium detachments). Seafan pattern of subretinal small vessel may be visible. Retinal and subretinal cicatrisation (disciform scar) ultimately develops in treated and evolved lesions.

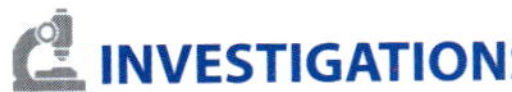 INVESTIGATIONS

Fluorescein Angiography

Indications of Fluorescein Angiography

- Diagnosis of choroid neovascularization prior to commencing treatment.
- When an alternative diagnosis to wet AMD (Polypoidal choroidal vasculopathy, PCV or retinal angiomatous proliferation, RAP) is suspected.
- To guide treatment with photodynamic therapy (PDT)
- Though previously it was used for monitoring as well, it is now done with the help of OCT.

The macular photocoagulation study gave the terminology that is used to describe the FA patterns of choroid neovascularization.[14] It has been classified as follows:

Classic Choroid Neovascularization

It appears as a discrete, well-demarcated focal area of hyperfluorescence (lacy pattern) in the early phases of the angiogram. It increases in intensity and extends beyond the boundaries of the hyper fluorescent area identified in earlier phases of the angiogram through mid- and late-phase frame. The fluorescence fades after several minutes.[14] It can be subfoveal, juxtafoveal (<200 μm from foveal avascular zone, FAZ) or extrafoveal (>200 μm from FAZ) in location.

Occult Choroid Neovascularization

Two hyper fluorescent patterns have been observed. The first pattern is termed fibrovascular pigment epithelial detachment (FVPED) which is best appreciated after 1–2 min of dye injection. It appears as stippled hyperfluorescent dots which may or may not show leakage in the late-phase. The second pattern is late leakage of an undetermined source in which there is no clearly identifiable classic CNV or FVPED in the early or mid-phase of the angiogram to account for an area of leakage in the late phase. It appear as speckled hyperfluorescence and the boundaries of this type of CNV cannot be determined precisely.[14]

Predominantly and Minimally Classic Choroid Neovascularization

It is based on the presence of classic component greater or less than 50% of the total lesion respectively.
- Indocyanine green angiography
  - The property of ICG being more protein-bound than sodium fluorescein and that it shows fluorescence in the near-infrared wavelength makes it more sensitive in the detection of CNV (especially in presence of hemorrhage, fluid or pigment). It can also delineate an occult CNV well. Three basic patterns of fluorescence have been observed in ICGA of CNV which are occult on FA.[15,16]
  - Small, focal *hot spot* (bright area of fluorescence > 1 disc area by the mid-phase of the angiogram)
  - A plaque (a well-demarcated area of fluorescence more than one disc area in size that emerges relatively late in the angiogram)
  - Ill-defined fluorescence
- Optical coherence tomography
  - It is mostly used for monitoring the response to treatment and sometimes as an aid in diagnosis of CNV. It typically appears as thickening and fragmentation of the RPE and choriocapillaris. Associated CMO, subretinal fluid, blood, scarring and outer retinal tubulations may be visible.
- Optical coherence tomography angiography
  It is a new enfaces OCT imaging that gives the vascular status of different layers of the retina, subretinal space and sub-RPE area and presence of any new vessels within them very clearly. It uses an optimized long wavelength

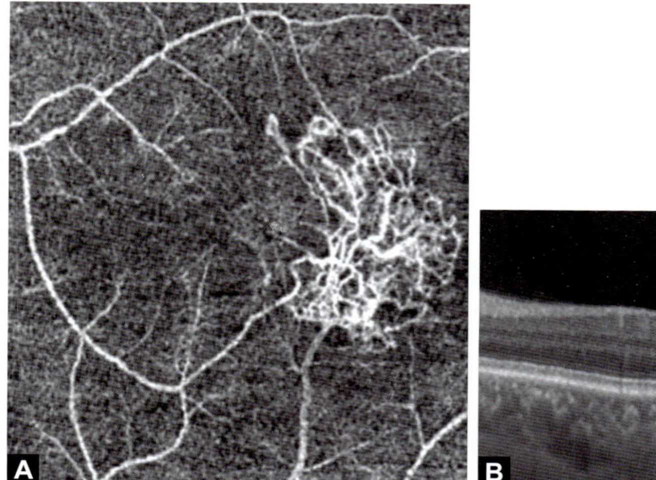
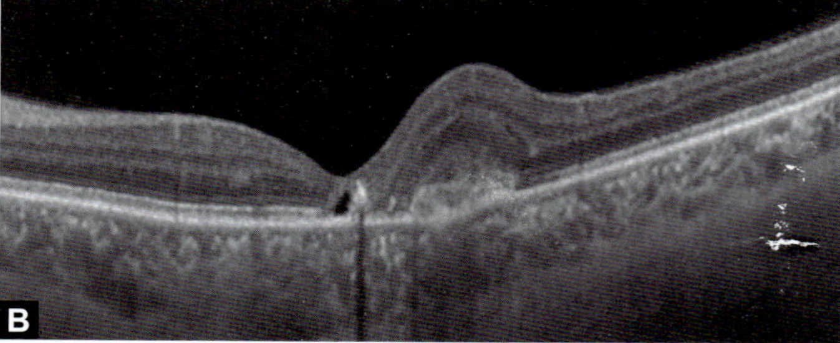

Figs. 12.1A and B: (A) Subretinal choroid neovascularization seen on optical coherence tomography angiography as an irregular hyper-reflective neovascular network, which is also seen in the same space on cross-sectional optical coherence tomography scan (B).

(1,050 nm), which achieves a better penetration of deeper layers of the eye and can pass through media opacities such as cataracts, hemorrhages, vitreous opacities, pigment, among others. It can also configure three-dimensional analysis of the chorioretinal and vascular lesions.

Type 1 choroid neovascularization is observed by OCT-A as a neovascular complex originating in the choroid and lying in the sub-RPE space. On higher resolution, CNV is visualized as an arborescent network of new vessels. Type 2 choroid neovascularization is present in the subretinal space primarily originating from there (Figs. 12.1A and B). Type 3 is identified as an intra- and subretinal bleeding correlated on OCT-A with an intraretinal neovascular network originating in the deep capillary plexus of the retina. OCTA enables imaging of the retinal and choroidal vascular structure by detecting the reflectance phase and amplitude variation of blood flow over time to distinguish vessels from static tissue. It has thus provided us with new insights to better understand and manage retinal and choroidal pathologies.

MYOPIC CHOROID NEOVASCULARIZATION

Myopic choroid neovascularization is one of the most common complication that results in reduced central vision in patients with pathologically myopia (Figs. 12.2 and 12.3). Contrary to the belief that myopic CNV occurs in eyes with pathological myopia only, it is now evident that it can occur in any degree of myopia and even in eyes without typical myopic degenerative fundus changes.[17,18] Lacquer cracks are thought to be the predisposing lesion. Myopic CNV develops in 10% of high myopes and 30% of these patients who have a CNV in one eye eventually develop CNV in the other eye.[19] As the retina is thin and stretched bleeding usually does not overlie the CNV and thus, CNV is easily observed on fundus evaluation and OCT as shown in Figures 12.2A and B. FA is used for

its diagnosis. Myopic CNV are mostly classic CNV with well-defined hyperfluorescence in the early phases and leakage of fluorescein dye during the late phases.[20,21] There are three stages of myopic CNV. In the initial phase, there is direct damage to the photoreceptors, causing central visual loss. Then, as the CNV regresses, a fibrous pigmented scar forms, referred to as Forster–Fuchs' retinal spot. Finally, atrophy develops around the regressed CNV, which results in poor long-term visual outcome.[22] Intravitreal anti-VEGF therapy remains the mainstay of treatment. Prior to the anti-VEGF era and laser photocoagulation, verteporfin photodynamic therapy (PDT) and surgical excision or macular translocation used to be performed to treat CNV.

Intravitreal anti-VEGF

Currently, Ranibizumab is the only Food and Drug Administration (FDA) approved drug for myopic CNV. REPAIR and RADIANCE study showed its efficacy and safety in this condition.[23,24] The pro Re Nata (PRN) dosing of Ranibizumab was found to be superior to PDT in RADIANCE study.[23] MYRROR study for Aflibercept in myopic CNV in Asian population has found it to be safe and effective. Bevacizumab is also used but its intraocular use is not FDA approved.

- Laser photocoagulation was used widely to treat extrafoveal myopic CNV prior to the anti-VEGF era. It has been found that laser causes retinal tissue damage with atrophy. Long-term visual acuity maintenance is a concern and a high rate of recurrence is seen.[25]
- Photodynamic therapy: It is approved for the treatment of subfoveal myopic CNV. The Verteporfin Photodynamic Therapy (VIP trial) showed that visual acuity stabilized although did not improve.[26] The most important limitation of PDT is long-term chorioretinal atrophy which may develop in some patients, contributing to vision loss.

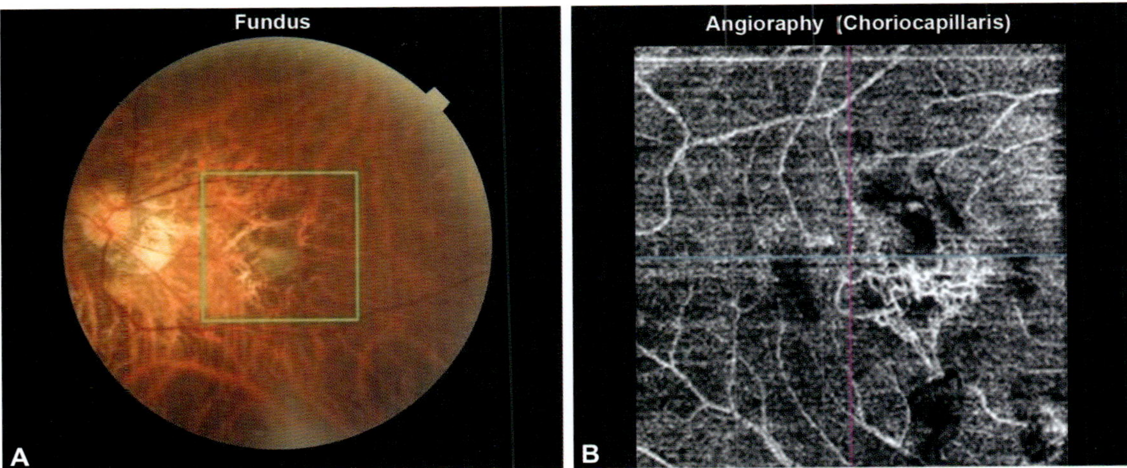

Figs. 12.2A and B: Myopic choroidal neovascular membrane. (A) Shows the fundus photograph of left eye of a myopic patient with tilted optic disc, temporal myopic crescent and diffuse chorioretinal atrophy. A dirty grayish-green lesion can be seen at the macula inferior to fovea. (B) Shows the optical coherence tomography angiography image of the area of interest with choroidal neovascular membrane at the level of retinal pigment epithelium and choriocapillaris.

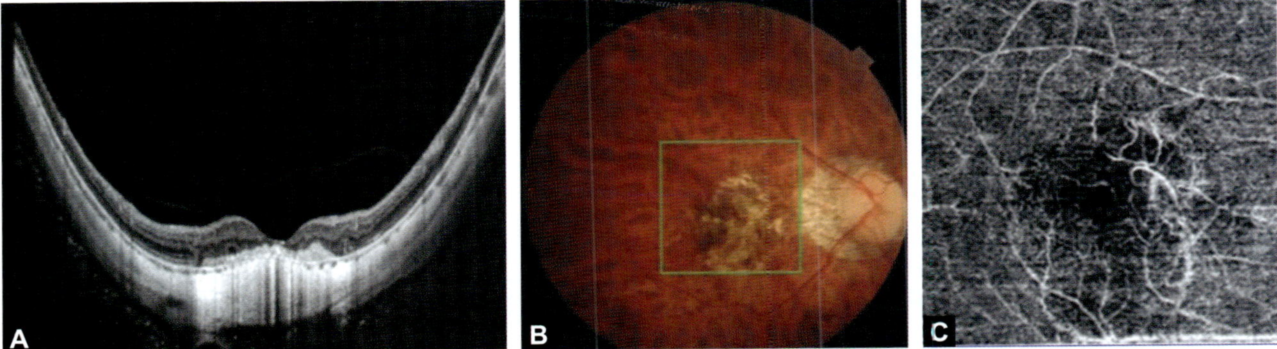

Figs. 12.3A to C: High myopic eye with choroid neovascularization on spectral domain–optical coherence tomography (A) and color fundus image (B), which is also visualized on optical coherence tomography angiography (C) as a type I neovascularization.

However, as atrophy is an important feature of myopic CNV, further studies are required to determine whether this atrophy is accelerated by PDT or is part of the disease's natural course.

CHOROID NEOVASCULARIZATION POST CHOROIDAL RUPTURE

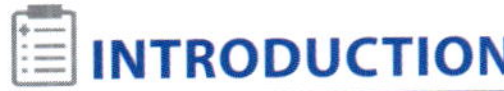 ### INTRODUCTION

Choroidal rupture is characterized by a breach in inner choroid and overlying RPE-Bruch's complex secondary to blunt trauma. Acute anteroposterior compression and subsequent equatorial expansion is the cause for rupture.[27,28] 5–10% of eyes with choroidal rupture develops CNV in the long term.[29-31] CNV develops in response to the break in relatively inelastic Bruch's membrane and is the cause for late loss of vision in such cases. The risk factors for CNV formation are older age, macular location of rupture and greater length of rupture.[29] FA helps in differentiating between posttraumatic healed macular scar and CNV as the scar stains slowly in the late phase without leakage while CNV shows characteristic early leakage which increases in late phase. Management options include observation, intravitreal anti-VEGF agents, laser photocoagulation, PDT and submacular surgery.[30,32,33] Subfoveal CNV is generally treated with anti-VEGF agents, although photodynamic therapy can also be used. Laser photocoagulation is used for extrafoveal lesions, that too rarely. Subfoveal surgery for choroidal rupture complicated by CNV is less commonly done.

ANGIOID STREAKS

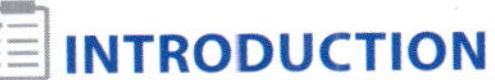 ### INTRODUCTION

Angioid streaks are irregular crack-like dehiscences in the collagenous and elastic portion of brittle and thickened Bruch's membrane (Figs. 12.4 to 12.6).[34] These are

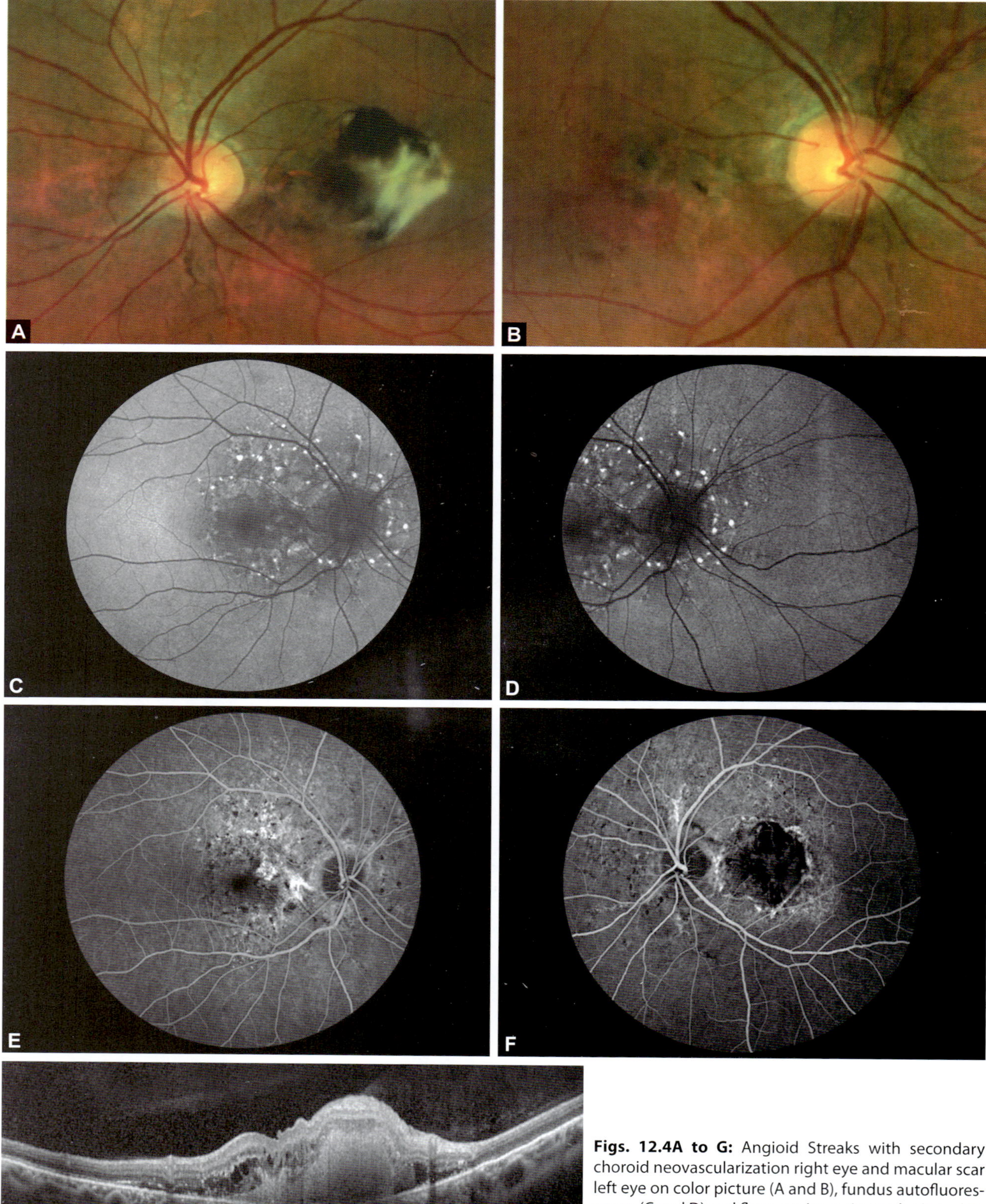

Figs. 12.4A to G: Angioid Streaks with secondary choroid neovascularization right eye and macular scar left eye on color picture (A and B), fundus autofluorescence (C and D) and fluorescein angiography (E and F). Wide field optical coherence tomography reveals subretinal choroid neovascularization(G).

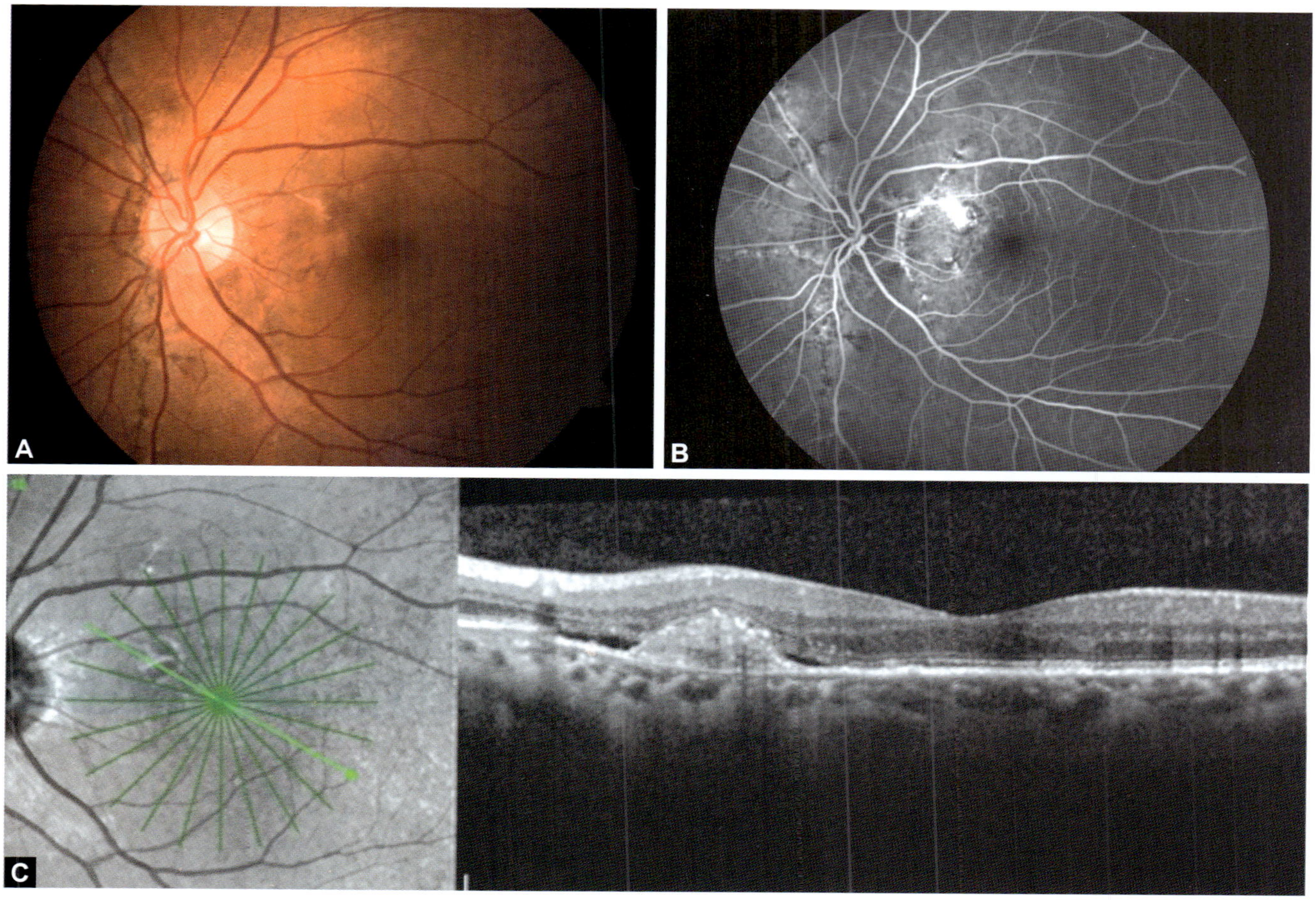

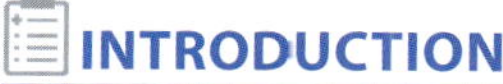

Figs. 12.5A to C: Angioid streaks with choroid neovascularization on color fundus image (A), which is hyperfluorescent on fluorescein angiography (B). Spectralis optical coherence tomography reveals the subretinal choroid neovascularization with fluid (C).

associated with overlying retinal pigment epithelium (RPE) atrophy and calcific degeneration. Around 50% of the patients with angioid streaks have associated systemic conditions such as pseudoxanthoma elasticum (Gronblad–Strandberg syndrome), osteitis deformans (Paget's disease), fibrodysplasia hyperelastica (Ehlers–Danlos syndrome), acromegaly, Marfan syndrome and blood dyscrasias.[35] Angioid streaks are usually asymptomatic. Choroidal neovascular growth may occur through the defect in Bruch's membrane in 72–86% of eyes with angioid streaks.[36] CNV is usually bilateral but asymmetric, with the fellow eye involvement occurring usually after 18 months of the initial eye.[37] Pseudoxanthoma patients have a higher risk of CNV development compared to patients with other systemic diseases. FA delineates the streaks and associated CNV very well. Laser photocoagulation for macular CNV carries a high recurrence rate and poor overall visual outcome.[38] Prophylactic treatment of streaks prior to development of CNV is not recommended.[39] PDT and macular translocation surgery for macular CNV shows variable visual outcomes.[40] Significant visual improvement has been noted with the use of anti-VEGF therapy with bevacizumab and ranibizumab.[41,42]

PRESUMED OCULAR HISTOPLASMOSIS SYNDROME

INTRODUCTION

Ocular histoplasmosis occurs as focal infection of the choroid at the time of systemic infection with Histoplasma capsulatum via the respiratory tract.[43,44] This results in an atrophic scar that disrupts the Bruch's membrane and provides access to the subretinal space for neovascularization.[45] Patients are usually asymptomatic unless an active CNV supervenes that results in sudden onset metamorphopsia or decrease in vision secondary to hemorrhage or exudation. Ocular histoplasmosis is diagnosed by presence of at least two of the following fundus lesions in one or both eyes in the absence of ocular inflammation:[46,47]

- Discrete, focal, atrophic (i.e. punched-out) choroidal scars in the macula or the periphery, smaller in size than the optic disc (histo spots).

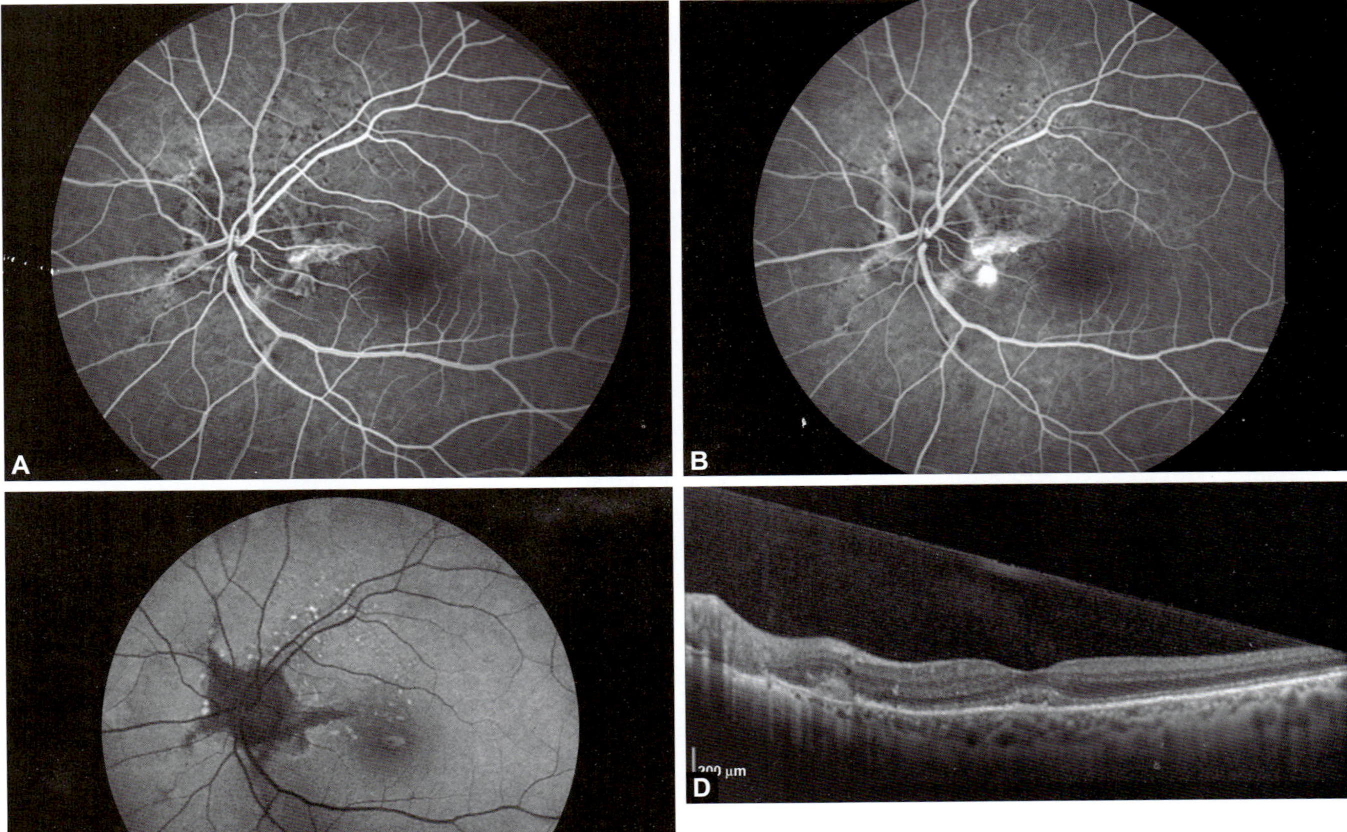

Figs. 12.6A to D: Shows peripapillary early choroid neovascularization in an angioid streaks patient with increasing hyperfluorescence on fluorescein angiography (A and B). However, fundus autofluorescence (C) and optical coherence tomography (D) show no active hyperfluorescence or any subretinal fluid on optical coherence tomography.

- Peripapillary chorioretinal scarring (i.e., peripapillary atrophy).
- Choroid neovascularization or associated sequelae (hemorrhagic retinal detachment, fibrovascular disciform scar).

60% cases have bilateral involvement but may not be symmetric at initial presentation. The risk of developing CNV is less than 5% in the affected eye but the risk increases up to 25% in the presence of macular histo spots. Investigations include HLA testing (HLA B7 and HLA DRw2), serological tests and fundus fluorescein angiography or optical coherence tomography when CNV is suspected. There is no treatment known to prevent an inactive lesion from giving rise to an exudative or hemorrhagic neovascular complex. Systemic corticosteroids have been suggested, particularly in cases of *active* histo spots and subfoveal CNV.[46] However, in the era of anti-VEGF and PDT the use of systemic corticosteroids even in subfoveal cases is now mainly of historical interest. Similarly, submacular surgery for CNV was an important treatment alternative earlier for patients with severe vision loss.[48,49] Currently intravitreal anti-VEGF is the treatment of choice in active CNV as it has shown good results in various studies.[50,51] An ongoing study is comparing efficacy and safety of aflibercept in POHS with CNV (HANDLE study). PDT can be considered in subfoveal CNV and is United States Food and Drug Administration approved for it. Combination therapy with anti-VEGF and PDT has also shown encouraging results.[52] Laser photocoagulation can be considered for extrafoveal and juxtafoveal CNV in view of good results shown in MPS study.

CHOROID NEOVASCULARIZATION IN WHITE DOT SYNDROMES AND OTHER NONINFECTIOUS POSTERIOR UVEITIS

The white dot syndromes are a heterogeneous group of disorders with multiple whitish-yellow inflammatory lesions affecting the outer retina, RPE and choroid. These disorders have active yellowish lesions with overlying serous detachment of neurosensory retina. These lesions depigment over time and change into chorioretinal scars. CNV may arise from the edge of old chorioretinal scars but frequently arise in inflamed areas (Figs. 12.7A and B). Low grade chronic widespread inflammation of choriocapillaris lead to nonperfusion, ischemia and subsequently neovascularization (Figs. 12.8A and B). ICGA shows large areas of nonperfusion and is essential for evaluation of choroidal status in such cases.[53,54]

CNV occurs very frequently, in about 32% to 46% cases of multifocal choroiditis, usually anterior to RPE in the macular or peripapillary area.[55,56] CNV develops in 17% to 40% eyes with punctate inner choroidopathy.[57,58] CNV is a well-known

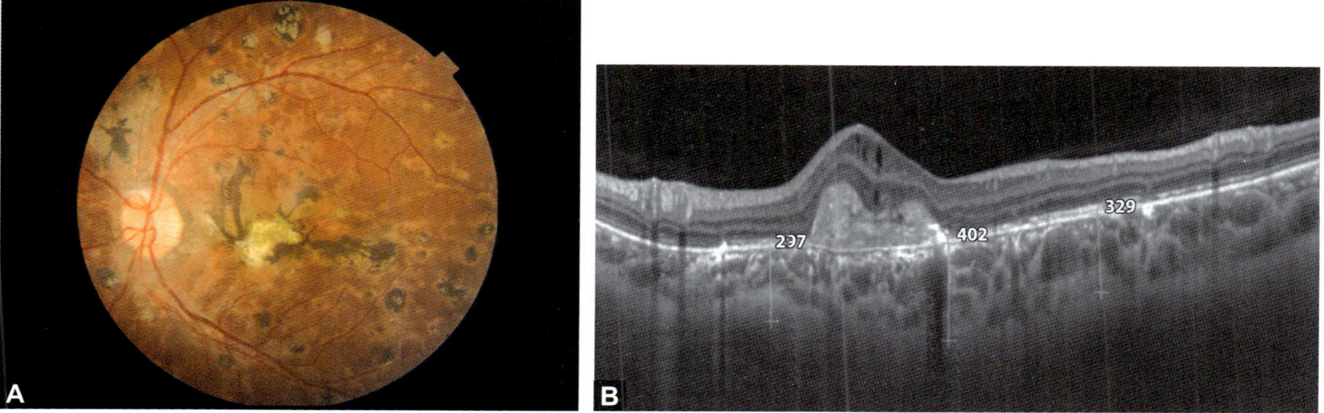

Figs. 12.7A and B: Case of serpiginous choroiditis with central subretinal choroid neovascularization scar on color fundus image and optical coherence tomography.

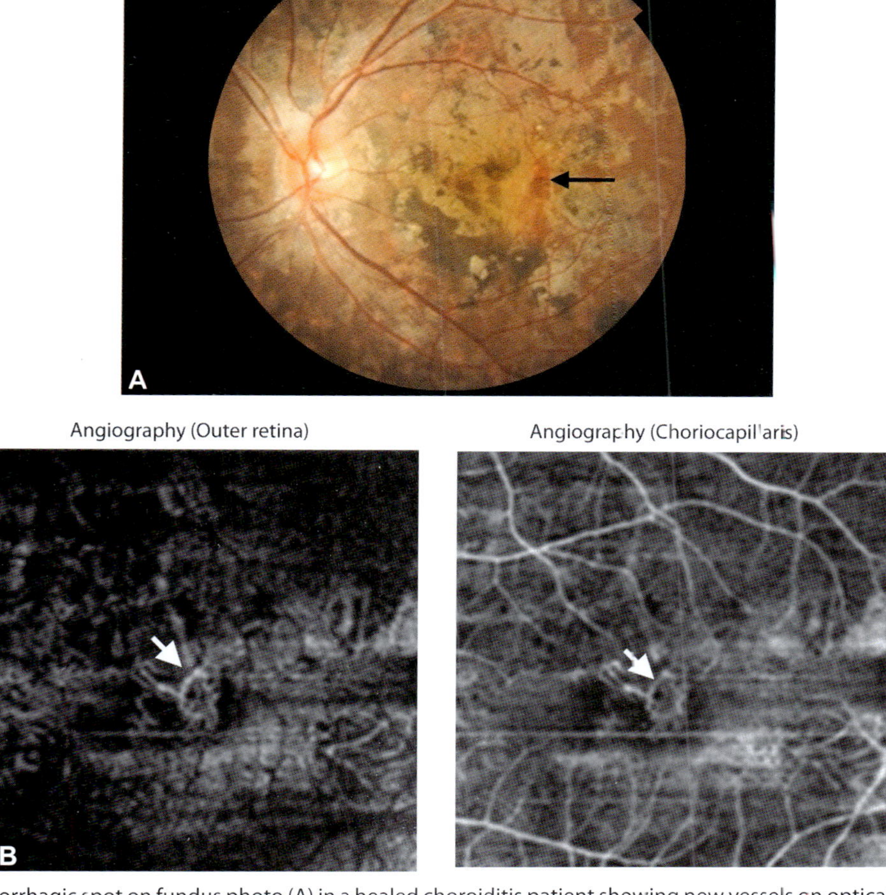

Figs. 12.8A and B: Hemorrhagic spot on fundus photo (A) in a healed choroiditis patient showing new vessels on optical coherence tomography angiography (B).

complication of serpiginous choroidopathy in 10% to 25% of affected patients, generally occurring close to the edge of chorioretinal lesions.[59,60] Subretinal fibrosis and uveitis syndrome (SFU),[61] acute posterior multifocal placoid pigment epitheliopathy (APMPPE),[62] birdshot retinochoroidopathy,[63] multiple evanescent white dot syndrome (MEWDS),[64] Vogt-Koyanagi-Harada (VKH),[65] sympathetic ophthalmia[66] and sarcoidisis[67] are some of the other noninfectious uveitis that can have CNV as a possible sequelae.

The first line of management in noninfectious inflammatory CNV is control of intraocular inflammation with steroids, usually given systemically but can also be used locally in unilateral disease. As the inflammatory process seems to involve the whole immune system, the use of systemic steroids should be considered.[68] Safety and efficacy of immunosuppression for the control of CNV in uveitis have been described.[69] Mycophenolate mofetil (MMF) has been found to improve arteriolopathy and decrease the soluble mediators involved in CNV pathophysiology.[70] For such reasons, MMF can be a promising drug for the long-term control of inflammatory CNV.[71] If steroids with or without immunosuppressive therapy show an insufficient response, additional therapies aimed directly at the neovascular process like anti-VEGF therapy should be rapidly introduced.[72] Surgical removal of CNV, laser photocoagulation and PDT have a marginal role in current scenario.

CHOROID NEOVASCULARIZATION IN INFECTIOUS UVEITIS

Toxoplasma gondii commonly affects the eye and association between retinochoroiditis and CNV is frequent.[73] CNV occurs close to the edge of an atrophic chorioretinal scar. In such cases, FA helps in distinguishing the neovascular lesion from the reactivation of retinochoroiditis. CNV can occur concomitantly with a reactivation of retinochoroiditis. CNV is managed by anti-VEGFs. CNV associated with recurrent retinochoroiditis is treated with the classical triple regimen of anti-toxoplasmic antibiotics with corticosteroids.[74]

Toxocara canis may lead to CNV which typically grows near an active or quiescent choroidal granuloma.[75]

IDIOPATHIC CHOROID NEOVASCULARIZATION

In a significant number of otherwise healthy young patients with CNV, no apparent cause can be found constituting idiopathic CNV (ICNV) (Figs. 12.9A to D).[76] The diagnosis

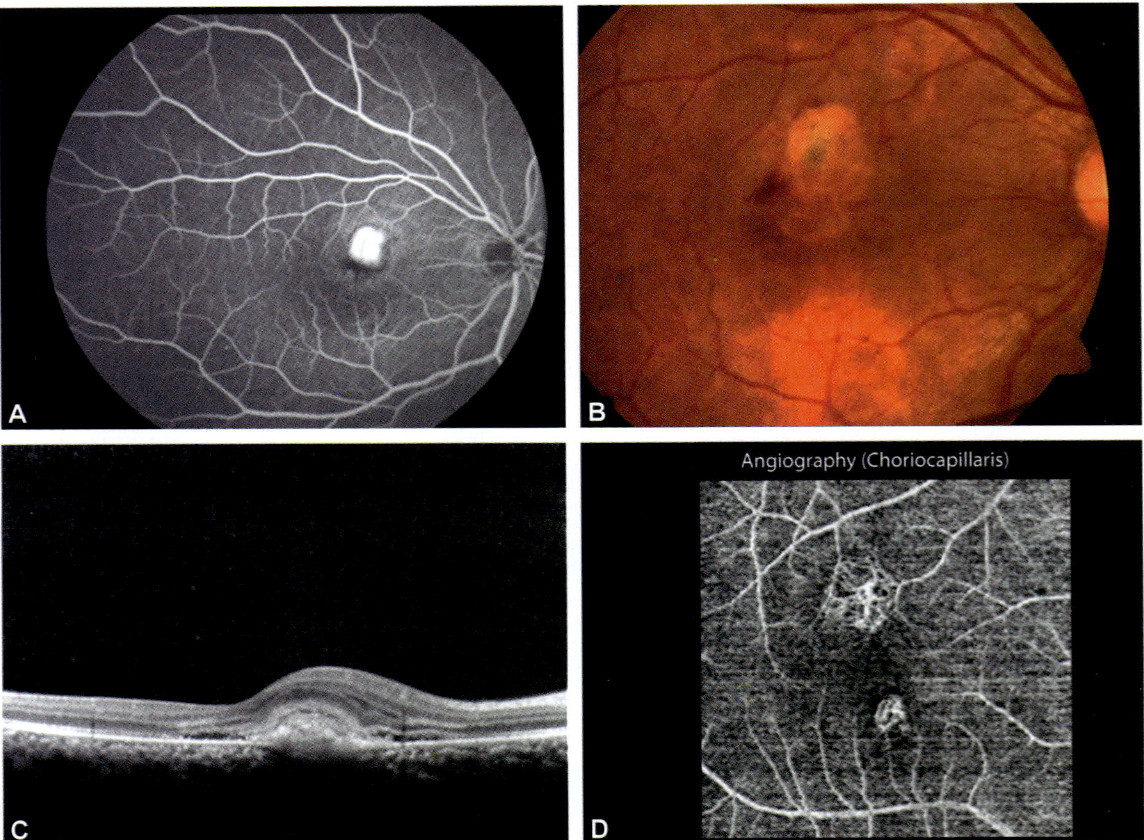

Figs. 12.9A to D: Idiopathic choroid neovascularization seen on fluorescein angiography (A), Fundus color photograph (B) spectral domain–optical coherence tomography (C) and also on optical coherence tomography angiography (D).

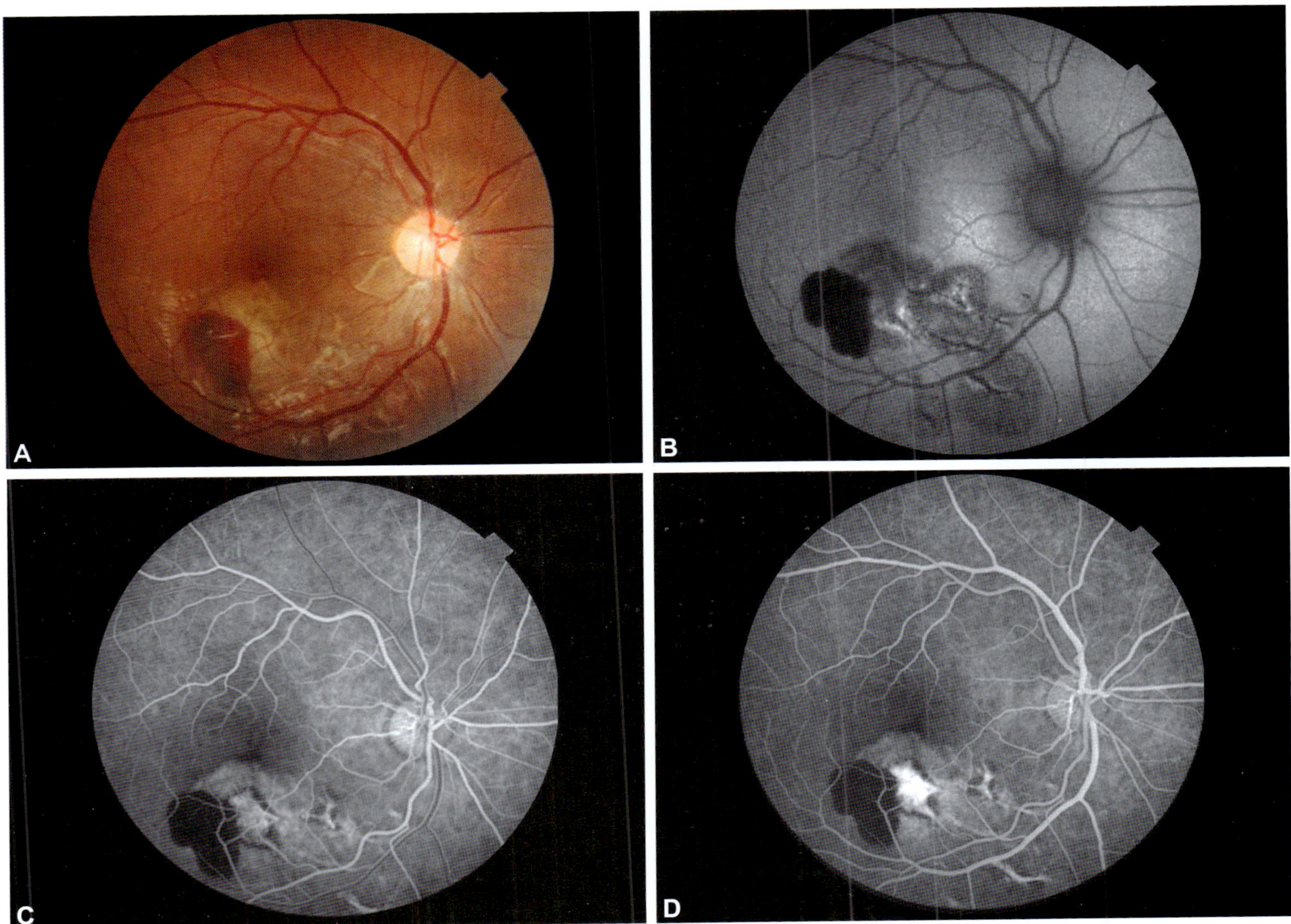

Figs. 12.10A to D: Multimodal imaging in a case of idiopathic choroid neovascularization. (A) Shows a fundus photograph with choroid neovascularization with subretinal bleed inferotemporal to fovea. (B) Shows fundus autofluorescence image with blocked autofluorescence due to subretinal hemorrhage and choroid neovascularization scar adjacent to it. (C and D) Show the early and late venous flow phases of fluorescein angiography with blocked fluorescence due to hemorrhage and adjacent hyperfluorescence which is increasing in intensity with time.

is one of exclusion of other possible associations of CNV. ICNV has been reported to constitute 17% of the cases of CNV in patients younger than 50 years.[77] An underlying low grade inflammation may be the likely possible cause. ICNV are typically type 2 CNV (subretinal) with the following characteristics: small, well-defined focal lesions extending above the RPE. These cases are usually unilateral and the natural history is better than that seen in AMD.[78] ICNV appears to be less diffuse in its extent than the lesions of AMD on fluorescein angiography (Figs. 12.10A to D). Multimodality imaging is shown in figure.

Macular Photocoagulation Study Group recommended laser photocoagulation for management of extrafoveal and juxtafoveal CNV lesions.[79,80] PDT has also been used.[81,82] Visual results with transpupillary thermotherapy[83] and submacular surgery or macular translocation are far from satisfactory.[84,85] Intravitreal anti-VEGF agents are safe and tolerable for managing subfoveal idiopathic choroid neovascularization (Figs. 12.11 and 12.12).[86-88]

CHOROID NEOVASCULARIZATION IN MACULAR TELANGIECTASIA

Choroidal neovascularization is a known complication of macular telangiectasia (Figs. 12.13A to D). It has been grouped under stage 5 of Gass and Blodi classification and Stage 2 (proliferative) of Yannuzzi classification of idiopathic parafoveal telangiectasia. It is postulated that due to chronic neurodegenerative process, occlusion, vascular changes and ectatic capillary changes, there is loss of outer retinal layers and formation of cavitations or cysts which will eventually lead to subretinal neovascularization, exudation and hemorrhages.[89] OCTA has emerged as an extremely important modality to scan macular telangiectasia.

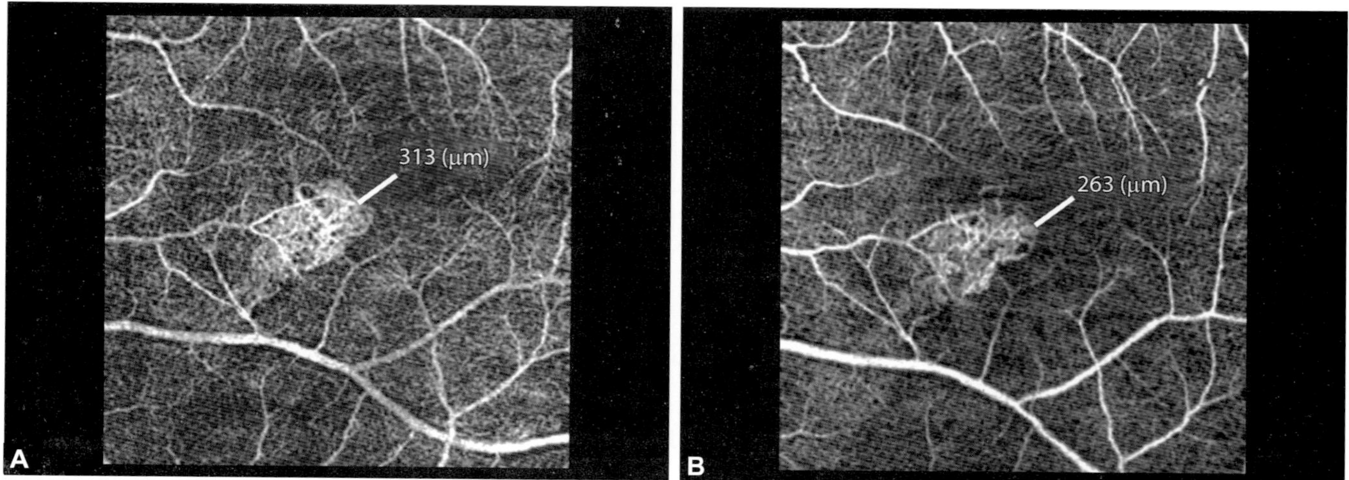

Figs. 12.11A and B: (A) Pre-injection idiopathic choroid neovascularization clearly delineated and close to fovea, (B) one month post ranibizumab the choroid neovascularization intensity and size is reduced on swept source–optical coherence tomography angiography.

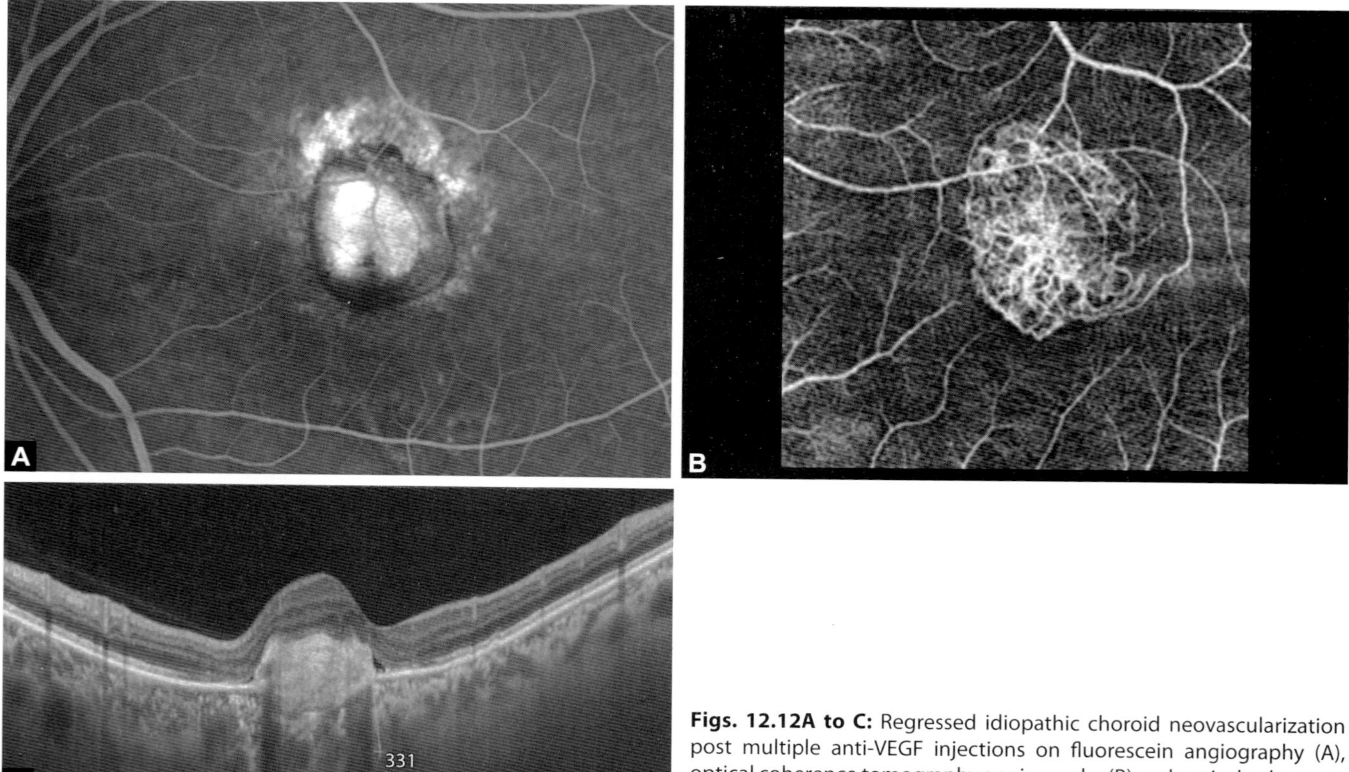

Figs. 12.12A to C: Regressed idiopathic choroid neovascularization post multiple anti-VEGF injections on fluorescein angiography (A), optical coherence tomography angiography (B) and optical coherence tomography (C) which show a scar formation with absence of SRF.

For extrafoveal lesions, laser photocoagulation is the treatment of choice. Transpupillary thermotherapy has also been reported with positive results. Juxtafoveal lesions warrant the use of PDT or intravitreal anti-VEGFs. Macular surgery has also been reported, but the results are not satisfactory.[90-94]

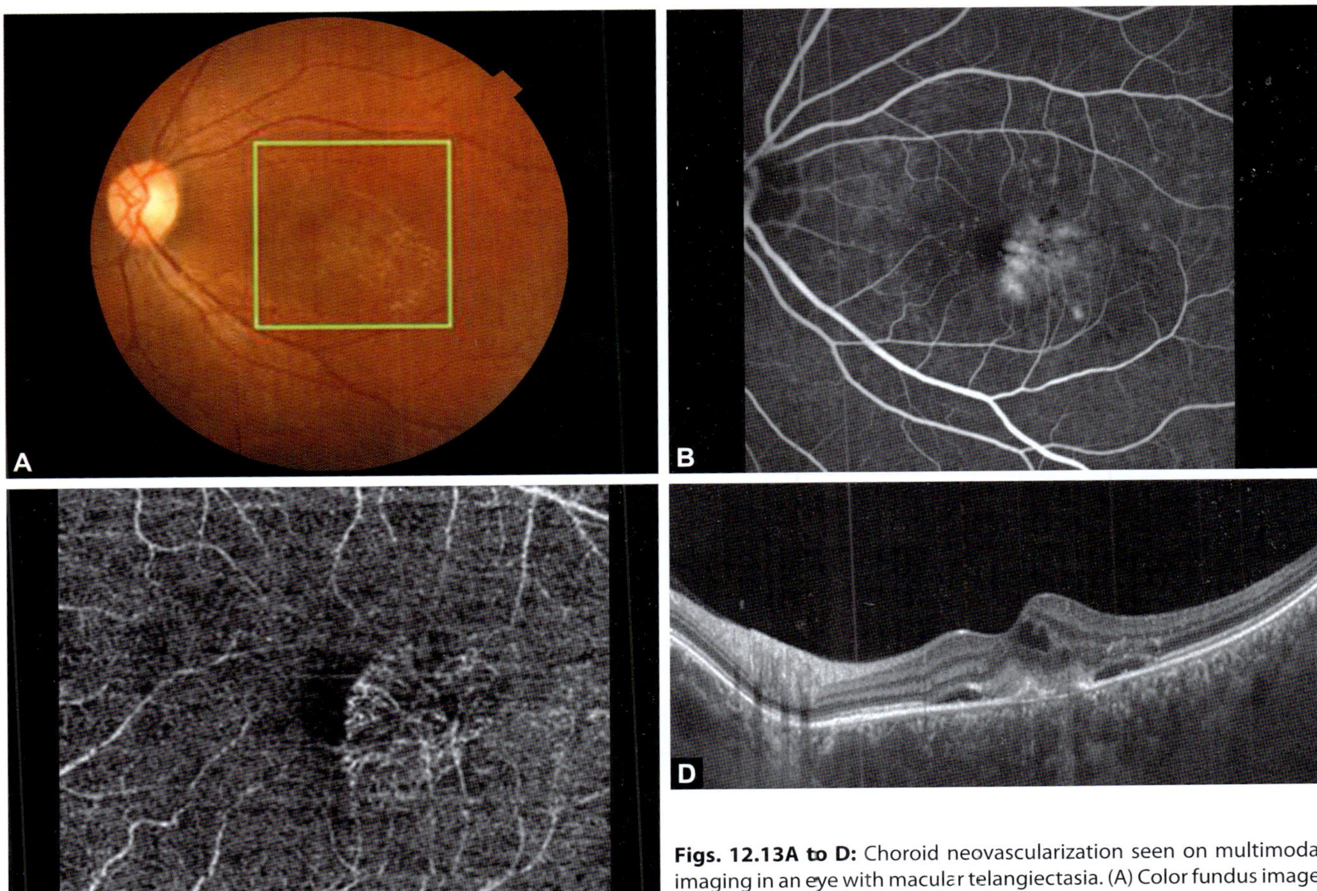

Figs. 12.13A to D: Choroid neovascularization seen on multimodal imaging in an eye with macular telangiectasia. (A) Color fundus image, (B) Fluorescein angiography. (C) Optical coherence tomography angiography and (D) optical coherence tomography.

REFERENCES

1. Grossniklaus HE, Greer WR. Choroidal neovascularization. Am J Ophthalmology. 2004;137(3):496-503.
2. Yannuzzi LA, Freund KB, Takahashi BS. Review of retinal angiomatous proliferation or type 3 neovascularization. Retina. 2008;28(3):375-84.
3. Liu Y, Cox SR, Morita T, et al. Hypoxia regulates vascular endothelial growth factor gene expression in endothelial cells. Identification of a 5' enhancer. Circ Res. 1995;77(3):638-43.
4. Maxwell PH, Dachs GU, Gleadle JM, et al. Hypoxia-inducible factor-1 modulates gene expression in solid tumors and influences both angiogenesis and tumor growth. Proc Natl Acad Sci USA. 1997;94(15):8104-9.
5. Tsuzuki Y, Fukumura D, Oosthuyse B et al. Vascular endothelia growth factor (VEGF) modulation by targeting hypoxia-inducible factor-1alpha—hypoxia response element—VEGF cascade differentially regulates vascular response and growth rate in tumors. Cancer Res. 2000;60(22):624-852.
6. Ryan SJ. Subretinal neovascularization after argon laser photocoagulation. Albrecht Von Graefes Arch Klin Exp Ophthalmology. 1980;215(1):29-42.
7. Wallow I, Johns K, Chandra BS, et al. Chorioretinal and choriovitreal neovascularization after photocoagulation for proliferative diabetic retinopathy. A clinicopathologic correlation. Ophthalmology. 1985;92(4):523-32.
8. McNeil PL, Muthukrishnan L, Warder E, et al. Growth factors are released by mechanically wounded endothelial cells. J Cell Biol.1989;109(2):811-22.
9. Tombran-Tink J, Shivaram SM, Chader GJ, et al. Expression, secretion, and age-related downregulation of pigment epithelium-derived factor, a serpin with neurotrophic activity. J Neurosci. 1995;15(7 Pt 1):4992-5003.
10. Tomita M, Yamada H, Adachi Y, et al. Choroidal neovascularization is provided by bone marrow cells. Stem Cells. 2004;22(1):21-6.
11. Bressler NM, Bressler SB, Fine SL. Age-related macular degeneration. Surv Ophthalmology. 1988;32(6):375-413.
12. Fine AM, Elman MJ, Ebert JE, et al. Earliest symptoms caused by neovascular membranes in the macula. Arch Ophthalmology. 1986; 104(4):513-4.
13. Loewenstein A, Bressler NM, Bressler SB. Epidemiology of RPE disease. In: Marmor MF, Wolfensberger TJ (Eds). Retinal pigment epithelium current aspects of function and disease. New York: Oxford University Press;1999
14. Macular Photocoagulation Study Group. Subfoveal neovascular lesions in age-related macular degeneration: guidelines for evaluation and treatment in the Macular Photocoagulation Study. Arch Ophthalmology. 1991;109(9):124-257.

15. Regillo CD, Benson WE, Maguire JI, et al. Indocyanine green angiography and occult neovascularization. Ophthalmology. 1994; 101(2):28-08.

16. Yannuzzi LA, Slakter JS, Sorenson JA, et al. Digital indocyanine green videoangiography and choroidal neovascularization. Retina. 1992;12:191-223.

17. Leveziel N, Yu Y, Reynolds R, et al. Genetic factors for choroidal neovascularization associated with high myopia. Invest Ophthalmology Vis Sci. 2012;53(8):5004-9.

18. Ikuno Y, Jo Y, Hamasaki T, et al. Ocular risk factors for choroidal neovascularization in pathologic myopia. Invest Ophthalmology Vis Sci. 2010;51(7):3721-5.

19. Ohno-Matsui K, Yoshida T, Futagami S, et al. Patchy atrophy and lacquer cracks predispose to the development of choroidal neovascularisation in pathological myopia. Br J Ophthalmology. 2003; 87(5):570-3.

20. Neelam K, Cheung CM, Ohno-Matsui K, et al. Choroidal neovascularization in pathological myopia. Prog Retin Eye Res. 2012; 31(5):495-525.

21. Chan WM, Ohji M, Lai TY, et al. Choroidal neovascularisation in pathological myopia: an update in management. Br J Ophthalmology. 2005;89(11):1522-8.

22. Yoshida T, Ohno-Matsui K, Yasuzumi K, et al. Myopic choroidal neovascularization: a 10-year follow-up. Ophthalmology. 2003; 110(7):1297-305.

23. Wolf S, Balciuniene VJ, Laganovska G, et al. RADIANCE: a randomized controlled study of ranibizumab in patients with choroidal neovascularization secondary to pathologic myopia. Ophthalmology. 2014;121(3):682-92.

24. Tufail A, Narendran N, Patel PJ, et al. Ranibizumab in myopic choroidal neovascularization: the 12-month results from the REPAIR study. Ophthalmology. 2013;120(9):1944-5.

25. Secretan M, Kuhn D, Soubrane G, et al. Long-term visual outcome of choroidal neovascularization in pathologic myopia: natural history and laser treatment. Eur J Ophthalmology. 1997;7(4):307-16.

26. Verteporfin in Photodynamic Therapy Study Group. Photodynamic therapy of subfoveal choroidal neovascularization in pathologic myopia with verteporfin. 1-year results of a randomized clinical trial—VIP report no. 1. Ophthalmology. 2001;108(5):841-52.

27. Youssri AI, Young LH. Closed-globe contusion injuries of the posterior segment. Int Ophthalmology Clin. 2002;42(3):79-86.

28. Aguilar JP, Green WR. Choroidal rupture: a histopathologic study of 47 eyes. Retina. 1984;4(4):269-75.

29. Ament CS, Zacks DN, Lane AM, et al. Predictors of visual outcome and choroidal neovascular membrane formation after traumatic choroidal rupture. Arch Ophthalmology. 2006;124(7):957-66.

30. Francis JH, Freund KB. Photoreceptor reconstitution correlates with visual improvement after intravitreal bevacizumab treatment of choroidal neovascularization secondary to traumatic choroidal rupture. Retina. 2011;31(2):422-4.

31. Arrim ZI, Simmons IG. Traumatic choroidal rupture. Emerg Med J. 2009;26(12):880.

32. Yadav NK, Bharghav M, Vasudha K, et al. Choroidal neovascular membrane complicating traumatic choroidal rupture managed by intravitreal bevacizumab. Eye (Lond). 2009;23(9):1872-3.

33. Harissi-Dagher M, Sebag M, Gauthier D, et al. Photodynamic therapy in young patients with choroidal neovascularization following traumatic choroidal rupture. Am J Ophthalmology. 2005; 139(4):726-8.

34. Klein BA. Angioid streaks: a clinical and histopathologic study. Am J Ophthalmology. 1947;30(8):955-68.

35. Clarkson JG, Altman RD. Angioid streaks. Surv Ophthalmology. 1982;26(5):235-46.

36. Georgalas I, Papconstantinou D, Koutsandrea C, et al. Angioid streaks, clinical course, complications, and current therapeutic management. Ther Clin Risk Manag. 2009;5(1):81-9.

37. Connor PJ jr, Juergens JL, Perry HO, et al. Pseudoxanthoma elasticum and angioid streaks: A review of 106 cases. Am J Med. 1961;30:537-43.

38. Gelisken O, Hendriskse F, Deutman AF. A long-term follow-up study of laser coagulation of neovascular membranes in angioid streaks. Am J Ophthalmology. 1988;105(3):299-303.

39. Gass HD. Stereoscopic atlas of macular diseases: Diagnosis and treatment. 4th edition. St Louis: Mosby 1997;118-25.

40. Chan WM, Lim TH, Pece A, et al. Verteporfin PDT for nonstandard indications: a review of current literature. Graefes Arch Clin Exp Ophthalmology. 2010;248(5):613-26.

41. Finger RP, Issa PC, Schmitz-Valckenberg S, et al. Long-term effectiveness of intravitreal bevacizumab for choroidal neovascularization secondary to angioid streaks in pseudoxanthoma elasticum. Retina. 2011;10:1-11.

42. Myung J, Bhatnagar P, Spaide RF, et al. Long-term outcomes of intravitreal antivascular endothelial growth factor therapy for the management of choroidal neovascularization in pseudoxanthoma elasticum. Retina. 2010;30(5):748-55.

43. Schlaegel TF. Ocular histoplasmosis. New York: Grune & Stratton.1977:1-301.

44. Wong VG, Kwon-Chung KJ, Hill WB. Koch's postulates and experimental ocular histoplasmosis. Int Ophthalmology Clin.1975; 15(3):139-45.

45. Weingeist TA, Watzke RC. Ocular involvement by Histoplasma-capsulatum. Int Ophthalmology Clin. 1983;23(2):33-47.

46. Gass JDM. Stereoscopic atlas of macular diseases. Diagnosis and treatment. St Louis, Mosby; 1987.

47. Patz A, Fine SL. Presumed ocular histoplasmosis. In: Yannuzzi LA, Gitter KA, Schatz H (Eds). The macula: a comprehensive text and atlas. Baltimore: Williams & Wilkins; 1979.

48. Thomas MA, Kaplan HJ. Surgical removal of subfoveal neovascularization in the presumed ocular histoplasmosis syndrome. Am J Ophthalmology. 1991;111(1):1-7.

49. Thomas MA, Grand MG, Williams DF, et al. Surgical management of subfoveal choroidal neovascularization. Ophthalmology. 1992; 99(6):952 68.

50. Adan A, Navarro M, Casaroli-Marano RP, et al. Intravitreal bevacizumab as initial treatment for choroidal neovascularization associated with presumed ocular histoplasmosis syndrome. Graefes Arch Clin Exp Ophthalmology. 2007;245(12):1873-5.

51. Heier JS, Brown D, Ciulla T, et al. Ranibizumab for choroidal neovascularization secondary to causes other than age-related macular degeneration: a phase I clinical trial. Ophthalmology. 2011;118(1):111-8.

52. Han DP, McAllister JT, Weinberg DV, et al. Combined intravitreal anti-VEGF and verteporfin photodynamic therapy for juxtafoveal and extrafoveal choroidal neovascularization as an alternative to laser photocoagulation. Eye (Lond). 2010;24(4)713-6.

53. Slakter JS, Giovannini A, Yannuzzi LA, et al. Indocyanine green angiography of multifocal choroiditis. Ophthalmology. 1997; 104(11):1813-9.

54. Altan-Yaycioglu R, Akova YA, Akca S, et al. Inflammation of the posterior uvea: Findings on fundus fluorescein and indocyanine green angiography. Ocult Immunol Inflamm. 2006;14(3):171-9.

55. Dreyer RF, Gass DJ. Multifocal choroiditis and panuveitis. A syndrome that mimics ocular histoplasmosis. Arch Ophthalmology. 1984;102(12):1776-84.

56. Morgan CM, Schatz H. Recurrent multifocal choroiditis. Ophthalmology. 1986;93(9):1138-47.

57. Watzke RC, Packer AJ, Folk JC, et al. Punctate inner choroidopathy. Am J Ophthalmology. 1984;98(5):572-84.

58. Reddy CV, Brown J Jr, Folk JC, et al. Enlarged blind spots in chorioretinal inflammatory disorders. Ophthalmology. 1996; 103(4):606-17.

59. Kuo IC, Cunningham ET Jr. Ocular neovascularization in patients with uveitis. Int Ophthalmology Clin. 2000;40(2):111-26.

60. Jampol LM, Orth D Daily MJ, et al. Subretinal neovascularization with geographic (serpiginous) choroiditis. Am J Ophthalmology. 1979;88(4):683-9.

61. Brown J Jr, Folk JC, Reddy CV, et al. Visual prognosis of multifocal choroiditis, punctate inner choroidopathy, and the diffuse subretinal fibrosis syndrome. Ophthalmology. 1996;103(7):1100-5.

62. Pagliarini S, Piguet B, Ffytche TJ, et al. Foveal involvement and lack of visual recovery in APMPPE associated with uncommon features. Eye. 1995;9(Pt 1):42-7.

63. Brucker AJ, Deglin EA, Bene C, et al. Subretinal choroidal neovascularization in birdshot retinochoroidopathy. Am J Ophthalmology. 1985;99(1):40-4.

64. Rouvas AA, Ladas ID, Papakostas TD, et al. Intravitreal ranibizumab in a patient with choroidal neovascularization secondary to multiple evanescent white dot syndrome. Eur J Ophthalmology. 2007;17(6):996-9.

65. Read RW, Rechodouni A, Butani N, et al. Complications and prognostic factors in Vogt-Koyanagi-Harada disease. Am J Ophthalmology. 2001;131(5):599-606.

66. Kilmartin DJ, Forrester JV, Dick AD. Cyclosporine-induced resolution of choroidal neovascularization associated with sympathetic ophthalmia. Arch Ophthalmology. 1998;116(2):249-50.

67. Inagaki M, Harada T, Kiribuchi T, et al. Subfoveal choroidal neovascularization in uveitis. Ophthalmologica. 1996;210(4): 229-33.

68. Caicedo A, Espinosa-Heidmann DG, Piña Y, et al. Blood-derived macrophages infiltrate the retina and activate Muller glial cells under experimental choroidal neovascularization. Exp Eye Res. 2005;81(1):38-47.

69. Dees C, Arnold JJ, Forrester JV, et al. Immunosuppressive treatment of choroidal neovascularization associated with endogenous posterior uveitis. Arch Ophthalmology. 1998;116(11):1456-61.

70. Shihab FS, Bennett WM, Yi H, et al. Mycophenol atemofetil ameliorates arteriolopathy and decreases transforming growth factor-beta1 in chronic cyclosporine nephrotoxicity. Am J Transplant. 2003;3:1550-9.

71. Neri P, Manoni M, Fortuna C, et al. Association of systemic steroids and mycophenolate mofetil as rescue therapy for uveitic choroidal neovascularization unresponsive to the traditional immunesuppressants: Interventional case series. Int Ophthalmology. 2010;30(5):583-90.

72. Tran TH, Fardeau C, Terrada C, et al. Intravitreal bevacizumab for refractory choroidal neovascularization (CNV) secondary to uveitis. Graefes Arch Clin Exp Ophthalmology. 2008;246(12):1685-92.

73. Fine SL, Owens SL, Haller JA, et al. Choroidal neovascularization as a late complication of ocular toxoplasmosis. Am J Ophthalmology. 1981;91(3):318-22.

74. Bahia-Oliveira LM, Jones JL, Azevedo-Silva J, et al. Highly endemic, waterborne toxoplasmosis in north Rio de Janeiro state, Brazil. Emerg Infect Dis. 2003;9(1):55-62.

75. Lampariello DA, Primo SA. Ocular toxocariasis: A rare presentation of a posterior pole granuloma with an associated choroidal neovascular membrane. J Am Optom Assoc. 1999;70(4):245-52.

76. Ho AC, Yannuzzi LA, Piscicano K, et al. The natural history of idiopathic subfoveal choroidal neovascularisation. Ophthalmology. 1995;102(5):782-9.

77. Cohen SY, Laroche A, Leguen Y, et al. Etiology of choroidal neovascularization in young patients. Ophthalmology. 1996; 103(8):1241-4.

78. Lindblom B, Andersson T. The prognosis of idiopathic neovascularisation in persons younger than 50 years of age. Ophthalmology. 1998;105(10):1816-20.

79. Macular photocoagulation study group. Argon laser photocoagulation for idiopathic neovascularisation. Results of a randomized clinical trial. Arch Ophthalmology. 1983;101:1358-61.

80. Macular photocoagulation study group. Krypton laser photocoagulation for idiopathic neovascularisation. Results of a randomized clinical trial. Arch Ophthalmology. 1990;108:832-7.

81. Sickenberg M, Schmidt-Erfurth U, Miller JW, et al. A preliminary study of photodynamic therapy using verteporfin for choroidal neovascularisation in pathologic myopia, ocular histoplasmosis syndrome, angioid streaks, and idiopathic causes. Arch Ophthalmology. 2000;118(3):327-36.

82. Chan WM, Lam DS, Wong TH et al. Photodynamic therapy with verteporfin for subfoveal idiopathic choroidal neovascularization: one-year results from a prospective case series. Ophthalmology. 2003;110(12):2395-402.

83. Kumar A, Prakash G, Singh RP. Transpupillary thermotherapy for idiopathic subfoveal choroidal neovascularization. Acta Ophthalmology Scand. 2004;82(2):205-8.

84. Thomas MA, Dickinson JD, Melberg NS, et al. Visual results after surgical removal of subfoveal choroidal neovascular membranes. Ophthalmology. 1994;101(8):1384-96.

85. Fujii GY, Humayun MS, Pieramici DJ, et al. Initial experience of inferior limited macular translocation for subfoveal choroidal neovascularisation resulting from causes other than age-related macular degeneration. Am J Ophthalmology. 2001;131(1):90-100.

86. Mandal S, Garg S, Venkatesh P, et al. Intravitreal bevacizumab for subfoveal idiopathic choroidal neovascularisation. Arch Ophthalmology. 2007;125(11):1487-92.

87. Inoue M, Kadonosono K, Watanabe Y, et al. Results of 1-year follow-up examinations after intravitreal bevacizumab administration for idiopathic choroidal neovascularisation. Retina. 2010; 30(5):733-8.

88. Zhang H Liu ZL, Gu F. Intravitreal bevacizumab for treatment of subfoveal idiopathic choroidal neovascularization: results of a 1-year prospective trial. Am J Ophthalmology. 2012;153(2):300-6.

89. Wu L, Evans T, Arevalo JF. Idiopathic macular telangiectasia type 2 (idiopathic juxtafoveolar retinal telangiectasis type 2A, Mac Tel 2). Surv Ophthalmology. 2013;58(6):536-59.

90. Dave V, Chhablani J, Narayanan R. Different treatment modalities for choroidal neovascularization in two eyes of one patient with bilateral type 2A parafoveal telangiectasia. Indian J Ophthalmology. 2013;61(7):353-5

91. Jia Y, Bailey ST, Wilson DJ, et al. Quantitative optical coherence tomography angiography of choroidal neovascularisation in age-related macular degeneration. Ophthalmology. 2014;121(7): 1435-44.

92. Schwartz DM, Fingler J, Kim DY, et al. Phase-variance optical coherence tomography: a technique for noninvasive angiography. Ophthalmology. 2014;121(1):180-7.

93. Coscas GJ, Lupidi M, Coscas F, et al. Optical coherence tomography angiography versus traditional multimodal imaging in assessing the activity of exudative age-related macular degeneration: a new diagnostic challenge. Retina. 2015;35(11):2219-28.

94. Miyata M, Ooto S, Hata M, et al. Detection of myopic choroidal neovascularization using optical coherence tomography angiography. Am J Ophthalmology. 2016;165:108-14.

Chapter 13

Vitreomacular Interface and Anomalous Posterior Vitreous Detachment

Vineet Mutha, Yogita Gupta, Divya Agarwal, Atul Kumar

VITREORETINAL INTERFACE

Attachment of vitreous body with the inner retina is referred to as vitreoretinal interface which is composed of vitreous cortex, internal limiting membrane (ILM) and Muller cell foot plates. It is a complex structure leading to an array of disorders when it deviates from its normal anatomy. Vitreous is composed of 99% water and 1% other molecules like collagen, hyaluronan, fibroblasts and glycosaminoglycans. The vitreoretinal interface additionally has *laminocytes* along with laminin, fibronectin and heparin sulfate which play a key role in adhesions between retina and vitreous.[1,2] Furthermore, collagen types VI, VII and XVIII are present at this interface apart from the common vitreous collagen types II, V, IX and XI. These collagens are present in varying densities leading to varying strengths of adhesions with stronger attachments at optic disc, posterior pole (macula), equator, around blood vessels, lattice degenerations and the strongest attachment is at the vitreous base.[1,3]

Newer studies on vitreoretinal interface suggest that at the posterior pole, there are islands of collagen IV which lead to healing process forming epiretinal membranes while at the vitreous base collagen II is abundant with intraretinal penetrations and thus, very strong adhesions which grows posteriorly with age leading to increased incidence of horse shoe tears anterior to equator after posterior vitreous detachments.[1] Vitreous cortex at optic disc and fovea is thinner and vitreous is liquefied in a pocket above fovea known as premacular vitreous pocket. The latter is 6 mm × 0.6 mm in size on an average and its abnormalities may lead to vitreomacular traction, epiretinal membranes and various other interface disorders.[4]

POSTERIOR VITREOUS DETACHMENT

Phenomenon of separation of vitreous from the retina and the optic disc is known as Posterior Vitreous Detachment (PVD) (Fig. 13.1). Latter is commonly seen in aged individuals (more than 60 years) though studies suggest that the process starts much earlier.[5] Uchino et al. described the stages of PVD based on their OCT based study as:[5]

Stage 0: Absence of PVD.

Stage 1: Incomplete PVD around fovea in less than equal to three quadrants (Fig. 13.2).

Stage 2: Incomplete PVD around fovea in all quadrants with residual attachment at the fovea, optic nerve and mid-peripheral retina.

Stage 3: Incomplete PVD with full separation from fovea but residual attachment at the optic nerve and mid-peripheral retina (Fig. 13.3).

Stage 4: Complete PVD identified with biomicroscopy but not seen on OCT (Fig. 13.4).

The newer SSOCT based classifications takes status of precortical vitreous pocket into consideration:[6]

Stage 0: No PVD with an intact precortical pocket.

Stage 1: Paramacular PVD.

Stage 2: Perifoveal PVD.

Stage 3: Separation from fovea with persistent attachment to the optic disc. (A) Intact precortical vitreous pocket. (B) Break in precortical vitreous pocket.

Stage 4: *Complete PVD*—in this gradual process of vitreous separation, usually liquefaction (synchysis) and collapse (syneresis) go hand in hand. Sebag et al. introduced the concept of anomalous PVD in which liquefaction occurs without complete separation of vitreous from the retina and also may lead to splitting of vitreous cortex in two parts that is *vitreoschisis*.[7]

ANOMALOUS POSTERIOR VITREOUS DETACHMENT

Occurrence of liquefaction more than the vitreoretinal separation leads to anomalous PVD (APVD, Table 13.1 and Flowchart 13.1). If the peripheral adhesions are stronger, APVD leads to retinal tears while if the attachment is stronger at the macula, APVD causes vitreomacular traction syndrome, vitreoschisis, macular holes, epiretinal membrane, diabetic macular edema and new evidence suggests that even

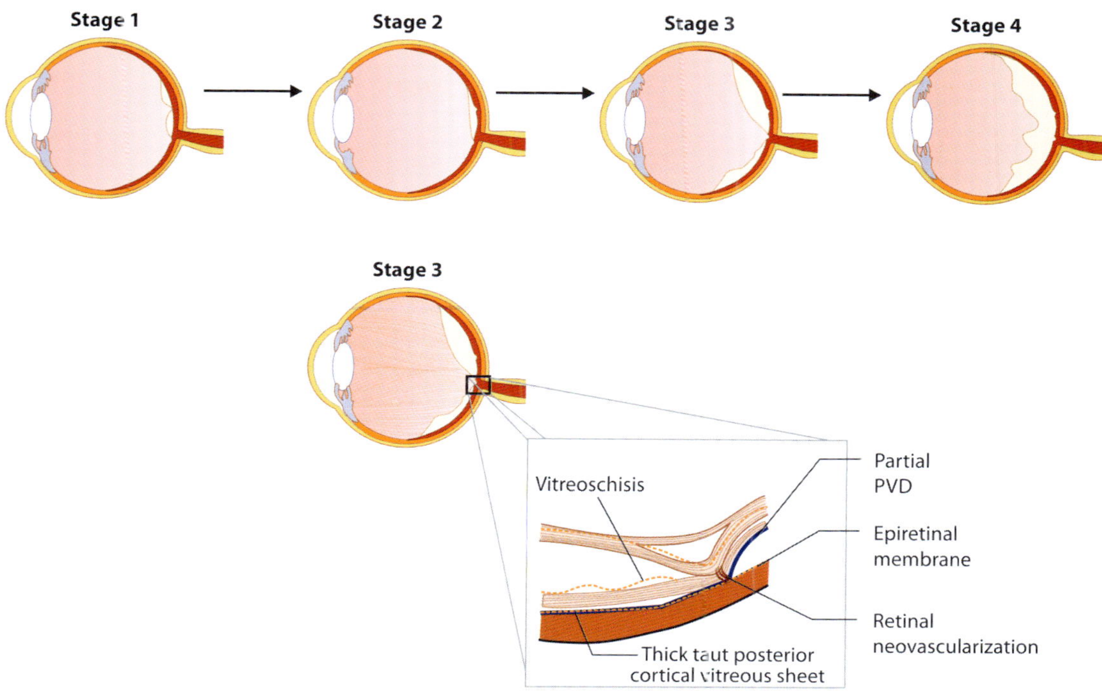

Fig. 13.1: Diagrammatic representation of stages of posterior vitreous detachment (PVD) and anomalous PVD.

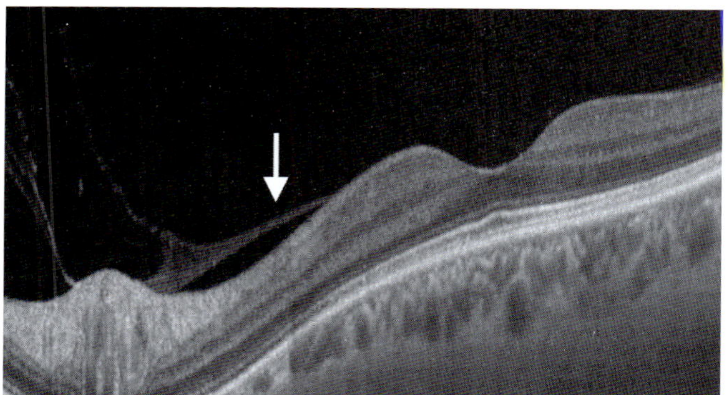

Fig. 13.2: Stage 1 posterior vitreous detachment (PVD) with vitreous separated from zone between disc and macula (white arrow).

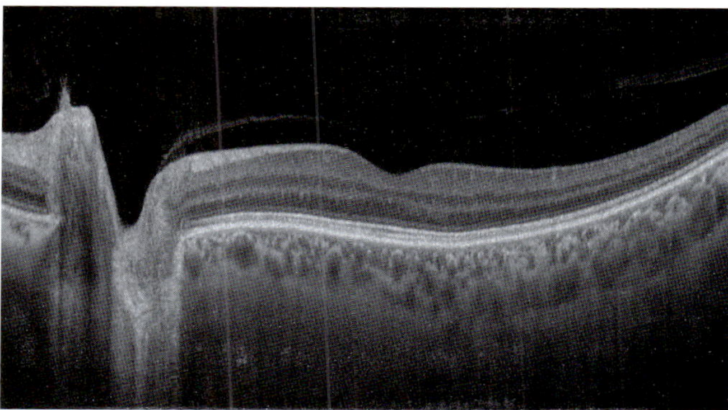

Fig. 13.3: Stage 3 posterior vitreous detachment (PVD) with vitreous separated from fovea but attached to disc.

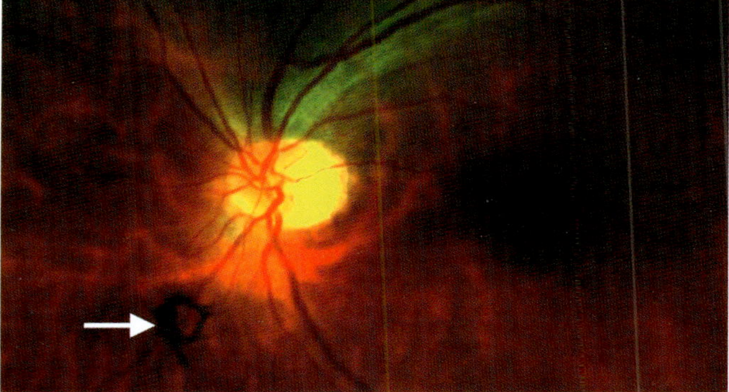

Fig. 13.4: Optomap pseudocolor image showing Stage 4 posterior vitreous detachment (PVD) with Weiss ring visible (white arrow).

Table 13.1: Manifestations of anomalous PVD.

	Possible mechanism	Manifestation of anomalous PVD
Vitreoschisis (Fig. 13.5) (Splitting of posterior vitreous cortex)	Premacular membrane Vitreopapillary adhesion Centrifugal contraction	Macular hole (Fig. 13.6)
	Premacular membrane No vitreopapillary adhesion Centripetal contraction	Macular pucker, ERM (Fig. 13.7)
Partial PVD (No splitting of posterior vitreous cortex)	Peripheral separation Macular traction	VMT syndrome: Focal (Figs. 13.8A and B) and broad based (Fig. 13.9) Exudative AMD (Fig. 13.10)
	Peripheral separation Optic disc traction	Vitreopapillary traction
	Posterior separation Peripheral traction	Retinal tears and detachment

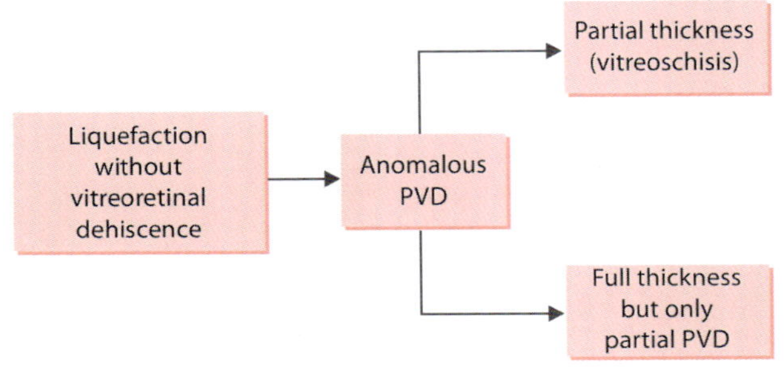

Flowchart 13.1: Classification of anomalous posterior vitreous detachment (PVD).

Source: Sebag J. Anomalous posterior vitreous detachment: a unifying concept in vitreoretinal disease. Graefes Arch Clin Exp Ophthalmol. 2004;242(8):690-8.

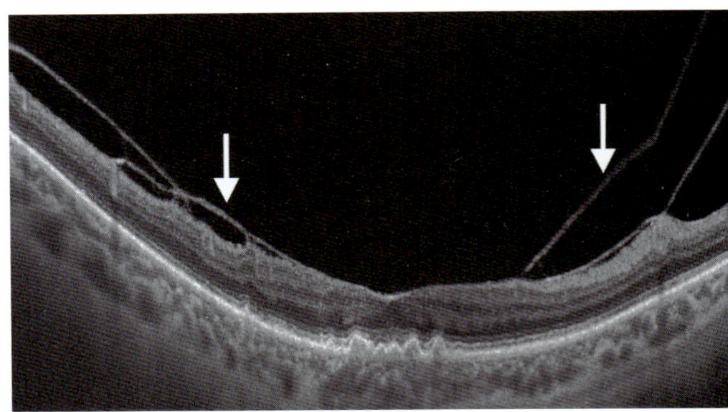

Fig. 13.5: Splitting of posterior vitreous cortex (white arrows)—Vitreoschisis.

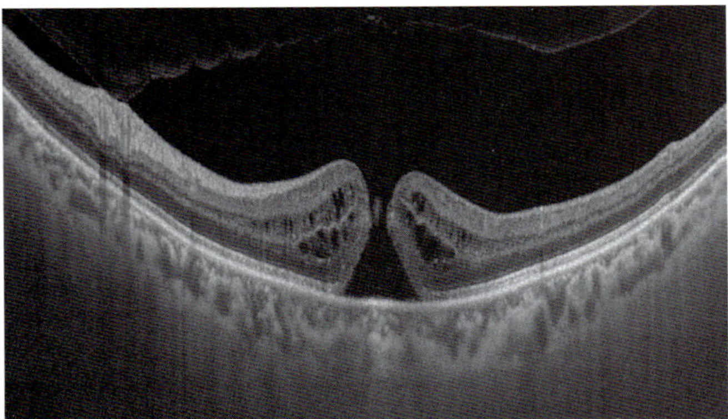

Fig. 13.6: Stage III full thickness macular hole with perifoveal vitreous detachment.

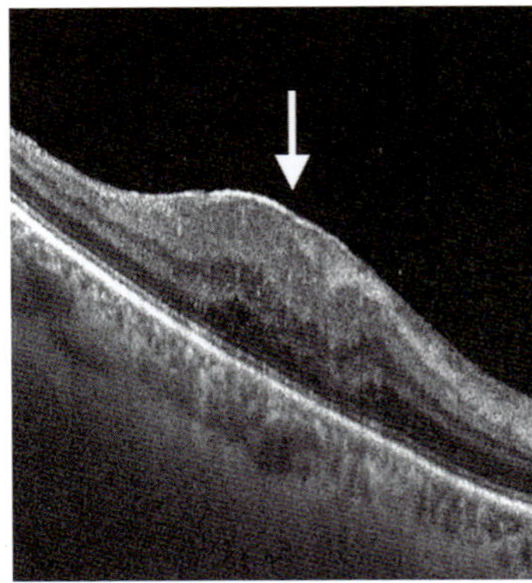

Fig. 13.7: Epiretinal membrane with distorted foveal contour (white arrow).

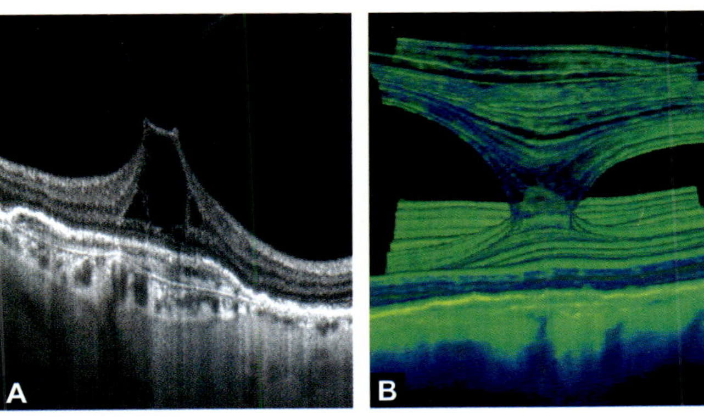

Figs. 13.8A and B: (A) Focal vitreomacular traction (<1,500 µm width). (B) 3-dimensional pseudocolor image of the same.

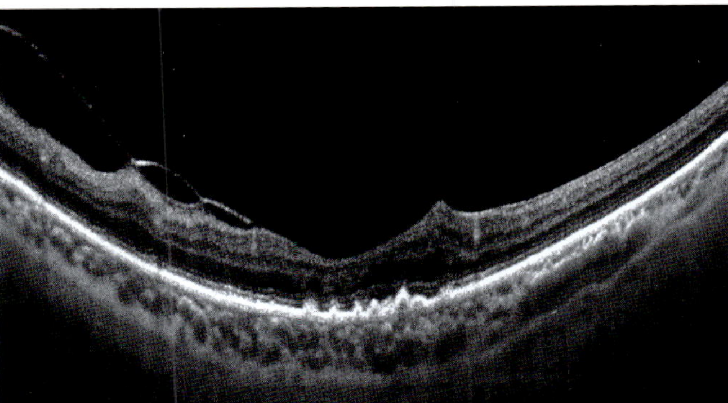

Fig. 13.9: Broad based vitreomacular traction (>1,500 µm width).

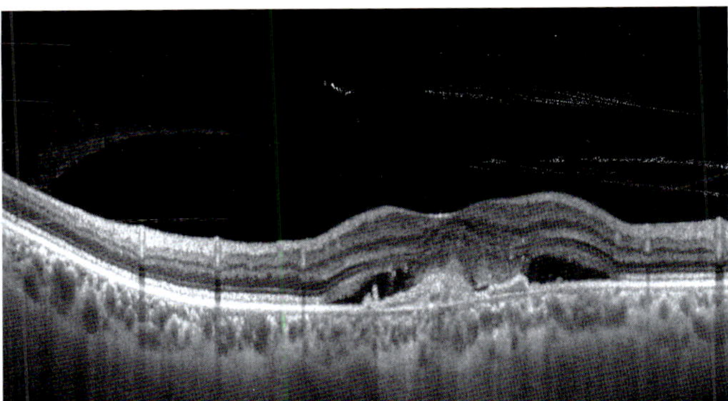

Fig. 13.10: Anomalous posterior vitreous detachment with neovascular age related macular degeneration.

age-related macular degeneration is associated. APVD at the optic disc causes vitreopapillary traction.[7]

MANIFESTATIONS OF ANOMALOUS PVD

The manifestations of anomalous PVD are given in Table 13.1.

ROLE OF OCRIPLASMIN

Ocriplasmin (Jetrea, Thrombogenics USA, 125 µg/0.1 mL) is a truncated form of human plasmin with a molecular weight of 27 KDa which helps in dissolution of laminin and fibronectin which are abundant at the vitreoretinal interface. Thus, helps in pharmacological posterior vitreous detachment. Recently, role of ocriplasmin has been proven in small macular holes and vitreomacular traction syndrome. This drug is yet unavailable in India owing to its high cost.[8] Ocriplasmin may lead

to unexplained visual loss, lens subluxation, alterations in ERG, dyschromatopsia and even, retinal detachments rarely.

KEY POINTS

- Vitreous is composed of 99% water.
- Most common collagen types found in vitreous are II, V, IX and XI.
- Posterior vitreous detachment starts around fovea.
- Vitreous is most strongly attached to retina at vitreous base and optic disc.
- Anomalous PVD is one in which liquefaction is more than vitreoretinal separation.

REFERENCES

1. Ponsioen TL, Hooymans JM, Los LI. Remodelling of the human vitreous and vitreoretinal interface—a dynamic process. Prog Retin Eye Res. 2010;29(6):580-95.
2. Snead MP, Snead DR, James S, et al. Clinicopathological changes at the vitreoretinal junction: posterior vitreous detachment. Eye (Lond). 2008;22(10):1257-62.
3. Mirza RG, Johnson MW, Jampol LM. Optical coherence tomography use in evaluation of the vitreoretinal interface: a review. Surv Ophthalmology. 2007;52(4):397-421.
4. Kishi S. Vitreous anatomy and the vitreomacular correlation. Jpn J Ophthalmology. 2016;60(4):239-73.
5. Uchino E, Uemura A, Ohba N. Initial stages of posterior vitreous detachment in healthy eyes of older persons evaluated by optical coherence tomography. Arch Ophthalmology. 1960. 2001;119(10):1475-9.
6. Itakura H, Kishi S. Evolution of vitreomacular detachment in healthy subjects. JAMA Ophthalmology. 2013;131(10):1348-52.
7. Sebag J. Anomalous posterior vitreous detachment: a unifying concept in vitreoretinal disease. Graefes Arch Clin Exp Ophthalmology. 2004;242(8):690-8.
8. Shaikh M, Miller JB, Papakostas TD, et al. The efficacy and safety profile of ocriplasmin in vitreomacular interface disorders. Semin Ophthalmology. 2017;32(1):52-5.

Chapter 14

Vitreomacular Traction

Atul Kumar, Vineet Mutha, Meghal Gagrani, Kabiruddin Molla

INTRODUCTION

The aging of the eye is associated with liquefaction of the vitreous gel and changes in its structure, leading to separation of the posterior vitreous and hyaloid from the optic nerve and macula. In the sequence of age-related events, the liquefaction of vitreous occurs forming fluid-pockets inside vitreous (synchysis) and the vitreous gel undergoes contraction or condensation (syneresis). This separation starts from the perifoveal region, proceeding to the superior and inferior vascular arcades, fovea, mid-peripheral retina and then, to the optic disc. Subsequently, it may detach anteriorly as far as the vitreous base. This is the course of a normal posterior vitreous detachment (PVD).[1,2] PVD becomes total when the posterior vitreous completely detaches from the optic disc.

The posterior cortical vitreous is bound to the retinal internal limiting membrane (ILM) at their interface by molecular attachment complexes comprising of laminin, fibronectin, chondroitin sulfate, several glycoproteins, various collagen types and other extracellular matrix constituents. However, the vitreoretinal interface is not uniform (Fig. 14.1). Only in certain areas is the vitreous firmly adherent to the underlying retina. The vitreous straddling the ora serrata is one such site

of firm adherence to the underlying retina and pars plana and is referred to as the vitreous base. Areas around the optic disc, fovea and over the posterior pole also have strong attachment of collagen fibers of the vitreous to the ILM.

When the PVD remains incomplete, an initial nonphysiologic asymptomatic persistence of the vitreous leads to vitreomacular adhesion (VMA) which is a transient phase. However, these adhesions can lead to sites of strong vitreoretinal and vitreopapillary attachments causing an anteroposterior traction on the retina by exerting a pull with the means of condensed bands of cortical vitreous. Concurrent condensation and shrinkage of the vitreous gel leads to a tangential traction on the retina. These tractional forces induced by abnormal vitreomacular adherence and incomplete detachment of the posterior vitreous at the macula lead to various morphologic and functional changes at the macula described as vitreomacular traction (VMT) syndrome, a term coined by Reese et al.[3] in 1970 based on their histopathological findings.

ANOMALOUS POSTERIOR VITREOUS DETACHMENT

Abnormal posterior vitreous detachment (PVD) results in premature vitreous liquefaction associated with insufficiently weakened vitreoretinal adhesion. This vitreoretinal traction exerts unequal forces to different places of the retina due to stronger adhesion at several points throughout the fundus where the ILM is thinnest, i.e. at the peripapillary area, along major vessels, at the location of lattice degeneration, enclosed ora bays, retinal tufts, at points of degenerative remodeling or areas of acquired changes such as postinflammatory lesions, at the vitreous base and mainly at the 500 μm foveolar zone and the margin of the 1,500 μm foveal zone.

Anomalous PVD is thus, a unifying concept explaining variety of possible manifestations (Flowchart 14.1) depending upon where the vitreous gel is liquefied and where vitreoretinal adhesion is strong.[3] Macular hole, epiretinal membrane with macular pucker, VMT syndrome, vitreopapillary traction, retinal tears and detachments are commonly encountered in clinical practice due to anomalous PVD.

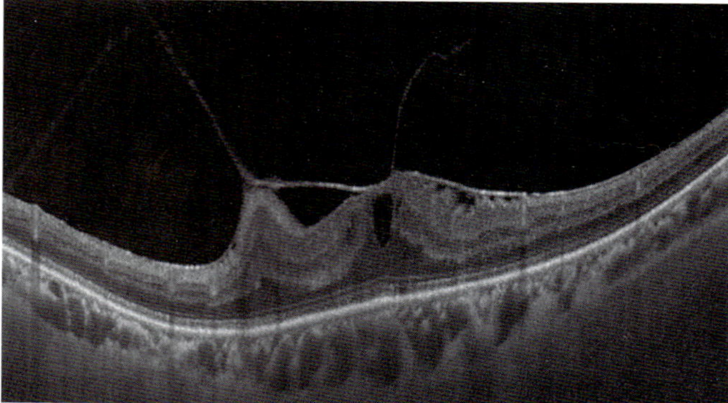

Fig. 14.1: Optical coherence tomography (OCT) shows multiple areas of vitreomacular traction in a diabetic retinopathy eye.

Flowchart 14.1: Schematic diagram demonstrating various manifestations of anomalous PVD.[3]

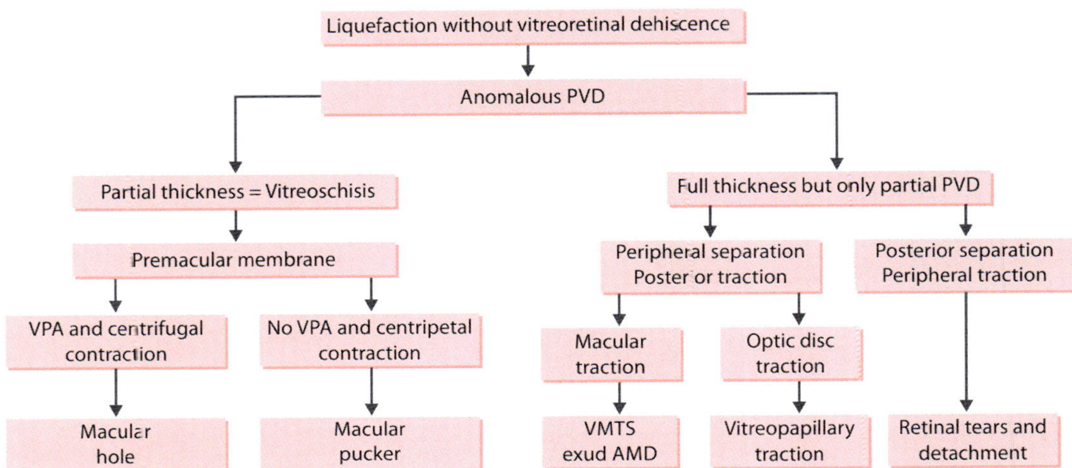

CLASSIFICATION OF DISORDERS OF VITREOMACULAR INTERFACE

Recently, the International Vitreomacular Traction Study (IVTS) Group[4] developed OCT based, strictly anatomic definitions and a classification system for diseases of the vitreomacular interface, like vitreomacular adhesion (VMA), vitreomacular traction (VMT) and macular hole (Tables 14.1 and 14.2).

Vitreomacular Adhesion

The VMA is a perifoveal vitreous detachment and is defined by elevation of the perifoveal cortical vitreous above the retina on at least one OCT B-scan image with persistent vitreous attachment within a 3 mm radius of the fovea in the absence of changes in the contour of the retina.[4] VMA may be subclassified by size of adhesion-focal (less than equal to 1,500 μm) or broad (more than 1,500 μm); and by the presence or absence of concurrent macular abnormalities.[4]

It can be thought to represent that stage in the natural course of PVD, in which the vitreous has partially detached from the perifoveal region but has not yet caused any contour abnormality of retinal surface. Generally, there are no visual symptoms in this stage. Asymptomatic patients found to have VMA are not candidates for any surgical therapy.

Vitreomacular Traction

As PVD progresses, excessive traction may be caused on the macula. Anatomic changes may result in the foveal contour, intraretinal pseudocyst formation, elevation of the fovea from the RPE, an epiretinal membrane (ERM) or a combination that typically results in reduced or distorted vision.[5]

The VMT is defined by these anatomic changes in the contour of the foveal surface without full thickness defects in the retinal layers due to vitreous traction on the macula. OCT findings include anatomic changes with perifoveal posterior vitreous detachment and macular attachment of the vitreous cortex within a 3 mm radius of the fovea. Like VMA, VMT may also be subclassified by size of adhesion—focal (less than equal to 1,500 μm) or broad (more than 1,500 μm); and by the presence or absence of concurrent macular abnormalities. The diameter of the VMA is inversely related to macular morbidity and foveal deformation. Tractional forces at macula are higher for narrower attachments. In diffuse attachments, the tractional forces are distributed beyond the border of the foveal region.[11] Based on this physical theory, focal VMT may lead to MH, tractional CME, and foveal retinal detachment, and broad VMT may lead to ERM and diffuse retinal thickening.

The International Vitreomacular Traction Study Group in 2013 coined an OCT based classification system for clinical evaluation of the vitreoretinal interface.[5]

CLINICAL FEATURES

The VMT syndrome can occur at any age and there is no racial predilection. It affects both sexes, although women show a slightly higher incidence because of premature vitreous liquefaction and an earlier onset of PVD favored by low estrogen postmenopausal state.[6,7]

Cases of VMA remain asymptomatic. The presenting symptoms of VMT include: reduced or blurred vision, metamorphopsia or scotoma. Symptoms have a gradual onset and progression, excepting sudden loss of vision in cases of foveal detachment. VMT was earlier considered an isolated

Table 14.1: OCT based definitions of VMA and VMT.

Entity	Definition (based on at least one OCT B-scan image)	Associated retinal findings	Symptoms
Vitreomacular adhesion (VMA)	Partial vitreous detachment as indicated by: • Elevation of cortical vitreous above the retinal surface in the perifoveal area • Persistent vitreous attachment to the macula within a 3mm radius from the center of the fovea • Acute angle between posterior hyaloid and inner retinal surface • Absence of changes in foveal contour or retinal morphology	None	None
Vitreomacular traction (VMT)	Partial vitreous detachment as indicated by: • Elevation of cortical vitreous above the retinal surface in the perifoveal area • Persistent vitreous attachment to the macula within a 3mm radius from the center of the fovea • Acute angle between posterior hyaloid and inner retinal surface • Presence of changes in foveal contour or retinal morphology (distortion of foveal surface, intraretinal structural changes, such as pseudocyst formation, elevation of fovea above the RPE, or a combination of any of these three features) • Absence of full thickness interruption of all retinal layers	Foveal pseudocyst, macular thickening, retinal capillary leakage, macular schisis, cystoid macular edema, retinal detachment	Reduced or distorted vision

Source: Sebag J. Anomalous posterior vitreous detachment: a unifying concept in vitreoretinal disease. Graefes Arch Clin Exp Ophthalmol. 2004;242(8):690-8.

Table 14.2: OCT based classification of VMA and VMT.[4]

Entity	OCT based classification
Vitreomacular adhesion (VMA)	By size of attachment area: • Focal: Width of attachment less than equal to 1500 µm • Broad: Width of attachment more than 1500 µm By presence of concurrent retinal conditions: • Concurrent: Associated with other macular abnormalities (e.g. age-related macular degeneration, retinal vein occlusion, diabetic macular edema) • Isolated: Not associated with other macular abnormalities
Vitreomacular traction (VMT)	By size of attachment area: • Focal: Width of attachment less than equal to150 µm • Broad: Width of attachment more than 1,500 µm By presence of concurrent retinal conditions: • Concurrent: Associated with other macular abnormalities (e.g. age-related macular degeneration, retinal vein occlusion, diabetic macular edema) • Isolated: Not associated with other macular abnormalities

pathology however, now it is believed to be present in a wide spectrum of macular diseases including MH, cystoid macular edema (CME), ERM, diabetic retinopathy and age-related macular degeneration. We have particularly observed the association of VMT in diabetic retinopathy eyes and surgical removal of the taut attached posterior hyaloid resulted in relief of foveal traction.

Clinically, following signs may be noted in VMT syndrome: cystic changes in the macula (including pseudocyst or macular edema), thick, taut posterior hyaloid membrane, glistening epiretinal membrane, retinal capillary leakage, subretinal or subfoveal fluid, tractional macular schisis, full thickness macular hole or retinal detachment. The detached posterior hyaloid can often be seen clinically. VMT syndrome may be found as an isolated finding or concurrently with macular diseases, such as age-related macular degeneration, retinal vein occlusion, and diabetic macular edema.

INVESTIGATIONS

Optical coherence tomography (OCT) is an excellent noninvasive imaging tool to visualize vitreoretinal interface and is useful for the diagnosis and management of VMT syndromes (Figs. 14.2A and B). A hyper-reflective and thickened band suggesting posterior hyaloid membrane is often seen posterior to hyporeflective vitreous. In VMT, partially detached posterior vitreous can be seen along with persistent vitreous attachment to the fovea or macula and/or the optic disc margin. Changes in the foveal contour may also be visualized on OCT imaging.

A round or diffuse hyper-reflective zone between the photoreceptor inner segment/outer segment junction line and the cone outer segment tip line at the center of the fovea

has been observed in the OCT images of eyes with VMT and ERM. This characteristic sign, termed as the *cotton ball sign* by Tsunoda et al.[8] indicates an inward traction on the fovea and may predict visual impairment.

Much before the present knowledge of OCT evolved, and before the IVTS group defined VMT, Yamada and Kishi[9] described 2 types of vitreous traction profiles in eyes of VMT as per the tomographic features:

- *V shaped*: The vitreous cortex is detached from the retina both temporal and nasal to the fovea, and attached only to the fovea, and this morphology majorly refers to focal VMT.
- *J shaped[6] or arc shaped*: The vitreous cortex is detached from the retina temporal to the fovea, but remains attached attached to the fovea and the retina nasal to the fovea. This mostly refers to broad VMT.

Focal VMT is pathogenic of macular hole formation, tractional cystoid macular edema and foveal detachment (Figs. 14.3A and E), while broad VMT has been seen to be associated with epiretinal membranes, diffuse retinal thickening and impaired foveal depression recovery.[6]

VMA in symptomatic patients has been graded based on SD-OCT[9] as following:

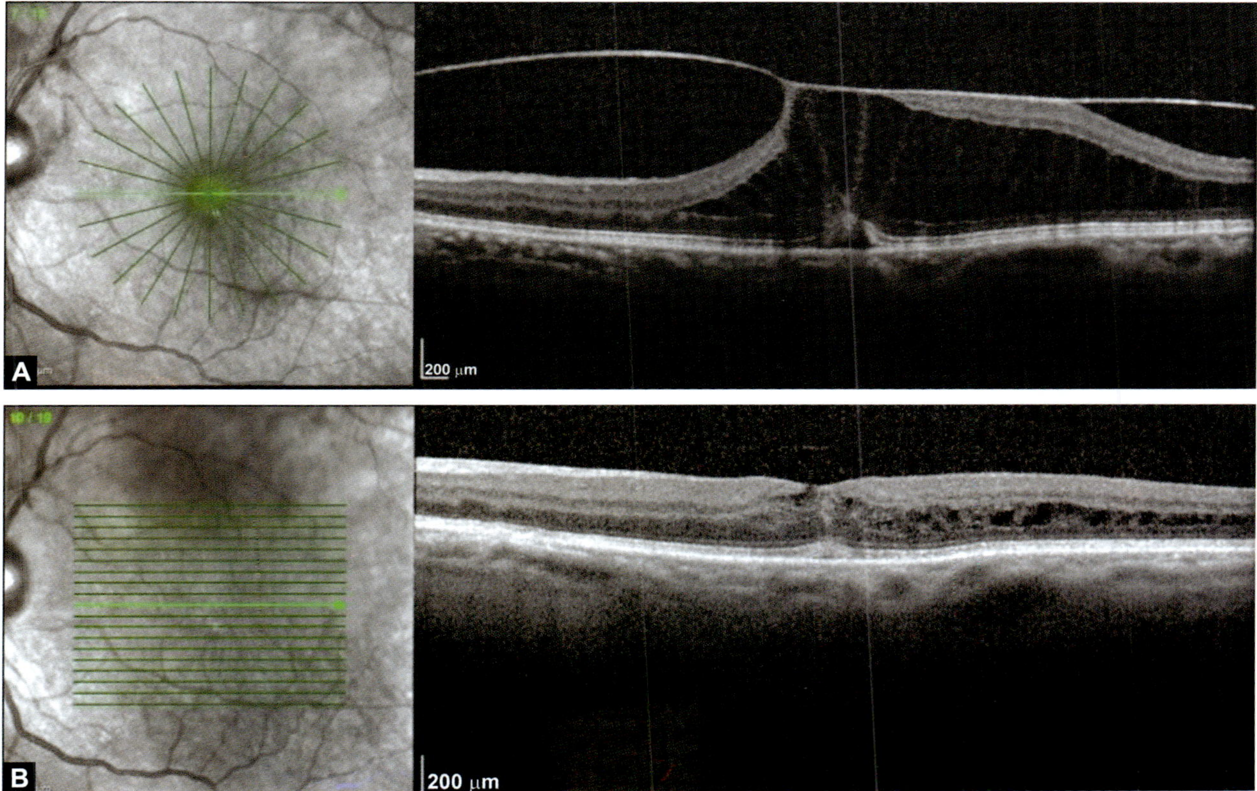

Figs. 14.2A and B: (A) Broad based vitreomacular traction (VMT) visible on optical coherence tomography (OCT) scan of a patient with presenting visual acuity of 4/60; (B) postoperative optical coherence tomography (OCT) findings of patient showing the restoration of normal macular contour with BCVA of 6/9.

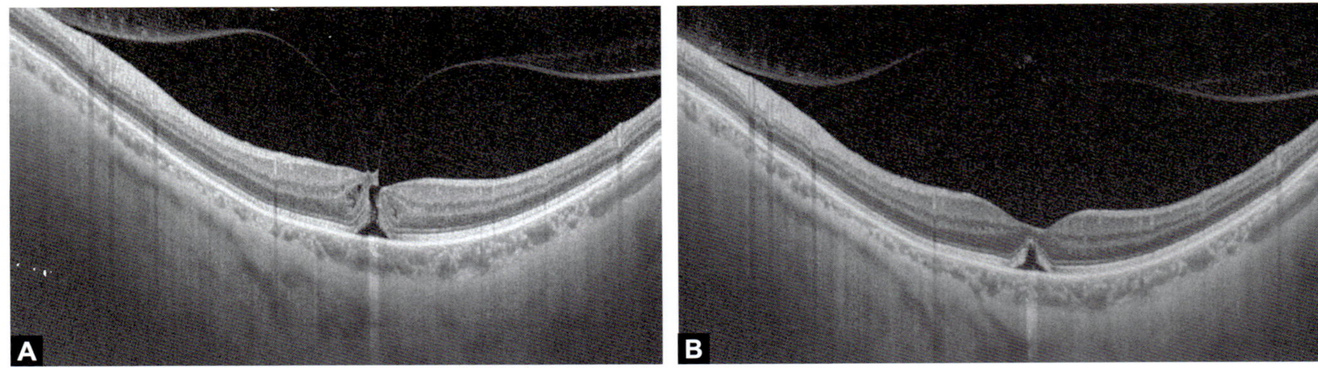

Figs. 14.3A and B: (A) Vitreomacular traction (VMT) with early macular hole formation seen in the initial SS-OCT. Following observation, 2 weeks later OCT revealed release of VMT and closure of hole (B).

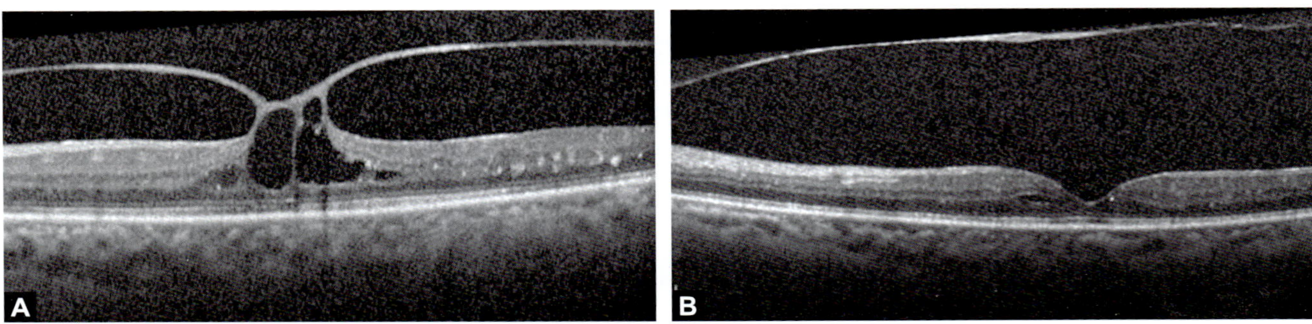

Figs. 14.4A and B: Spontaneous release of broad based vitreomacular traction (VMT) in the above OCT.

- *Grade 1*: Incomplete cortical vitreous separation with attachment at the fovea.
- *Grade 2*: Grade 1 findings plus intraretinal cysts or clefts.
- *Grade 3*: Grade 2 findings plus subretinal fluid.

The en-face OCT imaging technology is also useful for visualizing VMT as it provides not only longitudinal B-scan but also coronal C-scan images of the retina, which help define the lateral extent of the hyaloidal macular traction as sigmoid hyper-reflective bands inside the hyporeflective vitreous chamber.[10] Thus, the C-scan image shows the entire extent of posterior vitreomacular adherence and their relationship with the vascular arcades, the optic disc, and the fovea.[10]

Fluorescein angiography: Fluorescein angiography demonstrates sites of retinal capillary leakage in macula in case of chronic CME and leakage at the optic disc.[11] Fluorescein pooling may be seen in case of associated retinal detachment.[11]

B-scan ultrasonography: A thin, smooth membrane with minimal after-movements seen anterior to the retinal surface and having a focal attachment suggests a partial PVD.

MANAGEMENT

The VMT can be managed using pars plana vitrectomy, pneumatic vitreolysis, enzymatic vitreolysis, and observation.

Observation

Initial observation is generally offered to patients with mild symptoms with VMA/VMT features on SD-OCT, before going for surgical or medical options.[9] Cases with no significant macular changes are often kept under observation. A regular self-assessment using Amsler grid is recommended to such patients to watch for the disease progression. The clinical course of VMT based on observation only may be associated with spontaneous release of traction. Punjabi et al.[13] (2007) reported closure in *stage 2* idiopathic FTMH with VMT as documented by OCT (Figs. 14.4A and B).

Surgery

Pars plana vitrectomy (PPV) is the surgery of choice to relieve all the tractional forces at the vitreoretinal interface (Fig. 14.5). Asymptomatic patients do not have significant benefit from surgical therapy. Functional improvement occurs only after the reconstitution of foveal architecture, which may take months to years. Surgical outcomes vary with duration and type of VMT. PPV is often combined with careful peeling of ERM and ILM, peeling of posterior cortical vitreous, air-fluid exchange which is followed by air or gas tamponade.

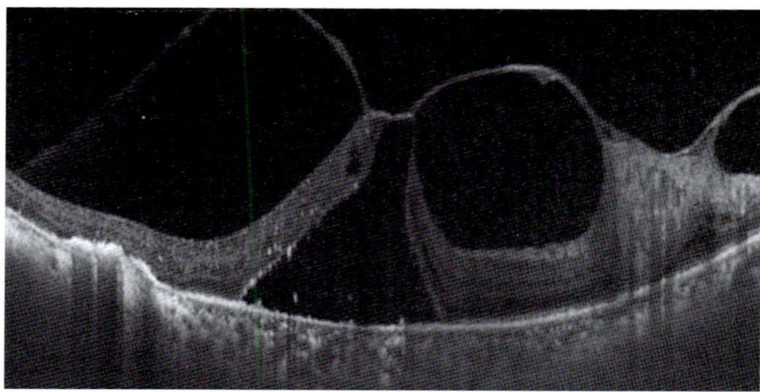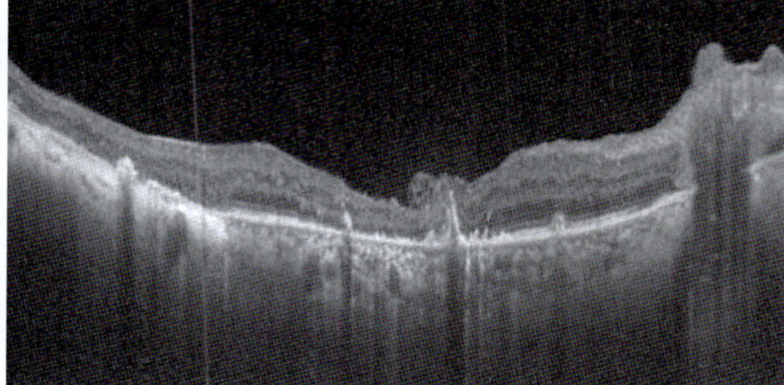

Fig. 14.5: Diabetic vitreomacular traction (VMT) with multiple attachments (A) show complete traction relief postoperatively (B). A small ruff of fibrous tissue over the fovea was left behind as removal could have risks of a macular hole formation. Vision improved from 2/60 to 6/60 at 2 weeks postoperatively.

Enzymatic Vitreolysis

Pharmacologic vitreolysis for VMT syndrome refers to use of enzymatic agents (Table 14.3) which cause induction of vitreous liquefaction and vitreoretinal separation, by creating a cleavage plane between posterior vitreous and retina, in a more safe manner than mechanical means.

These agents when administered in VMT eyes, target the proteins at the vitreoretinal interface which are the sites of action of ocriplasmin, namely laminin, fibronectin and collagen types VI, VII, XVIII.

Ocriplasmin (formerly microplasmin), a recombinant truncated molecular form of human plasmin with proteolytic activity against these anchoring proteins, is used for pharmacologic vitreolysis. It lacks activity against type IV collagen, explaining its targeted action at the vitreoretinal interface without significant toxic damage to the retinal surface. It has been highly expressed in the *Pichia pastoris* yeast expression system and has minimal effective dose of 125 µg.

MIVI-TRUST[12] trial (microplasmin for intravitreal injection-traction release without surgical treatment) is a large randomized controlled phase III clinical trial, comparing intravitreal injection of 125 µg/0.1 mL ocriplasmin versus placebo in patients with symptomatic VMA. Stalmans et al. found statistically significant higher rates of resolution of pathology with ocriplasmin injection, including resolution of VMA.[14] Floaters, photopsia, injection-related ocular pain, or conjunctival hemorrhage, macular hole, retinal tear/detachment and significant unexplained short-term vision loss are the reported side effects with intravitreal ocriplasmin injection. The US Food and Drug Administration (FDA) approved Jetrea (Ocriplasmin, ThromboGenics, Inc., Iselin, NJ) in 2012 for the treatment of patients with symptomatic VMA (i.e. VMT).[15]

Various adverse events with ocriplasmin which are unrelated to vitreous detachment include cataract, increased intraocular pressure and conjunctival hemorrhage. A self-resolving acute, transient visual dysfunction may occur in some patients, although its mechanism of action is not fully understood. Ocriplasmin may have a diffuse enzymatic effect on photoreceptors or the retinal pigment epithelium not limited to areas of VMA. Hence, proper informed consent needs to be taken before such a procedure.

Other pharmacological agents, include liquefactants, such as hyaluronidase and collagenase, act through vitreous liquefaction and interfactants, such as dispase or RGP (arginine-glycine-aspartate) peptides which act through vitreoretinal interface disruption. These agents are nonphysiological and may worsen the existing tractional pathology. Plasmin-based agents have shown some ability to synchronously liquefy vitreous and weaken the vitreoretinal adhesion.

PNEUMATIC VITREOLYSIS

An injection of a gas bubble can lead to syneresis (vitreous collapse) and synchysis (vitreous liquefaction) during the intravitreal gas bubble expansion stage and resulting PVD. A study by Steinle et al. comparing the options of C3F8 gas, SF6 gas and intravitreal ocriplasmin (ARVO 2016 Seattle, May 2 2016. Abstract Number: 1806) showed that C3F8 gas showed a VMT release of 84% compared to SF6 56% release and ocriplasmin 48%. A *dipping bird maneuver*, by bringing your head down repeatedly, accelerated the PVD induction. However, one must be particularly mindful, if one recommends what has not yet been proven (pneumatic vitreolysis), over a proven pharmacological option. We need to provide patients with a comprehensive review of treatment options that is based on the available evidence-based trials.

Table 14.3: Enzymes and effects of pharmacologic vitreolysis.	
Enzyme	*Target*
Chondroitinase	Chondroitin sulfate
Hyaluronidase	Hyaluronan
Dispase	Type IV collagen
Ocriplasmin (Formerly microplasmin)	Laminin and fibronectin

REFERENCES

1. Johnson MW. Posterior vitreous detachment: evolution and complications of its early stages. Am J Ophthalmology. 2010;149(3): 371-82.

2. Flynn HW Jr, Relhan N. The Charles Schepens Lecture: management options for vitreomacular traction: use an individualized approach. Ophthalmology Retina. 2017;1(1):3-7.

3. Reese AB, Jones IS, Cooper WC. Vitreomacular traction syndrome confirmed histologically. Am J Ophthalmology. 1970;69(6):975-7.

4. Sebag J. Anomalous posterior vitreous detachment: a unifying concept in vitreoretinal disease. Graefes Arch Clin Exp Ophthalmology. 2004;242(8):690-8.

5. Duker JS, Kaiser PK, Binder S, et al. The International Vitreomacular Traction Study Group classification of vitreomacular adhesion, traction, and macular hole. Ophthalmology. 2013;120(12):2611-9.

6. Johnson MW. Posterior vitreous detachment: evolution and role in macular disease. Retina. 2012;32(Suppl 2):S174-8.

7. Bottós J, Elizalde J, Arevalo JF, et al. Vitreomacular syndrome. J. Ophthalmic Vis Res. 2012;7(2):148-61.

8. Tsunoda K, Watanabe K, Akiyama K, et al. Highly reflective foveal region in optical coherence tomography in eyes with vitreomacular traction or epiretinal membrane. Ophthalmology. 2012;119(3):581-7.

9. Yamada N, Kishi S. Tomographic features and surgical outcomes of vitreomacular traction syndrome. Am J Ophthalmology 2005;139(1):112-7.

10. John VJ, Flynn HW, Smiddy WE, et al. Clinical course of vitreomacular adhesion managed by initial observation. Retina. 2013;34(3):442-6.

11. Forte R, Pascotto F, de Crecchio G. Visualization of vitreomacular tractions with en face optical coherence tomography. Eye (Lond). 2007;21(11):1391-4.

12. AAO. Diseases of the Vitreous and the Vitreoretinal Interface. In: Retina and Vitreous. Section 12. Basic and Clinical Science Course;2013:302-4.

13. Punjabi OS, Flynn HW Jr, Legarreta JE, et al. Documentation by spectral domain OCT of spontaneous closure of idiopathic macular holes. Ophthalmic Surg Lasers Imaging. 2007;38(4):330-2.

14. Stalmans P, Benz MS, Gandorfer A, et al. Enzymatic vitreolysis with ocriplasmin for vitreomacular traction and macular holes. N Engl J Med. 2012;367(7):606-15.

15. FDA. FDA approves Jetrea for symptomatic vitreomacular adhesion in the eyes. Maryland; US FDA; 2012.

Chapter 15

Epiretinal Membranes

Atul Kumar, Kavitha Duraipandi, Raghav Ravani, Nasiq Hasan

INTRODUCTION

An epiretinal membrane (ERM) is an accumulation of fibro-cellular tissue on the surface of internal limiting membrane of the central retina. Iwanoff first described them as abnormal proliferation of translucent and semi-vascular cellular membranes on the inner retinal surface in 1865.[1]

Since then, numerous other terms have been used to describe this entity including: epimacular membrane, macular pucker, cellophane maculopathy, preretinal macular gliosis/fibrosis and surface-wrinkling retinopathy. All these terms describe the clinicoanatomic morphology of pathologic lesions caused by epiretinal membranes of varying severity and morphological features. Macular epiretinal membranes are clinically considered as a separate entity as compared to proliferative vitreoretinopathy due to their location, clinical features and clinical course.

PATHOPHYSIOLOGY

An ERM develops on the inner retinal surface due to the abnormal fibrocellular proliferation. During the course of posterior vitreous detachment (PVD), schisis of the posterior vitreous may occasionally occur, leaving a sheet of posterior cortical vitreous still adhered to the macula (*vitreoschisis*), over which cellular membranes may proliferate, leading to formation of an ERM. Inflammatory mediators promote such membrane formation.

The origin of these cellular membranes has been debated for long. According to Iwanoff, endothelial cells were responsible for the formation of epiretinal membranes.[1] Smith proposed that the origin of the cells in the membranes was from either the pigmented or nonpigmented cells of the pars ciliaris, retinal pigment epithelium (RPE), mesodermal components of the vascular system, normal vitreous cells and inflammatory cells within the vitreous.[2]

Roth and Foos[3] gave a theory of idiopathic ERM, according to which during acute PVD, migration of glial cells of the superficial retina occurs through micro-breaks in the internal limiting membrane (ILM) at the macular region (where it has relatively tight adherence) followed by proliferation on the surface of the inner retina. Later, fibrocytes and macrophages get further added to these membranes.

In another theory, ERMs that form in eyes having retinal breaks have been thought to depict a milder form of proliferative vitreoretinopathy caused by liberation and proliferation of retinal pigment epithelial cells into the vitreous cavity, along with other cellular constituents to form contractile membranes on the surface of the retina.[4,5]

CLASSIFICATION OF EPIRETINAL MEMBRANES

Epiretinal membranes can either be idiopathic (idiopathic ERMs), which are hypothesized to be caused by an abnormality of the vitreoretinal interface in the setting of anomalous PVD (posterior vitreous detachment) (*see* Chapter 13) or secondary to primary intraocular diseases (secondary ERMs) like rhegmatogenous retinal detachment, vascular occlusions, uveitis, trauma and intraocular surgery (Box 15.1).

Gass proposed a clinical classification of ERM[6] in 1987, where he classified ERMs into three grades:

- *Grade 0: Cellophane maculopathy*, characterized by translucent membranes with no retinal distortion or obscuration of underlying vessels. There may be an irregular reflex, mild sheen or glint, without a distinct edge.
- *Grade 1: Crinkled cellophane maculopathy*, causing an irregular wrinkling of inner retina but underlying vessels are still visible. They show an increased vascular tortuosity, with perimacular vessels seen to be pulled towards an epicenter.
- *Grade 2: Macular pucker with opaque membranes*, causing obscuration of the underlying vessels, more prominent retinal distortion and arcuate vessels seen to be closer together, often leading to foveal ectopia, heterotopia or a shallow retinal detachment.

Another classification system (OCT-based) has been developed by Konicaris V et al.[7] (Box 15.2).

Box 15.1: Etiological classification of ERM.

- Idiopathic
- Secondary
  - Intraocular inflammation, e.g. uveitis
  - Trauma (blunt or penetrating)
  - Iatrogenic (any ocular surgery, laser or cryotherapy)
  - Retinal vascular diseases (vascular occlusions, diabetic retinopathy, etc.)
  - Vitreous hemorrhage
  - Retinal detachment, retinal tears
  - Intraocular tumors

EPIDEMIOLOGY

Idiopathic ERMs are most frequently found to affect individuals over the age of 50 years, with no sexual predilection. Various studies have found the prevalence of ERMs to range between 7–11.8%.[8,9] The incidence of bilaterality is approximately 10–20% and the membranes are usually asymmetric. Secondary ERMs have no correlation with age and sex and are seen in approximately 3–8.5% of patients.

 ## CLINICAL FEATURES

The symptoms vary greatly depending upon the location, nature of the membrane and the degree of architectural disruption of the underlying inner and outer retinal layers.

- Thin membranes outside the macula are often asymptomatic. Such ERMs are mostly nonprogressive or slowly progressive.
- Thick epiretinal membranes within the macula lead to a reduction in visual acuity.
- Anatomic alterations in the macular region lead to significant distortion, binocular diplopia or even macropsia.
- Can be associated with macular edema or (more rarely) a lamellar or full thickness macular hole. In such cases, there may be significant diminution of vision.

DIAGNOSIS

A +90 D slit-lamp biomicroscopy is often used to evaluate the ERM. It is seen as an irregular translucent, glistening layer over the macula, which is best detected by red-free light or monochromatic blue or green light. Retinal distortion can be visualized in the region of ERM. Full thickness retinal folds, macular edema or foveal ectopia may be seen associated with ERM. Advanced membranes are opaque and show distortion of the underlying retinal architecture causing retinal wrinkling, striae and tortuosity of arcade vessels.

Amsler grid may help in subjective evaluation and documentation of metamorphopsia caused by the retinal distortion or macular heterotopia secondary to ERM. The Amsler grid is a grid containing horizontal and vertical lines with a dot in the centre. It is done at 33cms distance. The patient fixates with one eye on the dot as it is a monocular test , and is asked if any of the lines show distortion or are wavy signifying metamorphopsia. Each small square in the grid subtends an

Box 15.2: OCT-based classification of epiretinal membranes.[7]

Category A: with posterior vitreous detachment (PVD)
A1: without contraction of the ERM
A2: with the presence of membrane contraction
- A2.1: with retinal folding
- A2.2: with edema
- A2.3: with cystoid macular edema
- A2.4: with lamellar macular hole

Category B: with no PVD
B1: without vitreomacular traction (VMT)
B2: with VMT
- B2.1: with edema
- B2.2: presenting with retinal detachment
- B2.3: with schisis

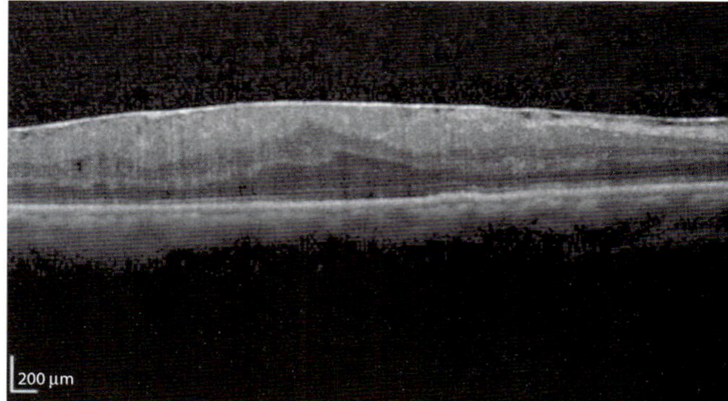

Fig. 15.1: Optical coherence tomography (OCT) showing hyper-reflective epiretinal membrane with distorted retinal architecture.

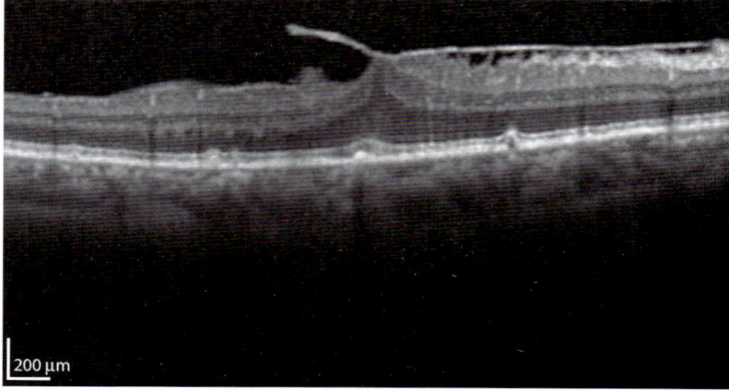

Fig. 15.2: Epiretinal membrane (ERM) with visible wrinkling of the retinal surface and traction at the macula.

angle of 1 degree at the macula. These charts have value in diagnosis, follow-up and deciding management of patients of ERM.

The OCT helps in the evaluation of cases of ERM and helps in deciding the surgical approach. OCT shows a hyper-reflective structure on the inner retinal surface (Fig. 15.1) which may be partially or globally adherent. Loss of foveal contour, cystoid macular edema, pseudohole, macular hole and vitreomacular traction may be delineated easily with the help of OCT (Figs. 15.2 to 15.4).

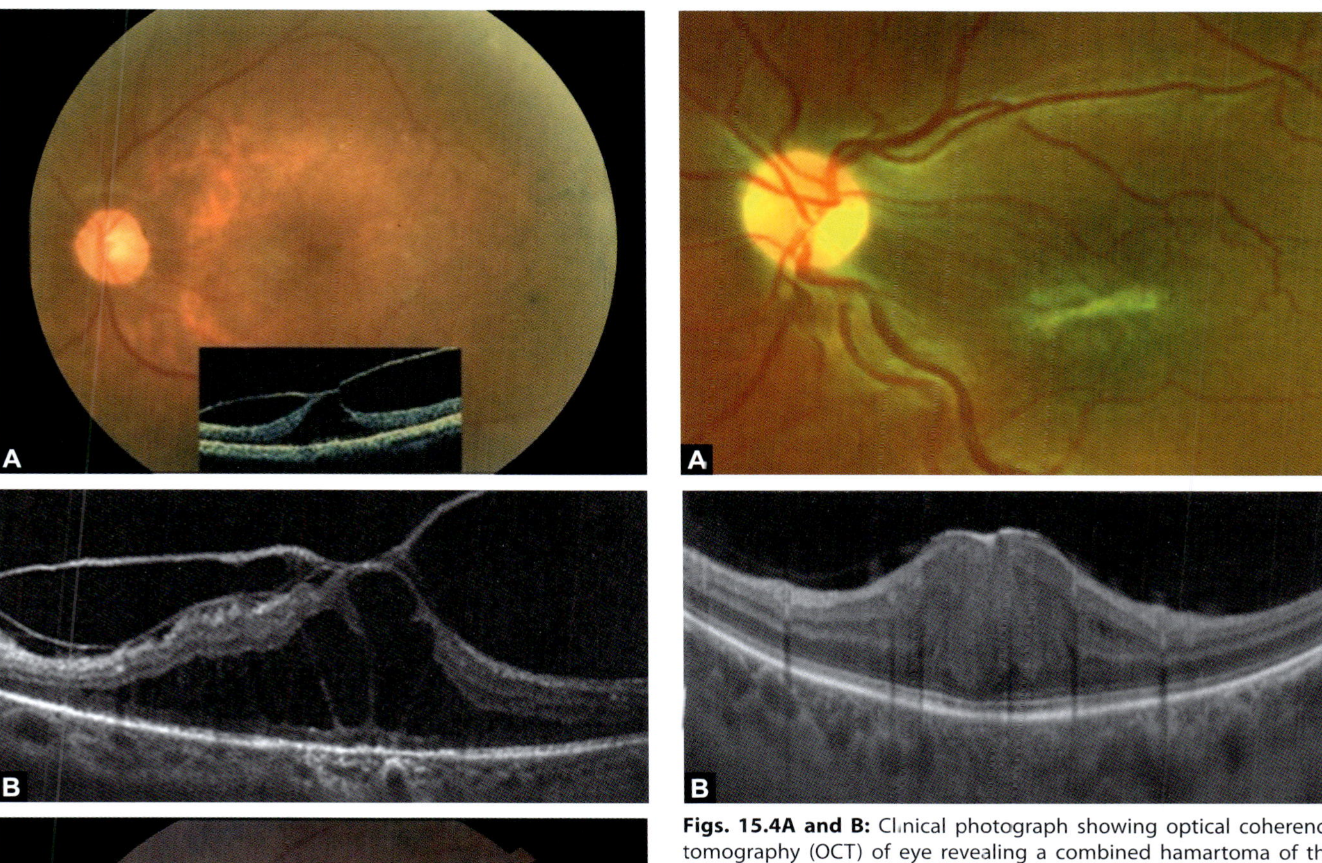

Figs. 15.4A and B: Clinical photograph showing optical coherence tomography (OCT) of eye revealing a combined hamartoma of the retina and retinal pigment epithelium (CHRRPE) with overlying taut epiretinal membrane (ERM) at the macula.

Figs. 15.3 A to C: (A) Fundus photograph of the patient with epiretinal membrane (ERM). Inset shows optical coherence tomography (OCT) image of the patient showing ERM with vitreomacular traction (VMT) with cystic spaces. (B) Preoperative SD-OCT image of the same patient showing ERM with VMT with cystic spaces. (C) Postoperative fundus photograph and SD-OCT image (inset) of the same patient showing restoration of normal foveal contour with resolution of cystic spaces ERM straddling the cystic macula with associated VMT.

On fluorescein angiography, macular leakage, the degree of vascular tortuosity and extent of wrinkling of the inner retina, can be assessed. Vascular leakage is irregular in the region of ERM and thus, helps define anatomic limits of ERM.

It can also help differentiate other differentials, such as subretinal neovascular membranes.

MANAGEMENT AND SURGICAL TECHNIQUES

The majority of patients with ERMs are asymptomatic and hence, no treatment is indicated. Often patients having asymptomatic epiretinal membrane are identified via OCT in primary care optometric and ophthalmologic practices and are referred for evaluation. Rouvas[10] et al. also recommended that monitoring of nontractional epiretinal membranes may be a safe option in patients who are not good surgical candidates thus besides the tractional ERM on OCT, surgery is advocated in patients with reduced visual acuity and metamorphopsia.

Surgical Management

Since the time, Machemer developed the concept of membrane peeling in the mid-1970s, many variations and refinements in techniques as well as instrumentation have been developed.

In this procedure, the outer edge of the membrane is identified and a dissection plane is created with the use of a blunt-tipped pick or a bent needle. Once the edge of the membrane is seen, it may be gently lifted off the retinal surface with the use of a fine forceps or a pick.

The membrane should be lifted tangentially rather than in an anteroposterior direction to avoid pulling on and tearing the underlying retina. This maneuver is relatively simple to perform, if the edge of the membrane is visible.

Presently, the surgical procedure of choice for ERM is: Pars Plana Vitrectomy (Microincision Vitrectomy Surgery or MIVS) with or without brilliant blue G(BBG) assisted peeling of the ERM followed by air/gas tamponade. There is negative staining as the ERM is not stained with BBG dye. However, repeat dye staining (double stain-double peel technique) after ERM removal stains the inner ILM which is then peeled to prevent recurrence of ERM formation over it.

A meta-analysis of epiretinal membrane surgery with and without ILM peeling was performed by Liu et al.,[14] and it was found that patients who underwent ILM peeling had better visual acuity 12 months postsurgery. However, 18 months postoperatively, the meta-analysis of two papers suggested that patients who did not undergo ILM peeling had marginally better visual acuity.[14]

Once the membrane is removed, it is essential for the surgeon to look for any breaks in the retina in the posterior pole as well as in the periphery. Any elegant maneuvers completed to remove the membranes become immaterial if the retina detaches because of a missed break. Indirect ophthalmoscopy combined with careful scleral depression of the anterior retina should be performed to detect peripheral breaks. Breaks which have no subretinal fluid accumulation can be treated by laser retinopexy or cryoretinopexy.

Postoperative Management

The most common postoperative complication that may be seen is the accelerated progression of nuclear sclerosis of the lens, which may occur in as many as 75% eyes over time. Most of these patients may require cataract extraction within 2 years to maximize the advantages afforded by membrane peeling.

Postoperative retinal detachment may be caused either by a missed break or by a new break that formed after further contraction of the remaining anterior vitreous. This detachment occurs in less than 5% patients. 5–10% of idiopathic cases may have recurrence of epiretinal membrane formation but this percentage may be higher in postinflammatory cases.

PROGNOSTIC FACTORS

Different studies have attempted to identify the prognostic factors affecting visual outcomes after surgical management of ERMs. The favorable factors[12] identified include:

- Good preoperative visual acuity.
- Smaller duration of symptoms before surgery.
- Intact foveal autofluoresence.
- Smaller central foveal thickness or central macular thickness at baseline.

- Maintained integrity of the photoreceptor inner/outer segment junction and integrity of cone outer segment tip line at baseline.

With the introduction of higher resolution OCTs, new structural details will be unveiled and other prognostic factors might be found, adding value for better patient counseling regarding decision to operate. However, one should never omit a comprehensive preoperative evaluation (with slit-lamp, indirect ophthalmoscopy, intraocular pressure, visual acuity evaluation and metamorphopsia and other symptoms evaluation) in the decision making.[11] Although improvement in visual acuity is achieved in most cases, it is often difficult to completely eliminate metamorphopsia.

Some surgeons have advocated membranectomy in non-vitrectomized eyes[13] for macular pucker. Since the rate of cataract formation after vitrectomy is very high, this technique aims to prevent cataract progression because the surgeon does not perform vitrectomy. Long-term safety and efficacy are still awaited. ERM recurrence rate was also found to be higher than normal.[12]

ROLE OF CHROMOVITRECTOMY IN ERM REMOVAL SURGERY (TABLE 15.1)

- *Triamcinolone acetonide*: Its crystals bind avidly to the vitreous gel, enabling visualization of a clear contrast between empty portions of the vitreous cavity and areas where vitreous is still present. Triamcinolone acetonide is injected into the vitreous cavity toward the area to be visualized [0.1–0.3 mL, 40 mg/mL (4%) concentration] and highlights posterior hyaloid very well.
- *Indocyanine green (ICG):* This is a water-soluble tricarbocyanine dye useful to stain the internal limiting membrane (ILM) as it provides adequate contrast between the stained ILM and the unstained underlying retina. Long exposure of retinal pigment epithelium (RPE) cells to ICG may have a RPE-damaging effect, which is a dose-dependent toxicity. It is advisable to use ICG only in low concentrations (0.5 mg/mL (0.05%) or less) and with an osmolarity of approximately 290 mOsm.
- *Infracyanine green:* Iodine and its derivatives may be toxic to the RPE. Therefore infracyanine green (IFCG), a dye free of iodine in its formulation and physiologic osmolarity is believed to have less potential for RPE toxicity than ICG. Due to its better safety profile, IFCG may represent an alternative to ICG during ILM peeling in chromovitrectomy.
- *Trypan blue*: Visualization of ERMs can also be made easy with the use of trypan blue 0.15% solution. The blue stained epiretinal membranes, against the unstained retina can then be atraumatically peeled off. This facilitates visualization of associated macular hole and improves safety of the surgical procedure. In order to enhance the staining properties of trypan blue, the dye is injected after fluid air exchange or it may be mixed with glucose 5-10% to create a *heavy* trypan blue, which is denser than bal-

Table 15.1: Agents currently used for chromovitrectomy during vitreoretinal surgery.

Dye (concentration)	Premacular membrane	ILM	Vitreous	Mode of application*	Comments
ICG (0.5–0.05%)	—	Selective +++	—	Usually fluid-filled globe	Question of toxicity, off-label
Brilliant blue G (0.025%)	—	Selective ++	—	Fluid-filled globe (if heavy BBG is used)	Approved in Europe
Trypan blue (0.15%)	+++	(+)	(+)	Fluid- or air-filled globe	Approved in Europe
Triamcinolone acetonide	—	Nonselective (+)	+++	Fluid-filled globe	Not a dye, pharmacologic properties
Fluorescein	—	—	+	Intravitreal, intra-venous, or perioral application	

*Surgical technique may vary depending on individual surgeon preference.

anced salt solution. However, higher glucose concentration should be avoided because glucose 50% has a highly toxic osmolarity of 2,020 mOsm/L. It is recommended that trypan blue be used mainly for ERM staining as it has particular affinity for epiretinal glial tissues such as the ERM. It is suggested to mix 0.3 mL of trypan blue with 0.1 mL of glucose 10%, resulting in a 1 mg/mL (0.1%) solution with an osmolarity of 300 mOsm.

- *Brilliant blue G (BBG or ILM-Blue):* This relatively safe dye helps to stain the ILM preferentially, though not the ERM. This helps in identifying the ILM as a negative stain and helps in its complete removal. In humans, brilliant blue causes adequate ILM staining (*see* Figs. 15.3A to C) in an iso-osmolar solution of 0.25 mg/mL (0.025%) to 0.50 mg/mL (0.05%) with good clinical results and no signs of toxicity on multifocal electroretinogram. This stain has become a good alternative to ICG and IFCG in chromo vitrectomy because of its remarkable affinity for the ILM. We consider this dye, the best one for ILM peeling in macular hole surgery. It thus provides a negative staining to an ERM by staining the adjacent ILM and hence aids in removal of the ERM also. Double staining can further be performed as described later.
- *Membrane Blue-Dual* (Membrane Blue-Dual™ DORC International, Zuidland, Netherlands) is a dye to stain both the ILM as well as the ERM and consists of a combination of trypan Blue 0.15%+ BBG 0.025% + 4% PEG. Due to a new integrated carrier 4% PEG solution, it can be injected in a BSS filled eye and sinks immediately as a cohesive ball without diffusion throughout the whole globe.

Double Staining Technique

The double staining technique described by Shimada and colleagues[15] involves negative staining of the overlying ERM, which does not actually stain but is visible against a sur-rounding blue stained ILM. The unstained ERM is first peeled off and then, BBG dye is injected a second time to stain the unstained ILM now, unmasked after peeling of ERM. This technique is effective in removal of both the ERM and the ILM. Various studies have found less recurrence of ERM with this technique as ILM provides a scaffold "causing" recurrence of macular pucker. Few surgeons prefer not to peel the ILM to improve visual outcomes and avoid mechanical damage to the retina.

Use of intraoperative optical coherence tomography system (Rescan 700 IOCT™, Carl Zeiss Meditech, Germany) gives real-time imaging of the membranes peeled and has revolutionized macular surgeries. It helps the surgeon to assess the area and strength of the vitreomacular adhesion. It enables one to identify and carefully peel the membranes without de-roofing any foveal cyst. Early normalization of the retinal contour can be seen after removal of the membranes.

REFERENCES

1. Iwanoff A. Beitrage zur normalen und pathologischen anatomie des auges. Graefes Arch Clin Exp Ophthalmology. 1865;11:135-70.
2. Smith TR. Pathologic findings after retina surgery. In: Schepens C (Ed). Importance of the vitreous body in retina surgery with special emphasis on reoperations. St Louis: CV Mosby; 1960. pp. 61-75.
3. Foos RY. Vitreoretinal juncture—simple epiretinal membranes. Graefes Arch Clin Exp Ophthalmology. 1974;189(4):231-50.
4. Cherfan GM, Smiddy WE, Michels RG, et al. Clinicopathologic correlation of pigmented epiretinal membranes. Am J Ophthalmology. 1988;106(5):536-45.
5. Smiddy WE, Maguire AM, Green WR, et al. Idiopathic epiretinal membranes. Ultrastructural characteristics and clinicopathologic correlation. Ophthalmology. 1989;96(6):811-20.
6. Gass JD. Stereoscopic Atlas of Macular Diseases: Diagnosis and treatment, 2nd edition. St Louis: CV Mosby; 1977.
7. Konidaris V, Androudi S, Alexandridis A, et al. Optical coherence tomography-guided classification of epiretinal membranes. Int Ophthalmology. 2015;35(4):495-501.

8. Klein R, Klein BE, Wang Q, et al. The epidemiology of epiretinal membranes. Trans Am Ophthalmology Soc. 1994;92:403-25.

9. Mitchell P, Smith W, Chey T, et al. Prevalence and associations of epiretinal membranes. The Blue Mountains Eye Study, Australia. Ophthalmology. 1997;104(6):1033-40.

10. Rouvas A, Chatziralli I, Androu A, et al. Long-term anatomical and functional results in patients undergoing observation for idiopathic nontractional epiretinal membrane. Eur J Ophthalmology. 2016;26(3):273-8.

11. Machemer R. Die chirurgische entfernung von epiretina en makul-amembranen (macular puckers). Klin Monatsbl Augenheilkd. 1978;173:36-42.

12. Miguel AI, Legris A. Prognostic factors of epiretinal membranes: A systematic review. J Fr Ophtalmol. 2017;40(1):61-79.

13. Sawa M, Ohji M, Kusaka S, et al. Nonvitrectomizing vitreous surgery for epiretinal membrane long-term follow-up. Ophthalmology. 2005;112(8):1402-8.

14. Liu H, Zuo S, Ding C, et al. Comparison of the effectiveness of pars plana vitrectomy with and without internal limiting membrane peeling for idiopathic retinal membrane removal: a meta-analysis. J Ophthalmology. 2015;97:45-68.

15. Shimada H, Nakashizuka H, Hattori T, et al. Double staining with brilliant blue G and double peeling for epiretinal membranes. Ophthalmology. 2009;116(7):1370-6.

Chapter 16

Macular Hole

Atul Kumar, Raghav Ravani, Manasa S, Aman Kumar, Ankita Srivastava

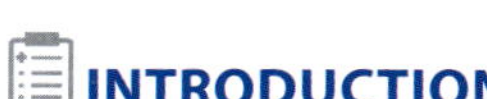

INTRODUCTION

Macular holes are characterized by the absence of neurosensory retinal tissue at the fovea. The peak incidence of idiopathic macular hole occurs in 6–8 decades of life, affecting women more frequently than men. It occurs earlier in myopic eyes. Most of the cases are idiopathic and age related. Other causes include trauma,[1] chronic cystoid macular edema (CME), laser treatment,[2] retinal vascular disease,[3] retinal detachment repair,[4] lightning, and electrocution.[5] A single case of live intravitreal cysticercosis with full thickness macular hole has also been reported recently.[6]

The Eye Disease Case-Control Study Group reported that the incidence of idiopathic macular holes are more in women (72%) and over 50% of patients are in 65–74 years age group.[7] The risk of involvement of the fellow eye is estimated to be ~10–15% at 5 years.[8,9] Once complete posterior vitreous detachment (PVD) occurs, the risk of occurrence of macular hole decreases.[10,11]

The first reported case of a macular hole was reported by Knapp in 1869 in a patient who had sustained a severe contusion.[1] These early reports were related only to traumatic cases. The first nontraumatic case was reported by Kuhnt.[12]

PATHOGENESIS

Vitreomacular traction has been said to be the factor behind idiopathic macular holes. Idiopathic macular hole results from the earliest stage of PVD. The age and sex prevalence of this disease are similar to those of PVD. Macular hole is a full thickness retinal defect at the fovea. The glial cells extend across the retinal surface along the margins of the hole in continuity with an adjacent epiretinal membrane (ERM). Cystic changes occur in the outer plexiform layer in the parafoveal retina.[13,14] The retinal pigment epithelial cells in the area of the hole accumulate lipofuscin and lose their apical microvillous processes.

Various theories have been proposed to explain the pathogenesis of macular hole formation.

Vascular Theory

This theory was given by Coats and Kuhnt. It relates macular hole to a degenerative process, possibly due to vascular insufficiency in the macular area.[15]

Traumatic Theory

It was very popular in late 19th century. It suggested that the mechanical waves caused by vitreous led to macular necrosis and laceration. Posttraumatic cystic degeneration and coalescence of the cysts was implicated in the pathogenesis of traumatic macular holes.

Vascular and Cystoid Degeneration Theory

It was proposed by Coats in 1907. It suggested cystic retinal changes caused by trauma and other mechanisms are responsible for the macular hole formation. Cystoid degeneration with secondary hole formation is described in various conditions like vascular occlusions, severe hypertension, and solar maculopathy.[14]

The Vitreous Theory

In 1912, Zeeman described the histopathology of premacular vitreous condensation. Aaberg and Lister noted that anteroposterior vitreous traction leads to tractional macular detachment, cystoid macular degeneration and subsequent macular hole formation.

Gass hypothesized that tangential traction from Müller cell proliferation and contraction of the vitreoretinal interface contributes to macular hole formation.[16]

Recent hypotheses suggest interplay between the oblique or anteroposterior traction via a persistent vitreofoveal attachment, tangential vitreoretinal traction and involutional changes in the inner retinal layers.

Jensen and Larsen suggested that the lateral displacement of foveal photoreceptors led to the development of macular holes by using binocular kinetic perimetry.[17] Lateral displacement of photoreceptors result in a "pin cushion" distortion in macular holes.

Morgan and Schatz have proposed a mechanism of involutional macular thinning which combines vitreous, vascular and cystic degeneration theories.[12] Gass and Johnson in 1988 gave a comprehensive classification for idiopathic macular holes.

CLINICAL STAGING OF MACULAR HOLE FORMATION

Clinical stages of idiopathic macular hole was originally described by Gass and Johnson and updated subsequently.[16] The stages of macular hole formation are described below (Figs. 16.1A to D):

Stage 1A (Impending Hole)

On slit lamp biomicroscopy, a yellow spot about 100–200 micron in diameter is seen on the foveola. The foveal contour is lost giving a foveal reflection. There is no vitreo-foveolar separation.

Anatomic interpretation: Spontaneous tangential traction of the prefoveal cortical vitreous causes foveolar detachment creating an intraretinal yellow spot. This finding is not pathognomonic of macular hole formation as this is also seen in cases of central serous chorioretinopathy, CME, and acute maculopathy resulting from sun gazing.

Stage 1B (Occult Hole)

On slit lamp biomicroscopy, a yellow ring approximately 200–300 micron in diameter is seen on the foveola. It is associated with loss of foveolar depression with no vitreo-foveolar separation.

Anatomic interpretation: The foveal serous detachment elevates the surrounding perifoveal retina elongating the periumbal fovea forming an impending hole. The centrifugal displacement of the photoreceptors, xanthophyll and radiating nerve fibers leads to a localized dehiscence in the deeper retinal layers. Since the overlying internal limiting membrane (ILM), horizontal processes of Muller cells, and prefoveolar vitreous remains intact, the hole is not appreciated on clinical examination (occult hole). This finding appears to be specific for macular hole formation.

Stage 2

Small full thickness retinal defect less than 400 microns is seen as a central circular defect with an elevated retinal rim.

Anatomic interpretation: A dehiscence occurs in the contracted prefoveolar vitreous bridging the occult retinal hole making the retinal defect clinically appreciable. Spontaneous separation of vitreous from fovea may occur forming a pseudo-operculum. There is no loss of foveolar retina and no PVD.

Stage 3

A full thickness retinal defect greater than 400 microns diameter with a rim of elevated retina is seen corresponding to

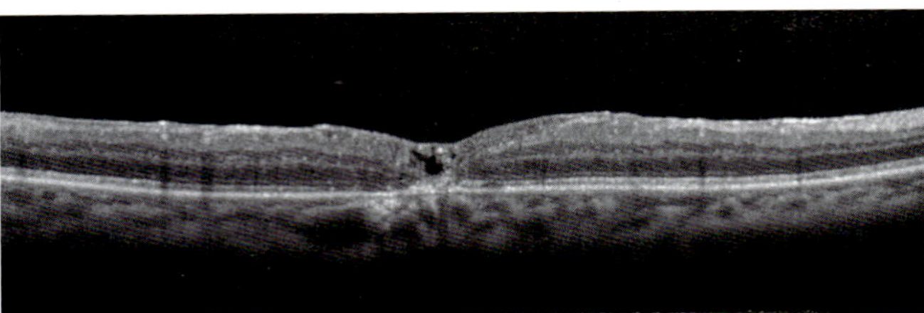

Fig. 16.1A: Spectral domain-optical coherence tomography scan of a stage 1 macular hole.

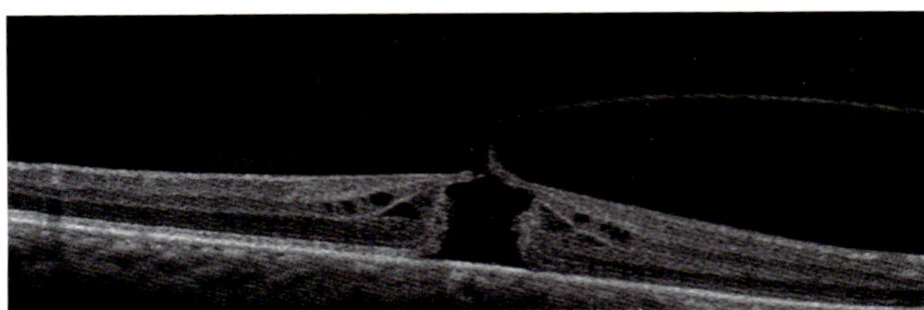

Fig. 16.1B: Spectral domain-optical coherence tomography scan of a stage 2 macular hole depicting a full thickness hole with an operculum and attached posterior hyaloid (Post vitreomacular traction early stage 2 macular hole).

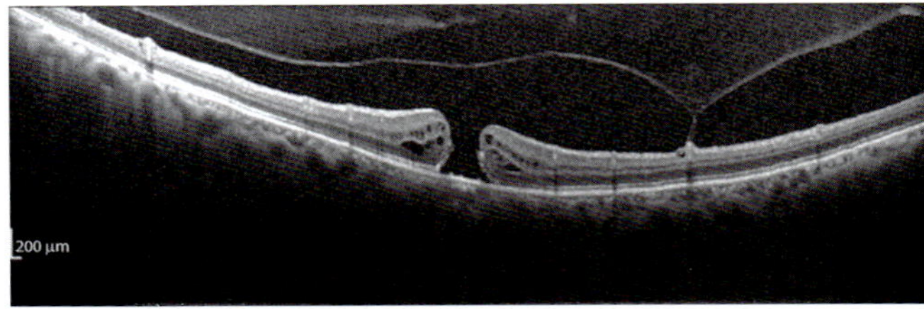

Fig. 16.1C: Spectral domain-optical coherence tomography scan of a stage 3 macular hole with incomplete posterior vitreous detachment.

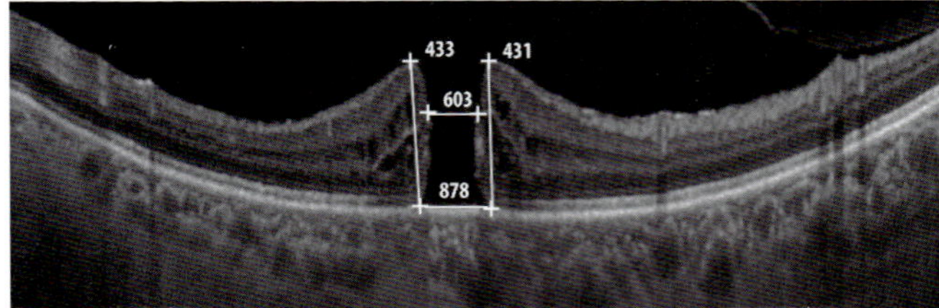

Fig. 16.1D: Spectral domain-optical coherence tomography image of a stage 4 macular hole depicting the completely detached posterior vitreous with detached operculum.

the surrounding cuff of fluid and edema. A prefoveolar opacity (pseudo-operculum) may or may not be associated.

Anatomic interpretation: A full thickness hole with vitreo-foveal separation with incomplete PVD.

Stage 4

Full thickness hole with a rim of elevated retina and a complete PVD is classified under stage 4. Anterior displacement of the pseudo-operculum may be noted in this stage.

Anatomic interpretation: A full thickness hole with complete PVD.

Based on their findings, Gass concluded that apart from anteroposterior traction, a tangential traction was also responsible in the pathogenesis of idiopathic macular hole.

The International Vitreomacular Traction Study Group has classified that macular holes as small, medium and large.[18] If the minimum linear dimension is less than or equal to 250 μm, it is classified as small macular hole. They are associated with 100% closure rate after vitrectomy and they are most responsive to pharmacological vitreolysis among all the full-thickness macular hole (FTMH). FTMH with minimum dimension between 250 μm and 400 μm are classified as medium and are associated with more than 90% closure rate with vitrectomy alone. FTMH with minimum linear dimension more than 400 μm at the time of diagnosis are classified as large. They have 90–95% closure rate with vitrectomy and ILM peeling and 75% with vitrectomy alone. They further classified macular holes depending on the presence or absence of vitreomacular traction as primary and secondary. Primary FTMH occurs due to vitreous traction on fovea from an anomalous PVD. Secondary FTMH is caused by pathologies other than vitreomacular traction including high myopia, blunt trauma, lightning strikes, macular schisis, best disease, macular telangiectasia, anti-vascular endothelial growth factor therapy in neovascular age-related macular degeneration, retinal vascular occlusions, diabetic macular edema, and uveitis.

 ## CLINICAL FEATURES

Symptoms

Patients with macular hole who are symptomatic present with a variable degree of central visual loss depending on the size of the hole, the location of the hole relative to the foveola, and the size of any associated neurosensory retinal detachment. Some patients are completely asymptomatic when the macular hole is diagnosed on routine ophthalmological examination. They may present with central scotoma and metamorphopsia as well.

Signs

The best way to examine a macular hole is on a slit lamp biomicroscopy using a contact or a noncontact lens. Biomicroscopy with 90D lens is the investigation of choice.

In patients with a stage 1 macular hole, a yellow spot (stage 1A) or yellow ring (stage 1B) is visualized in the center of the fovea. Stage 2 macular holes are characterized by a FTMH less than 400 μm in diameter. Stage 3 macular holes are larger than 400 μm in diameter and may have an associated cuff of subretinal fluid with no Weiss ring. Stage 4 macular holes are similar to stage 3 holes except that a total PVD (Weiss ring) is present (Fig. 16.2). The base of the hole may contain yellow-white deposits which may represent lipofuscin-laden macrophages or proliferation of retinal pigment epithelium (RPE). There may be overlying operculum suggesting a vitreofoveolar separation.

Traumatic macular holes can be identified by their irregular edges and absence of PVD (Fig. 16.3). It is usually associated with other injuries such as commotio retinae, massive vitreous hemorrhage, hyphema, chorioretinal atrophy, choroidal rupture, angle recession, peripheral retinal breaks, and traumatic retinal detachment.

Differentiating a true macular hole from a pseudo hole can be done with a slit beam or laser aiming beam test.

The Watzke-Allen test is performed on the slit lamp by placing the macular lens and by aiming a narrow slit beam centered over the macular hole. This beam in a case of

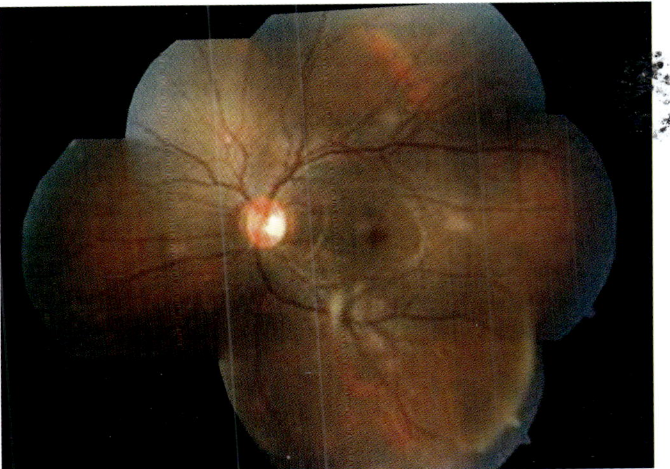

Fig. 16.2: Color fundus photograph of right eye of a patient with idiopathic macular hole depicting the full thickness foveal defect with bare retinal pigment epithelium and surrounding cuff of fluid.

Fig. 16.3: Color fundus montage depicting a traumatic macular hole. The choroidal rupture is visible in the montage and is an association with the traumatic hole.

macular hole will be perceived as being bent, pinched, or interrupted. This is reported as a positive test. If negative with vertical beam, a horizontal beam can be tried.

In the laser aiming beam test, a 50-μm laser aiming beam when projected into the macular hole will not be perceived.

INVESTIGATIONS AND DIAGNOSIS

Optical Coherence Tomography

It is a high resolution imaging technique that helps us to image both the neurosensory retina and vitreoretinal interface.[19] Optical coherence tomography (OCT) has specifically improved the visualization of very shallow detachments of the posterior hyaloid over the macula. Gaudric et al.[20] utilized OCT to study eyes with macular holes as well as the fellow eyes to detect the initial stages of vitreous separation. They found that initial stages of vitreous separation occurred in the peripheral portion of the macula which then later spread throughout the macula with the hyaloid attached to the foveola and the optic disc.

Optical coherence tomography helps us to differentiate true macular holes from pseudoholes, lamellar holes and cystic lesions of the macula (Figs. 16.4A and B). It helps us to know the status of the vitreoretinal interface helping us to plan our management. OCT has immensely improved visualization of very shallow detachments of the posterior hyaloid over the macula. Associated ERMs can be easily picked up.

Fundus Autofluorescence

Autofluorescence has more of a prognostic value in macular holes. A full thickness macular hole appears hyperautofluorescent at fovea due to the absence of macular pigments. An operculum if present would give rise to a shadow effect on fundus autofluorescence. The surrounding subretinal fluid appears hypoautofluorescent due to attenuation of light that reaches the RPE (Fig. 16.5). A healthy RPE on fundus autofluorescence indicates a better anatomical outcome after surgery. Successful surgical closure would result in the disappearance of the hyperautofluorescence as RPE is again covered by retinal/glial tissue.

Fluorescein Angiography

In stage 1, faint hyperfluorescence or no abnormality at all is seen on fluorescein angiography. In stage 2 hole, a round area of window defect may or may not be seen. Stage 3 and 4 holes typically produce a window defect with early transmission of fluorescence in phase with choroidal filling. No late leakage of the dye is seen.

B-scan Ultrasonography

Vitreoretinal surgical observations of eyes with stage 1 or stage 2 macular holes was done by Johnson and coworkers utilizing the B-scan ultrasonography[21] showing a shallow, localized detachment of perifoveal vitreous typically extending to the temporal vascular arcades. The findings of Gaudric and Johnson and coworkers on OCT and ultrasonography gave a new way to a modified theory of anteroposterior traction, not the tangential traction as suggested by Gass.

Microperimetry

It provides a topographic mapping of the retinal sensitivity and also aids in mapping of absolute and relative scotomas in macular holes both preoperatively and postoperatively.

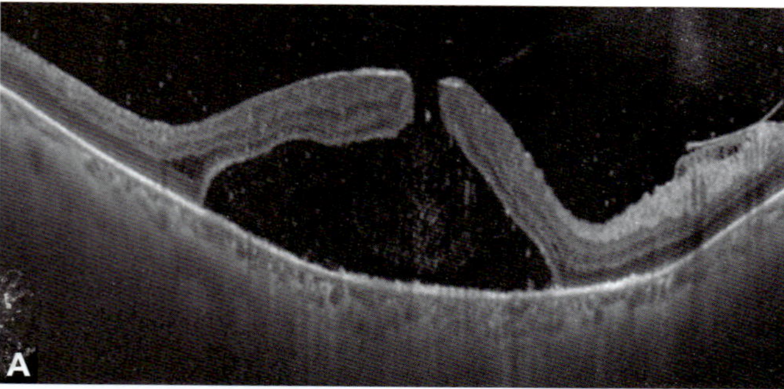

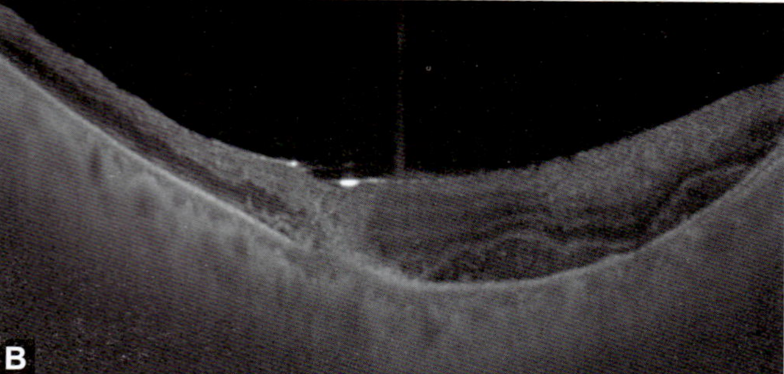

Figs. 16.4A and B: (A) Preoperative macular hole RD on OCT; and (B) OCT image showing closure postsurgery (under gas).
(RD: Retinal detachment; OCT: optical coherence tomography)

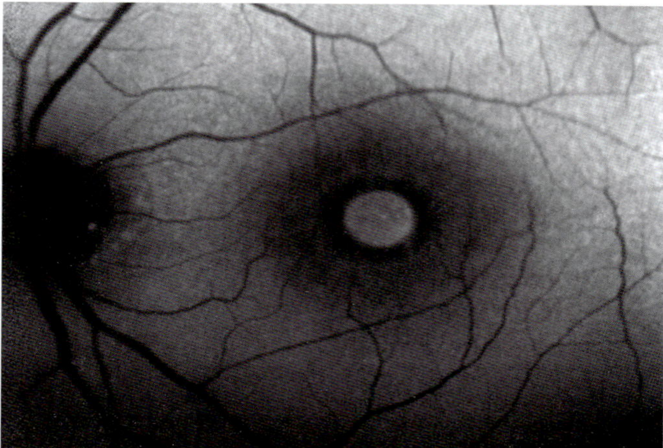

Fig. 16.5: Fundus autofluorescence of left eye depicting a full thickness macular hole seen as a hyper autofluorescent area and the surrounding hypoautofluorescence corresponding to the cuff of fluid.

Multifocal Electroretinography

It gives a topographic measure of the electrophysiological activity of retina. Multifocal electroretinography tests the local retinal function and is recorded from the cone driven retina under the light adapted condition. It can map the electrophysiological activity of the foveal area in macular holes preoperatively and also provides an objective measure of the functional outcome after surgery.

DIFFERENTIAL DIAGNOSIS

There are a number of entities that mimic macular hole in their clinical appearance.

Epiretinal Membrane and Pseudohole

An ERM that is discontinuous, contracted, located in or near the fovea may lead to a hole like partial-thickness tissue loss at the fovea with no actual tissue defect and has steep edges, and is referred to as a pseudohole. It may be often associated with an ERM. A true full thickness macular hole has a distinct and circular margin with a surrounding cuff of subretinal fluid with a pseudo-operculum. An ERM with a pseudohole will have a contracted or circumlinear edge in or near the fovea with macular puckering without any cuff of subretinal fluid around the hole, and fluorescein angiography shows no window defect (Fig. 16.6A).

Lamellar Hole

Aborted macular hole formation or some cases of chronic CME lead to the formation of partial thickness defects of macula known as lamellar macular holes. Pseudo-operculum may be present. Cuff of subretinal fluid or central window defect on fluorescein angiography are not seen. Lamellar hole borders are more sloping and ill-defined (Fig. 16.6B).

Cystoid Macular Edema

A large central macular cyst may simulate a full thickness macular hole (Fig. 16.7). The associated ocular conditions with CME such as ocular inflammatory disorders, ocular tumors, retinitis pigmentosa and fluorescein angiography helps in differentiation from a true macular hole. On fluorescein angiography, CME shows early superficial leakage and late accumulation in cystoid spaces.

Other Lesions

Other lesions mimicking a 'pre-hole' lesion include central serous chorioretinopathy with central yellow spot, subfoveal choroidal neovascularization (CNV) with foveal cyst, solar retinopathy, macular drusen in age-related macular degeneration,[22] or a pseudo-operculum.[23]

PROGNOSTIC FACTORS

The prognostic indicators for macular hole surgery include presenting visual acuity, duration of symptoms, the size of the

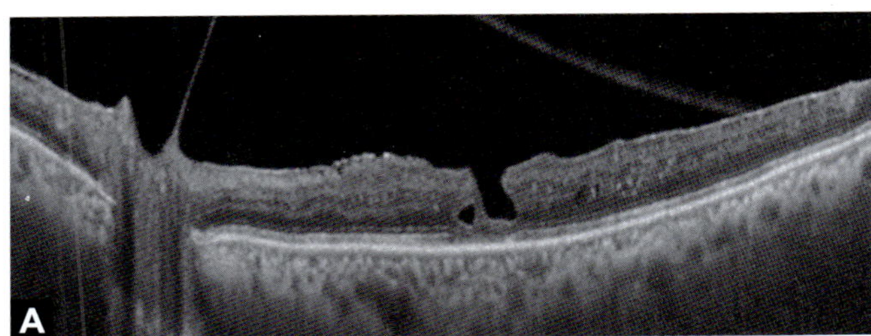
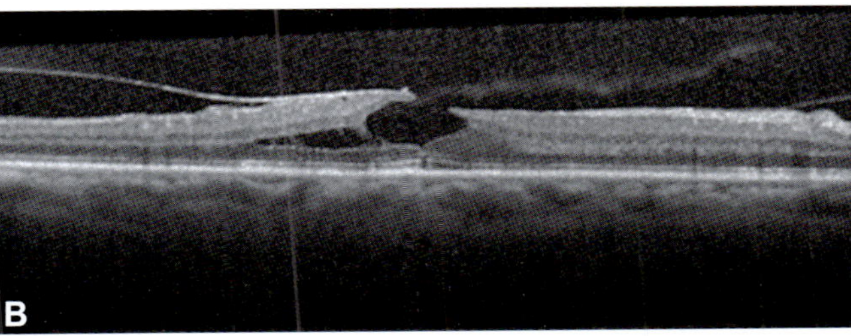

Figs. 16.6A and B: (A) Spectral domain-optical coherence tomography (SD-OCT) of a pseudohole where there is an absence of a full thickness defect and steep walls as opposed to a lamellar hole; and (B) SD-OCT scan of a lamellar macular hole with an intact operculum.

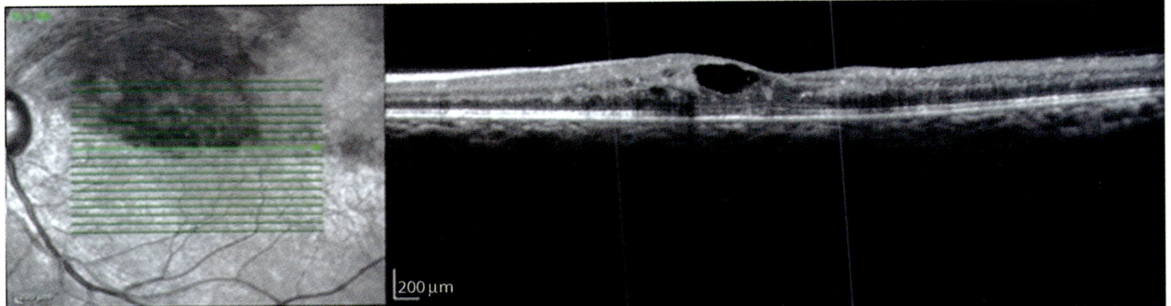

Fig. 16.7: Spectral domain-optical coherence tomography scan of a patient with cystoid macular edema.

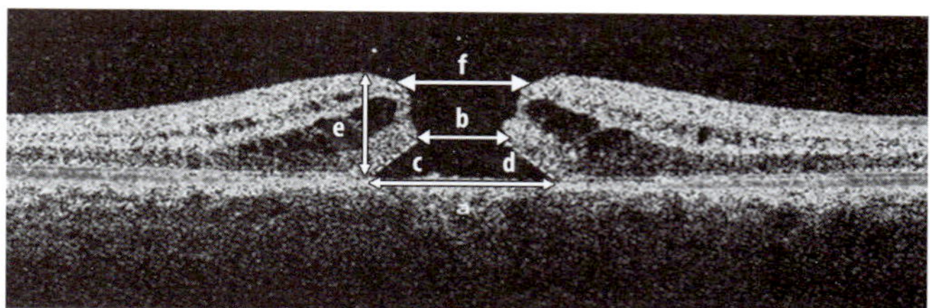

Fig. 16.8: Pictorial representation of the dimensions taken to calculate the different prognostic indicators of macular hole.

macular hole, macular hole indices, intraoperative adjuncts and repeat surgeries. Most surgeons indicate surgery for stage 2, 3, or 4 macular holes with lesser duration of presentation with visual acuity of at least 20/50 or worse.

In 2002, OCT was first used to analyze macular holes preoperatively.[24] The least horizontal diameter of the macular hole measurement divided holes into less than 400 μm (stage 2) and greater than 400 μm (stage 3). Preoperative morphological indices in full thickness macular hole that correlate with postoperative functional outcome include--macular hole height (MHH), base diameter (BD), minimum linear diameter (MLD), macular hole inner opening (MHIO), tractional hole index (THI), macular hole index (MHI), and hole form factor (HFF).

Macular hole indices were calculated from OCT images (Fig. 16.8).

- Macular hole height: Vertical length between the retinal pigment epithelium and the highest point of the hole (Fig. 16.8, measurement e)
- Base diameter: Measured at the level of RPE (Fig. 16.8, measurement a)
- Minimum linear diameter: Minimum dimension measurable (Fig. 16.8, measurement b)
- Macular hole inner opening: Distance between the innermost layer in the defect (Fig. 16.8, measurement f)
- Tractional hole index: e/b (e = MHH, b = MLD)
- Macular hole index: e/a (a= BD)
- Hole form factor: c + d / a [c = left arm length, d= right arm length, a= base diameter (Fig. 16.8)].

Small holes (<400 μm) showed better gain in visual outcome compared to larger holes as calculated by MLD and BD. The functional outcome is better with lesser MHI and THI. MLD and BD were predictive of anatomical closure while MHI predicted ELM restoration. Postoperative visual outcome has significant statistical correlation with BD, MLD, THI and MHI.

 ## SURGICAL MANAGEMENT AND TECHNIQUES

Historical Background

In 1991, Kelly and Wendel introduced and propagated pars plana vitrectomy, removal of the posterior cortical vitreous with strict face-down positioning after gas-fluid exchange for the repair of macular holes.[25] The original technique of Kelly

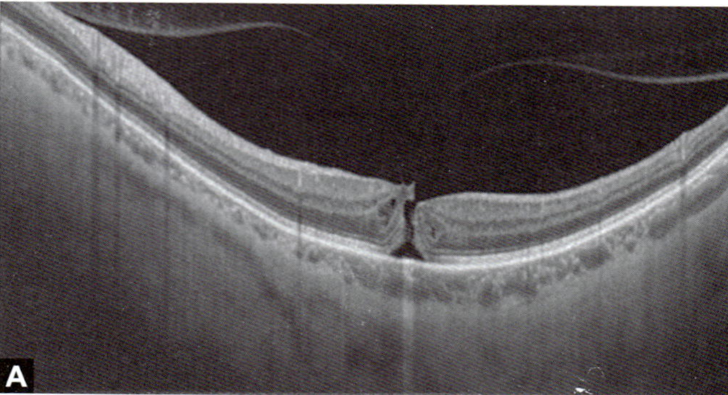

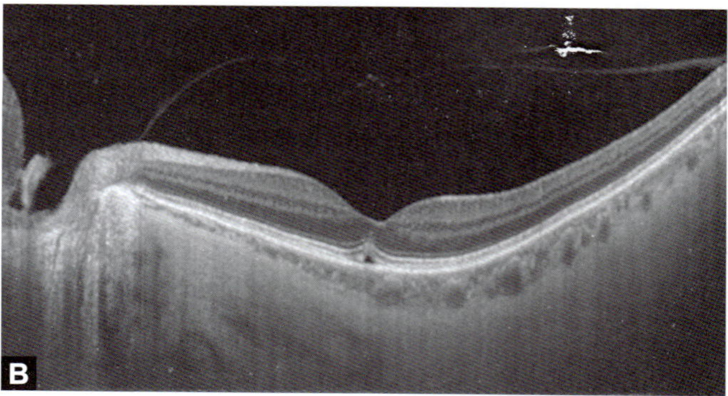

Figs. 16.9A and B: (A) Early post vitreomacular traction stage 2 macular hole (6/12) which (B) closed spontaneously (6/9) over 4 weeks.

and Wendel remains the basis of the surgical techniques till today.

In the initial report by Kelly and Wendel, 58% holes showed successful closure with improvement of visual acuity by two or more lines in 42%. In a second report, Wendel and coauthors reported 73% anatomic success and 55% visual improvement.[26] The greater success in holes of shorter duration has been confirmed by this and several other studies.

Surgery for Macular Hole

Early stage 2 macular holes and traumatic holes are known to spontaneously close over few weeks, hence a wait and watch policy is mandatory for such patients (Figs. 16.9A and B). If on serial visits, the hole enlarges in diameter and does not close, they should be considered for macular hole surgery (MHS).

Careful patient selection is important. Symptomatic patients with stage 2, 3 or 4 macular holes benefit from MHS. The aim of the surgery is to relieve vitreomacular traction and to provide retinal tamponade. Tangential traction is released by removal of the vitreous, ERMs and ILM surrounding the hole. Tamponade is usually provided by total gas fluid exchange (nonexpansile concentration of long-acting gas) and strict postoperative prone positioning.

A standard three port pars plana vitrectomy is performed followed by the induction of a complete PVD. The ILM is stained with vital dyes like indocyanine green (ICG), brilliant blue G and trypan blue (0.15%).

Vital stains enhance and display tissues such as ILM, posterior hyaloid and fine ERM. Staining of the ILM was essential in the successful closure of macular holes especially large macular holes (>400 μm). These stains make ILM peeling easier, faster, and less traumatic.

Tangential traction is relieved by identification and removal of the cortical vitreous or posterior hyaloid and removal of fine ERMs around the hole. Tamponade is provided by total gas-fluid exchange with air or 20–25% SF6 or 12–14% C3F8 gas mixture and strict face-down positioning for first 3 days postoperatively. In the standard ILM peel technique, the ILM is peeled completely about 2 disc diameter around the fovea.

Inverted Internal Limiting Membrane Flap Technique

Instead of peeling the ILM completely, one edge is left attached to the edge of the hole, trimmed and inverted over the hole with a soft tipped cannula or a diamond dusted membrane scraper (Figs. 16.10 and 16.11). Tucking the flap into the hole is not advised owing to its traumatic nature. The intraoperative OCT guided ILM peeling and inverting the flap augments the precision of surgery and aids in confirming the position of flap after air fluid exchange (Figs. 16.12A and B).

The technique of pars plana vitrectomy with ILM peeling has become the standard procedure of choice in the management of macular holes. The base diameter and the minimum diameter have an important role in the anatomical success of macular hole surgery. Larger diameter holes are associated with higher failure rates. In 2010, Michalewska et al.[27] did a prospective randomized study of 50 eyes comparing the inverted ILM flap technique with the standard ILM peel in large macular holes with least dimension more than

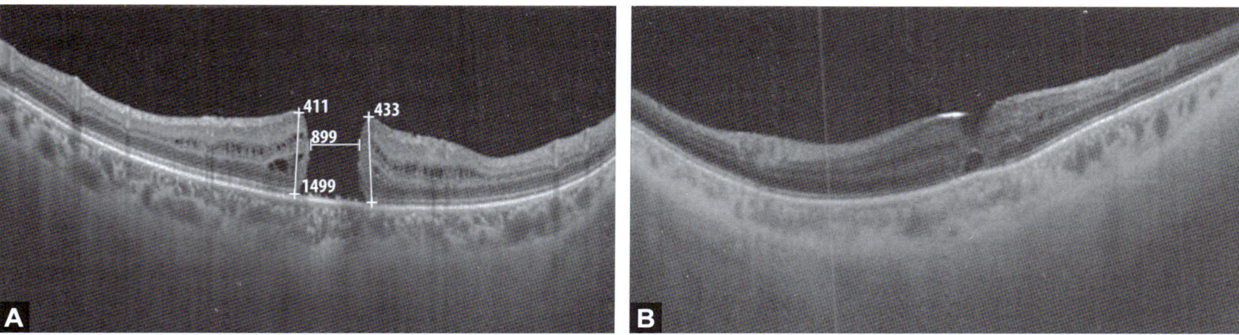

Figs. 16.10A and B: (A) Large macular hole preoperatively with base diameter of 1499 μm and MHI 0.28, (B) Macular hole closure in early postoperative follow up post inverted ILM flap surgery and gas injection. (MHI: macular hole index; ILM: internal limiting membrane)

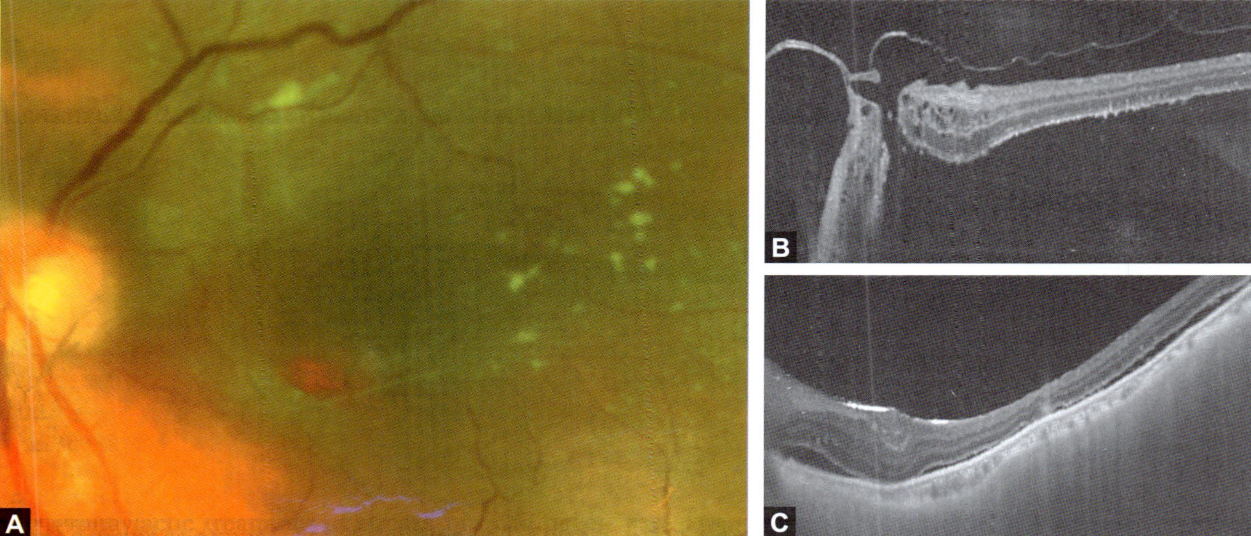

Figs. 16.11A to C: Post VMT macular hole RD seen on (A) color picture and (B) OCT; (C) Postoperatively, on first day in a C3F8 gas-filled eye, there is an evidence of hole closure with DSM.
(VMT: vitreomacular traction; RD: retinal detachment; OCT: optical coherence tomography; DSM: dome-shaped macula)

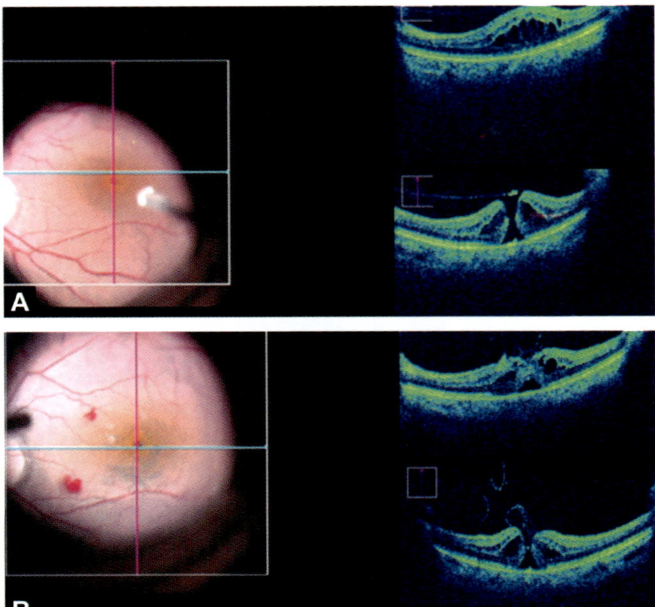

Figs. 16.12A and B: (A) The intraoperative optical coherence tomography scan depicting a full thickness macular hole during surgery with posterior hyaloid attached to one edge. (B) The intraoperative optical coherence tomography scan depicting an inverted internal limiting membrane (ILM) flap bridging the macular hole post-ILM peel.

or equal to 400 μm. They concluded that the former provided superior anatomical and functional outcomes.

The technique of placing inverted flap of ILM over large macular holes greater than 400 μm is an attempt to achieve type 1 closure of macular hole with no tissue defect or bare RPE has been proven to be effective in closing large macular holes.

The standard procedure of PPV and membrane peeling is associated with flat-closed macular holes, or flat-open macular holes in 19–39% cases. Flat-open closure is a type 2 closure. Though even this is considered a success, the functional outcome in terms of visual acuity is limited and recurrence of macular holes in noted more often in type 2 closure.

The mechanism of closure of macular hole in cases of large holes with inverted flap surgery is that the inverted flap provides a basement membrane that enables a better proliferation of glial cells and hence aids in the better alignment of photoreceptors in close proximity to the foveola. It has also been proposed that the peeled-off ILM over the macular hole seals off the macular hole and augments the tamponade and scaffold provided by the nonexpansile gas mixture. The residual fluid at the macular hole is pumped out by the RPE at the base of the hole which helps approximate the hole edges together. The ILM flap will prevent further seepage of fluid into the hole with the momentary change in position of the patient from prone to supine.

Prognostic Factors

The duration of symptoms may predict anatomic macular hole closure and visual improvement. Kelly and Wendel[25] reported that visual improvement was best for holes with symptoms of less than 6 months. Longstanding macular holes may show limited anatomic and functional benefits. Patients with uncertain duration of holes or holes present for more than 1 year or holes with a flatter morphology on OCT should be explained about the guarded prognosis for visual recovery even after post surgery anatomical closure of hole. With use of the inverted ILM flap technique, older holes are showing higher closure rates, also the continuity of the outer retinal bands including the ellipsoid band (EZ) and the interdigitation zone (IZ) play a major role in visual recovery in eyes with macular holes and even other macular pathologies.

Should ILM be Peeled in All Macular Hole Surgeries?

The ILM is the basal lamina of the inner retina and acts as a scaffold for proliferation of fibrocytes, myofibroblasts, and retinal pigment epithelial cells. Although ILM peeling leads to successful macular hole closure, it has been postulated that removal of this membrane could be functionally damaging to the retina because of its role in structural integrity.

A Cochrane review of four controlled trials[28] showed that there was no statistically significant benefit in visual outcome at 6 months or 12 months with ILM peeling. However, chances of primary macular hole closure was higher for all stages of macular holes with ILM peeling. When stratified by stage, the odds of the hole closure after ILM peeling was progressively higher at each of stage 2, 3, and 4.

Intraocular Tamponade

Air and longer-acting gases such as SF6 and C3F8 can be used as the postoperative intraocular tamponade. Advantages of air include less demanding positioning with potentially reduced risk of ulnar neuropathy, less risk of cataractogenesis and postoperative rise of intraocular pressure. Bovine and recombinant transforming growth factor (TGF-beta), autologous serum, autologous plasma, thrombin and fibrin, autologous platelet concentrate also have been used as adjunctive substances for encouraging healing response in holes.

Is Face-down Positioning Necessary with Intraocular Gas Tamponade?

Face-down or prone positioning can be bothersome for patients. Hu et al.[29] found overall lower macular hole closure rates in eyes which were not advised face-down positioning; however, this made no difference for holes lesser than 400 μm in size. The authors recommend additional studies to determine the necessity of positioning for larger holes. A multicenter randomized control trial is being undertaken to determine closure rates of large (>400 μm) macular holes with positioning.[30]

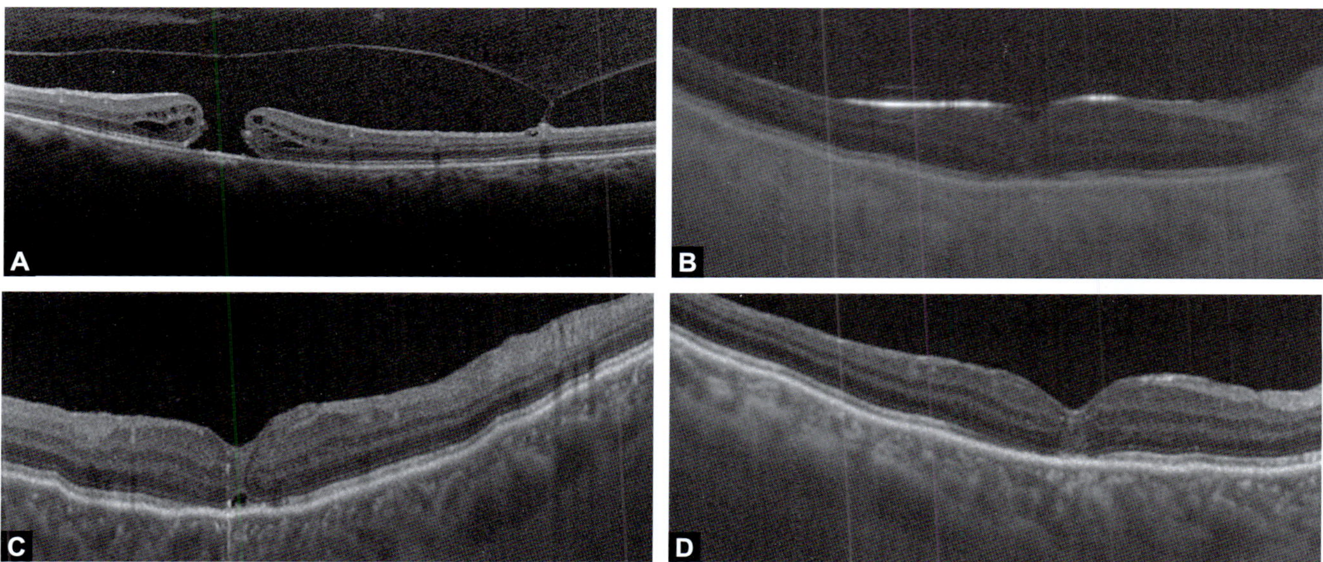

Figs. 16.13A to D: (A) Preoperative spectral domain-optical coherence tomography (SD-OCT) scan of a stage 3 full thickness macular hole; (B) Postoperative SD-OCT scan of the same patient after 1 week of inverted internal limiting membrane (ILM) flap technique depicting the hyper-reflective layer bridging the hole indicating the presence of the ILM flap; (C) Postoperative 1 month picture of the same patient depicting a type 1 closure with inner/outer segment (IS/OS) discontinuity and a cystic space in outer retina; and (D) Postoperative 3-month SD-OCT scan of the same patient depicting a type 1 closure with restoration of ellipsoid band continuity.

Macular hole surgery using silicone oil tamponade was done in a series of patients with chronic systemic illness such as arthritis who may be unable to carry out strict postoperative face-down posturing for 10–15 days thought necessary for the closure of macular holes. They found that the anatomical results (80%) in this series was similar to other studies using gas tamponade although the visual results were less rewarding.[31] A prospective study to compare treatment of persistently open macular holes with heavy silicone oil versus C2F6 found the former to be more efficacious.[32]

Figures 16.13A to D denote the spectral domain-OCT scan of a patient with full thickness macular hole with minimum linear dimension 664 µm who underwent inverted ILM flap technique with 25% SF6 tamponade.

Ocriplasmin in Macular Hole Surgery

Ocriplasmin intravitreal injection 2.5 mg/mL (Jetrea, ThromboGenics) is used for enzymatic vitreolysis for small (<400 µm) full thickness macular holes associated with vitreomacular traction (MIVI-TRUST Study Group). Stalmans and colleagues reported nonsurgical macular hole closure in 40.6% of eyes injected with ocriplasmin compared with 10.6% of placebo-injected eyes.[33] Alberti and la Cour reported a lower primary macular hole closure rate with ocriplasmin as compared to primary pars plana vitrectomy.[34] Visual acuity was slightly worse in eyes that had been treated with ocriplasmin only although median visual gain was equivalent. Vitrectomy is also a more cost-effective option.[35]

MANAGEMENT OF FAILED MACULAR HOLES

Internal Limiting Membrane Autograft for Failed Macular Holes

Failure of primary macular hole surgery may occur because of poor patient compliance or traction from a residual or recurrent ERM. But, a cause is not determined in most cases. An alternative available is ILM graft for patients who fail the first surgery involving ILM peeling (Figs. 16.14A and B). More evidence is awaited in this area of surgery.

A prospective study of 10 eyes with failed macular hole surgery at our center evaluated perfluorocarbon liquid assisted placement of an autologous fragment of ILM larger than the hole diameter taken from just outside the arcade. Intraocular tamponade with 14% C3F8 provided sufficient long-term tamponade with a prone position advised for 5 days. 90% of the holes closed with no neurosensory defect and the transplanted ILM flaps were visible as hyperreflective areas on swept-source OCT within 7 days of surgery. This disappeared within 3 months. The mean best corrected visual acuity (BCVA) was 0.99 ± 0.25 (range, 0.52–1.30) before surgery and 0.57 ± 0.36 (range, 0.15–1.05) at the final visit.

No major complication was observed. ILM graft could be a useful alternative for the treatment of macular holes which fail after the first surgery, when ILM peeling has already been performed. A higher number of patients is needed to further evaluate this new technique.

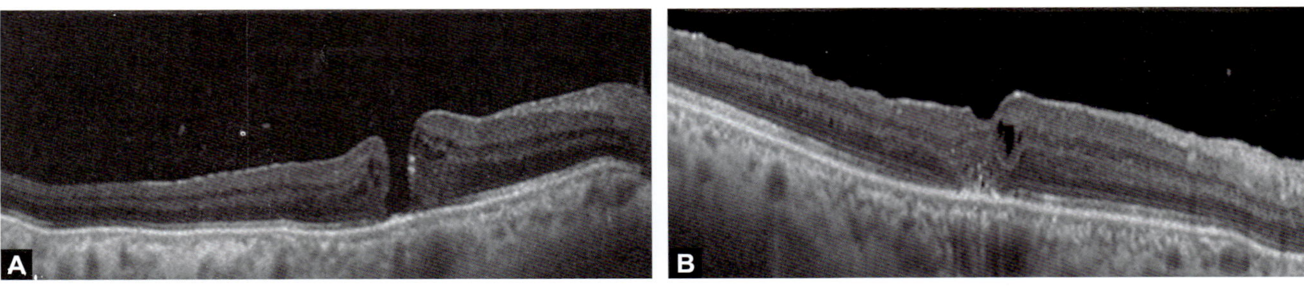

Figs. 16.14A and B: (A) Initial OCT shows failed MH closure after inverted ILM flap surgery with visual acuity of 6/60 at 1 month; and (B) Post ILM autograft surgery, the hole is closed with vision of 6/24 at 1 month. (OCT: optical coherence tomography; MH: macular hole; ILM: internal limiting membrane)

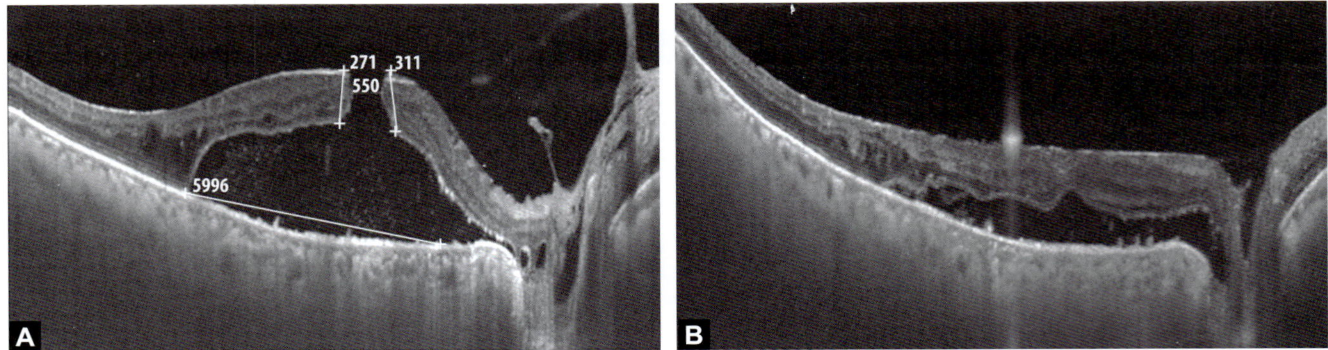

Figs. 16.15A and B: (A) Preexisting macular hole with localized RD; (B) After inverted ILM flap surgery shows settling macula under gas at 1 week postoperatively.
(RD: Retinal detachment; ILM: Internal limiting membrane)

CHALLENGES AND COMPLICATIONS

Challenges in Macular Hole Surgery

Despite the fact that the macular hole surgery is one of the most successful vitreoretinal surgeries, there are some situations where surgical success is still grim. These include large macular holes, traumatic macular holes, macular hole in detached retina and in high myopia (Figs. 16.15A and B). Various techniques including the earlier mentioned inverted ILM flap technique has been tried in these situations.

The macular hole tapping[36] and arcuate partial retinotomy[37] has been described for large idiopathic holes. Though they provide good anatomical outcomes, the functional outcomes were still poor owing to the traumatic nature of these procedures. Inverted ILM flap technique has also been tried in traumatic macular holes, macular hole in detached retina and in myopic macular holes[38]. Perfluorocarbon liquid (PFCL) and Viscoat assisted[39] inverted ILM flap technique is also described in literature. Microscope-integrated intraoperative OCT helps in identification of vitreoschisis and ensures proper placement of inverted ILM flap over macular hole which are difficult to visualise as in patients with pathological myopia with macular hole and retinal detachment, thereby increasing the anatomical and functional success.[40]

Complications of Macular Hole Surgery

The potential complications are similar to other vitreoretinal surgical cases such as iatrogenic retinal breaks and raised intraocular pressure. Late postoperative complications include reopening of macular holes, visual field defects, progressive nuclear sclerosis and retinal pigmentary changes. The etiology of anatomic failure may be because of poor case selection (extremely large holes often with ragged edges as in traumatic holes are unlikely to close), patient noncompliance in postoperative prone positioning, residual ERMs and retinal stiffening.

CHOROMOVITRECTOMY FOR MACULAR HOLE SURGERY

Dyes for Internal Limiting Membrane Peeling—To Use or Not to Use?

Brilliant blue G is the most frequently used dye introduced by Enaida et al. in 2006. It is nontoxic, either *in vivo* or *in vitro*, to retinal cells and consists of anionic aminotriarylmethane with 280 mOsm osmolarity, molecular weight of 854, and a 7.4 pH.

Brilliant blue G is a safe colorant to dye the ILM as no dose-dependent or time-dependent toxicity has been observed. At low concentrations, it has high affinity for ILM and obviates the need for fluid-air exchange. High molecular weight brilliant blue dye is also commercially available as ILM-Blue [0.025% brilliant blue G, 4% polyethylene glycol (PEG)] and Membrane Blue-Dual (0.15% trypan blue, 0.025% brilliant blue G, 4% PEG). Both dyes being heavy, sink onto the macula obviating the need of fluid-air exchange.[41,42]

Special Considerations

Internal limiting membrane is a semitransparent membrane and difficult to identify in lesser pigmented eyes and therefore, dyes have come into use to facilitate its visualization during surgery.

Toxicity of ICG dye has been reported with unknown mechanism, but involving atypical retinal pigment epithelial changes with a direct toxic effect to RPE. In vitro studies have shown that exposure of ICG to the cultured human RPE cells results in dose- and time-dependent damage to cellular structure. ICG dye is retained within the retinal tissue for months exposing it to potential phototoxicity. Brilliant blue G seems to be one of the most innocuous dye with small alterations in the retinal cells in animal tests. As far as our personal experience demonstrates, we have no evidence that brilliant blue G used for short periods of time during vitreoretinal surgery produces any structural or functional damage.[43-47]

Toxicity of retinal dyes is assessed on the basis of visual acuity after macular surgery but is difficult to evaluate as it depends it depends on many factors such as the patient's age, the severity of macular disease, and its time of appearance.

The surgical technique, the type of lighting, the distance of the light probe from the macula, and the time that the macula has been exposed are factors that also affect the BCVA and retinal cell damage after surgery.

POSTOPERATIVE ANATOMICAL OUTCOMES

Anatomical closure of macular hole is defined as reapproximation of the edges of the hole with a central foveal thickness greater than 100 µm and attachment of previously elevated cuff of retina surrounding the macular hole to the adjacent RPE.

Postoperative anatomical appearance can be classified as type 1 closure, type 2 closure and nonclosure.[48] If the macular hole was observed to close without a foveal defect in the neurosensory retina, it was considered as type 1 closure (Fig. 16.16). If the foveal defect of neurosensory retina persists postoperatively with flattening of surrounding cuff of fluid and the rim of the macular hole is attached to the underlying RPE with a reduction in hole diameter, it was considered to be a type 2 closure (Fig. 16.17). Type 1 closure corresponds to the 'u' and 'v' type of closure and type 2 corresponds to the 'w' pattern.[49] Nonclosure is termed when the rim of the macular hole remains detached from the RPE with everted edges and with no decrease in diameter postoperatively (Fig. 16.18). Nonclosure is also described as flat open appearance and is

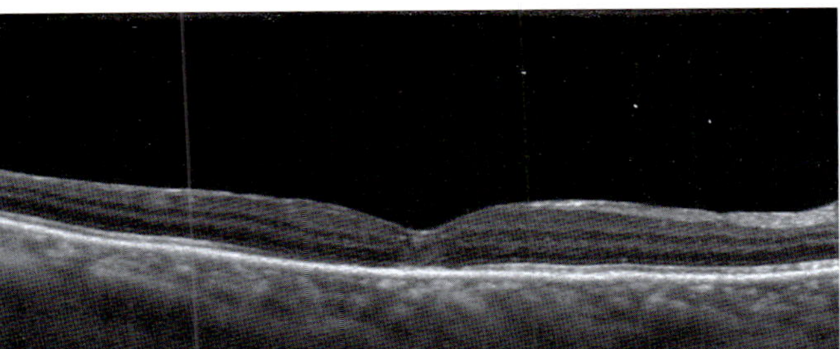

Fig. 16.16: Spectral domain-optical coherence tomography image of type 1 macular hole closure.

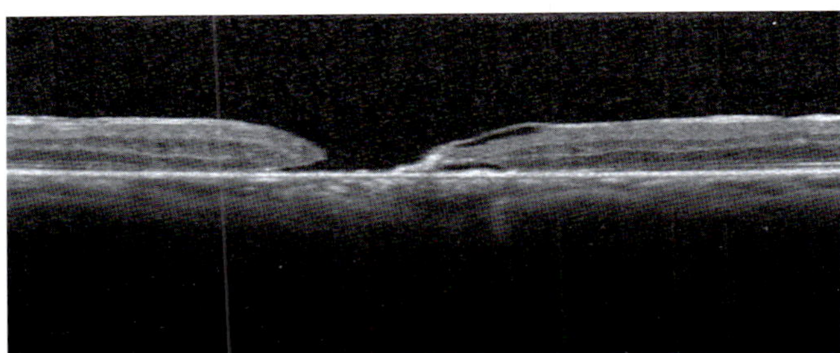

Fig. 16.17: Spectral domain-optical coherence tomography image of type 2 macular hole closure.

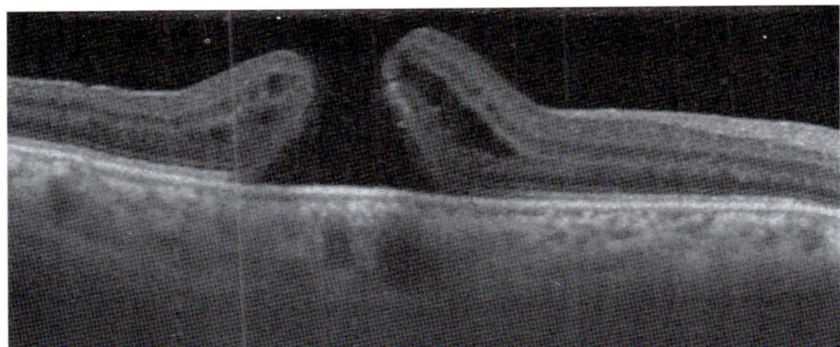

Fig. 16.18: Spectral domain-optical coherence tomography image of a nonclosure of macular hole following failed macular hole surgery.

different from type 2 closure/flat closed appearance of macular hole.

SHOULD WE OPERATE ON LAMELLAR HOLES?

Witkin et al.[50] presented four criteria for the diagnosis of lamellar holes (Fig. 16.19) using OCT:

- Irregular foveal contour
- Break in the inner fovea
- Dehiscence of inner foveal retina from outer retina
- Absence of a full thickness foveal defect and presence of intact foveal photoreceptors.

Good and stable visual acuity may allow observation of most lamellar holes. A case series reported that stable visual acuity remained stable in 78% of patients, and deterioration

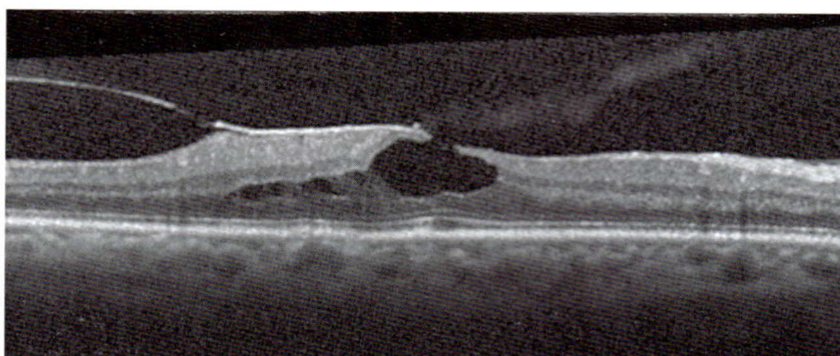

Fig. 16.19: Lamellar macular hole shows a break in the inner fovea and dehiscence of inner retina from outer retina besides absence of a full thickness defect.

in 22% of patients which ranged from 2 letters to 15 letters.[51] Surgical intervention may be indicated in cases with dropping visual acuity.

REFERENCES

1. Knapp H. Ueber isolerte zerreissungen der aderhaut in folge von traumen auf dem augapfel. Arch Augenklinik. 1869;1:6-29.
2. Vendantham V. Optical coherence tomography findings in macular hole due to argon laser burn. Arch Ophthalmology 2006;124(2):287-8.
3. Cohen SM, Gass JDM. Macular hole formation following severe hypertensive retinopathy. Arch Ophthalmology. 1994;112:878-9.
4. Brown GC. Macular hole following rhegmatogenous retinal detachment repair. Arch Ophthalmology. 1988;106:765-6.
5. Chavanne H. Pseudo–trou maculaire par electrocution. Bull Soc Ophthalmology Fr. 1958;271-5.
6. Karthikeya R, Ravani RD, Kakkar P, et al. Intravitreal cysticercosis with full thickness macular hole: management outcome and intraoperative optical coherence tomography features. BMJ Case Reports. 2017;2017.
7. Risk factors for idiopathic macular holes: The Eye Disease Case–Control Study Group. Am J Ophthalmology. 1994;118:754-61.
8. Ezra E, Wells JA, Gray RH, et al. Incidence of idiopathic full-thickness macular holes in fellow eyes. A 5-year prospective natural history study. Ophthalmology. 1998;105:353-9.
9. Lewis ML, Cohen SM, Smiddy WE, et al. Bilaterality of idiopathic macular holes. Graefes Arch Clin Exp Ophthalmology. 1996;234:241-5.
10. Fisher YL, Slakter JS, Yannuzzi LA, et al. A prospective natural history study and kinetic ultrasound evaluation of idiopathic macular holes. Ophthalmology. 1994;101:5-11.
11. Akiba J, Quiroz MA, Trempe L. Role of posterior vitreous detachment in idiopathic macular holes. Ophthalmology. 1990;97:1610-3.
12. Kuhnt H. Tber eine eigentumliche veranderung der netzhaut ad maculam (retinitis atrophicans sive rareficans centralis). Z Augenheilk. 1900;105(3):45-9.
13. Fuchs E. Zur veranderung der macula lutea nach contusion. Ztschr Augenheilkd. 1901;6:181-6.
14. Coats G. The pathology of macular holes. Roy London Hosp Report. 1907;17:69-96.
15. Duke-Elder S, Dobree JH. System of Ophthalmology: Diseases of the Retina. London: Henry Kimpton; 1967. pp. 1-878.
16. Gass JD. Idiopathic senile macular hole. Its early stages and pathogenesis. Arch Ophthalmology. 1988;106:629-39.
17. Jensen OM, Larsen M. Objective assessment of photoreceptor displacement and metamorphopsia: a study of macular holes. Arch Ophthalmology. 1998;116:1303-6.
18. Duker JS, Kaiser PK, Binder S, et al. The International Vitreomacular Traction Study Group classification of vitreomacular adhesion, traction, and macular hole. Ophthalmology. 2013;120(12):2611-9.
19. Hee MR, Puliafito CA, Wong C, et al. Optical coherence tomography of macular holes. Ophthalmology. 1995;102:748-56.
20. Gaudric A, Haouchine B, Massin P, et al. Macular hole formation. New data provided by optical coherent tomography. Arch Ophthalmology. 1999;117:744-51.
21. Johnson MW, Van Newkirk MR, Meyer KA. Perifoveal vitreous detachment is the primary pathogenic event in idiopathic macular hole formation. Arch Ophthalmology. 2001;119:215-22.
22. Gass JDM, Joondeph BC. Observations concerning patients with suspected impending macular holes. Am J Ophthalmology. 1990;109:638-646.
23. Gass JDM, VanNewkirk M. Xanthic scotoma and yellow foveolar shadow caused by a pseudo–operculum after vitreofoveal separation. Retina. 1992;12:242-4.
24. Ip MS, Baker BJ, Duker JS, et al. Anatomical outcomes of surgery for idiopathic macular hole as determined by optical coherence tomography. Arch Ophthalmology. 2002;120:29-35.
25. Kelly NE, Wendel RT. Vitreous surgery for idiopathic macular holes: results of a pilot trial. Arch Ophthalmology. 1991;109:654-9.
26. Wendel RT, Patel AC, Kelly NA, et al. Vitreous surgery for macular holes. Ophthalmology. 1993;100:1671-6.
27. Michalewska Z, Michalewski J, Adelman RA, et al. Inverted internal limiting membrane flap technique for large macular holes. Ophthalmology. 2010;117(10):2018-25.
28. Spiteri Cornish K, Lois N, Scott N, et al. Vitrectomy with internal limiting membrane (ILM) peeling versus with no peeling for idiopathic full-thickness macular hole (FTMH). Cochrane Database Syst Rev. 2013;6:CD009306.
29. Hu Z, Xie P, Ding Y, et al. Face-down or no face-down posturing following macular hole surgery: a meta-analysis. Acta Ophthalmology. 2016;94(4):326-33.
30. Pasu S, Bunce C, Hooper R, et al. PIMS (Positioning In Macular hole Surgery) trial––a multicentre interventional comparative randomized controlled clinical trial comparing face-down positioning, with an inactive face-forward position on the outcome of surgery for large macular holes: study protocol for a randomized controlled trial. Trials. 2015;16(1):527.
31. Karia N, Laidlaw A, West J, et al. Macular hole surgery using silicone oil tamponade. Br J Ophthalmology. 2001;85(11):1320-3.
32. Cillino S, Cillino G, Ferraro LL, et al. Treatment of persistently open macular holes with heavy silicone oil (Densiron 68) versus C2F6. A prospective randomized study. Retina. 2016;36(4):688-94.
33. Haller JA, Stalmans P, Benz MS, et al. MIVI-TRUST Study Group Efficacy of intravitral ocriplasmin for treatment of vitreomacular adhesion. Ophthalmology. 2015;122(1):117-22.
34. Alberti M, la Cour M. Is visual acuity non-inferior in full-thickness macular holes treated with ocriplasmin. Acta Ophthalmology. 2016;94(2):e166-7.
35. Chang JS, Smiddy WE. Cost evaluation of surgical and pharmaceutical options in treatment of vitreomacular adhesions and macular holes. Ophthalmology. 2014;121(9):1720-6.
36. Kumar A, Tinwala SI; Gogia V, et al. Tapping of Macular Hole Edges: The Outcomes of a Novel Technique for Large Macular Holes. Asia Pac J Ophthalmology (Phila). 2013;2(5):305-9.
37. Charles S, Randolph JC, Neekhra A, et al. Arcuate retinotomy for the repair of large macular holes. Ophthalmic Surg Lasers Imaging Retina. 2013;44(1):69-72.

38. Kuriyama S, Hayashi H, Jingami Y, et al. Efficacy of inverted internal limiting membrane flap technique for the treatment of macular hole in high myopia. Am J Ophthalmology. 2013;156(1): 125-31.

39. Song Z, Li M, Liu J, et al. Viscoat assisted inverted internal limiting membrane flap technique for large macular holes associated with high myopia. J Ophthalmology. 2016;2016:8283062.

40. Kumar A, Kakkar P, Ravani R, et al. Utility of microscope integrated optical coherence tomography (MIOCT) in the treatment of myopic macular hole retinal detachment. BMJ Case Rep. 2017;2017.

41. Enaida H, Hisatomi T, Goto, Y, et al. Brilliant Blue G selectively stains the internal limiting membrane/brilliant blue G-assisted membrane peeling. Retina. 2006;26:631-6.

42. Marc Veckeneer, Andreas Mohr, Essam Alharthi, et al. Novel 'heavy' dyes for retinal membrane staining during macular surgery: multicenter clinical assessment. Acta Ophthalmology. 2014;92:339-44.

43. Ando F, Sasano K, Ohba N, et al. Anatomic and visual outcomes after indocyanine green-assisted peeling of the retinal internal limiting membrane in idiopathic macular hole surgery. Am J Ophthalmology. 2004;137:609-14.

44. Horio N, Horiguchi M. Effect on visual outcome after macular hole surgery when staining the internal limiting membrane with indocyanine green dye. Arch Ophthalmology. 2004;122:992-6.

45. Haritglou C, Gandorfer A, Gass CA, et al. Indocyanine green-assisted peeling of the internal limiting membrane in macular hole surgery affects visual outcome: A clinicophathologic correlation. Am J Ophthalmology. 2002;134:836-41.

46. Haritoglou C, Gandorfer A, Gass CA, et al. The effect of indocyanine green on functional outcome of macular pucker surgery. Am J Ophthalmology. 2003;135:328-37.

47. Engelbrecht NE, Freeman J, Sternberg Jr P, et al. Retinal pigment epithelial changes after macular hole surgery with indocyanine green-assisted internal limiting membrane peeling. Am J Ophthalmology. 2002;133:89-94.

48. Kang SW, Ahn K, Ham DI. Types of macular hole closure and their clinical implications. Br J Ophthalmology. 2003;87(8):1015-9.

49. Imai M, Iijima H, Gotoh T, et al. Optical coherence tomography of successfully repaired idiopathic macular holes. Am J Ophthalmology. 1999;128(5):621-7.

50. Witkin AJ, Ko TH, Fujimoto JG, et al. Redefining lamellar holes and the vitreomacular interface: an ultrahigh-resolution optical coherence tomography study. Ophthalmology. 2006;113(3): 388-97.

51. Theodossiadis PG, Grigoropoulos VG, Emfietzoglou I, et al. Evolution of lamellar macular hole studied by optical coherence tomography. Graefes Arch Clin Exp Ophthalmology. 2009;247(1): 13-20.

Myopic Foveoschisis

Atul Kumar, Raghav Ravani, Aditi Mehta, Sriram Simakurthy

INTRODUCTION

Myopic foveoschisis is one of the macular pathologies seen in patients with high/pathological myopia. The prevalence of pathologic myopia varies in different geographic regions, with highest prevalence in Asian population.[1,2] Increased degenerative changes in the retina due to mechanical stretching and thinning of the choroid and retinal pigment epithelium may be seen as a result of the excessive elongation of the eye. High myopes are predisposed to numerous macular pathologies like lacquer cracks, retinal pigment epithelium (RPE) atrophy or hyperplasia, choroidal neovascularization, myopic macular hole, myopic foveoschisis, chorioretinal atrophy, etc.[3-5]

Myopic macular retinoschisis, also referred to as myopic foveoschisis or myopic traction maculopathy is characterized by splitting of the layers of retina at macula, leading to localized accumulation of intraretinal and subretinal fluid, in the absence of a full-thickness macular hole.[6] This was first described by Phillips in 1958 as an elevation within the posterior pole without a macular hole.[7] Identification and documentation of this entity using optical coherence tomography (OCT) was first done by Takano and Kishi in 1999.[6]

INCIDENCE AND COURSE

Myopic foveoschisis is seen in about 9% of high myopes with posterior staphyloma.[8] Myopic foveoschisis may remain anatomically and functionally stable for a long duration, with case reports of spontaneous resolution over time.[9-11] Within two years, about half of the patients may develop serious complications leading to vision loss like full-thickness macular hole and macular retinal detachment, though the functional and anatomical status may not directly correlate.[12,13] A retrospective study of myopic foveoschisis showed worsening of visual acuity in 69% and stable vision in 31% over a mean follow-up of 31.2 months.

PATHOGENESIS

With advent and advancement of optical coherence tomography (OCT), the pathoanatomical features of myopic foveoschisis have been better characterized and its pathogenesis is better understood. Various possible mechanisms for pathogenesis of myopic foveoschisis have been postulated.

Myopic foveoschisis almost always occurs within the posterior staphyloma. There is gradual stretching and splitting of the retina due to inner retinal noncompliance with inner retina being less flexible than the outer retina. This is one of the most likely hypothesis.[14] Various factors leading to limitation of inner retinal flexibility include persistent adherence of vitreous cortex to inner retinal layer after posterior vitreous detachment, presence of epiretinal membranes, internal limiting membrane rigidity, etc (Fig. 17.1).[15] Collagen fibers and cell debris along with fibrous glial cells on the inner surface of the excised internal limiting membrane (ILM) samples has been noted on electron microscopy in 70% of the patients with myopic foveoschisis.[16]

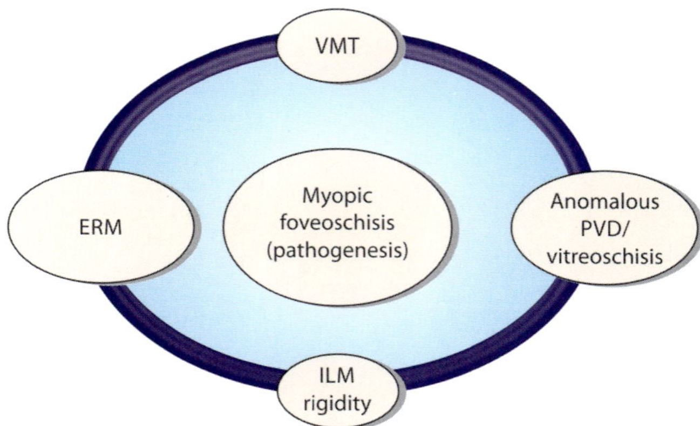

Fig. 17.1: Possible pathogenic mechanisms of myopic foveoschisis. (VMT: Vitreomacular traction; ERM: Epiretinal membrane; ILM: Internal limiting membrane; PVD: Posterior vitreous detachment).

CLINICAL FEATURES

Though it is difficult to accurately diagnose or rule out myopic foveoschisis without OCT in high myopia with posterior staphyloma, clinical examination may reveal mild elevation of posterior retina in presence of other signs of pathological myopia. Thus, OCT along with fundus autofluorescence, plays an important role in diagnosis, complete assessment of extent of retinoschisis and layers involved, presence of macular hole or macular hole detachment, etc. thereby influencing surgical planning (Figs. 17.2A and B).

INVESTIGATIONS

Imaging

Optical Coherence Tomography

Myopic foveoschisis, as the name suggests, presents with splitting of retinal layers at fovea. In atrophic retina, it is important to distinguish retinoschisis from retinal detachment by presence of bridging columns within the schisis layers and by presence of the ellipsoid layer (inner segment/outer segment junction) of photoreceptors, both of which are suggestive of schisis.[17] OCT may show presence, extent and layers involved in foveoschisis, presence and size of macular hole, presence and extent of detachment (Figs. 17.3A and B). It may also depict features suggestive of traction.

For example, internal limiting membrane separation from the retinal layer (called ILM detachment) is suggestive of tractional forces of ILM (Fig. 17.3A).[18] Similarly, microvascular traction is seen on vertical scan in OCT as tent-like peak of inner retina coincident with retinal vessels (Fig. 17.4).[19] Shimada et al. described four stages in the natural course of macular retinoschisis in myopes without macular hole and retinal detachment which includes the following:[9]

- *Stage 1*: Focal irregularity and thickening of external retina.
- *Stage 2*: An outer lamellar hole developed within the thickened area with a small retinal detachment (RD).
- *Stage 3*: Vertical enlargement of outer lamellar hole.
- *Stage 4*: Elevation of the upper edge of the external retina while being attached to the upper part of the retinoschisis layer accompanied by further enlargement of the retinal detachment (RD).

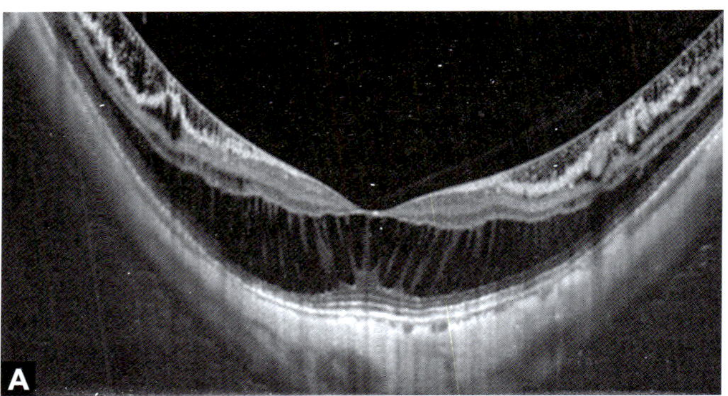
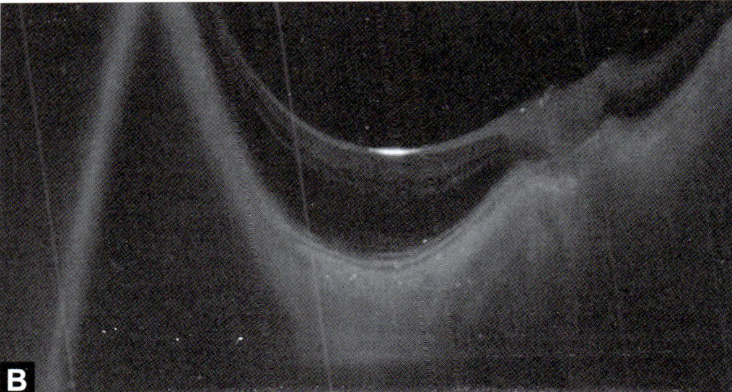

Figs. 17.2A and B: (A) Pathological myopia eye depicting myopic foveoschisis with foveal thinning and an epiretinal membrane (ERM). Note the near absence of the degenerated choroid with scleral tissue abutting onto retinal pigment epithelium (RPE) layer. (B) Postoperatively in the gas filled eye, the schisis is shallower.

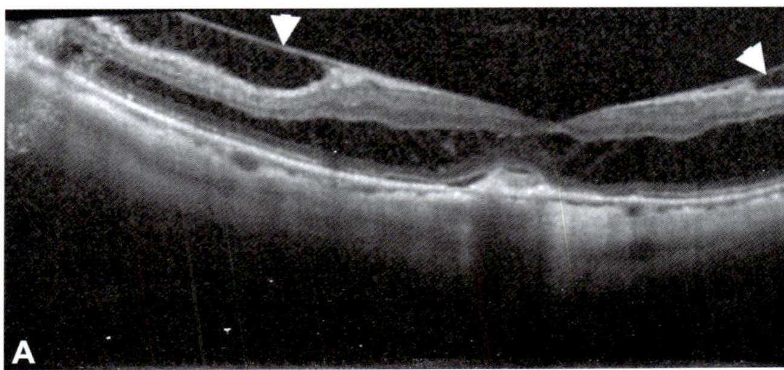
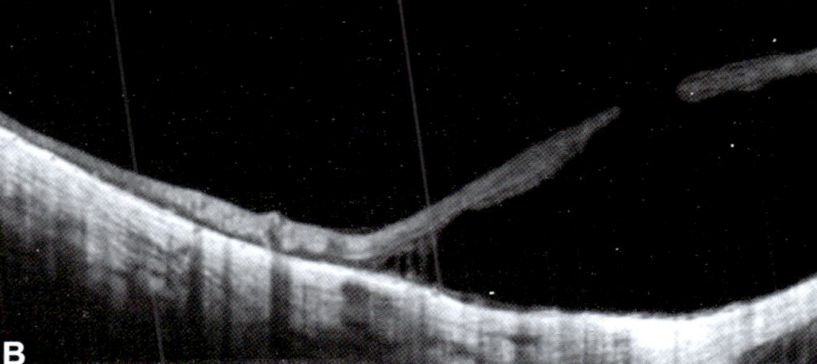

Figs. 17.3A and B: Swept-source optical coherence tomography (SS-OCT) image: (A) Myopic traction maculopathy (MTM) with foveoschisis. Note the rigid internal limiting membrane (ILM) seen as ILM detachment (white arrowheads). (B) SS-OCT of myopic macular hole retinal detachment in a patient with myopic foveoschisis.

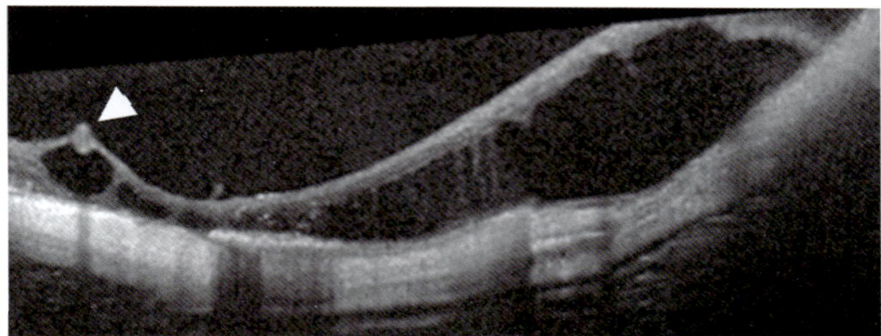

Fig. 17.4: Optical coherence tomography (OCT) image of a patient with myopic foveoschisis showing traction along retinal arteriole with tenting of inner retina (white arrowhead).

Fundus autofluorescence helps to differentiate detachment from schisis, as loss of contact between photoreceptors and RPE results in hypoautofluorescence suggestive of retinal detachment.[20] This may be used to monitor progression of myopic foveoschisis. The disappearance of hyperautofluorescence or presence of hypoautofluorescence on follow-up may suggest need for surgical intervention.

TREATMENT OF MYOPIC FOVEOSCHISIS

Asymptomatic patients with minimal foveoschisis could be followed up closely with serial optical coherence tomography scans.

As discussed earlier, the proposed mechanisms for myopic foveoschisis include anterior-posterior traction or vitreomacular traction (VMT), vitreoretinal interface abnormalities like epiretinal membrane (ERM) or rigidity of internal limiting membrane (ILM). The surgical intervention is aimed at removal of these traction forces responsible for the foveoschisis. Pars plana vitrectomy (PPV) has been proposed to eliminate the tractional forces and thus for the treatment of the disorder.[21,22,13] Other treatment option includes macular buckling.[23-25]

Pars plana vitrectomy with or without ILM peeling has been shown to be effective in resolution of myopic foveoschisis. ILM peeling has been recommended in various studies to eliminate all residual traction on the inner retina, thereby allowing the inner retinal surface to adapt to the shape of the posterior staphyloma.[21,22,13,26-32] (Figs. 17.5A and B).

However, good anatomical and visual outcomes has also been reported after PPV alone without ILM peeling.[33-36] ILM peeling in these high myopes can be challenging in view of poor contrast despite ILM staining due to severe chorioretinal degeneration over the posterior pole. Surgical complications like macular hole and retinal detachment has been reported.[36,37] Fovea-sparing ILM peeling for myopic traction maculopathy has shown good anatomical and visual outcome without occurrence of macular hole without risk of creating an iatrogenic macular hole in such eyes (Figs. 17.6A and B).[38]

Use of gas tamponade in eyes with myopic tractional maculopathy (MTM) following PPV remains debatable. Some studies have shown faster resolution of MTM with gas tamponade with variable visual acuity, which however is not consistent in other studies.[27,30]

A study by Kumar A et al. demonstrating outcomes of microscope integrated intraoperative OCT with center-sparing ILM peeling showed good functional and anatomical success with low intraoperative and postoperative complications.[39] The use of microscope-integrated optical coherence tomography allows seamless, high-resolution, real-time imaging of ILM peeling and traction removal. This also allows visualization of ILM, especially in cases of myopic foveoschisis wherein ILM visibility is difficult due to poor contrast. Microscope-integrated OCT also allows visualization of thinned out retina or cystic changes, and thereby helps guide

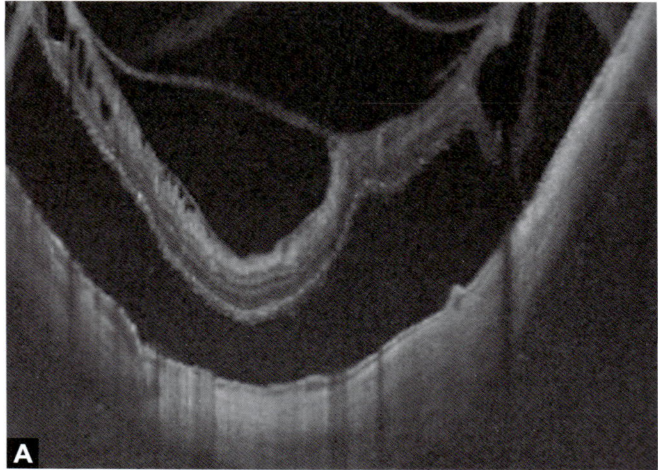

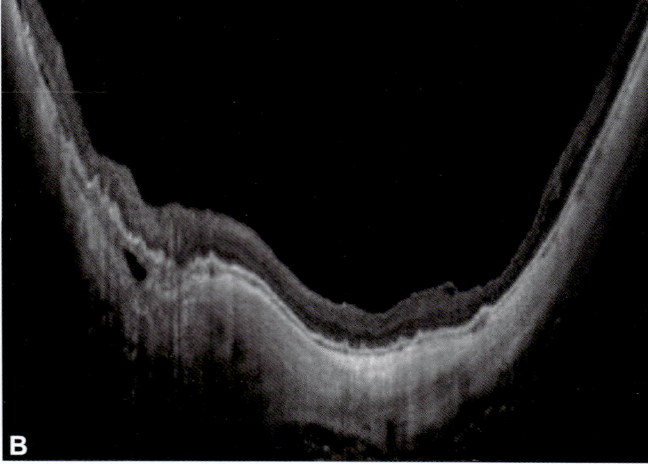

Figs. 17.5A and B: (A) Preoperative swept-source optical coherence tomography (SS-OCT) reveals an eye with myopic foveoschisis and retinal detachment. Hyaloid traction is visible. (B) Postoperative OCT shows a settled retina with relief of traction.

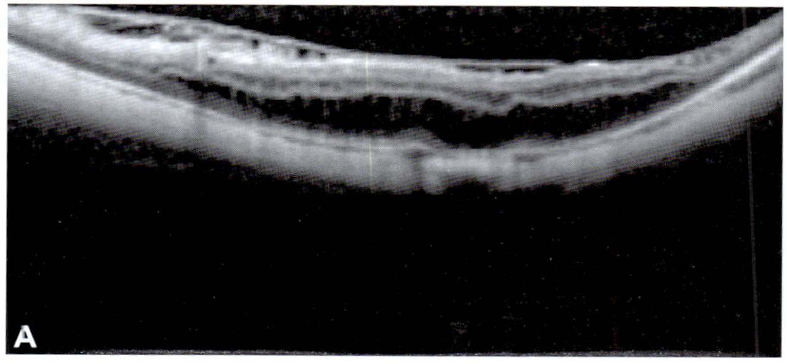 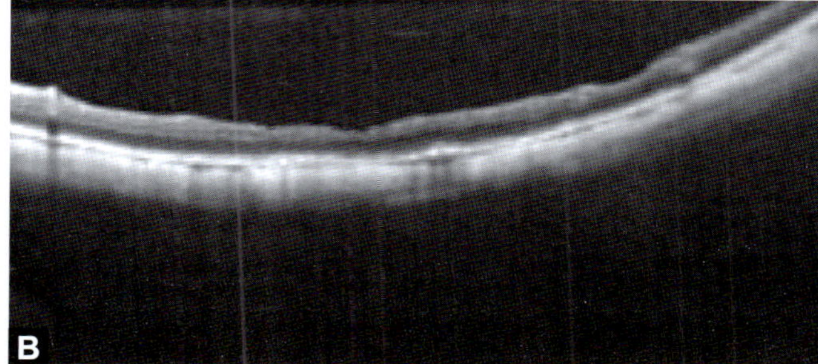

Figs. 17.6A and B: (A) Preoperative swept-source optical coherence tomography (SS-OCT) of a patient with myopic foveoschisis. (B) Postoperative SS-OCT image following pars plana vitrectomy with fovea sparing internal limiting membrane (ILM) peeling.

ILM peeling to avoid intraoperative macular hole formation with improved surgical outcome. At our center, we prefer pars plana vitrectomy with triamcinolone-assisted posterior vitreous detachment (PVD) induction, followed by intraoperative OCT guided center-sparing ILM peeling and gas tamponade for cases of myopic foveoschisis.

In such patients with pathological myopia undergoing surgery for myopic foveoschisis, presence of refractive surgery like phakic intraocular lens (phakic IOL) may pose intraoperative challenges during critical steps like PVD induction and ILM peeling under high magnification lenses due to aberrations and formation of ghost images.[40] Thus, a thorough posterior segment evaluation including posterior segment OCT should be done during refractive workup in high myope individuals before a decision for a refractive procedure is made.[40]

SUMMARY

Macular abnormalities are frequent in patients with degenerative myopia. Vitreoretinal interface abnormalities and traction are important in pathophysiology of myopic foveoschisis. Optical coherence tomography contributes significantly in diagnosis of these patients and is an important investigation in examination of eyes with pathological myopia. Myopic foveoschisis may be missed on clinical examination alone, hence it is prudent to get an OCT done in all cases of pathological myopia.

REFERENCES

1. Sperduto RD, Seigel D, Roberts J, et al. Prevalence of myopia in the United States. Arch Ophthalmology. 1983;101(3):405-7.
2. Wong TY, Ferreira A, Hughes R, et al. Epidemiology and disease burden of pathologic myopia and myopic choroidal neovascularization: an evidence-based systematic review. Am J Ophthalmology. 2014;157(1):9-25.
3. Neelam K, Cheung CM, Ohno-Matsui K, et al. Choroidal neovascularization in pathological myopia. Prog Retina Eye Res. 2012;31(5):495-525.
4. Silva R. Myopic maculopathy: a review. Ophthalmologica. 2012;228(4):197-213.
5. Mitry D, Zambarakji H. Recent trends in the management of maculopathy secondary to pathological myopia. Graefes Arch Clin Exp Ophthalmology. 2012;250(1):3-13.
6. Takano M, Kishi S. Foveal retinoschisis and retinal detachment in severely myopic eyes with posterior staphyloma. Am J Ophthalmology. 1999;128(4):472-6.
7. Phillips CI. Retinal detachment at the posterior pole. Br J Ophthalmology. 1958;42(12):749-53.
8. Baba T, Ohno-Matsui K, Futagami S, et al. Prevalence and characteristics of foveal retinal detachment without macular hole in high myopia. Am J Ophthalmology. 2003;135(3):338-42.
9. Shimada N, Ohno-Matsui K, Baba T, et al. Natural course of macular retinoschisis in highly myopic eyes without macular hole or retinal detachment. Am J Ophthalmology. 2006;142(3):497-500.
10. Benhamou N, Massin P, Haouchine B, et al. Macular retinoschisis in highly myopic eyes. Am J Ophthalmology. 2002;133(6):794-800.
11. Akiba J, Konno S, Sato E, et al. Retinal detachment and retinoschisis detected by optical coherence tomography in a myopic eye with macular hole. Ophthalmic Surg Lasers. 2003;31(3):240-2.
12. Polito A, Lanzetta P, Del Borrello M, et al. Spontaneous resolution of a shallow detachment of the macula in a highly myopic eye. Am J Ophthalmology. 2003;135(4):546-7.
13. Kanda S, Uemura A, Sakamoto Y, et al. Vitrectomy with internal limiting membrane peeling for macular retinoschisis and retinal detachment without macular hole in highly myopic eyes. Am J Ophthalmology. 2003;136(1):177-80.
14. Ikuno Y. Pathogenesis and treatment of myopic foveoschisis. Nippon Ganka Gakkai Zasshi. 2006;110(11):855-63.
15. Bando H, Ikuno Y, Choi JS, et al. Ultrastructure of internal limiting membrane in myopic foveoschisis. Am J Ophthalmology. 2005;139(1):197-9.
16. Tang J, Rivers MB, Moshfeghi AA, et al. Pathology of macular foveoschisis associated with degenerative myopia. J Ophthalmology 2010.
17. Ip M, Garza-Karren C, Duker JS, et al. Differentiation of degenerative retinoschisis from retinal detachment using optical coherence tomography. Ophthalmology. 1999;106(3):600-5.
18. Sayanagi K, Ikuno Y, Tano Y. Tractional internal limiting membrane detachment in highly myopic eyes. Am J Ophthalmology. 2006;142(5):850-2.
19. Ikuno Y, Gomi F, Tano Y. Potent retinal arteriolar traction as a possible cause of myopic foveoschisis. Am J Ophthalmology. 2005;139(1):462-7.

20. Sayanagi K, Ikuno Y, Tano Y. Different fundus autofluorescence patterns of retinoschisis and macular hole retinal detachment in high myopia. Am J Ophthalmology. 2007;144(2):299-301.

21. Kobayashi H, Kishi S. Vitreous surgery for highly myopic eyes with foveal detachment and retinoschisis. Ophthalmology. 2003;110(9):1702-7.

22. Ikuno Y, Sayanagi K, Ohji M, et al. Vitrectomy and internal limiting membrane peeling for myopic foveoschisis. Am J Ophthalmology. 2004;137(4):719-24.

23. Baba T, Tanaka S, Maesawa A, et al. Scleral buckling with macular plombe for eyes with myopic macular retinoschisis and retinal detachment without macular hole. Am J Ophthalmology. 2006; 142(3):483-7.

24. Ando F, Ohba N, Touura K, et al. Anatomical and visual outcomes after episcleral macular buckling compared with 1842 Retina, the journal of retinal and vitreous diseases 2015 volume 35 number 9 those after pars plana vitrectomy for retinal detachment caused by macular hole in highly myopic eyes. Retina. 2007;27(1):37-44.

25. Mateo C, Burés-Jelstrup A, Navarro R, et al. Macular buckling for eyes with myopic foveoschisis secondary to posterior staphyloma. Retina. 2012;32(6):1121-8.

26. Kumagai K, Furukawa M, Ogino N, et al. Factors correlated with postoperative visual acuity after vitrectomy and internal limiting membrane peeling for myopic foveoschisis. Retina 2010;30(6): 874-80.

27. Zheng B, Chen Y, Chen Y, et al. Vitrectomy and internal limiting membrane peeling with perfluoropropane tamponade or balanced saline solution for myopic foveoschisis. Retina. 2011;31(4): 692-701.

28. Shin JY, Yu HG. Visual prognosis and spectral-domain optical coherence tomography findings of myopic foveoschisis surgery using 25-Gauge transconjunctival sutureless vitrectomy. Retina. 2012;32(3):486-92.

29. Lim SJ, Kwon HY, Kim HS, et al. Vitrectomy and internal limiting membrane peeling without gas tamponade for myopic foveoschisis. Graefes Arch Clin Exp Ophthalmology. 2012;250(11):1573-7.

30. Kim KS, Lee SB, Lee WK. Vitrectomy and internal limiting membrane peeling with and without gas tamponade for myopic foveoschisis. Am J Ophthalmology. 2012;153(2):320-6.

31. Uchida A, Shinoda H, Koto T, et al. Vitrectomy for myopic foveoschisis with internal limiting membrane peeling and no gas tamponade. Retina. 2014;34(3):455-60.

32. Sepulveda G, Chang S, Freund B, et al. Late recurrence of myopic foveoschisis after successful repair with primary vitrectomy and incomplete membrane peeling. Retina 2014;34(9):1841-7.

33. Kwok AK, Lai TY, Yip WW. Vitrectomy and gas tamponade without internal limiting membrane peeling for myopic foveoschisis. Br J Ophthalmology. 2005;89:1180-3.

34. Gaucher D, Haouchine B, Tadayoni R, et al. Long-term follow-up of high myopic foveoschisis: natural course and surgical outcome. Am J Ophthalmology. 2007;143(3):455-62.

35. Yeh SI, Chang WC, Chen LJ. Vitrectomy without internal limiting membrane peeling for macular retinoschisis and foveal detachment in highly myopic eyes. Acta Ophthalmology. 2008;86(2):219-24.

36. Spaide R, Fisher Y. Removal of adherent cortical vitreous plaques without removing the internal limiting membrane in the repair of macular detachments in highly myopic eyes. Retina. 2005;25(3):290-5.

37. Gao X, Ikuno Y, Fujimoto S, et al. Risk factors for development of full thickness macular hole after pars plana vitrectomy for myopic foveoschisis. Am J Ophthalmology. 2013;155(6):1021-7.

38. Shimada N, Sugamoto Y, Ogawa M, et al. Fovea-sparing internal limiting membrane peeling for myopic traction maculopathy. Am J Ophthalmology. 2012;154(4):693-701.

39. Kumar A, Ravani R, Mehta A, et al. Outcomes of microscope integrated intraoperative optical coherence tomography guided center sparing internal limiting membrane peeling for myopic traction maculopathy: a novel technique. Int Ophthalmology 2017.

40. Kumar A, Mehta A, Ravani RD, et al. Management of a case of myopic foveoschisis with phakic intraocular lens (pIOL) in situ: intraoperative challenges. BMJ Case Rep. 2017.

Chapter 18

Optic Nerve Head Pit with Maculopathy

Atul Kumar, Karthikeya R, Raghav Ravani, Yogita Gupta

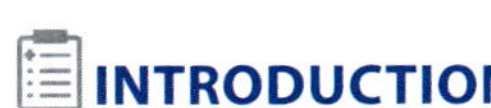 INTRODUCTION

Optic nerve head pits or optic disc pits (ODP) are congenital localized excavations present commonly on the inferotemporal aspect of the optic disc. They can be oval or round in shape and may vary in color from gray, white to yellow. They usually measure less than one half of a disc diameter in width.[1] They can be located anywhere on the nerve head, but most commonly they are located on the temporal aspect of the disc. Optic nerve pits are often asymptomatic and only when macular involvement is observed in the form of macular schisis, neurosensory detachment (NSD), outer or inner lamellar holes does vision drop and central blurring of vision occurs necessitating treatment in about 25% to 75% of eyes. These are usually associated with macular schisis. Pits located centrally on the optic disc are not associated with retinal detachment. ODP associated maculopathy can rarely resolve spontaneously but most cases require treatment to prevent permanent visual loss.

EPIDEMIOLOGY, PATHOGENESIS AND GENETICS

Incidence of optic disc pits is rare and occurs in about 1 per 11,000 patients.[2] Most cases are unilateral with only about 5% of the cases being bilateral. About one-half of the patients have either a current or a past evidence of a neurosensory detachment.[3] Reports of more than one pit in the same disc exists in literature.

Various theories have been proposed explaining the pathogenesis of optic disc pits but exact cause of their development is still uncertain (Flowchart 18.1). Most of them are associated with a posterior vitreous detachment. The origin of the submacular fluid and the embryological defect leading to optic disc pit are still debatable.

Optic pits associated with retinochoroidal colobomas have been proposed to occur secondary to the defect in closure of the embryonic fissure. Some authors have proposed that optic disc pits are actually colobomas. The finding of optic nerve pits associated with colobomas in few cases

Flowchart 18.1: Pathogenesis of fluid accumulation within the retina in optic nerve head pit maculopathy eyes.

supports this conclusion, where the pits are considered as atypical form of the anomaly.[4-6] But contrary to this, most pits occur in the temporal or inferotemporal location, suggesting that the optic disc pits are not true colobomas.[4]

Mann suggested that the pits occur as a result of failure of closure of only the upper end of the embryonic fissure while others hypothesize it to result from disturbances in the development of the primitive epithelial papilla.[7]

In 1908, Reis first reported maculopathy associated with optic disc pits.[6,8] There are multiple speculations about the likely source of the fluid in cases of ODP associated maculopathy-fluid from the vitreous cavity,[1] subarachnoid space,[9] choroid vasculature, vessels at the base of the optic disc pit and through macular holes. A small diaphanous tissue overlying congenital optic pits and the intravitreal traction on the optic pit by an anomalous Cloquet's canal may play a role in the development of macular detachment.[10]

Optic disc pits are isolated, nonfamilial malformations.[11] Few reports of familial origin have been reported. Mostly congenital, but an acquired nature of these anomalies has also been described.[12]

CLASSIFICATION

Based on the optical coherence tomography (OCT) findings of the disc pit and associated changes over the macula, different stages have been proposed (Figs. 18.1A to C and Table 18.1).[13-16]

CLINICAL FEATURES

Most optic disc pits (ODPs) are asymptomatic. They become symptomatic only when associated with macular changes, such as neurosensory detachment (serous) over macula (25% to 75% of cases) which generally presents in the 3rd or 4th decade (Figs. 18.1 and 18.2).[4,17] The involved disc is usually larger than that of the contralateral side.[1] The detachments are usually shallow, and may be associated with subretinal deposits with are macrophages that have engulfed retinal pigment epithelial cells. Retinal detachment is often associated with larger and temporally located pits. ODPs may be associated with splitting of retinal layers, called retinoschisis. Usually, the area of schisis is larger than the area of neurosensory detachment. Even ILM detachments are known to occur with this condition (Fig. 18.1C).

Within 2 weeks of development of retinal detachment, approximately one-fourth of eyes develop macular hole.[3] Such macular holes usually have an intact ILM overlying it (Figs. 18.3A and B). They are associated with visual field defects like enlarged blind spots due to the optic disc per se and retinal detachment secondary to the pit. Centrally and eccentrically located pits are associated with other visual field defects like nasal and temporal steps, paracentral scotomas, localized constriction, etc. Optic disc pit complicated by detachment of outer layers may lead to a dense central scotoma.

The pits can appear in different colours from gray being the most common to yellow and back. Eccentrically located pits are associated with RPE changes in peripapillary region or atrophy of choroid, predisposing to choroidal neovascularization.

SYSTEMIC ASSOCIATIONS

There are no known systemic associations of congenital optic disc pits. However, an association with basal encephalocele has been described.[18]

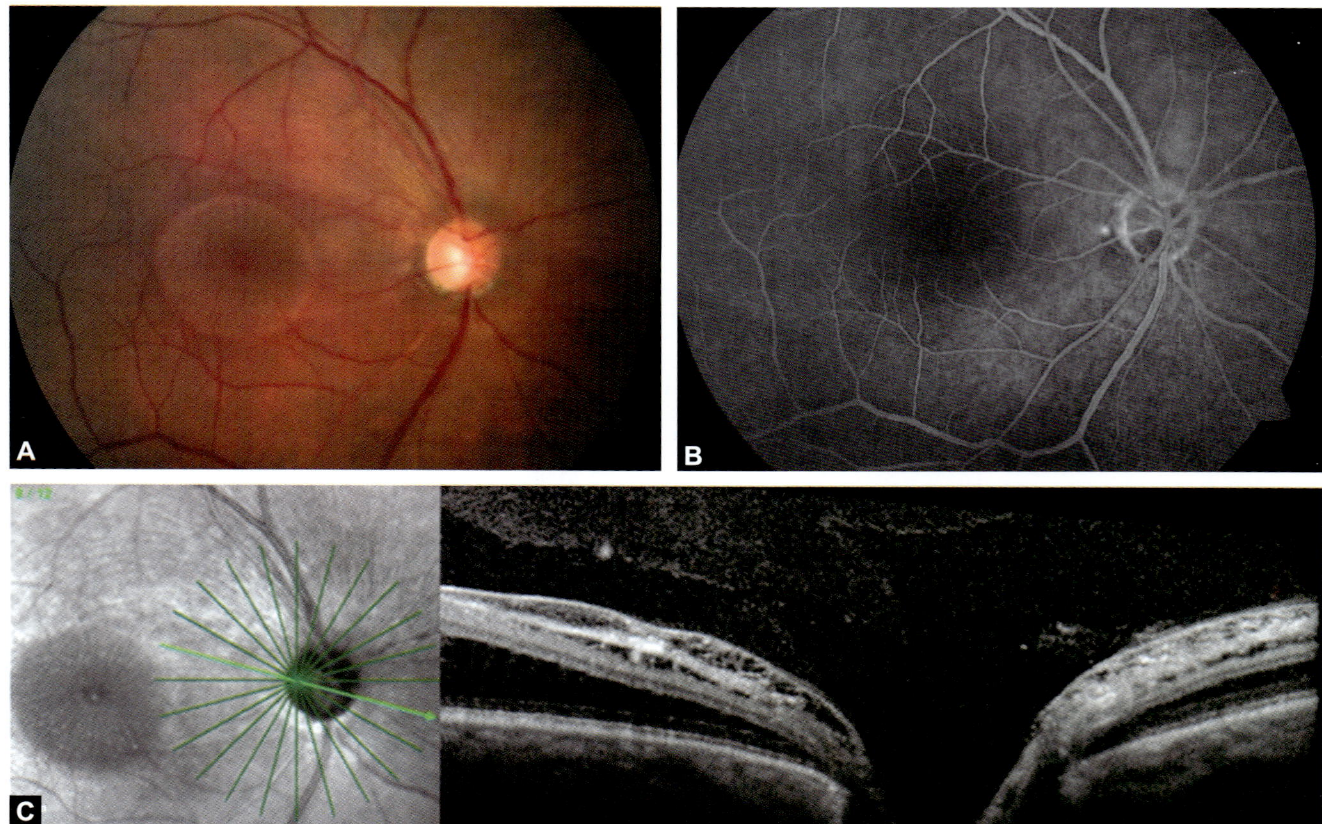

Figs. 18.1A to C: (A) Stage 3 optic disc pit with serous detachment mimicking central serous retinopathy (CSR). (B) On fundus fluorescein angiography (FFA), no dye pooling is visible within the serous detachment. (C) Optical coherence tomography (OCT) shows a multilayered schisis extending till the disc head.

Table 18.1: Stages of optic disc pit.

Stage 1	Isolated asymptomatic pits
Stage 2	Development of a schisis cavity
Stage 3	Development of a serous macular detachment
Stage 4	Development of macular cysts and/or outer layer holes
Burnt stage	Temporal optic disc pit with macular pigmentary changes indicating previous macular detachment or a similar therapeutic intervention.

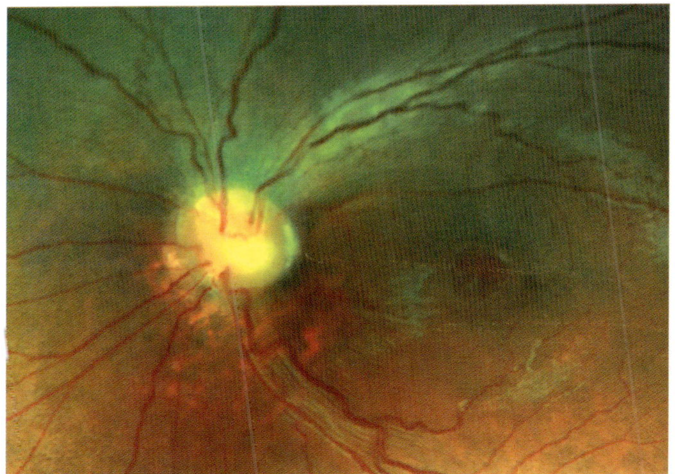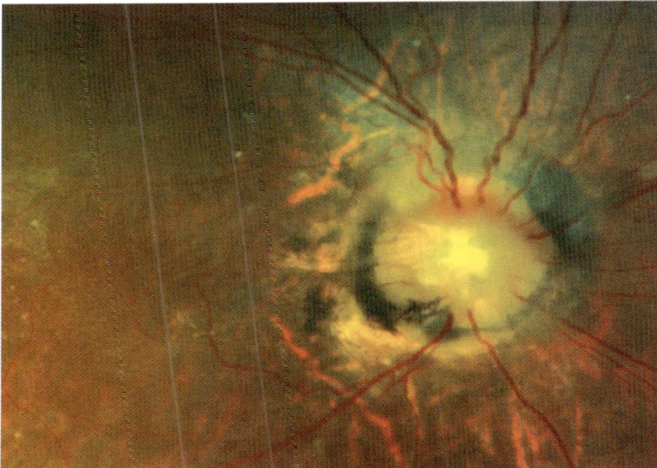

Fig. 18.2: Morning glory disc with optic disc pit.

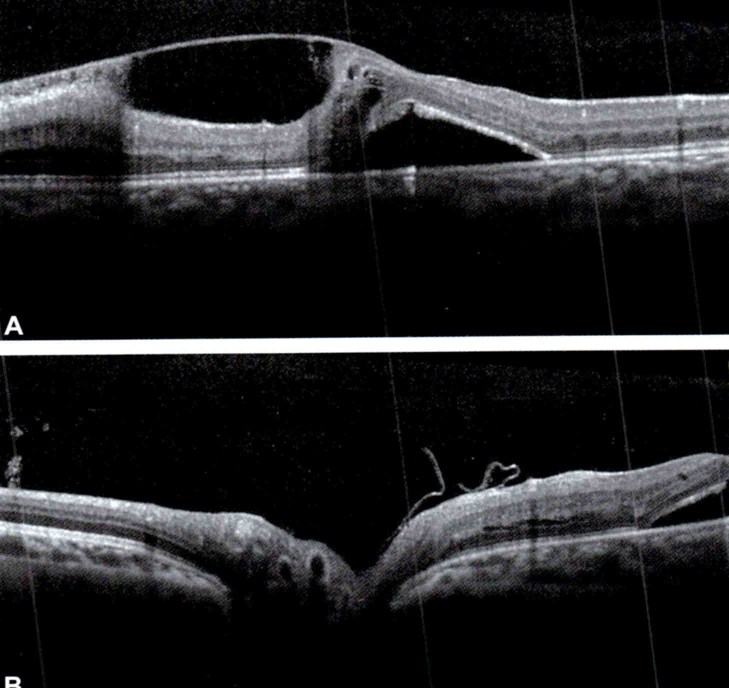

Figs. 18.3A and B: (A) Optic nerve head (ONH) pit with serous detachment and ILM detachment (B) Postsurgery, at 2 weeks the serous detachment is settling, and the ILM remnants stuffed into the pit are visible.

DIAGNOSIS AND DIAGNOSTIC AIDS (FIGS. 18.4 AND 18.5)

Fundus fluorescein angiography (FFA) in an eye with optic pit generally reveals hypofluorescence in early stages and hyperfluorescence in late stages.[19,20] This is because of leakage from the blood vessels in the base of optic pit, or diversion of the dye from the vitreous cavity to the pit.[21] The optic disc pit appear hypofluorescent on indocyanine green angiography and late hyperfluorescence corresponding to the area of macular detachment. OCT can reveal macular schisis, cystic changes over the macula, macular neurosensory detachment, and lamellar and outer retinal holes.[13-15]

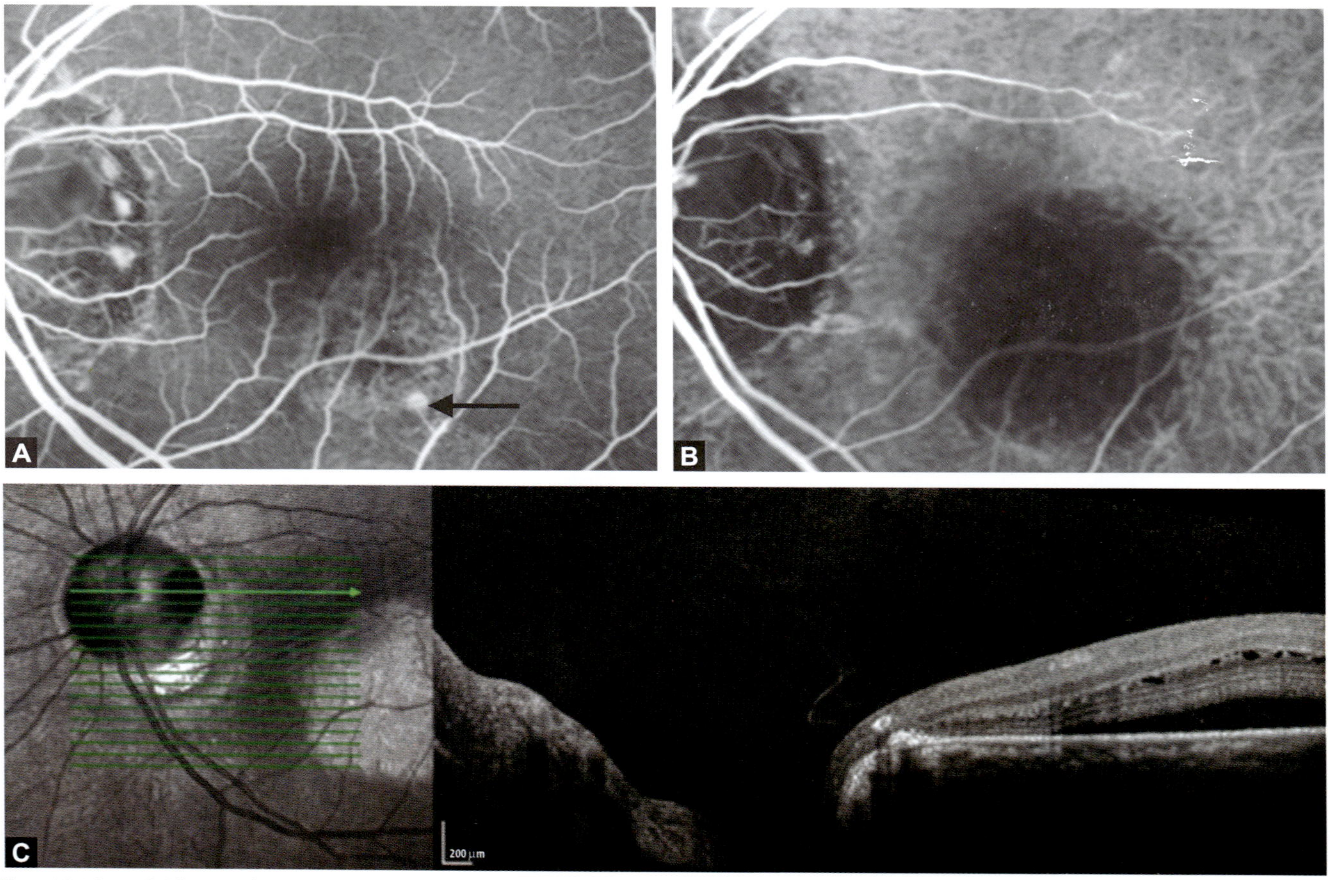

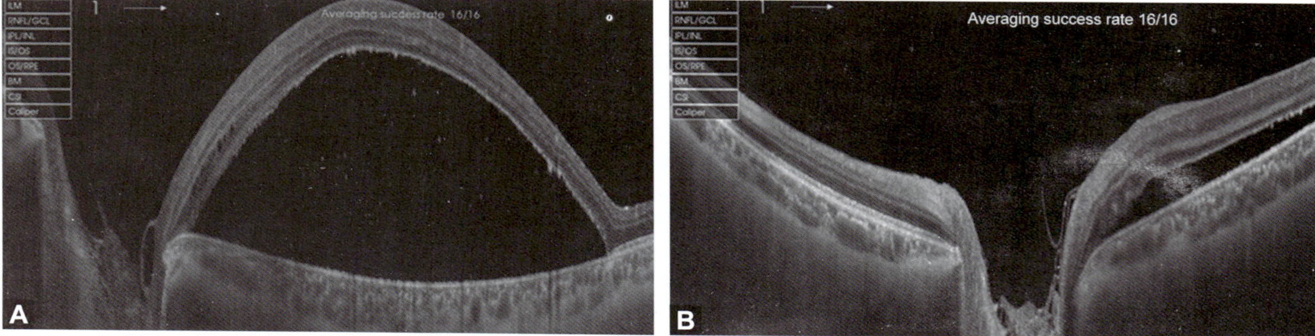

Figs. 18.4A to C: This eye had an optic nerve head pit with subretinal fluid not extending till the temporal edge of the disc. FA revealed an extrafoveal central serous chorioretinopathy (CSC) leak (black arrow) (A) and corresponding hypofluorescence on ICGA (B). OCT is confirmatory with macular detachment not extending till the edge of the disc (C).

Figs. 18.5A and B: (A) Pre- and (B) postoperative optical coherence tomography (OCT) images of an optical disc pit-maculopathy eye. ILM remnants are visible within the pit-sac

TREATMENT, COURSE AND OUTCOMES

The natural course of untreated retinal macular retinal detachment is variable. Retinal detachments associated with optic pits may occasionally resolve without need of any intervention. But in about 50% of the cases subretinal fluid may not resolve with time, leading to vision loss.[3]

A variety of treatment modalities have been described for the treatment of the macular detachment including observation, mannitol,[22] steroids,[23] diathermy,[24] photocoagulation along the edges of the area of detachment or laser along the temporal edge of the optic nerve head,[25] intravitreal injection of expanding gas without vitrectomy,[26] and macular scleral buckling.[27]

Steroids cause temporary resorption of fluid and the fluid invariably reappears on discontinuation of therapy. Laser photocoagulation of the peripapillary retina also has been described for ODP associated maculopathy. The laser reaction and subsequent scar between neurosensory retina and RPE causes closure of the communication between the pit and the subretinal space causing resorption of fluid and preventing subsequent collection. Two to three rows of laser spots carefully placed not closer than 500 µm to the disc margins in the temporal retina adjacent to the ODP has been shown to cause resolution in several cases.[28] Adverse effects of this modality includes paracentral scotomas, reduction in final visual acuity and failure of the procedure. Laser also causes slow resorption of the fluid, sometimes over 6–9 months.

Pars plana vitrectomy along with endolaser of the disc pit margin and gas tamponade is an alternate approach. Combination of laser photocoagulation with or without intravitreal tamponade using gas or silicone oil has also been tried.[13,29-31] Macular buckling has also been reported by a group to be highly successful anatomically and functionally with good long term outcomes but it is technically challenging procedure to perform and has not been widely tested.[32]

The current standard of care for ODP associated maculopathy is pars plana vitrectomy with internal limiting membrane peeling and gas tamponade (Figs. 18.5A and B). Promising results have been seen with a modified operative technique of ILM stuffing (intraoperative OCT i.e. iOCT-assisted) performed at our centre. A brilliant blue G dye assisted ILM peeling is done in a peripheral to central fashion so that the free edge of the ILM flap is near the disc edge. This flap is then stuffed gently within the disc pit using a Tano's diamond dusted membrane scraper.[33] Fluid-air exchange is then performed followed by C_8F_8 gas injection and intermittent head own position for 3–5 days. The gas keeps the ILM flap stuffed within the pit and closes off the passage. Alternatively tiny scleral graft has also been described which can be stuffed into the pit.[33] Hirakata et al[34] have described pars plana vitectomy (PPV) with or without ILM peel and closure of ports under fluid with encouraging results too.[35,36]

REFERENCES

1. Gass JD. Serous detachment of the macula. Secondary to congenital pit of the optic nervehead. Am J Ophthalmology. 1969;67(6):821-41.
2. Brown GC, Shields JA, Goldberg RE. Congenital pits of the optic nerve head. II. Clinical studies in humans. Ophthalmology. 1980;87(1):51-65.
3. Kranenburg EW. Crater-like holes in the optic disc and central serous retinopathy. Arch Ophthalmology. 1960;64:912-24.
4. Brown GC, Tasman WS. Congenital anomalies of the optic disk. New York, Grune and Stratton, 1983. 95-91.
5. Brown GC, Augsburger JJ. Congenital pits of the optic nerve head and retinochoroidal colobomas. Can J Ophthalmology. 1980;15(3):144-6.
6. Neilsen J. Pits on the optic disc. Acta Ophthalmology. 1924;2:291-3.
7. Reis W. Eine wenig bekannte typische missbildung am Sehnerveneintritt: Umschriebene Grubenbildung auf der Papilla n. optici. Ztschr Augen. 1908;19:505-28.
8. Mann, I. Developmental Anomalies of the Eye. British Medical Association, London. 2nd edition;1957.pp. 113-6.
9. Petersen HP. Pits or crater-like holes in the optic disc. Arch Ophthalmology. 1958;36:435-43.
10. Irvine AR, Crawford JB. Sullivan JH. The pathogenesis of retinal detachment with morning glory disk and optic pit. Retina. 1986;6(3):146-50.
11. Akiba J, Kakehashi A, Hikichi T, et al. Vitreous findings in cases of optic nerve pits and serous macular detachment. Am J Ophthalmology. 1993;116(1):38-41.
12. Veugelen D Leys, A. Autosomal dominant heredity of optic pits: a report of two families. Bull Soc Belge Ophthalmology. 1987;223(2):75-81.
13. Morgan OG. Acquired hole in the disk. Br J Ophthalmology. 1951;35(7):437-9.
14. Lincoff H, Kreissig I. Optical coherence tomography of pneumatic displacement of optic disk pit maculopathy. Br J Ophthalmology. 1998;82(4):367-72.
15. Rutledge BK, Puliafito CA, Duker JS, et al. Optical coherence tomography of macular lesions associated with optic nerve head pits. Ophthalmology. 1996;103(7):1047-53.
16. Krivoy D, Gentile R, Liebmann JM, et al. Imaging congenital optic disk pits and associated maculopathy using optical coherence tomography. Arch Ophthalmology. 1996;114(2):165-70.
17. Lincoff H, Schiff W, Krivoy D, et al. Optic coherence tomography of optic disk pit maculopathy. Am J Ophthalmology. 1996;122(2):264-6.
18. Brodsky MC. Congenital optic disk anomalies. Surv Ophthalmology. 1994;39:89-112.
19. Van Nouhuys JM, Bruyn GW. Nasopharyngeal trans-sphenoidal encephalocele, crater-like hole in the optic disk and agenesis of the corpus callosum, pneumoencephalographic visualization in a case. Psychiat Neurol Neurochir. 1964;67:243-58.
20. Gass JD. Serous detachment of the macula. Secondary to congenital pit of the optic nervehead. Am J Ophthalmology. 1969;67(6):821-41.
21. Gordon R, Chatfield RK. Pits in the optic disk associated with macular degeneration. Br J Ophthalmology. 1969;53(7):481-9.
22. Brown GC, Augsburger JJ. Congenital pits of the optic nerve head and retinochoroidal colobomas. Can J Ophthalmology. 1980;15(3):144-6.
23. Goldberg RE. Optic nerve pit and associated coloboma with serous detachment. Arch Ophthalmology. 1974;91(2):160-1.
24. Mustonen E, Varonen T. Congenital pit of the optic nerve head associated with serous detachment of the macula. Acta Ophthalmology (Copenh). 1972;50(5):689-98.

25. Mizuno K, Ozawa K. Central flat detachment and pseudohole with optic pit treated with diathermy. Nihon Ganka Kiyo. 1970;21(5):378-83.

26. Majima Y, Niimi K, Hasegawa Y. Light coagulation therapy in pit of the optic nerve with detachment of the maculae luteae. Nippon Ganka Gakkai Zasshi. 1973;77(2):99-104.

27. Bonnet M. Serous macular detachment associated with optic nerve pits. Graefes Arch Clin Exp Ophthalmology. 1991;229(6):526-32.

28. Georgopoulos GT, Theodossiadis PG, Kollia AC, et al. Visual field improvement after treatment of optic disk pit maculopathy with the macular buckling procedure. Retina.1999;19(5):370-7.

29. Brockhurst RJ. Optic pits and posterior retinal detachment. Trans Am Ophthalmology Soc. 1975;73:264-91.

30. Postel EA, Pulido JS, McNamara JA, et al. The etiology and treatment of macular detachment associated with optic nerve pits and related anomalies. Trans Am Ophthalmology Soc. 1998;96:73-88.

31. Cox MS, Witherspoon CD, Morris RE, et al. Evolving techniques in the treatment of macular detachment caused by optic nerve pits. Ophthalmology. 1988;95(7):889-96.

32. Georgalas I, Petrou P, Koutsandrea C, et al. Optic disk pit maculopathy treated with vitrectomy, internal limiting membrane peeling, and gas tamponade: a report of two cases. Eur J Ophthalmology. 2009;19(2):324-6.

33. Theodossiadis GP, Theodossiadis PG. The macular buckling technique in the treatment of optic disk pit maculopathy. Semin Ophthalmology. 2000;15(2):108-15.

34. Kumar A, Gogia V, Nagpal R, et al. Minimal gauge vitrectomy for optic disk pit maculopathy: our results. Indian J Ophthalmology. 2015;63(12):924-6.

35. Hirakata A, Inoue M, Hiraoka T, et al. Vitrectomy without laser treatment or gas tamponade for macular detachment associated with an optic disk pit. Ophthalmology. 2012;119(4):810-8.

36. Ooto S, Mittra RA, Ridley ME, et al. Vitrectomy with inner retinal fenestration for optic disk pit maculopathy. Ophthalmology. 2014;121(9):1727-33.

Submacular Hemorrhage

Atul Kumar, Dheepak Sundar, Raghav Ravani, Farin Shaikh

INTRODUCTION

Submacular hemorrhage (SMH) frequently results from a choroidal neovascular membrane (CNVM) secondary to age-related macular degeneration (AMD) or more commonly from polypoidal choroidal vasculopathy (PCV). Other conditions associated with CNVM, including myopia, trauma, ocular histoplasmosis and angioid streaks, can also lead to submacular hemorrhage.[1-3] A small, thin SMH can be observed, while massive submacular hemorrhages often have a poor prognosis regardless of intervention.

In patients with SMH, there is accumulation of blood between the retinal pigment epithelium (RPE) and the neurosensory retina and/or under the retinal pigment epithelium. This can lead to substantial vision loss if it involves the center of the macula.[1-3] Once considered to be highly devastating, this condition is now increasingly being managed using anti-vascular endothelial growth factor (VEGF) agents, pneumatic displacement and fibrinolytics with modest success. Yet it still continues to be an important cause of vision loss, especially in the population of patients with neovascular AMD.[4]

Small and thin films of subretinal blood less than 1 disc diameter (DD) in size are not considered as SMH and are part of the clinical manifestation of neovascular AMD. SMH greater than 1 DD but less than 4 DD is considered as small SMH, one that is larger than 4 DD but is confined within the temporal arcades is classified as a medium sized SMH (Figs. 19.1A and B) and the one that crosses temporal arcade is considered as a massive SMH (hemorrhagic retinal detachment) (Fig. 19.2). Also, SMHs in which foveal thickness exceeds 500 μm are labeled as thick SMH. Sub-RPE hemorrhage is also a part of SMH.[5]

ETIOLOGY

Submacular hemorrhage is most commonly seen in patients with CNVM secondary to neovascular AMD. In Asian population, polypoidal choroidal vasculopathy (PCV) is an important cause of SMH. Anticoagulant and antiplatelet therapy

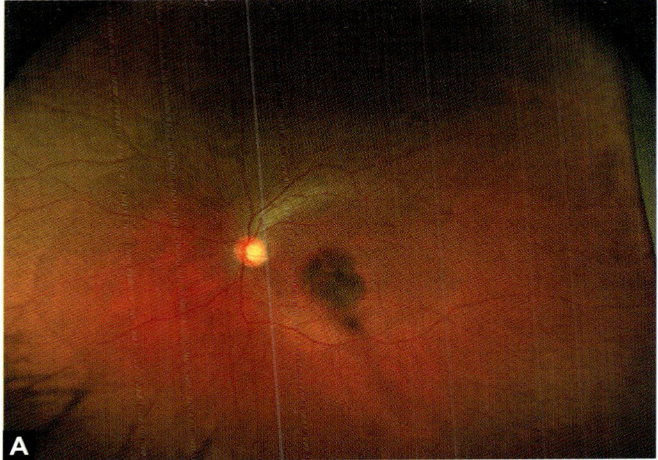

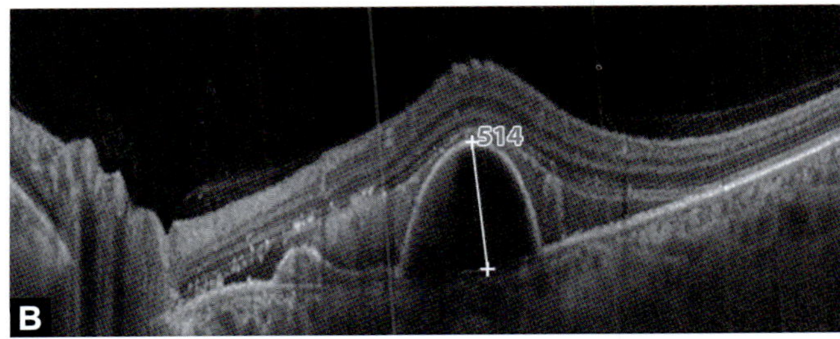

Figs. 19.1A and B: Ultrawide field fundus photograph showing medium-sized submacular hemorrhage with scalloped margins. Swept-source optical coherence tomography (SS-OCT) reveals subretinal with subpigment epithelial detachment (PED) blood secondary to a polypoidal choroidal vasculopathy (PCV) lesion.

increases the risk of large SMH in hypertensive patients with AMD.[6] Other risk factors are hypertension, treatment with photodynamic therapy and treat-and-extend regimens of anti-VEGF therapy.[5] Other causes of CNVM like pathological myopia, presumed ocular histoplasmosis syndrome, choroidal rupture, angioid streaks can also lead to SMH. Trauma is

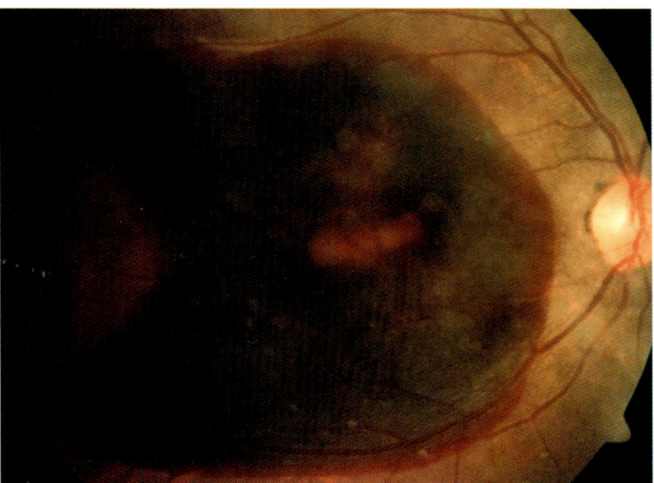

Fig. 19.2: Fundus photograph of a patient with massive submacular hemorrhage extending beyond the arcades.

another important cause of SMH, immediate in cases of choroidal rupture and late CNVM. Retinal artery macroaneurysm (RAM), coagulopathies, tumors like choroidal melanoma, choroidal metastasis and retinal cavernous hemangioma, terson syndrome, iatrogenic (surgical or laser induced) and rarely Valsalva retinopathy and diabetic retinopathy can cause SMH.[3] Idiopathic cases have also been reported.

PATHOPHYSIOLOGY

Glatt and Machemer[7] were the first to study the ultrastructural changes in retina after a subretinal hemorrhage in a rabbit eye and proposed three important mechanisms causing permanent tissue damage—(1) shearing effect on the photoreceptors, (2) toxic effect of iron and (3) the barrier effect of the clot. The study suggested that irreversible damage to the retina occurred as early as 24 hours and photoreceptors were almost absent by 7 days.

The fibrin strands in the clot interdigitate with the photoreceptors as early as 25 minutes after the onset of hemorrhage and when the clot retracts, contraction of these fibrin strands cause tearing of the photoreceptor outer and inner segment in sheets. Toth CA et al. noted this to occur within one hour in two thirds of their experimental model of subretinal hemorrhage in cats. It was also noted that, if subretinal tissue plasminogen activator (tPA) was present, the fibrin strands did not form and there was no photoreceptor damage. The blood in subretinal space is later engulfed by macrophages, RPE and Müller cells; and the hemosiderin from the breakdown of red blood cells gets converted into ferritin which is toxic to the retina, RPE and choriocapillaris. Gradually over time, iron causes atrophy of all the layers of retina and choriocapillaris. Damage also occurs due to the diffusion barrier formed by the clot. Retinal circulation supplies only as far as the inner

nuclear layer of the retina. The photoreceptor-RPE complex receives its blood supply from the choriocapillaris through diffusion. A clot in the subretinal/sub-RPE space leads to lack of nutrient diffusion to the photoreceptors and subsequent atrophy. Also blood in the subretinal space attracts macrophages and fibroblasts that cause fibrosis and scarring.

Subretinal pigment epithelium bleeds cause more severe vision loss and are associated with a worse prognosis because sub-RPE blood cuts off the RPE along with the photoreceptors from receiving nutrition from choriocapillaris and causes severe RPE and photoreceptor degeneration and atrophy.

Patients of pathological myopia may develop submacular bleeds which may be spontaneous, secondary to lacquer cracks or secondary to a choroidal neovascular membrane.[9]

CLINICAL FEATURES

Patients with a subfoveal bleed experience sudden painless diminution of vision associated with a central scotoma and metamorphopsia. But in those with an extrafoveal bleed or bleed at macula with a preexisting disciform scar, symptoms may be minimal. Logically, thin and smaller SMHs lead to milder symptoms as opposed to thicker and larger SMHs. On examination, there is an elevation of the neurosensory retina caused by blood under it. The subretinal nature of blood is ascertained by the unobscured visibility of the overlying retinal vessels. The color of the blood may vary from fresh bright red or dark red to green in thick hemorrhages.[3] Old SMHs get dehemoglobinized and turn yellow in color. The color of the underlying blood is also important to differentiate a subretinal bleed from a sub-RPE bleed (discussed below). If the subretinal blood is thick, the underlying RPE details like hyperplasia, atrophy, drusen may not be visible. The borders of the SMH are usually irregular and scalloped. When there is liquefaction, there may be layering of the liquefied blood in a gravity dependent manner giving rise to a pseudohypopyon appearance. Associated findings like soft drusen, disciform scar, pathological myopia, RAM, histospots, angioid streaks leading toward the etiology may be noted in either eye. Large dome-shaped SMHs can be confused with choroidal melanomas. RAM and retinal cavernous hemangioma can result in simultaneous preretinal, intraretinal and subretinal bleeding. In these cases, the intraretinal blood dissects through the layers of the retina leading to subretinal bleeding. The overlying preretinal and intraretinal blood may obscure the subretinal blood in these cases and lead to delayed diagnosis.

Subretinal pigment epithelium bleed is also considered a part of SMH, although this behaves differently from the regular subretinal bleed. This involves blood between the RPE and the Bruch's membrane. This often coexists with a subretinal bleed or it may occasionally occur as a stand-alone condition. Sub-RPE bleeds usually present with a worse visual acuity (VA), are usually deep red or green to black in color, with regular borders and visible overlying details of RPE hyperplasia or drusen.

Fluorescein angiography usually shows blocked fluorescence by the subretinal blood. A leaking CNVM can be seen at the margin of the subretinal blood or through the blood, if the blood layer is thin. Indocyanine angiography is of greater help in such cases since it uses infrared light which can penetrate RPE and blood better leading to the visualization of CNVM through the hemorrhage.

Optical coherence tomography (OCT) can help in localizing the level of bleed and estimating the thickness of the blood, both of which are of prognostic significance. It also helps in assessing the status of the overlying neurosensory retina by examination of the continuity of the various zones and lines of the outer retina [like the ellipsoid zone, formerly called as inner and outer segments (IS-OS) junction] and thickness of the foveal retina. Subretinal bleed can be identified on OCT by elevation of the neurosensory retina from RPE, the space being filled with a hyper-reflective material producing a dense shadow beyond it. Sub-RPE blood causes elevation of the RPE from the Bruch's membrane by a hyper-reflective substance which causes shadowing effect on the underlying structures.

NATURAL HISTORY

Literature on the natural history of SMH generally concludes that they have poor prognosis, especially in patients with AMD and large subfoveal bleeds. Scupola et al.[10] observed 60 eyes with submacular hemorrhage due to AMD over a mean duration of 24 months and noted that VA was worse in 80% of eyes with final mean VA of 20/1250. Natural history of SMH was studied in submacular surgery group-B trial in 168 patients and it was found that only 11% had a best corrected visual acuity (BCVA) better than 20/200 as compared to 38% at baseline. Also, 40% had BCVA of 20/800 or worse at the 24-month examination, even though only 18% of eyes had this level of VA at baseline.[11]

PROGNOSTIC FACTORS IN SUBMACULAR BLEEDS

Subretinal hemorrhage damages tissue through a variety of mechanisms: The presence of iron, hemosiderin and fibrin in the blood has toxic effects on the overlying photoreceptors; clot retraction can cause shearing stress and damage the photoreceptors; and finally, physical separation of the photoreceptors from the RPE causes both to atrophy and can result in disciform scar formation. As the mechanisms of damage are time-dependent, early intervention is generally better.

Prognosis primarily depends on three factors: (1) Etiology, (2) volume (horizontal extent and thickness) and (3) duration of the hemorrhage. AMD-related SMH usually fares poorly as compared to trauma, myopia or RAM causing SMH. Histopathological studies indicate that there is usually atrophy of photoreceptors in both early and late stages of CNV with or without associated subretinal hemorrhage which precludes good vision gain in these cases even if SMH

is timely displaced.[3] In a study by Bennet et al. it was found that patients with AMD fared worst and patients with choroidal rupture fared better than others.[12] Foveal involvement is an obvious poor prognostic factor. Thicker hemorrhages occupying a larger area are also generally associated with poorer prognosis. As previously discussed, subretinal blood starts causing damage to the photoreceptors as early as after 25 minutes and therefore early displacement is of paramount importance. A favorable outcome has been suggested if the blood is displaced within 14 days of onset but the earlier it is displaced, the better are the results.[13,14]

Other variables like recurrent hemorrhage, sub-RPE hemorrhage, baseline visual acuity and other ocular comorbidities are also important.[13,14]

 TREATMENT

Since the publication of the results of the submacular surgery group B trial, mechanical removal of clot with membrane has fallen out of favor in cases of SMH.[11] It was shown in this trial that surgery to mechanically remove the clot versus observation led to comparable outcomes (56% of operated patients had greater than or equal to two line loss vs 59% of observed eyes) and that there were higher risk of complications like retinal detachment and cataract in the operated group.[11] The goals of treatment currently are to displace the subretinal blood from macular area, so as to prevent the damage of the RPE and photoreceptors and to be able to visualize and treat the underlying primary pathology that has caused the SMH. The following options either individually by themselves or in various combinations are the modalities in current use for achieving this goal:

- Pneumatic displacement
- Fibrinolysis
- Anti-VEGF agents
- Macular translocation surgery.

Pneumatic Displacement

Pneumatic displacement of SMH (with and without tPA) was first described by Heriot who was the first to report the use of an intravitreal gas bubble for such a purpose.[15] It is a simple office procedure involving minimal risks and has been reported to produce displacement of blood in 65% of the cases and leads to results better than the natural history of the condition.[5] Undiluted volume of 0.3 mL of perfluoropropane or 0.5 mL of sulfur hexafluoride is injected into the vitreous cavity by an aseptic method and prone position is advised for up to 2 weeks (Figs. 19.3A to D). Anterior chamber paracentesis helps prevent acute intraocular pressure rise and subsequent vascular complications. It has also been suggested by Stopa and Lincoff[16] that a more optimum displacement can be achieved by a straight-ahead position postoperatively instead of the prone position.

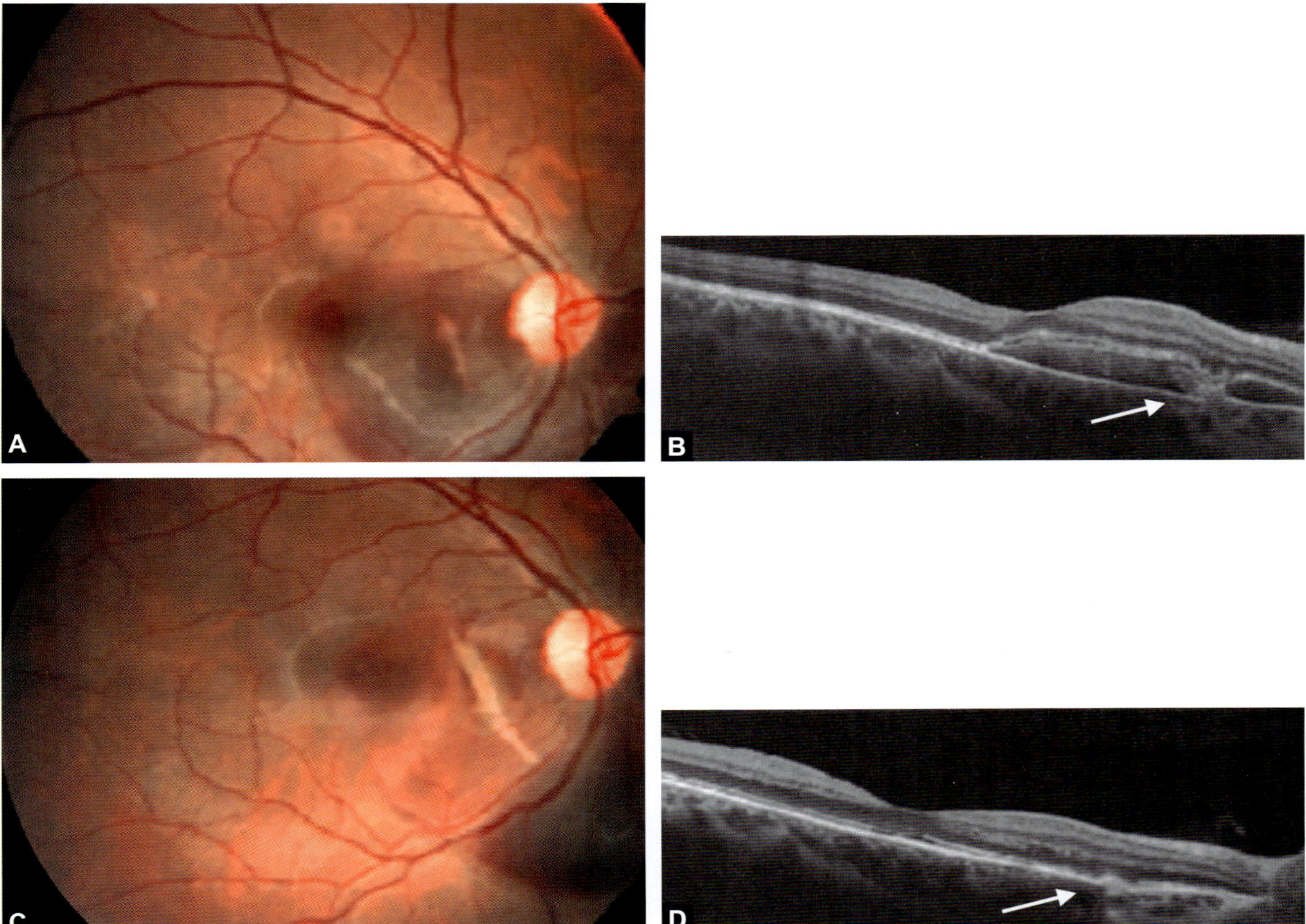

Figs. 19.3A to D: Clinical fundus image and optical coherence tomography showing (A and B) Submacular hemorrhage (SMH) secondary to trauma with choroidal rupture (arrow). (C and D) Postintravitreal gas injection showing resolution of the SMH (white arrow).

Subretinal pneumatic displacement[17] was first described by Martel and Mahmoud for more efficient and rapid displacement of the SMH. In this method, air is injected into the subretinal space after recombinant tPA (rtPA) and anti-VEGF injection to alter the buoyant and gravitational forces acting on the clot and to cause its early inferior displacement.

Tissue plasminogen activator is an endogenous serine protease with a fibrin specific thrombolytic activity which causes clot lysis by the activation of plasminogen to plasmin which in turn breaks down the fibrin meshwork in the clot. It is secreted by endothelial cells in-vivo as a response to injury. Currently, tPA is produced through recombinant DNA technology. Peyman et al. were first to report using tPA in two cases to evacuate SMH due to RAM by subretinal injection through a micropipette and then extracting the dissolved clot through the retinotomy after about 60 minutes.[18]

Dissolution of a fibrin clot is thought to reduce the damage caused to the photoreceptors by the contracting fibrin network within the clot and liquefaction aids in easy displacement. The usual dose is 12.5–50 µg for subretinal use. Subsequently, intravitreal use of rtPA was also found to aid in the dissolution and displacement of SMH in animal and human studies and is also widely used nowadays for achieving clot lysis and displacement. In doses over 50 micrograms for intravitreal use and subretinal use, retinal toxicity has been noted in the form for exudative RD, RPE hyperplasia and pigmentation and reduced b-wave amplitude on ERG. Recurrent hemorrhage is a theoretical risk of using rtPA, especially in recent onset (<72 hours) hemorrhage.

Anti-Vascular Endothelial Growth Factor

Fibrinolysis and pneumatic displacement do not address the primary pathology, which is neovascular AMD in the majority of cases. Anti-VEGFs are the first line and currently the most effective treatment for neovascular AMD and they also reduce the risk of recurrent SMH. Anti-VEGF monotherapy has

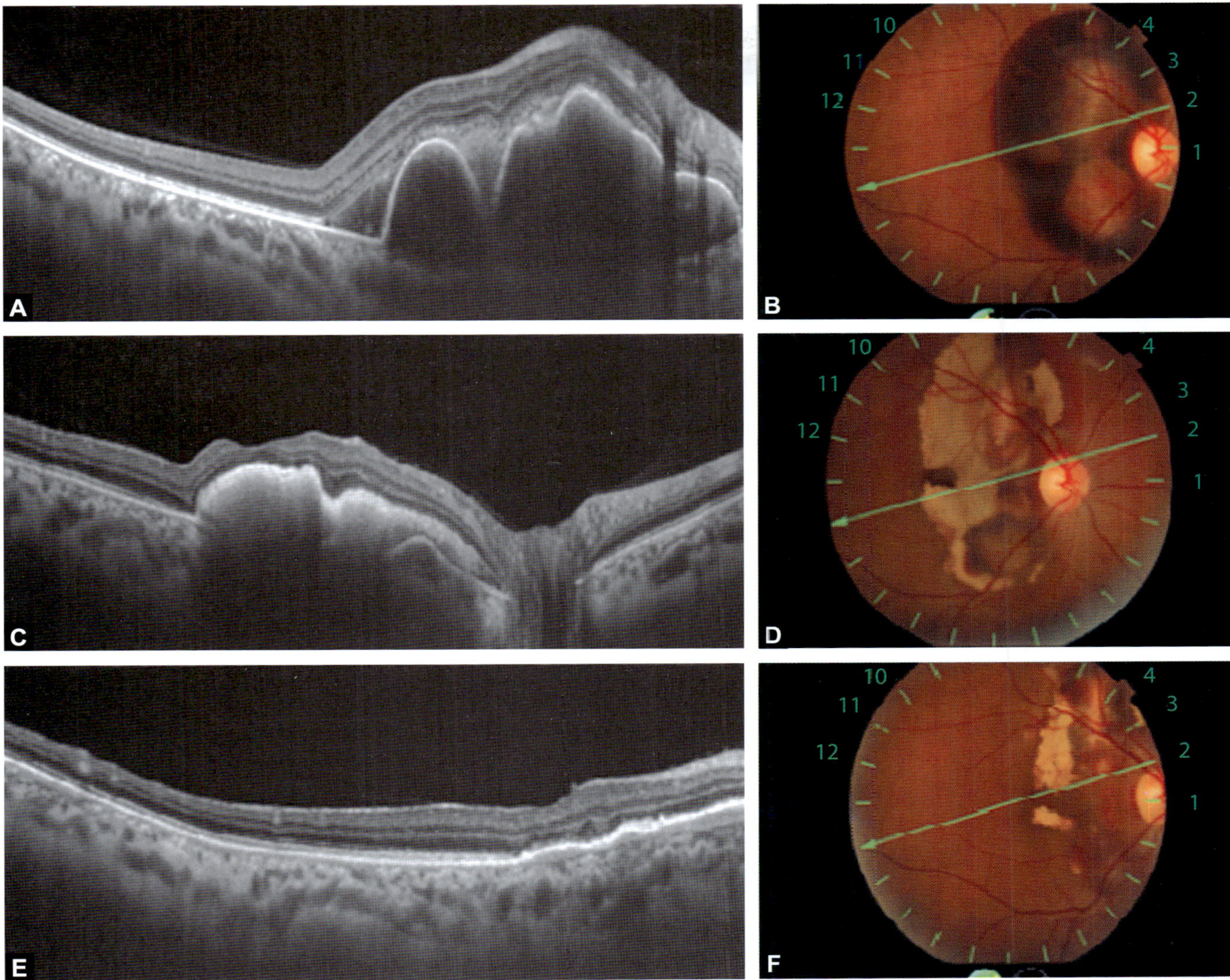

Figs. 19.4A to F: Thumb-shaped hemorrhagic pigment epithelial detachments (PEDs) secondary to polypoidal choroidal vasculopathy, showing rapid resolution with monthly injections of intravitreal aflibercept (2 mg in 0.05 mL). The subretinal blood, however, organizes over time with change in color.

also been shown to be effective in reducing the size of SMH (Figs. 19.4A to F). They are especially useful in cases with a SMH superior to fovea where pneumatic displacement can cause foveal involvement.

Combination Therapy

Copious literature exists today on the management of SMH[5] but most of them are retrospective case series and without a control group. Randomized control trials are difficult to conduct in this rare and devastating condition. Available literature shows that the above three primary modalities have been used in all combinations.[5] Intravitreal rtPA and gas is a widely reported method as it is simple, minimally invasive and an efficient method for displacing the blood (Figs. 19.5 to 19.8). It is reported to successfully displace SMH in about 71% of cases.[5]

It is especially useful in traumatic and idiopathic causes of SMH which do not require anti-VEGF and usually present early. The tPA liquefies the clot and prevents further damage to the retina during displacement of the clot which is adherent to the neurosensory retina and RPE by the gas bubble. Vitrectomy with subretinal rtPA and gas as well as vitrectomy with subretinal rtPA and aspiration of the clot are also reported methods. All the above modalities can be combined with intravitreal anti-VEGF administration to treat the primary pathology. Combination of intravitreal rtPA, gas and

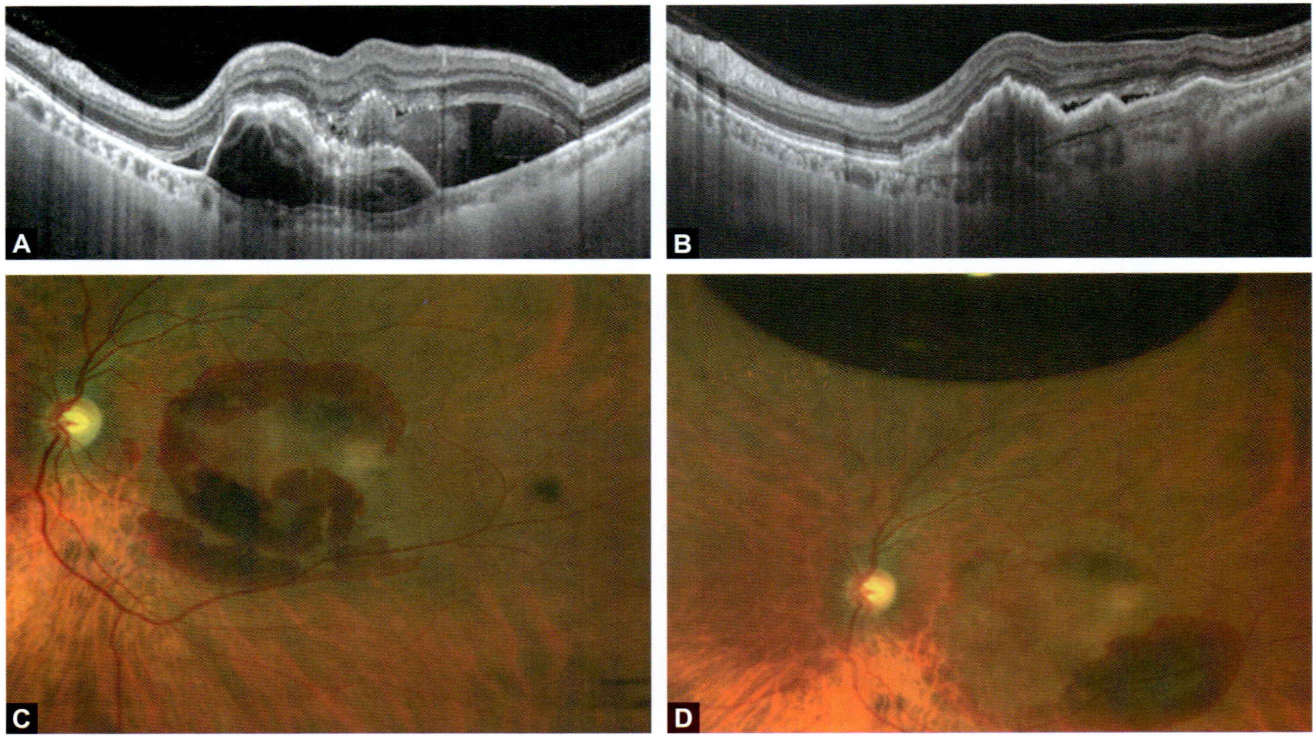

Figs. 19.5A to D: (A and C) Preoperative picture and optical coherence tomography (OCT) showing combined subretinal pigment epithelium (RPE) and subretinal blood. (B and D) Postsubretinal recombinant tissue plasminogen activator (rtPA) treatment reveals displacement of subretinal blood mostly with minimal movement of sub-RPE blood.

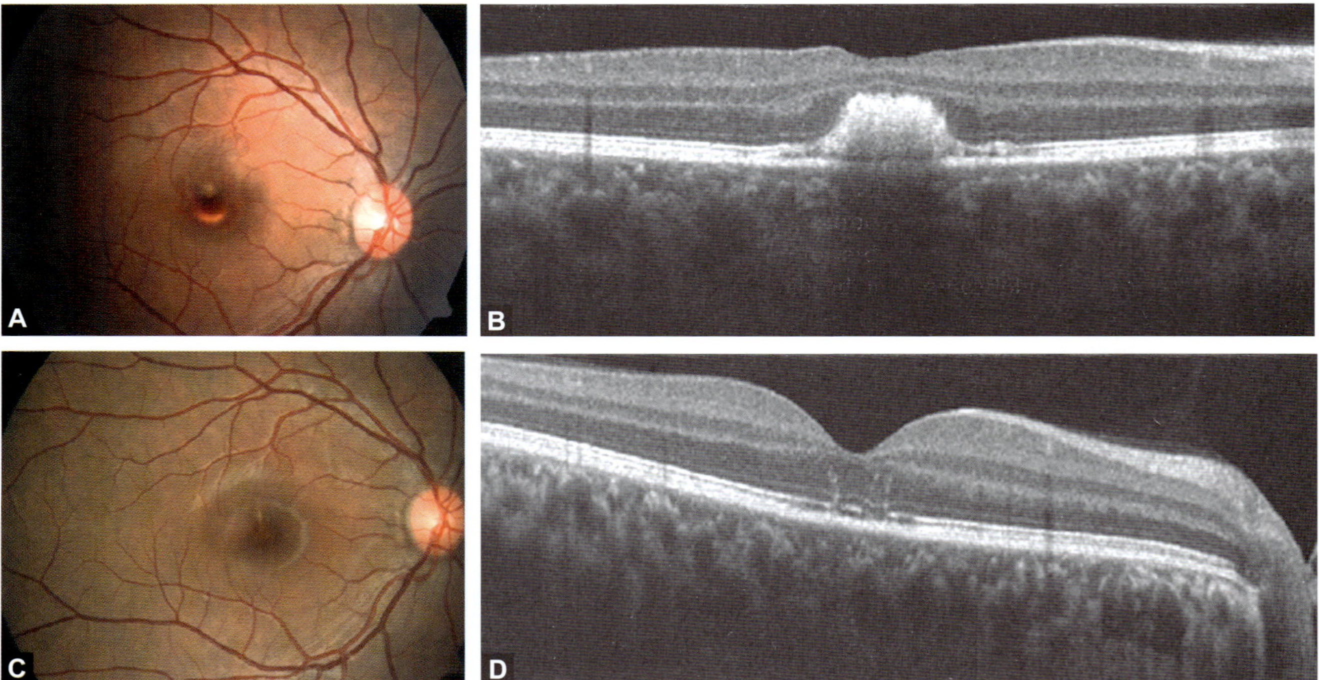

Figs. 19.6A to D: (A and B) Fundus photograph and optical coherence tomography (OCT) showing submacular hemorrhage secondary to trauma, best corrected visual acuity (BCVA-5/60). (C and D) showing displacement of submacular hemorrhage (SMH) at 3 months postintravitreal recombinant tissue plasminogen activator (rtPA) + gas (BCVA-6/18).

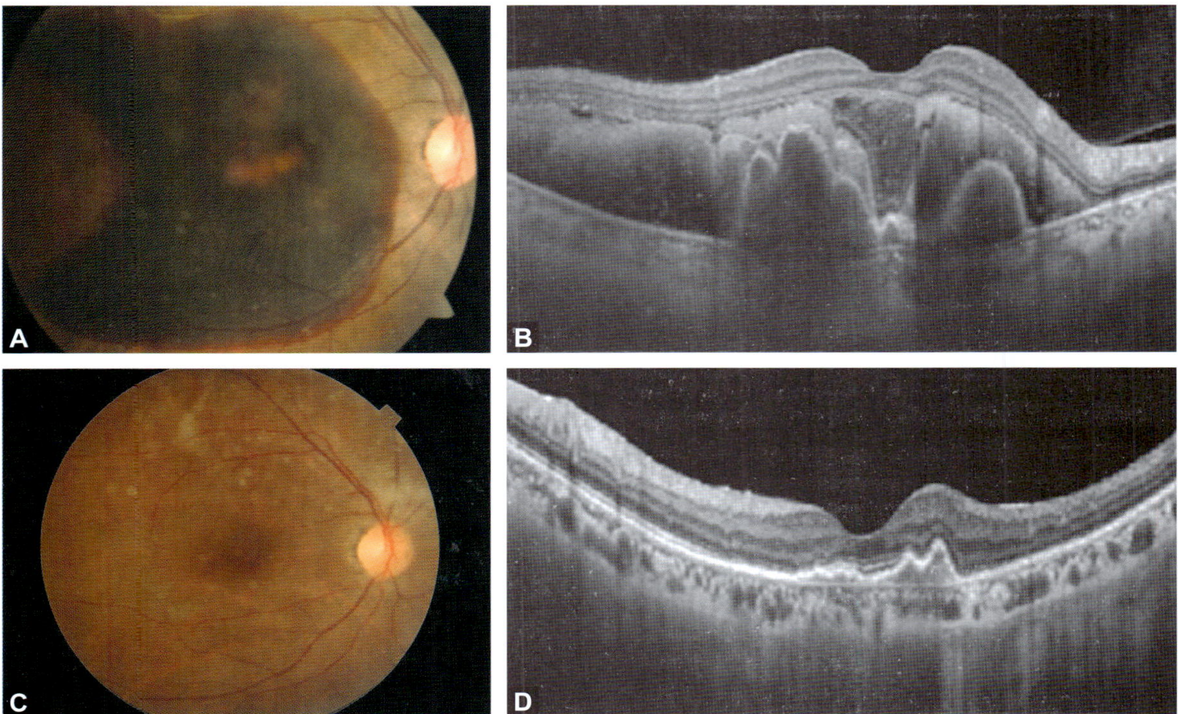

Figs. 19.7A to D: (A) Preoperative fundus photograph of a massive submacular hemorrhage (SMH) secondary to polypoidal choroidal vasculo-pathy, best corrected visual acuity-hand movement close to the face (BCVA-HMCF). (B) Swept source optical coherence tomography (SS-OCT) of the same showing thumb-shaped pigment epithelial detachments (PEDs) and SMH. (C and D) Postoperative subretinal recombinant tissue plasminogen activator (r-tPA) and gas 8th month showing resolution of SMH (BCVA-6/18).

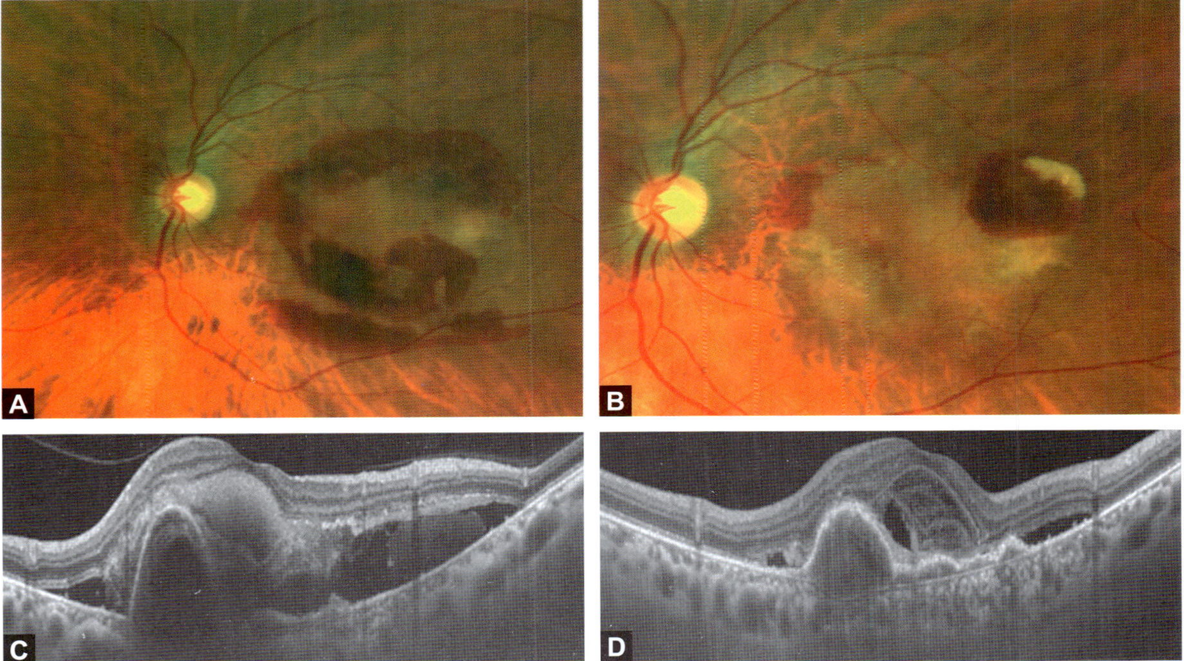

Figs. 19.8A to D: Pre- (A and C) and post (B and D) submacular tissue plasminogen activator (tPA) 50 u with 0.1 cc Avastin and 0.4 cc air. There is displacement of the submacular bleed in this polypoidal choroidal vasculopathy (PCV) eye.

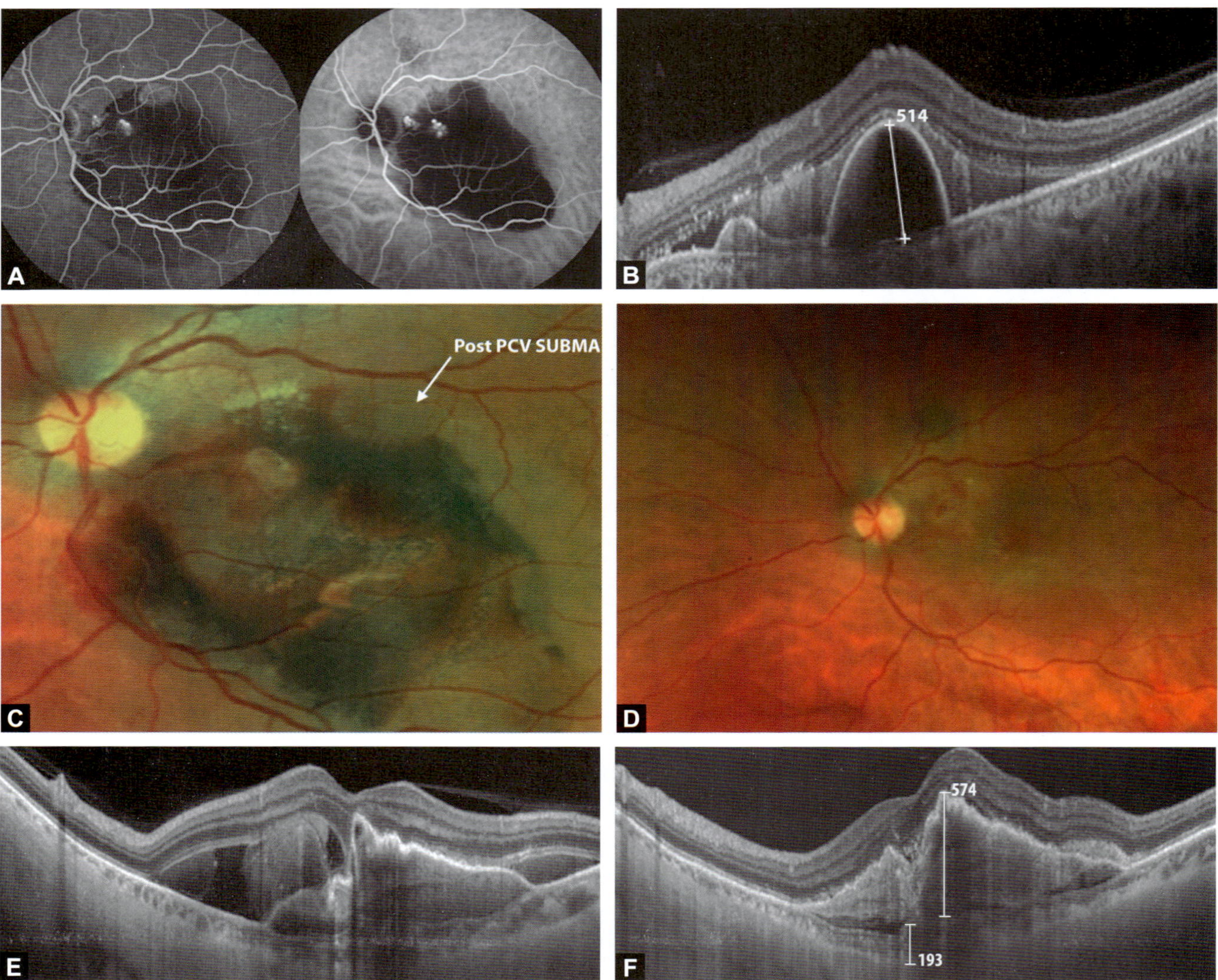

Figs. 19.9A to F: Large submacular bleed preoperatively (A-C) and postoperatively (D-F) on color picture and swept source optical coherence tomography (SSOCT). (A) Fluorescein angiography (FA) and indocyanine-green angiography (ICGA) imaging reveal large polyps within the bleed. Postsubmacular injection of recombinant tissue plasminogen activator (rtPA) (12.5 ug/0.1) + Injection avastin (2.50 mg) and 3 cc air, the bleed liquefied and was displaced inferiorly (D), with OCT showing absence of hemorrhage though the pigment epithelial detachments (PEDs) persist (F).

anti-VEGF is known as "triple therapy" for SMH. Intravitreal anti-VEGF alone or intravitreal gas alone can also be used in resource limited settings. Vitrectomy with subretinal injection of a "therapeutic cocktail"[17] which consists of 0.4 mL of rtPA (12.5 µg/0.1 mL), 2.5 mg/0.1 mL of bevacizumab and 0.3 mL of air using a 41-gauge needle followed by gas in the vitreous cavity and propped up positioning is the modality of choice used by the author in cases of SMH due to AMD[1] (Figs. 19.9A to F).

Macular Translocation Surgery

In extremely large subretinal bleeds literally extending anterior to the equator and close to ora, invasive surgeries like macular translocation, in which retina is cut along the ora and the resulting iatrogenic large retinal flap is reflected back, allowing for cutter and forceps removal of the trapped blood.

CONCLUSION

Submacular hemorrhage is a condition with a poor natural history leading to profound vision loss if untreated, hence it requires early and prompt treatment. Treatment with rtPA, pneumatic displacement and anti-VEGFs either intravitreal or subretinal, can lead to favorable results compared to the natural history. Even with surgery, the underlying disease must be managed and the postsurgical addition of anti-VEGF agents appears to help preserve vision and prevent rebleeds over time.

REFERENCES

1. Kumar A, Roy S, Bansal M, et al. Modified Approach in Management of Submacular Hemorrhage Secondary to Wet Age-Related Macular Degeneration. Asia Pac J Ophthalmology (Phila). 2016;5(2):143-6.
2. Lauritzen DB, Weiter JJ. Management of subretinal hemorrhage. Int Ophthalmology Clin. 2002;42(3):87-95.
3. Hochman MA, Seery CM, Zarbin MA. Pathophysiology and management of subretinal hemorrhage. Surv Ophthalmology. 1997;42(3):195-213.
4. Malik FF, Poulaki V. Management of submacular hemorrhage. Int Ophthalmology Clin. 2014;54(2):51-9.
5. Stanescu-Segall D, Balta F, Jackson TL. Submacular hemorrhage in neovascular age-related macular degeneration: A synthesis of the literature. Surv Ophthalmology. 2016;61(1):18-32.
6. Ying GS, Maguire MG, Daniel E, et al. Association between Antiplatelet or Anticoagulant Drugs and Retinal or Subretinal Hemorrhage in the Comparison of Age-Related Macular Degeneration Treatments Trials. Ophthalmology. 2016;123(2):352-60.
7. Glatt H, Machemer R. Experimental subretinal hemorrhage in rabbits. Am J Ophthalmology. 1982;94(6):762-73.
8. Toth CA, Morse LS, Hjelmeland LM, et al. Fibrin directs early retinal damage after experimental subretinal hemorrhage. Arch Ophthalmology Chic. 1991;109(5):723-9.
9. Kumar A, Chawla R, Kumawat D, et al. Insight into high myopia and the macula. Indian J Ophthalmology. 2017;65(2):85-91.
10. Scupola A, Coscas G, Soubrane G, et al. Natural history of macular subretinal hemorrhage in age-related macular degeneration. Ophthalmologica. 1999;213(2):97-102.
11. Bressler NM, Bressler SB, Childs AL, et al. Surgery for hemorrhagic choroidal neovascular lesions of age-related macular degeneration: ophthalmic findings: SST report no. 13. Ophthalmology. 2004;111(11):1993-2006.
12. Bennett SR, Folk JC, Blodi CF, et al. Factors prognostic of visual outcome in patients with subretinal hemorrhage. Am J Ophthalmology. 1990;109(1):33-7.
13. Lewis H. Intraoperative fibrinolysis of submacular hemorrhage with tissue plasminogen activator and surgical drainage. Am J Ophthalmology. 1994;118(5):559-68.
14. Rishi E, Gopal L, Rishi P, et al. Submacular hemorrhage: A study amongst Indian eyes. Indian J Ophthalmology. 2012;60(6):521-5.
15. Heriot W. Intravitreal gas and TPA: an outpatient procedure for submacular hemorrhage. In: American Academy of Ophthalmology Annual Vitreoretinal Update. Chicago, IL; 1996.
16. Stopa M, Lincoff A, Lincoff H. Analysis of forces acting upon submacular hemorrhage in pneumatic displacement. Retina. 2007;27(3):370-4.
17. Martel JN, Mahmoud TH. Subretinal pneumatic displacement of subretinal hemorrhage. JAMA Ophthalmology. 2013;131(12):1632-5.
18. Peyman GA, Nelson NC Jr, Alturki W, et al. Tissue plasminogen activating factor assisted removal of subretinal hemorrhage. Ophthalmic Surg. 1991;22(10):575-82.

Chapter 20

Cystoid Macular Edema

Pranita Sahay, Raghav Ravani, Atul Kumar

DEFINITION

Cystoid macular edema (CME) is the thickening of retina at the macula due to accumulation of intraretinal fluid following breakdown of any of the blood retinal barriers. The fluid mostly collects in the outer plexiform layer (OPL) of the macula in the form of honeycomb-like cystic spaces.

CAUSES

Cystoid macular edema can be attributed to metabolic changes, ischemia, hydrostatic forces, inflammatory and toxic mechanisms, or mechanical forces acting at the macula (Table 20.1).

PATHOGENESIS

Loss of blood retinal barrier (BRB) integrity causes retinal thickening which in turn leads to extracellular (or vasogenic) edema. The BRB is composed of an inner and outer barrier constituted by vascular endothelium and retinal pigment epithelium (RPE) layer, respectively. The breakdown of BRB results from disruption of the tight junctions between these cells.[1] Increased hydrostatic pressure gradient between retinal capillaries and retinal interstitial tissue causes macular edema. This could occur either with elevated intravascular capillary pressure or with excessive protein accumulation in retinal interstitial tissue.[2]

The underlying pathogenesis of the above-mentioned causes is given in Table 20.2.

Inflammation is the key pathogenetic factor in almost all causes of CME. This is substantiated by clinically associated iritis, cyclitis, vitritis and retinal phlebitis.

HISTOPATHOLOGY

The fluid originates from the perifoveal capillaries and accumulates in Henle's layer and inner nuclear layer (INL) of the retina. This fluid accumulation around the neuronal and glial cells gives rise to honeycomb cystoid appearance. This pooling forms a flower-petal pattern accumulation due to radial arrangement of both glia and Henle's inner fibers at the fovea.[3] Occasionally, subretinal fluid can also be present.

Table 20.1: Causes of cystoid macular edema (CME).

Category	Causes
Metabolic	• Diabetic retinopathy • Radiation retinopathy
Ischemic	• Retinal vascular occlusion • Diabetic retinopathy • Severe hypertensive retinopathy • Vasculitis • Collagen disorders
Mechanical	• Vitreomacular traction (VMT) • Epiretinal membrane (ERM)
Inflammatory	• Uveitis • Postsurgical CME (cataract surgery, retinal detachment surgery, vitrectomy, filtration surgery, penetrating keratoplasty, cryotherapy, laser photocoagulation) • Choroidal inflammatory disorders (sarcoidosis, Vogt-Koyanagi-Harada syndrome, birdshot chorioretinopathy)
Hydrostatic	• Hypotony • Venous occlusion
Others	• Retinal macroaneurysm • Macular telangiectasia • Choroidal neovascularization • Choroidal hemangioma • Drugs (epinephrine, betaxolol, latanoprost) • Retinitis pigmentosa
Pseudo CME	• X-linked retinoschisis • Nicotinic acid maculopathy • Optic disc pit maculopathy • Goldmann Favre disease

Table 20.2: Pathogenesis of cystoid macular edema (CME).

Cause	Key pathogenetic features
Diabetic macular edema (DME)	Leukostasis, endothelial apoptosis, pericyte loss, inflammatory cytokines, capillary hypoperfusion, vascular endothelial growth factors, vitreomacular traction (VMT)
Retinal vascular occlusion	Capillary hypoperfusion, increased intravascular pressure
Intermediate uveitis	T-cell mediated cytokines, prostaglandins mediated tight junction disruption
Postsurgical CME	Perivascular leukocytic infiltrates
Drug toxicity	Prostaglandin mediated
Vasculitis	Capillary ischemia, inflammatory cytokines
Retinitis pigmentosa	Failure of the pumping activity of diseased retinal pigment epithelium (RPE)

 ## CLINICAL FEATURES

Symptoms

Visual loss, metamorphopsia, micropsia and central visual field defect are the usual clinical presentations..

Signs

Slit-lamp biomicroscopy may reveal foveal thickening and loss of foveal reflex (Fig. 20.1). Vitritis (vitreous cells) and optic nerve head swelling can be seen in severe cases. In chronic cases, epiretinal membrane (ERM) or lamellar/full thickness macular hole may also form. In addition, subretinal fluid may also be present.

 ## INVESTIGATIONS

Optical Coherence Tomography

Optical coherence tomography (OCT) shows diffuse retinal thickening with cystic spaces, which is more prominent in the INL and OPL (Figs. 20.2A and B).[4] Occasionally subretinal fluid accumulation can be seen as a nonreflective area beneath the neurosensory retina.

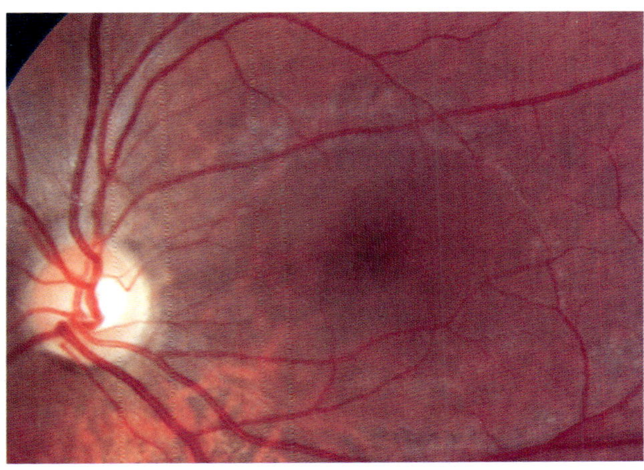

Fig. 20.1: Fundus color photograph of cystoid macular edema.

Optical coherence tomography is a faster and noninvasive imaging technique which can also provide quantitative measurement of the macular thickness that can be used to monitor the clinical course and to make therapeutic decisions. Optical coherence tomography can also detect vitreomacular traction (VMT) or ERM associated with CME.

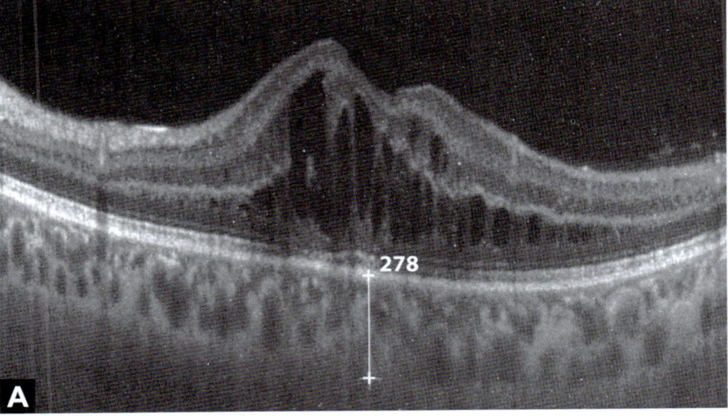

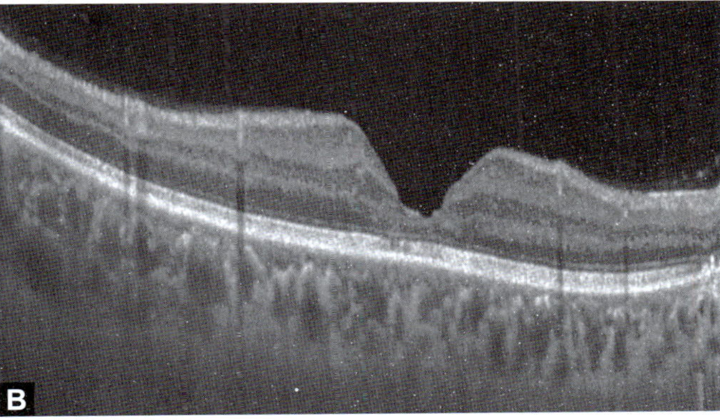

Figs. 20.2A and B: (A) Preoperative (B) Postoperative optical coherence technology (OCT) image of a patient having cystoid macular edema.

Fluorescein Angiography

Most cases of CME are mild and asymptomatic; it is relevant to distinguish between symptomatic or clinical CME and edema apparent only on fluorescein angiography (angiographic CME).

On fluorescein angiography multiple small focal fluorescein leaks and late pooling of the dye in extracellular cystoid spaces can be seen which points toward abnormal perifoveal retinal capillary permeability as the source of edema.[5,6] The pooling forms a flower-petal pattern due to radial foveal arrangement of both glia and Henle's inner fibers (Figs. 20.3 and 20.4).

PSEUDOPHAKIC CYSTOID MACULAR EDEMA

Pseudophakic CME, also known as Irvine-Gass syndrome, is a common cause of visual loss following cataract surgery (Figs. 20.5A to C).[7,8] Angiographic edema have been reported in 60% of intracapsular surgeries, 15–30% of extracapsular surgeries and in 4–11% of phacoemulsification surgeries.[9,10]

Clinically significant macular edema occurs in about 1–2% of patients undergoing cataract surgery.[11,12] This occurs likely due to surgery-induced inflammation and vitreous disturbances which exert a mechanical force at the macula.[13,14] The peak incidence occurs approximately 6–10 weeks postoperatively with spontaneous resolution occurring clinically in approximately 95% of uncomplicated cases, usually within 6 months.

Risk factors for post-cataract surgery CME include:
- Increased surgical manipulation
- Iris chafing
- Iris prolapse
- Anterior chamber intraocular lens (IOL) implantation
- Iris fixated IOL/scleral fixated IOL
- Posterior capsule rupture
- Vitreous loss
- Vitreous wick syndrome
- Retained cortical matter
- Dropped nuclear and/or cortical lens matter
- Systemic vascular disorders like diabetes
- Preexisting epiretinal membrane/uveitis
- Postoperative topical medication [prostaglandin (PG) analogs, preservatives]

PSEUDOCYSTOID MACULAR EDEMA

Rare cases such as X-linked hereditary retinoschisis, Goldmann-Favre disease, some cases of retinitis pigmentosa, vitreomacular traction, taxane and nicotinic acid maculopathy have clinical macular edema but lacks leakage into cystic spaces on fluorescein angiography. These are thus known as nonleaking CME or nonangiographic CME or noninflammatory CME. Toxicity to the Müllerian glial cells with subsequent intracellular edema and subclinical extracellular leakage has been proposed as the cause in cases of drug toxicities.[15] High prevalence of antiretinal autoantibodies in patients with retinitis pigmentosa (RP) suggests an inflammatory autoimmune-like process for leakage at RPE level.[16]

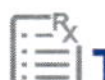TREATMENT

Cystoid macular edema resolves spontaneously in most of the cases even without treatment.[17] However, it is impossible to predict which cases may become chronic. Risk of ultrastructural changes can be induced in chronic macular edema causing transition from treatable to untreatable and ischemic forms of macular edema. Hence, early treatment is beneficial.

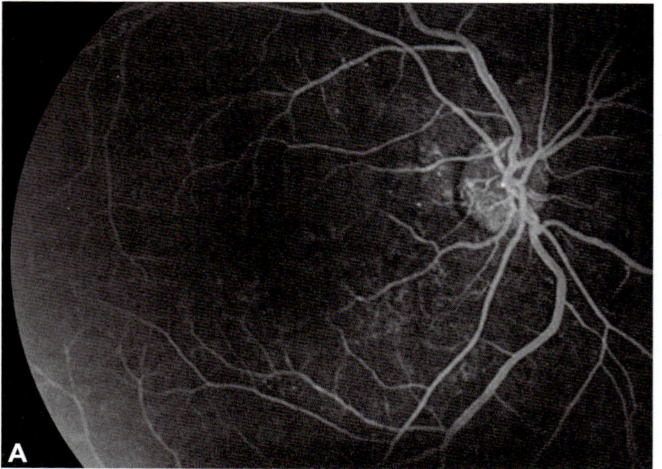
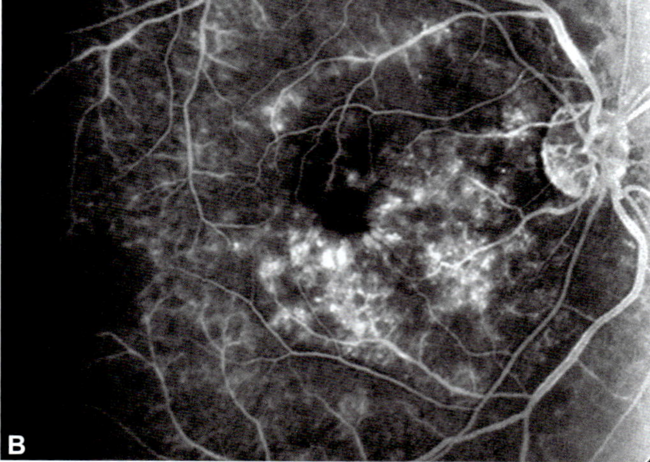

Figs. 20.3A and B: (A) Fluorescein angiography (FA) of right eye of patient with long standing central retinal vein occlusion (CRVO). (B) Right frame shows the characteristic petaloid appearance.

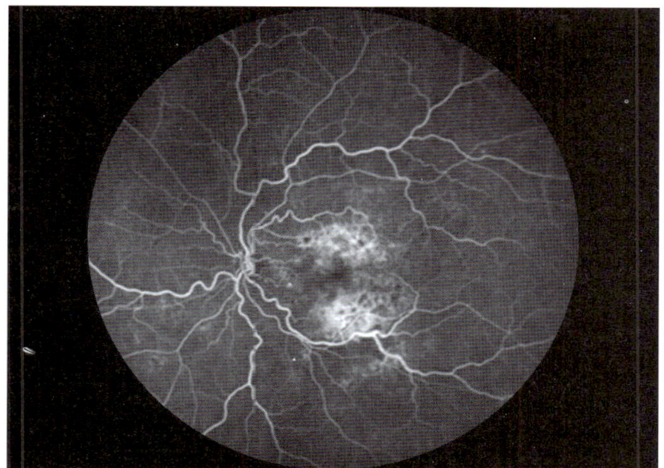

Fig. 20.4: Fluorescein angiogram of left eye with nonischemic central retinal vein occlusion (CRVO) with cystoid macular edema (CME).

Medical Management

Medical management for macular edema includes four groups of drugs: (1) carbonic anhydrase (CA) inhibitors, (2) COX inhibitors, (3) corticosteroids and (4) vascular endothelial growth factor (VEGF) inhibitors.

Carbonic anhydrase inhibitors like acetazolamide alters the polarized distribution of CA at the level of the RPE and improve the ability of the RPE to pump fluid out of the retina.[18] Under physiological conditions, the subretinal fluid is removed by metabolic transport to the choroid by around 70%. Active ion transport is enhanced by acetazolamide through the RPE which drives the fluid efflux.[19,20] Nonrandomized studies have shown improved visual function in eyes with postsurgical macular edema.[21,22] However, there are no randomized studies to support their role. Also, tachyphylaxis and on-off effect adds to their limitations.[22]

COX inhibitors like nonsteroidal drugs inhibits the enzyme cyclooxygenase, which blocks the synthesis and release of prostaglandins.[23] Thus, inflammatory mediators responsible for the edema formation are targeted by nonsteroidal anti-inflammatory drugs (NSAIDs). Topical NSAIDs are the mainstay in the treatment of inflammatory CME.[24] Topical NSAIDs are efficacious both in the prevention[25-27] and treatment[28,29] of inflammatory CME, particularly after cataract surgery. However, they have limited role in ischemic insult and chronic edema as in diabetic macular edema (DME).

Corticosteroids have multiple mechanisms by which they decrease macular edema. These include inhibition of enzyme COX,[30] stabilization and increase in number of endothelial tight junctions,[31,32] decrease in the production of the VEGF,[33] and increased RPE resorption of fluid by unknown ways. Potency levels of corticosteroids differ depending on their chemical composition.

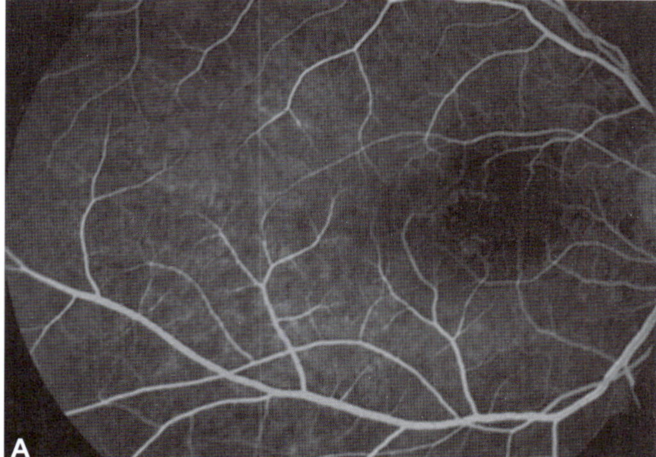

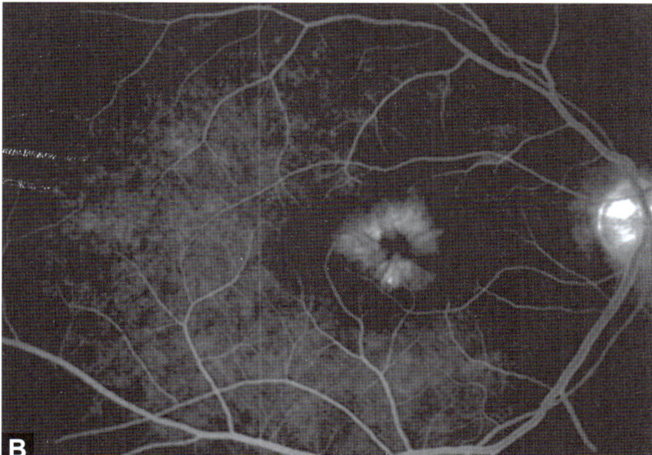

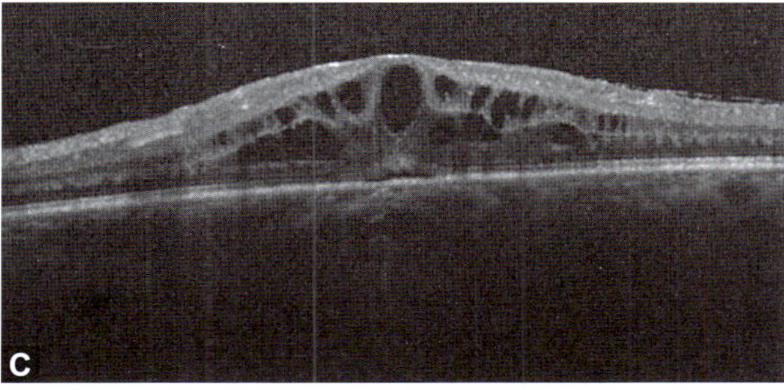

Figs. 20.5A to C: (A and B) Fluorescein angiography of the right eye with pseudophakic cystoid macular edema (CME). Note the petaloid hyperfluorescence seen. (C) Spectral domain optical coherence tomography (SD-OCT) shows cystic changes within the central retina and loss of foveal dip.

Topical, periocular, intraocular, oral and intravenous routes are the different routes of administration of steroids to treat CME. CME that fails to respond to conventional treatment might benefit from intravitreal triamcinolone acetonide.[34] However, its shortcomings include risk of cataract, secondary glaucoma and sometimes a need for repeated injections. Dexamethasone and fluocinolone intravitreal implants overcome some of these limitations and have been found to be safe and efficacious in macular edema associated with retinal venous occlusion as well as posterior uveitis.[35-37] The multicenter uveitis steroid treatment trial (MUST) found no significant differences in systemic steroid versus intraocular steroid implant (fluocinolone acetonide).

Vascular endothelial growth factor inhibitors (pegaptanib, ranibizumab and bevacizumab) act by decreasing VEGF-mediated inner BRB breakdown (endothelial tight junction disruption). Marked reduction in macular edema have been noted in various studies with a significant improvement in visual function.[38-41] Ranibizumab has been approved for use in macular edema following retinal venous occlusions and diabetic retinopathy.

Steroid sparing immunosuppressive drugs are frequently used as additional second line agents, particularly in patients with severe intraocular inflammation and CME.[42]

Interferon α2,[43] cyclosporine A[44] and anti-TNF therapy[45] have provided promising results as a treatment for long-standing refractory CME in uveitis. Somatostatin analogs such as octreotide which act by blocking the local and systemic production of growth hormone, insulin like growth factor and VEGF have also found to be effective in the treatment of CME.[46]

Surgical Management

Laser Photocoagulation

Laser photocoagulation for the treatment of DME has been supported by multiple studies in the past[47-49] but in the current era of VEGF inhibitors and steroids, use of grid laser application has reduced.

Yttrium Aluminum Garnet Vitreolysis

Neodymium yttrium aluminum garnet (Nd: YAG) mediated lysis of vitreous strands to cataract surgery wound, on slit lamp may reduce vitreous traction leading to resolution of CME.[50]

Pars Plana Vitrectomy

Vitreoretinal traction has been found to be a significant contributor to macular edema in diabetic retinopathy, Irvine-Gass syndrome and in VMT syndrome. Surgical removal of such traction has been found to be beneficial.[51-53] Internal limiting membrane (ILM) peeling ensures complete traction release, diffusional barrier is removed, and reproliferation of fibrous astrocytes is inhibited.[54]

The beneficial effect of vitrectomy for nontractional edema is due to two likely mechanisms. First, oxygen diffusion within the posterior segment increases with vitrectomy.[55-57] Second, excess of growth factors (VEGF, interleukin 6, platelet-derived growth factor, etc.) will be mechanically removed with vitrectomy with restitution of the BRB especially in ischemic retinopathies, such as diabetic retinopathy and retinal venous occlusions.[58,59]

Prophylaxis

Minimal surgical manipulation is an important prophylactic measure for macular edema.[60] Several studies have shown the effect of postoperative prophylactic treatment with topical NSAIDs (ketorolac tromethamine 0.5%, indomethacin 1% and diclofenac 1%) in preventing CME.[61,62] Prophylaxis must be considered especially for patients with risk factors, especially uveitis, diabetes, venous retinal occlusions and intraoperative complications.

REFERENCES

1. Tranos PG, Wickremasinghe SS, Stangos NT, et al. Macular edema. Surv Ophthalmology. 2004;49:470-90.
2. Stefánsson E. Physiology of vitreous surgery. Graefes Arch Clin Exp Ophthalmology. 2009;247(2):147-63
3. Scholl S, Augustin A, Loewenstein A, et al. General pathophysiology of macular edema. Eur J Ophthalmology. 2011;21:S10-19.
4. Kim SJ, Bressler NM. Optical coherence tomography and cataract surgery. Curr Opin Ophthalmology. 2009;20(1):46-51.
5. Staurenghi G, Invernizzi A, de Polo L, et al. Macular edema. Diagnosis and detection. Dev Ophthalmology. 2010;47:27-48.
6. Shetty N. Cystoid macular edema. Atlas of fundus fluorescein angiography. New York, Informa Healthcare; 2004. pp. 130-4.
7. Irvine SR. A newly defined vitreous syndrome following cataract surgery. Am J Ophthalmology. 1953;36(5):599-619.
8. Flach AJ. The incidence, pathogenesis and treatment of cystoid macular edema following cataract surgery. Trans Am Ophthalmology Soc. 1998;96:557-634.
9. Belair ML, Kim SJ, Thorne JE, et al. Incidence of cystoid macular edema after cataract surgery in patients with and without uveitis using optical coherence tomography. Am J Ophthalmology. 2009;148(1):128-35.e2.
10. Perente I, Utine CA, Ozturker C, et al. Evaluation of macular changes after uncomplicated phacoemulsification surgery by optical coherence tomography. Curr Eye Res. 2007;32(3):241-7.
11. Henderson BA, Kim JY, Ament CS, et al. Clinical pseudophakic cystoid macular edema. Risk factors for development and duration after treatment. J Cataract Refract Surg. 2007;33(9):1550-8.
12. Wolf EJ, Braunstein A, Shih C, et al. Incidence of visually significant pseudophakic macular edema after uneventful phacoemulsification in patients treated with nepafenac. J Cataract Refract Surg. 2007;33(9):1546-9.
13. Irvine SR. A newly defined vitreous syndrome following cataract surgery. Am J Ophthalmology. 1953;36(5):499-619.
14. Schepens CL, Avila MP, Jalkh AE, et al. Role of the vitreous in cystoid macular edema. Surv Ophthalmology. 1984;28(Suppl):499-504.
15. Smith SV, Benz MS, Brown DM. Cystoid macular edema secondary to albumin-bound paclitaxel therapy. Arch Ophthalmology. 2008;126(11):1605-6.
16. Heckenlively JR, Solish AM, Chant SM, et al. Autoimmunity in hereditary retinal degenerations, II: clinical studies: antiretinal antibodies and fluorescein angiogram findings. Br J Ophthalmology. 1985;69(10):758-64
17. Henderson BA, Kim JY, Ament CS, et al. Clinical pseudophakic cystoid macular edema. Risk factors for development and duration after treatment. J Cataract Refract Surg. 2007;33(9):1550-8.
18. Marmor MF, Maak T. Enhancement of retinal adhesion and subretinal fluid absorption by acetazolamide. Invest Ophthalmology Vis Sci. 1982;23:121-4.

19. Wolfensberger TJ, Chiang RK, Takeuchi A, et al. Inhibition of membrane bound carbonic anhydrase enhances subretinal fluid absorption and retinal adhesiveness. Graefes Arch Clin Exp Ophthalmology. 2000;238(1):76-80.

20. Marmor MF, Negi A. Pharmacologic modification of subretinal fluid absorption in the rabbit eye. Arch Ophthalmology. 1986;104(11):1674-7.

21. Cox SN, Hay E, Bird AC. Treatment of chronic macular edema with acetazolamide. Arch Ophthalmology. 1988;106(9):1190-5.

22. Weene LE. Cystoid macular edema after scleral buckling responsive to acetazolamide. Ann Ophthalmology. 1992;24(11):423-4.

23. Colin J. The role of NSAIDs in the management of postoperative ophthalmic inflammation. Drugs. 2007;67(9):1291-308.

24. Wolfensberger TJ, Herbort CP. Treatment of cystoid macular edema with nonsteroidal anti-inflammatory drugs and corticosteroids. Doc Ophthalmology. 1999;97(3-4):381-6.

25. Flach AJ, Stegman RC, Graham J, et al. Prophylaxis of aphakic cystoid macular edema without corticosteroids. A pairedcomparison, placebocontrolled doublemasked study. Ophthalmology. 1990;97:1253-8.

26. Almeida DR, Johnson D, Hollands H, et al. Effect of prophylactic nonsteroidal anti-inflammatory drugs on cystoid macular edema assessed using optical coherence tomography quantification of total macular volume after cataract surgery. J Cataract Refract Surg. 2008;34(1):64-9.

27. DeCroos FC, Afshari NA. Perioperative antibiotics and anti-inflammatory agents in cataract surgery. Curr Opin Ophthalmology. 2008;19(1):22-6.

28. Nelson ML, Martidis A. Managing cystoid macular edema after cataract surgery. Curr Opin Ophthalmology. 2003;14(1):39-43.

29. Sivaprasad S, Bunce C, Patel N. Nonsteroidal anti-inflammatory agents for treating cystoid macular oedema following cataract surgery. Cochrane Database Syst Rev. 2005;1:CD004239.

30. Nehmé A, Edelman J. Dexamethasone inhibits high glucose, TNFα, and IL1βinduced secretion of inflammatory and angiogenic mediators from retinal microvascular pericytes. Invest Ophthalmology Vis Sci. 2008;49(5):2030-8.

31. Romero IA, Radewicz K, Jubin E, et al. Changes in cytoskeletal and tight junctional proteins correlate with decreased permeability induced by dexamethasone in cultured rat brain endothelial cells. Neurosci Lett. 2003;344(2):112-6.

32. Antonetti DA, Wolpert EB, DeMaio L, et al. Hydrocortisone decreases retinal endothelial cell water and solute flux coincident with increased content and decreased phosphorylation of occludin. J Neurochem. 2002;80:667-77.

33. Edelman JL, Lutz D, Castro MR. Corticosteroids inhibit VEGF-induced vascular leakage in a rabbit model of blood–retinal and blood-aqueous barrier breakdown. Exp Eye Res. 2005;80(2):249-58.

34. Martidis A, Duker JS, Greenberg PB, et al. Intravitreal triamcinolone for refractory diabetic macular edema. Ophthalmology. 2002;109(5):920-7.

35. Haller JA, Bandello F, Belfort R Jr, et al. Randomized, sham-controlled trial of dexamethasone intravitreal implant in patients with macular edema due to retinal vein occlusion. Ophthalmology. 2010;117(6):1134-46.e3.

36. Lowder C, Belfort R Jr, Lightman S, et al. Dexamethasone intravitreal implant for noninfectious intermediate or posterior uveitis. Arch Ophthalmology. 2011;129:545-53.

37. Boyer DS, Faber D, Gupta S, et al. Dexamethasone intravitreal implant for treatment of diabetic macular edema in vitrectomized patients. Retina. 2011;31(5):915-23.

38. Arimura N, Otsuka H, Yamakiri K, et al. Vitreous mediators after Intravitreal bevacizumab or triamcinolone acetonide in eyes with proliferative diabetic retinopathy. Ophthalmology. 2009;116(5):921-6.

39. Ghasemi Falavarjani K, Parvaresh MM, Modarres M, et al. Intravitreal bevacizumab for pseudophakic cystoid macular edema: a systematic review. J Ophthalmic Vis Res. 2012;7(3):235-9.

40. Rotsos TG, Moschos MM. Cystoid macular edema. Clin Ophthalmology. 2008;2(4):919-30.

41. Cervera E, Diaz-Llopis M, Udaondo P, et al. Intravitreal pegaptanib sodium for refractory pseudophakic macular oedema. Eye (Lond). 2008;22(9)1180-2.

42. Tranos PG, Wickremasinghe SS, Stangos NT, et al. Macular edema. Surv Ophthalmology. 2004;49(5):470-90.

43. Deuter CM, Koetter I, Guenaydin I, et al. Interferon alfa2a: a new treatment option for long lasting refractory cystoid macular edema in uveitis? A pilot study. Retina. 2006;26(7):786-91.

44. Nussenblatt RB, Palestine AG, Chan CC, et al. Randomized, doublemasked study of cyclosporine compared to prednisolone in the treatment of endogenous uveitis. Am J Ophthalmology. 1991;112:138-46.

45. Theodossiadis PG, Markomichelakis NN, Sfikakis PP. Tumor necrosis factor antagonists: preliminary evidence for an emerging approach in the treatment of ocular inflammation. Retina. 2007;27(4):399-413.

46. Rothova A. Inflammatory cystoid macular edema. Curr Opin Ophthalmology. 2007;18(6):487-92.

47. Blankenship GW. Diabetic macular edema and argon laser photocoagulation: a prospective randomized study. Ophthalmology. 1979;86(1):69-76.

48. Early Treatment Diabetic Retinopathy Study research group. Photocoagulation for diabetic macular edema. Early Treatment Diabetic Retinopathy Study report number 1. Arch Ophthalmology 1985;103(12):1796-806.

49. Weiter JJ, Zuckerman R. The influence of the photoreceptor–RPE complex on the inner retina. An explanation for the beneficial effects of photocoagulation. Ophthalmology. 1980;87(11):1133-9.

50. Katzen LE, Fleischman JA, Trokel S. YAG laser treatment of cystoid macular edema. Am J Ophthalmology. 1983;95(5):589-92.

51. Lewis H, Abrams GW, Blumenkranz MS, et al. Vitrectomy for diabetic macular traction and edema associated with posterior hyaloidal traction. Ophthalmology. 1992;99(5):753-9.

52. Fung WE. Vitrectomy for chronic aphakic cystoid macular edema. Results of a national, collaborative, prospective, randomized investigation. Ophthalmology. 1985;92(8):1102-11.

53. Margherio RR, Trese MT, Margherio AR, et al. Surgical management of vitreomacular traction syndromes. Ophthalmology. 1989;96(9):1437-45.

54. Gandorfer A, Messmer EM, Ulbig MW, et al. Resolution of diabetic macular edema after surgical removal of the posterior hyaloid and the inner limiting membrane. Retina. 2000;20(2):126-33.

55. Stefansson E, Novack RL, Hatchell DL. Vitrectomy prevents retinal hypoxia in branch retinal vein occlusion. Invest Ophthalmology Vis Sci. 1990 31(2):284-9.

56. Holekamp NM, Shui YB, Beebe DC. Vitrectomy surgery increases oxygen exposure to the lens: a possible mechanism for nuclear cataract formation. Am J Ophthalmology. 2005;139(2):302-10.

57. Giblin FJ, Quiram PA, Leverenz VR, et al. Enzyme induced posterior vitreous detachment in the rat produces increased lens nuclear pO_2 levels. Exp Eye Res. 2009;88(2):286-92.

58. Stefánsson E. The therapeutic effects of retinal laser treatment and vitrectomy. A theory based on oxygen and vascular physiology. Acta Ophthalmology Scand. 2001;79(5):435-40.

59. Stefánsson E. Ocular oxygenation and the treatment of diabetic retinopathy. Surv Ophthalmology. 2006;51(4):364-80.

60. Ersoy L, Caramoy A, Ristau T, et al. Aqueous flare is increased in patients with clinically significant cystoid macular oedema after cataract surgery. Br J Ophthalmology. 2013;97(7):862-5.

61. Rossetti L, Autelitano A. Cystoid macular edema following cataract surgery. Curr Opin Ophthalmology. 2000;11(1):65-72.

62. Almeida DR, Khan Z, Xing L, et al. Prophylactic nepafenac and ketorolac versus placebo in preventing postoperative macular edema after uneventful phacoemulsification. J Cataract Refract Surg. 2012;38(9):1537-43.

Chapter 21

Low Vision Management in Retinal Diseases

Anu Sharma

DEFINITION

In the practice of eye care, low vision has a specific meaning as defined by World Health Organization (WHO). This is as follows:

"A person with low vision is one who has impairment of visual functioning even after treatment and/or standard refractive correction, and has a visual acuity of less than 6/18 to light perception, or a visual field of less than 10 degrees from the point of fixation, but who uses, or is potentially able to use, vision for planning and/or execution of a task for which vision is essential."

In 1975, WHO used the term "Low Vision" to collectively describe the ICD-9 categories of visual impairment (VI) to include all those with visual acuity less than 6/18 and equal to or better than 3/60 in the better eye.

However, the current ICD-10 revision, replaced the term Low Vision by two categories (1 and 2) of VI.[1] Category 1 referred to the presenting VI <6/18–6/60 in the better eye (moderate VI) and Category 2 referred to the presenting VI <6/60–3/60 in the better eye (severe VI).

MAGNITUDE

- Worldwide, about 253 million people are estimated to be visually impaired (Global Vision Impairment Data 2015 from IAPB Vision Loss Expert Group), of which, 36 million are blind and 217 million are moderate-severe visually impaired (MSVI)
- About 90% of the world's visually impaired population live in developing countries.
- Currently, India has around 12 million blind people which makes India home to one-third of the world's blind population.

CAUSES

Uncorrected refractive errors are the major cause of visual impairment (about 49%). Other causes include cataract (25.8%) and glaucoma (2.8%). Other potential causes include conditions like age-related macular degeneration (ARMD), corneal opacity, trachoma and diabetic retinopathy. According to the Global Vision Impairment Facts, 65% of visually impaired and 82% of blind people are over 50 years of age.

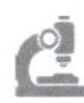 INVESTIGATIONS AND EVALUATION OF LOW-VISION PATIENT

- *Observation*: This can yield significant preliminary information about visual status that can be used to plan examination and rehabilitation strategies. The postural abnormalities, mobility, and appearance should be assessed on the patient's first visit to clinic.
- *History*: Patient history is essential pre-requisite for low vision examination. It should include chief complaints, nature, onset, progression and duration of presenting problem, visual difficulties encountered, complete visual and ocular history, ocular history of family members, social history, information about education, vocational training, mobility and previous use of low vision devices. An initial perception helps to a tailored visual and psychosocial rehabilitation to correspond to individual's expectations.
- *Measuring visual performance*: An appropriate test must be selected carefully to assess the performance in the practical tasks simulating day-to-day real settings.[2]
- *Initial evaluation should include*:
  - Visual acuity assessment: Distance and near visual acuity
  - Refraction
  - Ocular motility and Binocular vision assessment
  - Visual field assessment
  - Ocular health assessment.

Supplemental testing may include glare testing, contrast sensitivity, color vision testing and electrophysiological tests.

Measurement of Visual Acuities

In case of low vision patients, the conventional methods should not be followed and customized charts are necessary.[3] The measurement of the poorer seeing eye should be done followed by the better eye. This sequence provides the patient with a positive experience, as it emphasizes the increased amount of residual vision in the better seeing eye. Recently, Berkeley Rudimentary Vision Test (BRVT) is found to be effective for evaluating low vision patients with poor levels of visual acuity, worse than 2.0 logMAR (logarithm of the minimum angle of resolution) (commensurate with decimal visual acuity 0.01).[4] Both monocular and binocular acuities should be recorded along with unaided and aided acuities.

Distance Acuity

Snellen, Bailey-Lovie, LogMAR or Feinbloom charts can be used for distance acuity measurement. LogMAR chart is considered to be ideal as there is a uniform progression of letter sizes with a standardized separation of letters. Ferris and colleagues modified the Bailey-Lovie chart for Early Treatment of Diabetic Retinopathy Study (ETDRS).[5] This ETDRS chart is recommended at the testing distance of 4, 2 or 1 meter and can be translated into Snellen 20 ft equivalent (Fig. 21.1). The ETDRS chart is available in Landolt C configuration as well as in numeric optotypes. There is also an LEA Symbol Test System and HOTV chart for pediatric patients.

- *Distance Visual Acuity Testing Procedure*: Initial testing distance should be typically 10 ft. If not resolved, the chart can be moved to 5ft, 2ft and 1ft and 4 m, 2 m, and 1 m, respectively, in ETDRS chart.
- It is not recommended to record acuities as fingers counting as it might be demoralizing to the patient and it is appropriate to bring the chart to the equivalent viewing distance.
- The clock-dial technique is used to determine the optimal EV angle both monocularly and binocularly.
- The isolated optotypes may also be used as contour interaction is eliminated.
- Visual acuity should also be measured with any telescopic devices brought by the patient in the clinic.

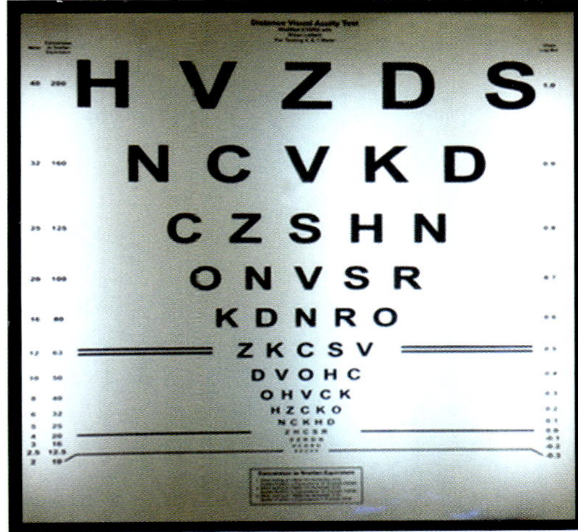

Fig. 21.1: ETDRS Chart maintains a consistent number of letters in each row. The separation between the letters (in a row) and between rows is standardized.

- The standard photopic levels of illumination should be at least 85 cd/m² and mesopic levels should be at least 2 cd/ m².
- It is important to evaluate the reproducibility of visual acuity in retinal conditions like ARMD,[6] by testing in simulated real life conditions.
- Specific activities customized as per the need of profession of the patient should be checked.
  - Blackboard/TV for school going children
  - Recognizing faces or reading bus number or metro stations for adults
  - Photophobia from sunlight, glare from car light in night must be recorded.
  - Need for different lights in different environments must be checked for proper low vision aid trial.

Near Acuity

Types of near acuity charts:
- Single-letter charts: The single-letter charts include Reduced Snellen's chart, Lighthouse near visual acuity chart, and Reduced Ferris-Bailey ETDRS charts. The ETDRS chart maintains a constant number of letters in each row. The logarithmic progression and proportional spacing of optotypes enables an accurate evaluation of visual acuity. It may be used at any distance and provides Snellen equivalent acuities for 40 cm and 20 cm.
- LEA numbers low-vision book (LNLVB).
- Feinbloom chart.
- Word and continuous text charts:
  There are word and continuous text charts such as Jaeger, Lighthouse Game Card for children and Lighthouse Continuous text card for adults.
  - MNRead Card (The Lighthouse, Inc.) (Fig. 21.4).
  Designation of near visual acuity can be as: M units (as measure of print size by indicating distance in meters at which the height of smaller letters subtend 5 min of arc), N notation (as smallest print size of standard Times New Roman font that can be read denoted in points), Snellen Equivalent notation (to express the distance visual acuity value that is mathematically equal to near acuity value at 40 cm). Conversion is possible by remembering that: 1.0 M units = 1.45 mm = 8 points (N or Times New Roman font size) = typical newsprint size. Continuous text charts of M (Fig. 21.2) and N (Fig. 21.3) notation are available. The reading performance is shown to correlate well with the psychophysical measures and the quality of life as studied by Murro et al.[7] in patients with Stargardt's disease.

There are newer logarithimic reading charts, which have been developed according to the standards of the International Council of Ophthalmology. These reading charts are: the Bailey-Lovie Word Reading Chart, the Colenbrander English Continuous Text Near Vision Cards, the Oculus Reading Probe II, the MNRead Charts, the SKread Charts, and the RADNER Reading Charts.[8]

MNREAD Card (The Lighthouse Inc.): The test combines a quick reading performance assessment with a reading acuity

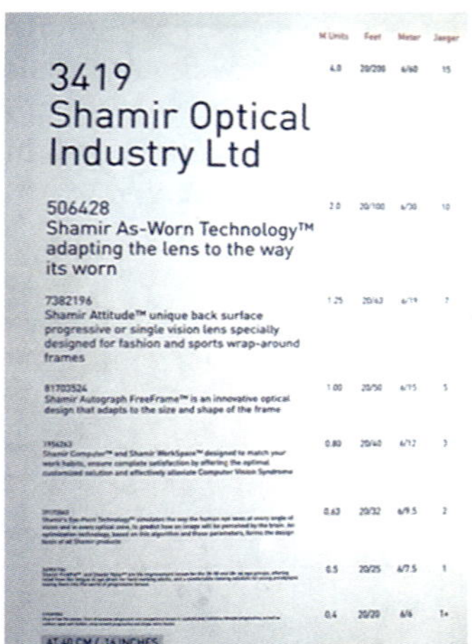

Fig. 21.2: M Notation chart.

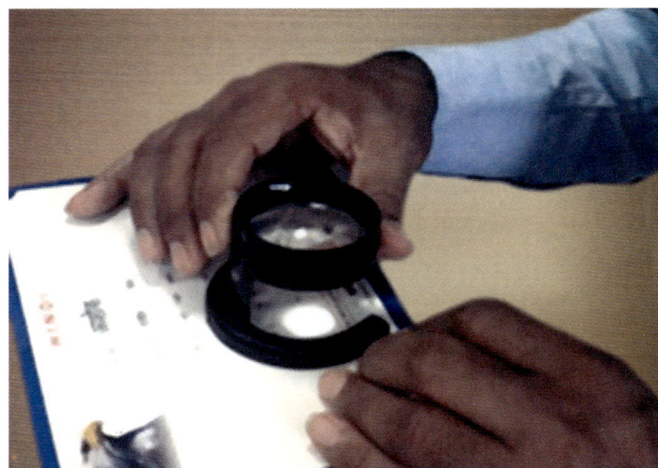

Fig. 21.3: N Notation chart.

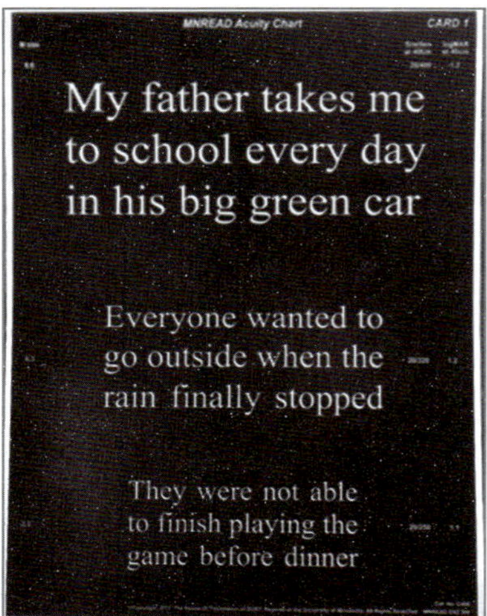

Fig. 21.4: MNRead chart for assessment of reading speed.

- Isolation of letters and words through the use of a typoscope should be demonstrated to determine, if resolution is enhanced. Typoscope also reduces contour interaction as in macular disorders and reduces background glare and enhances quality of image.

The visual acuities are recorded at the test distance from the spectacle plane. The distance at which it is measured should always be mentioned.

Amount of magnification can be calculated based on the present visual acuity and the required visual acuity:

(a) If VA is measured in a LogMAR notation:

Magnification = (1. 25)n

Where, n = number of steps

If the present acuity = 0.5 and the required acuity = 0.1

Then, magnification = (1.25)4 = 2.44×

(b) Magnification required = Required VA/ Present VA

In Snellen notation to improve from 6/60 to 6/6

Magnification required = (6 × 60)/(6 × 6).

Illumination

The illumination of acuity chart should be uniform and glare free for the estimation of the correct visual acuity. There should be facility to vary the levels of illumination as the better response can be recorded in low illumination levels in cases of rod monochromatism and at high illumination levels in cases of retinitis pigmentosa and macular degenerations. Both mesopic high contrast and low contrast visual acuity should be checked and repeatability should be assessed with the ETDRS charts.[9]

Refraction

It is an essential component and may be especially helpful for patients who have central scotomas with normal peripheral fields. The peripheral vision is instrumental in EV as well as during mobility-related visual activities. It is particularly important in patients who have congenital disorders, such

assessment (Fig. 21.4). The passages are printed in decreasing M sizes in logarithmic progression from 8.0 M to 0.12 M. This test is unique in that each three-line sentence has an identical number of characters (letters and spaces). The test can be used to estimate the smallest print for which good reading efficiency can be obtained in addition to noting the smallest print that can just be read.[8]

- *Near Visual Acuity Testing Procedure*: Single-letter and continuous text acuity both should be evaluated at distances within arm's length (standard testing distance of 40 cm).
- Continuous text acuities should also be evaluated.
- Eccentric fixation positions should be explored and recorded, if present.
- The clock-dial technique should be used to explore any optimal eccentric viewing (EV) angle.

as albinism, monochromatism or retinopathy of prematurity. Keratometry should be done to obtain idea of corneal toricity and integrity such as albinism, aniridia, and congenital pendular nystagmus.

Retinoscopy: A phoropter is generally not used when evaluating the low-vision patient. Instead, a trial frame or clips (Halberg, Janelli) and lenses are used. The large aperture lenses enable the patient to assume a habitual eccentric fixation. It also aids in observation of head turns and eye movements and reduces retinoscopy time. A radical retinoscopy should be performed followed by careful subjective refraction.

Subjective refraction: It should be performed with properly illuminated chart placed perpendicular to the patient and *not* propped up against the wall. This positioning reduces glare and minimizes differences in testing distances as the patient reads each line on the chart.

The refractive error determination is done by doing the Bracketing technique,[2] in which plus and minus lenses of equal powers are compared until a favorable response is elicited. Besides, previous glasses can be good starting point of refraction. Retinoscopy, is the most useful tool for refraction for low vision, especially if the patient is a poor responder. Autorefractors have limited use, due to media problems or eccentric viewing.

It is important to provide reassurance and encouragement whenever needed. A short period of rest is recommended while examining elderly subjects.[10] In case low vision subjective refraction is done with the telescopes, Stenopaic slit can be used to estimate the astigmatism. Arc perimetry and bowl perimetry should be performed to explore peripheral field constriction using various targets.

Binocularity

For those patients who have acuities that differ no more than a factor of 1.5, investigation of binocularity is important.

Binocularity for distance and near can be checked using Worth's four-dot test, Red filter test, Bagolini's striated glasses, Synaptophore or tests with prisms.[11] The low vision patients use monocular cues present in the visual environment in the absence of binocularity.

The following tests measure the psychophysical, sensory, electrical, or structural aspects of the patient's visual system. These are performed when the patients cannot achieve an expected level of function.

Visual Field Status

The visual field status is one of the important baseline investigation. The size and location of the scotoma can affect reading ability, despite appropriate magnification and visual acuity improvement. It is helpful to explore EV and fixation skills. Any apparent *EV* angle should be recorded using a clock-dial designation. It is important to mention here that different eccentric fixation and viewing strategies for the distance and

the near may be employed to enhance visual discrimination. This is the adaption, which enables the patient to maintain his or her place while reading much of the line of print unobscured by the scotoma. Sometimes there can be multiple eccentric fixation points. Hence, distance acuity should not be used to determine magnification needs for near-point acuities.[12]

The single-letter visual acuity is considered better than continuous text acuity in individuals with central scotomas or metamorphopsia. They may consistently omit letters at the end or the beginning of lines. During testing, they may repeat the lines and tend to show higher visual acuity when optotypes are isolated than when presented within a row of optotypes as the contour interaction effects are more significant in macular disorders. In cases of visual field constriction, resolution may actually appear to improve as optotypes decrease in size thereby improving the visual performance.

Visual Field Testing in Low Vision

It is done for following reasons:
- Characterize patient's visual loss
- Determining legal blindness
- Deciding on vocational and mobility training
- Calculating compensation for functional loss
- To guide patient for preferred retinal fixation or environmental modifications
- To design devices and strategies that allow the patients to achieve their maximum visual potential.

Assessment can be done using:
- Confrontation method—for gross field defect
- Amsler grid testing—The presence of significant distortion may hamper the quality of vision
- Goldmann Perimetry—It is very useful to quantitatively locate the size and extent of scotoma and to evaluate tunnel vision or peripheral visual field loss.

The majority of low vision patients have some loss in macular function often resulting in eccentric fixation.

Contrast Sensitivity (CS) Testing

It should be done routinely when the patient's performance does not match the expected results. CS related to visual functioning more closely than visual acuity. When a patient reports that he is having greater difficulty seeing in the rain and fog, while the measurement of visual acuity gives a consistent value on each visit to clinic, loss of CS is suspected. The contrast threshold (CT) is defined as an object with the lowest contrast that a patient can recognize.

Contrast sensitivity is the compliment (reciprocal) of CT and is usually expressed as a logarithm of 1/CT, where CT is expressed as a percentage. It is measured using a letter contrast chart with letters of the same size but decreasing contrast. Contrast assessment can be done with Pelli-Robson contrast sensitivity chart (Fig. 21.5) at one meter, Lea contrast flip chart, Hiding Heidi contrast test chart. A patient with low contrast acuity will have to be prescribed a low vision aid

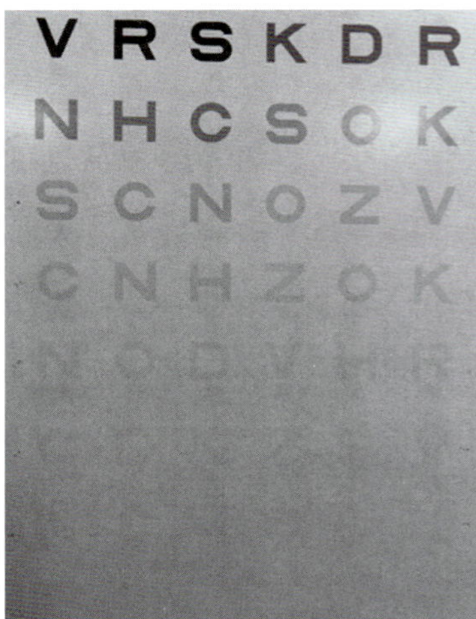

Fig. 21.5: Pelli-Robson contrast sensitivity chart.

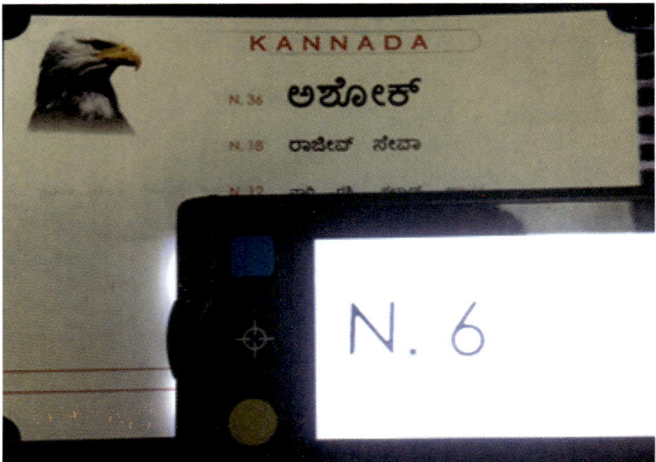

Fig. 21.6: Print enhancement systems for computers that enlarge print and enhance print contrast.

with higher than expected magnification, higher illumination and/or absorptive filters or typoscopes.

INTERVENTIONS THAT INCREASE THE CONTRAST RESERVES

Contrast reserves can be increased and performance can be enhanced by either decreasing the threshold or increasing the sensitivity or increasing the contrast of the objects to be recognized.

CCTV (Closed-Circuit Television or Computer Displays)

They are the special print enhancement systems for computers that not only enlarge print but also enhance print contrast to better than 95%. These devices could be hand held (Fig. 21.6) or desktop magnifiers. These systems are also able to enlarge text substantially, sometimes even up to 60× larger than the original text. A patient may often choose to magnify text 6–10 times above his or her acuity threshold. Magnification usually increases contrast reserve because CS tends to improve as objects increase in size. It is especially important to provide glare free screens when patients with poor CS use a CCTV or computer display.

Modifications in the Environment

A patient's home and work environment may be modified to compensate for poor CS. Utensils, furniture, doorways, light switches, and steps can be modified, so that they stand out with high contrast by marking with reflective tapes or lights. One can use furniture covers, slipcovers, doilies, and table cloths to lighten or darken a background to enhance contrast. Dangerous objects should have sufficient contrast to attract the patient's attention. In most cases, it is best to recommend that the patient's home or work environment be evaluated by

a low vision rehabilitation specialist and that both verbal and written recommendations be provided to the patient.

Lighting Evaluation and Instruction

It can be critical factor in patients with reduced CS. The best light levels are a matter of individual preference. A minimal lighting evaluation should include testing with directional and diffuse incandescent and fluorescent lights. Directional lights should be shaded and positioned to the side or above the objects in the room, so that the bulb is never in the patient's field of view.

Mobility Instruction

Patients with CS loss of greater than 20%, CT should be routinely referred for mobility training because their personal safety is at risk. The ability to detect low-contrast obstacles (encountered as curbs, steps, irregularities in the streets, and sidewalk surfaces) is essential for safe and independent travel. Patients with severe CS loss would be good candidate for a CCTV for all reading needs and should use books on tape for casual reading. They would be poor candidates for optical magnification than initially predicted. They would have special lighting needs and would require mobility instructions and an assessment of the home and work environment to ensure that utensils, tools, furniture and light switches, among other objects, have high contrast.

Standard Amsler Grid Testing

The Amsler grid tests the central 20° of visual field centred on the fixation. There are seven types of charts. The standard chart (Fig. 21.7) consists of a central white horizontal and vertical grid, with each line 0.5 mm apart. The square grid is 10 cm on each side of the fixation target. The chart is held at 33 cm with the reading aid. The patient occludes one eye, while looking at the center of the grid, is asked, if any of the ver-

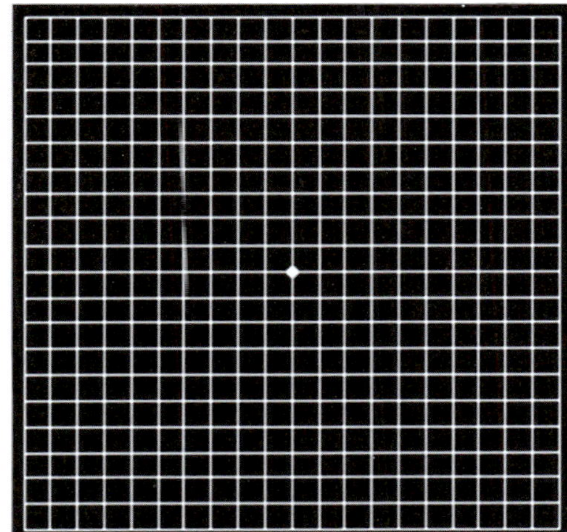

Fig. 21.7: Amsler grid chart.

tical or horizontal lines are missing or distorted. Distortions of the Amsler's grid reflect the presence of metamorphopsia, caused by macular elevations or depressions.[13] The patient should also be asked, if the actual white grid seems to have any color or tint which may be due to hemorrhages.

Threshold Amsler's Grid Testing

A variation on standard Amsler's grid testing is threshold Amsler's grid testing (Stereo Optical Co, Chicago, IL). The crossed polarized filters are used to reduce the contrast of a standard Amsler's grid and is available as an Amsler's grid kit, which comprises of threshold Amsler's polarizers, a black plastic Amsler's grid, and a white Amsler's grid pad.

SUBJECTIVE TESTING OF PATIENTS WITH MEDIA OPACITIES

Fundus examination is difficult in the cases of cataracts, vitreous opacities, and corneal scars.

It is imperative to perform the following investigations in such cases.

- *Potential acuity meter (PAM)*: The PAM unit, manufactured by Mentor (Norwell, MA), is called the Guyton-Minkowski Potential Acuity meter. It measures the retinal visual acuity behind mild to moderate media opacities. Retinal pathology should be considered if PAM test reveals a true loss of visual acuity despite the presence of a media opacity.
- *White light and laser interferometry*: The examples are the Rodenstock laser retinometer (Rodenstock USA, Inc., Danbury, CT) and the Visometer (Haag-Streit, Bern, Switzerland). These project stripes of coherent light through media opacities.
- *Photostress recovery test*: It helps to distinguish disruption of normal macular physiology from early optic nerve disease.

- *Glare testing*: The brightness acuity test (BAT) is used in measuring the reduction of visual acuity in the presence of glare when a cataract or corneal opacity is present. Glare can be caused by intraocular light scattering and is more specific in evaluating anterior segment media opacities. The glare acuity measurement is also available in various auto-refractometers.
- *Color vision testing*: The most commonly used tests are the color plate tests, such as Ishihara pseudoisochromatic or Dvorine color plates and the color arrangements tests such as Farnsworth dichotomous test. The Nagel anomaloscope is more sophisticated test and is used to help in the diagnosis of both congenital and acquired color vision deficiencies.
- *Dark adaptometry*: The standard instrument used is Goldmann-Weekers dark adaptometer (Haag-Streit, Bern, Switzerland). The change in sensitivity is measured in log units which correspond to their rods and cones system.

Low vision is often due to complicated ocular conditions requiring a variety of tests to determine the diagnosis, prognosis, or functional implications of vision loss. These investigations assist the practitioner in providing the most efficient and comprehensive services.

Objective Testing of Retinal Function

- Optical coherence tomography (OCT) to assess any macular edema, if present.
- Fundus fluorescein angiography/indocyanine green angiography (FFA/ICG) to rule out any activity in macular lesions.
- B-scan ultrasonography: It can help detect retinal detachment, retinoschisis, staphyloma, buried drusens or retinal tumors.
- Electrodiagnostic testing: The electroretinography (ERG) and visually evoked response (VER) are used in assessing the electrical processing of the ocular structures in low vision patients.

Scanning laser ophthalmoscope-based microperimetry assesses the preferred retinal locus to estimate the fixation which is eccentric in most of the conditions.

Microperimetry

It is used to find the preferred retinal location in cases of geographic atrophy with fixed eccentric fixation[14] and thus helps the low vision therapist in guiding the patient to use this preferred retinal location (Fig. 21.8)

Figure 21.9 shows a case of an elderly female patient having disciform scar seen on fundus photographs (Figs. 21.9A and B) and OCT scan (Figs. 21.9C and D). The microperimetry (Figs. 21.9E and F) done on MAIA show the preferred retinal locus on the map along with reduced sensitivity of the macula.

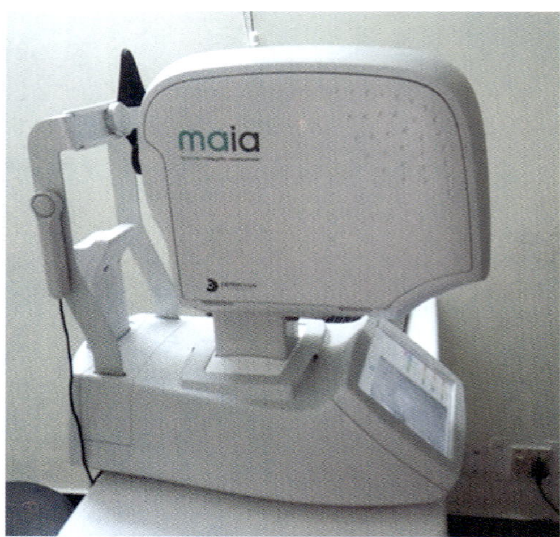

Fig. 21.8: Microperimetry using Macular Integrity assessment, MAIA.

MAGNIFICATION ASSOCIATED WITH LOW VISION SYSTEMS

The components of retinal image magnification (RIM) are relative size magnification (RSM), relative distance magnification (RDM), and lens vertex magnification (LVM).

$$RIM = (RSM)\,(RDM)\,(LVM)$$

The depth of field impacts on the final RIM. It allows the use of magnifiers in ways that produce images on the retina that are usable and functional, although not in perfect focus.

Low Vision Distance Systems

- Spectacles and contact lenses
- Absorptive lenses and coatings
- Pinhole lenses
- Telescopes
- Field expanders and awareness systems for patients with extremely reduced peripheral fields.

Spectacles

Low vision patients typically rely on magnification and they may function better in spectacles. Two special needs may exist, one is that of protection from glasses and the other is the correction of high refractive errors.

The recommendations are:
- The frame should be relatively round, with adjustable nose pads for the proper vertical alignment and not oversized so that the interpupillary distance should be as close as possible.
- High-index lenses should be recommended when prescribing for high refractive errors.
- Antireflective coatings with the scratch resistant coatings help in improving the quality of the image.
- Lens design may be lenticular glasses for aphakics (Fig. 21.10) or myodiscs or blended myodisc for high myopics.

Aspheric design reduces the aberrations and removes the ring scotoma.

GLARE AND PHOTOPHOBIA

Glare and photophobia are the two very common complaints of patients with low vision. Visual function often improves with the help of nonoptical aids[15] by reducing glare and enhancing contrast and eliminating abnormal sensitivity to the light. The options available are:
- Coatings and tints
- Polaroid filters
- Yellow or amber filters
- Photochromatic lenses.

Corning Photochromatic (Glare Control) Filters

Corning photochromatic filter (CPF), designed by Corning Medical Optics, Elmira, NY, is a filter and is an aid to protect eyes with progressive retinal degenerations. In 1981, Corning introduced the CPF-550-S lens specifically for retinitis pigmentosa as the cut-off wavelength is 550 nm. Another latest addition are the Glare Cutter lenses (Fig. 21.11) with more transmittance in 390–410 nm. The advantage is it causes minimum color distortion and blocks 100% ultraviolet B (UVB) and greater than 99% UVA.

The Essilor's Xperio is a polarized lens which gives 100% UV protection from harmful UV rays and is available in gray-green tints. Its quite thin and has refractive index of 1.502. Airwear is another thinner, lighter, and tougher lens suitable in case of high refractive errors.

Typoscope (Fig. 21.12) is a small rectangular card that has a horizontal slot to allow for the viewing of two to three lines of printed text. It is a masking device with a line cut out from an opaque, nonreflecting, black plastic or thick paper.

NOIR sunfilters (NOIR, Medical Technologies, South Lyon, MI) (Figs. 21.13A to C) are commonly prescribed.[16] They are the plastic filters of several transmission in both goggle and frame styles. The retrospective studies of NOIR filters have shown that Models 101 is preferred by glaucoma, retinitis pigmentosa and ARMD patients, and 102 by diabetics.

CONTACT LENSES

- They can be prescribed for high refractive errors for optimum vision and wider field of view as there are fewer spherical aberrations and aniseikonia is also reduced with contact lenses.
- *Tinted and opaque lenses for albinism and aniridia (Fig. 21.14)*: They are made with an opaque periphery and clear pupil (4 mm) to reduce photophobia. Adventures in Color (Golden, CO) and Custom Color Contacts (New York, NY) customize the tints. Also available are Illusion lens from CIBA Vision (Duluth, GA).
- *X-chrome lenses for the color deficits*: These lenses transmit light in the red zones (590–700 nm). They enhance color perception or make things more vivid.[17]

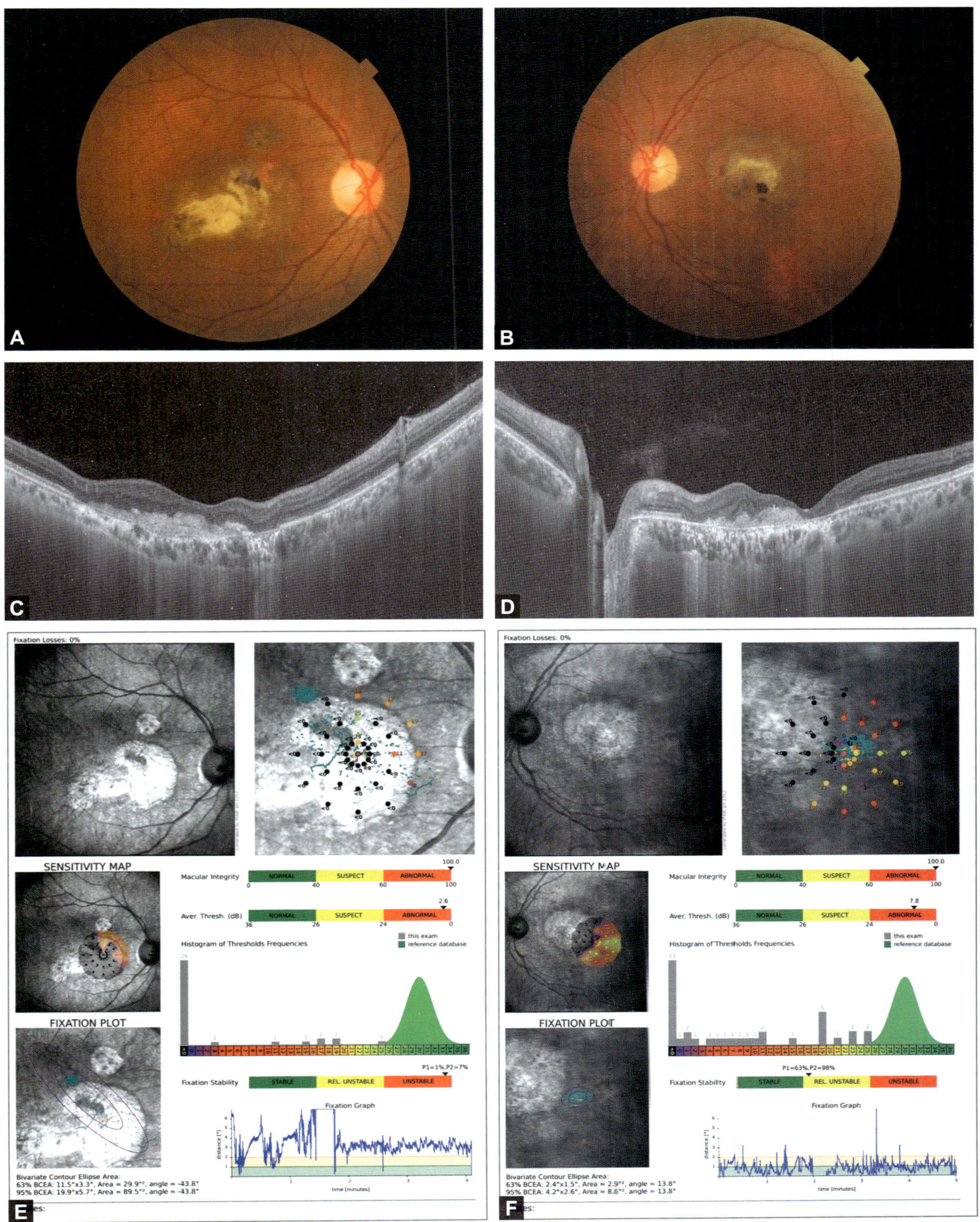

Figs. 21.9A to F: Microperimetry of a patient with disciform macular scar in both eyes, having reduced contrast sensitivity.

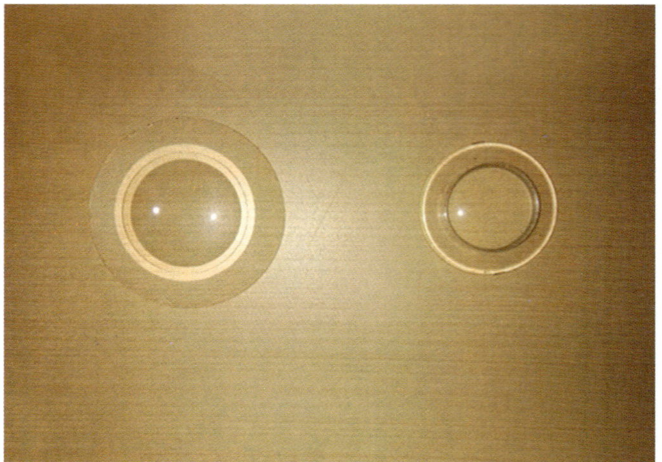

Fig. 21.10: Lenticular lenses for aphakes.

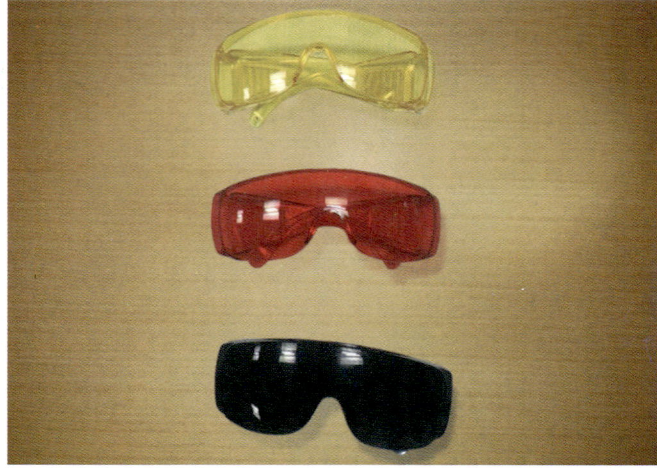

Fig. 21.11: Glare cutter (390–410 nm).

Fig. 21.12: Typoscope to reduce glare and enhance contrast.

- *Contact lens telescopic system*: It may be used in the design of a Galilean telescopic system. The ocular eyepiece is a high powered concave contact lens and the objective is a lower powered convex spectacle lens. This produces a relatively large field of view as compared to an equivalent powered Galilean handheld or spectacle-mounted telescope. However, only up to 1.8× magnification can be achieved.

TELESCOPE

It is an optical instrument used to magnify the apparent size of a distant object. Most telescopes are refracting type. As it uses a converging lens as the objective lens. It can be used to amplify light, enabling faint distant point sources of light to be seen.[18] Telescopes make distant objects appear closer to the patient than they actually are.

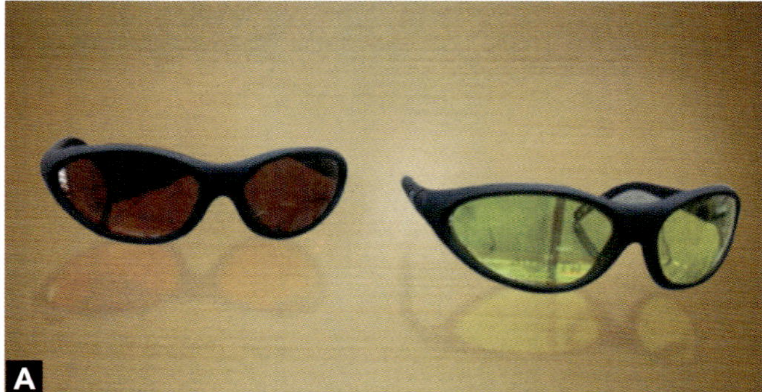

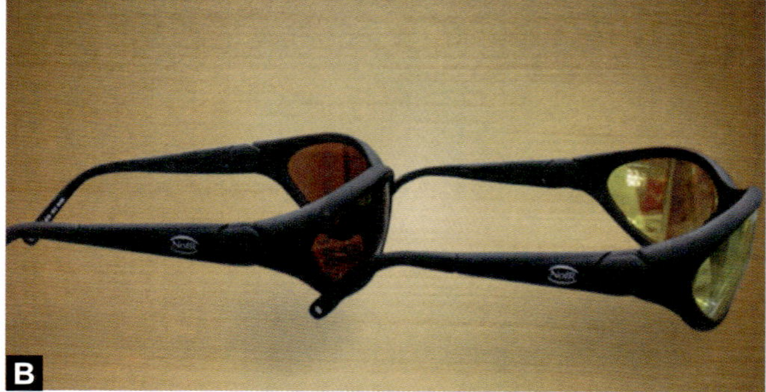

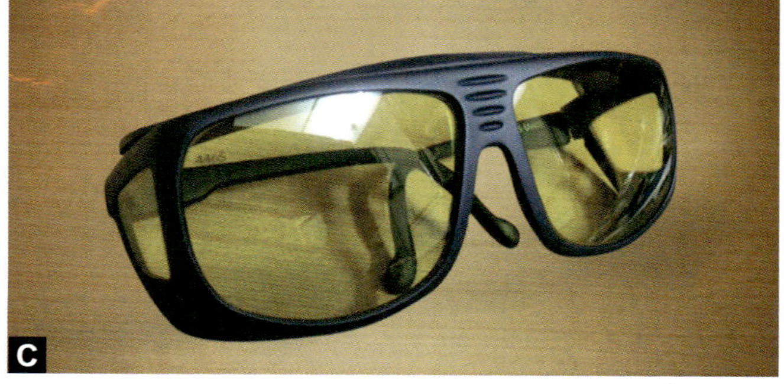

Figs. 21.13A to C: NOIR Filter glasses.

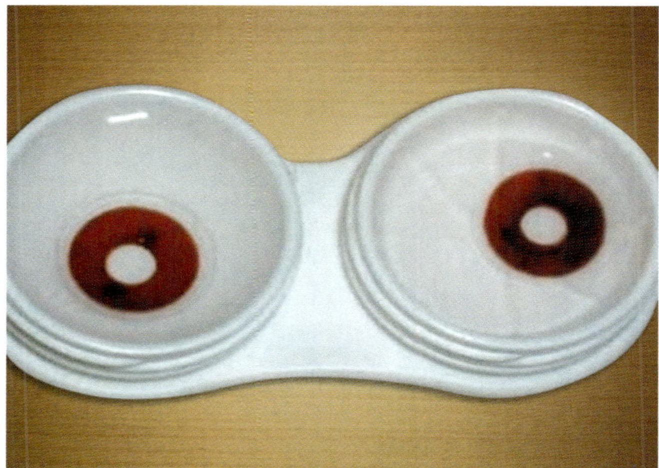

Fig. 21.14: Tinted and opaque lenses.

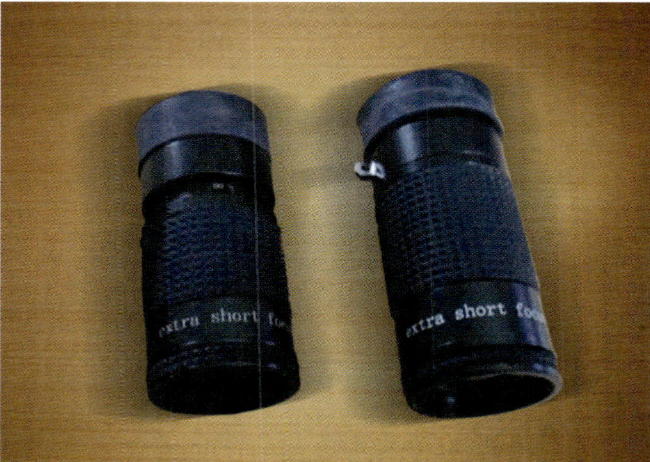

Fig. 21.15: Handheld monocular telescope.

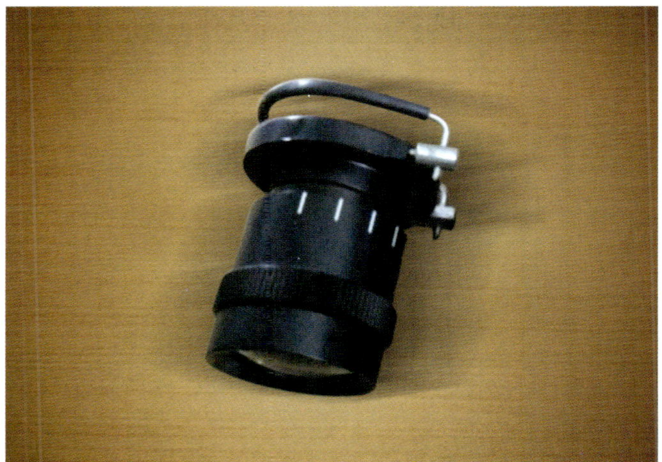

Fig. 21.16: Clip on telescope.

There are two basic designs based on the principle of angular magnification.

1. *Galilean telescope*: The eyepiece is a negative lens and the objective is a positive lens. The quality of the image is relatively poor.
2. *Keplerian telescope*: It is heavier in weight. Both the eyepiece and the objective lens are positive with the incorporated prisms to upright the image.

Types of Telescopes

These are available in 3×, 4×, 6×, and 8× magnifications. The field of view decreases with the magnification.

- *Handheld monocular*: These can be easily removed, allow hand-free use, and are less expensive (Fig. 21.15)
- *Clip-on*: This telescope allows to be flipped up out of the patient's line of sight when it is not being used and flipped back down when it needs to be used (Fig. 21.16).

- *Spectacle mounted, monocular or binocular*: These are generally involved with activities that demand more prolonged viewing (watching TV, or a movie) or for which hands have to be free (Fig. 21.17).
- *SEETV 2× aspheric binocular lens*: The "SEETV" glasses focus on objects from 10 feet to infinity with clarity on the enlarged image (Figs. 21.18 and 21.19). The "SEETV" glasses are specially designed for watching TV. It is one of the easiest to fit apparatus. It is ideal for watching movies, and provides 2.1 to 3× magnification. The lenses are scratch resistant, which is optimum even for pediatric use.

Bioptic Design

The term was coined by Designs for Vision Inc., (Ronkonkoma, NY) to describe its miniature Galilean telescopes, which were prescribed for driving. It describes the telescope mounted on the upper portion of the carrier lens, which allows viewing under the telescope (through the carrier lens) when the telescopic magnification is not required (Figs. 21.20A and B). When telescope is mounted on lower position of the carrier lens (similar to bifocal), it is said to be in the reading or surgical position. It is available in 1.7× and 2.2× magnifications, recommended for individuals with mild vision loss of 20/100, and as a 0.5× field expander for individuals with tunnel vision. The SightScope is lighter in weight and is better cosmetically. The sharp optics provide a broad range of clear vision without focusing and can be flipped out of the way when not needed.

Ocutech, Inc. (Chapel Hill, NC)

It is a horizontal light path vision enhancing system and is a Keplerian telescope that appears as a horizontal periscope lying across top of a spectacle frame (Fig. 21.21). The optics include a right angle prism, an achromatic doublet objective (which is movable to focus the system), a roof-pentaprism, and a Kellner two-lens, three-element eyepiece. The telescope has the ability to correct for refractive errors from +12.00 D to −12.00 D by focusing the telescope.

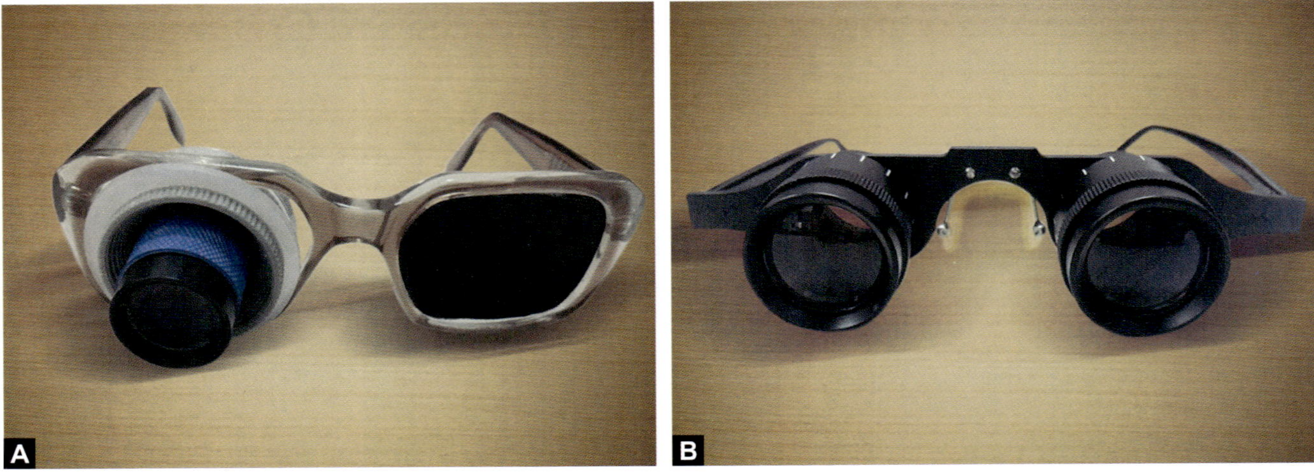

Figs. 21.17A and B: Spectacle mounted—(A) Monocular and (B) Binocular telescopes.

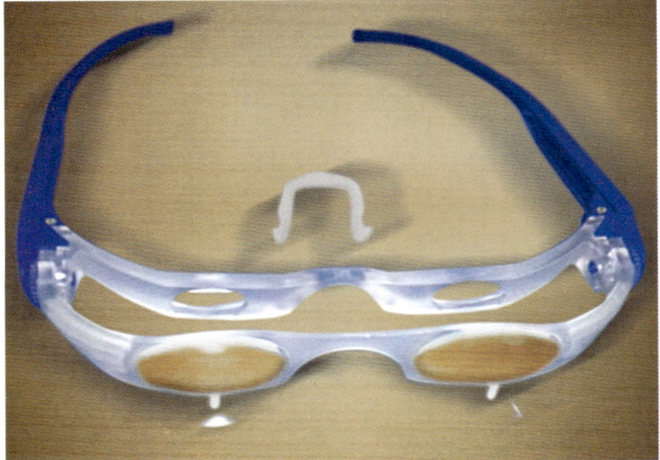

Fig. 21.18: SEETV glasses.

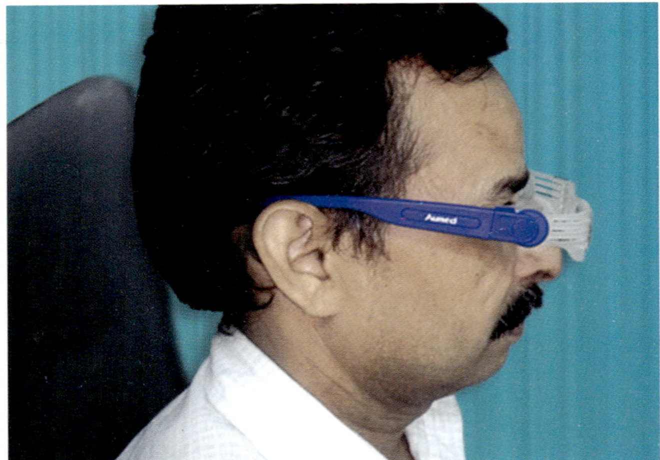

Fig. 21.19: Patient wearing SEETV glasses.

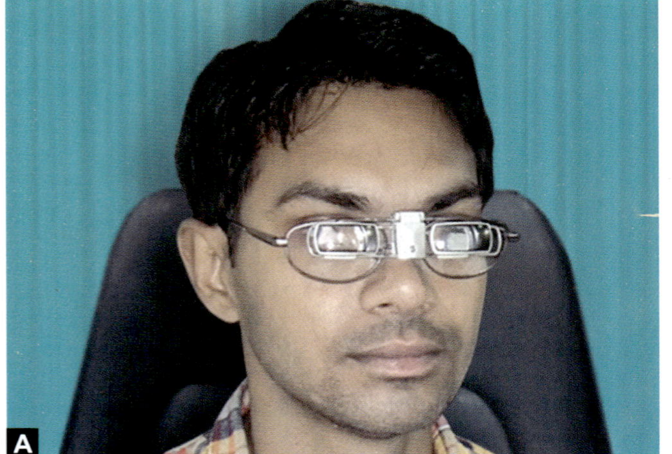

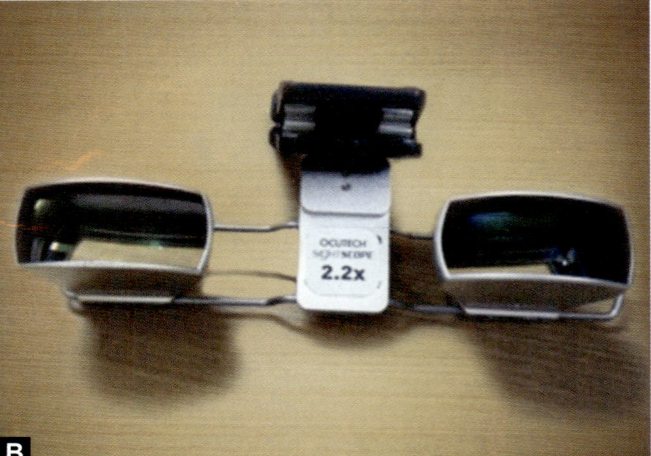

Figs. 21.20A and B: (A) Bioptic design; (B) SightScope flip.

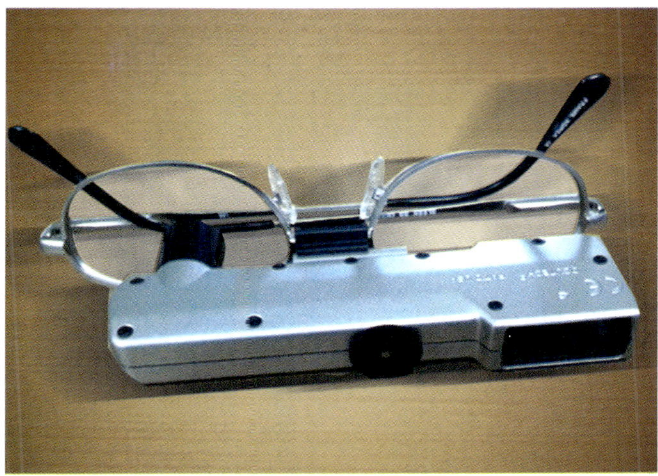

Fig. 21.21: Ocutech low vision aid.

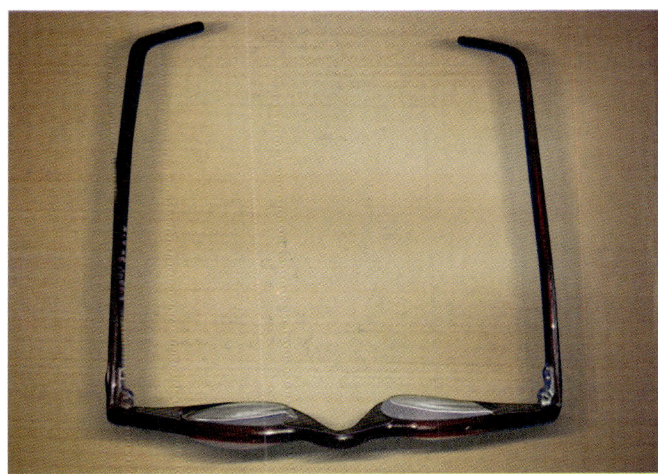

Fig. 21.22: Magnifying glasses.

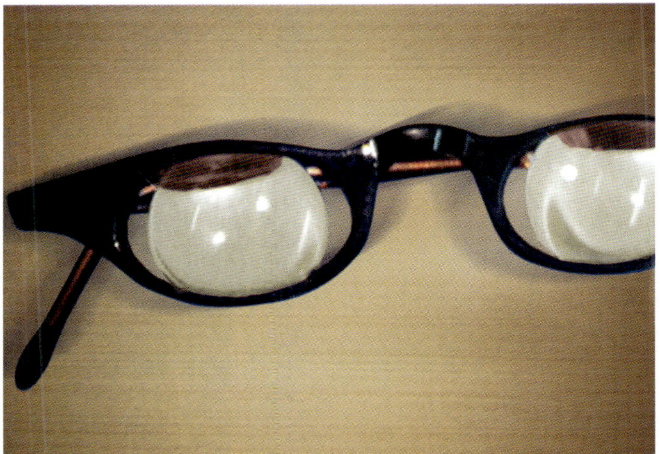

Fig. 21.23: Prismatic spherical lenses.

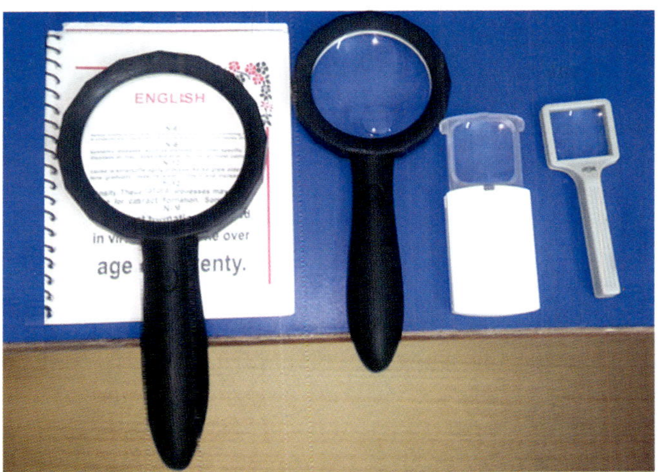

Fig. 21.24: Hand magnifiers.

LOW VISION NEAR SYSTEMS

Magnifying Glasses

These are the high plus reading glasses with powers ranging from +4.0 D to +24.0 D (Fig. 21.22). These are the plastic lenses of high refractive index lenses. The patient has to read at the focal point according to the addition.

- *Prismatic glasses (Fig. 21.23)*: When binocular corrections are required, base in prisms are added to aid the binocularity with powers ranging from +4.0D to +18.0 D.
- Aspheric design to improve the quality of the image by reducing the aberrations.

The advantages of the spectacles are that the hands are free, reading time can be prolonged, and is the most comfortable. The disadvantage is that it cannot be of use in certain macular conditions, such as macular scars post neovascular ARMD.

Hand Magnifiers

These are the convex lenses held in front of the spectacle plane and are used for reading signs, labels, price tags, and identifying money (Fig. 21.24). The available magnifications are +4.0 D to +68.0 D. They can be aspheric, bi-aspheric or aplanatic designs. Aplanatic designs provide better image quality and distortion-free field. The magnifiers with LEDs (light-emitting diode), the illuminated ones, work better in conditions like ARMD.

Stand Magnifiers

These are the fixed focused, easy to use, and are used by elderly with tremors, arthritis, and constricted fields (Figs. 21.25A and B). They may be self-illuminated and are available in range from 2× to 16×.

The reading material should be placed on the flat surface. The patient is instructed to use the reading glasses, so that the

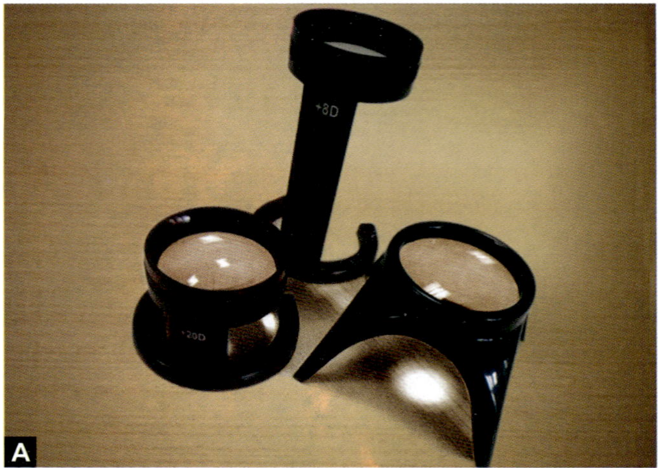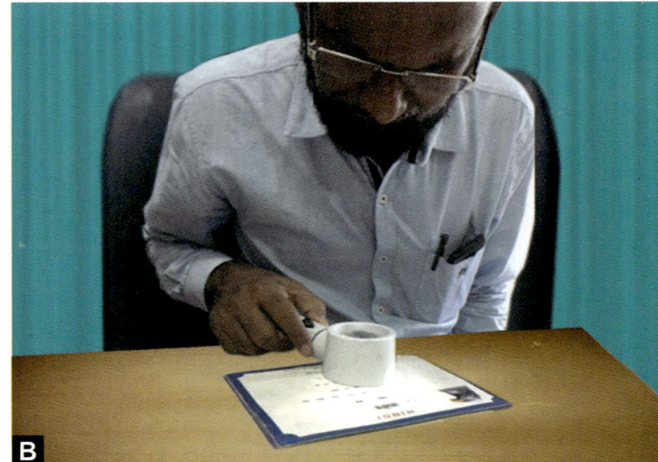

Figs. 21.25A and B: Stand magnifiers.

diverging rays coming from the magnifying lens converge and a virtual image is formed behind the lens.

A patient may have many different near demands, one magnifier may not solve all the visual concerns and might need several magnifiers to meet his or her needs. The factors affecting the field of view include lens power and lens size.

The practitioner should always be positive and provide appropriate encouragement.

Dome Magnifier

They are the dome-shaped visual aids used for reading (Fig. 21.26). It is made of optical grade acrylic and are available in 3×, 4× and 6× magnification with the diameter of 2 inch to 4.5 inch. It is commonly used by patients having macular degenerations, dystrophies, Stargardt disease and patients having retinitis pigmentosa.

Bar Magnifier

It is also made up of acrylic and is available in 3× to 6× magnifications and magnifies the entire line of the text (Fig. 21.27).

NONOPTICAL DEVICES

The function of nonoptical device is to enhance the visibility of retinal image and optimize the use of magnifiers.

- Reading lamps and stands
- Signature guides
- Bold line note books
- Notex guide for the currency
- Signature guide
- Cane stick for mobility and orientation
- Dog guides, sighted guides
- Filters
- Pinhole glasses (Fig. 21.28)
- CCTV—portable video magnifier (Fig. 21.29). It assists in providing the optimum near vision in all cases of macular degenerations, glaucoma, retinitis pigmentosa and

diabetic retinopathy and dry as well as wet ARMD.[19] It is a combination of a customized camera and a viewing screen/monitor and can provide a magnification of up to 82×.

Adjustable Table

It is used to relieve strain on the neck and back while readiytng (Fig. 21.30).

Signature Guide

It helps to sign the document and is useful in cases of ARMD[17] (Fig. 21.31).

Cane Stick

It provides assistance for mobility. It has an advantage of being highly maneuverable, reliable, and requires virtually no maintenance. Pioneering work was done by Dr Richard Hoover in 1940 at the Valley Forge Army Hospital.

Typoscope

It enhances the image by decreasing the glare and enhancing contrast (*see* Fig. 21.12).

Desktop Electronic Magnifier (Fig. 21.32)

It is an electronic magnifier with 20 inches monitor with magnification up to 85× with adjustable brightness and contrast. It benefits in the cases of some severely impaired low vision patients like those having ARMD.

Low Vision Enhancement Systems

It was initially developed by a team of doctors and researchers at John Hopkins School of Medicine along with NASA. It is a head mounted electronic magnification system. It provides a monochrome image and has automatic focus capabilities at distance, intermediate and near distances.

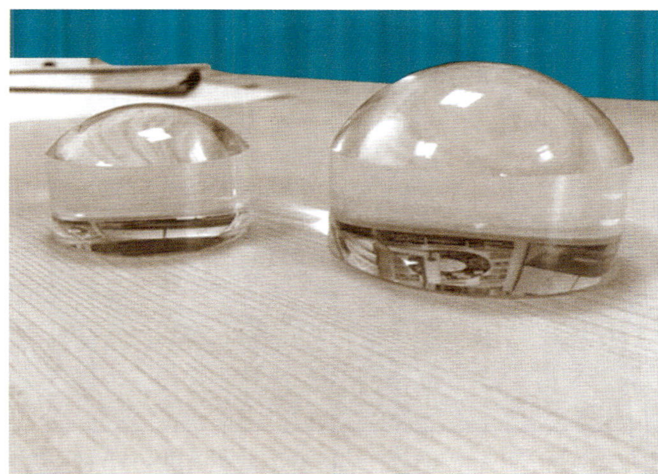

Fig. 21.26: Dome magnifiers.

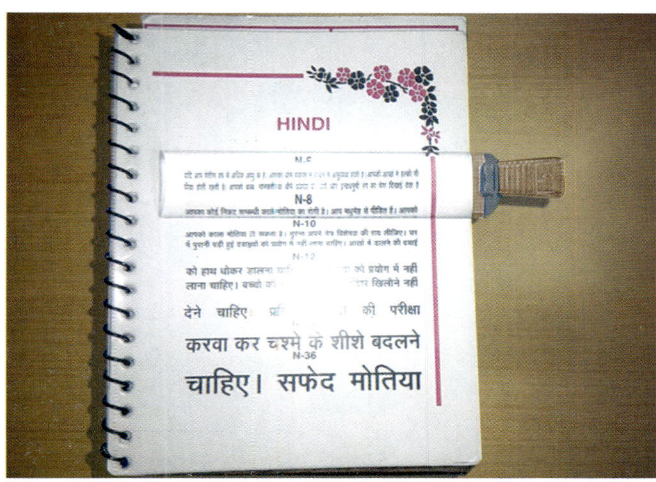

Fig. 21.27: Bar magnifier.

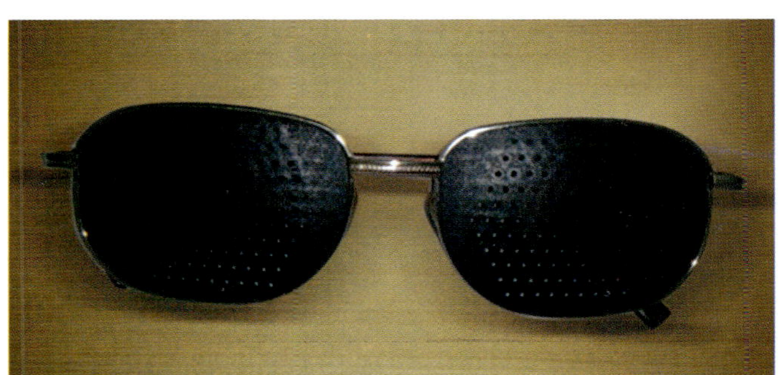

Fig. 21.28: Pinhole glasses.

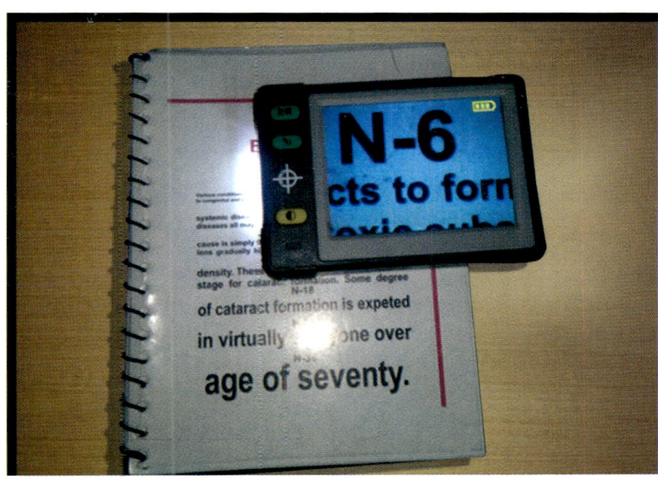

Fig. 21.29: CCTV.

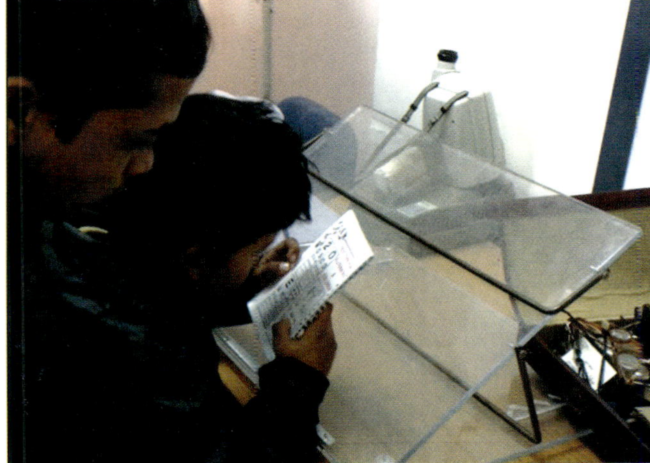

Fig. 21.30: Adjustable table.

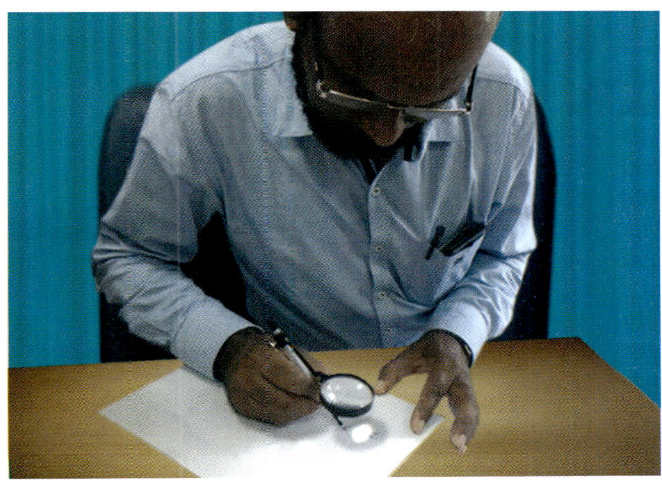

Fig. 21.31: Signature guide.

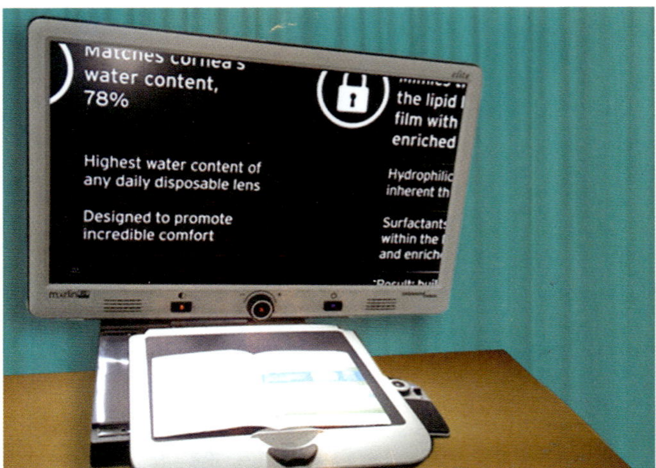

Fig. 21.32: Merlin desktop magnifier.

eSight

It is lightweight LVES. It has a high speed, high definition camera that captures, enhances and displays it on LED screens in front of the user's eyes.

Low vision rehabilitation is a new emerging sub-specialty that aims to improve the functionality and independence of patients with visual impairment using a multi-disciplinary approach. Despite the advances in the field, uptake of low vision services still remain low due lack of awareness amongst the patients as well as the ophthalmologists. Hence, a low vision clinician should be aware of the range of specialists, vocational services and community based services needed by people with low vision.

REFERENCES

1. World Health Organization. List of Official ICD-10 Updates Ratified October 2006. Geneva: WHO; 2006. Available from: http://www.who.int/classifications/icd/2006Updates.pdf.
2. Gilbert C, van Dijk K. When someone has low vision. Community Eye Health. 2012;25(77):4-11
3. Bonavolonta P, Travade I, Forte R, et al. A chart for low visual acuities: experience in a centre for low vision and rehabilitation. J Fr Ophthalmology. 2010;33(6):391-6
4. Miwa M, Iwanami M, Oba MS, et al. Comparison of LogMAR charts with angular vision for visually impaired: the Berkeley rudimentary vision test vs LogMAR One target Landolt Ring Eye chart. Graefes Arch Clin Exp Ophthalmology. 2013;251(12):2761-7.
5. Ferris L, Kassoff A, Bresnick GH, et al. New visual acuity charts for research purposes. Am J Ophthalmology. 1982;94:91-6.
6. Barteselli G, Gomez ML, Doede AL, et al. Visual; function assessment in simulated real-life situations in patients with age related macular degeneration compared to normal subjects. Eye (Lond). 2014;28(10):1231-8.
7. Murro V, Sodi A, Giacomelli G, et al. Reading ability and quality of life in Stargardt disease. Eur J Ophthalmology. 2017;14:0.
8. Radner W. Reading charts in ophthalmology. Graefes Arch Clin Exp Ophthalmology. 2017;255(8):1-8.
9. Barrio A, Antona B, Puel MC. Repeatability of mesopic visual acuity measurements using high and low contrast ETDRS letter charts. Graefes Arch Clin Exp Ophthalmology 2015;253(5):791-5.
10. Bailey II. The optometric examination of the elderly patient. In: Rosenbloom AA, Morgan MW (Eds). Vision and Aging. Boston: Butterworth-Heinemann; 1993.
11. Cao KY, Markowitz SN. Residual stereopsis in age-related macular degeneration patients and its impact on vision-related abilities: A pilot study. J Optom. 2014;7(2):100-5.
12. Rosenthal BP. The structured low vision evaluation. In: BP Rosenthal, Cole RG (Eds). Problems in Optometry. A Structured Approach to Low Vision Care. Hagerstown, MD: Lippincott; 1991.
13. Faye EE. Evaluating near vision: The Amsler grid and field defects. In: Faye EE (Ed). Clinical Low Vision. Boston: Little, Brown; 1984.
14. Parcella E, Parcella F, Mazzeo F, et al. Effectiveness of vision rehabilitation treatment through MP1 microperimeter in patients with visual loss due to macular diseases. Clin Ter. 2012;163(6):e 423-8.
15. Rosenberg EA, Sperazza LC. The visually impaired patient. Am Fam Physician. 2008;77(10):1431-6.
16. Ding C, Sun B, ZhengY. Contrast sensitivity of several blindness-inducing eye diseases and the influence of tinted filter lens. 1997;33(4):286-8.
17. Severinsky B, Yahalom C, Florescu Sebok T, et al. Red tinted contact lenses may improve quality of life in retinal diseases. Optom Vis Sci. 2016;93(4): 445-50.
18. Ackuaku-Dogbe EM, Baidoo BA, Braimah ZI, et al. Causes of low vision and their management at Korle Bu Teaching Hospital, Accra, GHANA. J West Afr Coll Surg. 2016;6(3):105-22.
19. Lovie-Kitchen JE, Bowman KJ. Senile Macular Degeneration. Boston: Butterworth; 1985.

Retinal Vascular Disorders

Chapter 22

Retinal Arterial Occlusion

Raghav Ravani, Sahil Agrawal, Yogita Gupta, Vineet Mutha

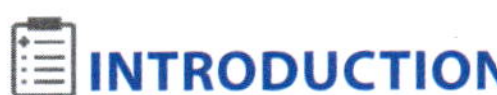 INTRODUCTION

The central retinal artery supplies blood to the inner retina. The cilioretinal artery arising from choroidal circulation also contributes in 15–30% of eyes. Arterial occlusive disease affecting the retina may involve afferent vessels anywhere from the common carotid artery to the intraretinal arterioles. The amount of retinal ischemia and symptoms depends on the vessel involved ranging from an asymptomatic peripheral arteriolar occlusion to total blindness in cases of ophthalmic artery occlusion. For the purpose of discussion, the arterial occlusive disease in this chapter has been divided into:

- Branch retinal artery occlusion (BRAO)
- Central retinal artery occlusion (CRAO)

BRANCH RETINAL ARTERY OCCLUSION

Branch retinal artery occlusion, as the name suggests results due to occlusion of branches arising from the central retinal artery.

Epidemiology

As with other systemic vascular disorders, BRAO is commonly found in older age group, though occasionally can be seen in young adults. BRAOs may comprise about 38% of all acute retinal artery obstructions.[1]

Pathophysiology

Arterial occlusion at any site may result either from embolization from a distant foci or from thrombosis of the affected vessel. The most common cause of nonarteritic retinal arterial occlusion is retinal emboli.[2] Retinal emboli may be visible on ophthalmoscopy around 62% of the time in BRAO[3] and in about 20–40% cases of CRAO[4,5] (Fig. 22.1). Retinal emboli consist of the following:[6]

- Cholesterol (74% of cases)
- Calcified material (15.5%)
- Platelet and fibrin (15.5%).

Other rare causes of emboli include those comprising of fat or septic emboli from fracture of bones following trauma or infective carditis respectively.

The yellow refractile embolus of cholesterol (also called as Hollenhorst plaque) is the most common embolus (Fig. 22.1). These are usually small, and are seen at site of bifurcation of vessels and usually originate from carotid arteries and less commonly from other proximal arteries in patients with atherosclerosis.

Calcific emboli are less common, larger and completely obstruct the blood flow, thus leading to more severe manifestations. The origin is commonly from the cardiac valves.[7,8]

Clinical Features

Patient presents with monocular sudden onset painless diminution of vision, especially in a particular part of the visual field. Nearly three-fourths of the patients present with a presenting acuity of 20/40 or better.[3,9]

Ophthalmoscopic examination in acute phase reveals retinal opacification in a sectoral pattern at macula and edema along the distribution of the obstructed artery (Fig. 22.2). Probable pathophysiologic mechanism is the blocked axo-

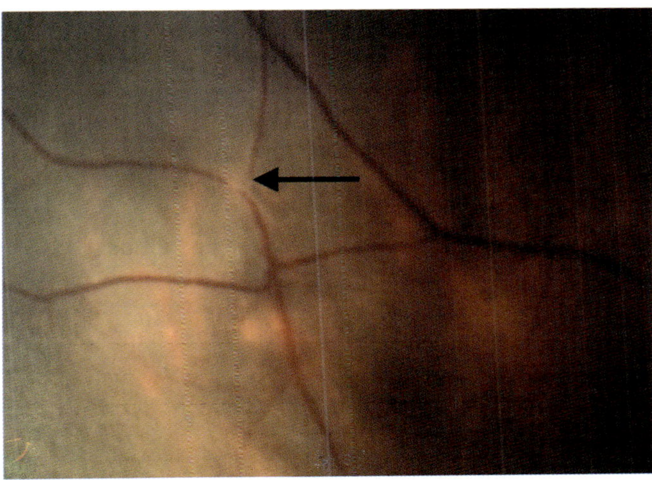

Fig. 22.1: Color fundus picture showing retinal emboli/Hollenhorst plaque (black arrow) at the bifurcation site of retinal artery.

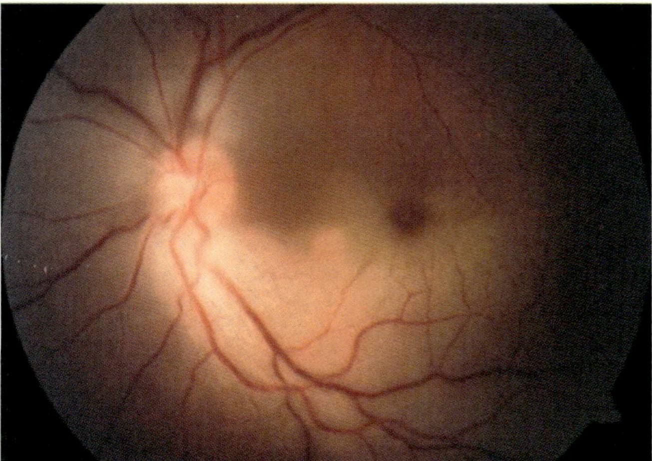

Fig. 22.2: Inferotemporal sectoral pattern of retinal opacification with edema and pallor along the inferotemporal arterial arcade.

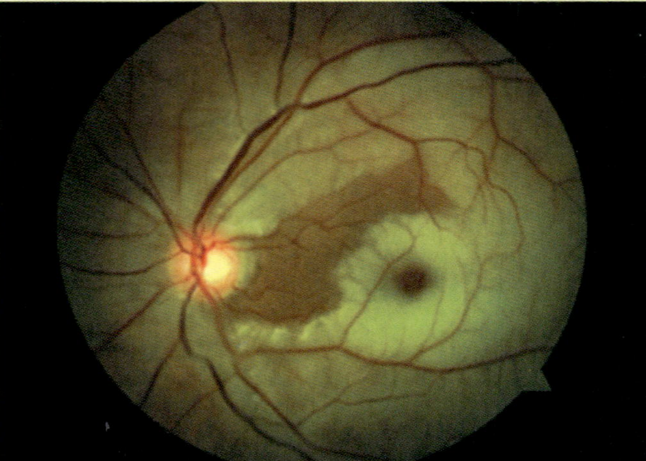

Fig. 22.3: Central retinal artery occlusion (CRAO) with cilioretinal artery sparing.

plasmic flow in the nerve fiber layer in the ischemic area. Fundoscopically, chronic stage of BRAO is characterized by arterial attenuation, sectoral nerve fiber layer loss, posterior-segment neovascularization and rarely iris neovascularization. Pathognomonic for BRAO is the presence of artery-to-artery collaterals. Visual field examination shows sectoral defects in 49%. Other common field defects include presence of central scotoma in 20% and central altitudinal defect in 13%.[9]

Investigations

Since, CRAO and BRAO have similar risk factors and pathophysiology, an evaluation similar to that described under the section of CRAO is recommended.

Treatment and Visual Outcome

Branch retinal artery occlusion being less severe with good visual prognosis, aggressive therapy is recommended in cases with significant foveal involvement. Visual acuity often improves to 20/40 or better in 80%.[10] Long-term follow-up for possibility of development of neovascularization of the iris (though uncommon) and neovascular glaucoma is recommended.

CENTRAL RETINAL ARTERY OCCLUSION

Von Graefe first described CRAO in the setting of endocarditis causing multiple systemic emboli in a report in 1859.

Epidemiology

Incidence of CRAO in general population is as low as approximately 8.5 cases per 100,000.[11] CRAO is mostly seen in elderly age group, however few case reports suggest occurrence in

children and younger patients as well.[10,12] It occurs more frequently in males compared to females. Bilateral manifestation is seen in 1–2% of cases. CRAO may occur sequentially in both eyes.[13]

Clinical Features

Sudden, painless and severe loss of vision in the involved eye, with or without history of amaurosis fugax is the usual presenting symptom. History of amaurosis fugax has higher correlation with stroke than retinal emboli alone.[14] Estimated risk of CRAO after amaurosis fugax is about 1% per year.[15] Presenting visual acuity may range from counting fingers to perception of light in majority of the patients.[16,17] Central visual sparing is seen with presence of cilioretinal artery supplying the fovea (Fig. 22.3). In cases with absence of light perception, concomitant involvement of optic nerve or impairment of the choroidal circulation due to ophthalmic artery occlusion should be considered.[16] On examination, afferent pupillary defect is seen irrespective of macular sparing.[10] Intraocular pressure remains normal in the acute phase but may rise in cases which develop rubeosis iridis and subsequent neovascular glaucoma. Rubeosis in CRAO tends to occur earlier with average of around 4–5 weeks after onset of occlusion with incidence of 16.6–18.8%,[18-20] compared to 3–5 months after onset in CRVO. The chances of rubeosis are higher in more severe obstruction and chronic obstruction.

Ophthalmoscopic findings (Figs. 22.4A to C) in the acute phase predominantly involve the posterior pole and include appearance of cherry-red spot at the fovea, posterior pole retinal opacity/whitening, box-caring of retinal vessels, arterial attenuation, edema of optic disc or optic nerve pallor. The appearance of a cherry-red spot at the posterior pole decreases with time since onset of CRAO. Also, there is resolution of retinal thickening over a period of 4–6 weeks. Patent cilioretinal artery is seen in about 15–30% of patients. In such

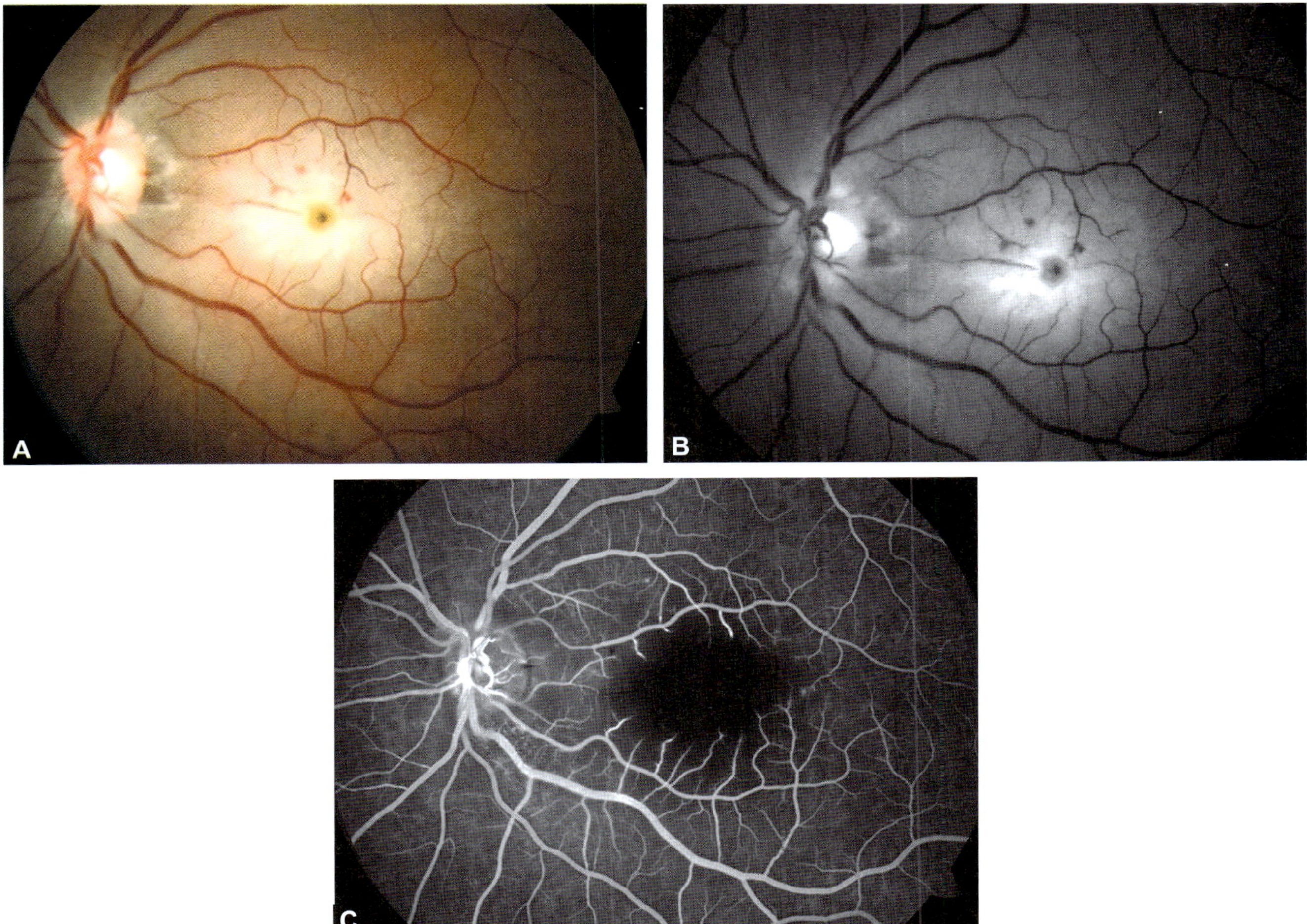

Figs. 22.4A to C: Central retinal artery occlusion (CRAO) showing (A) Cherry red spot. (B) Fundus autofluorescence image of the same patient. (C) Fundus fluorescein angiography image showing enlarged foveal avascular zone.

cases, the papillomacular bundle perfused by the cilioretinal artery remains sharply demarcated from the surrounding retinal whitening (*see* Fig. 22.3).

The visual acuity in such cases depends on location and extent of the area perfused by the cilioretinal artery.[1,17,21,22]

In cases of arteritic CRAO, the optic disc edema is seen due to associated anterior ischemic optic neuropathy.

Chronic CRAO is characterized by optic atrophy, arterial attenuation, cilioretinal collaterals around the disc and macular RPE changes. Neovascularization at optic disc is rare since elaboration of angiogenic factors is rare in nonviable or infarcted retina compared to viable ischemic retina.

Although rare, combined CRVO and CRAO (Figs. 22.5A and B), has frequently been reported associated with inflammatory, infectious or coagulation disorders.

Ancillary Tests

Fundus fluorescein angiography in CRAO shows delayed and sluggish filling of the retinal vasculature (Fig. 22.6). There is a significant delay in appearance of dye in retinal arterial branches as compared to central retinal artery. Typically, there is a delay in appearance of dye in the central retinal artery by 5–20 seconds. In eyes with acute CRAO, there may be areas of delayed choroidal perfusion in about 11% of cases.[16]

Optical coherence tomography (OCT) in acute stages shows increased reflectivity of inner retina with irregular macular contour due to intracellular edema. Chronic stages of CRAO show thinning and atrophy of the inner retina on OCT (Figs. 22.7A and B).

Visual field analysis shows central scotoma followed by paracentral scotoma as the most common field defect in CRAO. Preservation of central island of vision corresponding to the perfused retina with peripheral constriction of field is seen in patients with cilioretinal sparing.[17]

Electroretinography (ERG) in CRAO typically shows negative waveform characterized by attenuation of b-wave more than a-wave.

During autofluorescence imaging in acute stage of CRAO, the thickened inner layer of retina blocks the normal autoflu-

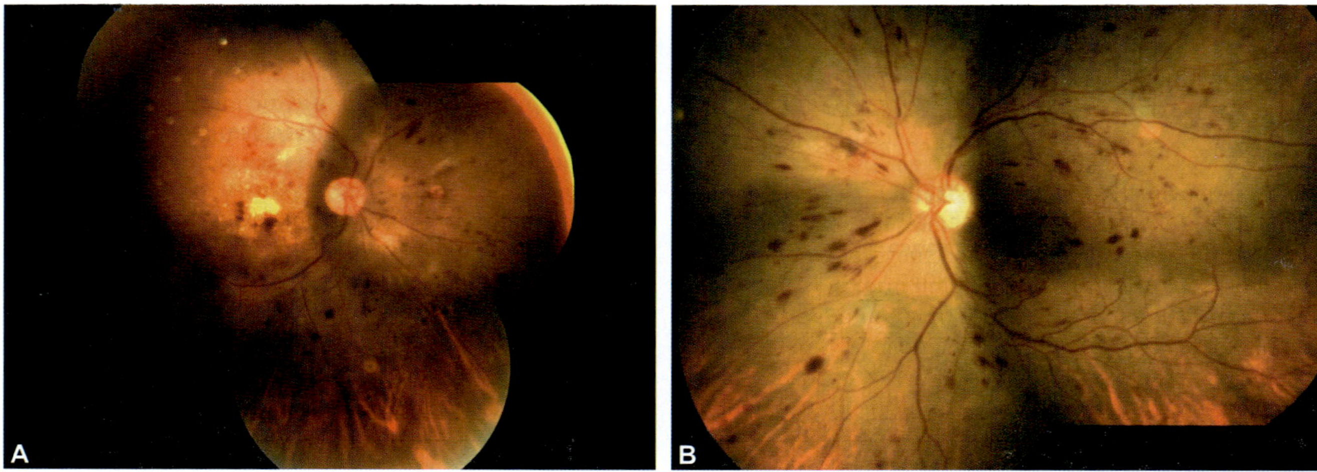

Figs. 22.5A and B: Bilateral central retinal vein occlusion with central artery occlusion.

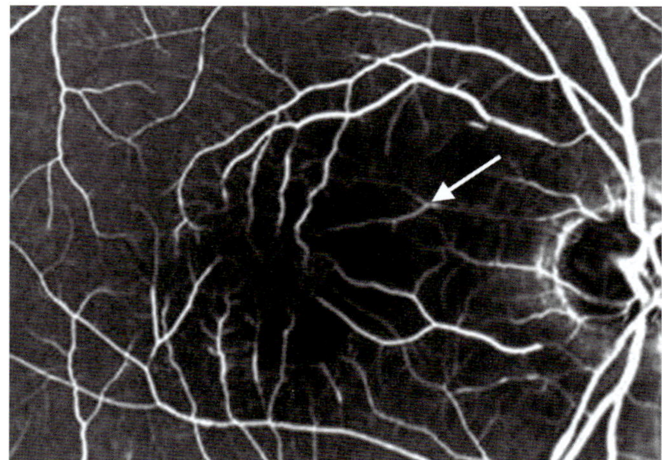

Fig. 22.6: Fundus fluorescein angiography in a patient with central retinal artery occlusion (CRAO) showing pruning of vessels (white arrow) and emboli at the site of occlusion.

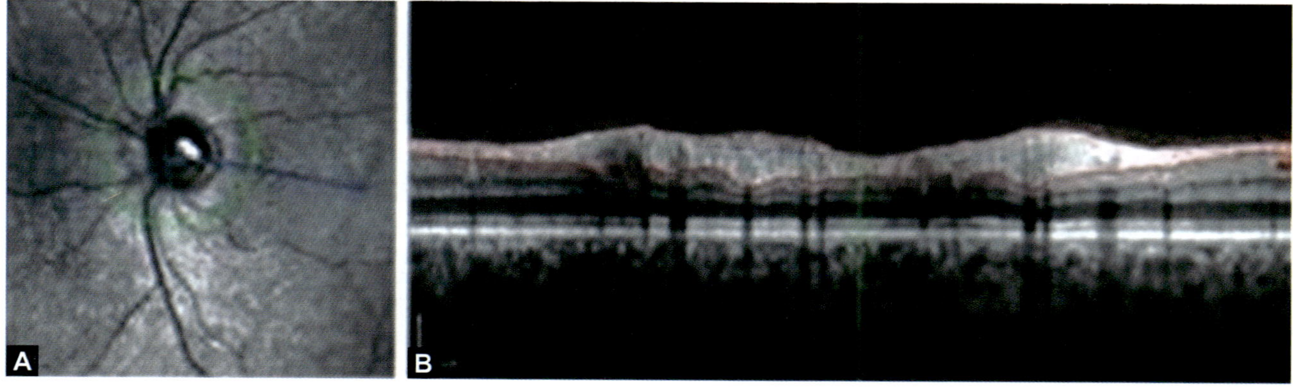

Figs. 22.7A and B: Optical coherence tomography of a patient with central retinal artery occlusion (CRAO) showing irregular foveal contour with increased reflectance from inner retinal layers due to retinal edema.

orescence of the RPE leading to decreased autofluorescence. In chronic stages of CRAO with atrophy of inner retinal layer, autofluorescence imaging reveals window defect.[23]

Evaluation

Central retinal artery occlusion is an ophthalmic emergency and treatment should not be delayed. Yet, it is necessary to find the cause of CRAO and targeted workup is required. It is essential to rule out giant cell arteritis in elderly patients by evaluating complete blood count with erythrocyte sedimentation rate (ESR) and C-reactive proteins. The patient with relevant history and increased CRP should be started immediately on steroid therapy to prevent involvement of the other eye and should be considered for temporal artery biopsy, if required.

In embolic CRAO, investigations should be done to look for potential source of embolus. This includes carotid artery Doppler and echocardiography. Positive investigation entails consultation with cardiologist for appropriate intervention or chronic anticoagulation therapy. Transesophageal echocardiography is more sensitive and has a higher yield than transthoracic approach, but requires proper case selection and is done in patients with high suspicion and negative transthoracic echocardiography.

In young patients, it is necessary to evaluate for hypercoagulable states with proper history taking and investigations. This includes tests for serum homocysteine levels, sickle-cell disease, factor V Leiden mutation, protein C, protein S, antithrombin III, and antiphospholipid antibody.

Treatment

Central retinal artery occlusion is an ophthalmic emergency when presented early in course of disease. The treatment of CRAO continues to be a challenge in absence of a set treatment protocol with variable outcomes. Spontaneous resolution has been reported in 22% of patients.[24] The visual outcomes, however, have been unsatisfactory with less than 10% having meaningful visual recovery.[25,26] The damage to the retina and visual recovery depends on the duration of ischemic insult. Retina can withstand ischemia without significant damage up to 97 minutes after acute CRAO. However, there is irreversible damage after about 4 hours of the onset of acute CRAO. Thus providing a very narrow window period from onset of complete obstruction to the time after which there is irreversible damage and no intervention might help. Since complete obstruction is rarely seen, treatment of CRAO should be within 24 hours of onset of symptoms.

The principle of treatment for CRAO consists of dislodging emboli or lysing the thrombus, maintaining retinal oxygenation, vasodilatation of the ocular blood supply, reducing the intraocular pressure and increasing retinal blood flow.[27-30]

Treatment options can be conservative or surgical intervention. Various conservative modalities include ocular massage, inhalation of carbogen, hyperbaric oxygen, vasodilating medications like pentoxifylline and sublingual isosorbide dinitrate, intravenous mannitol or oral glycerol, anterior-chamber paracentesis, intravenous steroids (in arteritic CRAO), or thrombolytics.

Various surgical modalities have been used for treatment of CRAO.

Neodymium-doped yttrium aluminum garnet (Nd-YAG) laser arteriotomy has been reported to result in extrusion of embolus and re-establishment of circulation in patients with CRAO.

Thrombolytics, either intravenous or intra-arterial have been considered for treatment of CRAO including streptokinase, urokinase, tissue plasminogen activator (t-PA), but requires a thorough work-up and a checklist of systemic risks and contraindications has to be ruled out. The European Assessment Group for Lysis in the Eye (EAGLE) study, a prospective, randomized clinical trial evaluating effect of intra-arterial t-PA with conservative management showed no significant difference in the improvement of vision, with slight better outcome with conservative management and increased rate of cerebral hemorrhage in intervention group.

CILIORETINAL ARTERY OCCLUSION

Cilioretinal artery is clinically seen as a separate artery from central retinal artery in about 20% of eyes and in 32% of eyes on fluorescein angiography that fill with choroidal circulation.[21] CLRAO accounts for about 5% of all retinal arterial occlusions.[31] CLRAO may occur either alone or in association with CRVO or with anterior ischemic optic neuropathy.

Fundoscopically, CLRAO is seen as an area of retinal whitening along the distribution of cilioretinal artery. Visual field defect may vary from centrocecal scotoma to central, or altitudinal defect depending on isolated CLRAO or in association with other disorder. Detailed systemic evaluation and workup needs to be done as in cases of other retinal arterial occlusion

Prognosis depends on whether CLRAO occurs in isolation or in association with CRVO or anterior ischemic optic neuropathy. Prognosis is the best in isolated CLRAO and worst with associated anterior ischemic optic neuropathy, especially in cases with underlying giant cell arteritis involving posterior ciliary artery. Concomitant CRVO is seen in about 40% of CLRAO (Fig. 22.8), and concomitant CLRAO is seen in 5% of eyes with CRVO.[32,33]

Generally no treatment is required in cases with isolated CLRAO. Cases with underlying giant cell arteritis needs to treated actively for it.

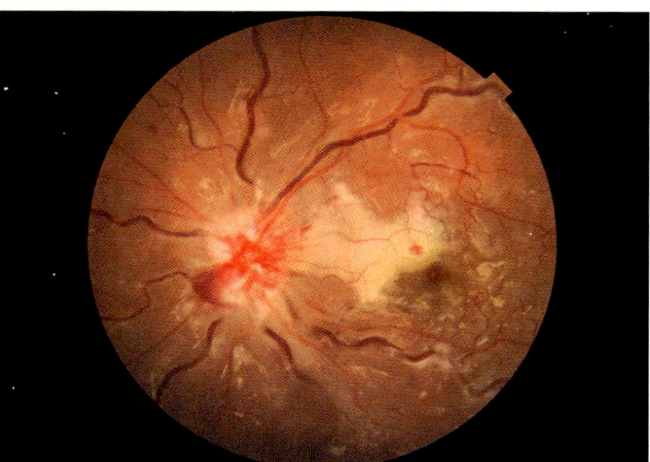

Fig. 22.8: Central retinal vein occlusion (CRVO) with cilioretinal artery occlusion.

REFERENCES

1. Brown GC, Shields JA. Cilioretinal arteries and retinal arterial occlusion. Arch Ophthalmology. 1979;97:84-92.
2. Hayreh SS. Acute retinal arterial occlusive disorders. Prog Retin Eye Res. 2011;30:359-94.
3. Ros MA, Magargal LE, Uram M. Branch retinal-artery obstruction: a review of 201 eyes. Ann Ophthalmology. 1989;21:103-7.
4. Brown GC, Magargal LE, Shields JA, et al. Retinal arterial obstruction in children and young adults. Ophthalmologyogy. 1981;88:18-25.
5. Sharma S, ten Hove MW, Pinkerton RM, et al. Interobserver agreement in the evaluation of acute retinal artery occlusion. Can J Ophthalmology. 1997;32:441-4.
6. Arruga J, Sanders MD. Ophthalmologyogic findings in 70 patients with evidence of retinal embolism. Ophthalmologyogy. 1982;89:1336-47.
7. Gold D. Retinal arterial occlusion. Trans Sect Ophthalmology Am Acad Ophthalmology Otolaryngol. 1977;83:OP392-408.
8. Ramakrishna G, Malouf JF, Younge BR, et al. Calcific retinal embolism as an indicator of severe unrecognised cardiovascular disease. Heart. 2005;91:1154-7.
9. Hayreh SS, Podhajsky PA, Zimmerman MB. Branch retinal artery occlusion: natural history of visual outcome. Ophthalmology. 2009;116:1188-94. e1-4.
10. Brown GC, Magargal LE, Shields JA, et al. Retinal arterial obstruction in children and young adults. Ophthalmology. 1981;88:18-25.
11. Rumelt S, Dorenboim Y, Rehany U. Aggressive systematic treatment for central retinal artery occlusion. Am J Ophthalmology. 1999;128:733-8.
12. Greven CM, Slusher MM, Weaver RG. Retinal arterial occlusions in young adults. Am J Ophthalmology. 1995;120:776-83.
13. Appen RE, Wray SH, Cogan DG. Central retinal artery occlusion. Am J Ophthalmology. 1975;79:374-81.
14. Breen LA. Atherosclerotic carotid disease and the eye. Neurol Clin. 1991;9:131-45.
15. Kline L. The natural history of patients with amaurosis fugax. Ophthalmology Clin North Am. 1996;9:351-7.
16. Brown GC, Magargal LE. Central retinal artery obstruction and visual acuity. Ophthalmology. 1982;89:14-9.
17. Hayreh SS, Zimmerman MB. Central retinal artery occlusion: visual outcome. Am J Ophthalmology. 2005;140:376-91.
18. Duker JS, Brown GC. Iris neovascularization associated with obstruction of the central retinal artery. Ophthalmology. 1988;95:1244-50.
19. Duker JS, Sivalingam A, Brown GC, et al. A prospective study of acute central retinal artery obstruction. The incidence of secondary ocular neovascularization. Arch Ophthalmology. 1991;109:339-42.
20. Hayreh SS, Rojas P, Podhajsky P, et al. Ocular neovascularization with retinal vascular occlusion–II. Incidence of ocular neovascularization with retinal vein occlusion. Ophthalmology. 1983;90:488-506.
21. Justice Jr J, Lehmann RP. Cilioretinal arteries. A study based on review of stereo fundus photographs and fluorescein angiographic findings. Arch Ophthalmology. 1976;94:1355-8.
22. Singh S, Dass R. The central artery of the retina. II. A study of its distribution and anastomoses. Br J Ophthalmology. 1960;44:280-99.
23. Mathew R, Papavasileiou E, Sivaprasad S. Autofluorescence and high definition optical coherence tomography of retinal artery occlusions. Clin Ophthalmology. 2010;4:1159-63.
24. Duker JS, Brown GC. Recovery following acute obstruction of the retinal and choroidal circulations. A case history. Retina. 1988;8:257-60.
25. Meyer CH, Holz FG. Images in clinical medicine. Blurred vision after cardiac catheterization. N Engl J Med. 2009;361:2366.
26. Rasmussen KE. Retinal and cerebral fat emboli following lymphography with oily contrast media. Acta Radiol Diagn (Stockh). 1970;10:199-202.
27. Biousse V, Calvetti O, Bruce BB, et al. Thrombolysis for central retinal artery occlusion. J Neuroophthalmol. 2007;27:215-30.
28. Brown GC, Magargal LE, Shields JA, et al. Retinal arterial obstruction in children and young adults. Ophthalmology. 1981;88:18-25.
29. Kim RW, Juzych MS, Eliott D. Ocular manifestations of injection drug use. Infect Dis Clin North Am. 2002;16:607-22.
30. Charawanamuttu AM, Hughes-Nurse J, Hamlett JD. Retinal embolism after hysterosalpingography. Br J Ophthalmology. 1973;57:166-9.
31. Brown GC, Magargal LE, Sergott R. Acute obstruction of the retinal and choroidal circulations. Ophthalmology. 1986;93:1373-82.
32. Brown GC, Moffat K, Cruess A, et al. Cilioretinal artery obstruction. Retina. 1983;3:182-7.
33. Fong AC, Schatz H, McDonald HR, et al. Central retinal vein occlusion in young adults (papillophlebitis). Retina. 1992;12:3-11.

Ocular Ischemic Syndrome

Chapter 23

Raghav Ravani, Suman Lata, Rohan Chawla, Atul Kumar

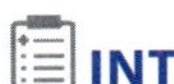 INTRODUCTION

Ocular ischemic syndrome comprises of a constellation of ocular symptoms and signs secondary to chronic, severe carotid artery obstruction. Kearns and Hollenhorst[1] reported these symptoms and signs due to carotid obstruction as "venous stasis retinopathy"

DEMOGRAPHY

Patients with ocular ischemic syndrome generally present between 5th and 8th decade of life with a mean age of about 65 years, which is same as for other systemic arterial occlusive disease. It occurs twice as common in males than in females with no racial predilection. It is usually unilateral, with bilateral involvement seen in 20% of patients.

ETIOPATHOGENESIS

High-grade carotid stenosis: This leads to chronic ophthalmic artery insufficiency thereby resulting in a decreased oxygen supply to the eye.

Most commonly, ipsilateral carotid artery occlusion is seen in patients with ocular ischemic syndrome. Occasionally, it may also be secondary to ipsilateral ophthalmic artery occlusion.[2-4] Atherosclerosis is responsible for carotid artery occlusion in most of the patients with ocular ischemic syndrome.[2] Other reported causes includes giant cell arteritis,[5] dissecting aneurysm of carotid artery[6] and Eisenmenger syndrome. Inflammatory conditions like trauma[7], Behçets disease,[8] and fibromuscular dysplasia[9] may also lead to obstruction of carotid artery that may cause ocular ischemic syndrome.

 CLINICAL PRESENTATION

Most common presentation in more than 90% of cases is visual loss. Usually, the visual loss is insidious that occurs over a period of weeks to months, however, it may be sudden in about 12% of cases. Other symptoms include prolonged recovery following light exposure,[10] localized pain over the orbital area of the affected eye[2] (also called "ocular angina") due to ischemia of the globe and/or ipsilateral dura or due to neovascular glaucoma. There could be history of amaurosis in about 10% of cases.[2]

Ocular Findings

Anterior Segment Signs

At the initial presentation itself, about two-thirds of eyes with ocular ischemic syndrome have neovascularization of the iris.[2] Despite the presence of angle closure due to fibrous membrane IOP rise is seen in not more than 50% of patients. This is due to impaired ciliary body perfusion. About 20% of these eyes have anterior chamber cellular reaction.[2] In advanced cases, cataractous lens may also be seen.

Posterior Segment Signs

Typical fundoscopic findings include attenuation of retinal arteries with dilated but nontortuous retinal veins (Figs. 23.1A to C). This helps to differentiate ocular ischemic syndrome from central retinal vein occlusion. Mid peripheral, nonconfluent retinal hemorrhages are seen in about 80% of eyes. Neovascularization of disc (35%) and retina (8%) can be found in patients with ocular ischemic syndrome with incidence of vitreous hemorrhage reported as much as 4%.[2] About 12% of these eyes have a cherry-red spot. Other posterior segment signs include cotton-wool spots, spontaneous retinal arterial occlusion extending one or more disc diameter away from the disc and anterior ischemic optic neuropathy.[2,11,12]

ANCILLARY TESTS

Fluorescein Angiography

Fluorescein angiography typically shows delayed arm-to-choroid and arm-to-retina circulation times, delayed and/or patchy choroidal filling, prolonged retinal arteriovenous transit time, retinal vascular staining, macular edema,[13]

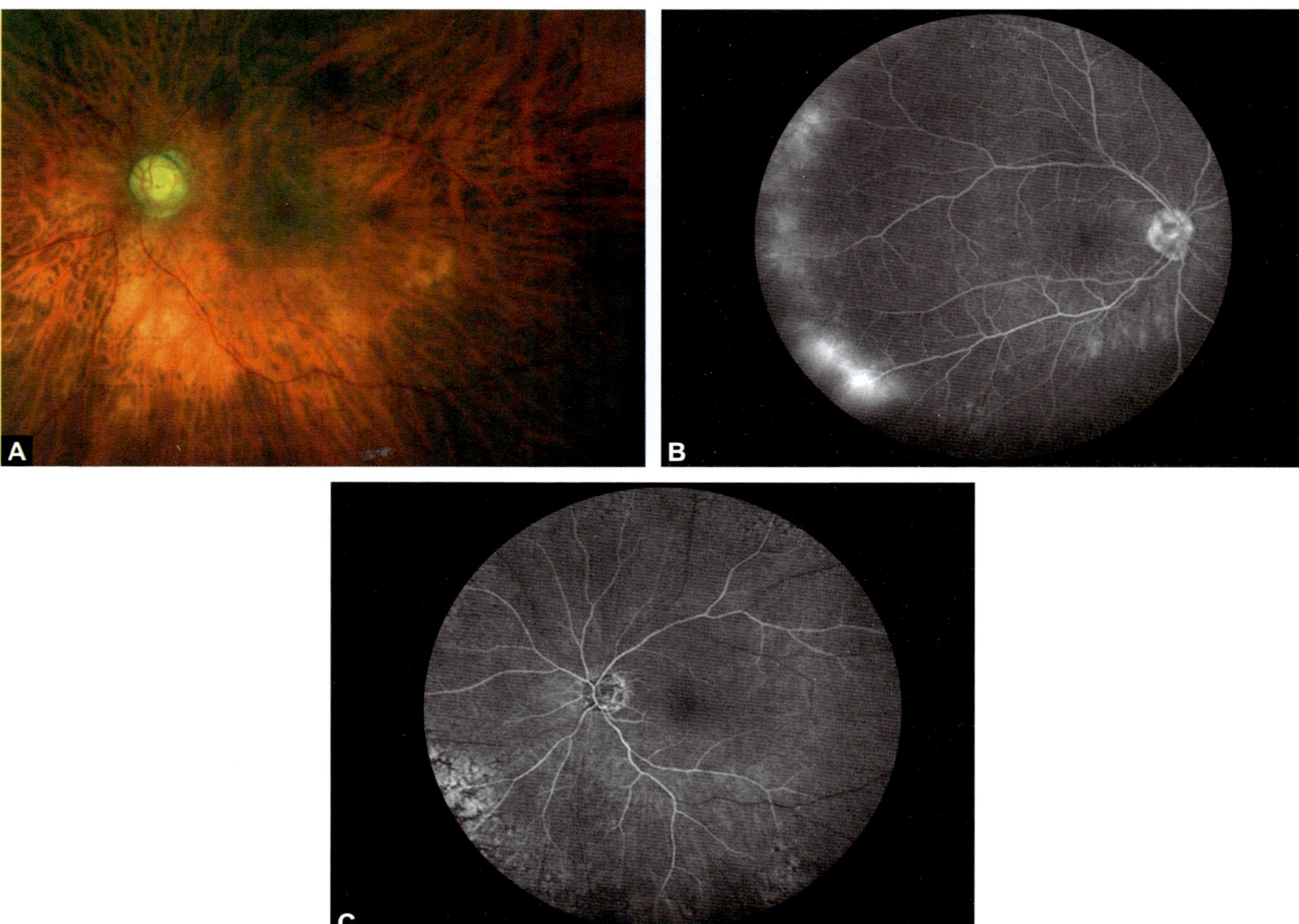

Figs. 23.1A to C: Threadlike arterioles with pale disc in an eye with ocular ischemic syndrome. Fluorescein angiography (FA) shows NVE in the right eye with optic nerve head hyperfluorescence and left eye on FA reveals delayed filling of dye in the veins. (NVE: Neovascularisation elsewhere).

retinal capillary nonperfusion,[14-16] optic nerve head hyperfluorescence and microaneurysmal leak.

Electroretinography

Since ocular ischemic syndrome leads to ischemia of both inner as well as outer retina, electroretinography (ERG) shows decreased amplitude or even a total loss of both a- and b- waves. Patients with retinal ischemia secondary to carotid artery stenosis show decreased amplitude of the oscillatory potential on ERG.[17]

Other tests like visual evoked potential (VEP) may be useful in follow-up of cases undergoing endarterectomy.[18] It may show improvement of recovery time of the amplitude of major positive peak after photostress. Ophthalmodynamometry can also be of some benefit.[19,20]

Systemic tests should include color Doppler imaging, MRA imaging and carotid angiography.

SYSTEMIC ASSOCIATIONS

Systemic arterial hypertension (73%) and diabetes mellitus (56%) are commonly associated with ocular ischemic syndrome.[21] Other associated conditions may include peripheral vascular disease,[21] stroke,[22] and giant cell arteritis.[23]

Differential Diagnoses

- Central retinal vein occlusion
- Giant cell arteritis.

TREATMENT

Ocular ischemic syndrome has an uncertain natural course, with poor long-term visual outcome in most of the patients in advanced disease and more than 90% of patients with rubeosis iridis develop legal blindness.

Various treatment options include extracranial to intracranial bypass surgery in cases with total carotid artery obstruction[24-29] with poor visual outcomes at one year after surgery. Endarterectomy may be done in patients with partial carotid artery obstruction with fair results especially in patients without rubeosis iridis.[30,31] Endarterectomy may lead to increased aqueous formation and severe rise in intraocular pressure (IOP) in eyes with rubeosis iridis and fibrovascular angle closure with low or normal IOP.[32,33] The North American Symptomatic Carotid Endarterectomy trial[34] noted decreased risk of ipsilateral stroke with endarterectomies as compared to medical treatment.

In patients with neovascularization of iris or neovascularization at disc or elsewhere, full scatter panretinal laser photocoagulation has been advocated.[35] Glaucoma filtering surgeries along with panretinal photocoagulation have also been performed. Macular edema may respond to intravitreal triamcinolone acetonide or anti-VEGF agents.[36,37] Medical therapy should be targeted toward risk factors like atherosclerosis, systemic arterial hypertension, diabetes mellitus, etc.

Besides the ocular treatment, therapy, systemic therapy should include antiplatelet and anticoagulant therapy.

REFERENCES

1. Kearns TP, Hollenhorst RW. Venous stasis retinopathy of occlusive disease of the carotid artery. Proc Mayo Clin. 1963;38:304-12.
2. Brown GC, Magargal LE. The ocular ischemic syndrome. Clinical, fluorescein angiographic and carotid angiographic features. Int Ophthalmology. 1988;11:239-51.
3. Bullock J, Falter RT, Downing JE, et al. Ischemic ophthalmia secondary to an ophthalmic artery occlusion. Am J Ophthalmology. 1972;74:486-93.
4. Madsen PH. Venous-stasis insufficiency of the ophthalmic artery. Acta Ophthalmology. 1965;40:940-7.
5. Hamed LM, Guy JR, Moster ML, et al. Giant cell arteritis in the ocular ischemic syndrome. Am J Ophthalmology. 1992;113:702-5.
6. Duker JS, Belmont JB. Ocular ischemic syndrome secondary to carotid artery dissection. Am J Ophthalmology. 1988;106:750-2.
7. Sadun AA, Sebag J, Bienfang DC. Complete bilateral internal carotid artery occlusion in a young man. J Clin Neuroophthalmol. 1983;3:63-6.
8. Dhobb M, Ammar F, Bensaid Y, et al. Arterial manifestations in Behçet's disease: four new cases. Ann Vasc Surg. 1986;1:249-52.
9. Effeney DJ, Krupski WC, Stoney RJ, et al. Fibromuscular dysplasia of the carotid artery. Austral NZ J Surg. 1983;53:527-31.
10. Donnan GA, Sharbrough FW. Carotid occlusive disease. Effect of bright light on visual evoked response. Arch Neurol. 1982;39:687-9.
11. Brown GC. Anterior ischemic optic neuropathy occurring in association with carotid artery obstruction. J Clin Neuroophthalmol. 1986;6:39-42.
12. Waybright EA, Selhorst JB, Combs J. Anterior ischemic optic neuropathy with internal carotid artery occlusion. Am J Ophthalmology. 1982;93:42-7.
13. Brown GC. Macular edema in association with severe carotid artery obstruction. Am J Ophthalmology. 1986;102:442-8.
14. Kahn M, Green WR, Knox DL, et al. Ocular features of carotid occlusive disease. Retina. 1986;6:239-52.
15. Michelson PE, Knox DL, Green WR. Ischemic ocular inflammation. A clinicopathologic case report. Arch Ophthalmology. 1971;86:274-80.
16. Dugan JD, Green WR. Ophthalmic manifestations of carotid occlusive disease. Eye. 1991;5:226-38.
17. Coleman K, Fitzgerald D, Eustace P, et al. Electroretinography, retinal ischaemia and carotid artery disease. Eur J Vasc Surg. 1990;4:569-73.
18. Banchini E, Franchi A, Magni R, et al. Carotid occlusive disease. An electrophysiological investigation. J Cardiovasc Surg. 1987;28:524-7.
19. Kearns TP. Ophthalmology and the carotid artery. Am J Ophthalmology 1979;88:714-22.
20. Kearns TP. Differential diagnosis of central retinal vein obstruction. Ophthalmology. 1983;90:475-80.
21. Sivalingam A, Brown GC, Magargal LE, et al. The ocular ischemic syndrome II. Mortality and systemic morbidity. Int Ophthalmology. 1989;13:137-91.
22. Duker JS, Brown GC, Bosley TM, et al. Asymmetric proliferative diabetic retinopathy and carotid artery disease. Ophthalmology. 1990;97:859-74.
23. Casson RJ, Fleming FK, Shaikh A, et al. Bilateral ocular ischemic syndrome secondary to giant cell arteritis. Arch Ophthalmology. 2001;119:306-7.
24. Edwards MS, Chater NL, Stanley JA. Reversal of chronic ischaemia by extracranial-intracranial arterial by-pass. Neurosurgery. 1980;7:480-3.
25. Higgins RA. Neovascular glaucoma associated with ocular hypoperfusion secondary to carotid artery disease. Austral J Ophthalmology. 1984;12:155-62.
26. Katz B, Weinstein FR. Improvement of photostress recovery testing after extracranial–intracranial bypass surgery. Br J Ophthalmology. 1986;70:277-80.
27. Kearns TP, Younge BR, Peipgras PG. Resolution of venous stasis retinopathy after carotid artery bypass surgery. Proc Mayo Clin. 1980;55:342-6.
28. Kiser WD, Gonder J, Magargal LE, et al. Recovery of vision following treatment of the ocular ischemic syndrome. Ann Ophthalmology. 1983;15:305-10.
29. Shibuya M, Suzuki Y, Takayasu M, et al. Effects of STA-MCA anastomosis for ischaemic oculopathy due to occlusion of the internal carotid artery. Acta Neurochir. 1990;103:71-5.
30. Sivalingam A, Brown GC, Magargal LE. The ocular ischemic syndrome. III. Visual prognosis and the effect of treatment. Int Ophthalmology. 1991;15:15-20.
31. Johnston ME, Gonder JR, Canny CL. Successful treatment of the ocular ischemic syndrome with panretinal photocoagulation and cerebrovascular surgery. Can J Ophthalmology. 1988;23:114-9.
32. Coppeto JR, Wand M, Bear L, et al. Neovascular glaucoma and carotid artery obstructive disease. Am J Ophthalmology. 1985;99:567-70.
33. Melamed S, Irvine J, Lee DA. Increased intraocular pressure following endarterectomy. Ann Ophthalmology. 1987;19:304-6.
34. North American Symptomatic Carotid Endarterectomy Trial Collaborators, Barnett HJM, Taylor DW, et al. Beneficial effect of carotid endarterectomy in symptomatic patients with high-grade carotid stenosis. N Engl J Med. 1991;325:445-53.
35. Allen RC, Bellows AR, Hutchinson BT, et al. Filtration surgery in the treatment of neovascular glaucoma. Ophthalmology. 1982;89:1181-7.
36. Klais CM, Spaide RF. Intravitreal triamcinolone acetonide injection in ocular ischemic syndrome. Retina. 2004;24:459-61.
37. Amselem L, Montero J, Diaz-Llopis M, et al. Intravitreal bevacizumab (Avastin) injection in ocular ischemic syndrome. Am J Ophthalmology. 2007;144:122-4.

Chapter 24

Retinal Vein Occlusion

Prateek Kakkar, Siddhi Goel, Atul Kumar, Alisha Kishore

BRANCH RETINAL VEIN OCCLUSION

 ### Introduction

Retinal vein occlusion (RVO) comprises of conditions caused due to blockade of small or large caliber vessels carrying blood away from the retina. These may present clinically as an asymptomatic condition to as severe as complete visual loss. It is one of the most common retinal pathology worldwide causing visual loss.

Pathogenesis

One of the most important risk factor for branch retinal vein occlusion (BRVO) is arteriolosclerosis.[1,2] The vein and the retinal arteriole have a common adventitial sheath[3] so thickening of the retinal arteriole leads to compression of the underlying vein.[4] Due to this, various secondary changes including venous endothelial cell loss, thrombus formation and potential occlusion may occur.[4-6] Figure 24.1 demonstrates the typical appearance of BRVO involving the inferotemporal quadrant of the left eye. Similarly, central retinal vein occlusion (CRVO) may occur when atherosclerotic changes of the artery lead to compression of the vein as the central retinal vein and artery have a common adventitial sheath at arteriovenous crossings posterior to the lamina cribrosa.[7] Due to the impeded drainage of blood, there is a stagnation of vascular contents that leads to hypoxia in the surrounding retina. This leads to capillary endothelial damage, further obstruction and hypoxia. Hence, a vicious cycle results causing increased tissue perfusion pressure and further obstruction.[8,9]

Predisposing Factors[10-18]

Common

1. The most important factor being age; more than 50% of cases occur in patients older than 65 years.
2. *Hypertension* is present in up to 73% of RVO patients older than age of 50 years and in 25% of younger patients. It is most prevalent in patients with BRVO, especially when

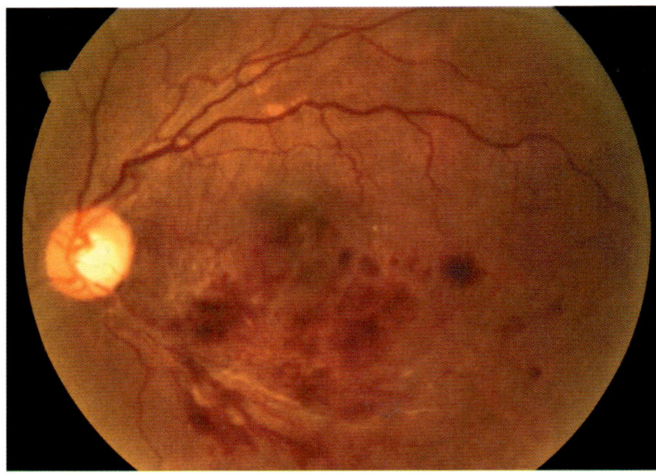

Fig. 24.1: Fundus photograph of left eye with inferotemporal branch retinal vein occlusion (BRVO) with extensive hemorrhages.

the site of obstruction is at an arteriovenous crossing. Predisposition to recurrence of RVO in the same or fellow eye occurs, if the blood pressure is uncontrolled.[12-16]

3. *Hyperlipidemia* (total cholesterol >6.5 mmol/L) is present in 35% of patients.[17,18]
4. *Diabetes mellitus* is seen in 10% of patients older than 50 years but is uncommon in younger patients. About 70% of type 2 diabetics have other cardiovascular risk factors like hypertension.[12,14-17]
5. *Oral contraceptive pills*: In young female patients, oral contraceptive pills are the most common underlying association with an increased risk, if the patient has underlying thrombophilia.[11]
6. *Raised intraocular pressure* (IOP) can increase the risk of CRVO especially in cases with obstruction at the edge of optic disc.[11]
7. *Smoking* may increase the risk of RVO, although inconsistent results have been reported.[11-13]

Uncommon

Uncommon predispositions may assume more importance in patients under the age of 50 years.[11]

1. Myeloproliferative disorders:
- Polycythemia
- Abnormal plasma proteins (e.g. myeloma, macroglobulinemia).

2. Acquired hypercoagulable states:
- Hyperhomocysteinemia
- Lupus anticoagulant and antiphospholipid antibodies
- Dysfibrinogenemia

3. Inherited hypercoagulable states:
- Activated protein C resistance (factor V Leiden mutation)
- Protein C deficiency
- Protein S deficiency
- Antithrombin deficiency
- Prothrombin gene mutation
- Factor XII deficiency.

4. Inflammatory disease associated with occlusive periphlebitis:
- Behçet syndrome
- Sarcoidosis
- Wegener granulomatosis
- Goodpasture syndrome.

5. Miscellaneous:
- Chronic renal failure
- Causes of secondary hypertension (e.g. Cushing syndrome) or hyperlipidemia (e.g. hypothyroidism)
- Orbital disease
- Dehydration.

Systemic Assessment

All patients must undergo following systemic assessment to reveal the underlying systemic associations:
1. Blood pressure.
2. Erythrocyte sedimentation rate (ESR) or plasma viscosity (PV).
3. Complete blood count (CBC).
4. Random blood glucose. Further assessment for diabetes if indicated.
5. Random total and high-density lipoprotein (HDL) cholesterol. Additional lipid testing may be considered.
6. Plasma protein electrophoresis—to detect dysproteinemias such as multiple myeloma.
7. Urea, electrolytes and creatinine. Chronic renal failure is a rare cause of RVO, but renal disease may occur in association with hypertension.
8. Thyroid function tests. Patients with RVO have a higher prevalence of thyroid disease than the general population. Thyroid dysfunction is also associated with dyslipidemia.
9. Electrocardiography (ECG)—to detect left ventricular hypertrophy secondary to hypertension. Also, required for the Framingham equation for calculation of cardiovascular risk.

Following selected investigations are to be ordered in patients according to their clinical indication,[19-23] especially in patients younger than 50 years, past history or family history of thrombosis, those with bilateral RVO, and in patients when an etiological factor cannot be found.
1. Chest X-ray—sarcoidosis, tuberculosis, left ventricular hypertrophy in hypertension.
2. C-reactive protein (CRP)—sensitive indicator of inflammation.
3. Thrombophilia screen—particularly indicated in cases of heritable thrombophilias; typically includes thrombin time, prothrombin time and activated partial thromboplastin time, antithrombin functional assay, protein C, protein S, activated protein C resistance, factor V Leiden mutation, prothrombin G20210A mutation; anticardiolipin antibody [immunoglobulin G (IgG) and immunoglobulin M (IgM)], lupus anticoagulant.
4. Autoantibodies—rheumatoid factor, antinuclear antibody, anti-DNA antibody.
5. Serum angiotensin-converting enzyme (ACE)—sarcoidosis.
6. Fasting plasma homocysteine level. To exclude hyperhomocysteinemia.
7. Treponemal serology. Local testing preference should be discussed with the microbiology team.
8. Carotid Doppler imaging. To exclude ocular ischemic syndrome.

Classification of Branch Retinal Vein Occlusion

Branch retinal vein occlusion is a focal occlusion of a retinal vein other than the central retinal vein. It may be classified as:
1. *Major BRVO*—involving first order temporal vessel at the disc or away from the disc.
2. *Macular BRVO*—involving only a macular branch.
3. *Peripheral BRVO*—not involving the macular circulation.

Ophthalmoscopic findings show characteristic segmental distribution of intraretinal hemorrhages (Fig. 24.2A). With time, the hemorrhages resolve and the retinal vascular abnormalities can be appreciated on fluorescein angiography (FA). FA demonstrates delayed filling of the occluded vein, varying areas of capillary nonperfusion (CNP), microaneurysms, macular leakage and ischemia (Fig. 24.2B). The presence of intraretinal fluid, subretinal fluid and cystoid macular edema (CME) is visible on optical coherence tomography (OCT) B-scans and retinal thickness maps can reveal areas of localized retinal thickening (Fig. 24.2C).

Diagnosis

Presentation: Patients present with sudden onset of blurred vision and metamorphopsia, or a relative visual field defect. Patients with peripheral occlusions may be asymptomatic.

Visual acuity is variable and is principally dependent on the extent of macular involvement.

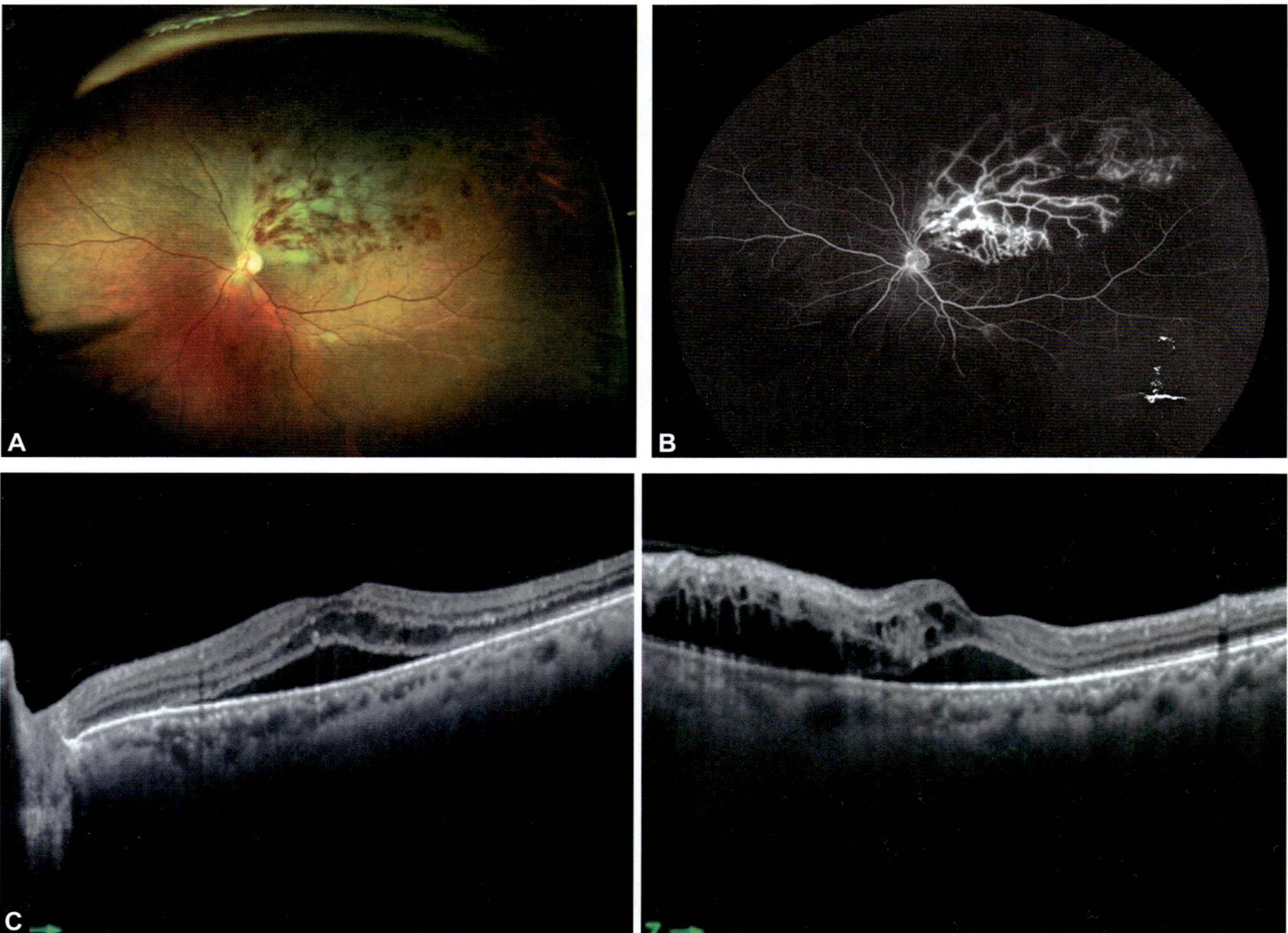

Figs. 24.2A to C: Presentation of a case of superotemporal branch retinal vein occlusion (BRVO). (A) Ultrawide field pseudocolor photograph showing multiple characteristic flame-shaped hemorrhages and soft exudates along with macular edema; (B) Fluorescein angiographic image of the same patient suggestive of dilated, tortuous superotemporal retinal vessels with adjoining capillary nonperfusion areas; (C) Swept-source optical coherence tomography (SS-OCT) reveals severe macular edema.

Fundus:
- Dilatation and tortuosity of the affected venous segment.
- The site of occlusion is often identifiable as an arterio-venous crossing point.
- Flame-shaped and dot/blot hemorrhages, retinal edema, sometimes cotton wool spots affecting the sector of the retina drained by the obstructed vein.

Fluorescein angiography shows variable delayed venous filling, blocked fluorescence due to retinal hemorrhages, staining of the vessel wall, hypofluorescence due to CNP and 'pruning' of the vessels in the ischemic areas (Figs. 24.3A and B). Ultra-widefield fluorescein angiography (UWFA) has been proven to be of benefit in BRVO patients and provides evidence of retinal vascular pathology in a majority of fellow eyes of patients with BRVO[24] (Figs. 24.4A and B).

OCT demonstrates and aids in quantification of the severity of macular edema and is a useful modality for monitoring the response to treatment (Figs. 24.5A and B).

OCT angiography is a new, noninvasive technology which can be a potential clinical tool for diagnosis and follow-up of retinal vascular occlusions. It can detect foveal avascular zone enlargement, retinal ischemia, microvascular abnormalities and signs of vascular congestion in both the superficial and deep capillary networks (Figs. 24.6 and 24.7).

Course: The acute features usually resolve within 6–12 months and may be replaced by the following:
- Exudates, venous sheathing and sclerosis peripheral to the site of obstruction, collaterals and variable residual hemorrhages.

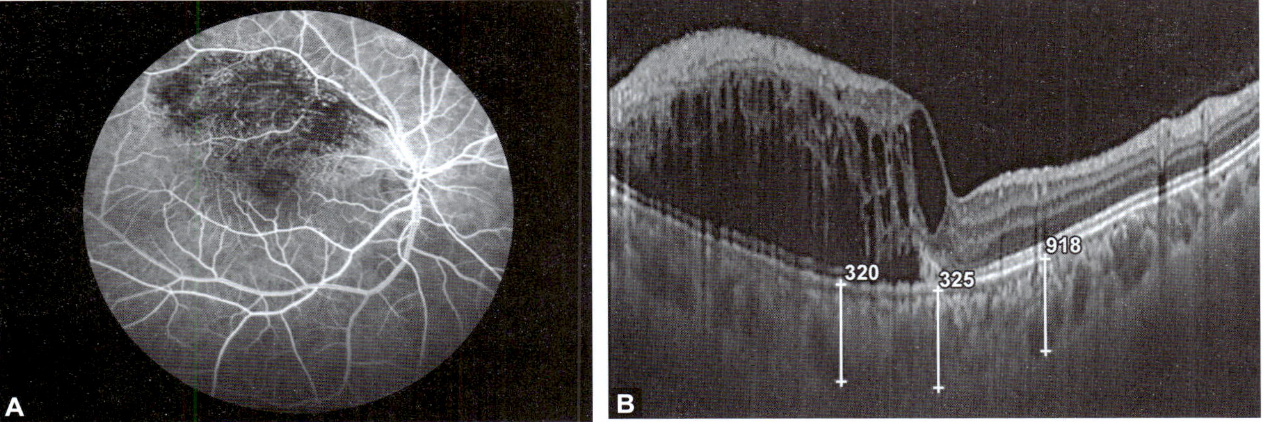

Figs. 24.3A and B: A hypertensive patient with vision 6/60 showing superotemporal branch retinal vein occlusion on fundus fluorescein angiography (A) with extensive macular edema on optical coherence tomography (B).

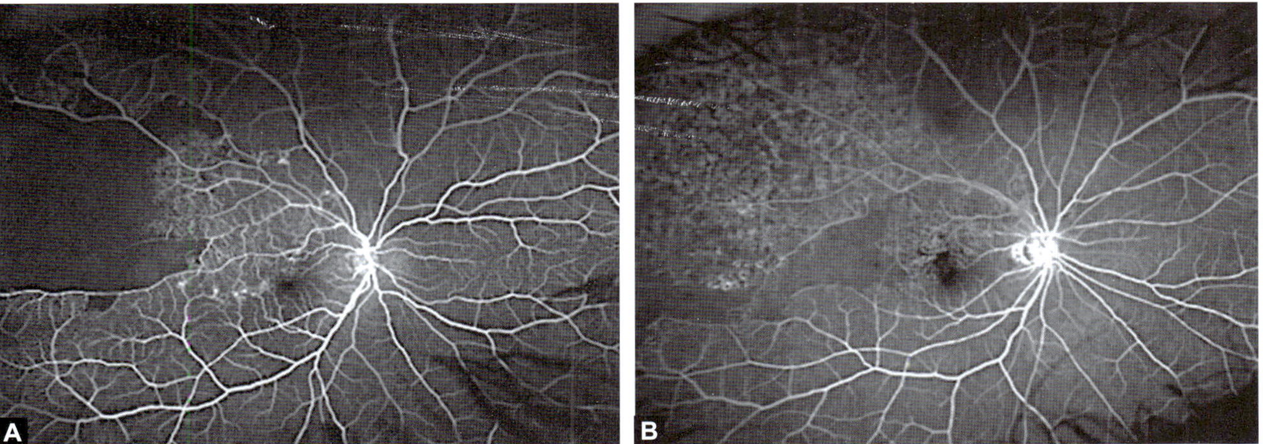

Figs. 24.4A and B: Ultra-widefield fluorescein angiography of a patient with superotemporal BRVO with areas of capillary nonperfusion (CNP) (A) which was subsequently lasered (B).

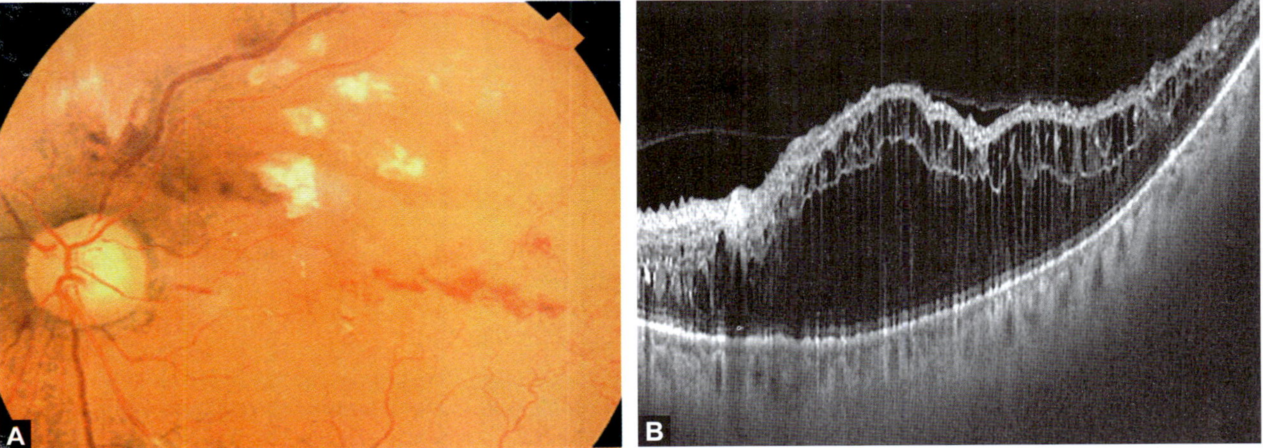

Figs. 24.5A and B: A case of ischemic superotemporal BRVO with retinoschisis on fundus photograph (A) and optical coherence tomography (B).

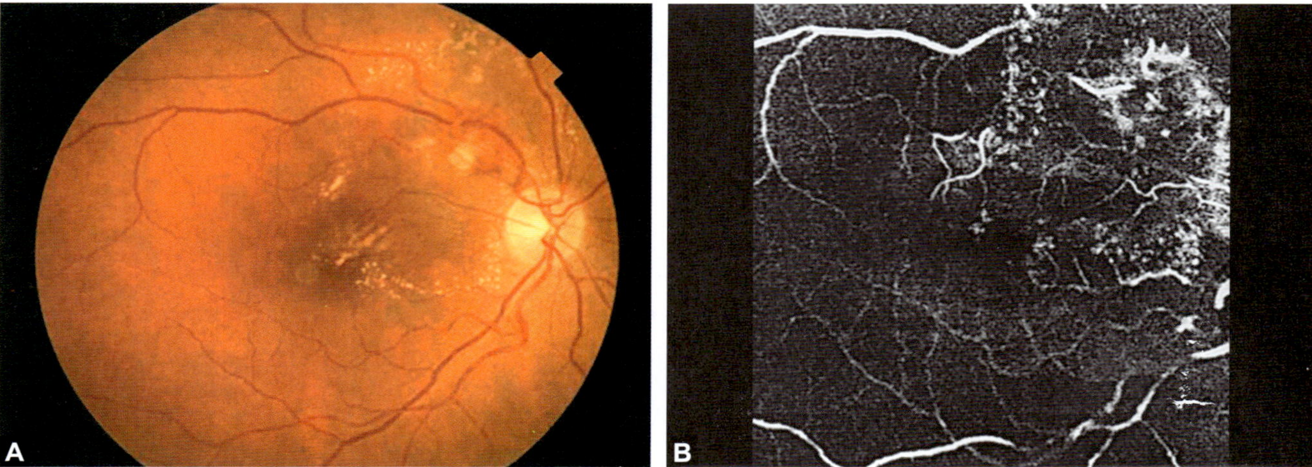

Figs. 24.6A and B: Superotemporal tributary branch retinal vein occlusion (BRVO) on color picture and optical coherence tomography angiography showing ischemic areas and numerous microaneurysms.

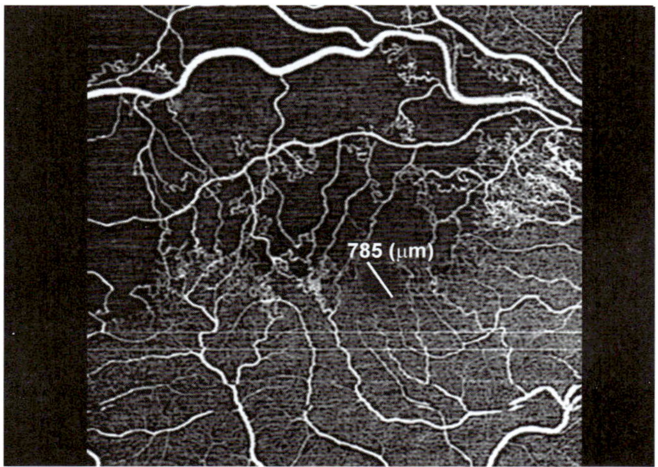

Fig. 24.7: Optical coherence tomography angiography reveals capillary dropout areas in an eye with superotemporal branch retinal vein occlusion.

- Collateral vessels are characterized by slightly tortuous veins that develop locally or across the horizontal raphe between the inferior and superior vascular arcades and are best detected on FA.
- The severity of residual signs is highly variable and may be subtle.

Prognosis

At 6 months, about 50% of eyes achieve visual acuity of 6/12 or better. Approximately 50% of untreated eyes with BRVO retain 6/12 or better while 25% will have visual acuity less than 6/60.[25,26] The three main vision-threatening complications are:

1. Chronic macular edema: It is the most common cause of persistent poor visual acuity after BRVO.[25,27] Patients with visual acuity of 6/12 or worse may benefit from laser photocoagulation provided the macula is not significantly ischemic.[25]
2. Macular ischemia
3. Neovascularization: Retinal neovascularization occurs in about 60% of eyes with more than 5 disc areas of nonperfusion and a third with less than 4 disc areas—about 40% overall.[25] Neovascularization elsewhere (NVE) is considerably more common than neovascularization of the disc (NVD). NVE usually develops at the border of the triangular sector of ischemic retina drained by the occluded vein. New vessels usually appear within 6–12 months but may develop at any time; they can lead to recurrent vitreous and preretinal hemorrhage, and occasionally tractional retinal detachment.

Treatment

Medical Treatment

Treatment of BRVO is centered on control of systemic risk factors and the management of vision-threatening complications. If a hypercoagulable state is present, anticoagulant therapy may be started in consultation with a hematologist. Although anticoagulant therapy may not be of any benefit in most cases for the prevention or management of BRVO. Such therapy may be associated with systemic complications and could also increase the risk of intraretinal hemorrhage, hence not recommended.

Laser Treatment

Branch retinal vein occlusion study for macular edema: The Branch Vein Occlusion Study (BVOS) was a multicenter randomized clinical trial, funded by the National Eye Institute, which reported that argon grid laser photocoagulation may reduce visual loss from macular edema.[25]

Important eligibility criteria for BVOS were:

- Fluorescein-proven perfused macular edema involving the foveal center
- Absorption of intraretinal hemorrhage from the foveal center
- Recent BRVO (usually 3–18 months' duration)
- No diabetic retinopathy
- Best-corrected visual acuity (BCVA) equal to 20/40 or worse.

In the BVOS, grid laser photocoagulation of leaking areas was done covering the whole of capillary-free zone and extending in the periphery up to the major vascular arcade. Recommended treatment parameters include:

- Duration of 100 ms
- Spot size of 100 μm diameter
- Power setting sufficient to produce a 'medium' white burn.

On 2–4 months follow-up FA was repeated, if any residual leakage was seen with persistence of reduced visual acuity, additional photocoagulation was applied. Gain in visual acuity was defined as improvement of two or more Snellen lines (beyond baseline) at two consecutive visits 4 weeks apart. After 3 years of follow-up, 63% of treated eyes gained two or more lines of vision compared to 36% of untreated eyes. The average gain in visual acuity for treated eyes was one Snellen line more compared to the untreated eyes.[25]

Grid pattern photocoagulation results in thinning of outer retina which leads to more oxygen delivery to inner layers and an overall decreased oxygen consumption. It has been hypothesized that this leads to reduction in macular edema by causing autoregulatory retinal vascular constriction in the areas of leakage. According to BVOS, it is advisable to defer laser therapy for initial 3–6 months and only observe. This also allows clearing of retinal hemorrhages to allow for good quality FA. Only if the macular perfusion is normal and vision is worsening or is worse than 20/40, grid laser therapy must be considered. It is not recommended in cases with macular ischemia.[25]

Branch Retinal Vein Occlusion study for neovascularization:[28] The BVOS suggested that the cases having CNP areas greater than 5 disc diameter are at risk of developing subsequent neovascularization (40%). Of these 40% eyes, about 60% eyes are prone to develop vitreous hemorrhage subsequently usually within first 6–12 months but may be seen up to 3 years.

It was seen that during the BVOS study, for neovascularization—photocoagulation is equally effective in preventing vitreous hemorrhage whether done before or after the development of neovascularization.[28] Peripheral scatter laser, therefore, is recommended in patients only after confirming neovascularization on FA. This has been seen to reduce the chances of vitreous hemorrhage by half in such patients.[28] The scatter laser photocoagulation can be applied with argon blue-green laser with a burn width of 200–500 μm spaced one burn width apart to achieve 'medium' white burns. The entire area of CNP, as defined by FA is covered but extending no closer than 2 disc diameters from the center of the fovea and extending at least to the equator in the periphery[28] (*see* Figs. 24.4A and B).

Steroid Treatment

Macular edema results from the breakdown in blood retinal barrier. This is mediated partly by an increase in vascular endothelial growth factor (VEGF) and partly by increased inflammatory cytokines.[29,30] Corticosteroids have anti-inflammatory effects and have also shown efficacy against VEGF.[31,32] Corticosteroids are, therefore, considered as a good option for the treatment of macular edema in BRVO.

SCORE (triamcinolone) study: The *Standard Care versus Corticosteroid for Retinal Vein Occlusion (SCORE) study* was a multicenter, randomized controlled study of 411 patients divided into three treatment arms. The three groups were treated by macular grid laser, 1 mg intravitreal triamcinolone acetonide (IVTA) and 4 mg IVTA, respectively. The trial allowed retreatment after every 4 months for each group wherever needed. It also evaluated the safety and efficacy of IVTA for the treatment of BRVO-associated macular edema.[33]

It concluded that at 12 months follow-up, no significant difference in vision or the reduction of macular edema measured by CCT between each group, being similar for pseudophakics or others. Only difference was in long-term maintenance of vision which was greater in lasered group at the end of 3 years. Significant dose-dependent ocular side effects of IVTA were noted like cataract and glaucoma.

Therefore, the use of IVTA is advised in only those cases where the treatment is refractory to other modalities, and especially preferred in pseudophakic patients.

GENEVA (dexamethasone implant) study: The *Global Evaluation of Implantable Dexamethasone in Retinal Vein Occlusion with Macular Edema (GENEVA) study* was a multicenter, randomized controlled study which evaluated sustained-release, biodegradable, dexamethasone intravitreal implant (Ozurdex, Allergan, Irvine, CA) for the treatment of macular edema in CRVO and BRVO patients[34] (Fig. 24.8). Ozurdex is a biode-

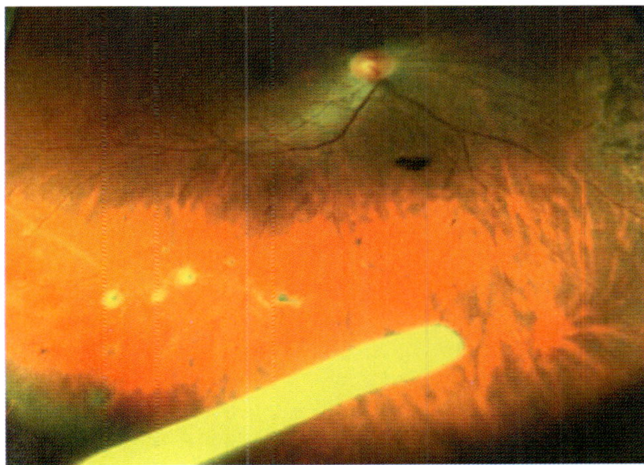

Fig. 24.8: Optos fundus photograph showing Ozurdex implant in vitreous cavity of a patient with branch retinal vein occlusion with macular edema.

gradable copolymer of poly (D,L-lactide-co-glycolide) acid (PLGA) containing micronized dexamethasone. Dexamethasone is gradually released over several months after breakdown of the PLGA into lactic and glycolic acid via Krebs cycle and finally into water and carbon dioxide. A 23-gauge custom injector is used to inject the drug intravireally through the pars plana route. Two doses of 0.7 mg and 0.35 mg were used in the study. An increase in BCVA of greater than or equal to 15 ETDRS letters was achieved in 30% of the Ozurdex 0.7 mg group, 26% of the 0.35 mg group, and 13% of the sham group 60 days after injection (peak response) in patients with BRVO (p <0.001 for each group versus sham).[34] A statistically significant difference in BCVA and central retinal thickness on OCT between both Ozurdex groups and sham was seen up to 90 days after injection.[34]

However, significantly greater complications were seen in the Ozurdex groups as compared with sham group. These included secondary rise in IOP and anterior chamber reaction which were mostly managed medically. Following this study, Ozurdex implants have been approved by The US Food and Drug Administration (USFDA) for the treatment of vein occlusions.

Anti-VEGF Treatment

Macular edema results due to increased levels of VEGF occurring because of ischemia in retinal layers. This leads to increased vascular permeability, vasodilation, migration of endothelial cells, and neovascularization.[29,30,35] There are several anti-VEGF agents in use currently for the treatment of RVOs—ranibizumab (Lucentis), bevacizumab (Avastin), pegaptanib (Macugen), and aflibercept (Eylea).

Branch retinal vein occlusion (ranibizumab) study: The Branch Retinal Vein Occlusion study was a prospective, multicenter, randomized controlled study to evaluate the efficacy and safety of ranibizumab for the treatment of macular edema in BRVO.[36] A total of 397 patients were randomized into three groups: (1) sham injection; (2) 0.3 mg ranibizumab; and (3) 0.5 mg ranibizumab. It concluded that ranibizumab is superior to traditional laser treatment for BRVO-associated macular edema with little risk of adverse events.

The BRIGHTER study is a recently published 24-month trial with patients randomized 2:2:1 to receive 0.5 mg ranibizumab (group 1), 0.5 mg ranibizumab plus laser (group 2), or laser alone (group 3) for the treatment of BRVO. The study confirmed that the efficacy of ranibizumab for BRVO with no additional benefit of laser. There was a mean gain of BCVA from the baseline of 14.4 letters in group 1; 14.8 letters in group 2; and 6.0 letters in group 3 (p <0.0001). Patients received an average of 4.8 injections in group 1 and 4.5 in group 2. There was no difference in visual acuity outcomes among patients who had ischemic versus nonischemic BRVO.[37]

Therefore, the current recommendation for patients diagnosed with macular edema from BRVO is to give monthly 0.5 mg ranibizumab injection for 3 months. If treatment fails after 3 months (<5 ETDRS letter gain, or improvement of <50 μm in central subfield thickness), then traditional grid macular laser should be performed.

Other anti-VEGF agents have also been tried for therapy of BRVO. These include bevacizumab (Avastin®) and aflibercept (Eylea®).

BERVOLT study: Bevacizumab treatment of macular edema in CRVO and BRVO study was a retrospective study to assess the efficacy and safety of intraocular injections of bevacizumab in patients with macular edema following RVOs. There was a significant change in BCVA in BRVO group and there were no adverse outcomes.[38] Therefore, bevacizumab may be used in that treatment of BRVO as a cheaper alternative to ranibizumab.

VIBRANT study: The double-masked trial randomly assigned 183 patients, in the ratio of 1:1 to monthly injections of aflibercept 2 mg or laser.[39] Eligible patients had center-involving macular edema diagnosed within 12 months of screening, BCVA between 20/40 and 20/320, sufficient clearing of intraretinal hemorrhages to allow for baseline laser treatment, and were treatment-naïve. The primary efficacy endpoint of greater than or equal to 15 letters improvement from baseline BCVA was met by 53% of aflibercept eyes and 27% of laser-treated eyes. Secondary efficacy data analyzing mean change from baseline visual acuity and mean decrease in central retinal thickness also showed superior results for aflibercept versus laser.[39]

To summarize the therapy for BRVO, the primary treatment includes observation especially for first 2–3 months followed by detailed evaluation of retinal perfusion and neovascularization. UWFA is advised whenever possible to look for capillary dropout regions and peripheral nonperfusion areas alongside macular edema. In cases wherever there is macular edema and no contraindication, an anti-VEGF injection is recommended. At least three injections are recommended at 4 weeks' interval, or until the central macular thickness (CMT) is less than or equal to 250 μm on OCT. The injections are repeated in patients with higher CMT until the same is achieved. Patients not responding to anti-VEGF therapy are given IVTA or steroid implant therapy. If there is still no response, then grid laser photocoagulation is the therapy of choice. For patients with focal leaks on FA, focal laser photocoagulation is done.

The CNP areas are lasered using the green laser therapy as described before. If the patient has macular edema along with CNP areas, then combined therapy of anti-VEGF followed by laser photocoagulation of the CNP regions usually delayed by 2 weeks is preferred. Patients are usually followed up 3–6 monthly once declared cured, along with UWFA and OCT evaluations done on follow-up visits.

A study done in Dr Rajendra Prasad Centre for Ophthalmic Sciences, compared the role of UWFA-guided peripheral laser along with intravitreal ranibizumab vs. ranibizumab only in BRVO with macular edema. The study demonstrated that UWFA-guided targeted retinal photocoagulation reduced

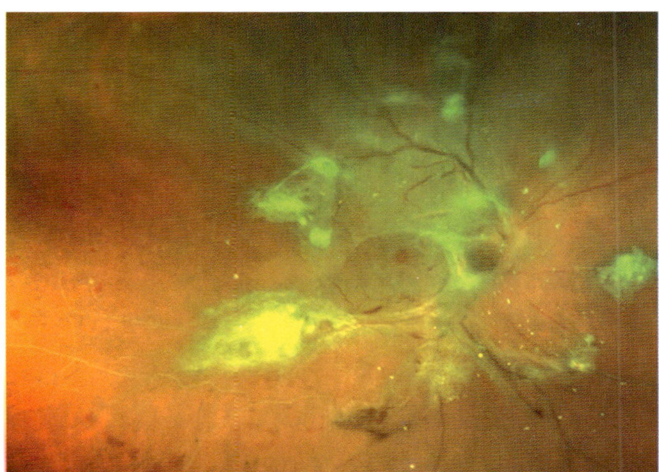

Fig. 24.9: Ultra-widefield image showing inferotemporal BRVO with tractional retinal detachment (TRD) involving macula.

the number of injections of anti-VEGF required in the treatment of BRVO with macular edema, while maintaining similar benefits in visual acuity, CMT and contrast sensitivity with ranibizumab alone. Targeted retinal photocoagulation is thus an effective adjuvant for the treatment of ischemic BRVO with macular edema (unpublished data).

Surgical Treatment

Eyes with BRVO are prone for vitreous hemorrhage and even tractional retinal detachment (Fig. 24.9) which may lead to secondary retinal break formation and eventual combined retinal detachment.

CENTRAL RETINAL VEIN OCCLUSION

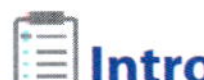 **Introduction**

Central retinal vein occlusion is a retinal condition occurring as a result of obstruction of blood flow in the central retinal vein. It is a cause of significant ocular morbidity.

Epidemiology

Population-based studies report the prevalence of CRVO at less than 0.1–0.4%.[17,40,41] Men and women are equally affected. Usual age of presentation is over 65 years,[13,17,21] although it may be found in younger population as well. While the former age groups are associated with systemic vascular conditions like diabetes or hypertension, latter age group patients usually have an underlying hypercoagulable or inflammatory etiology.[19,20] CRVO is occurs unilaterally usually. There is an annual risk of approximately 1% of developing any type of retinal vascular occlusion in the fellow eye. The 5-year risk of developing CRVO in the fellow eye is 7%.[42,43]

 **Pathophysiology**

The pathophysiology of CRVO is not clearly understood. It is hypothesized that during raised IOP, there is posterior bowing of the lamina cribrosa, the sieve-like opening in sclera, where the central retinal vein and artery are compressed. This leads to further compression of the central retinal vein in case of raised IOP, and can explain the correlation between CRVO and glaucoma. Occlusion of the central retinal vein may occur due to compression by an atherosclerotic central retinal artery or secondary to inflammation.

In acute occlusions, there is usually a thrombus sticking to the endothelium causing obstruction to blood flow which may get recanalized subsequently over 1–5 years.[7] Growth factors released from the ischemic retina following CRVO lead to retinal edema and neovascularization. VEGF has been found to be raised in such eyes along with other cytokines and growth factors, including interleukin-6 (IL-6), IL-8, interferon-induced protein-10, monocyte chemotactic protein-1, and platelet-derived growth factor-A.[29,44-46] The severity of neovascularization and vascular permeability correlates with level of intraocular VEGF levels prompting the development of anti-VEGF agents for the treatment of CRVO.[47]

Younger patients with CRVO may have associated hematologic abnormalities especially hypercoagulable states as previously described.[22]

Clinical Presentation and Diagnosis

Presentation: Usually there is a sudden onset, painless loss of vision, but may present as gradual decline in vision or a relative visual field defect. Less often a patient may be asymptomatic.

Visual acuity is variable, but approximately 40% patients have vision between 20/50–20/200. Rest about 30% have visual acuity better than 20/40 or worse than 20/200 each.[21,48] It is principally dependent on the extent of macular involvement.

Anterior segment:
- Undilated slit-lamp examination to rule out any evidence of neovascularization of the iris (NVI) or neovascularization of the angle (NVA) should be done in all cases. NVI usually starts at the pupillary border, although it may be present over the iris surface. Ectropion uvea may be noted. NVA is seen as fine vessels bridging across the scleral spur. NVI may be seen in 30–50% cases.[21,48] Undilated gonioscopy should be performed routinely in all cases at presentation as NVA may be present in up to 12% of patients not presenting with NVI.[21]
- Pupillary reaction to note presence of relative afferent pupillary defect (RAPD).
- Intraocular pressure must be recorded at each follow-up visit due to the risk of neovascular glaucoma.

Fundus:
- Dilatation and tortuosity of entire venous segment.

- Flame-shaped and dot/blot hemorrhages are present in all four quadrants of the retina usually in a radiating fashion from the optic nerve head giving the classic appearance of 'blood and thunder' or 'splashed tomato' (Figs. 24.10 and 24.11).
- Macular edema, cotton wool spots, splinter hemorrhages, optic disc swelling may be observed to a variable extent.
- Vitreous hemorrhage may be present to a variable extent, usually occurring as a consequence of breakthrough bleeding.
- Optociliary shunt vessels may be seen on the optic nerve head signifying collaterals between choroidal and retinal circulation.
- In late stages, NVD or NVE can develop. These can further lead to fibrovascular sequelae of vitreous hemorrhage or tractional retinal detachment.
- Rarely associated ciliary artery or central retinal artery occlusion may occur.[49,50] Hemispherical vein occlusion, a variant of CRVO may also be seen (Figs. 24.12A and B).

Fluorescein angiography shows variable delayed venous filling, blockage by blood, staining of the vessel wall, hypofluorescence due to CNP and 'pruning' of vessels in the ischemic areas. UWFA provides evidence of retinal vascular pathology in a majority of patients and is a useful tool to look for peripheral ischemic regions.

The *OCT* demonstrates and allows quantification of the severity of macular edema and is a useful way of monitoring its course or the response to treatment.

Course: The acute features usually resolve within 6–12 months and may be replaced by:
- Exudates, venous sheathing and sclerosis peripheral to the site of obstruction, collaterals and variable residual hemorrhages.
- Collaterals are characterized by slightly tortuous veins that develop locally or across the horizontal raphe between the inferior and superior vascular arcades and are best detected on FA (Fig. 24.13).
- As the retinal hemorrhages resolve with time, retinal pigment epithelial (RPE) alterations may be seen. Duration of resolution varies in accordance with extent of hemorrhage, although macular hemorrhages may persist. Epiretinal membrane (ERM) formation may follow.

Central Retinal Vein Occlusion Study

The Central Vein Occlusion Study (CVOS) is one of the most important studies on vein occlusions and has formulated important management protocols for the treatment of CRVO. A randomized, multicenter study was undertaken on 728 patients with CRVO to study its natural course.[21,50] One of the most important prognosticating factor was found to be visual acuity at presentation. Majority of the patients with visual acuity of 20/40 or better maintained their vision. Individuals with intermediate visual acuity (20/50–20/200) had a variable outcome: 21% improved to better than 20/50, 41% stayed in

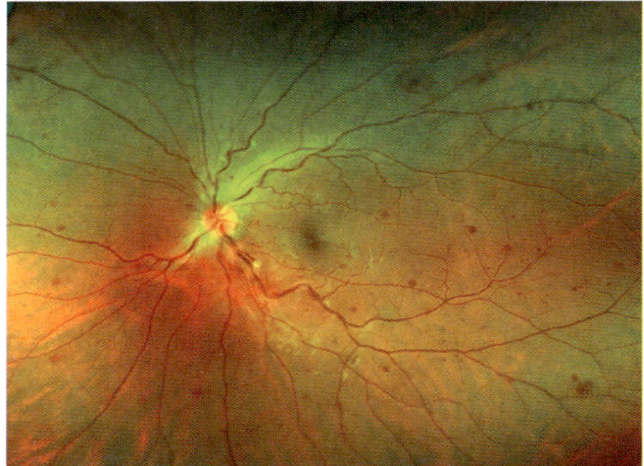

Fig. 24.10: Nonischemic central retinal vein occlusion in a young female (6/6) with multiple superficial hemorrhages.

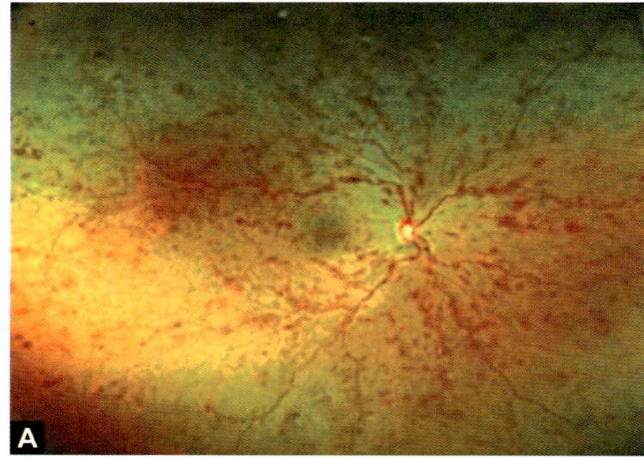

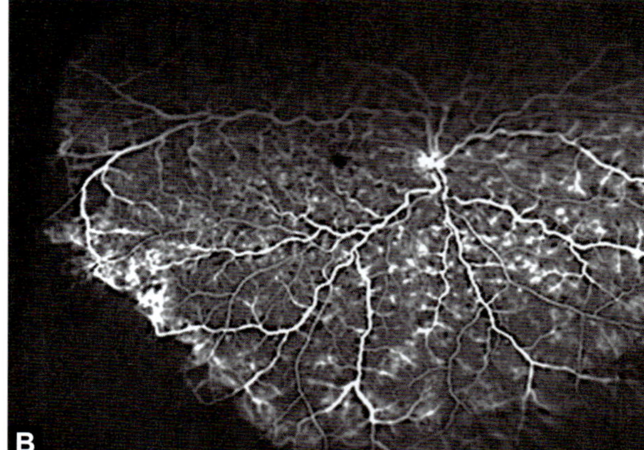

Figs. 24.11A and B: Clinical photograph and corresponding fluorescein angiography of a patient with ischemic central retinal vein occlusion. Clinical image showing multiple flame-shaped hemorrhages and hard exudates at the macula with tortuous, dilated veins. FA image shows extensive areas of peripheral nonperfusion with areas of blocked fluorescence due to overlying retinal hemorrhages.

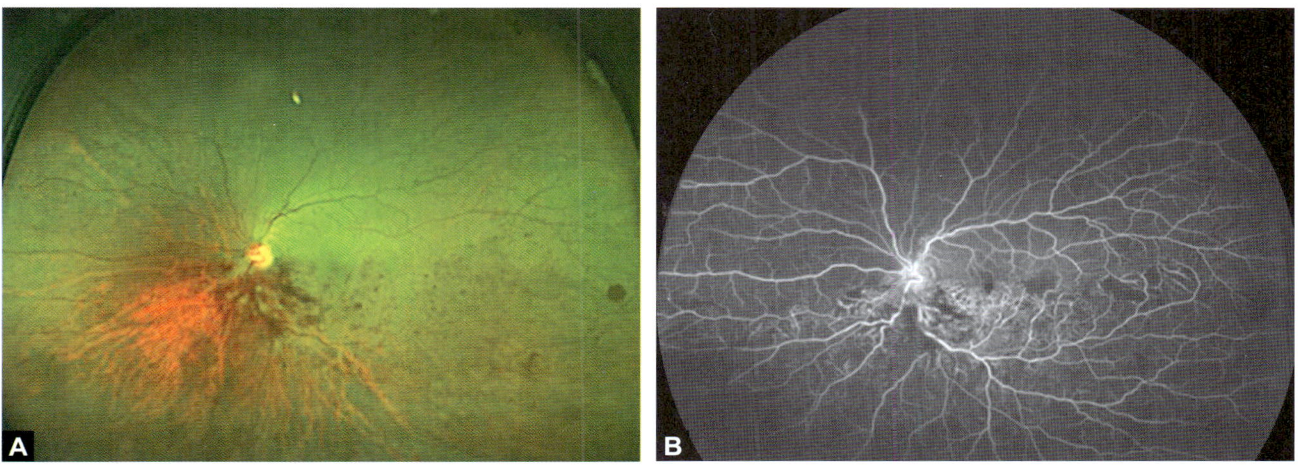

Figs. 24.12A and B: Inferior hemispherical vein occlusion, a variant of central retinal vein occlusion (CRVO).

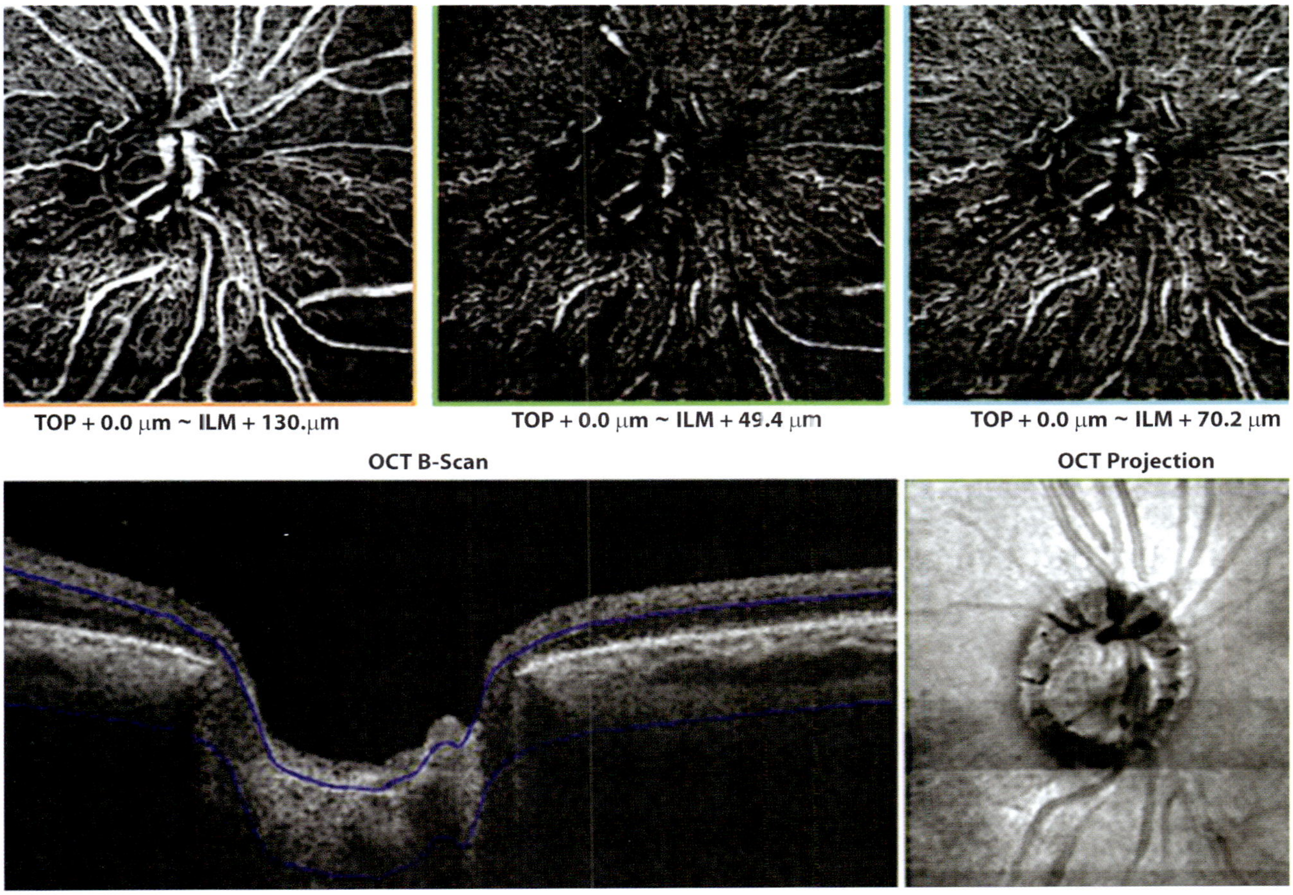

TOP + 0.0 μm ~ ILM + 130.μm   TOP + 0.0 μm ~ ILM + 49.4 μm   TOP + 0.0 μm ~ ILM + 70.2 μm

OCT B-Scan   **OCT Projection**

Fig. 24.13: Optical coherence tomography angiography of the optic disc showing dilated, tortuous vessels over the disc in an eye with central retinal vein occlusion.

the intermediate group and 38% became worse than 20/200. Persons with poor visual acuity at onset (<20/200) had only a 20% chance of improvement.[50,51] NVI and NVA were important anterior segment findings noted by the study group. NVA may develop without any NVI in 6–12% of eyes with CRVO.[21,45] The CVOS used an index defined by 2 or more clock-hours of

Table 24.1: Comparison between perfused and nonperfused central retinal vein occlusion.

Features	Perfused	Nonperfused
Prevalence	75–80%	20–25%
Initial visual acuity	Better than 6/60	Worse than 6/60
RAPD	Slight to nil	Marked
Fundus	Less hemorrhages and cotton wool spots	Extensive hemorrhages and cotton wool spots
Fluorescein angiography	≤10 DD of CNP areas	≥10 DD of CNP areas
visual field defects	Rare	Common
ERG	Normal	Reduced b-wave amplitude, reduced b:a ratio
Prognosis	≤10% develop NVI/NVA	≥35% develop NVI/NVA
Other names	Nonischemic, incomplete, partial	Ischemic, hemorrhagic, complete

(CNP: Capillary nonperfusion; DD: Disc diameter; ERG: Electroretinography; NVI: Neovascularization of the iris; NVA: Neovascularization of the angle; RAPD: Relative afferent pupillary defect).

NVI or any NVA as an evidence of significant anterior-segment neovascularization which was seen in 52% of eyes with 75 disc areas or more of angiographic nonperfusion and 16% of eyes with 10–29 disc areas of angiographic nonperfusion.[51]

The CVOS classified the perfusion status of a CRVO as perfused, nonperfused, or indeterminate based on fluorescein angiographic characteristics. The perfusion status in CRVO is assessed by conventional wide angle fundus FA using photographic protocol from the CVOS (Table 24.1).

A CRVO is categorized as indeterminate when the perfusion status cannot be determined on angiography due to sufficient intraretinal hemorrhages.[13,21]

The CVOS concluded that the patients with good initial visual acuity and perfusion status on fundus FA have better visual outcomes as compared to those with severe visual loss (<20/200) or nonperfused status on fundus FA. More than 80% patients with indeterminate perfusion were later declared nonperfused, and correlated with initial visual acuity. Eyes with nonperfused CRVO were much more likely to have poor visual acuity at initial presentation and at final visit than those with perfused CRVO.[8,21]

Ultra-widefield imaging (Optos Tx200, Optos Inc.) is capable of capturing a 200° field allowing for simultaneous view of the posterior pole, mid-periphery and periphery. It helps to visualize the peripheral nonperfused areas that cannot be identified with conventional angiography (Figs. 24.14A and B). This can be used to guide the therapy in patients with vein occlusions.[52,53]

Treatment

Primary Treatment

After thorough evaluation of the cause of CRVO, therapy must be first directed at seeking treatment for the primary systemic or ocular pathology, wherever possible. Patients

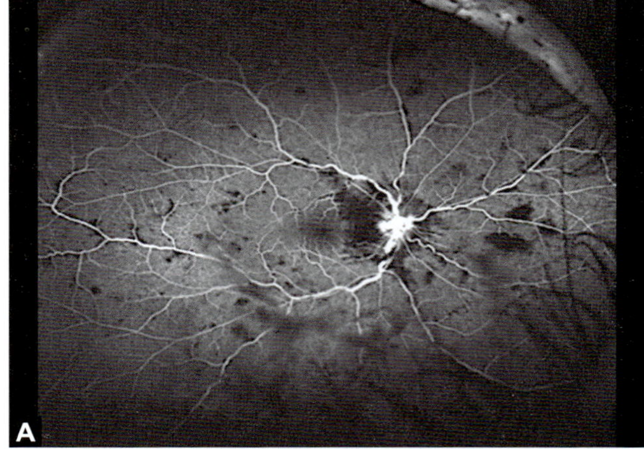

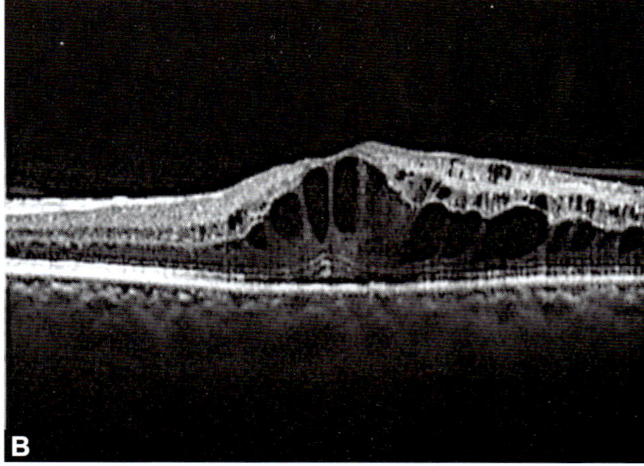

Figs. 24.14A and B: Ultra-widefield fluorescein angiography (UWFA) of a patient with nonischemic central retinal vein occlusion with associated macular edema as seen on swept-source optical coherence tomography.

with systemic hypertension or diabetes must be started on appropriate systemic drugs and these parameters must be closely monitored regularly. Those with hypercoagulable states must be treated with appropriate systemic anticoagulants. Patients with raised IOP or other risk factors must be started on antiglaucoma therapy or treatment wherever necessary. This is necessary not only as treatment of primary disease, but also as a prophylaxis for the prevention of a similar disorder in the fellow eye.

Rheological Therapy

Hyper or isovolemic hemodilution can be performed. The latter is more easy to control and allows for significantly lower hematocrit values in the capillary bed. Hemodilution acts by reducing blood viscosity and improving retinal blood flow. Isovolemic hemodilution is performed by simultaneous venesection and replacement of the lost volume by a plasma substitute usually hydroxyethyl starch or dextran.[54] Good visual outcomes have been described in various studies.[55-58] However, these results have been debatable due to the small study populations and combined therapies were applied in some of the studies. Nevertheless, isovolemic hemodilution is accepted as a first-line treatment within the first 8 weeks after CRVO, as it increases retinal perfusion. The therapy is usually well tolerated. Nonetheless, patients have to be carefully selected and should not have any severe cardiorespiratory or renal disease.

Late treatment has negligible effect on ischemia and in prevention of secondary glaucoma; therefore, eyes showing established neovascularization need additional laser photocoagulation.[59] Other rheologically active substances which have been tested for the treatment of RVO include troxerutin and pentoxifylline. The first is thought to improve microcirculation in capillaries and venules by inhibiting erythrocyte and platelet aggregation improving erythrocyte deformability.[60] Pentoxifylline causes vasodilation and improves retinal flow.[61] Both substances have been used in the treatment of peripheral vein occlusions of the extremities. However, no prospective studies are available in evaluating the efficacy of these drugs in RVO.

Secondary Treatment

These therapies are mainly directed to deal with the sequelae of the CRVO rather than the acute ocular illness particularly retinal edema and neovascularization. Retinal edema becomes a problem only when the macula is involved. Neovascularization is known to occur in eyes with CRVO within a span of first 3 months after the vein occlusion leading to neovascular glaucoma, thereby also popularly described as '100-day glaucoma'.[21] The main goals of treatment are to minimize macular edema, maintain central visual acuity, reduce the risk of vitreous hemorrhage and prevent neovascular glaucoma. In addition to the time-tested therapeutic option of retinal laser photocoagulation, newer modalities like anti-VEGF agents and IVTA have gained popularity in the last two decades for both macular edema and neovascularization in RVOs.

Treatment of macular edema:
1. Observation: The CVOS does not recommend grid laser photocoagulation for CRVO-associated macular edema as they did not find any significant improvement in visual acuity of treated or untreated eyes.[62] Observation is advised especially for the initial few weeks.
2. Corticosteroid therapy: Corticosteroids have been found to stabilize the blood-retinal barrier along with modulating cytokine levels of inflammatory mediators especially via local route of administration.[34,63] Systemic steroids help in cases of vein occlusion secondary to systemic inflammatory diseases.[64] Intravitreal corticosteroids provide targeted treatment while reducing potential systemic toxicity and aid in resolution of macular edema in CRVO.[62,35-67]

The *SCORE* study compared the efficacy and safety of two doses of preservative-free IVTA (1 mg and 4 mg) versus standard of care (i.e. observation per CVOS) for the treatment of CME in 271 eyes with CRVO.[63] It was a randomized, multicenter clinical trial comparing 4 mg IVTA, 1 mg IVTA and observation as therapeutic options. Retreatment was advised with IVTA every 4 months for 1 year unless there was significant improvement defined as:

- Central subfield OCT thickness less than or equal to 225 µm, or
- Visual acuity greater than or equal to 20/25, or
- Significant interval improvement with presumed potential for continued improvement without treatment.

Therapy was discontinued if significant adverse effects such as significant rise in IOP occurred or if there was no improvement following two consecutive injections.

The SCORE study showed significant improvement in visual acuity with IVTA compared to observation. At 1 year, there was a gain of greater than or equal to 15 letters in 26% of eyes in the 4 mg group and 27% of eyes in the 1 mg group as compared to 7% of untreated eyes. Mean change in visual acuity was a loss of only 1.2 letters in both IVTA groups as compared to a loss of 12.1 letters in the observation group. In pseudophakic eyes, there was a mean gain in visual acuity of 2 letters in the 1-mg group and a mean loss of visual acuity of 1 letter in the 4-mg group as compared to a mean loss of 14 letters in the observation group.[63]

Main ocular side effects included cataract formation and elevated IOP.[63] Cataract was observed in 26% in the 1 mg group and 33% of eyes in 4 mg IVTA group, compared to 18% in the observation group. Elevated IOP was observed in 20% and 35% of eyes in the 1 mg and 4 mg IVTA groups, respectively, compared to 8% in the observation group. At 12 months, no cases of endophthalmitis or retinal detachment were noted in any group.[63]

To counter the limited duration of treatment efficacy of IVTA, sustained-release steroid implants have been advocated including Retisert[34] and Ozurdex.[29,34] Retisert is a sustained-release fluocinolone acetonide implant and has been found to be efficacious up to 1 year after administration for CME due to CRVO.[34] Adverse effects were manly cataract formation which required surgical intervention.

In 2009, the FDA approved a sustained-release intravitreal dexamethasone delivery system, Ozurdex, for the treatment of macular edema is secondary to CRVO. The Ozurdex implant has been seen to improve mean visual acuity and lower rate of less than or equal to 15 letters loss according to few studies.[34] Although there are minimal adverse effects reported it has also been questioned regarding the efficacy lasting up to 6 months. It has been found to be effective best till 3 months after injection.[34]

3. Intravitreal anti-VEGF therapy: High level of VEGF has been found in ischemic CRVO eyes and it is hypothesized that VEGF aids in endothelial cell proliferation. This may further lead to blockade of vessels and in turn lead to ischemia.[29,68] Therefore, a targeted therapy against VEGF is advocated. Several intravitreal anti-VEGF agents have been developed including ranibizumab (Lucentis), bevacizumab (Avastin), and pegaptanib (Macugen).

Ranibizumab: Ranibizumab is a 48 kDa fully humanized recombinant monoclonal antibody antigen-binding fragment (Fab) that binds and neutralizes all known active forms of VEGF-A. The *CRUISE* trial was a double-masked, multicenter, randomized phase III trial that prospectively compared monthly intravitreal injections of 0.3 mg or 0.5 mg ranibizumab to sham-injected controls in the treatment of 392 patients with macular edema after CRVO.[69] The results of both treatment arms were significant over the sham group but mostly equivalent to each other. Only systemic adverse events noted were one case each of transient ischemic attack and myocardial infarction throughout the study.[69] The results of this study prompted FDA approval of ranibizumab for the treatment of CRVO. However, the long-term effects of ranibizumab studied by the RETAIN study at 4 years concluded that the effects of ranibizumab are maintained in approximately less than half patients and rest of the patients require repeated subsequent injections for therapy.[70]

Aflibercept: Also known as VEGF trap, it is a pharmacologically engineered protein that binds VEGF and thus prevents VEGF binding to its cellular receptor. The VEGF trap is composed of two different binding domains from VEGF receptor 1 and 2, and is designed to bind the VEGF-A isoform with higher affinity than pegaptanib or ranibizumab hence, offering a theoretically longer time interval time between treatments.[71]

COPERNICUS and *GALILEO* were two randomized, multicenter, double-masked, sham-controlled studies that assessed the safety and efficacy of aflibercept in the treatment of macular edema following CRVO.[69,72-74] Both the studies compared 2 mg intravitreal aflibercept injection (IAI) to sham treatment initially for 6 months period, with injections being repeated every 4 weeks. After 6 monthly injections, patients continued to receive aflibercept treatment during 24–52 weeks if they met prespecified retreatment criteria [pro re nata (PRN)], except for patients in the sham control group in the GALILEO study who continued to receive sham injections through week 52. In the COPERNICUS study, after 6 months, 56% of patients receiving aflibercept 2 mg monthly gained at least 15 letters of BCVA from baseline as measured by ETDRS, compared to 12% of patients receiving sham injections (p <0.01), the primary endpoint of the study.[72] During weeks 52–100, patients were evaluated at least quarterly and received IAI PRN. It concluded that the visual and anatomic improvements after fixed dosing through week 24 and PRN dosing with monthly monitoring from weeks 24 to 52 were diminished after continued PRN dosing with a reduced monitoring frequency from weeks 52 to 100.[73]

In the GALILEO study, after 6 months, 60% of patients receiving IAI 2 mg monthly for the first 6 months, gained at least 15 letters of BCVA from baseline as compared to 22% of patients receiving sham injections (p <0.01) during this time, the primary endpoint of the study. Patients receiving aflibercept 2 mg monthly gained on average 18 letters of vision compared to a mean gain of 3.3 letters with sham control injections (p <0.01), a secondary endpoint.[69] From weeks 52 to 76, patients were monitored every 8 weeks, and both groups received intravitreal aflibercept PRN. It was found that the anatomic and visual outcomes were fixed after extended treatment intervals.[74]

Both the studies recommended the early use of IAI for CME following CRVO and that the results are largely maintained. Following this FDA granted approval to Eylea® (Regenron Pharma, NY) use for macular edema in vein occlusions.

Pegaptanib: It is popularly known by the brand name Macugen. It is an oligonucleotide aptamer, a 28-base RNA oligonucleotide with two branched 20-kDa polyethylene glycerol moieties which binds selectively to the VEGF-165 isoform and prevents its binding to the VEGF receptor. It received FDA approval for use in neovascular age-related macular degeneration but was used off-label for vein occlusion.

Its use in CRVO patients has been attempted and has been found to prevent visual loss in doses of 0.3 mg and 1 mg, when given monthly. Also it has been found to decrease the mean central retinal thickness significantly more than the untreated patients.[75] With the development of newer broad spectrum anti-VEGF agents, its use has declined overall in the management of retinal disorders.

Bevacizumab: It is a full-length recombinant humanized monoclonal antibody with a molecular weight of 149 kDa. It binds to and inhibits all isoforms of VEGF-A.[76,77] It is used as off-label for vein occlusions due to its low cost and reported efficacy.

Bevacizumab has been shown to decrease retinal thickness and improve visual acuity in eyes with CRVO-associated macular edema in various stuides.[68,78-81] Treatment with bevacizumab is given at 4- to 8 week intervals to avoid recurrence of CME in both ischemic and nonischemic CRVO. Its additional effect includes rapid resolution of anterior-segment neovascularization indicating that neovascular complications of CRVO including neovascular glaucoma may respond well to anti-VEGF agents. The most common adverse events are conjunctival hyperemia and subconjunctival hemorrhage at the injection site. Rare cases of endophthalmitis have been reported.[79,80]

The early use of anti-VEGF agents or IVTA is preferred over observation as the standard of care in current times. Due to the worse adverse effect profile of intravitreal steroids compared with anti-VEGF agents, the latter are preferred wherever possible. The overall efficacy has been found to be fairly similar between the two. IVTA has the advantage of fewer injections with repeat injections being required at 3 monthly intervals. Use of combined therapy is still being studied and their clinical use shall be clearer in near future.

Treatment of ocular neovascularization:

1. Laser photocoagulation: The CVOS recommended that panretinal photocoagulation (PRP) be delivered promptly after the development of NVI/NVA but not prophylactically in eyes with nonperfused CRVO.[82] In approximately 90% of cases, the regression of NVI/NVA occurs within 1–2 months of PRP. PRP augmentation may be done in cases where the progression continues. Patients with NVD/NVE should be treated immediately with PRP to avoid anterior-segment neovascularization. Prophylactic PRP is advised only in high-risk cases like:
   - Male gender
   - Short duration of CRVO
   - Extensive retinal nonperfusion
   - Extensive retinal hemorrhages
   - In cases where frequent ophthalmologic follow-up is not possible.

2. Medical therapy: Topical or systemic antiglaucoma agents help to reduce elevated IOP. Cycloplegic agents are required to prevent posterior synechia formation. Topical corticosteroids helps in reducing exudation by stabilizing tight junctions in neovascular tissue and also help in reducing inflammation. Surgical intervention for control of IOP may be required in the cases not responding to medical management. Anti-VEGF agents may be used as adjunct before PRP for definitive treatment as it helps to reduce neovascularization temporarily. Laser must be delivered within 3–7 days of anti-VEGF administration.

Alternative Treatments

Oral pentoxifylline: Oral pentoxifylline is a potent vasodilator which is postulated to improve retinal circulation and has shown reduction in mean CMT by about 10% of baseline in CRVO patients with CME at 5 months by volumetric analysis.[83] Usual dose of oral pentoxifylline used for retinal condition is 400 mg three times a day.[83]

Chorioretinal venous anastomosis: It has been attempted to create a chorioretinal anastomosis between a nasal retinal vein branch and choroidal circulation as it is expected that it will allow venous blood to flow out from the eye and prevent retinal ischemia and associated complications.

This may be achieved either by using argon or neodymium: yttrium aluminum garnet (Nd:YAG) laser delivery directly at a branch retinal vein to rupture the posterior vein wall and Bruch's membrane,[84,85] or surgically via transretinal venipuncture technique.[86,87] Studies report approximately two-line improvement after successful therapy.[88] Complications may be intraretinal, subretinal, or vitreous hemorrhage which may be nonclearing, ERM formation, fibrovascular proliferation, secondary neovascularization and tractional retinal detachment.[34,89,90] Even after successful anastomosis visual recovery may be limited due to thrombosis of the treated vein with progressive retinal ischemia and development of macular pigment abnormalities following resolution of chronic macular edema.[84]

Tissue plasminogen activator (tPA): Local thrombolysis with rtPA (recombinant tPA)—either by intravitreal injection or, during vitreoretinal surgery by direct injection into the occluded vessel has been shown to be effective in patients with CRVO.[9,92] rtPA is a synthetic fibrinolytic agent that helps in destabilizing intravascular thrombi by converting plasminogen to plasmin. Reduction in size of clot may lead to entire dislodgment of the clot and subsequent recanalization of the vein. However, there may be serious complications like vitreous hemorrhage and increase in macular edema and systemic toxcitiy.[57,93] Systemic administration of rtPA has been attempted at various doses with moderate success in a few studies, but the risk of intraocular hemorrhage or fatal stroke limits its use.[94-97] Its use is therefore very limited, although intravitreal use prevents any systemic risks.

Vitrectomy: Pars plana vitrectomy is required in eyes with nonclearing vitreous hemorrhage from secondary retinal neovascularization. A complete endolaser is done along with epiretinal or fibrovascular membranes removal, wherever necessary.

Radial optic neurotomy: It was hypothesized that transvitreal incision of the nasal scleral ring to release pressure on the central retinal vein may help in improving perfusion of the retina. Various studies have reported high rates of adverse outcomes, along with low to moderate success rates.[98-101] With newer treatment modalities at hand, its use has gone out of vogue.

REFERENCES

1. Bowers DK, Finkelstein D, Wolff SM, et al. Branch retinal vein occlusion. A clinicopathologic case report. Retina. 1987;7:252-9.
2. Frangieh GT, Green WR, Barraquer-Somers E, et al. Histopathologic study of nine branch retinal vein occlusions. Arch Ophthalmology. 1982;100:1132-40.

3. Seitz R. The Retinal Vessels. St. Louis: CV Mosby; 1964. pp. 20-74.

4. Bandello F, Tavola A, Pierro L, et al. Axial length and refraction in retinal vein occlusions. Ophthalmologica. 1998;212:133-5.

5. Kumar B, Yu DY, Morgan WH, et al. The distribution of angioarchitectural changes within the vicinity of the arteriovenous crossing in branch retinal vein occlusion. Ophthalmology. 1998;105:424-7.

6. Clemett RS. Retinal branch vein occlusion. Changes at the site of obstruction. Br J Ophthalmology. 1974;58:548-54.

7. Green WR, Chan CC, Hutchins GM, et al. Central retinal vein occlusion: a prospective histopathologic study of 29 eyes in 28 cases. Retina. 1981;1:27-55.

8. Hayreh SS, Podhajsky PA, Zimmerman MB. Natural history of visual outcome in central retinal vein occlusion. Ophthalmology. 2011;118(1):119-33.

9. Christoffersen NL, Larsen M. Pathophysiology and hemodynamics of branch retinal vein occlusion. Ophthalmology. 1999;106: 2054-62.

10. Risk factors for branch retinal vein occlusion. The Eye Disease Case-control Study Group. Am J Ophthalmology. 1993;116:286-96.

11. The Eye Disease Case-Control Study Group. Risk factors for central retinal vein occlusion. Arch Ophthalmology. 1996;114:545-54.

12. Elman MJ, Bhatt AK, Quinlan PM, et al. The risk for systemic vascular diseases and mortality in patients with central retinal vein occlusion. Ophthalmology. 1990;97:1543-8.

13. Hayreh SS, Zimmerman B, McCarthy MJ, et al. Systemic diseases associated with various types of retinal vein occlusion. Am J Ophthalmology. 2001;131:61-77.

14. Koizumi H, Ferrara DC, Brue C, et al. Central retinal vein occlusion case control study. Am J Ophthalmology. 2007;144:858-63.

15. Cheung N, Klein R, Wang JJ, et al. Traditional and novel cardiovascular risk factors for retinal vein occlusion: the multiethnic study of atherosclerosis. Invest Ophthalmology Vis Sci. 2008;49:4297-302.

16. Di Capua M, Coppola A, Albisinni R, et al. Cardiovascular risk factors and outcome in patients with retinal vein occlusion. J Thromb Thrombolysis. 2010;30:16-22.

17. Mitchell P, Smith W, Chang A. Prevalence and associations of retinal vein occlusion in Australia. The Blue Mountains Eye Study. Arch Ophthalmology. 1996;114:1243-7.

18. O'Mahoney PR, Wong DT, Ray JG. Retinal vein occlusion and traditional risk factors for atherosclerosis. Arch Ophthalmology. 2008;126:692-9.

19. Gutman FA. Evaluation of a patient with central retinal vein occlusion. Ophthalmology. 1983;90:481-3.

20. Fong AC, Schatz H. Central retinal vein occlusion in young adults. Surv Ophthalmology. 1993;37:393-417.

21. The Central Vein Occlusion Study Group. Natural history and clinical management of central retinal vein occlusion. Arch Ophthalmology. 1997;115:486-91.

22. Lahey JM, Tunc M, Kearney J, et al. Laboratory evaluation of hypercoagulable states in patients with central retinal vein occlusion who are less than 56 years of age. Ophthalmology. 2002;109:126-31.

23. Cahill MT, Stinnett SS, Fekrat S. Meta-analysis of plasma homocysteine, serum folate, serum vitamin B(12), and thermolabile MTHFR genotype as risk factors for retinal vascular occlusive disease. Am J Ophthalmology. 2003;136:1136-50.

24. Prasad PS, Oliver SC, Coffee RE, et al. Ultra-wide-field angiographic characteristics of branch retinal and hemi central retinal vein occlusion. Ophthalmology. 2010;117(4):780-4.

25. Argon laser photocoagulation for macular edema in branch vein occlusion. Branch Vein Occlusion Study Group. Am J Ophthalmology. 1984;98:271-82.

26. Rehak J, Rehak M. Branch retinal vein occlusion: pathogenesis, visual prognosis, and treatment modalities. Curr Eye Res. 2008;33(2):111-31.

27. Magargal LE, Sanborn GE, Kimmel AS, et al. Temporal branch retinal vein obstruction: a review. Ophthalmic Surg. 1986;17:240-6.

28. Argon laser scatter photocoagulation for prevention of neovascularization and vitreous hemorrhage in branch vein occlusion. A randomized clinical trial. Branch Vein Occlusion Study Group. Arch Ophthalmology. 1986;104:34-41.

29. Aiello LP, Avery RL, Arrigg PG, et al. Vascular endothelial growth factor in ocular fluid of patients with diabetic retinopathy and other retinal disorders. N Engl J Med. 1994;331:1480-7.

30. Noma H, Minamoto A, Funatsu H, et al. Intravitreal levels of vascular endothelial growth factor and interleukin-6 are correlated with macular edema in branch retinal vein occlusion. Graefes Arch Clin Exp Ophthalmology. 2006;244:309-15.

31. Zhang X, Bao S, Lai D, et al. Intravitreal triamcinolone acetonide inhibits breakdown of the blood-retinal barrier through differential regulation of VEGF-A and its receptors in early diabetic rat retinas. Diabetes. 2008;57:1026-33.

32. McAllister IL, Vijayasekaran S, Chen SD, et al. Effect of triamcinolone acetonide on vascular endothelial growth factor and occludin levels in branch retinal vein occlusion. Am J Ophthalmology. 2009;147:838-46.

33. Scott IU, Ip MS, VanVeldhuisen PC, et al. A randomized trial comparing the efficacy and safety of intravitreal triamcinolone with standard care to treat vision loss associated with macular edema secondary to branch retinal vein occlusion: the Standard Care vs Corticosteroid for Retinal Vein Occlusion (SCORE) study report 6. Arch Ophthalmology. 2009;127:1115-28.

34. Haller JA, Bandello F, Belfort Jr R, et al. Randomized, sham-controlled trial of dexamethasone intravitreal implant in patients with macular edema due to retinal vein occlusion. Ophthalmology. 2010;117:1134-46.e3.

35. Bates DO. Vascular endothelial growth factors and vascular permeability. Cardiovasc Res. 2010;87:262-71.

36. Campochiaro PA, Heier JS, Feiner L, et al. Ranibizumab for macular edema following branch retinal vein occlusion: six-month primary end point results of a phase III study. Ophthalmology. 2010;117:1102-12.e1.

37. Mones JM. BRIGHTER and CRYSTAL studies. Paper presented at: American Academy of Ophthalmology 2014 Annual Meeting; October 17-21, 2014; Chicago, Illinois.

38. Kornhauser T, Schwartz R, Goldstein M, et al. Bevacizumab treatment of macular edema in CRVO and BRVO: long-term follow-up. (BERVOLT study: bevacizumab for RVO long-term follow-up). Graefes Arch Clin Exp Ophthalmology. 2015;254(5): 835-44.

39. Campochiaro PA, Clark WL, Boyer DS, et al. Intravitreal aflibercept for macular edema following branch retinal vein occlusion: the 24-week results of the VIBRANT study. Ophthalmology. 2015; 122(3):538-44.

40. Klein R, Klein BE, Moss SE, et al. The epidemiology of retinal vein occlusion: the Beaver Dam Eye Study. Trans Am Ophthalmology Soc. 2000;98:133-43.

41. Rogers S, McIntosh RL, Cheung N, et al. The prevalence of retinal vein occlusion: pooled data from population studies from the United States, Europe, Asia, and Australia. Ophthalmology. 2010;117(2):313-9.

42. Deramo VA, Cox TA, Syed AB, et al. Vision-related quality of life in people with central retinal vein occlusion using the 25-item National Eye Institute Visual Function Questionnaire. Arch Ophthalmology. 2003;121:1297-302.

43. Fekrat S, Shea AM, Hammill BG, et al. Resource use and costs of branch and central retinal vein occlusion in the elderly. Curr Med Res Opin. 2010;26(1):223-30.

44. Pe'er J, Folberg R, Itin A, et al. Vascular endothelial growth factor upregulation in human central retinal vein occlusion. Ophthalmology. 1998;105(3):412-6.

45. Funk M, Kriechbaum K, Prager F, et al. Intraocular concentrations of growth factors and cytokines in retinal vein occlusion and the effect of therapy with bevacizumab. Invest Ophthalmology Vis Sci. 2009;50:1025-32.

46. Noma H, Funatsu H, Mimura T, et al. Vitreous levels of interleukin-6 and vascular endothelial growth factor in macular edema with central retinal vein occlusion. Ophthalmology. 2009;116:87-93.

47. Boyd SR, Zachary I, Chakravarthy U, et al. Correlation of increased vascular endothelial growth factor with neovascularization and permeability in ischemic central vein occlusion. Arch Ophthalmology. 2002;120:1644-50.

48. Schatz H, Fong AC, McDonald HR, et al. Cilioretinal artery occlusion in young adults with central retinal vein occlusion. Ophthalmology. 1991;98:594-601.

49. Brown GC, Duker JS, Lehman R, et al. Combined central retinal artery-central vein obstruction. Int Ophthalmology. 1993;17:9-17.

50. Decroos FC, Fekrat S. The natural history of retinal vein occlusion: what do we really know? Am J Ophthalmology. 2011;151:739-41.

51. Browning DJ, Scott AQ, Peterson CB, et al. The risk of missing angle neovascularization by omitting screening gonioscopy in acute central retinal vein occlusion. Ophthalmology. 1998;105:776-84.

52. Tsui I, Kaines A, Havunjian MA, et al. Ischemic index and neovascularization in central retinal vein occlusion. Retina. 2011;31:105-10.

53. Spaide RF. Peripheral areas of nonperfusion in treated central retinal vein occlusion as imaged by wide-field fluorescein angiography. Retina. 2011;31:829-37.

54. Chen HC, Wiek J, Gupta A, et al. Effect of isovolaemic haemodilution on visual outcome in branch retinal vein occlusion. Br J Ophthalmology. 1998;82:162-7.

55. Hansen LL, Wiek J, Arntz R. Randomized study of the effect of isovolemic hemodilution in retinal branch vein occlusion (in German). Fortschr Ophthalmology. 1988;85:514-6.

56. Poupard P, Elecjam JJ, Dupeyron G, et al. Role of acute normovolemic hemodilution in treating retinal venous occlusions (in French). Ann Fr Anesth Reanim. 1986;5:229-33.

57. Shahid H, Hossain P, Amoaku WM. The management of retinal vein occlusion: is interventional ophthalmology the way forward? Br J Ophthalmology. 2006;90:627-39.

58. Glacet-Bernard A, Coscas G, Chabanel A, et al. A randomized, double-masked study on the treatment of retinal vein occlusion with troxerutin. Am J Ophthalmology. 1994;118:421-9.

59. De Sanctis MT, Cesarone MR, Belcaro G, et al. Treatment of retinal vein thrombosis with pentoxifylline: a controlled, randomized trial. Angiology. 2002;53(Suppl 1):35-8.

60. Evaluation of grid pattern photocoagulation for macular edema in central vein occlusion. The Central Vein Occlusion Study Group M report. Ophthalmology. 1995;102:1425-33.

61. Hayreh SS. Management of central retinal vein occlusion. Ophthalmologica 2003;217:167-88.

62. Ip MS, Scott IU, VanVeldhuisen PC, et al. A randomized trial comparing the efficacy and safety of intravitreal triamcinolone with observation to treat vision loss associated with macular edema secondary to central retinal vein occlusion: the Standard Care vs Corticosteroid for Retinal Vein Occlusion (SCORE) study report 5. Arch Ophthalmology. 2009;127:1101-14.

63. Ramchandran RS, Fekrat S, Stinnett SS, et al. Fluocinolone acetonide sustained drug delivery device for chronic central retinal vein occlusion: 12-month results. Am J Ophthalmology. 2008;146:285-91.

64. Jonas JB, Kreissig I, Degenring RF. Intravitreal triamcinolone acetonide as treatment of macular edema in central retinal vein occlusion. Graefes Arch Clin Exp Ophthalmology. 2002;240:782-3.

65. Ip MS, Kumar KS. Intravitreous triamcinolone acetonide as treatment for macular edema from central retinal vein occlusion. Arch Ophthalmology. 2002;120:1217-9.

66. Greenberg PB, Martidis A, Rogers AH, et al. Intravitreal triamcinolone acetonide for macular oedema due to central retinal vein occlusion. Br J Ophthalmology. 2002;86:247-8.

67. Park CH, Jaffe GJ, Fekrat S. Intravitreal triamcinolone acetonide in eyes with cystoid macular edema associated with central retinal vein occlusion. Am J Ophthalmology. 2003;136:419-25.

68. Ferrara DC, Koizumi H, Spaide RF. Early bevacizumab treatment of central retinal vein occlusion. Am J Ophthalmology. 2007;144:864-71.

69. Brown DM, Campochiaro PA, Singh RP, et al. Ranibizumab for macular edema following central retinal vein occlusion: six-month primary endpoint results of a phase III study. Ophthalmology. 2010;117:1124-33.e1.

70. Campochiaro PA, Sophie R, Pearlman J, et al. Long-term outcomes in patients with retinal vein occlusion treated with ranibizumab: the RETAIN study. Ophthalmology. 2014;121(1):209-19.

71. Nguyen QD, Shah SM, Hafiz G, et al. A phase I trial of an IV-administered vascular endothelial growth factor trap for treatment in patients with choroidal neovascularization due to age-related macular degeneration. Ophthalmology. 2006;113:1522.e1-14.

72. Haller JA, Boyer DS, Heier JS, et al. VEGF trap-eye in CRVO. Primary endpoint results of the phase 3 COPERNICUS study. Invest Ophthalmology Vis Sci. 2011;52:6643.

73. Heier JS Clark WL Boyer DS, et al. Intravitreal aflibercept injection for macular edema due to central retinal vein occlusion: two-year results from the COPERNICUS study. Ophthalmology. 2014;121(7):1414-20.

74. Ogura Y, Roider J, Korobelnik JF, et al. Intravitreal aflibercept for macular edema secondary to central retinal vein occlusion: 18-month results of the phase 3 GALILEO study. Am J Ophthalmology. 2014;158(5):1032-8.

75. Wroblewski JJ, Wells 3rd JA, Adamis AP, et al. Pegaptanib sodium for macular edema secondary to central retinal vein occlusion. Arch Ophthalmology 2009;127:374-80.

76. Ferrara N, Hillan KJ, Gerber HP, et al. Discovery and development of bevacizumab, an anti-VEGF antibody for treating cancer. Nat Rev Drug Discov. 2004;3:391-400.

77. Presta LG, Chen H, O'Connor SJ, et al. Humanization of an anti-vascular endothelial growth factor monoclonal antibody for the therapy of solid tumors and other disorders. Cancer Res. 1997;57:4593-9.

78. Costa RA, Jorge R, Calucci D, et al. Intravitreal bevacizumab (Avastin) for central and hemicentral retinal vein occlusions: IBeVO study. Retina. 2007;27:141-9.

79. Pai SA, Shetty R, Vijayan PB, et al. Clinical, anatomic, and electrophysiologic evaluation following intravitreal bevacizumab for macular edema in retinal vein occlusion. Am J Ophthalmology. 2007;143:601-6.

80. Stahl A, Agostini H, Hansen LL, et al. Bevacizumab in retinal vein occlusion results of a prospective case series. Graefes Arch Clin Exp Ophthalmology. 2007;245:1429-36.

81. Kriechbaum K, Michels S, Prager F, et al. Intravitreal Avastin for macular oedema secondary to retinal vein occlusion: a prospective study. Br J Ophthalmology. 2008;92:518-22.

82. A randomized clinical trial of early panretinal photocoagulation for ischemic central vein occlusion. The Central Vein Occlusion Study Group N report. Ophthalmology. 1995;102:1434-44.

83. Park CH, Scott AW, Fekrat S. Effect of oral pentoxifylline on cystoid macular edema associated with central retinal vein occlusion. Retina. 2007;27:1020-5.

84. McAllister IL, Constable IJ. Laser-induced chorioretinal venous anastomosis for treatment of non-ischemic central retinal vein occlusion. Arch Ophthalmology. 1995;113:456-62.

85. Fekrat S, Goldberg MF, Finkelstein D. Laser-induced chorioretinal venous anastomosis for non-ischemic central or branch retinal vein occlusion. Arch Ophthalmology. 1998;116:43-52.

86. Fekrat S, de Juan E Jr. Chorioretinal venous anastomosis for central retinal vein occlusion: transvitreal venipuncture. Ophthalmic Surg Lasers. 1999;30:52-5.

87. Peyman GA, Kishore K, Conway MD. Surgical chorioretinal venous anastomosis for ischemic central retinal vein occlusion. Ophthalmic Surg Lasers. 1999;30:605-14.

88. McAllister IL, Gillies ME, Smithies LA, et al. The Central Retinal Vein Bypass Study: a trial of laser-induced chorioretinal venous anastomosis for central retinal vein occlusion. Ophthalmology. 2010;117:954-65.

89. McAllister IL, Douglas JP, Constable IJ, et al. Laser-induced chorioretinal venous anastomosis for nonischemic central retinal vein occlusion: evaluation of the complications and their risk factors. Am J Ophthalmology. 1998;126:219-29.

90. Bavbek T, Yenice O, Toygar O. Problems with attempted chorioretinal venous anastomosis by laser for non-ischemic CRVO and BRVO. Ophthalmologica. 2005;219:267-71.

91. Lahey JM, Fong DS, Kearney J. Intravitreal tissue plasminogen activator for acute central retinal vein occlusion. Ophthalmic Surg Lasers. 1999;30;427-34.

92. Weiss JN, Bynoe LA. Injection of tissue plasminogen activator into a branch retinal vein in eyes with central retinal vein occlusion. Ophthalmology. 2001;108:2249-57.

93. Sharma A, D'Amico DJ. Medical and surgical management of central retinal vein occlusion. Int Ophthalmology Clin. 2004;44:1-16.

94. Hattenbach LO, Steinkamp G, Scharrer I, et al. Fibrinolytic therapy with low-dose recombinant tissue plasminogen activator in retinal vein occlusion. Ophthalmologica. 1998;212:394-8.

95. Hattenbach LO, Wellermann G, Steinkamp GW, et al. Visual outcome after treatment with low-dose recombinant tissue plasminogen activator or hemodilution in ischemic central retinal vein occlusion. Ophthalmologica. 1999;213:360-6.

96. Hattenbach LO, Friedrich Arndt C, Lerche R, et al. Retinal vein occlusion and low-dose fibrinolytic therapy (R.O.L.F.): a prospective, randomized, controlled multicenter study of low-dose recombinant tissue plasminogen activator versus hemodilution in retinal vein occlusion. Retina. 2009;29:932-40.

97. Elman MJ. Thrombolytic therapy for central retinal vein occlusion: results of a pilot study. Trans Am Ophthalmology Soc. 1996;94:471-504.

98. Opremcak EM, Rehmar AJ, Ridenour CD, et al. optic neurotomy for central retinal vein occlusion: 117 consecutive cases. Retina. 2006;26:297-305.

99. Weizer JS, Stinnett SS, Fekrat S. Radial optic neurotomy as treatment for central retinal vein occlusion. Am J Ophthalmology. 2003;136:814-9.

100. Arevalo JF, Garcia RA, Wu L, et al. Radial optic neurotomy for central retinal vein occlusion: results of the Pan-American Collaborative Retina Study Group (PACORES). Retina. 2008;28:1044-52.

101. Martinez-Jardon CS, Meza-de Regil A, Dalma-Weiszhausz J, et al. Radial optic neurotomy for ischaemic central vein occlusion. Br J Ophthalmology. 2005;89:558-61.

Chapter 25

Hypertensive Retinopathy and Choroidopathy

Vineet Mutha, Raghav Ravani, Yamini Attiku, Chirakshi Dhull

INTRODUCTION

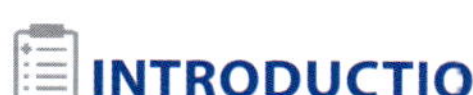

Hypertension is one of the major causes of morbidity and mortality across the world.[1] It affects directly or indirectly, almost all the organs in the body, especially heart, kidneys, brain, and eye as target organs. Various structural and functional changes are seen in the eye vasculature secondary to systemic hypertension depending on the severity and duration of hypertension. Hypertension may affect retinal, choroidal, and optic nerve circulations resulting in varied clinical presentation. Various clinical conditions associated with hypertension include hypertensive retinopathy, hypertensive choroidopathy, optic neuropathy, retinal vein occlusion, progression of diabetic retinopathy, retinal arterial macroaneurysm, etc.[2-5]

HYPERTENSIVE RETINOPATHY

Retinopathy is the most common ocular manifestation of hypertension. Pathophysiologically, hypertensive retinopathy can be divided into various stages.[6] "Vasoconstrictive" phase is the initial vasospasm and increased vasomotor tone which occurs due to elevated blood pressure with consequent diffuse retinal arteriolar narrowing. "Sclerotic phase" pathologically includes intimal thickening, medial wall hyperplasia and hyaline degeneration. Clinically focal retinal arteriolar narrowing (Figs. 25.1A and B), arteriolar wall opacification ("silver or copper wiring"), banking of veins distal to arteriovenous crossing (Bonnet sign), right-angled deflection of veins (Salus sign) and tapering of veins on either sides of the crossing (Gunn sign) can be seen in the sclerotic phase. "Exudative" phase due to sustained rise in blood pressure is characterized by disruption of blood-retinal barrier. Pathologically, this includes necrosis of endothelial cells and smooth muscles (leading to microaneurysms), exudation of blood and lipids (causing hemorrhages and hard exudates), and nerve fiber layer infarcts (seen as cotton wool spots). "Malignant hypertension" may result in optic disc swelling (Figs. 25.2A and B).

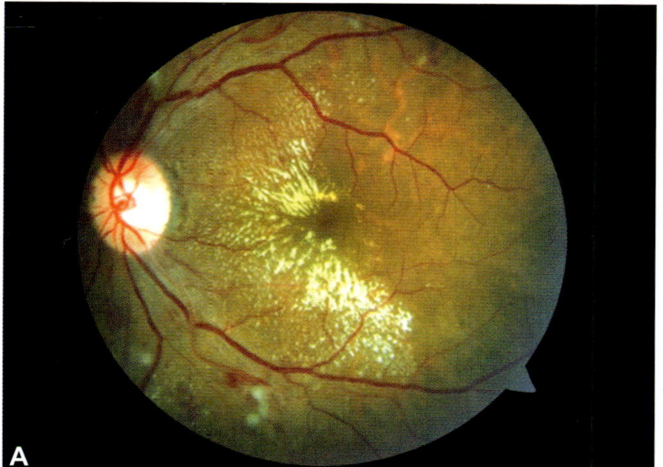
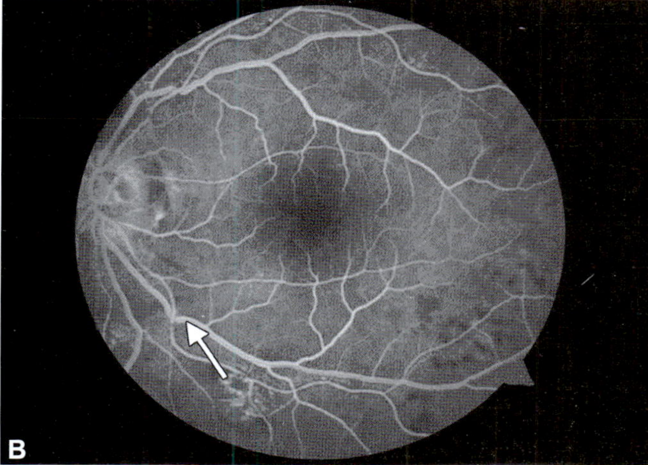

Figs. 25.1A and B: Color fundus picture (A) and fluorescein angiography (B) of a patient with hypertensive retinopathy reveals diffuse and focal arteriolar narrowing with hard exudates (macular star) and marked arteriovenous (AV) nicking (arrow) in an eye with hypertensive retinopathy.

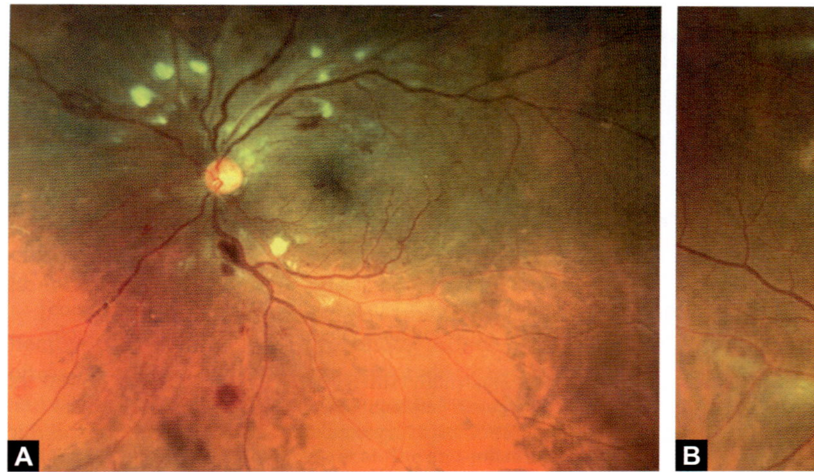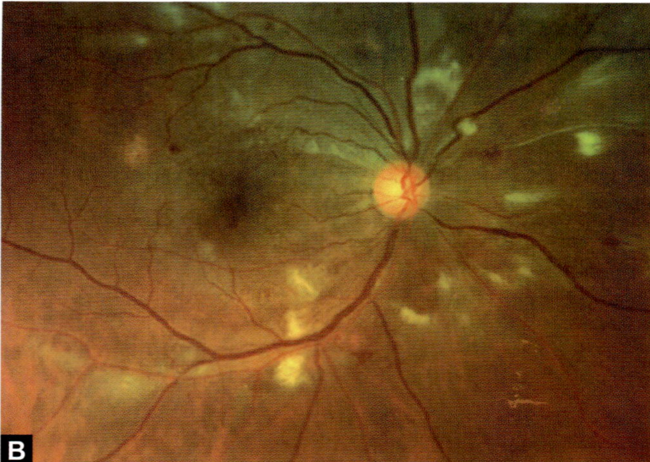

Figs. 25.2A and B: Ultrawide field pseudocolor images of an eye with hypertensive retinopathy showing marked arteriovenous (AV) crossing changes and soft exudates.

CLASSIFICATION

Various classifications for hypertensive retinopathy have been described.[7-12] While classifying hypertensive retinopathy, it is important to consider the superimposed changes caused by arteriosclerosis which may be accelerated by hypertension. The Scheie classification[7] addresses the arteriosclerotic and hypertensive changes separately (Tables 25.1 to 25.3).

The Keith-Wagener-Barker (KWB) classification[8] divides the retinal changes into the following four groups with increasing grades of severity (Table 25.1).

Based on correlation of different signs with prognosis from a population-based data, a new simplified classification of hypertensive retinopathy has been proposed by Wong and Mitchell (2004) (Table 25.4).[9]

Anterior ischemic optic neuropathy, characterized by unilateral swelling of the optic disc, visual loss, and sectoral visual-field loss, should be ruled out.

A study compared the traditional KWB classification to the simplified three-grade classification for hypertensive retinopathy. They assessed the interobserver and intraobserver grading reliability of the KWB system to the proposed Mitchell-Wong "simplified" three-grade classification. The findings indicated that the simplified classification of hypertensive retinopathy was both reliable and repeatable.

Table 25.1: Keith-Wagener-Barker classification.

Grade	Features
I	Mild generalized retinal arteriolar narrowing
II	Definite focal narrowing and arteriovenous nipping
III	The above and retinal hemorrhages, exudates, and cotton-wool spots
IV	Grade III and papilledema

Table 25.2: Scheie classification—hypertensive changes.

Stage	Features
0	No visible changes
1	Diffuse arteriolar narrowing. No focal constriction.
2	More pronounced arteriolar narrowing with focal constriction
3	More severe narrowing (diffuse and focal) and retinal hemorrhages
4	In addition to all features described above, retinal edema, disc edema, and hard exudates are observed

Table 25.3: Scheie classification—arteriosclerotic changes.

Stage	Features
0	Normal
1	Broadening of light reflex along the blood vessel
2	More prominent crossing and light reflex changes
3	Copper wire appearance and more pronounced arteriovenous (AV) compression
4	Silver wire appearance and most severe AV crossing changes. The vessel appears white but can be shown to be patent on fluorescein angiography.

Table 25.4: Wong-Mitchell classification.

Grade of retinopathy	Retinal signs	Systemic associations*
None	No detectable signs	None
Mild	Generalized arteriolar narrowing, focal arteriolar narrowing, arteriovenous nicking, opacity (copper wiring) of arteriolar wall, or a combination of these signs	Modest association with risk of clinical stroke, subclinical stroke, coronary heart disease and death
Moderate	Aneurysm, cotton-wool spot, hard exudate, or a combination of these signs	Strong association with risk of clinical stroke, subclinical stroke, cognitive decline and death from cardiovascular causes
Malignant	Signs of moderate retinopathy plus swelling of the optic disc	Strong association with death

*A modest association is defined as an odds ratio of greater than 1 but less than 2. A strong association is defined as an odds ratio of 2 or greater.

The advantage of the simplified method over the KWB system in correlating retinal microvascular signs to incident cardiovascular risk supports its adoption in clinical practice.[10]

SYSTEMIC RELATIONSHIP OF HYPERTENSIVE RETINOPATHY

Stroke

Various studies have been reported that suggest strong relationship between presence of hypertensive retinopathy and presence of cerebrovascular conditions including subclinical/clinical stroke. A large multicenter study showed that otherwise healthy people with signs of moderate hypertensive retinopathy are more likely to have subclinical MRI-defined cerebral infarction, white matter lesion or atrophy than those without hypertensive retinopathy signs.[13-16] Some studies have found association of specific signs hypertensive retinopathy with certain types of strokes.[17] For example retinal arteriolar narrowing with lacunar stroke, retinal hemorrhages association with cerebral hemorrhages.

Coronary Artery Disease

Hypertensive retinopathy has been associated with increased risk of mortality associated with coronary heart disease and stroke.[17-19] Hypertensive retinopathy can be predictive of clinical coronary artery disease events and congestive heart failure.[20-22]

End-organ Damage

Retinopathy signs have been recognized as risk factor for various renal condition including microalbuminuria and renal impairment.[23-25]

HYPERTENSIVE CHOROIDOPATHY

Choroidal ischemia acts as an underlying mechanism for hypertensive choroidopathy, which affects retinal pigment epithelium and the retina. As compared to hypertensive retinopathy, hypertensive choroidopathy is a less recognized entity. Pathophysiology of choroidopathy is similar to hypertensive retinopathy and involves fibrinoid necrosis of choriocapillaris due to elevated blood pressure leading to patchy choroidal infarcts and other signs of hypertensive choroidopathy like Elschnig spots and Siegrist streaks.

Elschnig's spots is the term used to describe deep, round, gray-yellow patches at sites of occluded choriocapillaris that leak profusely on fluorescein angiography. On healing, these become pigmented and do not leak on fluorescein angiography.

Siegrist's streaks are linear hyperpigmented lesions along choroidal arteries. In cases with accelerated hypertension, localized areas of retinal and retinal pigment epithelial detachments may occur secondary to RPE dysfunction, occlusion of choriocapillaris and due to breakdown in blood retinal barrier.

MALIGNANT HYPERTENSIVE RETINOPATHY

Malignant hypertension (accelerated hypertension) is the term used to describe sudden increase in blood pressure. Ocular features of malignant hypertension include bilateral disc swelling, retinal hemorrhages, and soft exudates. Hypertensive choroidopathy is typically seen in accelerated hypertension. Optic disc swelling in accelerated hypertension may occur due to ischemia of the axons, raised intracranial pressure, and hypertensive encephalopathy.[26]

REFERENCES

1. Lawes CM, Vander HS, Rodgers A. Global burden of blood-pressure-related disease, 2001. Lancet. 2008;371:1513-8.
2. Wong TY, Mitchell P. The eye in hypertension. Lancet. 2007;369:425-35.
3. Cheung N, Mitchell P, Wong TY. Diabetic retinopathy. Lancet. 2010;376:124-36.

4. Wong TY, Scott IU. Clinical practice. Retinal-vein occlusion N Engl J Med. 2010;363:2135-44.

5. Panton RW, Goldberg MF, Farber MD. Retinal arterial macroaneurysms: risk factors and natural history. Br J Ophthalmology. 1990; 74:595-600.

6. Tso MO, Jampol LM. Pathophysiology of hypertensive retinopathy. Ophthalmology. 1982;89:1132-45.

7. Scheie, HG. Evaluation of ophthalmoscopic changes of hypertension and arteriolar sclerosis. AMA Arch Ophthalmology. 1953;49:117-38.

8. Keith NM, Wagener HP, Barker NW. Some different types of essential hypertension: their course and prognosis. Am J Med Sci. 1939;197:332-43.

9. Wong TY, Mitchell P. Current concepts; Hypertensive Retinopathy. N Engl J Med. 2004;351:2310-7.

10. Downie LE, Hodgson LA, Dsylva C, et al. Hypertensive retinopathy: comparing the Keith-Wagener-Barker to a simplified classification. J Hypertens. 2013;31(5):960-5.

11. Chopra A, Sharma A, Singh S, et al. Changing Perspectives in Classifications of Hypertensive Retinopathy. IOSR J Dent Med Sci. 2014;13:51-54.

12. Dodson PM, Lip GY, Eames SM, et al. Hypertensive retinopathy: a review of existing classification systems and a suggestion for a simplified grading system. J Hum Hypertens. 1996;10:93-8.

13. Kawasaki R, Cheung N, Mosley T, et al. Retinal microvascular signs and 10-year risk of cerebral atrophy: the Atherosclerosis Risk in Communities (ARIC) Study. Stroke. 2010;41:1826-8.

14. Wong TY, Klein R, Sharrett AR, et al. Cerebral white matter lesions, retinopathy, and incident clinical stroke. JAMA. 2002;288:67-74.

15. Cooper LS, Wong TY, Klein R, et al. Retinal microvascular abnormalities and MRI-defined subclinical cerebral infarction: the Atherosclerosis Risk in Communities Study. Stroke. 2006;37:82-6.

16. Cheung N, Mosley T, Islam A, et al. Retinal microvascular abnormalities and subclinical magnetic resonance imaging brain infarct: a prospective study. Brain. 2010;133:1987-93.

17. Wong TY, Klein R, Klein BE, et al. Retinal microvascular abnormalities and their relationship with hypertension, cardiovascular disease, and mortality. Surv Ophthalmology. 2001; 46:59-80.

18. Liew G, Wong TY, Mitchell P, et al. Retinopathy predicts coronary heart disease mortality. Heart. 2009;95:391-4.

19. Wong TY, Klein R, Nieto FJ, et al. Retinal microvascular abnormalities and 10-year cardiovascular mortality: a population-based case–control study. Ophthalmology. 2003;110:933-40.

20. Michelson EL, Morganroth J, Nichols CW, et al. Retinal arteriolar changes as an indicator of coronary artery disease. Arch Intern Med. 1979;139:1139-41.

21. Wong TY, Klein R, Sharrett AR, et al. Retinal arteriolar narrowing and risk of coronary heart disease in men and women. The Atherosclerosis Risk in Communities Study. JAMA. 2002;287:1153-9.

22. Duncan BB, Wong TY, Tyroler HA, et al. Hypertensive retinopathy and incident coronary heart disease in high risk men. Br J Ophthalmology. 2002;86:1002-6.

23. Gunn RM. Ophthalmoscopic evidence of (1) arterial changes associated with chronic renal diseases and (2) of increased arterial tension. Trans Ophthalmology Soc UK. 1982;12:124-5.

24. Saitoh M, Matsuo K, Nomoto S, et al. Relationship between left ventricular hypertrophy and renal and retinal damage in untreated patients with essential hypertension. Intern Med. 1998;37:576-80.

25. Wong TY, Coresh J, Klein R, et al. Retinal microvascular abnormalities and renal dysfunction: the atherosclerosis risk in communities study. J Am Soc Nephrol. 2004;15:2469-76.

26. Chatterjee S, Chattopadhyay S, Hope-Ross M, et al. Hypertension and the eye: changing perspectives. J Hum Hypertens. 2002;16:667-75.

Chapter 26

Retinal Artery Macroaneurysm

Raghav Ravani, Yogita Gupta, Abhidnya Surve, Atul Kumar

OVERVIEW

An aneurysm is a localized widening or dilatation of vascular structure (artery, vein or capillary). Aneurysms less than or equal to 100 µ are termed as microaneurysms and those between 100 µ and 250 µ are termed as macroaneurysms. The clinical entity retinal arterial macroaneurysm was formally described by Robertson[1] in 1973 though in literature it has been mentioned earlier.[1,2]

Cousins and colleagues[3] have classified macroaneurysms involving the retinal vasculature into four types. These are: (1) typical retinal artery macroaneurysm, (2) retinal venous aneurysms, (3) retinal capillary macroaneurysm, and (4) collateral-associated macroaneurysm. The later three types are more common and usually seen secondary to disease like (i) diabetes mellitus, (ii) retinal vein obstruction, and (iii) hematological conditions like sickle cell retinopathy or radiation retinopathy. In contrast retinal artery macroaneurysm is usually an isolated finding with characteristic clinical features.[2]

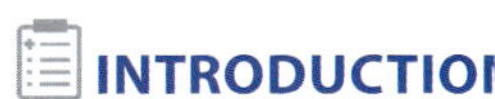 INTRODUCTION

Retinal arterial macroaneurysm is a fusiform or saccular dilatation of the retinal arterioles that usually arises within the first three orders of bifurcation. Their diameter ranges from 100 µm (lower limit for defining macroaneurysm) to 250 µm.

The most common site of occurrence is at arteriolar bifurcation or at arteriovenous crossing, especially in vessels with documented history of embolic damage.[4-6] The most common site of occurrence reported in patients presenting with visual symptoms is along superotemporal arcade.[1] These are usually solitary and unilateral. They can however be multiple in 20% (Fig. 26.1) and bilateral in 10% of cases. At presentation, about 10% of macroaneurysms are pulsatile.

EPIDEMIOLOGY

Retinal artery macroaneurysm typically occurs in elderly hypertensive women (especially in sixth decade). Females are three times more commonly affected than males, (M:F =

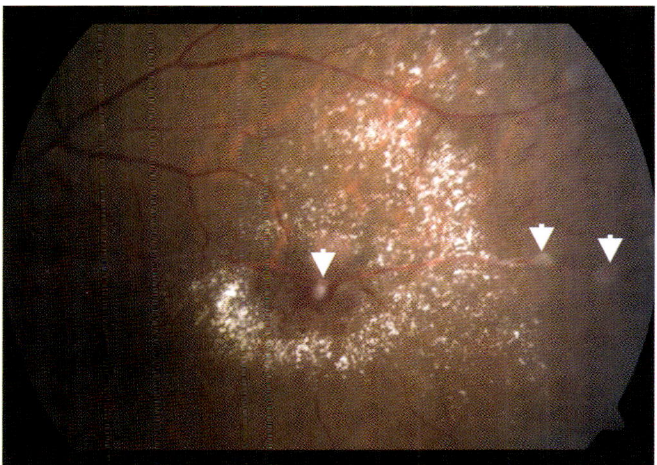

Fig. 26.1: Fundus photograph (50°) showing multiple retinal artery macroaneurysms (white arrowheads) with surrounding hard exudates.

1:3).[1,7,8] History of hypertension may be present in approximately 75% of patients. Abnormalities of serum lipid and lipoproteins have also been reported to be associated with the condition.[9]

 CLINICAL FEATURES

Clinically, two forms of presentation may be seen: (1) acute and (2) chronic. Often, retinal arterial macroaneurysms may be found in asymptomatic patients on routine examination. In acute form, patient presents with a sudden loss of vision due to retinal or vitreous hemorrhage. Hemorrhage may be seen at various levels like subretinal space, intraretinal, the subinternal limiting membrane space, the retrohyaloid space or the vitreous. Diagnosis in acute form may be difficult due to obscuration of macroaneurysm due to hemorrhage. A characteristic, though, not consistent feature during the acute stage is the presence of an "hour-glass hemorrhage" consisting of simultaneous subretinal and preretinal collections of

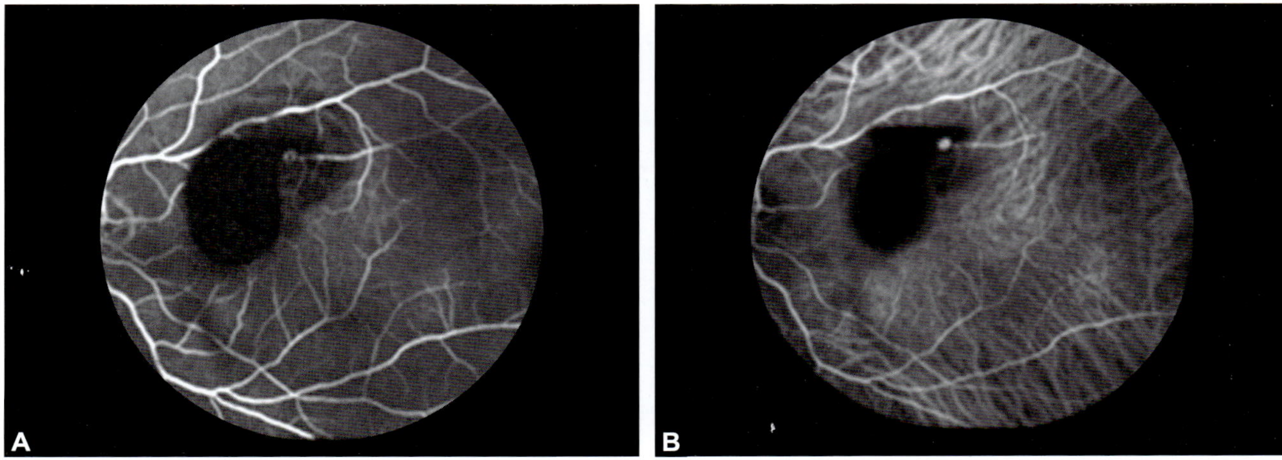

Figs. 26.2A and B: (A) Fundus fluorescein angiography (FFA); and (B) Indocyanine green (ICG) of a case of macroaneurysm. The macroaneurysm is seen better on ICG due to better penetration of infrared light through hemorrhage. The hour-glass hemorrhage is apparent on the FFA.

blood. The patient in chronic form may present with a gradual loss of vision due to collection of serous fluid or hard exudates within the retina leading to focal, diffuse or cystoid macular edema; or accumulation in the subretinal space leading to serous macular detachment.

Even after spontaneous resolution of hemorrhage, exudation and resolution of macroaneurysm itself, persistent decreased visual acuity may result from secondary epiretinal membranes. In some cases, large macroaneurysm at arteriovenous crossing may produce a branch retinal vein occlusion and symptoms secondary to it.

Macular hole formation following rupture of macroaneurysm have also been reported.[10,11]

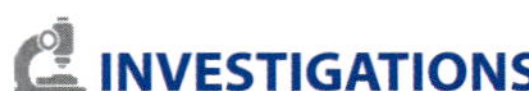

INVESTIGATIONS

Fundus Fluorescein Angiography

The typical fluorescein angiography appearance of a retinal arterial macroaneurysm consists of uniform filling in the early arterial phase. The late phase angiogram may show either staining of the vessel wall or leakage. There may be narrowing of the involved artery proximal and distal to the aneurysm. Obliteration of the distal part of the involved artery has also been reported.[9] Other angiographic findings include leakage from the surrounding dilated capillaries, areas of nonperfusion, and intraretinal microvascular abnormalities. There may be blocked fluorescence in acute form due to presence of hemorrhage (Fig. 26.2A).

Indocyanine Green Angiography

As the absorption and emission peak is in the near-infrared spectrum, this may allow better penetration through hemorrhage and especially helpful in cases with dense hemorrhage (Fig. 26.2B). Macroaneurysm in indocyanine green (ICG) angiography may be demonstrated as a pulsatile lesion con-

tiguous with the arterial wall. This is pathognomonic of retinal artery macroaneurysm.[12]

Optical Coherence Tomography

Initial examination may reveal intact retinal structures, but slowly deterioration of the foveal outer photoreceptor layer may develop due to chronic edema.[13]

With the advent of optical coherence tomography angiography (OCTA) the macroaneurysms which fall in the scanning limits of OCTA can also be imaged noninvasively (Fig. 26.3).

Histopathological studies have revealed gross distention of the involved arteriole. It may show thickened arterial walls secondary to fibrin-laminated clot along with muscular layer hypertrophy. A thrombus may be seen within the macroaneurysm. Other changes in the surrounding correlating

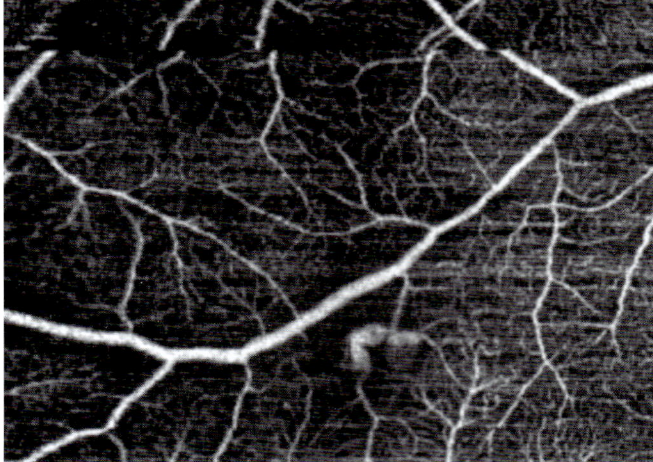

Fig. 26.3: Optical coherence tomography angiography (OCTA) image showing a patent macroaneurysm.

with the clinical presentation include extravasated blood and hemosiderin deposits in acute form and lipoidal exudates in the chronic form. Other findings may include proliferation of fibroglial tissue and dilated capillaries in the surrounding retina.

Systemic Evaluation

Association of systemic hypertension, cardiovascular disease and altered serum lipoprotein levels warrants thorough systemic and cardiac evaluation in patients with retinal artery macroaneurysm.

PATHOGENESIS

Various hypotheses related to development of macroaneurysm have been proposed. They include:

- *Focal damage to the arterial wall*: This may be secondary to embolic damage,[4-6] or periarteritis (e.g. from toxoplasmic inflammation),[14] or previous vascular damage (e.g. branched retinal vein occlusion).[15]
- *Chronic hypertensive vascular damage*: Since hypertension and arteriosclerosis are commonly associated with the condition, it is postulated that chronic hypertension and the associated arteriosclerosis in presence of increased intraluminal pressure predispose the vessels for focal dilatation and thus macroaneurysm.
- *Inherent structural defects in the blood vessels*: Less support to arterial wall at arteriovenous crossing due to common coat and lack of adventitia,[9] associated with increased intraluminal pressure in hypertensive patients may predispose to aneurysmal dilatation of the arterial wall.

NATURAL HISTORY

The natural history of retinal arterial macroaneurysm has been studied extensively.[7-9,16-18] The natural history of macroaneurysm depends largely on its clinical presentation, i.e. acute form or chronic form.

Acute form as discussed earlier consists of hemorrhage at various levels. After rupture of arterial aneurysm, arterial perforation may close leaving an intact aneurysm at risk of rebleed. Some aneurysms close spontaneously and the involved arteriole develops a kink at previous aneurysmal site or may become heavily sheathed. Chronic form may show resolution, either spontaneous or following photocoagulation leaving a kink in the vessel with occasional closure/constriction of the proximal vessel. Distal arterial sheathing may be seen but distal closure is rare. Many investigators have shown better prognosis with acute decompensation (hemorrhage) as compared to chronic forms. A study by Cleary and colleagues[9] concluded that macroaneurysms almost always resolve spontaneously after acute hemorrhage but rarely in cases with macular edema as the presentation. The prognosis depends on both the duration and severity of macular edema.

Some reports have shown arterial closure or branched retinal artery occlusion in cases of aneurysms, more frequent in cases after treatment (16% in treated v/s 8% in untreated cases).[15] The presence of pulsatile macroaneurysm as a sign of imminent rupture in the natural course of disease is controversial.[7,9,19,20]

⊕ DIFFERENTIAL DIAGNOSIS

In cases with a chronic form or those with a clear view of fundus, the diagnosis may be easily established. The fundus view may often be obscured by hemorrhage at various levels and thereby cause diagnostic dilemma. Many clinical entities may resemble retinal arterial macroaneurysm. It has been called another "masquerade" syndrome by Splatter.[21] Large capillary macroaneurysms secondary to retinal venous obstruction may appear similar to retinal arterial macroaneurysm but these originate from the venous side of the capillary bed.[22] All four types of macroaneurysm as described by Cousins and associates[3] may be seen after vein occlusion. Intraretinal hemorrhage at arteriovenous crossing in a case of branch retinal vein occlusion may simulate a macroaneurysm. This is known as Bonnet sign.[23] Small angiomas initially may be confused with macroaneurysms as they are small, without any tortuous feeder or draining vessels. Cases with acute subretinal hemorrhage in the macula with surrounding lipid exudates may obscure retinal macroaneurysm and thus mimic neovascular age-related macular degeneration. In cases with large subretinal or subretinal pigment epithelial hemorrhage, the condition may mimic a choroidal melanoma.

▤ MANAGEMENT

Treatment of retinal artery macroaneurysm depends on the clinical presentation. Patients with asymptomatic aneurysm without leakage should be treated conservatively with close follow-up. Macroaneurysms that have regressed/fibrosed spontaneously with or without rupture and hemorrhage could be observed without active intervention as these macroaneurysms rarely rebleed.[24] In the chronic form of disease where aneurysms leak leads to macular edema or those that threaten to involve the central macula, the macroaneurysms should be treated to shorten the duration of patency of macroaneurysm and to shorten the duration of macular edema, thereby affecting the visual prognosis of the patients.

Intervention in cases with retinal artery macroaneurysm include treatment targeted to the macroaneurysm, treatment for macular edema and treatment of secondary complications like vitreous hemorrhage, subhyaloid hemorrhage, sub-ILM hemorrhage or subretinal hemorrhage.

Laser Photocoagulation

Treatment of macroaneurysms with laser photocoagulation involves direct photocoagulation[7] of the aneurysm/the artery or perianeurysmal[6] technique/indirect photocoagulation (photocoagulation of area with microvascular changes surrounding the aneurysm) or both.[8] This may be associated with early increase in lipid exudation.[16] Complete resolution of these exudates may take several months. Various lasers have been studied for retinal artery macroaneurysm including argon laser,[7] xenon arc,[7] yellow dye laser[25,26] with partially overlapping burns, etc. Some of the studies suggest that direct laser treatment may be harmful and indirect treatment may lower the complication rate with better prognosis.[27] Possible complication with laser photocoagulation may include risk of hemorrhage due to rupture of aneurysm, branch retinal artery occlusion,[15,27] retinochoroidal anastomoses[28] and choroidal neovacularization.[28]

Treatment for Hemorrhage

Treatment depends on the retinal layer where hemorrhage occurs. Laser therapy like Q-switched neodymium: yttrium-aluminium garnet laser could be used to disperse retrohyaloid hemorrhage[29] (YAG hyaloidotomy) or to disperse sub-internal limiting membrane hemorrhage[30] into the vitreous thus enhancing spontaneous resorption of the blood from the vitreous. Surgical techniques have been described for removal of subfoveal and nonresolving vitreous hemorrhage. With advances in vitrectomy techniques, drainage of submacular hemorrhage resulting from ruptured retinal arterial macroaneurysm have been attempted[31-36] with or without the use of tissue plasminogen activator. Pneumatic displacement is also a treatment option in cases with small subfoveal hemorrhage. Pars plana vitrectomy is highly effective surgical treatment modality in cases of retinal artery macroaneurysm with dense, nonresolving vitreous hemorrhage.[36]

Anti-Vascular Endothelial Growth Factor

Recent studies on use of anti-vascular endothelial growth factor (VEGF) agents (bevacizumab and ranibizumab) for retinal macroaneurysm have shown promising results in patients with macroaneurysm-associated macular edema by improving visual acuity and central macular thickness.[37,38]

REFERENCES

1. Robertson DM. Macroaneurysms of the retinal arteries. Trans Am Acad Ophthalmology. Otolaryngol. 1973;77:OP55-67.
2. Rabb MF, Gagliano DA, Teske MP. Retinal arterial macroaneurysms. Surv Ophthalmology. 1988;33:73-96.
3. Cousins SW, Flynn HW Jr, Clarkson JG. Macroaneuryms associated with retinal branch vein occlusion. Am J Ophthalmology. 1990;109:567-70.
4. Wiznia RA. Development of a retinal artery macroaneurysm at the site of a previously detected retinal artery embolus. Am J Ophthalmology. 1982;114:642-3.
5. el-Asrar AM, Awad A, Tabbara KF. Retinal artery macroaneurysm in a patient with congenital heart disease. Br J Ophthalmology. 1993; 77:606-7.
6. Lewis RA, Norton MH, Wise GN. Acquired arterial macroaneurysms of the retina. Br J Ophthalmology. 1976;60:21.
7. Abdel-Khalek MN, Richardson J. Retinal macroaneurysm: natural history and guidelines for treatment. Br J Ophthalmology. 1986;70:2-11.
8. Lavin MJ, Marsh RJ, Peart S, et al. Retinal arterial macroaneurysms: a retrospective study of 40 patients. Br J Ophthalmology. 1987;71:817-25.
9. Cleary PE, Kohner EM, Hamilton AM, et al. Retinal macroaneurysms. Br J Ophthalmology. 1975;59:355-61.
10. Mitamura Y, Terashima H, Takeuchi S. Macular hole formation following rupture of retinal arterial macroaneurysm. Retina. 2002;22:113-15.
11. Sato R, Yasukawa T, Hirano Y, et al. Early-onset macular holes following ruptured retinal arterial macroaneurysms. Graefes Arch Clin Exp Ophthalmology. 2008;246:1779-82.
12. Schneider U, Wagner AL, Kreissig I. Indocyanine green video-angiography of hemorrhagic retinal arterial macroaneurysms. Ophthalmologica. 1997;211:115-8.
13. Tsujikawa A, Sakamoto A, Ota M, et al. Retinal structural changes associated with retinal arterial macroaneurysm examined with optical coherence tomography. Retina. 2009;29:782-92.
14. Ohga H, Egi K, Katayama T, et al. A case of retinal macroaneurysm with congenital ocular toxoplasmosis. Folia Ophthalmology Jpn. 1990;41:898.
15. Panton RW, Goldberg MF, Farber MD. Retinal arterial macroaneurysms: risk factors and natural history. Br J Ophthalmology. 1990;74:595-600.
16. Palestine AG, Robertson DM, Goldstein BG. Macroaneurysms of the retinal arteries. Am J Ophthalmology. 1982;93:164-71.
17. McCabe C, Flynn HW, McLean WC, et al. Nonsurgical management of macular hemorrhage secondary to retinal artery macroaneurysms. Arch Ophthalmology. 2000;118:780-5.
18. Yang CS, Tsai DC, Lee FL, et al. Retinal arterial macroaneurysms: risk factors of poor visual outcome. Ophthalmologica. 2005;219:366-72.
19. Psinakis A, Kokolakis PG, Theodossiadis C, et al. Pulsatile retinal arterial macroaneurysm: treatment with argon laser photocoagulation. J Fr Ophtalmol. 1989;12:673-6.
20. Yokoi N, Tohsaka S, Yamamoto T. A case of pulsating retinal arterial macroaneurysm. Folia Ophthalmology Jpn. 1990;41:584.
21. Spalter HF. Retinal macroaneurysms: a new masquerade syndrome. Trans Am Ophthalmology Soc. 1982;80:113-30.
22. Schulman J, Jampol LM, Goldberg MF. Large capillary aneurysms secondary to retinal venous obstruction. Br J Ophthalmology. 1981;65:36-41.
23. Kimmel AS, Magargal LE, Morrison DL, et al. Temporal branch retinal vein obstruction masquerading as a retinal arterial macroaneurysm: the Bonnet sign. Ann Ophthalmology. 1989;21:251-2.
24. Nadel AJ, Gupta KK. Macroaneurysms of the retinal arteries. Arch Ophthalmology. 1976;94:1092-6.
25. Joondeph BC, Joondeph HC, Blair NP. Retinal macroaneurysms treated with the yellow dye laser. Retina. 1989;9:187-92.
26. Mainster MA, Whitacre MM. Dye yellow photocoagulation of retinal arterial macroaneurysms. Am J Ophthalmology. 1988;105:97-8.
27. Brown DM, Sobol WM, Folk JC, et al. Retinal arteriolar macroaneurysms: long-term visual outcome. Br J Ophthalmology. 1994;78:534-8.
28. Chaum E, Greenwald MA. Retinochoroidal anastomoses and a choroidal neovascular membrane in a macular exudate following treatment for retinal macroaneurysms. Retina. 2002;22:363-6.
29. Tassignon MJ, Stempels N, Van Mulders L. Retrohyaloid premacular hemorrhage treated by Q-switched Nd-YAG laser. Graefes Arch Clin Exp Ophthalmology. 1989;227:440-2.
30. Raymond LA. Neodymium:YAG laser treatment for hemorrhages under the internal limiting membrane and posterior hyaloid face in the macula. Ophthalmology. 1995;102:406-11.

31. Hanscom TA, Diddie KR. Early surgical drainage of macular subretinal hemorrhage. Arch Ophthalmology. 1987;105:1722-3.

32. Peyman GA, Nelson NC, Alturki W, et al. Tissue plasminogen activating factor assisted removal of subretinal hemorrhage. Ophthalmic Surg. 1991;22:575-82.

33. Moriarty AP, McAllister IL, Constable IJ. Initial clinical experience with tissue plasminogen activator (tPA) assisted removal of submacular hemorrhage. Eye (Lond). 1995;9:582-8.

34. Lim JI, Drews-Botsch C, Sternberg P Jr, et al. Submacular hemorrhage removal. Ophthalmology. 1995;102:1393-9.

35. Ibanez HE, Williams DF, Thomas MA, et al. Surgical management of subretinal hemorrhage. A series of 47 consecutive cases. Arch Ophthalmology. 1995;113:62-9.

36. Brent BD, Gonce M, Diamond JG. Pars plana vitrectomy for complications of retinal arterial macroaneurysms—a case series. Ophthalmic Surg. 1993;24:534-6.

37. Tsakpinis D, Nasr MB, Tranos P, et al. The use of bevacizumab in a multilevel retinal hemorrhage secondary to retinal macroaneurysm: a 39-month follow-up case report. Clin Ophthalmology. 2011;5:1475-7.

38. Pichi F, Morara M, Torrazza C, et al. Intravitreal bevacizumab for macular complications from retinal arterial macroaneurysms. Am J Ophthalmology. 2013;155:287-94.

Chapter 27

Diabetic Retinopathy: Epidemiology, Pathogenesis, Classification and Clinical Trials

Neha Goel, Vinod Kumar, Atul Kumar

EPIDEMIOLOGY

Diabetic retinopathy (DR) is the most common microvascular complication of diabetes mellitus (DM) and the leading cause of visual loss in working aged adults around the world.[1] Apart from the effects on vision, the presence of DR and diabetic macular edema (DME) is a marker of concomitant diabetes complications in other organ systems. Population-based epidemiologic data are important in developing approaches to preventing DR. Clinical trials over the past 30 years have provided data on the prevalence, incidence and natural history of DR, and its associated risk factors. Asia has emerged as the global epicenter of the diabetes epidemic, especially China and India.

PREVALENCE OF DIABETIC RETINOPATHY AND DIABETIC MACULAR EDEMA

Varying rates of prevalence of DR have been reported in population-based samples, depending on the population and study methodology. A pooled individual participant meta-analysis involving 35 studies conducted worldwide from 1980 to 2008, estimated that the overall prevalence of any DR was 35.4%, proliferative diabetic retinopathy (PDR) was 7.2%, DME was 7.4%, and vision-threatening diabetic retinopathy (VTDR) was 11.7% among individuals with diabetes.2 The prevalence estimates of any DR and VTDR were similar in men and women and were highest in African Americans and lowest in Asians. Prevalence rates were substantially higher in those with type 1 diabetes and increased with duration of diabetes, and values for glycated hemoglobin (HbA1c), blood pressure, and cholesterol.[2]

In a study conducted at Chennai, DR prevalence was reported to be higher in urban (18%)[3] compared to rural areas (10.8%),[4] possibly due to the increasing affluence accompanied by changes in diet in the urban regions and selective mortality of those with diabetes-related complications in rural regions because of poor access to healthcare.

INCIDENCE OF DIABETIC RETINOPATHY AND DIABETIC MACULAR EDEMA

Most population-based cohort studies that have investigated the incidence of DR are based in the United States of America (USA) or the United Kingdom (UK). In the USA, the Wisconsin Epidemiologic Study of Diabetic Retinopathy (WESDR) found that among patients presumed to have type 1 diabetes, the 4-year cumulative incidence of DR was 59.0%.[5] At 10 years and 25 years, the cumulative incidence of DR rose to 89.3% and 97%, respectively.[6,7] However, the participants of this study were recruited between 1979 and 1980, thus the incidence today might be lower owing to advances in diagnostic techniques for DR and risk factor management in the last 3 decades. About 20% of type 1 diabetes and 14–25% of type 2 diabetes developed DME over a 10-year follow-up period.[8]

Data from the annual diabetic retinopathy screening program in England showed that the 5-year cumulative incidences of any DR, PDR and clinically significant DME were 36%, 0.7% and 0.6% among people with type 2 diabetes who were free of retinopathy at baseline. After 10 years of follow-up, the respective cumulative incidences rose to 66%, 1.5% and 1.2%.[9]

PROGRESSION AND REGRESSION OF DIABETIC RETINOPATHY

Several cohort studies have investigated the progression and regression of DR. Progression was more common than regression. Four to six year cumulative incidence of 2-step progression among the studies ranged from 24.1% to 38.9%, which increased to 64.1% and 83.1% in studies with 16-year or 25-year follow-up.[10]

While there is evidence that the prevalence and incidence of severe DR, including PDR and DME, may be decreasing in people more recently diagnosed with type 1 diabetes as a result of improved diabetes management, there is less certainty as to whether there has been a similar decline in type 2 diabetics.[11]

Table 27.1: Risk factors for diabetic retinopathy.

Nonmodifiable	Puberty, pregnancy
Modifiable	Hyperglycemia, dyslipidemia, obesity, hypertension
Novel	Apolipoprotein, inflammation, hormones, oxidative stress, vitamin D, genetic factors

RISK FACTORS

Risk Factors for Diabetic Retinopathy and Diabetic Macular Edema (Table 27.1)

Nonmodifiable Risk Factors

- *Puberty*: It is a well-established risk factor for type 1 diabetes mellitus. While prepubertal years of diabetes exposure may contribute to added risk of DR,[12] progression of DR may be more rapid in the postpubertal years.[13]
- *Pregnancy*: Both DR and DME are known to progress during pregnancy, especially in type 1 diabetics. But the changes regress in the postpartum period without any long-term consequences.[14]

Modifiable Risk Factors

- *Hyperglycemia*: The level of glycemic control is one of the most important predictive factors for DR and DME. Diabetes Control and Complications Trial (DCCT, type 1 DM) and the United Kingdom Prospective Diabetes Study (UKPDS, type 2 DM) are landmark clinical trials which provide strong evidence of reducing the risk of development and progression of retinopathy with tighter blood sugar control (HbA1c less than or equal to 7%).[15] The DCCT showed almost three-fourth reduction in incidence of DR and 54% reduction in progression from early to advanced stages.[16] There was 46% reduction in the incidence of DME compared to the conventional group.[17] Although there is a small risk of early worsening in DR in the first year of treatment, the overall long-term beneficial effects of intensive treatment outweigh this risk. Glycemic control should be achieved early in the disease course and maintained for as long as possible, since its protective effect is sustained even if tight glycemic control is lost. This is the "metabolic memory" effect observed after the DCCT.

  However, in the Action in Diabetes and Vascular Disease (ADVANCE)[18] and Action to Control Cardiovascular Risk in Diabetes (ACCORD)[19] trials, aggressive glycemic control (HbA1c <6.5%) was not found to significantly reduce the risk of DR development or progression in type 2 DM. In ACCORD, it was found that such an aggressive glycemic control might in fact be associated with increased mortality.

- *Hypertension*: Epidemiologic studies support hypertension as an important modifiable risk factor for DR and DME. In the UKPDS, tight blood pressure control (defined as target blood pressure <150/85 mm Hg) in patients with type 2 DM reduced the rate of progression of DR by 34%, and the risk of deterioration of visual acuity by 47%.[20] However, unlike hyperglycemia, the protective effect of blood pressure control waned quickly upon stopping intensive control.
- *Dyslipidemia*: Results of population-based studies regarding the role of dyslipidemia in DR are inconclusive, with no single lipid measure being consistently associated with DR. A large clinical trial of the Fenofibrate Intervention and Event Lowering in Diabetes (FIELD) study showed that fenofibrate, a lipid modifying agent, reduced the frequency for laser treatment for DME by 31% and for PDR by 30% in patients with type 2 DM.[21] Patients with DR benefit most from fibrate therapy if they have hypertriglyceridemia and low serum high-density lipoprotein (HDL)-cholesterol, and hence treatment can be justified in this subset of patients, with the hopes of slowing progression to PDR.
- *Obesity*: The influence of obesity on DR has been well studied but with conflicting results. In the EURODIAB Prospective Complications Study of individuals with type 1 diabetes, larger waist-to-hip ratio was associated with incidence of DR after more than 7 years of follow-up.[22] In contrast, a cross-sectional study in type 2 diabetes, performed in Asia, found an inverse relationship between obesity and DR.[23] To explain this discrepancy, it has been postulated that weight loss may be a feature of advanced and severe type 2 diabetes, hence, the observation that nonobese type 2 diabetics have greater risk of DR.

Novel Risk Factors

- *Apolipoproteins*: Apolipoprotein A1 (Apo-A1) is an HDL constituent while apolipoprotein B (Apo-B) is present in low-density lipoprotein (LDL), very low-density lipoprotein (VLDL), intermediate-density lipoprotein, and lipoprotein (a). Both these are independent of the prandial status and may be more relevant to the biophysical changes in DR than conventional lipids. It has been shown that the Apo-A1 level was inversely associated with the presence and severity of DR, whereas Apo-B and the Apo-B/Apo-A1 ratio were positively associated with DR.[24] Further population-based longitudinal studies are required to state if these can replace traditional lipid measures as biomarkers of DR.
- *Inflammatory factors*: Retinal and vitreous inflammation has been observed in diabetes, both in animal models and in human studies, where levels of cytokines, chemokines, and adhesion molecules have been found to be elevated in the vitreous and serum of patients with DR.[25] Studies have shown the association between systemic inflammatory markers and risk of DR to be inconsistent.[1] Local

retinal inflammation forms the basis of intravitreal administration of corticosteroids.

- *Metabolic hormones*: Leptin and adiponectin have been implicated as potential risk factors in DR. Although these hormones are secreted by adipocytes which are known to regulate energy balance in the body, leptin has been shown to upregulate vascular endothelial growth factor (VEGF) permeability and adiponectin downregulates the VEGF.[10]
- *Oxidative stress*: Accumulation of free radicals has been linked to several histopathological changes of DR by causing oxidative damage to cells. Markers of oxidative stress markers like lipid peroxide (LPO) could be used as measures of disease severity and prognosis.[10] Oxidative stress leads to activation of multiple pathways simultaneously so treatment targeted towards a specific pathway would be ineffective.
- *Vitamin D*: Other than regulating calcium metabolism, vitamin D also has anti-inflammatory and anti-angiogenic actions. Subsequently, vitamin D deficiency has been found to be associated with increased severity of DR in cross-sectional studies.[26,27]
- *Genetic factors*: Disparity in the risk and severity of DR between different ethnic groups after controlling for diverse environmental attributes indicates a genetic predisposition in the development of DR. Various studies including DCCT have shown severe retinopathy to have a heritable tendency in both type 1 and type 2 diabetes mellitus independent of other risk factors.[28] Predisposing genes for DR are human leukocyte antigen-DR 3/0

and 4/0, *VEGF* gene on chromosome 6, aldose reductase gene (type 2 DM) while *RAGE* gene was associated with reduced risk.

PATHOPHYSIOLOGY OF DIABETIC RETINOPATHY

Diabetes mellitus has been recognized as a global epidemic and DR, one of the commonest microvascular complications of diabetes, has become a significant global public health and economic problem. It is imperative to understand the pathophysiology of DR (Flowchart 27.1) in order to develop newer therapeutic modalities for the treatment of DR, especially vision-threatening DR.

Pathways of Hyperglycemia-induced Damage

Hyperglycemia is a critical factor in the development and progression of DR, as demonstrated by the DCCT and UKPDS;[15-17] however, the exact mechanism remains unclear. Several inter-related biochemical pathways have been proposed as links between hyperglycemia and DR.

- *Polyol pathway*: It is a two-step metabolic pathway in which glucose is reduced to sorbitol by aldose reductase, which is the rate-limiting enzyme. Sorbitol is then converted to fructose (Flowchart 27.2).

  In both humans and experimental animals, all retinal cell types known to be affected by diabetes contain aldose reductase and increased aldose reductase activity is involved in the destruction of these cells. Metabolism through this pathway is accelerated by elevated cytoplasmic glucose concentrations induced by hyperglycemia. Sorbitol being impermeable to cell membranes gets accumulated within the retinal cells, leading to osmotic damage.[29] Reduction of glucose to sorbitol also consumes nicotinamide adenine dinucleotide phosphate (NADPH), since NADPH is required for regeneration of reduced glutathione which could exacerbate oxidative stress.[30]

  The administration of aldose reductase inhibitors (ARIs) to animal models of diabetes at the onset of diabetes has demonstrated some benefit in preventing DR;

Flowchart 27.1: Pathogenesis of diabetic retinopathy.

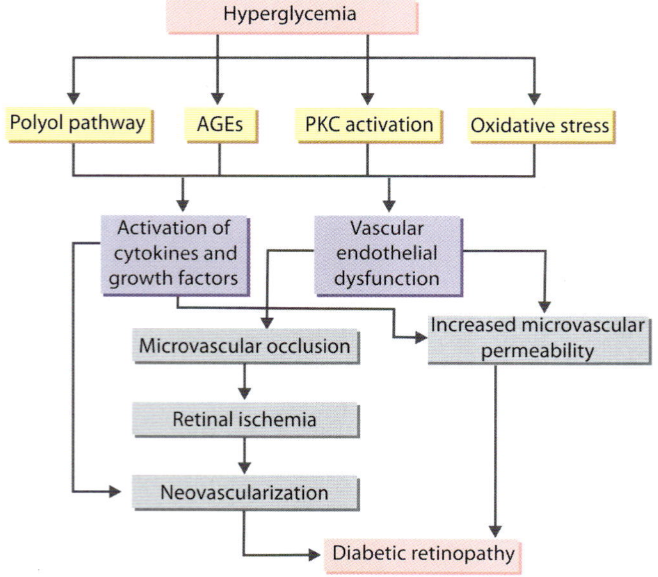

(AGEs: Advanced glycation end products; PKC: Protein kinase C).

Flowchart 27.2: Polyol pathway.

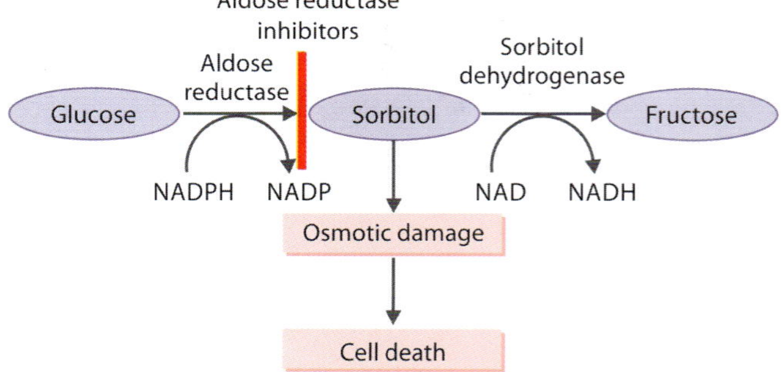

Flowchart 27.3: Advanced glycation end products (AGEs) formation.

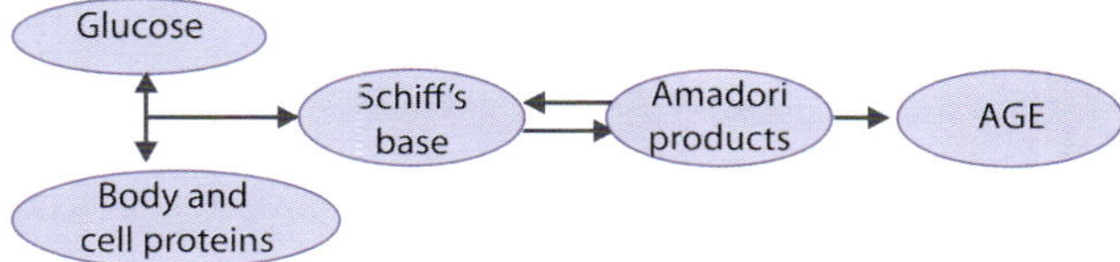

Flowchart 27.4: Protein kinase C (PKC) activation.

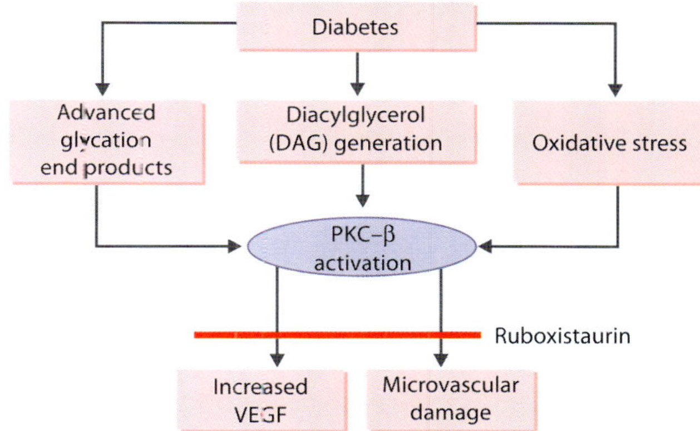

(VEGF: Vascular endothelial growth factor)

however, ARI clinical trials, such as the sorbinil retinopathy trial, have shown little clinical benefit.[31]

- *Nonenzymatic protein glycation*: Advanced glycation end products (AGEs) result from the nonenzymatic reaction of reducing sugars with free amino groups of proteins, lipids, and nucleic acids (Flowchart 27.3). Increased availability of glucose in diabetes accelerates their formation and levels in retinal blood vessels.

  Advanced glycation end product formation and activation of AGE receptors (RAGE) represent a key pathogenic mechanism in DR. Crosslinking by AGEs modify extracellular matrix proteins and alter their function. Interaction of AGEs with RAGE leads to cellular activation and pro-oxidant, proinflammatory events. The AGE inhibitor aminoguanidine has been shown to partially prevent microvascular damage in animal models and lowered urinary protein and slowed progression of DR in humans.[32]

- *Protein kinase C activation*: The protein kinase C (PKC) molecule is a serine/threonine kinase involved in signal transduction (Flowchart 27.4). Conventional and novel PKC isoforms are upregulated by diacylglycerol (DAG), which in turn is increased by intracellular hyperglycemia. In the retina, PKC-β activation leads to basement membrane and extracellular matrix alterations within the vasculature, increase in vascular permeability, enhanced release of angiogenic factors, endothelial and leukocyte dysfunction leading to capillary occlusion and leukostasis, and changes in blood flow to the retina.[33]

  Oral Ruboxistaurin mesylate, a specific inhibitor of PKC-β, has undergone phase 3 clinical trials in the PKC DR study (PKCDRS; 2005) and the Diabetic Macular Edema Study (PKCDMES, 2007). These studies reported that although PKC inhibition did not prevent DR, it significantly reduced the loss of vision and need for laser.[34]

- *Oxidative stress*: An increase in the steady state levels of reactive oxygen species (ROS) or a decrease in activity of endogenous enzymes that counter the oxidative stress such as superoxide dismutase (SOD), catalase, and glutathione peroxidase (GSH-Px) leads to cell and tissue damage. Oxidative stress induced by hyperglycemia is thought to be the key event in the pathogenesis of DR. Decreased levels of these endogenous enzymes have been seen in both clinical and experimental diabetes.[35]

Pathophysiological Process in Diabetic Retinopathy

The onset of DR is characterized by morphologic alterations of the small vessels, with early and selective loss of pericyte, thickening of the basement membrane, loss of inter-endothelial tight junctions, together with increased vascular permeability, capillary occlusions, microaneurysms and, later loss of endothelial cells. These changes are important, as they may be amenable to therapeutic interventions.

- *Pericyte loss*: Retinal pericyte control endothelial proliferation and the tightness of the blood retinal barrier, thus providing vascular stability. Retinal capillary coverage with pericyte is crucial for the survival of endothelial cells, particularly under stress conditions such as DM. Pericyte loss is considered one of the hallmarks of early DR. Hyperglycemia induces up regulation of angiopoietin-2 (Ang-2) which inhibits the pericyte-recruiting function of angiopoietin-1 (Ang-1). This suggests a novel, active, mechanism in pericyte loss rather than a passive mechanism in which pericyte loss is the result of toxic product accumulation and induction of destructive cellular signals generated within the pericyte.[36]

- *Capillary dropout*: Capillary dropout is a critical process in DR occurring due to functional derangement and structural changes in the retinal microvasculature, resulting in ischemia and release of angiogenic growth factors. Retinal ischemia in diabetes is postulated to occur by several mechanisms.[37]

  - *Retinal endothelial basement membrane thickening*: Early hyperglycemia causes an increase in the synthesis of basement membrane components in the retina.[38] At advanced stages, with the appearance of DR, there are qualitative alterations of specific basement membrane markers.

  - *Platelet aggregation*: Chronic hyperglycemia, via activation of PKC, causes production of platelet-activating factor (PAF) and subsequent increase in platelet-fibrin thrombi in the retinal capillaries compared to normal.[37]

- *Leukocyte activation/adherence:* Leukocytes are found to adhere to the retinal vascular endothelium early in experimental DR, although DR per se is not an inflammatory disease. Leukocytes are activated by PAF; β2 integrins present on activated leukocytes help them to adhere tightly to the endothelial cell via binding intercellular adhesion molecule-1 (ICAM-1).[39]

- *Angiogenesis:* It refers to the formation of new blood vessels from existing vessels. It occurs through a multistep process, including production of angiogenic growth factors by diseased tissue, binding of angiogenic growth factors to receptors on existing vascular endothelial cells (EC), activation of EC gene expression of pro-angiogenic molecules, EC invasion of surrounding tissue, *EC* migration and proliferation, formation of vascular tubes by EC, and stabilization of new blood vessels by mural cells. Each of these steps is potentially vulnerable to pharmacologic targeting, and antiangiogenic therapies directed at various steps are under investigation.

ROLE OF GROWTH FACTORS IN DIABETIC RETINOPATHY

A plethora of growth factors have been implicated in the development and progression of DR through regulation of the retinal vasculature. While these growth factors may act alone, more commonly, there is synergy between them and they interact with each other. Knockout studies have shown if a growth factor is deficient, then other growth factors are secreted to provide similar function.[37]

- *Vascular endothelial growth factor:* VEGF has potent angiogenic activity vasopermeability leading to the development of therapies targeting this growth factor. VEGF is physiologically required for regulating proliferation and assembling of EC, during vasculogenesis, as well as for their maintenance and survival throughout the lifetime of blood vessels. However, in diabetes, ischemia, oxidative stress and overactivation of PKC upregulate the expression of VEGF, leading to various pathological demonstrations such as angiogenesis, increased permeability of endothelium, decreased inhibition of proapoptotic proteins and activation of various other inflammatory mediators.[40]

  Vascular endothelial growth factor exerts its functions on EC via interaction with cellular receptors Flt-1 (VEGFR-1) and Flk-1/KDR (VEGFR-2), which are both receptor tyrosine kinases. This interaction initiates a signal transduction pathway leading to phosphorylation of proteins downstream in EC and inducing subsequent changes. While Flt-1 activation regulates metabolism of a large variety of cells, KDR specifically regulates the migration and proliferation of endothelial cells.[37]

  High levels of VEGF is seen in patients with PDR; however, it is also known to act in the pathophysiology of nonproliferative diabetic retinopathy (NPDR) causing increased vascular permeability, leakage and macular edema.

- *Other angiogenic factors:* Some other angiogenic factors have also been implicated in driving the retinal neovascularization. These growth factors might potentially have synergistic effects with VEGF or act at different steps in the neovascular process. These factors are briefly described below:

  - *Platelet-derived growth factor (PDGF):* It is strongly driven by retinal ischemia.[41] PDGF has been shown to promote migration and proliferation of EC along with an increase in the recruitment of pericytes, thus playing a key role in the angiogenesis cascade. PDGF also causes proliferation of vascularized connective tissue which can also be seen in retinal ischemia in the form of fibrovascular membranes.

  - *Basic fibroblast growth factors (bFGF or FGF2):* It acts indirectly by regulating the action of VEGF in retinal vascular cells.[37]

  - *Insulin-like growth factor-1 (IGF-1):* It binds to IGF-1 receptor (IGF-1R) on EC and induces all steps of angiogenesis.[37]

  - *Hepatocyte growth factor/scatter factor (HGF/SF):* It can also induce VEGF production and it seen to significantly increase in the vitreous of diabetics compared to normal controls.[37]

  - *Placenta growth factor (PIGF):* It is a member of the VEGF family, but binds only to VEGFR-1. In PDR, PIGF potentiates the effect of VEGF either via enhancing expression of VEGF or by forming a heterodimer with VEGF.[42]

  - *Erythropoietin:* It shows angiogenic activity in vascular endothelial cells by stimulating cell proliferation and migration through erythropoietin receptors expressed in these cells. Vitreous erythropoietin level has been found to be significantly higher among patients with PDR compared to those without diabetes.

  - *Angiopoietin-2:* It is shown to be upregulated during retinal development when angiogenesis occurs, thus it helps in vascular remodeling.

  - *Antiangiogenic factors:* Angiogenic and antiangiogenic factors interplay to maintain a guarded equilibrium in the normal physiology of the retinal vasculature. This balance is affected when the angiogenic factors outweigh endogenous inhibitors of angiogenesis in response to a pathological stimulus.

Pigment epithelium-derived factor (PEDF) inhibits neovascularization by promoting apoptosis of endothelial cells. It is downregulated in PDR.[43]

Thus, VEGF is well-recognized as a major stimulus in retinal neovascularization, and therapies directed against VEGF are currently being developed and used. However, a greater understanding of additional molecules regulating retinal neovascularization is emerging and the development of therapeutic strategies targeting these molecules may result in additional treatments for retinal neovascularization in DR.

CLINICAL TRIALS

In this era of evidence-based medicine, the impact of clinical trials on patient care cannot be underestimated. A large number of clinical trials have been conducted related to epidemiology and management of DR that shape current clinical practice in this field. The landmark clinical trials are briefly discussed below:

Clinical Trials Relating to Epidemiology of Diabetic Retinopathy

The DCCT[16] studied in patients with type 1 diabetes the effect of tight glycemic control on microvascular complications of diabetes. It recruited 1,441 patients and was done from 1983 to 1993. At baseline, 726 patients with no DR (the primary-prevention cohort) and 715 patients with mild DR (the secondary-intervention cohort) were randomly assigned to conventional or intensive therapy and followed for a mean of 6.5 years. The study found that the risk of developing DR in primary prevention group decreased by 76% in the intensive therapy (mean HbA1c 7.2%) as compared to the conventional therapy group. In the primary prevention cohort, intensive therapy reduced the risk for the development of DR by 76% as compared with conventional therapy (mean HbA1c 9.0%). In the secondary intervention cohort, intensive therapy slowed the progression of DR by 54% by intensive therapy and there was 47% reduction in development of proliferative or severe nonproliferative DR. The Epidemiology of Diabetes Interventions and Complications (EDIC)[44] determined the long-term effects of control of glycemic levels on micro- and macrovascular outcomes in the DCCT cohort of more than 1,400 patients followed up for 10 years. It showed no significant difference in mean HbA1c levels (8.07% vs 7.98%) between the original treatment groups. However, the former intensive group had significantly lower incidences of further retinopathy progression as compared to conventional group. Thus, difference in DR progression between the groups (metabolic memory) continues for at least 10 years but may be waning.

The United Kingdom Prospective Diabetes Study (UKPDS)[45]

The UKPDS was a prospective, multicenter cohort study, held across 23 hospitals in the UK over 20 years, examining the rates of micro- and macrovascular complications in patients with recently diagnosed type 2 diabetes mellitus in 1976.

It was designed to determine whether intensive blood glucose control can decrease, to determine whether the risk of macrovascular and microvascular complications in type 2 diabetes and whether intensive blood pressure control can reduce the complications in patients with hypertension. A total of 5,102 people with newly diagnosed type 2 diabetes were enrolled from 1977 to 1991.

- *Effect of initial retinopathy*: There was an "almost-linear" relationship between the initial number of microaneu- rysms and the risk of subsequent endpoints, i.e. photo- coagulation, cataract surgery, and vitreous hemorrhage.
- *Effect of initial glucose levels*: Patients with higher glucose levels (measured by HbA1c) at the beginning of the trial were more likely to have retinopathy. A 31% lowering of risk of retinopathy was seen with every 1% decrease in HbA1c level.
- *Effect of blood pressure control*: Hypertensive patients with type 2 diabetes were randomized to less tight (180/105 mm Hg) and tight blood pressure control (150/85 mm Hg). Patients assigned to tight control had a 34% reduction in progression of retinopathy and a 47% reduced risk of deterioration in visual acuity of three lines compared with the less tight control group.
- *Effect of glycemic control*: The progression of diabetic retinopathy was reduced by 21% and the need for laser photocoagulation by 29% in the intensive versus the con- ventional treatment group.

Importance of study: It established the importance of both good glycemic control and good blood pressure control in type 2 diabetics in reducing progression of diabetic retinopathy.

By better blood pressure control, almost a 33% reduction in risk occurs from death from long-term complications of diabetes, strokes and serious deterioration of vision. It also retards small blood vessel disease progression occurring in diabetics.

Action to Control Cardiovascular Risk in Diabetes Study

The ACCORD study was a randomized, controlled clinical trial (n = 10,251) from 2003 to 2009 that evaluated effect of intensive lowering of blood glucose, blood pressure and lipid lowering on cardiovascular disease (CVD) in patients with type 2 diabetes who had either established CVD or additional risk factors. HbA1c target in the intensive group was less than 6% and 7–7.9% in the control group. These participants were then enrolled into a lipid-lowering or blood-pressure lowering study. Over 10,000 patients were randomized to intensive glycemic control (targeting a glycosylated hemoglobin level below 6.0%) versus standard glycemic control (targeting a level from 7.0% to 7.9%). Half of them entered the blood pressure arm of the trial and were randomized to intensive blood pressure control, targeting a systolic pressure of less than 120 mm Hg or standard blood pressure control, targeting a systolic pressure of less than 140 mm Hg. The other half had a further randomization of the lipid arm of the trial to statins alone or statins plus fenofibrate. Thus, there were three trials within the ACCORD trial—the glycemia trial, the blood pressure trial, and the lipid trial. The original aim of the trial was to run for approximately 5 years, but the trial was stopped after 3.5 years in the intensive glycemia group because it found that the use of intensive therapy to target normal glycosylated hemoglobin levels increased mortality and did not significantly reduce major cardiovascular events.[19] The blood pressure trial found that targeting a systolic blood pressure of less than 120 mm Hg, as compared with less than 140 mm Hg, did not reduce the rate of a composite outcome of fatal and nonfatal major cardiovascular events.[46] The lipid trial concluded that the combination of fenofibrate and simvastatin did not reduce the rate of major cardiovascular events as compared with simvastatin alone.[47]

The results of the ACCORD eye study were published in the New England Journal of Medicine.[48] Intensive control decreased the progression of diabetic retinopathy from 10.4% to 7.3% over 4 years compared with standard treatment. Combination lipid therapy with fenofibrate plus simvastatin also reduced disease progression from 10.2% to 6.5% over 4 years compared to simvastatin therapy alone.

Although, in the blood pressure control arm of the study no difference in progression of diabetic retinopathy was seen between the groups, it is important to consider the differences between the ACCORD Eye Study population and the participants in the UKPDS and the target blood pressures. The UKPDS participants were newly diagnosed with diabetes without any established cardiovascular risk factors or lipid abnormalities while the ACCORD study population was older and at greater cardiovascular risk.

Action to Control Cardiovascular Risk in Diabetes Follow-On (ACCORDION) Eye Study Group

This follow on study post ACCORD study (2010–2014)[49] done in 1,310 participants included in the study, showed that diabetic retinopathy progressed in 5.8% with intensive glycemic treatment versus 12.7% with standard (95% CI 0.28–0.63, P <0.0001), 7.5% with intensive blood pressure treatment versus 6.0% for standard (95% CI 0.61–2.40, P = 0.59), and 11.8% with fenofibrate versus 10.2% with placebo (95% CI 0.71–1.79, P = 0.60).

Hence, tight glycemic control was beneficial in halting progression of retinopathy, though tight blood pressure and use of fenofibrate was not helpful.

Clinical Trials Relating to Classification and Management of Diabetic Retinopathy

The *Diabetic Retinopathy Study (DRS)*[50] was designed to determine if photocoagulation helps in preventing severe visual loss from PDR and to determine, if difference exists in the efficacy and safety of argon versus xenon photocoagulation for PDR. There were 1,758 patients who enrolled at 15 centers between 1972 and 1975. Patients were eligible, if they had best corrected visual acuity of 20/100 or better in each eye and the presence of PDR in at least one eye or severe NPDR in both eyes. The primary outcome measure was the development of severe vision loss (SVL), defined as visual acuity less than 5/200 at two consecutively completed 4-monthly follow-up visits. Both argon and xenon photocoagulation reduced the risk of SVL by 50% or more compared with no treatment. Based on this result, in 1976, the DRS protocol was modified to allow

eyes randomized to indefinite deferral of photocoagulation to receive photocoagulation. The study identified a stage of retinopathy, termed high-risk PDR, where the benefits of photocoagulation definitely outweighed the risks. No clear benefit was demonstrated for panretinal photocoagulation (PRP) in eyes with severe NPDR or in eyes with PDR without high-risk characteristics.

The *Diabetic Retinopathy Vitrectomy Study (DRVS)*[51,52] consisted of three arms which recruited patients between 1976 and 1983.

- *Group H*: Early vitrectomy for severe vitreous hemorrhage—616 patients who had SVL from recent (within 6 months prior to randomization) severe vitreous hemorrhage in at least one eye were randomly assigned either to early vitrectomy or to conventional management (vitrectomy carried out 1 year later, if hemorrhage persisted). It was found that early vitrectomy provided a greater chance of prompt recovery of visual acuity, especially in type 1 diabetics and if vision is poor in the fellow eye; although greater early risk of visual acuity of no light perception must be kept in mind.
- *Group N*: Course of visual acuity in severe PDR with conventional management—A total of 744 eyes of 622 patients with severe PDR were enrolled and followed over a 2-year period to determine their visual outcome.
- *Group NR*: Early vitrectomy for severe PDR in eyes with useful vision—381 patients were recruited from Group N, all of whom had extensive active neovascular or fibrovascular proliferations and visual acuity of 10/200 or better at least in one eye and assigned either to early vitrectomy or to conventional management (photocoagulation when indicated, with vitrectomy, if a severe vitreous hemorrhage occurred and failed to clear spontaneously during a 6-month waiting period or if retinal detachment involving the center of the macula occurred). It concluded that early vitrectomy is of benefit especially in those with both fibrous proliferations and at least moderately severe new vessels; in which extensive scatter photocoagulation has been carried out or is precluded by vitreous hemorrhage.

The *Early Treatment Diabetic Retinopathy Study (ETDRS)*[53,54] was a multi-center, randomized clinical trial designed to evaluate argon laser photocoagulation and aspirin treatment in the management of patients with moderate or severe NPDR or early PDR, issues that were not addressed by the DRS. A total of 3,711 patients were recruited between 1979 to 1985 and were to be followed for a minimum of 4 years.

- Eyes with moderate to severe NPDR or early PDR and no macular edema had one eye randomly assigned to immediate photocoagulation (further randomized to either full scatter or mild scatter PRP) and the other eye to deferral of photocoagulation (careful follow-up) until high-risk PDR developed. Results showed that scatter treatment is not indicated for eyes with mild-to-moderate NPDR, provided that careful follow-up could be maintained. As the retinopathy progresses to the severe NPDR or early PDR, scatter treatment should be considered, especially for patients with type 2 diabetes and it should be performed without delay for virtually all eyes with high-risk PDR.

- Eyes with diabetic macular edema and "less severe" retinopathy (mild or moderate NPDR) were assigned to immediate or deferred focal photocoagulation (direct laser for focal leaks and grid laser for diffuse leaks) with immediate or deferred mild scatter PRP. The most effective strategy was found to be immediate focal with delayed scatter initiated only when more severe retinopathy developed. Eyes with diabetic macular edema and "more severe" retinopathy (severe NPDR or early PDR) were assigned to immediate or deferred focal photocoagulation, with immediate mild scatter or full scatter PRP. The most effective strategy was found to be immediate focal combined with immediate mild scatter. The worst outcome strategy involved immediate full-scatter photocoagulation and deferred focal.
- Focal photocoagulation reduced the risk of moderate vision loss (defined as doubling of visual angle) by 50% or more and increased the chance of a small improvement in visual acuity, especially for those eyes with macular edema that involved or threatened the center of the macula. The principal benefit of focal treatment in clinically significant macular edema (CSME) was to reduce the risk of further visual loss rather than to improve vision.
- The trial use of aspirin therapy was based on clinical observation and on aspirin's possible mechanisms of action. Patients were assigned randomly to aspirin (650 mg daily) or placebo. It was found that aspirin had no clinically important beneficial effect on the progression of DR.

Diabetic Retinopathy Clinical Research Network (DRCR.net)

The DRCR Network (DRCR.net) is a collaborative network dedicated to facilitating multicenter clinical research of diabetic retinopathy, age-related macular degeneration (AMD), hereditary retinal degenerations and other retinal diseases. Principal emphasis is placed on clinical trials, but epidemiologic outcomes and other research may be supported as well. The DRCR.net was formed in September 2002 and currently includes over 115 participating sites with over 400 physicians throughout the United States.

The DRCR.net is funded by the National Eye Institute (NEI). The NEI is a part of the National Institutes of Health, which is the branch of government that funds medical research.

Its main protocols and their clinical relevance are described below:

PROTOCOL A[55] was a pilot study of laser photocoagulation for DME. It found that the current modified ETDRS (mETDRS) technique was more effective in reducing retinal thickening than a mild macular grid (MMG) technique, and should continue to be the standard approach.

PROTOCOL B[56] was a randomized trial comparing 1 mg and 4 mg doses of intravitreal triamcinolone acetonide (IVTA) and focal/grid photocoagulation (LP) for DME. It concluded that over a 2-year as well as 3-year period, LP was more effective and had fewer side effects than 1 mg or 4 mg doses of IVTA for most patients with DME.

PROTOCOL C[57] was designed to evaluate diurnal variation in optical coherence tomography (OCT) measuring retinal thickness in center involving DME. It found that most eyes with DME had little meaningful change in OCT central macular thickness (CMT) between 8 am and 4 pm.

PROTOCOL D[58] was to evaluate vitrectomy for DME in eyes with at least moderate vision loss and vitreomacular traction (VMT). Following vitrectomy, retinal thickening was reduced in most eyes. Between 28% and 49% of eyes were likely to have improvement of visual acuity, while between 13% and 31% are likely to have worsening. The results suggested that removal of epiretinal membrane (ERM) might favorably affect visual outcome after vitrectomy.

PROTOCOL E[59] was a randomized trial to provide data on the safety and efficacy of anterior or posterior subtenon's injections of triamcinolone acetonide (TA) either alone or in combination with focal photocoagulation in the treatment of mild DME. Results indicated that in cases of DME with good visual acuity, peribulbar TA, with or without focal photocoagulation, is unlikely to be of substantial benefit.

PROTOCOL F[60] was an observational study of the development of DME following scatter laser photocoagulation. It compared the effects of single-sitting versus four-sitting PRP on macular edema in subjects with severe NPDR or early PDR with relatively good visual acuity and no or mild center involved macular edema and found that clinically meaningful differences are unlikely in OCT thickness or visual acuity between the two groups.\

PROTOCOL G,[61] the subclinical DME study, determined the rate of progression of eyes with subclinical DME to clinically apparent DME or DME necessitating treatment during a 2-year period. Results indicated that the cumulative probability of meeting an increase in OCT CMT of at least 50 µm from baseline and a CMT of at least 300 µm, or treatment for DME was 27% by 1 year and 38% by 2 years. Thus, patients with subclinical DME should be monitored more closely for progression.

PROTOCOL H[62] was a phase 2 randomized clinical trial of intravitreal bevacizumab (IVB) for DME and demonstrated that IVB can reduce DME in some eyes, but the study was not designed to determine whether treatment is beneficial.

PROTOCOL I:[63] This study aimed at evaluating intravitreal 0.5 mg ranibizumab or 4 mg IVTA combined with focal/grid laser compared with focal/grid laser alone for treatment of DME involving the fovea. It enrolled 854 eyes of 691 participants with visual acuity of 20/32 to 20/320 that were randomized to sham injection + prompt laser (n = 293), 0.5 mg ranibizumab + prompt laser (n = 187), 0.5 mg ranibizumab + deferred (≥24 weeks) laser (n = 188), or 4 mg IVTA + prompt laser (n = 186). (Prompt laser was defined as being done 3–10 days post intravitreal injection, while deferred laser was ≥ 24 weeks post-intravitreal injection of either ranibizumab or IVTA).

It was found that intravitreal ranibizumab was more effective in treating DME involving center of macular compared to laser alone. In pseudophakic eyes, intravitreal triamcinolone along with prompt laser was more effective than laser alone but there was a risk of increase in intraocular pressure with triamcinolone.

PROTOCOL J[64] was titled Laser-Ranibizumab-Triamcinolone Study for DME + PRP. Its purpose was to evaluate the effects of intravitreal ranibizumab or TA in eyes receiving LP for DME and PRP. Mean changes in visual acuity from baseline were significantly better in the ranibizumab and triamcinolone groups compared with those in the sham group at the 14-week visit, mirroring retinal thickening results. Thus, the addition of 1 IVTA or 2 ranibizumab injections in eyes receiving LP for DME and PRP is associated with better visual acuity and decreased DME by 14 weeks.

PROTOCOL K[65] studied the course of response to focal photocoagulation for DME. It determined whether eyes with center involved DME, treated with LP, in which there is a reduction in CMT measured with OCT after 16 weeks, would continue to improve, if retreatment is deferred and found that 23% to 63% will continue to improve without additional treatment.

PROTOCOL L[66] compared visual acuity scores after auto-refraction versus research protocol manual refraction in diabetic patients with a wide range of visual acuity. It confirmed that with current instruments, autorefraction is not an acceptable substitute for manual refraction for most clinical trials with primary outcomes dependent on best-corrected visual acuity.

PROTOCOL M[67] was titled the Diabetes Education Study. It determined whether the point-of-care measurement of HbA1c and personalized diabetes risk assessments performed during retinal ophthalmologic visits improve glycemic control as assessed by HbA1c level. The study found that the addition of personalized education and risk assessment during retinal ophthalmologic visits did not result in a reduction in HbA1c level compared with usual care over 1 year.

PROTOCOL N[68] evaluated intravitreal ranibizumab compared with intravitreal saline injections on vitrectomy rates for vitreous hemorrhage from PDR. The cumulative probability of vitrectomy within 16 weeks was low in both groups. Short-term secondary outcomes including visual acuity improvement, increased PRP completion rates, and reduced recurrent vitreous hemorrhage rates suggested biologic activity of ranibizumab, however, long-term benefits remained unknown.

PROTOCOL O[69] evaluated reproducibility of retinal thickness measurements from OCT images obtained by time domain (TD) (Zeiss Stratus) and spectral-domain (SD) (Zeiss Cirrus and Heidelberg Spectralis) instruments and formulated equations to convert retinal thickness measurements from SD-OCT to equivalent values on TD-OCT. Reproducibility appeared better on Spectralis than Cirrus and Stratus. RTVue thickness reproducibility appeared similar to Stratus. Central subfield thickness changes greater than 10% when using the same machine or 20% when switching after conversion to equivalents were likely due to a true change beyond measurement error.

PROTOCOL P[70] was titled Cataract Surgery with Center-Involved DME Study. Low recruitment and heterogeneous pre- and postsurgical macular edema management in a cohort with DME limit definitive conclusions from this study.

PROTOCOL Q[71] was titled Cataract Surgery without Center-Involved DME Study. It estimated the incidence of central-involved macular edema at 16 weeks following cataract surgery in eyes with DR without definite central-involved DME preoperatively. The study concluded that in eyes with DR without concurrent central-involved DME, presence of noncentral DME immediately prior to cataract surgery, or history of DME treatment, might increase risk of developing central-involved macular edema 16 weeks after cataract extraction.

PROTOCOL R[72] was a phase 2 study to evaluate the effect of a topical, nonsteroidal anti-inflammatory drug, Nepafenac 0.1% 3 times a day for 12 months, in eyes with noncentral DME and good visual acuity. No meaningful effect on OCT-measured retinal thickness was found.

PROTOCOL S:[73] Untreated, PDR is a leading cause of blindness in the diabetic population. PRP has been an effective but inherently destructive treatment for 4 decades. Multiple trials of anti-VEGF therapy for DME have reproducibly demonstrated significant regression of retinopathy severity with VEGF inhibition. This observation led to considerable interest in comparing PRP to anti-VEGF therapy for preventing sight-threatening complications of PDR.

At the two-year primary endpoint, ranibizumab was non-inferior to PRP with a mean gain of +2.8 letters vs. +0.2 letters in the PRP group. In eyes with central DME at baseline, ranibizumab gave superior improvement in visual acuity with a gain of eight letters versus two letters in the PRP group, despite both arms receiving ranibizumab injections for the DME .

Important secondary outcomes also favored ranibizumab. Visual field loss, measured in decibels by Humphrey

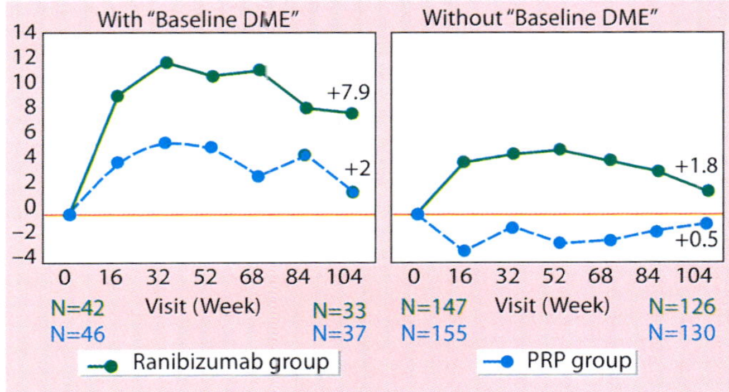

Fig. 27.1: Mean change in visual acuity stratified by baseline diabetic macular edema (DME).

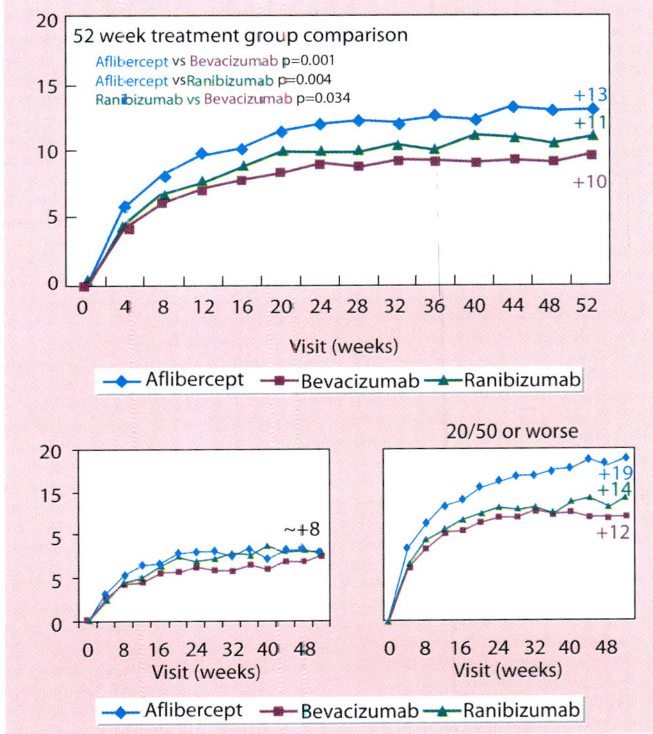

Fig. 27.2: Mean change in visual acuity over 2 years by baseline visual acuity subgroup.

Fig. 27.3: Protocol T results.

analyzers using the 30-2 and 60-4 programs, was significantly less in the ranibizumab arm. Eyes in the ranibizumab group had greater reductions in optical coherence tomography CST, and fewer eyes developed DME during the two years of the study (9 percent vs 28 percent in the PRP group). Also, rates of vitrectomy were less at 4 percent, vs 15 percent in the PRP group.

However, a major drawback was the fact, that patients in this protocol had to maintain their follow-up visits and the injection, or else they would progress in their PDR disease.

PROTOCOL T:[74,75] This important study compared the relative efficacy of three anti-VEGF agents to treat DME. 660 adults with center-involving DME were randomly assigned to receive intravitreal aflibercept 2.0 mg (n = 224), bevacizumab 1.25 mg (n = 218), or ranibizumab 0.3 mg (n = 218) as often as every 4 weeks, according to a protocol-specified algorithm. The study was conducted between August 2012 and August 2013 and analysis conducted from January 2015 to June 2015. The primary outcome was the mean change in visual acuity at 1 year. Results showed that intravitreal aflibercept, bevacizumab, or ranibizumab improved vision in eyes with center-involved DME, but the relative effect depended on baseline visual acuity. When the initial visual acuity loss was mild, there were no apparent differences; however, at worse levels of initial visual acuity (approximately 20/50 or worse), aflibercept was more effective at improving vision. Post hoc secondary findings suggested that for eyes with better initial visual acuity and thicker central subfield thickness, some visual acuity outcomes may be worse in the bevacizumab group than in the aflibercept and ranibizumab groups (Fig. 27.1).

Two-year results of the Diabetic Retinopathy Clinical Research Network Protocol T study showed that there was a 50% reduction in the number of injections required in the second year as compared to first year. The comparative effectiveness study showed similar vision gains at 2-year visit in all three drugs for center-involved DME.

At 2 years, aflibercept remained superior to bevacizumab, the advantage of aflibercept over ranibizumab noted at 1 year had decreased and was no longer statistically significant at 2 years. More interesting is that the percentage of eyes gaining three lines of vision favored aflibercept at 1 year but there was no difference at 2 years suggesting that in the long term, there may be little clinical difference in the effectiveness of these three agents (Figs. 27.2 and 27.3).

Focal/grid laser coagulation was administered in 41% of patients in the aflibercept group, 64% of patients in the bevacizumab group and 52% of patients in the ranibizumab group.

Protocol U: This recent protocol was designed to evaluate the comparison of ranibizumab only in one arm versus combination therapy of ranibizumab and dexamethasone implant (700 μg). The study enrolled 236 eyes, gave them three injections of ranibizumab (Lucentis, Genentech), and those who continued to have edema and vision loss were randomized into two arms. The combination arm included dexamethasone and ranibizumab, with ranibizumab given monthly and dexamethasone being able to be given a second time as early as 12 weeks later. The other arm just included ranibizumab every 4 weeks. No overall difference was found at the end of 24 weeks between the single or combined treatments. Primary outcome at 24 weeks revealed that there was an average of 2.7 letters gained in the combination arm, compared to 3.0 letters gained in the ranibizumab alone arm (P = 0.73).

Secondary outcomes showed that more subjects obtained 15 letters or more improvement in the combination group (11%), compared to the ranibizumab-only group (2%) (P = 0.03). Central subfoveal thickness decreased by 110 microns in the combination group compared to 62 microns in the ranibizumab only group (P > 0.001). 20% of patients developed ocular hypertension in the combination group (P > 0.001).

Concluding, Protocol U showed that based on the protocol's design, adding DEX to continued as-needed ranibizumab treatment did not improve visual acuity at 24 weeks, but it was more likely to reduce macular thickness.

On average, there was a greater reduction in retinal thickness in the dexamethasone plus ranibizumab group.

Clinical Trials Relating to Pharmacotherapy of Diabetic Retinopathy

The *READ-2 study* (Ranibizumab for Edema of the mAcula in Diabetes)[76] was a phase 2 prospective, randomized, interventional, multicenter clinical trial that compared ranibizumab with focal/grid laser or a combination of both in patients with DME, with an ETDRS visual acuity of 20/40 to 20/320 and baseline foveal thickness by OCT at least 250 μm. A total of 126 patients were randomized 1:1:1 to receive 0.5 mg of ranibizumab (group 1, 42 patients), focal/grid laser photocoagulation (group 2, 42 patients), or a combination of 0.5 mg of ranibizumab and focal/grid laser (group 3, 42 patients). Results showed that during a span of 6 months, ranibizumab injections had a significantly better visual outcome than focal/grid laser treatment. After the primary endpoint at month 6, most patients in all groups were treated only with ranibizumab. Intravitreal ranibizumab provided benefit for at least 2 years, and when combined with focal or grid laser treatments, the amount of residual edema was reduced, as were the frequency of injections needed to control edema, without impairment of visual acuity. The

2-year follow-up also showed that ranibizumab is associated with significant improvement in patients who previously received only laser photocoagulation. Thus, long-term visual outcomes for treatment of DME with ranibizumab are excellent, but many patients require frequent injections to optimally control edema and maximize vision.

The *RISE and RIDE*[77] were phase 3, double-masked, multicenter, 3-year clinical trials, which were sham-–treatment controlled for 24 months, to evaluate the efficacy and safety of intravitreal ranibizumab in DME. A total of 759 patients were randomized into three groups (1:1:1 randomization) to receive monthly treatment with 0.3 mg ranibizumab (n = 250), 0.5 mg ranibizumab (n = 252) or sham injection (control group, n = 257). At 24 months, significantly more ranibizumab-treated patients gained more than or equal to 15 ETDRS letters. Significant gains in average vision were observed 7 days after the first treatment.

The *RESTORE* study[78] was a 12-month, randomized, double-masked, multicenter phase 3 study to evaluate ranibizumab monotherapy or combined with laser versus laser monotherapy for DME. 345 patients were randomized to ranibizumab + sham laser, ranibizumab + laser or sham injections + laser. Ranibizumab or sham was given for 3 months then pro re nata (PRN); laser or sham laser was given at baseline then PRN. The main outcome measure was mean average change in visual acuity. Ranibizumab monotherapy and combined with laser provided superior visual acuity gain over standard laser in patients with visual impairment due to DME. At 1 year, no differences were detected between the ranibizumab and ranibizumab + laser arms.

The *BOLT* study[79] (A prospective randomized trial of intravitreal Bevacizumab or Laser Therapy in the management of DME) was a masked, single-center, 2-year, 2-arm clinical trial to compare repeated IVB and modified ETDRS macular laser therapy in patients with persistent CSME. A total of 80 eyes with center-involving CSME and at least 1 prior macular laser therapy were randomized to either IVB or macular laser therapy. The study provided evidence to support the use of bevacizumab in patients with center-involving CSME without advanced macular ischemia. Improvements in visual acuity and CMT seen with bevacizumab at 1 year were maintained over the second year with a mean of four injections, thus providing evidence supporting longer-term use of IVB for persistent center-involving CSME.

The *DA VINCI study*[80] (DME And VEGF Trap-Eye: INvestigation of Clinical Impact) was a randomized, double-masked, multicenter, phase 2 clinical trial that compared different doses and dosing regimens of VEGF Trap-Eye with laser photocoagulation in center-involved DME. Patients were randomized to 1 of 5 treatment regimens—VEGF Trap-Eye 0.5 mg every 4 weeks; 2 mg every 4 weeks; 2 mg every 8 weeks after 3 initial monthly doses; or 2 mg dosing as needed after 3 initial monthly doses, or macular laser photocoagulation. Intravitreal VEGF Trap-Eye produced a statistically significant improvement in visual acuity when compared with macular laser photocoagulation. Significant gains in visual acuity from baseline achieved at week 24 were maintained or improved at week 52 in all VEGF Trap-Eye groups.

The *VISTA DME and VIVID DME*[81] were two similarly designed, double-masked, randomized, active-controlled, 148-week, phase 3 trials to compare efficacy and safety of two dosing regimens of intravitreal aflibercept with macular laser photocoagulation for DME with central involvement. A total of 872 eyes were randomized in a 1:1:1 ratio to receive intravitreal aflibercept 2 mg every 4 weeks, intravitreal aflibercept 2 mg every 8 weeks after 5 initial monthly doses, or macular laser photocoagulation at baseline. At week 52, intravitreal aflibercept demonstrated significant superiority in functional and anatomic endpoints over laser, with similar efficacy in the two groups and this was sustained through week 100. In general, intravitreal aflibercept was well-tolerated.

The *FAME study*[82] (Fluocinolone Acetonide in Diabetic Macular Edema) consisted of two parallel, prospective, randomized, sham injection-controlled, double-masked, multicenter clinical trials that assessed the efficacy and safety of intravitreal inserts releasing 0.2 µg/day (low dose) or 0.5 µg/day (high dose) fluocinolone acetonide (FA) in patients with DME. Subjects with persistent DME despite at least one macular laser treatment were randomized 1:2:2 to sham injection (n = 185), low-dose insert (n = 375), or high-dose insert (n = 393). Both low- and high-dose FA inserts significantly improved visual acuity in patients with DME over 2 years, and the risk-to-benefit ratio was superior for the low-dose insert. This is the first pharmacologic treatment that can be administered by an outpatient injection to provide substantial benefit in patients with DME for at least 2 years.

The *MEAD study*[83] (Macular Edema: Assessment of implantable Dexamethasone in diabetes) consisted of two randomized, multicenter, masked, sham-controlled, phase 3 clinical trials that evaluated the safety and efficacy of dexamethasone intravitreal implant (Ozurdex, DEX implant) 0.7 mg and 0.35 mg in the treatment of DME. 1,048 eyes were randomized in a 1:1:1 ratio to study treatment with DEX implant 0.7 mg, DEX implant 0.35 mg, or sham procedure and followed for 3 years. The DEX implants 0.7 mg and 0.35 mg met the primary efficacy endpoint of achievement of more than or equal to 15-letter improvement in visual acuity from baseline. Rates of cataract-related adverse events in phakic eyes were 67.9%, 64.1%, and 20.4% in the DEX implant 0.7 mg, DEX implant 0.35 mg, and sham groups, respectively. Approximately one-third of patients in each DEX implant treatment group had a clinically significant increase in intraocular pressure and were usually controlled with medication or no therapy.

CLASSIFICATION

There is a need for consistent classification systems for DR and DME to enable categorization, classification and staging the severity of the disease in order to establish adequate therapy. This would also improve screening of individuals with diabetes, and improve communication between their healthcare providers.

Modified Airlie House Classification

In 1968, a group of experts developed a standardized classification for DR that was modified and used in the DRS and ETDRS. This was considered the gold standard for several years due to its satisfactory validity and reproducibility. It consisted of grading of stereo photographs in 7 standard fields and classified DR into 13 complex levels ranging from level 10 (absence of DR) to level 85 (severe vitreous hemorrhage or retinal detachment involving the macula).[84] While it was an excellent tool for research, its clinical application was limited by its complexity.

International Clinical Disease Severity Scale for Diabetic Retinopathy. In order to simplify the classification of DR, a group of 31 individuals from 16 countries, representing comprehensive ophthalmology, retina subspecialties, endocrinology, and epidemiology achieved a consensus regarding specific classification systems. Based on the ETDRS and WESDR publications, a five-stage disease severity classification for DR was agreed upon (Table 27.2):[85]

1. *No apparent retinopathy*: No abnormalities detected on dilated ophthalmoscopy.
2. *Mild NPDR*: Microaneurysms only, this corresponded to the EDRS stage 20.

Table 27.2: International clinical diabetic retinopathy disease severity scale.

Disease severity	Dilated ophthalmoscopy findings
No apparent retinopathy	No abnormality
Mild NPDR	Microaneurysms only
Moderate NPDR	More than just microaneurysms and less than severe disease
Severe NPDR	No signs of PDR and any of the following: • 20 intraretinal hemorrhages in each of the 4 quadrants • Venous beading in ≥2 quadrants • Prominent IRMA ≥1 quadrant
PDR	One or more of the following: • Neovascularization • Vitreous or preretinal hemorrhage

(NPDR: Nonproliferative diabetic retinopathy; PDR: Proliferative diabetic retinopathy; IRMA: Intraretinal microvascular abnormalities).

Source: Wilkinson CP, Ferris FL 3rd, Klein RE, et al Proposed international clinical diabetic retinopathy and diabetic macular edema disease severity scales. Ophthalmology. 2003;110(9): 1677-82.

3. *Moderate NPDR*: More than just microaneurysms but less than severe NPDR, this includes eyes with ETDRS levels 35 to 47.
4. *Severe NPDR*: This stage included ETDRS stages 53 and higher and carries the most ominous prognosis for progression to PDR. The diagnosis of severe NPDR is based on the 4:2:1 rule of the ETDRS. Using standard photographs 2A, 6A and 8A to compare with the fundus findings, severe NPDR can be diagnosed by the presence of any of the following and no signs of proliferative retinopathy:
   - Extensive (>20) intraretinal hemorrhages of at least the magnitude of standard photograph 2A in each of 4 quadrants.
   - Definite venous beading of the same magnitude or greater than standard photograph 6A in 2+ quadrants.
   - Prominent intraretinal microvascular abnormalities (IRMA) of the same magnitude or greater than standard photograph 8A in 1+ quadrant
5. *PDR*: One or more of the following:
   - Neovascularization of the disc, retina iris and/or angle
   - Vitreous or preretinal hemorrhage.

Thus, the levels of grading of retinopathy include three with relatively low risk and two with significant risk for visual loss. This new classification is simple to use, easy to remember and based on scientific evidence. This system is not intended as a guide for treatment of DR and DME, rather it is aimed that the identification of specific severity levels result in more appropriate and consistent referrals to treatment centers. Figures 27.4A to F illustrate clinical examples demonstrating different grades of DR.

With regards to DME (Figs. 27.5 to 27.7), it should be noted if DME is present or absent (No apparent retinal thickening or hard exudates in posterior pole). If it is present then it can be further classified as mild, moderate and severe depending on the distance of the exudates and thickening from the center of the fovea as follows:[85]

- *Mild DME*: The retinal thickening or hard exudates are located far from the center of the fovea.
- *Moderate DME*: Retinal thickening or hard exudates approaching the center of the macula but not involving the center.
- *Severe DME*: The center of the fovea is involved with hard exudate and thickening.

TELESCREENING FOR DIABETIC RETINOPATHY

The potential economic and social burden due to diabetes and DR necessitates an effective screening strategy, accurate case detection and treatment. The value of screening for DR is well established; since it has few visual or ocular symptoms until vision loss develops. With early detection, DR can be treated with modalities that can decrease the risk of SVL. The American Diabetes Association recommends DR screening with yearly retinal examination beginning at the time of diagnosis of diabetes for all patients aged 30 years and older.[86] Annual examinations are recommended

for patients under age 30 years beginning within 3–5 years after diagnosis of diabetes. Dilated, indirect ophthalmoscopy coupled with biomicroscopy or 7-standard field stereoscopic 30° fundus photography has been considered to be the screening techniques of choice. Because these techniques require a dedicated visit to an ophthalmologist, there is underutilization of this screening recommendation by at-risk members. The underuse has resulted in the exploration of remote retinal imaging, using film or digital photography, as an alternative to direct examination of the retina.

Advances in the fields of imaging and telecommunications have opened newer avenues for creation of efficient screening strategies for DR. Telemedicine allows evaluation of patient by a remotely located physician by exchange of medical data via electronic telecommunication.

For DR screening, at the physician or optometrist facility a nonmydriatic digital retinal camera to capture fundus images. The images are then transmitted electronically to a remote reading and grading center where a retinal expert reads them, generates a report of the status of retinopathy, with suggestions for follow-up. This report is returned by internet to the patient's location.[87] Smartphone-based cameras have emerged as cost-effective tools as well, however they require pupillary dilatation. Figure 27.8 displays the basic pathway for telescreening. Several digital camera and transmission systems are currently available:

- The Diabetic Retinopathy Digital Disease Detection and Tracking System (now called iScan™; Inoveon Corp., Oklahoma City, OK)
- DigiScope® (EyeTel Corp., Columbia, MD) in conjunction with the Wilmer Eye Institute at Johns Hopkins Medicine
- The Fundus AutoImager™ (Visual Pathways Inc., Prescott, AZ)
- ImageNet™ Digital Imaging System (Topcon Medical Systems Inc., Paramus, NJ)
- Zeiss FF450 Fundus Camera and the VISUPAC® Digital Imaging System (Carl Zeiss Meditech Inc., Dublin, CA).

The efficacy of digital image acquisition, as compared to film-based acquisition, has been reported.[88] On comparing high-resolution stereoscopic digital fundus photography to contact lens biomicroscopy, Rudnisky et al. found a high level of agreement regarding the detection of CSME and concluded that it is both sensitive and specific when identifying CSME.[89]

Guidelines for Diabetic Retinopathy Screening Program

The American Telemedicine Association (ATA) and Ocular Telehealth Special Interest Group have established the guidelines for DR telescreening in 2004.[90] The "Telehealth Practice Recommendations for Diabetic Retinopathy" divide DR telehealth program into four elements of care:
1. Image acquisition
2. Image review and evaluation
3. Patient care supervision
4. Image and data storage.

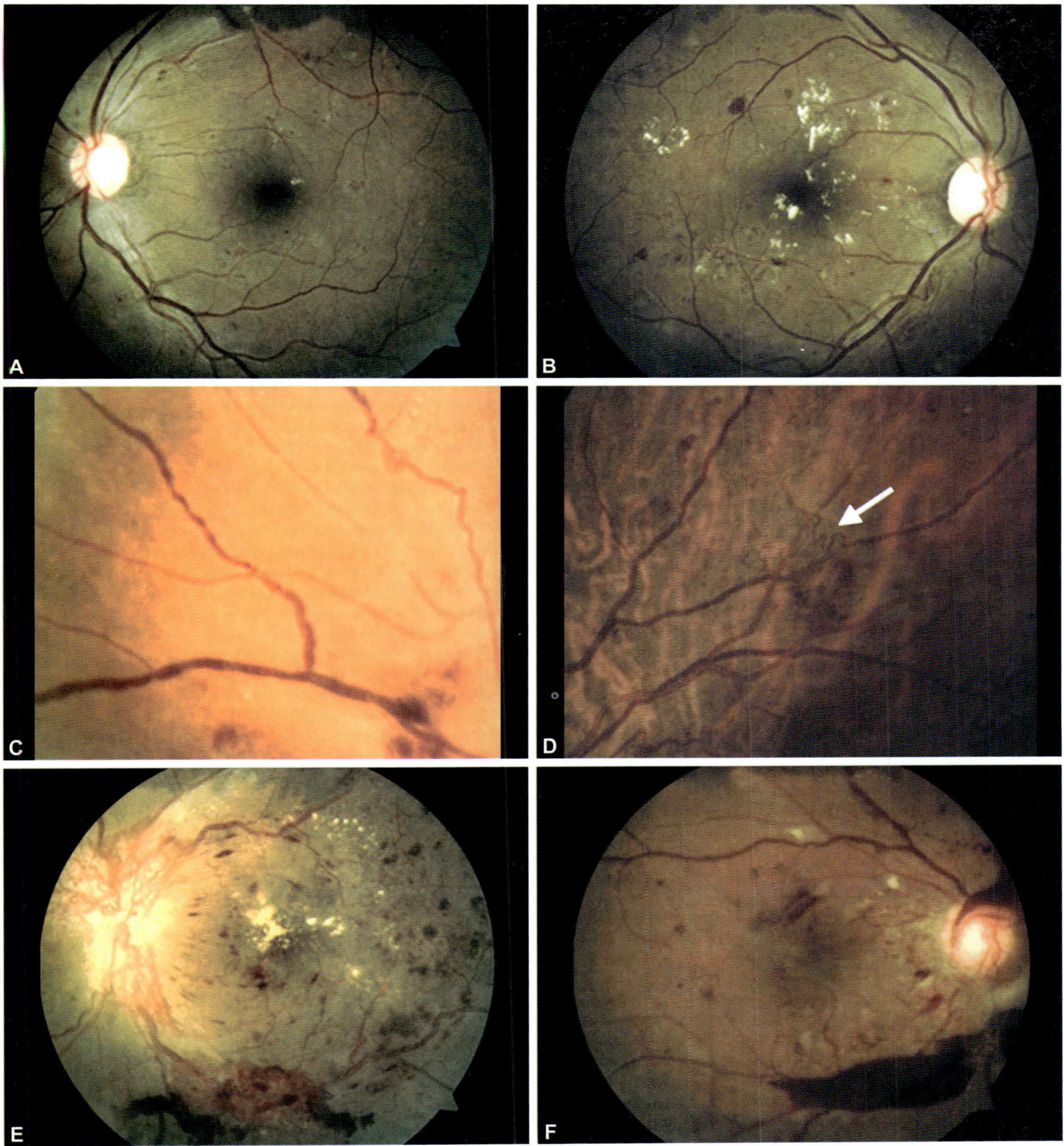

Figs. 27.4A to F: Clinical pictures showing grades of diabetic retinopathy. (A) Mild NPDR; (B) Moderate NPDR; (C) Venous beading (severe NPDR); (D) IRMA (severe NPDR); (E) Neovascularization (PDR); (F) Preretinal hemorrhage (PDR).
(NPDR: Nonproliferative diabetic retinopathy; IRMA: Intraretinal microvascular abnormalities; PDR: Proliferative diabetic retinopathy).

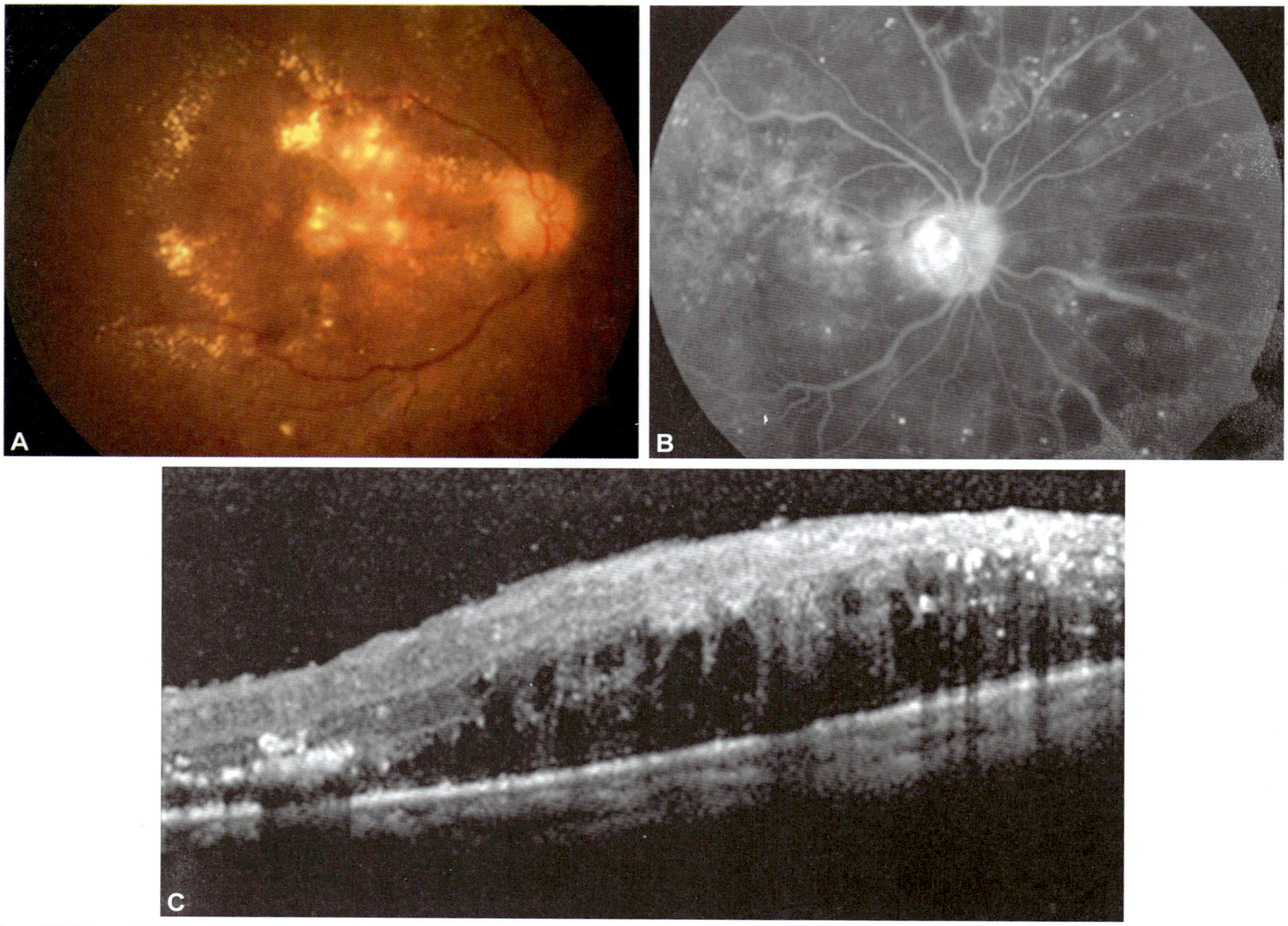

Figs. 27.5A to C: Clinical pictures showing severe DME with NVD. (A) Colored fundus picture showing severe DME with hard exudates and NVD; (B) FFA picture showing leakage suggestive of NVD; and (C) OCT picture showing severe DME with cystic changes. (DME: Diabetic macular edema; NVD: Neovascularization of the optic disc; FFA: Fluorescein fundus angiography; OCT: Optical coherence tomography).

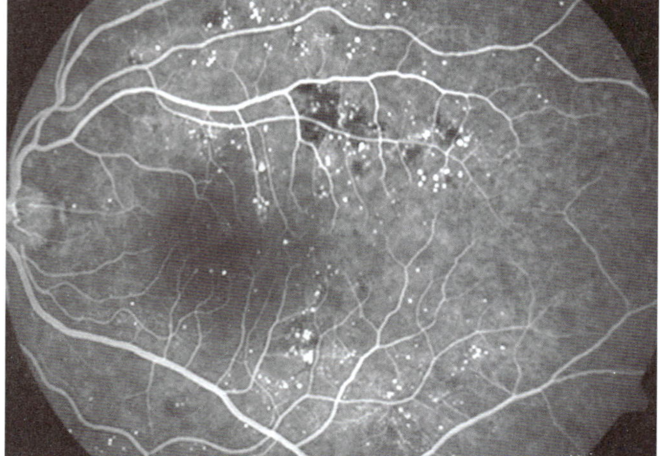

Fig. 27.6: Fluorescein fundus angiography picture showing multiple microaneurysms and intraretinal hemorrhages (blocked choroidal fluorescence) along superior arcade.

INDIAN SCENARIO

Seventy-four percent of India's population lives in rural areas with limited access to healthcare resources. In India, the ophthalmologist/population ratio is 1:10,700 and the distribution of ophthalmologists is more in urban areas compared to rural areas by a factor of ten. There can be ophthalmologist-based (screening in the presence of an ophthalmologist) and ophthalmologist-led (telescreening) models for DR screening. The number of ophthalmologists available is the limiting factor in initiating an ophthalmologist-based screening service in India. Because of this, the optimal screening model in India may be an ophthalmologist-led system.[91]

A mobile teleophthalmology model wherein real time consultation and examination of the patients in rural areas takes place by a mobile van with a satellite link to the central hub (main hospital) has been shown to be cost-effective in South India. A trained optometrist performs acquisition of

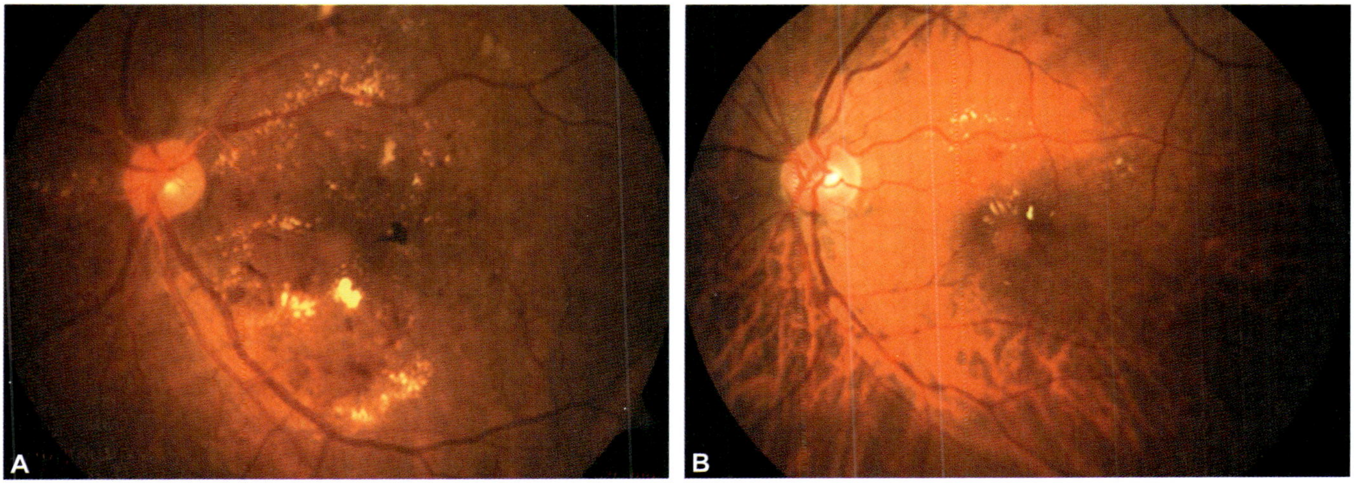

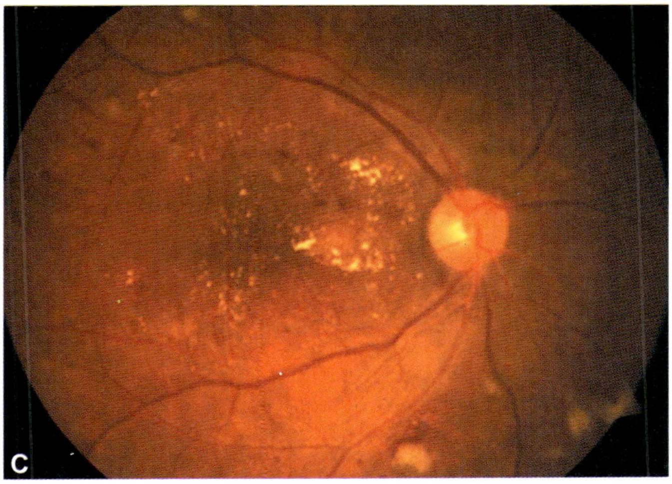

Figs. 27.7A to C: Colored fundus pictures of diabetic macular edema (DME). (A) Mild DME; (B) Moderate DME; and (C) Severe DME.

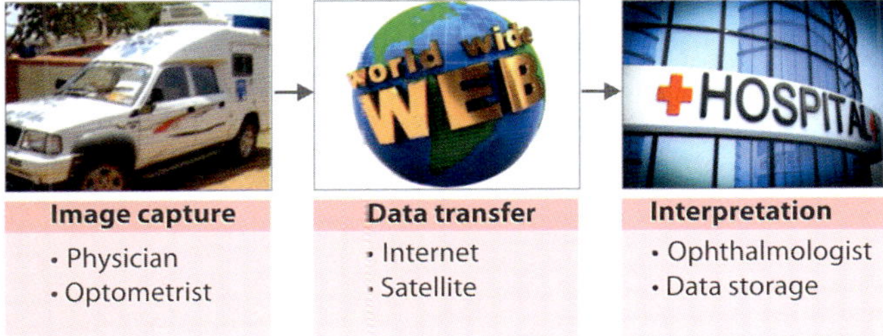

Fig. 27.8: Telescreening for diabetic retinopathy.

digital retinal images. The optometrist and the equipment are placed in a mobile van. The data and images are transferred to the hub where a vitreoretinal surgeon reviews the images and gives advice regarding management. Information is transferred through very small aperture terminal (VSAT) provided by the Indian Space Research Organization (ISRO).[92]

Teleophthalmology in DR care is both effective as well as cost-efficient.[91] To expand telescreening services to more remote areas newer technology like "cloud" storage, miniaturization of diagnostic equipment such as digital cameras, and automation of retinal image analysis can be used.

REFERENCES

1. Cheung N, Mitchell P, Wong TY. Diabetic retinopathy. Lancet. 2010;376(9735):124-36.
2. Yau JW, Rogers SL, Kawasaki R, et al. Global prevalence and major risk factors of diabetic retinopathy. Diabetes Care. 2012;35(3):556-64.
3. Raman R, Rani PK, Reddi Rachepalle S, et al. Prevalence of diabetic retinopathy in India: Sankara Nethralaya diabetic retinopathy epidemiology and molecular genetics study report 2. Ophthalmology. 2009;116(2):311-8.
4. Raman R, Ganesan S, Pal SS, et al. Prevalence and risk factors for diabetic retinopathy in rural India. Sankara Nethralaya Diabetic Retinopathy Epidemiology and Molecular Genetic Study III (SN-DREAMS III), report no 2. BMJ Open Diabetes Res Care. 2014;2(1):e000005.
5. Klein R, Klein BK, Moss SE, et al. The Wisconsin epidemiologic study of diabetic retinopathy: Ix. four-year incidence and progression of diabetic retinopathy when age at diagnosis is less than 30 years. Arch Ophthalmology. 1989;107(2):237-43.

6. Klein R, Klein BE, Moss SE, et al. The Wisconsin Epidemiologic Study of diabetic retinopathy. XIV. Ten-year incidence and progression of diabetic retinopathy. Arch Ophthalmology. 1994;112(9):1217-28.

7. Klein R, Knudtson MD, Lee KE, et al. The Wisconsin Epidemiologic Study of Diabetic Retinopathy: XXII the twenty-five-year progression of retinopathy in persons with type 1 diabetes. Ophthalmology. 2008;115(11):1859-68.

8. Klein R, Klein BE, Moss SE, et al. The Wisconsin Epidemiologic Study of Diabetic Retinopathy. XV. The long-term incidence of macular edema. Ophthalmology. 1995;102:7-16.

9. Jones CD, Greenwood RH, Misra A, et al. Incidence and progression of diabetic retinopathy during 17 years of a population based screening program in England. Diabetes Care. 2012;35: 592-6.

10. Lee R, Wong TY, Sabanayagam C. Epidemiology of diabetic retinopathy, diabetic macular edema and related vision loss. Eye Vis (Lond). 2015;2:17.

11. Klein R, Klein BE. Are individuals with diabetes seeing better? A long-term epidemiological perspective. Diabetes. 2010;59: 1853-60.

12. Donaghue KC, Fairchild JM, Craig ME, et al. Do all prepubertal years of diabetes duration contribute equally to diabetic complications? Diabetes Care. 2003;26:1224-9.

13. Klein BE, Moss SE, Klein R. Is menarche associated with diabetic retinopathy? Diabetes Care. 1990;13:1034-38.

14. Egan AM, McVicker L, Heerey A, et al. Diabetic retinopathy in pregnancy: a population-based study of women with pregestational diabetes. J Diabetes Res. 2015;2015:310239.

15. Mohamed Q, Gillies MC, Wong TY. Management of diabetic retinopathy: a systematic review. JAMA. 2007;298:902-16.

16. The Diabetes Control and Complications Trial Research Group, Nathan DM, Genuth S, et al. The effect of intensive treatment of diabetes on the development and progression of long-term complications in insulin-dependent diabetes mellitus. N Engl J Med. 1993;329(14):977-86.

17. The Diabetes Control and Complications Trial/Epidemiology of Diabetes Interventions and Complications Research Group, Lachin JM, Genuth S, et al. Retinopathy and nephropathy in patients with type 1 diabetes four years after a trial of intensive therapy. N Engl J Med. 2000;342(6):381-9.

18. Patel A, MacMahon S, Chalmers J, et al. Intensive blood glucose control and vascular outcomes in patients with type 2 diabetes. N Engl J Med. 2008;358:2560-72.

19. Gerstein HC, Miller ME, Byington RP, et al. Effects of intensive glucose lowering in type 2 diabetes. N Engl J Med. 2008;358: 2545-59.

20. UK Prospective Diabetes Study Group. Tight blood pressure control and risk of macrovascular and microvascular complications in type 2 diabetes: UKPDS 38. BMJ. 1998;317(7160):703-13.

21. Keech AC, Mitchell P, Summanen PA, et al. Effect of fenofibrate on the need for laser treatment for diabetic retinopathy (FIELD study): a randomised controlled trial. Lancet. 2007;370(9600):1687-97.

22. Chaturvedi N, Sjoelie AK, Porta M, et al. Markers of insulin resistance are strong risk factors for retinopathy incidence in type 1 diabetes. Diabetes Care. 2001;24(2):284-9.

23. Lu J, Hou X, Zhang L, et al. Association between body mass index and diabetic retinopathy in Chinese patients with type 2 diabetes. Acta Diabetol. 2015;52(4):701-8.

24. Sasongko MB, Wong TY, Nguyen TT, et al. Serum apolipoprotein AI and B are stronger biomarkers of diabetic retinopathy than traditional lipids. Diabetes Care. 2011;34:474-79.

25. Rangasamy S, McGuire PG, Das A. Diabetic retinopathy and inflammation: novel therapeutic targets. Middle East Afr J Ophthalmology. 2012;19:52-9.

26. Shimo N, Yasuda T, Kaneto H, et al. Vitamin D deficiency is significantly associated with retinopathy in young Japanese type 1 diabetic patients. Diabetes Res Clin Pract. 2014;106(2):e41-3.

27. He R, Shen J, Liu F, et al. Vitamin D deficiency increases the risk of retinopathy in Chinese patients with type 2 diabetes. Diabet Med. 2014;31(12):1657-64.

28. The Diabetes Control and Complications Trial Research Group. Clustering of long-term complications in families with diabetes in the diabetes control and complications trial. Diabetes. 1997;46:1829-39.

29. Gabbay KH. The sorbitol pathway and the complications of diabetes. N Engl J Med. 1973;288(16):831-6.

30. Lassègue B, Clempus RE. Vascular NAD(P)H oxidases: specific features, expression, and regulation. Am J Physiol Regul Integr Comp Physiol. 2003;285(2):R277-97.

31. Oates PJ, Mylari BL. Aldose reductase inhibitors: therapeutic implications for diabetic complications. Expert Opin Investig Drugs. 1999;8(12):2095-119.

32. Bolton WK, Cattran DC, Williams ME, et al. Randomized trial of an inhibitor of advanced glycation end products in diabetic nephropathy. Am J Nephrol. 2004;24:32-40.

33. Aiello LP, Clermont A, Arora V, et al. Inhibition of PKC beta by oral administration of ruboxistaurin is well tolerated and ameliorates diabetes-induced retinal hemodynamic abnormalities in patients. Invest Ophthalmology Vis Sci. 2006;47(1):86-92.

34. Aiello LP, Vignati L, Sheetz MJ, et al. Oral protein kinase C β inhibition using ruboxistaurin: efficacy, safety, and causes of vision loss among 813 patients (1,392 eyes) with diabetic retinopathy in the Protein Kinase C β Inhibitor-Diabetic Retinopathy Study and the Protein Kinase C β Inhibitor-Diabetic Retinopathy Study 2. Retina. 2011;31(10):2084-94.

35. Kern TS, Kowluru RA, Engerman RL. Abnormalities of retinal metabolism in diabetes or galactosemia: ATPases and glutathione. Invest Ophthalmology Vis Sci. 1994;35:2962-7.

36. Hammes HP. Pericytes and the pathogenesis of diabetic retinopathy. Horm Metab Res. 2005;37 Suppl 1:39-43.

37. Cai J, Boulton M. The pathogenesis of diabetic retinopathy: old concepts and new questions. Eye (Lond). 2002;16(3):242-60.

38. Stitt AW, Gardiner TA, Archer DB. Histological and ultrastructural investigation of retinal microaneurysm development in diabetic patients. Br J Ophthalmology. 1995;79:362-7.

39. Granger DN, Kubes P. The microcirculation and inflammation: modulation of leukocyte-endothelial cell adhesion. J Leukoc Biol 1994;55:662-75.

40. Behl T, Kotwani A. Exploring the various aspects of the pathological role of vascular endothelial growth factor (VEGF) in diabetic retinopathy. Pharmacol Res. 2015;99:137-48.

41. Freyberger H, Brocker M, Yakut H, et al. Increased levels of platelet-derived growth factor in vitreous fluid of patients with proliferative diabetic retinopathy. Exp Clin Endocrinol Diabetes. 2000;108:106-9.

42. Ziche M, Maglione D, Ribatti D, et al. Placenta growth factor-1 is chemotactic, mitogenic, and angiogenic. Lab Invest. 1997;76:517-31.

43. Mori K, Duh E, Gehlbach P, et al. Pigment epithelium-derived factor inhibits retinal and choroidal neovascularization. J Cell Physiol. 2001;188:253-63.

44. White NH, Sun W, Cleary PA, et al. Prolonged effect of intensive therapy on the risk of retinopathy complications in patients with type 1 diabetes mellitus: 10 years after the Diabetes Control and Complications Trial. Arch Ophthalmology. 2008;126:1707-15.

45. Turner RC. The UK Prospective Diabetes Study. A review. Diabetes Care. 1998;21 Suppl 3:C35-8.

46. ACCORD Study Group, Cushman WC, Evans GW, et al. The. Effects of intensive blood-pressure control in type 2 diabetes mellitus. N Engl J Med. 2010;362:1575-85.

47. ACCORD Study Group, Ginsberg HN, Elam MB, et al. The effects of combination lipid therapy in type 2 diabetes mellitus. N Engl J Med. 2010;362:1563-74.

48. ACCORD Study Group, ACCORD Eye Study Group, Chew EY, et al. Effects of medical therapies on retinopathy progression in type 2 diabetes. N Engl J Med. 2010;363:233-44.

49. Action to Control Cardiovascular Risk in Diabetes Follow-On (ACCORDION) Eye Study Group and the Action to Control Cardiovascular Risk in Diabetes Follow-On (ACCORDION) Study Group. Persistent Effects of Intensive Glycemic Control on Retinopathy in Type 2 Diabetes in the Action to Control Cardiovascular Risk in Diabetes (ACCORD) Follow-On Study. Diabetes Care. 2016;39(7):1089-100.

50. Photocoagulation treatment of proliferative diabetic retinopathy: Clinical applications of Diabetic Retinopathy Study (DRS) findings. DRS Report No. 8. The Diabetic Retinopathy Study Research Group. Ophthalmology. 1981;88:583-600.

51. Early vitrectomy for severe proliferative diabetic retinopathy in eyes with useful vision: Results of a randomized trial. Diabetic Retinopathy Vitrectomy Study Report Number 3. The Diabetic Retinopathy Vitrectomy Study Research Group. Ophthalmology. 1988;95:1307-20.

52. Early vitrectomy for severe vitreous hemorrhage in diabetic retinopathy: Four-year results of a randomized trial. Diabetic Retinopathy Vitrectomy Study Report Number 5. The Diabetic Retinopathy Vitrectomy Study Research Group. Arch Ophthalmology. 1990;108: 958-64.

53. Photocoagulation for diabetic macular edema. ETDRS Report Number 4. Early Treatment Diabetic Retinopathy Study Research Group. Int Ophthalmology Clin. 1987;27:265-72.

54. Early photocoagulation for diabetic retinopathy. ETDRS Report Number 9. Early Treatment of Diabetic Retinopathy Study. Ophthalmology. 1991;98:766-85.

55. Fong DS, Strauber SF, Aiello LP, et al. Writing Committee for the Diabetic Retinopathy Clinical Research Network. Comparison of the modified Early Treatment Diabetic Retinopathy Study and mild macular grid laser photocoagulation strategies for diabetic macular edema. Arch Ophthalmology. 2007;125(4):469-80.

56. Beck RW, Edwards AR, Aiello LP, et al. Diabetic Retinopathy Clinical Research Network. Three-year follow-up of a randomized trial comparing focal/grid photocoagulation and intravitreal triamcinolone for diabetic macular edema. Arch Ophthalmology. 2009;127:245-51.

57. Danis RP, Glassman AR, Aiello LP, et al. Diabetic Retinopathy Clinical Research Network. Diurnal variation in retinal thickening measurement by optical coherence tomography in center-involved diabetic macular edema. Arch Ophthalmology. 2006;124:1701-7.

58. Haller JA, Qin H, Apte RS, et al. Diabetic Retinopathy Clinical Research Network Writing Committee on behalf of the DRCR.net. Vitrectomy outcomes in eyes with diabetic macular edema and vitreomacular traction. Ophthalmology. 2010;117:1087-93.

59. Chew E, Strauber S, Beck R, et al. Diabetic Retinopathy Clinical Research Network. Randomized trial of peribulbar triamcinolone acetonide with and without focal photocoagulation for mild diabetic macular edema: a pilot study. Ophthalmology. 2007;114:1190-6.

60. Brucker AJ, Qin H, Antoszyk AN, et al. Diabetic Retinopathy Clinical Research Network. Observational study of the development of diabetic macular edema following pan-retinal (scatter) photocoagulation given in 1 or 4 sittings. Arch Ophthalmology. 2009;127:132-40.

61. Bressler NM, Miller KM, Beck RW, et al. Observational Study of Subclinical Diabetic Macular Edema. Eye (Lond). 2012;26:833-40.

62. Scott IU, Edwards AR, Beck RW, et al. Diabetic Retinopathy Clinical Research Network. A phase II randomized clinical trial of intravitreal bevacizumab for diabetic macular edema. Ophthalmology. 2007;114:1860-7.

63. Elman MJ, Bressler NM, Qin H, et al. Diabetic Retinopathy Clinical Research Network. Expanded 2-year Follow-up of Ranibizumab plus Prompt or Deferred Laser or Triamcinolone plus Prompt Laser for Diabetic Macular Edema. Ophthalmology. 2011;118: 609-14.

64. Googe J, Brucker AJ, Bressler NM, et al. Diabetic Retinopathy Clinical Research Network; Randomized trial evaluating short-term effects of intravitreal Ranibizumab or Triamcinolone Acetonide on macular edema following focal/grid laser for diabetic macular edema in eyes also receiving panretinal photocoagulation. Retina. 2011;31:1009-27.

65. Diabetic Retinopathy Clinical Research Network. The course of response to focal/grid photocoagulation for diabetic macular edema. Retina. 2009;29:1436-43.

66. Sun JK, Qin H, Aiello LP, et al. Evaluation of visual acuity measurements after autorefraction vs manual refraction in eyes with and without diabetic macular edema. Arch Ophthalmology. 2012;130(4):470-9.

67. Aiello LP, Ayala AR, Antoszyk AN, et al. Assessing the Effect of Personalized Diabetes Risk Assessments during Ophthalmologic Visits on Glycemic Control: A Randomized Clinical Trial. JAMA Ophthalmology. 2015;133(8):888-96.

68. Diabetic Retinopathy Clinical Research Network. Randomized clinical trial evaluating intravitreal ranibizumab or saline for vitreous hemorrhage from proliferative diabetic retinopathy. JAMA Ophthalmology. 2013;131(3):283-93.

69. Bressler SB, Edwards AR, Chalam KV, et al. Diabetic Retinopathy Clinical Research Network Writing Committee. Reproducibility of spectral-domain optical coherence tomography retinal thickness measurements and conversion to equivalent time-domain metrics in diabetic macular edema. JAMA Ophthalmology. 2014;132(9):1113-22.

70. Bressler SB, Baker CW, Almukhtar T, et al. Diabetic Retinopathy Clinical Research Network Authors/Writing Committee. Pilot study of individuals with diabetic macular edema undergoing cataract surgery. JAMA Ophthalmology. 2014;132(2):224-6.

71. Baker CW, Almukhtar T, Bressler NM, et al. Diabetic Retinopathy Clinical Research Network Authors/Writing Committee. Macular edema after cataract surgery in eyes without preoperative central-involved diabetic macular edema. JAMA Ophthalmology. 2013;131(7):870-9.

72. Friedman SM, Almukhtar TH, Baker CW, et al. Topical nepafenac in eyes with noncentral diabetic macular edema. Retina. 2015;35(5):944-56.

73. Gross JG, Glassman AR, Jampol LM, et al. Writing Committee for the Diabetic Retinopathy Clinical Research Network. Panretinal Photocoagulation vs Intravitreous Ranibizumab for Proliferative Diabetic Retinopathy: A Randomized Clinical Trial. JAMA. 2015;314(20):2137-46.

74. Wells JA, Glassman AR, Ayala AR, et al. Aflibercept, bevacizumab, or ranibizumab for diabetic macular edema. N Engl J Med. 2015;372(13):1193-203.

75. Wells JA, Glassman AR, Jampol LM, et al. Association of Baseline Visual Acuity and Retinal Thickness with 1-Year Efficacy of Aflibercept, Bevacizumab, and Ranibizumab for Diabetic Macular Edema. JAMA Ophthalmology. 2015;25:1-8.

76. Do DV1, Nguyen QD, Khwaja AA, et al. Ranibizumab for edema of the macula in diabetes study: 3-year outcomes and the need for prolonged frequent treatment. Arch Ophthalmology. 2012;8:1-7.

77. Nguyen QD, Brown DM, Marcus DM, et al. Ranibizumab for DME: Results from 2 phase III randomized trials: RISE and RIDE. Ophthalmology. 2012;119:789-801.

78. Mitchell P, Bandello F, Schmidt-Erfurth U, et al. The RESTORE study: ranibizumab monotherapy or combined with laser versus laser monotherapy for diabetic macular edema. Ophthalmology. 2011;118:615-25.

79. Rajendram R, Fraser-Bell S, Kaines A, et al. A 2-year prospective randomized controlled trial of intravitreal bevacizumab or laser therapy (BOLT) in the management of diabetic macular edema: 24-month data: report 3. Arch Ophthalmology. 2012;130:972-9.

80. Do DV1, Nguyen QD, Boyer D, et al. One-year outcomes of the DA VINCI Study of VEGF Trap-Eye in eyes with diabetic macular edema. Ophthalmology. 2012;119:1658-65.

81. Brown DM, Schmidt-Erfurth U, Do DV, et al. Intravitreal Aflibercept for Diabetic Macular Edema: 100-Week Results From the VISTA and VIVID Studies. Ophthalmology. 2015;122(10):2044-52.

82. Campochiaro PA, Brown DM, Pearson A, et al. Sustained delivery fluocinolone acetonide vitreous inserts provide benefit for at least 3 years in patients with diabetic macular edema. Ophthalmology. 2012;119:2125-32.

83. Boyer DS, Yoon YH, Belfort R Jr, et al. Ozurdex MEAD Study Group. Three-year, randomized, sham-controlled trial of dexamethasone intravitreal implant in patients with diabetic macular edema. Ophthalmology. 2014;121(10):1904-14.

84. Grading diabetic retinopathy from stereoscopic color fundus photographs—an extension of the modified Airlie House classification. ETDRS report number 10. Early Treatment Diabetic Retinopathy Study Research Group. Ophthalmology. 1991;98: 786-806.

85. Wilkinson CP, Ferris FL 3rd, Klein RE, et al. Global Diabetic Retinopathy Project Group. Proposed international clinical diabetic retinopathy and diabetic macular edema disease severity scales. Ophthalmology. 2003;110:1677-82.

86. American Diabetes Association. Position statement: Diabetic retinopathy. Clinical Practice Guidelines 2001. Diabetes Care. 2001;24(Supp 1):S73-6.

87. Liesenfeld B, Kohner E, Piehlmeier W, et al. A telemedical approach to the screening of diabetic retinopathy: digital fundus photography. Diabetes Care. 2000;23:345-8.

88. Fransen SR, Leonard-Martin TC, Feuer WJ, et al. Clinical evaluation of patients with diabetic retinopathy: accuracy of the Inoveon diabetic retinopathy-3DT system. Ophthalmology. 2002;109(3):595-601.

89. Rudnisky CJ, Hinz BJ, Tennant MT, et al. High-resolution stereoscopic digital fundus photography versus contact lens biomicroscopy for the detection of clinically significant macular edema. Ophthalmology. 2002;109(2):267-74.

90. Cavallerono J, Lawrence MG, Zimmer-galler I, et al. American Telemedicine Association, Ocular Telehealth Special Interest Group; National Institute of Standards and Technology Working Group. Telehealth practice recommendations for diabetic retinopathy. Telemed J E Health. 2004;10:469-82.

91. Raman R, Bhojwani DN, Sharma T. How accurate is the diagnosis of diabetic retinopathy on telescreening? The Indian scenario. Rural Remote Health. 2014;14(4):2809.

92. Sudhir RR, Frick KD, Raman R, et al. Mobile teleophthalmology: a cost effective screening tool for diabetic retinopathy in rural south India. eHealth Int. 2005;1:2-8.

Chapter 28

Diabetic Macular Edema

Stanford C Taylor, Cynthia Montana, Manthan Shah, Rajendra S Apte

INTRODUCTION

Diabetic macular edema (DME) is a leading cause of vision loss from diabetic retinopathy. The long-term incidence of DME is 17% in individuals with type 1 diabetes[1] and 28% in those with type 2 diabetes.[2,3] While DME is a disease complication that frequently affects diabetic patients over time, recent studies suggest the incidence of diabetes-related visual impairment from DME is less today than that seen 25 years ago.[4,5] Many postulate this improvement is due to advances in the management of diabetic retinopathy. The following sections explore how current therapeutic advances have reduced the deleterious effects of DME on visual function.

Disorganization of Inner Retinal Layers (DRIL), A New Biomarker may predict treatment response in DME

In many patients, eyes treated with an anti-VEGF agent for diabetic macular edema (DME) resolve the edema and improve their vision. However, there are eyes where the edema resolves over the course of anti-VEGF therapy but the vision remains the same or worsens, even leading to worsening edema with excellent visual acuity outcomes.

There is an inexact correlation between central subfield thickness and visual acuity, so researchers are looking into using biomarkers of vision, which might improve methods for evaluating potential new therapies.

Jennifer K Sun, MD, MPH and colleagues at the Joslin Diabetes Center, Boston, have identified a new biomarker called disorganization of the retinal inner layers (DRIL). The researchers looked for DRIL within the central 1 mm foveal zone (Fig. 28.1).

They found that even when adjusting for central retinal thickness and outer layer characteristics, DRIL was still the most robust SD-OCT parameter associated with visual acuity change over time. Though DRIL can worsen and persist, it can also resolve, and reverse. Concluding, DRIL change within the central foveal zone is a stronger predictive biomarker for both visual acuity and retinal sensitivity, than either retinal thickness, or outer layer changes.

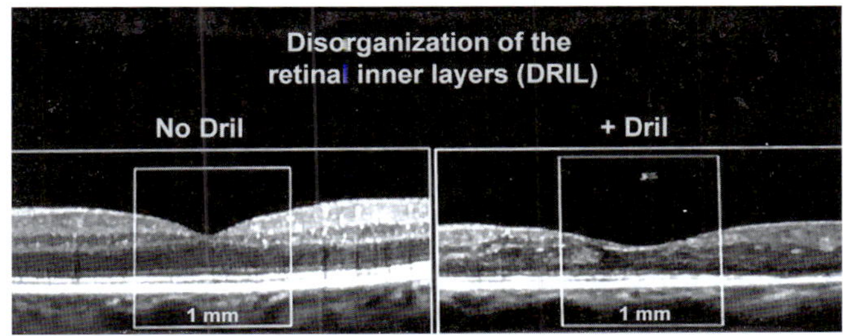

Fig. 28.1: The left OCT shows that the inner layers can be segmented, while DRIL is present in the right OCT and no definite inner layers of the retina can be perceived in the central 1 mm zone.

LASER FOR DIABETIC MACULAR EDEMA

While studied previously,[6-9] laser photocoagulation in the treatment of DME did not gain attention until the publication of the Early Treatment Diabetic Retinopathy Study (ETDRS) trial in 1985. This large, multicenter, randomized clinical trial (RCT) defined clinically significant macular edema (CSME) (Box 28.1 and Figs. 28.2A and B), characterized treatable lesions (Box 28.2 and Figs. 28.3A and B), and showed the beneficial effect of direct laser photocoagulation in the treatment of DME (Table 28.1, Figs. 28.4 and 28.5). 2,244 participants were assigned to focal laser photocoagulation versus deferral of photocoagulation groups for CSME. Most individuals were followed for 1–3 years following initial randomization. Patients with a baseline visual acuity worse than 20/200, high-risk proliferative diabetic retinopathy, or any neovascularization with hemorrhage were not eligible for the study. Multiple findings from the ETDRS trial demonstrated a beneficial effect of laser photocoagulation in the management of CSME. Investigators showed that vision loss of greater than 15 or more ETDRS letters occurs half as often in the focal photocoagulation group than the observation group at 3 years follow-up. Furthermore, eyes with a baseline visual acuity worse than 20/40 undergoing photocoagulation were more likely to have a visual gain of six or more letters than those in

Box 28.1: Clinically significant macular edema as defined by Early Treatment Diabetic Retinopathy Study (ETDRS).

Clinically significant macular edema (any of the following)
- Retinal thickening at or within 500 µm of the center of the macula.
- Hard exudates at or within 500 µm of the center of the macula associated with retinal thickening (residual hard exudates remaining after retinal thickening disappears is not included).
- Any zone of retinal thickening 1 disc area or larger, any part of which lies within one disc diameter of the center of the macula

Note: Classically, the diagnosis of macular edema is made clinically using contact-lens biomicroscopy.

Box 28.2: Characteristics of treatable lesions as defined by Early Treatment Diabetic Retinopathy Study (ETDRS).

- 'ETDRS characteristics of treatable lesion on fluorescein angiography.'
- Discrete points of retinal hyperfluorescence or leakage
- Areas of diffuse leakage within the retina
- Microaneurysms
- Intraretinal microvascular abnormalities
- Diffusely leaking retinal capillary bed
- Retinal avascular zones

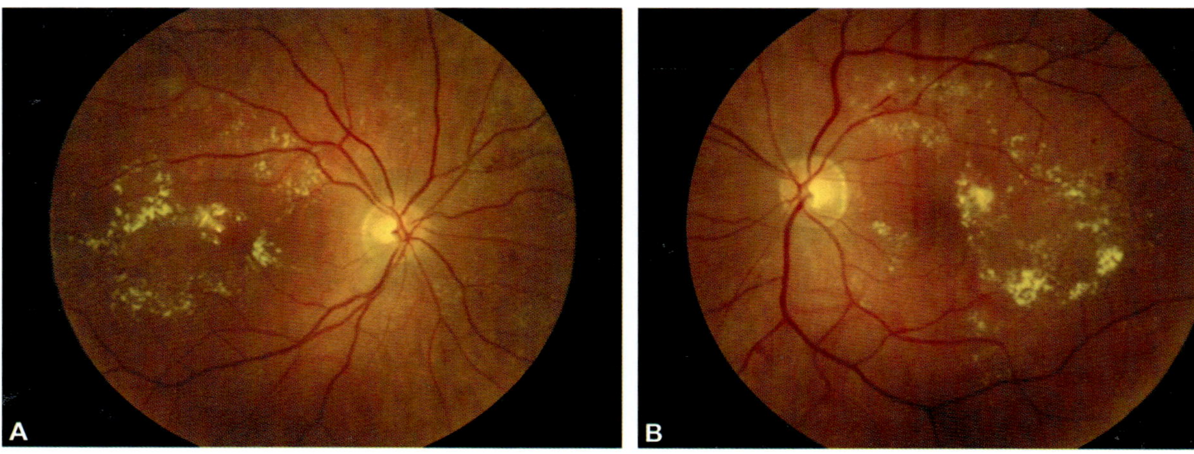

Figs. 28.2A and B: Fundus photographs of moderate nonproliferative diabetic retinopathy with associated hard exudates and diabetic macular edema in the right (A) and left (B) eye.

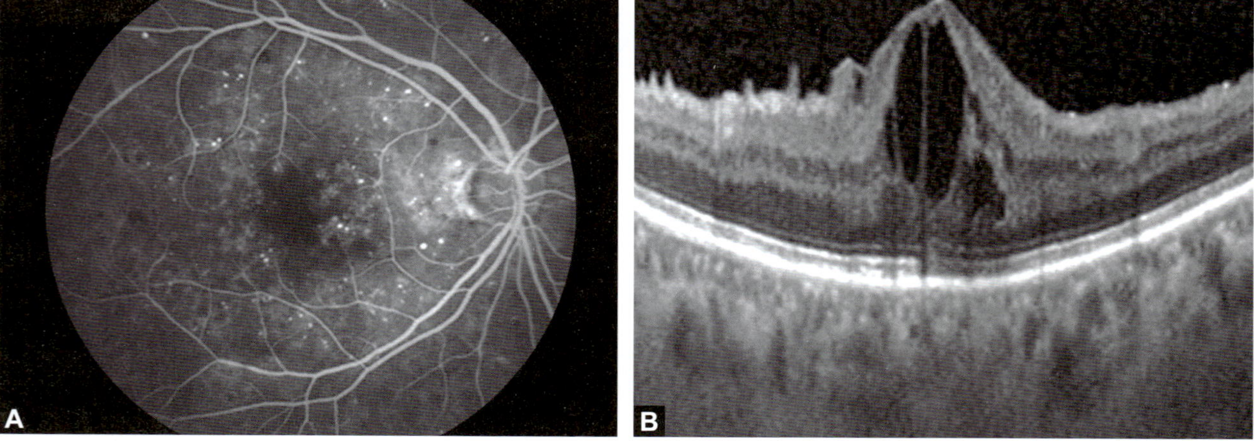

Figs. 28.3A and B: (A) Fluorescein angiography image of a patient with diabetic macular edema (DME) in the right eye. (B) Optical coherence tomography (OCT) picture of the same patient showing cystic center-involving DME.

the observation group. It was also shown that CSME decreases 65% in eyes treated with photocoagulation compared to 37% in the observation group.[10,11] Subsequent studies have also noted that focal laser therapy improves fixation behavior.[12]

Table 28.1: Modified Early Treatment Diabetic Retinopathy Study (ETDRS) technique (direct/grid photocoagulation).

Burn characteristic	Modified ETDRS technique
Direct treatment	Direct treatment of all leaking microaneurysms in areas of retinal thickening 500–3,000 µm from the center of the macula but not within 500 µm of the disc
Change in microaneurysm color with treatment	Not required, but at least a mild gray-white burn should be evident beneath all microaneurysms
Burn size for direct treatment	50 µm
Burn duration for direct	0.05–0.10 seconds
Grid treatment	Areas of diffuse leakage or non-perfusion area considered for grid treatment
Area considered for grid treatment	500–3,000 µm superiorly, nasally, and inferiorly from the center of macula
	500–3,500 µm temporally from macular center
	No burns are placed within 500 µm of the disc
Burn size for grid treatment	50 µm
Burn duration for grid treatment	0.05–0.10 sec
Burn intensity for grid treatment	Barely visible (light gray)
Burn separation for grid treatment	2 visible burn widths apart
Wavelength (grid and focal treatment)	Green to yellow

More recently, ETDRS investigators identified factors that predict who will respond positively to focal laser therapy. As would be expected, poor baseline visual acuity prior to initiating therapy is significantly associated with visual acuity improvement 2 years after laser photocoagulation. Surprisingly, though, optical coherence tomography (OCT) morphologic assessments (cystoid abnormalities, subretinal fluid, vitreoretinal abnormalities) and fundus photographic assessments (retinopathy severity, hemorrhage, microaneurysms, exudates, surface wrinkling) did not significantly predict individuals who would positively respond to laser.[13]

Mechanism of Action

Photocoagulation improves retinal edema through variable mechanisms of action. It is becoming apparent that the thermal burn augments retinal pigment epithelial (RPE) cell function via activation of intracellular signaling pathways.[14,15] RPE cells also have a variety of angiogenic functions and it is believed the new population of cells that arises following photocoagulation results in more efficacious fluid removal,[16,17] leading to improvement in retinal edema. Alternatively, in focal procedures targeted at individual microaneurysms, the thermal energy leads to thrombosis and subsequent closure of the leaking vascular abnormality, resulting in decreased retinal swelling. The disappearance of microaneurysms is a delayed process, often taking from 2 weeks to months following therapy to achieve closure.[18-20]

Changes to Focal Laser Technique since the Original ETDRS Trial

Treatment of CSME using the technique employed by the ETDRS investigators set the standard for conventional photocoagulation. In the years following the publication of the initial ETDRS results, multiple investigators have studied how to modify laser parameters to maximize the therapeutic effect of decreasing macular edema while minimizing the unwanted complications of macular laser.

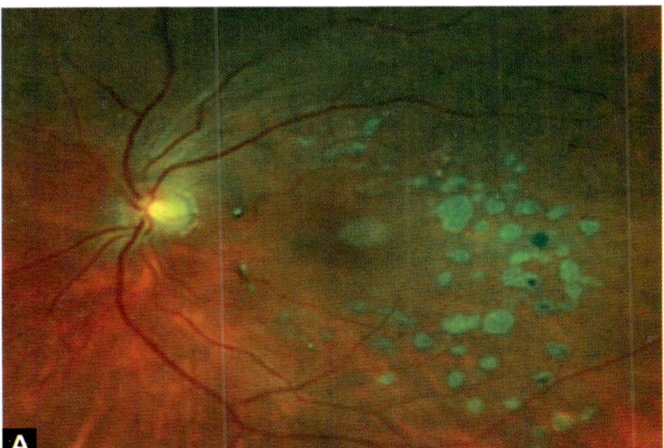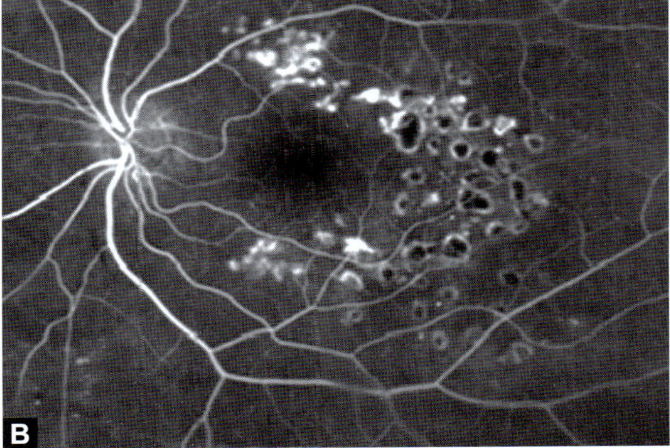

Figs. 28.4A and B: (A) Colored fundus picture showing macular grid laser spots. (B) Fluorescein angiography (FFA) picture of the same individual showing staining of grid laser spots in the late phase.

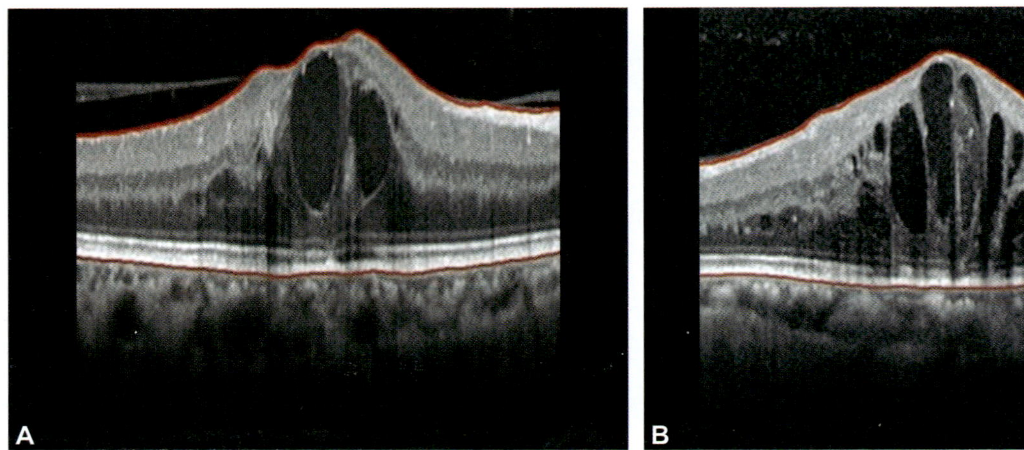

Figs. 28.5A and B: Optical coherence tomography image showing severe diabetic macular edema with cystoid changes at fovea.

Effect of Varying Laser Wavelength in Photocoagulation

Since the publication of the original ETDRS study, clinicians have moved away from using blue-green lasers in focal photocoagulation procedures. This was done for concern that blue lasers may be more phototoxic to the fovea because xanthophyll pigment in the inner retina at the fovea preferentially absorbs blue wavelengths of light. Today, the most commonly used wavelength is green, but laser of red,[21-23] infrared,[24-28] and yellow wavelengths[29-31] have all been shown to be noninferior to green wavelengths in treating DME.

Effect of Varying the Pattern of Laser Application in Photocoagulation

Macular grid laser photocoagulation (Figs. 28.4A and B) has been explored as an alternative to the directed laser therapy as investigated by the ETDRS. Rather than treating discrete lesions, macular grid photocoagulation typically follows a protocol of applying laser burns throughout the paracentral macula in a grid pattern. Microaneurysms are not treated directly and areas of focal edema are not treated differently than the rest of the macula. Some investigators spare the papillomacular bundle while others apply laser to this area. Study results show grid photocoagulation techniques are also beneficial in the treatment of DME,[32-36] but the Diabetic Retinopathy Clinical Research Network (DRCR.net) suggests that directed photocoagulation is more efficacious.[37]

Others have employed an approach of increasing the precision of targeted photocoagulation by using computer assisted navigation.[38-40] One study shows the rates of retreatment with navigated macular laser are less than in conventional photocoagulation.[41] However, few prospective studies exist directly comparing the results of modified ETDRS photocoagulation to navigated laser photocoagulation, so it is yet to be determined what other advantages navigated laser has over conventional techniques.

Effect of Varying Burn Intensity in Photocoagulation

Another modification to ETDRS photocoagulation technique that has been investigated is varying the burn intensity applied. A 532 nm pattern scan laser system (PASCAL) has been used to deliver a subthreshold laser grid throughout the macula and is shown to have noninferior visual acuity and central macular edema outcomes compared to conventional therapy.[42] This method is becoming increasingly popular and recent evidence suggests that subthreshold laser by decreasing the power, so the burn is lighter to barely clinically evident, is as effective in the treatment of DME and reduces clinically apparent retinal damage.[24-28,31,37,43,44]

Focal Laser Photocoagulation Today

Probably the most common approach to focal laser photocoagulation employed today in clinical practice follows the guidelines of the modified ETDRS technique (*see* Figs. 28.4A and B).[37] As explained above, subthreshold laser photocoagulation has also been extensively studied and many clinicians are trending towards decreasing the burn intensity in macular photocoagulation. With the advent of OCT imaging, the manner in which physicians identify treatable lesions has also changed since the publication of the original ETDRS article, and care must be taken when extrapolating the results of the original ETDRS to how patients are most often diagnosed and followed for DME today.[45] In addition, laser monotherapy is largely limited to noncenter involving DME while in center involving DME, the role of laser is described below in the context of anti-vascular endothelial growth factor (VEGF) pharmacotherapy.

Complications

Progressive enlargement of laser scars, also called as laser creep, is a potential complication of focal photocoagulation therapy. In one study, 5% of eyes undergoing conventional grid laser photocoagulation had enlargement of laser scars that progressed into the central fovea.[46] The resulting vision loss from subfoveal fibrosis and RPE atrophy can be worse than 20/200.[46-48] Subfoveal fibrosis likely occurs less frequently today as modified grid photocoagulation has replaced conventional grid laser. However, modified grid photocoagulation has been shown to result in a mild generalized loss of threshold sensitivity (3.44 dB after the first treatment and 6.86 dB after the second treatment) across the central five degrees of the visual field.[49] Case reports have further demonstrated that subretinal neovascularization can rarely occur as a complication of focal laser, originating from the edge of laser scars.[50]

ANTI-VEGF THERAPY

Development of Anti-VEGF Therapy

In 1983, Senger and Dvorak described a tumor-secreted factor that increased microvascular permeability in animal models.[51] This factor was isolated and cloned several years later by two groups independently[52,53] and termed vascular endothelial growth factor or VEGF. Subsequent work established the central role of VEGF in hypoxia-induced tumor angiogenesis,[54,55] and systemic VEGF inhibition eventually gained US Food and Drug Administration (FDA) approval as first- or second-line therapy for a variety of malignancies (reviewed in).[56]

Vascular endothelial growth factor was first implicated in ocular neovascularization in 1994, when Miller and colleagues discovered upregulation of VEGF in a primate model of retinal ischemia.[57] Later that year, a study of human patients found that intraocular VEGF is detectable in a significantly larger proportion of eyes with ischemic disease (proliferative diabetic retinopathy and ischemic central retinal vein occlusion) relative to nonischemic controls.[58] Multiple studies in quick succession demonstrated the efficacy of VEGF inhibition in the prevention of iris,[59] retinal[60-62] and choroidal[63] neovascularization in animal models of ischemic retinopathy. The first large randomized clinical trial of ocular VEGF inhibition was the VISION study published in 2004, where patients with neovascular age-related macular degeneration (AMD) were treated with intravitreal injection of the VEGF inhibitor pegaptanib (Macugen™). Patients who received pegaptanib had a significantly lower risk of visual acuity loss compared to sham-injected controls.[64]

VEGF and Diabetic Macular Edema

The pathogenesis of DME ultimately involves a complex interplay of angiogenesis and inflammation (reviewed in),[65] and abundant research has implicated VEGF signaling in both of these processes. While VEGF is required in a normal physiologic context for vasculogenesis and endothelial cell survival,[66,67] hyperglycemia and subsequent oxidative stress trigger VEGF overexpression.[68] VEGF stimulates increased nitrous oxide production via the calcineurin/NFAT pathway, with resultant activation of endothelial progenitor cells and angiogenesis.[69,70] Additionally, VEGF activates the NF-kappa–B complex which upregulates transcription of inflammatory mediators, including ICAM-1, VCAM-1 and MCP-1;[71-73] these factors in turn promote leukostasis, blood-retinal barrier breakdown and edema.[74-77] There is also evidence that VEGF may increase matrix metalloproteinase expression[78-81] with resulting damage to the retinal microvasculature via mitochondrial dysfunction and apoptosis.[82,83]

Importantly, the level of intraocular VEGF has been shown to correlate with DME severity in human subjects,[84-87] as well as with increased breakdown of the blood-retinal barrier in diabetic animal models.[88,89] Animal experiments have also suggested a causative relationship between elevated VEGF and DME-like pathology, wherein release of exogenous VEGF into the vitreous cavity of rabbits, primates and mice causes increased vascular permeability.[90,91]

Anti-VEGF Therapy for Diabetic Macular Edema (Figs. 28.6A to D)

The experimental data supporting a key role for VEGF in DME pathogenesis, as well as the success of anti-VEGF therapy in other clinical contexts,[92-94] paved the way for clinical trials testing the efficacy of VEGF inhibition for DME. At the time the earliest studies commenced, the standard of care for DME was focal laser photocoagulation as per the landmark ETDRS trial.[11] Following is a review of the major clinical trials for anti-VEGF agents in the treatment of DME (Table 28.2).

Pegaptanib (Macugen™)

In the late 1990s, researchers developed an aptamer, or 2'-F-pyrimidine RNA oligonucleotide ligand, with affinity for human VEGF (specifically, the proinflammatory VEGF-165 isoform).[55] The molecule was formulated for intravitreal delivery by Eyetech Pharmaceuticals™ and passed a phase I safety evaluation. A phase II, randomized, double-masked clinical trial was conducted by the Macugen™ Diabetic Retinopathy Study Group,[96] enrolling 172 patients with center-involving DME and best-corrected visual acuity (BCVA) between 20/50 and 20/320. Treatment involved intravitreal injection of pegaptanib (0.3 mg, 1 mg or 3 mg) or sham injection at weeks 0, 6 and 12, with additional injections every 6 weeks at the discretion of the investigators. Laser photocoagulation was deferred for all patients for the first 16 weeks of the study. For the primary endpoint measured at 36 weeks, patients treated with pegaptanib had significantly greater visual acuity relative to sham (gain of 4.7 ETDRS letters in the 0.3 mg group compared to loss of 0.4 letters in the sham group, $P = 0.04$). In a follow-up analysis, retinal neovascularization was found to have regressed in 8/13 of the pegaptanib patients compared to 0/3 of the sham patients.[97] A larger phase II/III randomized clinical trial, similar in design to the first study but comparing only the 0.3 mg pegaptanib dose to sham injection, was published in 2011.[98] After 1 year of injections as frequently as every 6 weeks, the pegaptanib group was 2.38 times more likely than the sham group to have experienced

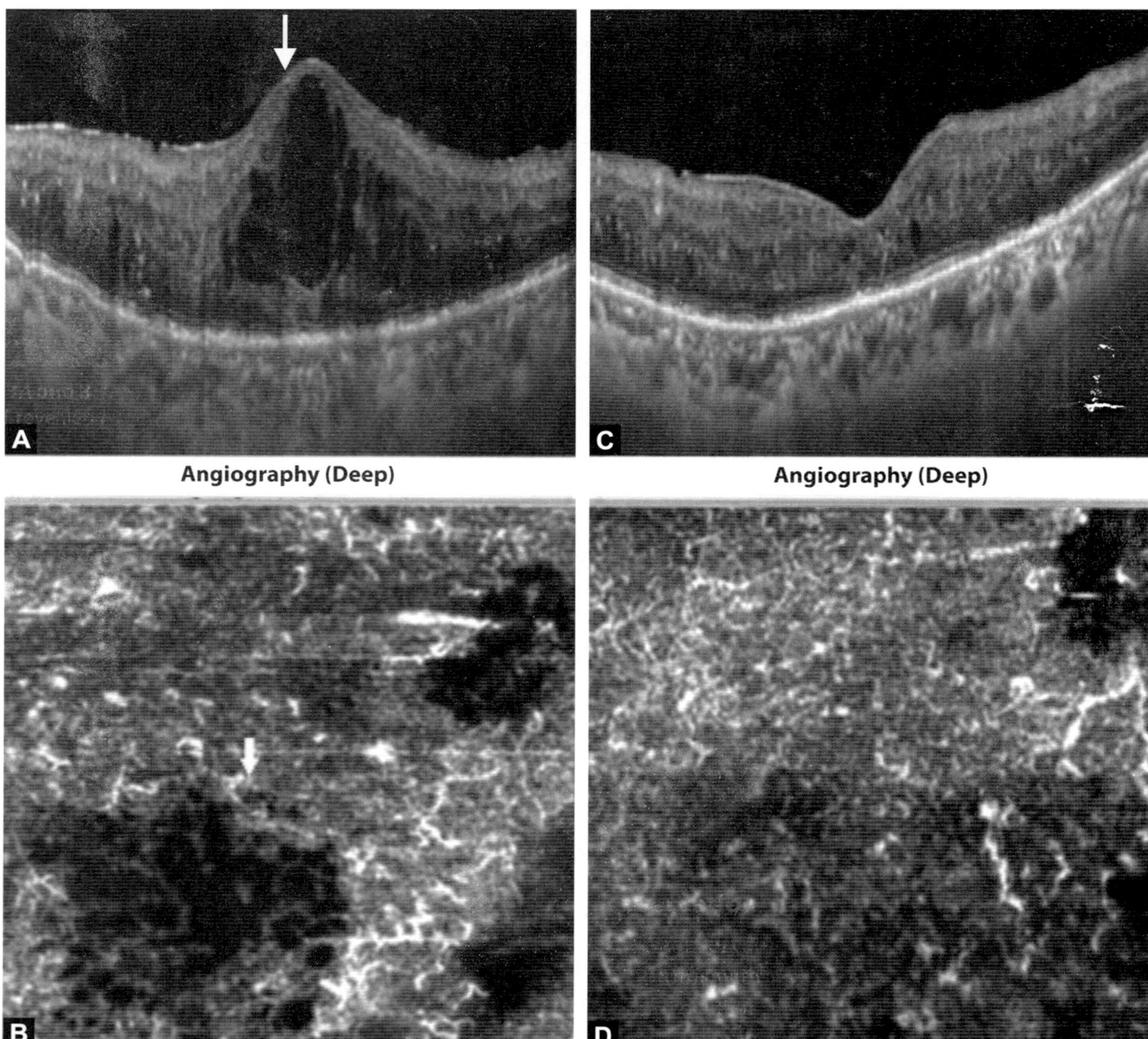

Figs. 28.6A to D: A case of diabetic retinopathy showing resolution of center involving diabetic macular edema (DME) (White arrow) after a single anti-VEGF injection. (A and C) on SSOCT images. (B) OCTA images showing DME (white arrow). (D) OCTA images showing 3 months post anti-VEGF status with resolved DME.

an improvement in BCVA of at least 10 letters ($P = 0.0047$). The average gain in BCVA after 2 years of therapy was 6.1 letters for the pegaptanib group versus 1.3 for sham ($P < 0.01$).

A noncontrolled, longitudinal study of 30 DME patients treated with 0.3 mg intravitreal pegaptanib (injections at weeks 0, 6 and 12) corroborated the vision improvement seen in the earlier controlled trials, with significant increases in BCVA (18.2–25.5 letters, $P < 0.005$), macular sensitivity (8.6–10.6 dB, P < 0.001) and Farnsworth-Munsell color discrimination (376.1 to 116 TES, $P = 0.0001$) at treatment completion relative to baseline.[99]

Bevacizumab (Avastin™)

Bevacizumab was the first anti-VEGF monoclonal antibody developed for therapeutic use by Genentech™ in the 1990s.

Consisting of humanized anti-VEGF Fab and IgG1 regions, it was shown to bind all VEGF-A isoforms and block activation of the receptor.[100] Its first published ophthalmologic use was for the treatment of neovascular AMD, wherein patients showed improvement in visual acuity, central retinal thickness and choroidal neovascular (CNV) leakage after 2–3 intravenous infusions.[101] These data were followed closely by two noncomparative studies of intravitreal bevacizumab for the treatment of DME. The first study was prospective and enrolled 51 patients with diffuse DME; each participant received at least one intravitreal injection of bevacizumab (1.25 mg).[102] Of the 23 patients who completed 12-week follow-up, mean retinal thickness was significantly decreased (501 ± 163 μm to 377 ± 117 μm, $P = 0.001$) although no significant change in ETDRS letter acuity was detected. The second study was retrospective

Table 28.2: Common anti-VEGF agents used for diabetic macular edema (DME).

Anti-VEGF drug	Mechanism	Dose	Major clinical trials	Comments
Pegaptanib (Macugen™)	Aptamer Binds the VEGF-165 isoform	0.3 mg	Cunningham et al.[36] Sultan et al.[98]	No longer in widespread use
Bevacizumab (Avastin™)	Monoclonal anti-VEGF-A antibody Binds all VEGF-A isoforms	1.25 mg	PACORES[103] DRCR.net Protocol H[107] BOLT[108,109] READ-2[115,116]	Least expensive of the anti-VEGF therapies Use for DME is off-label
Ranibizumab (Lucentis™)	Fab fragment of anti-VEGF-A antibody Binds all VEGF-A isoforms	0.3 mg/0.5 mg	RESOLVE[171] DRCR.net Protocol I[117-119] RESTORE[120,121] RISE/RIDE[122,123]	Faster clearance from the systemic circulation compared to other anti-VEGF agents[145,149]
Aflibercept (Eylea™)	Fusion of VEGFR1 and VEGFR2 Ig domains Binds VEGF-A, VEGF-B and PIGF	2 mg	DA VINCI[130,131] VISTA/VIVID[132,133] DRCR.net Protocol T[134]	Most expensive of the anti-VEGF therapies Superior BCVA outcomes compared to bevacizumab and ranibizumab for DME patients with baseline acuity 20/50 or worse[134]

and published by the Pan-American Collaborative Retina Study Group (PACORES).[103] 78 eyes from 64 consecutive patients with DME were included; treatment entailed at least one intravitreal injection of 1.25 or 2.5 mg bevacizumab. At an average 6-month follow-up interval, mean central macular thickness had decreased (387.0 ± 182.8 µm to 275.7 ± 108.3 µm, $P < 0.0001$) and BCVA had either stabilized or improved in the majority of eyes (41.4% and 55.1%, respectively).

Over the next several years, numerous randomized, controlled trials were published comparing intravitreal bevacizumab to other therapies for DME, including focal laser photocoagulation and combination therapy with intravitreal triamcinolone.[104-107] While study design and results varied somewhat, intravitreal bevacizumab was generally associated with significant improvement in BCVA over laser photocoagulation alone, with variable improvement in central retinal thickness. Addition of intravitreal triamcinolone to bevacizumab did not provide any additional benefit over bevacizumab alone, and there were no significant differences between two doses of bevacizumab (1.25 mg vs 2.5 mg).

One of the major studies was the Bevacizumab or Laser Therapy (BOLT) trial published in 2010,[108] enrolling 80 patients with clinically-significant macular edema, history of prior macular laser photocoagulation and baseline BCVA between 35 and 69 ETDRS letters. Patients were randomized to either intravitreal bevacizumab [1.25 mg injections given at weeks 0, 6 and 12, with subsequent injections as per central macular thickness (CMT)-based retreatment protocol] or macular laser photocoagulation (via the modified ETDRS

guidelines). For the primary endpoint at 12 months, ETDRS BCVA was significantly increased in the bevacizumab group (61.3 ± 10.4) compared to the laser group (50.0 ± 16.6, $P = 0.0006$) (Figs. 28.7A to F). Secondary outcomes also favored bevacizumab treatment over laser, with the former intervention associated with a greater likelihood of gaining at least 10 ETDRS letters (31% vs 7.9%, $P = 0.01$) and greater likelihood of losing fewer than 15 ETDRS letters (97.6% vs 73.7%, $P = 0.002$). There were also nonsignificant trends towards greater reduction in CMT with bevacizumab compared to laser (–130 ± 122 µm versus –38 ± 171 µm, $P = 0.06$), as well as greater reduction in ETDRS retinopathy severity. The improvement in BCVA was maintained out to 24 months, at which point the study participants had received a median number of 13 bevacizumab injections or 4 laser treatments.[109] Interestingly, the authors demonstrated with a post-hoc analysis that patients with persistent edema after 12 months of therapy ("late responders") still had the potential to respond to further treatment. By 24 months, 20% of the late responders had achieved a dry macula and 50% had gained more than 15 ETDRS letters.[110]

Ranibizumab (Lucentis™)

In the wake of the success of bevacizumab, Genentech™ developed a variant of this monoclonal antibody consisting of only the antigen-binding portion or Fab fragment. With a molecular weight of 48.3 kD compared to 148 kD for the full-length antibody, ranibizumab was hypothesized to penetrate more deeply into the retina following intravitreal administration. Radiolabeling studies comparing the distribution of the

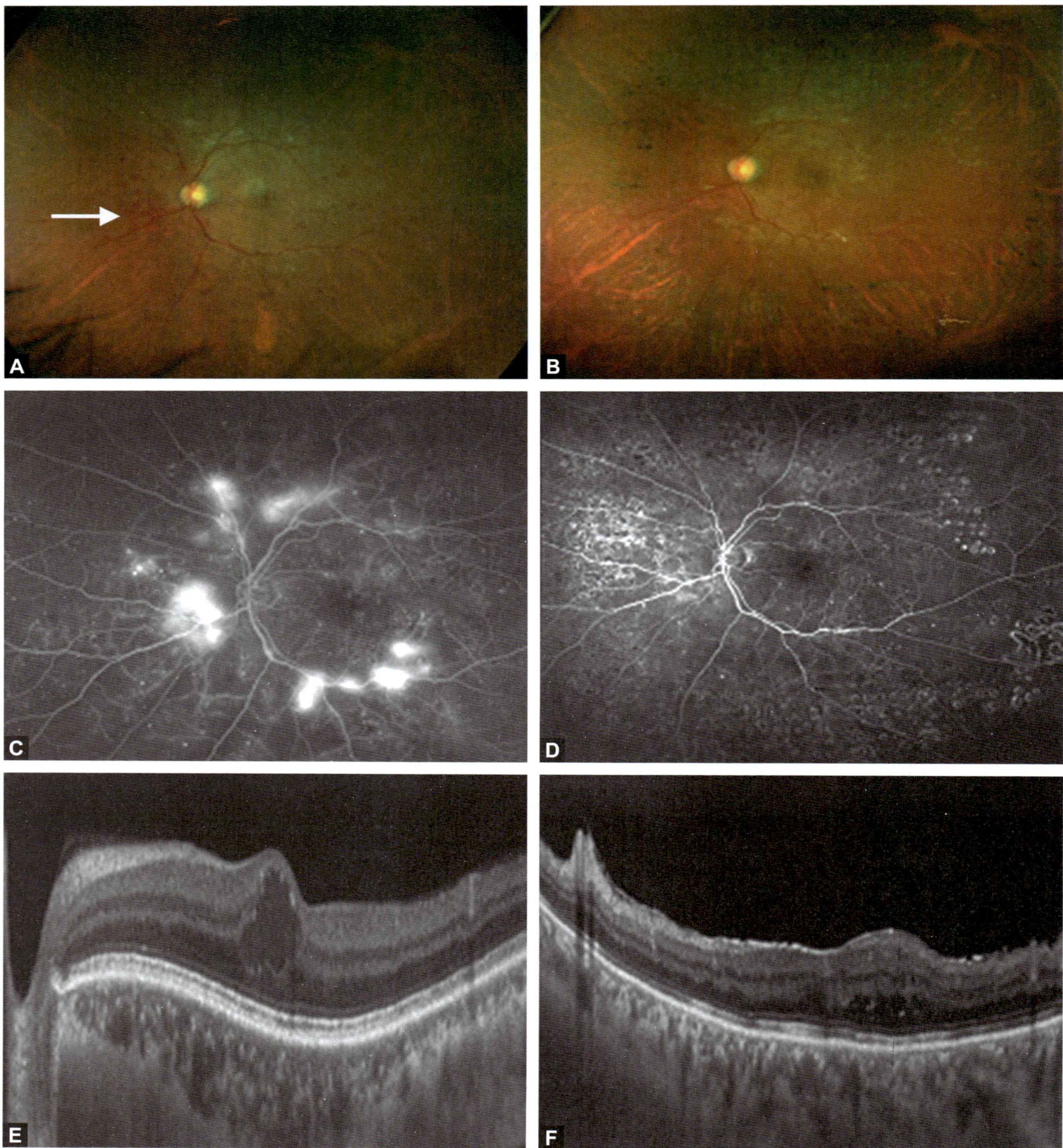

Figs. 28.7A to F: (A) Ultrawidefield fundus photography showing NVE (white arrow). (C) Corresponding fluorescein angiography (FFA) image showing leakage. (E) Optical coherence tomography (OCT) image of the same patient showing center involving DME. (B, D and F) 1 month follow-up pictures post-AntiVEGF and scatter laser showing resolution of diabetic macular edema (DME) and NVE.
(NVE: Neovascularization elsewhere; DME: Diabetic macular edema; VEGF: Vascular endothelial growth factor).

VEGF Fab fragment to the full-length HER2 monoclonal antibody supported this hypothesis, with the former but not latter detectable in deep retinal tissue and RPE after intravitreal administration to rhesus monkeys.[110] Following initial safety and efficacy studies in non-human primates,[63,112] the first human trials of ranibizumab were performed in the context of neovascular AMD.[113,114]

The Ranibizumab for Edema of the macula in Diabetes (READ-2) study was the first published prospective, randomized clinical trial of ranibizumab for the treatment of DME.[115] 126 patients with DME and baseline acuity between 20/40 and 20/320 were enrolled in this phase II study, and randomized to one of three arms: intravitreal ranibizumab (0.5 mg at baseline and months 1, 3 and 5), focal/grid laser photocoagulation (at baseline and month 3 if needed), and a combination of ranibizumab plus laser photocoagulation (both at baseline and month 3). For the primary outcome at 6 months, mean gain in BCVA was 7.24 ETDRS letters in ranibizumab-only group compared to mean loss of 0.43 letters in the laser-only group ($P = 0.0001$); the ranibizumab plus laser group gained an average of 3.8 letters (not statistically different than the drug-only group). Superiority of the ranibizumab and ranibizumab/laser groups over laser alone was also supported by secondary outcomes, including percentage of patients with at least 2 or 3 lines improvement in BCVA and mean change in central subfield thickness (CST) compared to baseline. The READ-2 study was continued for 24 months with retreatment criteria based on CST, with all three groups eligible for ranibizumab injections every 2–3 months.[115] By 24 months, each group had significant improvement in BCVA compared to baseline, with no significant differences among the three groups.

DRCR.net Protocol I was first published in 2010.[117] This phase III, multicenter trial randomized 854 eyes with fovea-involving DME to one of the four groups: (1) prompt focal/grid laser photocoagulation (within 3–10 days) plus sham injection, (2) prompt laser plus 0.5 mg intravitreal ranibizumab, (3) ranibizumab plus deferred (>24 weeks) laser, or (4) 4 mg intravitreal triamcinolone plus prompt laser. All eyes were injected at the baseline visit and every 4 weeks through week 12; starting at week 16, a retreatment protocol was instituted based on BCVA and CST. A laser retreatment protocol was also implemented for edema involving or threatening the center of the macula. For the 1-year primary outcome, there was a significant increase in ETDRS letter score for the two ranibizumab groups (9 ± 11, $P < 0.001$) but no significant increase in the triamcinolone group (4 ± 13, $P = 0.31$), relative to the sham injection group (3 ± 13). An important exception was a subgroup of pseudophakic patients, who fared comparably well with both ranibizumab and triamcinolone.[118] In terms of comparing prompt versus deferred laser treatment in conjunction with ranibizumab, 5-year follow-up data showed a mixed picture.[119] Although prompt laser was associated with a small reduction in total injections required over 5 years, there was no significant difference in mean visual acuity change and 56% of the deferred laser group never met criteria for any laser treatment at all. Thus, Protocol I demonstrated superiority of ranibizumab (plus or minus prompt laser) over triamcinolone plus laser in phakic patients.

The RESTORE trial was similar to Protocol I as it compared ranibizumab to macular laser, with re-treatment criteria following three initial monthly injections.[120] The study enrolled 345 patients randomly assigned to three interventions: 0.5 mg intravitreal ranibizumab, ranibizumab plus macular laser photocoagulation and laser alone. At 1 year, both groups receiving ranibizumab had significantly greater improvements in BCVA (+6.1 and +5.9 letters, $P < 0.0001$) relative to laser alone (+0.8 ETDRS letters, $P < 0.0001$); no significant difference was found between ranibizumab monotherapy and combined ranibizumab-laser therapy. Importantly, the as-needed retreatment protocol (based on change in BCVA) resulted in fewer ranibizumab injections over time, with an average of 2.7 injections in the 3rd year of the extended study compared to 7.4 in the 1st year.[121] This study also examined the safety of intravitreal ranibizumab. Although five ocular serious adverse events (SAEs) were reported for the ranibizumab groups over 36 months, none were thought by the investigator to be attributable to the drug or injection procedure.

The 2012 FDA approval for ranibizumab in the treatment of DME was based on two phase III clinical trials, RISE and RIDE. Conducted in parallel with identical methodology, these studies enrolled a total of 759 DME patients randomized to three treatment arms: sham injection, 0.3 mg ranibizumab and 0.5 mg ranibizumab.[122] Injections were given monthly, and patients were eligible for supplementation with macular laser (based on central foveal thickness) and/or panretinal photocoagulation (PRP) starting in the 3rd month. For the primary outcome at 24 months, both ranibizumab doses in both studies had a higher proportion of patients gaining at least 15 ETDRS letters compared to sham treatment (RISE, 44.8% for 0.3 mg and 39.2% for 0.5 mg versus 18.1% for sham, $P < 0.0001$ and $P = 0.0002$ respectively; RIDE, 33.6% for 0.3 mg and 45.7% for 0.5 mg vs 12.3% for sham, $P < 0.0001$). Nearly twice as many ranibizumab patients achieved a Snellen equivalent of 20/40 compared to sham. The proportions of patients with central foveal thickness more than 250 µm, leakage on fluorescein angiography (FA) or progression to proliferative diabetic retinopathy (PDR) were all significantly lower following ranibizumab treatment. Moreover, the average numbers of required macular laser and PRP treatments were significantly lower in the ranibizumab groups. The study was continued for another 12 months after the primary outcome, during which sham patients were eligible to cross over to monthly 0.5 mg ranibizumab (91% of the original sham group).[123] Interestingly, these crossover patients did not achieve the same magnitude of gain in BCVA after 1 year of treatment compared to the patients treated with ranibizumab initially, suggesting that delay in pharmacologic management of DME might cause loss of potential vision recovery.

Aflibercept (VEGF Trap-eye™; Eylea™)

At the same time, the anti-VEGF-A antibodies were being vetted in clinical trials, scientists were experimenting with alternate mechanisms of blocking VEGF activity. One such strategy was deployment of soluble decoy VEGF receptors,[124] with the theoretical advantage of sequestering all ligands—not only VEGF-A but also other structurally similar cytokines such as VEGF-B and PIGF—capable of activating the proangiogenic signaling cascade.[125] In 2002, researchers at Regeneron™ unveiled VEGF-Trap™ (aflibercept), a soluble decoy VEGF receptor engineered by fusing Ig domains from both VEGFR1 and VEGFR2 (the two best characterized VEGF receptors) with the constant region (Fc) of human IgG1.[126] In vitro assays confirmed the superiority of VEGF-Trap over ranibizumab and bevacizumab with regard to binding affinity for VEGF-A and PIGF, association kinetics with these ligands, and blockage of VEGF receptor activation.[127] In animal models, VEGF-Trap was shown to reduce choroidal neovascularization and blood-retinal barrier breakdown.[128] The biologic was reformulated for intravitreal injection and named VEGF Trap-eye™ or Eylea™.

After a small exploratory study in which intravitreal aflibercept was well tolerated and possibly efficacious for DME,[129] the first phase II controlled trial was designed. The DA VINCI study randomized 221 patients with center-involving DME to five treatment regimens, including four variations of aflibercept dosing (0.5 mg every 4 weeks, 2 mg every 4 weeks, 2 mg every 8 weeks after 3 initial monthly doses, 2 mg as-needed dosing after 3 initial monthly doses) and a macular laser control group. At the primary endpoint of 24 weeks, all aflibercept groups had significantly greater improvement in BCVA relative to laser.[130] These results were mirrored in the 52-week data, along with significantly greater reduction in mean central retinal thickness for aflibercept relative to laser.[131]

The VISTA and VIVID studies were conceived as a head-to-head comparison of aflibercept to macular laser photocoagulation.[132] Similar in design, these phase III trials randomized 872 patients with central-involving DME to three treatment arms: 2 mg intravitreal aflibercept every 4 weeks (2q4), 2 mg aflibercept every 8 weeks after 5 initial monthly doses (2q8), and macular laser. The mean improvement in BCVA at 52 weeks was significantly greater for the aflibercept groups relative to laser in both studies. Secondary outcomes also favored aflibercept over laser, including proportion of patients gaining more than 10 or 15 ETDRS letters from baseline, proportion of patients losing any letters from baseline, improvement in the Diabetic Retinopathy Severity Scale (DRSS) score and reduction in CST from baseline. The two aflibercept dosing regimens (2q4 and 2q8) were similarly efficacious, at both the primary 52-week endpoint and the recently published 100-week endpoint.[133] Results from VISTA and VIVID formed the basis for FDA approval of Eylea™ in 2014 for the treatment of DME (*see* Figs. 28.7A to F).

Comparison of anti-VEGF Agents

Bevacizumab, ranibizumab and aflibercept are currently the three most widely utilized pharmacologic therapies for DME, bevacizumab being used off-label. However, controversy has persisted since the introduction of these drugs due to their huge discrepancy in the cost. According to the Centers for Medicare and Medicaid Services (cms.gov), the 2016 average sales price is $71 for a single 10-mg vial of bevacizumab (typical intravitreal dose 1.25 mg), $1164 for a single 0.3-mg dose of bevacizumab and $1960 for a single 2-mg dose of aflibercept. Thus, there has been great interest in the relative efficacy of these drugs for DME treatment.

The most significant trial to date comparing the three anti-VEGF agents in DME is the DRCR.net Protocol T.[134] Funded by the National Institute of Health (albeit with ranibizumab and aflibercept provided by the drug manufacturers), all data collection and analysis were performed by the DRCR investigators. The study enrolled 660 patients with center-involving DME who had not received any anti-VEGF treatment within the previous 12 months. Participants were randomized to intravitreal injections of 1.25 mg bevacizumab, 0.3 mg ranibizumab or 2.0 mg aflibercept, with an injection given at baseline and then every four weeks according to re-treatment protocol. All patients with persistent DME were eligible for laser photocoagulation starting at week 24, and patients meeting treatment failure criteria were allowed to switch therapy regimens. For the primary outcome of change in visual acuity from baseline to 1 year, aflibercept—with an average gain of 13.3 letters—outperformed both bevacizumab (9.7 letter gain, $P < 0.001$) and ranibizumab (11.2 letter gain, $P = 0.03$). This superiority, however, was driven mainly by letter gains in a predefined subgroup of patients with poor baseline acuity (letter score less than 69, or Snellen equivalent 20/50). For patients with a baseline letter score of 78 to 69 (Snellen equivalent 20/32 to 20/40), all three drugs were similarly efficacious. Bevacizumab was noninferior to ranibizumab in both baseline acuity subgroups. In the follow-up study showing 2-year results, findings demonstrated persistent visual acuity improvements from baseline and a decreased number of injections in the 2nd year of treatment in all three groups. Aflibercept maintained superior visual acuity outcomes among eyes with worse baseline visual acuity in comparison to bevacizumab, but the superiority of aflibercept over ranibizumab noted at 1 year, was no longer demonstrated.[135] Another interesting comparative study, for which results have not yet been published, is the BRDME trial comparing the efficacy and cost of bevacizumab to ranibizumab in the treatment of DME.[136] This study will include a number of interesting secondary outcomes, including comparison of cost in terms of quality-adjusted life-years for the two drugs.

Anti-VEGF Therapy Today

Despite the valuable guidance provided by high-quality clinical trials, clinicians must ultimately integrate multiple variables—such as baseline visual acuity and CMT, response to previous treatment, and ocular or systemic comorbidities—when devising individualized treatment plans for DME. Physician surveys[137] have identified certain practices with near-complete consensus, such as the use of visual acuity and CRT in assessing treatment response, as well as more controversial practices such as the treat-and-extend scheme or the use of another anti-VEGF agent in nonresponders. The AAO Preferred Practice Pattern™ for Diabetic Retinopathy (aao.org) defers most treatment specific to clinicians, stating only that anti-VEGF therapy should be the initial treatment of choice for center-involving macular edema (with focal/grid laser as possible adjunctive therapy, as well as primary therapy for noncenter-involving DME).

There have been several interesting analyses of factors contributing to prescribing patterns for specific anti-VEGF agents. The use of intravitreal bevacizumab, for example, decreased 33% over the course of 1 year in Ohio after the FDA began mandating patient-specific prescriptions (PSPs) for compounded medications in 2013.[138] In a small survey, most physicians indicated that the increased regulatory burden shifted them away from bevacizumab. Financial incentives (Taylor et al., unpublished data) and safety/liability concerns[139-141] also likely contribute to physicians' individual prescribing habits.

Complications

Morbidity related to anti-VEGF therapy for DME can be secondary to effects of the drug itself and also to the intravitreal injection procedure (Figs. 28.8A to D). Systemic VEGF inhibition has well-established associations with thromboembolic events, hypertension, proteinuria and impaired wound healing (reviewed in).[142] Intravitreal VEGF inhibition had long been considered immune to these systemic complications, due to much smaller drug doses. However, intravitreally-injected anti-VEGF agents do in fact cross the blood-retinal barrier into the systemic circulation,[143] and human studies have shown that these drugs suppress serum VEGF levels for sustained periods of time.[144-146] Crossover studies and meta-analyses have raised concerns that intravitreal VEGF increases risk for systemic events, such as ischemic stroke and myocardial infarction.[147,148] While preliminary studies have demonstrated faster systemic clearance of ranibizumab compared to bevacizumab and aflibercept,[145,149] there are no high-quality data currently to indicate a safety advantage for any particular anti-VEGF agent.

Intraocular VEGF inhibition might also result in undesired effects, including tractional retinal detachment (TRD) and sterile ocular inflammation. One retrospective case series[150] reported the development/progression of TRD in 11 out of 211 patients who had received intravitreal bevacizumab as adjunctive therapy to vitrectomy for severe proliferative diabetic retinopathy (PDR). While the authors could not exclude natural progression of disease as the cause of TRD in these patients, they hypothesized that VEGF inhibition might have stimulated rapid neovascular involution and fibrosis with subsequent posterior hyaloid contraction and TRD.

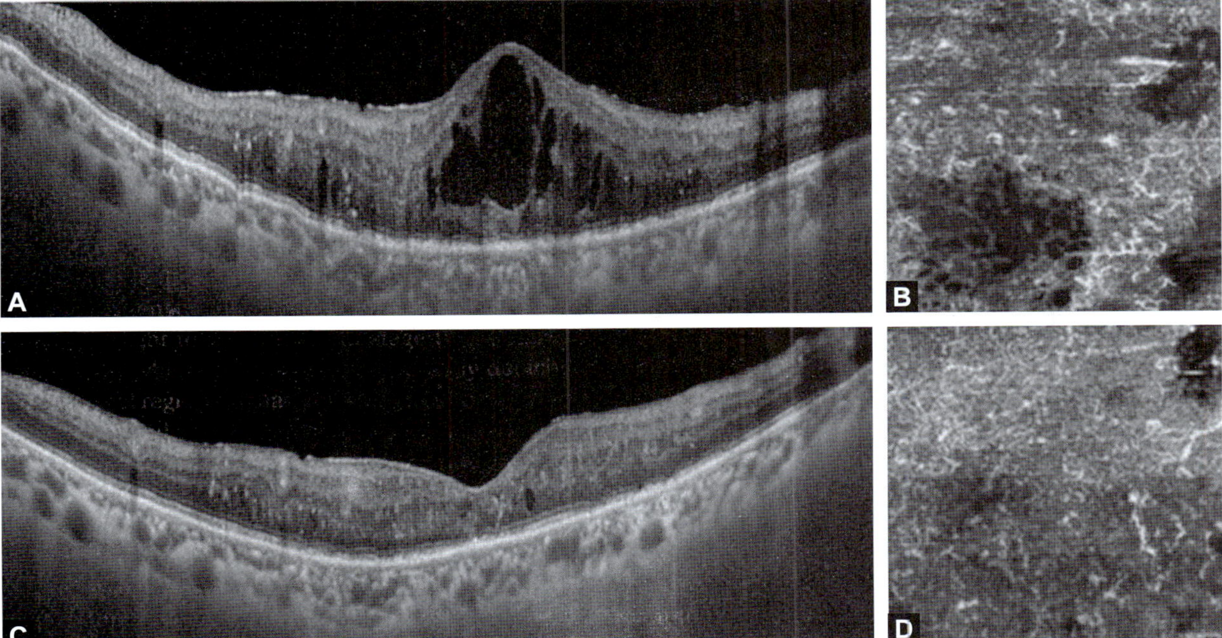

Figs. 28.8A to D: Center-involving DME with cystic fluid on OCT (A) and OCTA (B) imaging; after three initial doses of anti-VEGF injections, shows resolution (C and D). Note slight presence of DRIL in the parafoveal region (C).
(DME: Diabetic macular edema; OCT: Optical coherence tomography; OCTA: OCT Angiography; DRIL: Disorganization of retinal inner layer).

Notably, however, the recently-published DRCR.net Protocol S did not find any significant difference in the occurrence of retinal detachment (tractional or rhegmatogenous) between patients with PDR who were treated with PRP versus intravitreal ranibizumab.[151] With regard to sterile intraocular inflammation, the incidence in the literature following anti-VEGF therapy ranges between 0.033% and 2.9%.[152] All three drugs have been associated with cases, most of which are mild and respond to topical steroid therapy with good visual outcomes (reviewed in).[152,153]

Due to the sheer volume of intravitreal injections performed yearly—numbering 2.3 million among Medicare beneficiaries alone in 2012 (RBRVS DataManager Online, ©American Medical Association)—the risks associated with this procedure have been well-documented (reviewed in).[154,155] Endophthalmitis is one of the most feared complications due to its potentially devastating visual outcome. The incidence of postinjection endophthalmitis varies widely in literature, as does the injection technique, but several recent case series of office-based injections suggests an incidence around 0.01–0.05%.[156-158] The most commonly isolated microorganisms are coagulase-negative Staphylococcus spp. and Streptococcus spp.[158-160] Many clinicians incorporate procedures suggested to decrease the risk of endophthalmitis and/or ocular surface bacterial load, including topical 5% povidone-iodine and a face mask or no-talking policy during the injection; current evidence does not support the routine use of pre-, peri-, or postinjection antibiotics.[161,162] Other documented complications following intravitreal injection include secondary retinal detachment, intraocular hemorrhage and cataract, although these outcomes are often attributed to underlying ocular pathology or drug effects rather than the injection itself.[163]

In conclusion, VEGF inhibition has revolutionized the treatment of DME within the last decade and is currently the standard of care. Future directions may include the delivery of anti-VEGF agents by non-invasive and/or sustained-release methods,[164,165] the development of small-molecule inhibitors of the VEGF signaling pathway,[166,167] and VEGF inhibition via gene therapy.[168-171]

INTRAVITREAL TRIAMCINOLONE

The DRCR.net protocol B investigated the role of intravitreal steroids in the treatment of DME.[172-174] Specifically, triamcinolone was compared to focal/grid photocoagulation in a multicenter randomized clinical trial with 840 eyes of 693 subjects with fovea involving DME. All eyes were randomized to either focal/grid laser, 1 mg intravitreal triamcinolone or 4 mg intravitreal triamcinolone, and eyes were treated initially and retreated for persistent or new edema at 4 month intervals. At the 4 month mark, the 1 mg and 4 mg triamcinolone groups had better visual acuity compared to the laser group but that advantage disappeared at 1 year. Beyond 1 year, the laser monotherapy group showed superior visual acuity results, a trend that persisted through the duration of the 2-year study.[175-177] The OCT thickness results of the study were generally found to mirror the visual acuity results when comparing the three groups. Complication rates were also higher in the triamcinolone group, specifically cataract formation and intraocular pressure rise. At 2 years, a greater than 10 mm mercury intraocular pressure rise from baseline in 4%, 16% and 33% of eyes and a cataract surgery rate of 13%, 23% and 51% in the laser, 1 mg and 4 mg groups, respectively, was noted. Although the pseudophakic subgroup for the triamcinolone arm(s) did show better results than their respective overall group(s), the visual acuity differences between laser and triamcinolone could not solely be attributed to cataract formation.[178]

A 3-year follow-up study for protocol B confirmed the initial results. Change in visual acuity score from baseline was plus five for the laser group in comparison to zero in each triamcinolone group at 3 years. The rates of cataract formation were also significantly higher at 3 years with 46% and 83% of patients needing cataract surgery in the 1 mg and 4 mg groups versus only 31% in laser group.[179]

IMPLANTS

As illustrated earlier, intravitreal triamcinolone has two specific shortcomings that make it less than ideal as a primary agent: short-lasting effect and increased side-effect profile. One of those shortcomings has been eliminated with the advent of extended-release intravitreal steroid devices. Dexamethasone (Ozurdex™ Allergan) and fluocinolone (Retisert™ Bausch and Lomb) (Iluvien™ Alimer Sciences) are the two corticosteroid formulations currently employed. The dexamethasone implant delivers a low dose of medication over a period of 6 months[179] and the fluocinolone devices for up to 36 months,[181] which provides an advantage over anti-VEGF therapies that require more frequent administration.

The dexamethasone implant was the first intraocular steroid FDA approved for use in DME (Figs. 28.9A and B). In the Macular Edema: Assessment of Implantable Dexamethasone in Diabetes (MEAD) study, 1,048 patients with DME, vision between 20/50 to 20/200, and a central retinal thickness of greater than 300 μm were randomly assigned to treatment with a 0.7 mg dexamethasone implant, 0.35 mg implant, or sham procedure and followed for 3 years. Retreatments were allowed no more frequently than every 6 months and required evidence of residual edema on OCT. The primary endpoint of greater than 15 letters visual acuity improvement from baseline was achieved in 22% and 18% in the dexamethasone groups (0.7 mg and 0.35 mg, respectively) compared to 12% in the control group. Furthermore, subjects in the experimental groups required only an average of four treatments over those 3 years. The rates of cataract related events were higher in the treatment groups (67.9% and 64.1% in the 0.7 mg and 0.35 mg groups compared to 20% in the sham group) as were rates of intraocular pressure rise above baseline (27.7% and 24.8% in the 0.7 mg and 0.35 mg groups versus only 3.7% in the sham group). However, most of the cases of IOP rise in the study

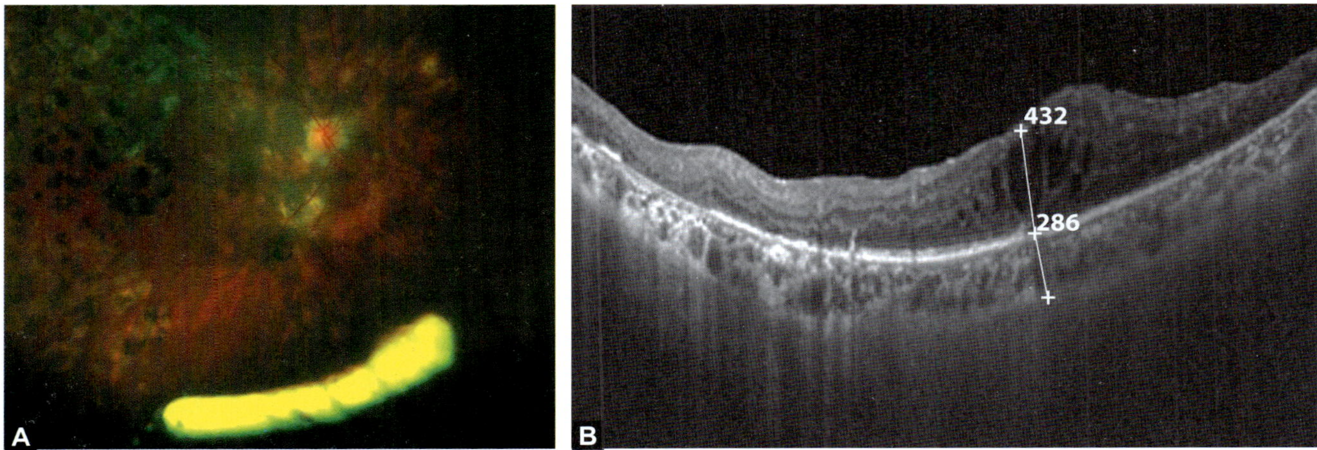

Figs. 28.9A and B: Widefield fundus image (A) showing dexamethasone implant in diabetic macular edema (DME) eye with recalcitrant edema, as seen on optical coherence tomography (OCT) (B).

were able to be controlled with intraocular pressure lowering medications alone and only two patients in the 0.7 mg group and one patient in the 0.35 mg group required trabeculectomy.[180]

Fluocinolone acetonide intravitreal implants provide a longer sustained delivery of steroid compared to the dexamethasone implant. The Retisert™ implant is currently FDA approved for use in posterior noninfectious uveitis but has also been studied for its efficacy in diabetic macular edema. In a prospective randomized controlled trial, 196 eyes with refractory DME were randomized to receive a 0.59-mg fluocinolone acetonide implant or focal/grid photocoagulation. The primary outcome measure was a greater than 15 letter gain from baseline at 6 months. 16.8% of the treatment group achieved this primary outcome in comparison to only 1.4% of patients in the focal/grid photocoagulation group (P = 0.0012). The trial lasted 4 years and at the 3 year mark, 31.1% of the treatment group had achieved greater than three lines visual acuity improvement from baseline compared to 20.0% of the comparison group. The adverse events profile for the treatment group, however, was significantly higher compared to the control group. 33.8% of eyes in the treatment group required incisional glaucoma surgery by 4 years and 91% required cataract surgery compared to only 20% in the focal/grid group.[182]

In contrast to the Retisert™ implant which requires a surgical procedure, Iluvien™ is a fluocinolone acetonide insert that is placed within the vitreous cavity via a 25-gauge needle. Its FDA approval for DME was based on the results of the Fluocinolone Acetonide for Macular Edema (FAME) study where two doses of fluocinolone acetonide, 0.2 µg/day (low dose) and 0.5 µg/day (high dose), were compared to sham injections over 2 years. 953 patients were randomized to sham injections and low and high dose fluocinolone treatments. Visual acuity improvement of 15 letters or more occurred at the 2-year mark in 28.7% and 28.6% of the low and high dose groups compared to 16.2% of the sham group. This visual acuity benefit of both treatment groups was seen as early as 3 weeks into the study and the advantage remained consistent at all subsequent time points. With regards to safety, the low and high dose injectables had a 3.7% and 7.6%, respectively, rate of incisional glaucoma surgery compared to 0.5% in the sham group at 2 years. The requirement for cataract surgery was also significantly higher in both implant groups but the visual improvement of these patients was similar to that of patients who were pseudophakic at baseline.[181]

When to Consider Steroids

As described, intraocular corticosteroids are frequently associated with cataract formation and intraocular pressure rise. Consequently, they are most often used in cases of macular edema refractory to other therapeutic modalities or in patients without glaucoma who have previously undergone cataract extraction.[182-184] As an example, in protocol B, subgroup analysis of the patients with the worst baseline visual acuity (20/200–20/320) showed that 77% of the 4 mg triamcinolone group had a greater than 10 letter improvement at 2 years compared to only 42% for laser while 0% had a greater than 10 letter loss compared to 17% for the laser group.[178] Some studies also suggest that DME in vitrectomized eyes may become refractory to anti-VEGF treatments due to the change in pharmacokinetics, and a dexamethasone implant may provide a more consistent drug dosage necessary to treat chronic DME.[185] The evidence for this is not uniform, as the DRCR network analysis of the number of anti-VEGF injections and visual outcomes of DME therapy are no different in vitrectomized versus non-vitrectomized eyes.[186]

Steroids have also proven useful when used in combination with other therapies. DRCR protocol I subgroup analysis demonstrated that triamcinolone combined with laser can be quite effective in improving visual acuity in pseudophakic patients with results comparable to ranibizumab with laser.[117] And, although protocol B demonstrated that laser is better than intravitreal triamcinolone at long term follow-up, there is strong evidence to suggest that the combination of intravitreal triamcinolone and laser would result in even better long term visual acuity outcomes than laser alone.[118,187]

In most cases, intravitreal steroids will not be considered as first line agents in treating DME. However, some physicians when treating patients with significant cardiac risk or recent cerebrovascular events may elect intravitreal steroids over anti-VEGF injections given the reported increased risk for all-cause mortality and hemorrhagic stroke in patients receiving intravitreal anti-VEGF therapy.[188] Overall, corticosteroids can be an effective option for the treatment of DME as long as the potential for its two main side effects (cataract formation and ocular hypertension) are properly taken into account and adjusted for.

MEDICAL THERAPIES FOR DIABETIC MACULAR EDEMA

Glycemic Control

The most important consideration in the management of diabetic retinopathy and DME is glycemic control. The Diabetes Control and Complications Trial (DCCT) was a large, randomized clinical trial that demonstrated intensive glycemic control resulted in a 76% reduction in the risk of developing diabetic retinopathy compared to conventional therapy in patients with type 1 diabetes. This trial also showed that patients in the intensive therapy group had a 23% risk reduction in the development of DME compared to the conventional therapy cohort.[189] A separate study, the United Kingdom Prospective Diabetes Study (UKPDS), confirmed that type 2 diabetics can also slow progression of diabetic retinopathy with intensive glucose control.[190] In both studies, the intensive glucose control groups had an average hemoglobin A1c (HbA1c) value of 7% compared to approximately 8% in the conventional therapy groups. The results of the DCCT and UKPDS highlight the importance for ophthalmologists to be aware of and assist patients and their primary care providers in maintaining optimum blood glucose levels.

While the DCCT and UKPDS showed the dramatic effect of intensive glycemic control on diabetic retinopathy and DME, caution must be taken to not be overly aggressive in lowering blood glucose levels. Two large randomized clinical trials have now demonstrated higher mortality, presumably related to hypoglycemia-related complications, in patients where intensive glucose control was pursued.[191,192] These studies show that the beneficial effects of intensive glucose control on the eye must be weighed against the increased risk of hypoglycemia-related adverse events.

Hyperglycemia damages the retinal circulation in multiple ways. High blood glucose levels lead to enhanced protein kinase C (PKC) activation, and PKC activity is associated with increased vascular permeability, angiogenesis and cytokine activation.[193] Animal models also demonstrate that inhibiting PKC in diabetic mice ameliorates retinal microvascular complications.[194] Hyperglycemia also leads to increased oxidative stress by increasing advanced glycation end products that then result in the formation of reactivation oxygen species.[195] The final common pathway of these intracellular, hyperglycemia-mediated biochemical processes is often retinal capillary endothelium and pericyte apoptosis.[196]

Fenofibrates

Fenofibrates are another systemic therapy that decreases the progression of diabetic retinopathy. The Fenofibrate Intervention and Event Lowering in Diabetes (FIELD) study found that long-term lipid lowering therapy with fenofibrate reduces the requirement for laser treatment for both DME and proliferative diabetic retinopathy.[197] This large, multinational, prospective study also demonstrated that the effect of fenofibrate reducing the need for laser therapy was independent of the effect of fenofibrate on plasma lipid concentrations. The results of the FIELD study were subsequently confirmed when the ACCORD-eye group found that fenofibrate reduced the progression of diabetic retinopathy over 4 years to 6.5% compared to 10.2% in the placebo group. As in the FIELD study, the ACCORD eye trial did not show an association between the lipid effects of fenofibrate and the progression of diabetic retinopathy.[198] While the results of these two trials are convincing, treating type 2 diabetics with fibrates as standard therapy for preventing retinopathy progression is yet to be adopted in most settings.

Several mechanisms have been proposed in attempt to explain how fibrates slow the progression of diabetic retinopathy. Experimental models demonstrate that fibrates work as agonists to peroxisome proliferator activated receptors (PPARs) and increase amounts of apoA-1, leading to a protective effect on retinal tissue.[199,200] ApoA-1 also functions as a scavenger of reactive oxygen species, and its increased levels in patients taking fibrates could result in decreased oxidative stress.[201] Fenofibrate-driven agonism to the alpha PPAR isoform has also been shown to alter lipid and triglyceride levels and produce an inhibitory environment to angiogenesis and inflammation.[202,203]

Thiazolidinediones

Pioglitazone and rosiglitazone are thiazolidinedione medications used to treat type 2 diabetes and they also act as agonists to the PPAR receptor. However, investigators have discovered that, in some patients, thiazolidinedione use is associated with the development of DME.[204-206] This can be considered as a contributing factor leading to DME, especially in patients who develop DME soon after initiating glitazone therapy. However, not all studies agree there is a causative link and the ACCORD eye study found no association between thiazolidinediones and DME.[207] More studies are being conducted to further clarify this potential link.

TOPICAL THERAPY FOR DME

The current standard of care for DME is intravitreal anti-VEGF therapy, with focal laser photocoagulation and/or intravitreal steroids serving as adjunctive or second-line therapy. While anti-VEGF drugs have substantially reduced vision impairment secondary to DME,[208-210] the treatment burden is high for patients, physicians and insurers. Thus, there is a strong incentive to develop less invasive therapies.[211] Following is a review of topical medications that have been studied in terms of efficacy for DME.

Topical NSAIDs

Nepafenac is a nonsteroidal anti-inflammatory drug (NSAID) prodrug converted to its active metabolite amfenac by intraocular hydrolases.[212] Studies in animal models[213-215] and human patients undergoing vitrectomy[216] have demonstrated good penetration to the posterior segment following topical instillation, with reduction in PGE2 levels in the retina, choroid and vitreous. In several case reports, DME patients treated with topical 0.1% nepafenac for at least 6 months showed improvement in BCVA and retinal/foveal thickness relative to baseline.[217,218] There is also evidence that topical nepafenac might reduce the incidence or severity of postcataract surgery macular edema, in both diabetic and nondiabetic patients.[219,220] Due to these promising results, a phase II, double-blind, randomized clinical trial was recently undertaken by the DRCR Network to study the effect of nepafenac on DME in a nonsurgical context (Protocol R).[221] This study enrolled 125 patients with noncenter involving DME; exclusion criteria included recent treatment of DME with focal/grid laser (in the previous 6 months or other treatment in the previous 4 months), as well as systemic steroid, NSAID, or anti-VEGF therapy. Patients were randomized to treatment with 0.1% nepafenac versus placebo. At the primary outcome of 12 months, there were no significant changes in BCVA or retinal volume between the two groups. Therefore, while nepafenac may be efficacious in the prevention or treatment of post-surgical DME, high-quality evidence currently argues against its routine use for noncenter involving DME. Other topical NSAIDs including ketorolac and bromfenac have likewise shown efficacy in the prevention and treatment of postoperative macular edema, when used in conjunction with topical steroids.[222-224] However, these drugs have not been studied in DME outside the context of cataract surgery. A recent Cochrane review emphasized the dearth of high-quality clinical trials studying the effects of topical NSAIDs on DME.[225]

Topical Steroids

In contrast to the abundance of data supporting intravitreal steroid therapy for DME, relatively few trials have studied the efficacy of topically instilled steroids. Topical delivery presents unique pharmacokinetic challenges,[226] and much basic research has focused on optimizing steroid formulations for posterior segment penetration. One strategy uses cyclodextrins—hydrophilic oligosaccharides[227]—to form water-soluble complexes with lipophilic dexamethasone. After promising pharmacokinetic results in an animal model,[228] the formulation was administered topically to a series of 19 patients with

DME.[229] Over a 4-week treatment period, BCVA significantly improved (logMAR 0.52 ± 0.41 at baseline to 0.37 ± 0.40 at 4 weeks, $P = 0.0025$) and CST decreased (512 ± 164 μm to 399 ± 154 μm, $P = 0.0016$). Both parameters reverted towards baseline after an additional 4 weeks of observation only, suggesting a steroid-related effect rather than the natural course of disease. Of note, intraocular pressure did increase an average of 2 points during the treatment period, and this parameter was also reversible after treatment cessation.

Difluprednate is another topical steroid which has been tested for efficacy in DME. In a small non-controlled study,[230] 20 patients with refractory DME were treated with 0.05% difluprednate emulsion TID for 3 months. By the end of the treatment period, BCVA had improved significantly relative to baseline (logMAR 0.88 ± 0.203 to 0.61 ± 0.175, $P < 0.001$), and central macular thickness had also significantly decreased (423 ± 72 μm to 346 ± 69 μm, $P < 0.001$).

However, these effects were accompanied by a significant elevation in IOP (13.9 ± 2.1 to 17.3 ± 4.9, $P = 0.007$), and 4 of 20 patients required anti-glaucoma medications with tapering of the steroid. In another small, controlled but non randomized study,[231] 19 eyes in 15 patients with DME were treated with 0.05% difluprednate 4 times daily for 1 month followed by twice daily for 2 months. Comparison was made to a control group of 22 eyes in 11 patients with DME who could not receive steroids due to history of steroid response. After 3 months of treatment, there was a trend towards improved visual acuity and decreased mean retinal thickness in the difluprednate group relative to controls, but the differences were not statistically significant. Ultimately, larger controlled studies with longer follow-up will be necessary in order to prove any efficacy (or lack thereof) of topical steroids for DME.[232]

Other Drug Classes

Due to the complexity of DME pathophysiology, there are many potential targets for pharmacologic modulation.[233] Nicotinic acetylcholine receptors are one such target; activation of these receptors on vascular endothelial cells stimulates proliferation and neovascularization in cell cultures and animal models.[234-235] Mecamylamine is a nonspecific nicotinic AChR blocker. Currently approved as an oral antihypertensive, it has been reformulated as a 1% topical ophthalmic solution (CoMentis™). Preliminary testing in patients with DME has found the drug to be safe and well-tolerated at BID dosing; the study was not powered to assess efficacy for DME.[236] The current development status of this drug for DME is unknown.

Molecules involved in leukostasis are also attractive drug targets. ICAM-1, for example, is a capillary endothelial cell surface ligand that mediates leukocyte adhesion; it is upregulated in the retinal/choroidal vasculature of diabetics.[238] Blocking the interaction of ICAM-1 with the leukocyte surface integrin LFA-1[239] is hypothesized to prevent retinal leukostasis and subsequent capillary obstruction, endothelial cell damage and vascular leakage.[75,77] SAR 1118 was developed as a small-molecule antagonist of the LFA-1/ICAM-1 interaction.[240] Topical administration to a diabetic rat model reduced retinal vasculature leukostasis and blood-retinal barrier breakdown.[241] It subsequently passed a phase Ib safety study in human patients; however, drug levels were undetectable in the vitreous so further investigations of DME efficacy were put hold.[242] As an aside, the drug manufacturer is currently seeking FDA approval for SAR 1118 (Lifitegrast™) as a treatment for dry eye.[243]

In conclusion, efforts to treat DME with topical agents have met with lackluster results so far. Future therapies will likely benefit from technological advances that increase drug distribution to the posterior segment.[244-247]

SURGICAL MANAGEMENT OF DIABETIC MACULAR EDEMA

Persistent DME despite therapy with ranibizumab occurs in 40% of patients after 24 weeks of therapy. While continued anti-VEGF therapy is effective in many, 40% of these individuals still have chronic persistent DME over 3 years of regular treatments.[248] This implies there may be VEGF-independent molecular mechanisms that are involved in the development and sustenance of macular edema, and the need for multitargeted pharmacotherapeutic strategies is still highly relevant.[249] The role of vitreous surgery in treating persistent DME in these settings has been studied by a number of investigators.

Termed "triple therapy," vitrectomy has been coupled with intravitreal triamcinolone and postoperative macular photocoagulation in cases of intractable non-tractional DME. Significant improvement in macular thickness as well as BCVA has been noted that extends beyond 1 year of postoperative follow-up.[250,251] Notably, over 75% of eyes in one series remained without recurrence of DME at 3-year follow-up.[252]

Sometimes, macular edema occurs in individuals with vitreomacular traction (VMT) and DME. The DRCR network investigated the impact of vitrectomy on 87 eyes with concurrent VMT and DME. Perioperative interventions such as epiretinal membrane peeling, intravitreal steroids or retinal photocoagulation were not standardized. At 6 months postvitrectomy, 68% of patients had at least a 50% reduction in CMT and BCVA improved by more than 10 letters in 38% of the cohort. 22% of individuals had worse vision than prior to vitrectomy.[253] When eyes with tractional DME were retrospectively compared to eyes with nontractional DME, both groups demonstrated similar visual acuity improvements and CMT improvements.[254]

In part, vitrectomy alleviates nontractional macular edema by removing the vitreous barrier adjacent to the retina and thus allowing for improved oxygenation. The vitreous cortex is also thought to serve as a collector of proangiogenic factors, so excision of the hyaloid removes that depository.[255,256] The literature for vitreous surgery in DME is still in the early stages and studies have been fraught with design, technique

or analysis flaws. Perhaps this is why vitrectomy has been advocated in DME only when accompanied by VMT.[257] However, with constantly evolving surgical techniques, outcomes are continually improving and vitreous surgery for the treatment of persistent DME will likely assume a more prominent role in the future.

REFERENCES

1. Klein R, Knudtson MD, Lee KE, et al. The Wisconsin Epidemiologic Study of Diabetic Retinopathy XXIII: the twenty-five-year incidence of macular edema in persons with type 1 diabetes. Ophthalmology. 2009;116:497-500.
2. Romero-Aroca P. Managing diabetic macular edema: the leading cause of diabetes blindness. World J Diab. 2011;2:98-104.
3. Klein R, Lee KE, Knudtson MD, et al. Changes in visual impairment prevalence by period of diagnosis of diabetes: the Wisconsin Epidemiologic Study of Diabetic Retinopathy. Ophthalmology. 2009;116:1937-42.
4. Romero-Aroca P, Fernandez-Balart J, Baget-Bernaldiz M, et al. Changes in the diabetic retinopathy epidemiology after 14 years in a population of Type 1 and 2 diabetic patients after the new diabetes mellitus diagnosis criteria and a more strict control of the patients. J Diab Comp. 2009;23:229-38.
5. Blankenship GW. Diabetic macular edema and argon laser photocoagulation: a prospective randomized study. Ophthalmology. 1979;86:69-78.
6. Patz A, Schatz H, Berkow JW, et al. Macular edema—an overlooked complication of diabetic retinopathy. Trans Am Acad Ophthalmology Otolaryngol. 1973;77:OP34-42.
7. Merin S, Yanko L, Ivry M. Treatment of diabetic maculopathy by argon-laser. Br J Ophthalmology. 1974;58:85-91.
8. Photocoagulation for diabetic maculopathy. A randomized controlled clinical trial using the xenon arc. British Multicentre Study Group. Diabetes. 1983;32:1010-6.
9. Photocoagulation for diabetic macular edema. Early Treatment Diabetic Retinopathy Study report number 1. Early Treatment Diabetic Retinopathy Study research group. Arch Ophthalmology. 1985;103:1796-806.
10. Treatment techniques and clinical guidelines for photocoagulation of diabetic macular edema. Early Treatment Diabetic Retinopathy Study Report Number 2. Early Treatment Diabetic Retinopathy Study Research Group. Ophthalmology. 1987;94:761-74.
11. Raman R, Santhanam K, Gella L, et al. Morphological and functional outcomes following modified early treatment diabetic retinopathy study laser in diabetic macular edema. Oman J Ophthalmology. 2015;8:92-6.
12. Aiello LP, Edwards AR, Beck RW, et al. Factors associated with improvement and worsening of visual acuity 2 years after focal/grid photocoagulation for diabetic macular edema. Ophthalmology. 2010;117:946-53.
13. Han JW, Lyu J, Park YJ, et al. Wnt/beta-catenin signaling mediates regeneration of retinal pigment epithelium after laser photocoagulation in mouse eye. Invest Ophthalmology Vis Sci. 2015;56:8314-24.
14. Tababat-Khani P, Berglund LM, Agardh CD, et al. Photocoagulation of human retinal pigment epithelial cells in vitro: evaluation of necrosis, apoptosis, cell migration, cell proliferation and expression of tissue repairing and cytoprotective genes. PLoS One. 2013;8:e70465.
15. Glaser BM, Campochiaro PA, Davis JL Jr, et al. Retinal pigment epithelial cells release an inhibitor of neovascularization. Arch Ophthalmology. 1985;103:1870-5.
16. Weiter JJ, Zuckerman R. The influence of the photoreceptor-RPE complex on the inner retina. An explanation for the beneficial effects of photocoagulation. Ophthalmology. 1980;87:1133-9.

17. Gogi D, Gupta A, Gupta V, et al. Retinal microaneurysmal closure following focal laser photocoagulation in diabetic macular edema. Ophth Surg Las. 2002;33:362-7.

18. Lee SN, Chhablani J, Chan CK, et al. Characterization of microaneurysm closure after focal laser photocoagulation in diabetic macular edema. Am J Ophthalmology. 2013;155:905-12.

19. Sachdev N, Gupta V, Abhiramamurthy V, et al. Correlation between microaneurysm closure rate and reduction in macular thickness following laser photocoagulation of diabetic macular edema. Eye. 2008;22:975-7.

20. Olk RJ. Argon green (514 nm) versus krypton red (647 nm) modified grid laser photocoagulation for diffuse diabetic macular edema. Ophthalmology. 1990;97:1101-12; discussion 12-3.

21. Khairallah M, Brahim R, Allagui M, et al. Comparative effects of argon green and krypton red laser photocoagulation for patients with diabetic exudative maculopathy. The Br J Ophthalmology. 1996;80:319-22.

22. Freyler H. Laser therapy of diabetic maculopathy. A comparative study of the argon green laser and dye red laser. Klinische Monatsblatter fur Augenheilkunde. 1990;197:176-81.

23. Figueira J, Khan J, Nunes S, et al. Prospective randomised controlled trial comparing sub-threshold micropulse diode laser photocoagulation and conventional green laser for clinically significant diabetic macular oedema. Br J Ophthalmology. 2009;93:1341-4.

24. Sivaprasad S, Sandhu R, Tandon A, et al. Subthreshold micropulse diode laser photocoagulation for clinically significant diabetic macular oedema: a three-year follow up. Clin Exp Ophthalmology. 2007;35:640-4.

25. Othman IS, Eissa SA, Kotb MS, et al. Subthreshold diode-laser micropulse photocoagulation as a primary and secondary line of treatment in management of diabetic macular edema. Clin Ophthalmology. 2014;8:653-9.

26. Friberg TR. Infrared micropulsed laser treatment for diabetic macular edema—subthreshold versus threshold lesions. Semin Ophthalmology. 2001;16:19-24.

27. Laursen ML, Moeller F, Sander B, et al. Subthreshold micropulse diode laser treatment in diabetic macular oedema. Br J Ophthalmology. 2004;88:1173-9.

28. Browning DJ, Antoszyk AN. The effect of the surgeon and the laser wavelength on the response to focal photocoagulation for diabetic macular edema. Ophthalmology. 1999;106:243-8.

29. Bressler SB, Almukhtar T, Aiello LP, et al. Green or yellow laser treatment for diabetic macular edema: exploratory assessment within the Diabetic Retinopathy Clinical Research Network. Retina. 2013;33:2080-8.

30. Kwon YH, Lee DK, Kwon OW. The short-term efficacy of subthreshold Micropulse yellow (577-nm) laser photocoagulation for diabetic macular edema. Korean J Ophthalmology. 2014;28:379-85.

31. McNaught EI, Foulds WS, Allan D. Grid photocoagulation improves reading ability in diffuse diabetic macular oedema. Eye. 1988;2 (Pt 3):288-96.

32. Olk RJ. Modified grid argon (blue-green) laser photocoagulation for diffuse diabetic macular edema. Ophthalmology. 1986;93:938-50.

33. McDonald HR, Schatz H. Grid photocoagulation for diffuse macular edema. Retina 1985;5:65-72.

34. Scott IU, Danis RP, Bressler SB, et al. Diabetic Retinopathy Clinical Research Network. Effect of focal/grid photocoagulation on visual acuity and retinal thickening in eyes with non-center-involved diabetic macular edema. Retina. 2009;29(5):613-7.

35. Lee CM, Olk RJ. Modified grid laser photocoagulation for diffuse diabetic macular edema. Long-term visual results. Ophthalmology. 1991;98:1594-602.

36. Shimura M, Yasuda K, Nakazawa T, et al. Effective treatment of diffuse diabetic macular edema by temporal grid pattern photocoagulation. Ophthalmic Surg Lasers Imaging. 2004;35:270-80.

37. Writing Committee for the Diabetic Retinopathy Clinical Research;Fong DS, Strauber SF. Comparison of the modified Early Treatment Diabetic Retinopathy Study and mild macular grid laser photocoagulation strategies for diabetic macular edema. Arch Ophthalmology. 2007;125:469-80.

38. Liegl R, Langer J, Seidensticker F, et al. Comparative evaluation of combined navigated laser photocoagulation and intravitreal ranibizumab in the treatment of diabetic macular edema. PloS One. 2014;9:e113981.

39. Kozak I, Oster SF, Cortes MA, et al. Clinical evaluation and treatment accuracy in diabetic macular edema using navigated laser photocoagulator NAVILAS. Ophthalmology. 2011;118:1119-24.

40. Kernt M, Cheuteu RE, Cserhati S, et al. Pain and accuracy of focal laser treatment for diabetic macular edema using a retinal navigated laser (Navilas). Clin Ophthalmology. 2012;6:289-96.

41. Neubauer AS, Langer J, Liegl R, et al. Navigated macular laser decreases retreatment rate for diabetic macular edema: a comparison with conventional macular laser. Clin Ophthalmology. 2013;7:121-8.

42. Pei-Pei W, Shi-Zhou H, Zhen T, et al. Randomised clinical trial evaluating best-corrected visual acuity and central macular thickness after 532-nm subthreshold laser grid photocoagulation treatment in diabetic macular oedema. Eye. 2015;29:313-21.

43. Ohkoshi K, Yamaguchi T. Subthreshold micropulse diode laser photocoagulation for diabetic macular edema in Japanese patients. Am J Ophthalmology. 2010;149:133-9.

44. Lavinsky D, Cardillo JA, Melo LA Jr, et al. Randomized clinical trial evaluating mETDRS versus normal or high-density micropulse photocoagulation for diabetic macular edema. Invest Ophthalmology Vis Sci. 2011;52:4314-23.

45. Virgili G, Menchini F, Murro V, et al. Optical coherence tomography (OCT) for detection of macular oedema in patients with diabetic retinopathy. Cochrane Database Of SystRev. 2011:CD008081.

46. Schatz H, Madeira D, McDonald HR, et al. Progressive enlargement of laser scars following grid laser photocoagulation for diffuse diabetic macular edema. Arch Ophthalmology. 1991;109:1549-51.

47. Guyer DR, D'Amico DJ, Smith CW. Subretinal fibrosis after laser photocoagulation for diabetic macular edema. Am J Ophthalmology. 1992;113:652-6.

48. Han DP, Mieler WF, Burton TC. Submacular fibrosis after photocoagulation for diabetic macular edema. Am J Ophthalmology. 1992;113:513-21.

49. Striph GG, Hart WM Jr, Olk RJ. Modified grid laser photocoagulation for diabetic macular edema. The effect on the central visual field. Ophthalmology. 1988;95:1673-9.

50. Lewen RM. Subretinal neovascularization complicating laser photocoagulation of diabetic maculopathy. Ophth Surg. 1988; 19:734-7.

51. Senger DR, Galli SJ, Dvorak AM, et al. Tumor cells secrete a vascular permeability factor that promotes accumulation of ascites fluid. Science. 1983;219:983-5.

52. Keck PJ, Hauser SD, Krivi G, et al. Vascular permeability factor, an endothelial cell mitogen related to PDGF. Science. 1989;246:1309-12.

53. Leung DW, Cachianes G, Kuang WJ, et al. Vascular endothelial growth factor is a secreted angiogenic mitogen. Science. 1989; 246:1306-9.

54. Shweiki D, Itin A, Soffer D, et al. Vascular endothelial growth factor induced by hypoxia may mediate hypoxia-initiated angiogenesis. Nature. 1992;359:843-5.

55. Plate KH, Breier G, Weich HA, et al. Vascular endothelial growth factor is a potential tumour angiogenesis factor in human gliomas in vivo. Nature. 1992;359:845-8.

56. Zhao Y, Adjei AA. Targeting angiogenesis in cancer therapy: moving beyond vascular endothelial growth factor. Oncologist. 2015;20:660-73.

57. Miller JW, Adamis AP, Shima DT, et al. Vascular endothelial growth factor/vascular permeability factor is temporally and spatially correlated with ocular angiogenesis in a primate model. Am J Pathol. 1994;145:574-84.

58. Aiello LP, Avery RL, Arrigg PG, et al. Vascular endothelial growth factor in ocular fluid of patients with diabetic retinopathy and other retinal disorders. N Engl J Med. 1994;331:1480-7.

59. Adamis AP, Shima DT, Tolentino MJ, et al. Inhibition of vascular endothelial growth factor prevents retinal ischemia-associated iris neovascularization in a nonhuman primate. Arch Ophthalmology. 1996;114:66-71.

60. Aiello LP, Pierce EA, Foley ED, et al. Suppression of retinal neovascularization in vivo by inhibition of vascular endothelial growth factor (VEGF) using soluble VEGF-receptor chimeric proteins. Proc Natl Acad Sci USA. 1995;92:10457-61.

61. Robinson GS, Pierce EA, Rook SL, et al. Oligodeoxynucleotides inhibit retinal neovascularization in a murine model of proliferative retinopathy. Proc Natl Acad Sci USA. 1996;93:4851-6.

62. Ozaki H, Seo MS, Ozaki K, et al. Blockade of vascular endothelial cell growth factor receptor signaling is sufficient to completely prevent retinal neovascularization. Am J Pathol 2000;156:697-707.

63. Krzystolik MG, Afshari MA, Adamis AP, et al. Prevention of experimental choroidal neovascularization with intravitreal anti-vascular endothelial growth factor antibody fragment. Arch Ophthalmology. 2002;120:338-46.

64. Gragoudas ES, Adamis AP, Cunningham ET Jr, et al. Pegaptanib for neovascular age-related macular degeneration. N Engl J Med. 2004;351:2805-16.

65. Fogli S, Mogavero S, Egan CG, et al. Pathophysiology and pharmacological targets of VEGF in diabetic macular edema. Pharmacol Res. 2016;103:149-57.

66. Senger DR. Vascular endothelial growth factor: much more than an angiogenesis factor. Mol Biol Cell. 2010;21:377-9.

67. Ferrara N. Role of vascular endothelial growth factor in regulation of physiological angiogenesis. Am J Physiol Cell Physiol. 2001;280:C1358-66.

68. Behl T, Kotwani A. Exploring the various aspects of the pathological role of vascular endothelial growth factor (VEGF) in diabetic retinopathy. Pharmacol Res. 2015;99:137-48.

69. Liu X, Li Y, Liu Y, et al. Endothelial progenitor cells (EPCs) mobilized and activated by neurotrophic factors may contribute to pathologic neovascularization in diabetic retinopathy. Am J Pathol. 2010;176:504-15.

70. Yang L, Guan H, He J, et al. VEGF increases the proliferative capacity and eNOS/NO levels of endothelial progenitor cells through the calcineurin/NFAT signalling pathway. Cell Biol Int. 2012;36:21-7.

71. Kim I, Moon SO, Kim SH, et al. Vascular endothelial growth factor expression of intercellular adhesion molecule 1 (ICAM-1), vascular cell adhesion molecule 1 (VCAM-1), and E-selectin through nuclear factor-kappa B activation in endothelial cells. J Biol Chem. 2001;276:7614-20.

72. Marumo T, Schini-Kerth VB, Busse R. Vascular endothelial growth factor activates nuclear factor-kappa B and induces monocyte chemoattractant protein-1 in bovine retinal endothelial cells. Diabetes 1999;48:1131-7.

73. Lu M, Perez VL, Ma N, et al. VEGF increases retinal vascular ICAM-1 expression in vivo. Invest Ophthalmology Vis Sci. 1999;40:1808-12.

74. Barouch FC, Miyamoto K, Allport JR, et al. Integrin-mediated neutrophil adhesion and retinal leukostasis in diabetes. Invest Ophthalmology Vis Sci. 2000;41:1153-8.

75. Schroder S, Palinski W, Schmid-Schonbein GW. Activated monocytes and granulocytes, capillary nonperfusion, and neovascularization in diabetic retinopathy. Am J Pathol. 1991;139:81-100.

76. Joussen AM, Poulaki V, Le ML, et al. A central role for inflammation in the pathogenesis of diabetic retinopathy. FASEB J. 2004;18:1450-2.

77. Miyamoto K, Khosrof S, Bursell SE, et al. Prevention of leukostasis and vascular leakage in streptozotocin-induced diabetic retinopathy via intercellular adhesion molecule-1 inhibition. Proc Natl Acad Sci USA. 1999;96:10836-41.

78. Rodrigues M, Xin X, Jee K, et al. VEGF secreted by hypoxic Muller cells induces MMP-2 expression and activity in endothelial cells to promote retinal neovascularization in proliferative diabetic retinopathy. Diabetes. 2013;62:3863-73.

79. Hoffmann S, He S, Ehren M, et al. MMP-2 and MMP-9 secretion by rpe is stimulated by angiogenic molecules found in choroidal neovascular membranes. Retina. 2006;26:454-61.

80. Noda K, Ishida S, Shinoda H, et al. Hypoxia induces the expression of membrane-type 1 matrix metalloproteinase in retinal glial cells. Invest Ophthalmology Vis Sci. 2005;46:3817-24.

81. Abu El-Asrar AM, Mohammad G, Nawaz MI, et al. Relationship between vitreous levels of matrix metalloproteinases and vascular endothelial growth factor in proliferative diabetic retinopathy. PloS One. 2013;8:e85857.

82. Kowluru RA. Role of matrix metalloproteinase-9 in the development of diabetic retinopathy and its regulation by H-Ras. Invest Ophthalmology Vis Sci. 2010;51:4320-6.

83. Kowluru RA, Mohammad G, dos Santos JM, et al. Abrogation of MMP-9 gene protects against the development of retinopathy in diabetic mice by preventing mitochondrial damage. Diabetes. 2011;60:3023-33.

84. Funatsu H, Yamashita H, Noma H, et al. Increased levels of vascular endothelial growth factor and interleukin-6 in the aqueous humor of diabetics with macular edema. Am J Ophthalmology. 2002;133:70-7.

85. Funatsu H, Yamashita H, Ikeda T, et al. Angiotensin II and vascular endothelial growth factor in the vitreous fluid of patients with diabetic macular edema and other retinal disorders. Am J Ophthalmology. 2002;133:537-43.

86. Funatsu H, Yamashita H, Ikeda T, et al. Vitreous levels of interleukin-6 and vascular endothelial growth factor are related to diabetic macular edema. Ophthalmology. 2003;110:1690-6.

87. Funatsu H, Yamashita H, Sakata K, et al. Vitreous levels of vascular endothelial growth factor and intercellular adhesion molecule 1 are related to diabetic macular edema. Ophthalmology. 2005;112:806-16.

88. Murata T, Ishibashi T, Khalil A, et al. Vascular endothelial growth factor plays a role in hyperpermeability of diabetic retinal vessels. Ophthalmic Res. 1995;27:48-52.

89. Murata T, Nakagawa K, Khalil A, et al. The relation between expression of vascular endothelial growth factor and breakdown of the blood-retinal barrier in diabetic rat retinas. Lab Invest. 1996;74:819-25.

90. Ozaki H, Hayashi H, Vinores SA, et al. Intravitreal sustained release of VEGF causes retinal neovascularization in rabbits and breakdown of the blood-retinal barrier in rabbits and primates. Exp Eye Res. 1997;64:505-17.

91. Derevjanik NL, Vinores SA, Xiao WH, et al. Quantitative assessment of the integrity of the blood-retinal barrier in mice. Invest Ophthalmology Vis Sci. 2002;43:2462-7.

92. Yang JC, Haworth L, Sherry RM, et al. A randomized trial of bevacizumab, an anti-vascular endothelial growth factor antibody, for metastatic renal cancer. New Engl J Med. 2003;349:427-34.

93. Kabbinavar F, Hurwitz HI, Fehrenbacher L, et al. Phase II, randomized trial comparing bevacizumab plus fluorouracil (FU)/ leucovorin (LV) with FU/LV alone in patients with metastatic colorectal cancer. J Clin Oncol. 2003;21:60-5.

94. Hurwitz H, Fehrenbacher L, Novotny W, et al. Bevacizumab plus irinotecan, fluorouracil, and leucovorin for metastatic colorectal cancer. New Engl J Med. 2004;350:2335-42.

95. Ruckman J, Green LS, Beeson J, et al. 2'-Fluoropyrimidine RNA-based aptamers to the 165-amino acid form of vascular endothelial growth factor (VEGF165). Inhibition of receptor binding and VEGF-induced vascular permeability through interactions requiring the exon 7-encoded domain. J Biol Chem. 1998;273:20556-67.

96. Cunningham ET Jr, Adamis AP, Altaweel M, et al. A phase II randomized double-masked trial of pegaptanib, an anti-vascular endothelial growth factor aptamer, for diabetic macular edema. Ophthalmology. 2005;112:1747-57.

97. Adamis AP, Altaweel M, Bressler NM, et al. Changes in retinal neovascularization after pegaptanib (Macugen) therapy in diabetic individuals. Ophthalmology. 2006;113:23-8.

98. Sultan MB, Zhou D, Loftus J, et al. A phase 2/3, multicenter, randomized, double-masked, 2-year trial of pegaptanib sodium for the treatment of diabetic macular edema. Ophthalmology. 2011;118:1107-18.

99. Rinaldi M, Chiosi F, dell'Omo R, et al. Intravitreal pegaptanib sodium (Macugen®) for treatment of diabetic macular oedema: a morphologic and functional study. Br J Clin Pharmacol. 2012;74:940-6.

100. Presta LG, Chen H, O'Connor SJ, et al. Humanization of an anti-vascular endothelial growth factor monoclonal antibody for the therapy of solid tumors and other disorders. Cancer Res. 1997;57:4593-9.

101. Michels S, Rosenfeld PJ, Puliafito CA, et al. Systemic bevacizumab (Avastin) therapy for neovascular age-related macular degeneration twelve-week results of an uncontrolled open-label clinical study. Ophthalmology. 2005;112:1035-47.

102. Haritoglou C, Kook D, Neubauer A, et al. Intravitreal bevacizumab (Avastin) therapy for persistent diffuse diabetic macular edema. Retina. 2006;26:999-1005.

103. Arevalo JF, Fromow-Guerra J, Quiroz-Mercado H, et al. Primary intravitreal bevacizumab (Avastin) for diabetic macular edema: results from the Pan-American Collaborative Retina Study Group at 6-month follow-up. Ophthalmology. 2007;114:743-50.

104. Soheilian M, Ramezani A, Bijanzadeh B, et al. Intravitreal bevacizumab (avastin) injection alone or combined with triamcinolone versus macular photocoagulation as primary treatment of diabetic macular edema. Retina. 2007;27:1187-95.

105. Wang YS, Li X, Wang HY, et al. Intravitreal bevacizumab combined with/without triamcinolone acetonide in single injection for treatment of diabetic macular edema. Chin Med J (Engl). 2011;124:352-8.

106. Lim JW, Lee HK, Shin MC. Comparison of intravitreal bevacizumab alone or combined with triamcinolone versus triamcinolone in diabetic macular edema: a randomized clinical trial. Ophthalmologica. 2012;227:100-6.

107. Stockdale CR, Scott IU, Edwards AR. A phase II randomized clinical trial of intravitreal bevacizumab for diabetic macular edema. Ophthalmology. 2007;114:1860-7.

108. Michaelides M, Kaines A, Hamilton RD, et al. A prospective randomized trial of intravitreal bevacizumab or laser therapy in the management of diabetic macular edema (BOLT study) 12-month data: report 2. Ophthalmology. 2010;117:1078-86 e2.

109. Rajendram R, Fraser-Bell S, Kaines A, et al. A 2-year prospective randomized controlled trial of intravitreal bevacizumab or laser therapy (BOLT) in the management of diabetic macular edema: 24-month data: report 3. Arch Ophthalmology .2012;130:972-9.

110. Sivaprasad S, Crosby-Nwaobi R, Heng LZ, et al. Injection frequency and response to bevacizumab monotherapy for diabetic macular oedema (BOLT Report 5). Br J Ophthalmology. 2013;97:1177-80.

111. Mordenti J, Cuthbertson RA, Ferrara N, et al. Comparisons of the intraocular tissue distribution, pharmacokinetics, and safety of 125I-labeled full-length and Fab antibodies in rhesus monkeys following intravitreal administration. Toxicol Pathol. 1999;27:536-44.

112. Husain D, Kim I, Gauthier D, et al. Safety and efficacy of intravitreal injection of ranibizumab in combination with verteporfin PDT on experimental choroidal neovascularization in the monkey. Arch Ophthalmology. 2005;123:509-16.

113. Rosenfeld PJ, Schwartz SD, Blumenkranz MS, et al. Maximum tolerated dose of a humanized anti-vascular endothelial growth factor antibody fragment for treating neovascular age-related macular degeneration. Ophthalmology. 2005;112:1048-53.

114. Heier JS, Antoszyk AN, Pavan PR, et al. Ranibizumab for treatment of neovascular age-related macular degeneration: a phase I/II multicenter, controlled, multidose study. Ophthalmology. 2006;113:633 e1-4.

115. Nguyen QD, Shah SM, Heier JS, et al. Primary End Point (Six Months) Results of the Ranibizumab for Edema of the mAcula in diabetes (READ-2) study. Ophthalmology. 2009;116:2175-81 e1.

116. Nguyen QD, Shah SM, Khwaja AA, et al. Two-year outcomes of the ranibizumab for edema of the mAcula in diabetes (READ-2) study. Ophthalmology. 2010;117:2146-51.

117. Elman MJ, Aiello LP, Beck RW, et al. Randomized trial evaluating ranibizumab plus prompt or deferred laser or triamcinolone plus prompt laser for diabetic macular edema. Ophthalmology. 2010;117:1064-77 e35.

118. Gillies MC, McAllister IL, Zhu M, et al. Intravitreal triamcinolone prior to laser treatment of diabetic macular edema: 24-month results of a randomized controlled trial. Ophthalmology. 2011;118 866-72.

119. Elman MJ, Ayala A, Bressler NM, et al. Intravitreal Ranibizumab for diabetic macular edema with prompt versus deferred laser treatment: 5-year randomized trial results. Ophthalmology. 2015;122:375-81.

120. Mitchell P, Bandello F, Schmidt-Erfurth U, et al. The RESTORE study: ranibizumab monotherapy or combined with laser versus laser monotherapy for diabetic macular edema. Ophthalmology. 2011;118:615-25.

121. Schmidt-Erfurth U, Lang GE, Holz FG, et al. Three-year outcomes of individualized ranibizumab treatment in patients with diabetic macular edema: the RESTORE extension study. Ophthalmology. 2014;121:1045-53.

122. Brown DM, Nguyen QD, Ehrlich JS, et al. Ranibizumab for diabetic macular edema (Author reply). Ophthalmology. 2013;120:221-2.

123. Brown DM, Nguyen QD, Marcus DM, et al. Long-term outcomes of ranibizumab therapy for diabetic macular edema: the 36-month results from two phase III trials: RISE and RIDE. Ophthalmology. 2013;120:2013-22.

124. Ferrara N, Chen H, Davis-Smyth T, et al. Vascular endothelial growth factor is essential for corpus luteum angiogenesis. Nat Med. 1998;4:336-40.

125. Carmeliet P, Moons L, Luttun A, et al. Synergism between vascular endothelial growth factor and placental growth factor contributes to angiogenesis and plasma extravasation in pathological conditions. Nat Med. 2001;7:575-83.

126. Holash J, Davis S, Papadopoulos N, et al. VEGF-Trap: a VEGF blocker with potent antitumor effects. Proc Natl Acad Sci USA. 2002;99 11393-8.

127. Papadopoulos N, Martin J, Ruan Q, et al. Binding and neutralization of vascular endothelial growth factor (VEGF) and related ligands by VEGF Trap, ranibizumab and bevacizumab. Angiogenesis. 2012;15:171-85.

128. Saishin Y, Saishin Y, Takahashi K, et al. VEGF-TRAP(R1R2) suppresses choroidal neovascularization and VEGF-induced breakdown of the blood-retinal barrier. J Cell Physiol 2003;195:241-8.

129. Do DV, Nguyen QD, Shah SM, et al. An exploratory study of the safety, tolerability and bioactivity of a single intravitreal injection of vascular endothelial growth factor Trap-Eye in patients with diabetic macular oedema. Br J Ophthalmology. 2009;93:144-9.

130. Do DV, Schmidt-Erfurth U, Gonzalez VH, et al. The DA VINCI Study: phase 2 primary results of VEGF Trap-Eye in patients with diabetic macular edema. Ophthalmology. 2011;118:1819-26.

131. Do DV, Nguyen QD, Boyer D, et al. One-year outcomes of the da Vinci Study of VEGF Trap-Eye in eyes with diabetic macular edema Ophthalmology. 2012;119:1658-65.

132. Korobelnik JF, Do DV, Schmidt-Erfurth U, et al. Intravitreal aflibercept for diabetic macular edema. Ophthalmology. 2014;121:2247-54.

133. Brown DM, Schmidt-Erfurth U, Do DV, et al. Intravitreal Aflibercept for Diabetic Macular Edema: 100-Week Results From the VISTA and VIVID Studies. Ophthalmology. 2015;122:2044-52.

134. Wells JA, Glassman AR, Ayala AR, et al. Aflibercept, bevacizumab, or ranibizumab for diabetic macular edema. N Engl J Med 2015;372:1193-203.

135. Wells JA, Glassman AR, Ayala AR, et al. Aflibercept, bevacizumab, or ranibizumab for diabetic macular edema: two-year results from a comparative effectiveness randomized clinical trial. Ophthalmology 2016;123(6):1351-9.

136. Schauwvlieghe AM, Dijkman G, Hooymans JM, et al. Comparing the effectiveness and costs of Bevacizumab to Ranibizumab in patients with Diabetic Macular Edema: a randomized clinical trial (the BRDME study). BMC Ophthalmology. 2015;15:71.

137. Bandello F, Midena E, Menchini U, et al. Recommendations for the appropriate management of diabetic macular edema: light on DME survey and consensus document by an expert panel. Eur J Ophthalmology. 2016:26(3):193-282.

138. Holfinger S, Miller AG, Rao LJ, et al. Effect of Regulatory Requirement for Patient-Specific Prescriptions for Off-Label Medications on the Use of Intravitreal Bevacizumab. JAMA Ophthalmology. 2016;134: 45-8.

139. Kaiser PK, Cruess AF, Bogaert P, et al. Balancing risk in ophthalmic prescribing: assessing the safety of anti-VEGF therapies and the risks associated with unlicensed medicines. Graefes Arch Clin Exp Ophthalmology. 2012;250:1563-71.

140. Sigford DK, Reddy S, Mollineaux C, et al. Global reported endophthalmitis risk following intravitreal injections of anti-VEGF: a literature review and analysis. Clin Ophthalmology. 2015;9:773-81.

141. Kwong TQ, Mohamed M. Anti-vascular endothelial growth factor therapies in ophthalmology: current use, controversies and the future. Br J Clin Pharmacol. 2014;78:699-706.

142. Kamba T, McDonald DM. Mechanisms of adverse effects of anti-VEGF therapy for cancer. Br J Cancer. 2007;96:1788-95.

143. Dinc E, Yildirim O, Necat Yilmaz S, et al. Intravitreal bevacizumab effects on VEGF levels in distant organs: an experimental study. Cutan Ocul Toxicol. 2014;33:275-82.

144. Wu WC, Lien R, Liao PJ, et al. Serum levels of vascular endothelial growth factor and related factors after intravitreous bevacizumab injection for retinopathy of prematurity. JAMA Ophthalmology. 2015;133:391-7.

145. Zehetner C, Kirchmair R, Huber S, et al. Plasma levels of vascular endothelial growth factor before and after intravitreal injection of bevacizumab, ranibizumab and pegaptanib in patients with age-related macular degeneration, and in patients with diabetic macular oedema. Br J Ophthalmology. 2013;97:454-9.

146. Rogers CA, Chakravarthy U, Harding SP, et al. Ranibizumab versus bevacizumab to treat neovascular age-related macular degeneration: one-year findings from the IVAN randomized trial. Ophthalmology. 2012;119:1399-411.

147. Schlenker MB, Thiruchelvam D, Redelmeier DA. Intravitreal anti-vascular endothelial growth factor treatment and the risk of thromboembolism. Am J Ophthalmology. 2015;160:569-80 e5.

148. Avery RL, Gordon GM. Systemic safety of prolonged monthly anti-vascular endothelial growth factor therapy for diabetic macular edema: a systematic review and meta-analysis. JAMA Ophthalmology. 2016;134:21-9.

149. Avery RL, Castellarin AA, Steinle NC, et al. Systemic pharmacokinetics following intravitreal injections of ranibizumab, bevacizumab or aflibercept in patients with neovascular AMD. Br J Ophthalmology. 2014;98:1636-41.

150. Arevalo JF, Maia M, Flynn HW Jr, et al. Tractional retinal detachment following intravitreal bevacizumab (Avastin) in patients with severe proliferative diabetic retinopathy. Br J Ophthalmology. 2008; 92:213-6.

151. Gross JG, Glassman AR, Jampol LM, et al. Panretinal Photocoagulation vs Intravitreous Ranibizumab for Proliferative Diabetic Retinopathy: A Randomized Clinical Trial. JAMA. 2015;314: 2137-46.

152. Agrawal S, Joshi M, Christoforidis JB. Vitreous inflammation associated with intravitreal anti-VEGF pharmacotherapy. Mediators Inflamm. 2013;2013:943409.

153. Marticorena J, Romano V, Gomez-Ulla F. Sterile endophthalmitis after intravitreal injections. Mediators Inflamm. 2012;2012:928123.

154. Sampat KM, Garg SJ. Complications of intravitreal injections. Curr Opin Ophthalmology. 2010;21:178-83.

155. Shikari H, Silva PS, Sun JK. Complications of intravitreal injections in patients with diabetes. Semin Ophthalmology. 2014;29:276-89.

156. Domalpally A, Ip MS, Ehrlich JS. Effects of intravitreal ranibizumab on retinal hard exudate in diabetic macular edema: findings from the RIDE and RISE phase III clinical trials. Ophthalmology. 2015;122:779-86.

157. Englander M, Chen TC, Paschalis EI, et al. Intravitreal injections at the Massachusetts Eye and Ear Infirmary: analysis of treatment indications and postinjection endophthalmitis rates. Br J Ophthalmology. 2013;97:460-5.

158. Gregori NZ, Flynn HW Jr, Schwartz SG, et al. Current infectious endophthalmitis rates after intravitreal injections of anti-vascular endothelial growth factor agents and outcomes of treatment. Ophthal Surg Lasers Imaging Retina. 2015;46:643-8.

159. Dossarps D, Bron AM, Koehrer P, et al. Endophthalmitis after intravitreal injections: incidence, presentation, management, and visual outcome. Am J Ophthalmology. 2015;160:17-25 e1.

160. Garg SJ, Dollin M, Storey P, et al. Microbial spectrum and outcomes of endophthalmitis after intravitreal injection versus pars plana vitrectomy. Retina. 2016;36:351-9.

161. Avery RL, Bakri SJ, Blumenkranz MS, et al. Intravitreal injection technique and monitoring: updated guidelines of an expert panel. Retina. 2014;34(Suppl 12):S1-S18.

162. Schwartz SG, Flynn HW, Grzybowski A. Controversies in Topical Antibiotics Use with Intravitreal Injections. Curr Pharm Des. 2015;21:4703-6.

163. Jager RD, Aiello LP, Patel SC, et al. Risks of intravitreous injection: a comprehensive review. Retina. 2004;24:676-98.

164. Shen HH, Chan EC, Lee JH, et al. Nanocarriers for treatment of ocular neovascularization in the back of the eye: new vehicles for ophthalmic drug delivery. Nanomedicine (Lond). 2015;10: 2093-107.

165. Schwartz SG, Scott IU, Flynn HW Jr, et al. Drug delivery techniques for treating age-related macular degeneration. Expert Opin Drug Deliv. 2014;11:61-8.

166. Landry JP, Fei Y, Zhu X, et al. Discovering small molecule ligands of vascular endothelial growth factor that block VEGF-KDR binding using label-free microarray-based assays. Assay Drug Dev Technol. 2013;11:326-32.

167. Titchenell PM, Antonetti DA. Using the past to inform the future: anti-VEGF therapy as a road map to develop novel therapies for diabetic retinopathy. Diabetes. 2013;62:1808-15.

168. Pechan P, Wadsworth S, Scaria A. Gene Therapies for neovascular age-related macular degeneration. Cold Spring Harb Perspect Med. 2015;5:a017335.

169. Rakoczy EP, Lai CM, Magno AL, et al. Gene therapy with recombinant adeno-associated vectors for neovascular age-related macular degeneration: 1 year follow-up of a phase 1 randomised clinical trial. Lancet. 2015;386:2395-403.

170. MacLaren RE. Gene therapy for age-related macular degeneration. Lancet 2015;386:2369-70.

171. Massin P, Bandello F, Garweg JG, et al. Safety and efficacy of ranibizumab in diabetic macular edema (RESOLVE Study): a 12-month, randomized, controlled, double-masked, multicenter phase II study. Diabetes Care. 2010;33:2399-405.

172. Antonetti DA, Klein R, Gardner TW. Diabetic retinopathy. New Engl J Med. 2012;366:1227-39.

173. Joussen AM, Doehmen S, Le ML, et al. TNF-alpha mediated apoptosis plays an important role in the development of early diabetic retinopathy and long-term histopathological alterations. Mol Vision. 2009;15:1418-28.

174. El-Asrar AM. Role of inflammation in the pathogenesis of diabetic retinopathy. Middle East African J Ophthalmology. 2012;19:70-4.

175. Miyamoto K, Hiroshiba N, Tsujikawa A, et al. In vivo demonstration of increased leukocyte entrapment in retinal microcirculation of diabetic rats. Invest Ophthalmology Vis Sci. 1998;39:2190-4.

176. Miyamoto K, Ogura Y. Pathogenetic potential of leukocytes in diabetic retinopathy. Semin Ophthalmology. 1999;14:233-9.

177. Ayalasomayajula SP, Ashton P, Kompella UB. Fluocinolone inhibits VEGF expression via glucocorticoid receptor in human retinal pigment epithelial (ARPE-19) cells and TNF-alpha-induced angiogenesis in chick chorioallantoic membrane (CAM). J Ocul Pharmacol Ther. 2009;25:97-103.

178. Diabetic Retinopathy Clinical Research Network. A randomized trial comparing intravitreal triamcinolone acetonide and focal/grid photocoagulation for diabetic macular edema. Ophthalmology. 2008;115:1447-9, 9 e1-10.

179. Beck RW, Edwards AR, Aiello LP, et al. Three-year follow-up of a randomized trial comparing focal/grid photocoagulation and intravitreal triamcinolone for diabetic macular edema. Arch Ophthalmology. 2009;127:245-51.

180. Boyer DS, Yoon YH, Belfort R Jr, et al. Three-year, randomized, sham-controlled trial of dexamethasone intravitreal implant in patients with diabetic macular edema. Ophthalmology. 2014;121:1904-14.

181. Campochiaro PA, Brown DM, Pearson A, et al. Long-term benefit of sustained-delivery fluocinolone acetonide vitreous inserts for diabetic macular edema. Ophthalmology. 2011;118:626-35 e2.

182. Pearson PA, Comstock TL, Ip M, et al. Fluocinolone acetonide intravitreal implant for diabetic macular edema: a 3-year multicenter, randomized, controlled clinical trial. Ophthalmology. 2011;118:1580-7.

183. Zhioua I, Semoun O, Lalloum F, et al. Intravitreal Dexamethasone Implant in Patients with Ranibizumab Persistent Diabetic Macular Edema. Retina. 2015;35:1429-35.

184. Escobar-Barranco JJ, Pina-Marin B, Fernandez-Bonet M. Dexamethasone Implants in Patients with Naive or Refractory Diffuse Diabetic Macular Edema. Ophthalmologica. 2015;233:176-85.

185. Boyer DS, Faber D, Gupta S, et al. Dexamethasone intravitreal implant for treatment of diabetic macular edema in vitrectomized patients. Retina. 2011;31:915-23.

186. Bressler SB, Melia M, Glassman AR, et al. Ranibizumab Plus Prompt or Deferred Laser for diabetic macular edema in eyes with vitrectomy before anti-vascular endothelial growth factor therapy. Retina. 2015;35:2516-28.

187. Maia OO Jr, Takahashi BS, Costa RA, et al. Combined laser and intravitreal triamcinolone for proliferative diabetic retinopathy and macular edema: one-year results of a randomized clinical trial. Am J Ophthalmology. 2009;147:291-7e2.

188. Falavarjani KG, Nguyen QD. Adverse events and complications associated with intravitreal injection of anti-VEGF agents: a review of literature. Eye. 2013;27:787-94.

189. The effect of intensive treatment of diabetes on the development and progression of long-term complications in insulin-dependent diabetes mellitus. The Diabetes Control and Complications Trial Research Group. New Engl J Med. 1993;329:977-86.

190. UK Prospective Diabetes Study (UKPDS) Group. Intensive blood-glucose control with sulphonylureas or insulin compared with conventional treatment and risk of complications in patients with type 2 diabetes (UKPDS 33). Lancet. 1998;352:837-53.

191. Group AS, Gerstein HC, Miller ME, et al. Long-term effects of intensive glucose lowering on cardiovascular outcomes. New Engl J Med. 2011;364:818-28.

192. Finfer S, Chittock DRl. Intensive versus conventional glucose control in critically ill patients. New Engl J Med. 2009;360:1283-97.

193. Geraldes P, King GL. Activation of protein kinase C isoforms and its impact on diabetic complications. Circ Res. 2010;106:1319-31.

194. Ishii H, Jirousek MR, Koya D, et al. Amelioration of vascular dysfunctions in diabetic rats by an oral PKC beta inhibitor. Science. 1996;272:728-31.

195. Santos JM, Mohammad G, Zhong Q, et al. Diabetic retinopathy, superoxide damage and antioxidants. Curr Pharma Biotechnol. 2011;12:352-61.

196. Kowluru RA, Abbas SN. Diabetes-induced mitochondrial dysfunction in the retina. Invest Ophthalmology Vis Sci. 2003;44:5327-34.

197. Keech AC, Mitchell P, Summanen PA, et al. Effect of fenofibrate on the need for laser treatment for diabetic retinopathy (FIELD study): a randomised controlled trial. Lancet. 2007;370:1687-97.

198. Group AS, Group AES, Chew EY, et al. Effects of medical therapies on retinopathy progression in type 2 diabetes. New Engl J Med. 2010;363:233-44.

199. Ciucin A, Hernandez C, Simo R. Molecular implications of the PPARs in the Diabetic Eye. PPAR Research. 2013;2013:686525.

200. Sasongko MB, Wong TY, Nguyen TT, et al. Serum apolipoprotein AI and B are stronger biomarkers of diabetic retinopathy than traditional lipids. Diabetes Care. 2011;34:474-9.

201. Wong TY, Simo R, Mitchell P. Fenofibrate—a potential systemic treatment for diabetic retinopathy? Am J Ophthalmology. 2012;154:6-12.

202. Pozzi A, Capdevila JH. PPAR alpha ligands as antitumorigenic and antiangiogenic agents. PPAR Research. 2008;2008:906542.

203. Meissner M, Stein M, Urbich C, et al. PPAR alpha activators inhibit vascular endothelial growth factor receptor-2 expression by repressing Sp1-dependent DNA binding and transactivation. Circ Res. 2004;94:324-32.

204. Idris I, Warren G, Donnelly R. Association between thiazolidinedione treatment and risk of macular edema among patients with type 2 diabetes. Arch Int Med. 2012;172:1005-11.

205. Ryan EH Jr, Han DP, Ramsay RC, et al. Diabetic macular edema associated with glitazone use. Retina. 2006;26:562-70.

206. Fong DS, Contreras R. Glitazone use associated with diabetic macular edema. Am J Ophthalmology. 2009;147:583-6e1.

207. Ambrosius WT, Danis RP, Goff DC Jr, et al. Lack of association between thiazolidinediones and macular edema in type 2 diabetes: the ACCORD eye substudy. Arch Ophthalmology. 2010;128:312-8.

208. Hodgson N, Wu F, Ferreyra H, et al. Economic and quality of life benefits of anti-VEGF therapy. Mol Pharm. 2016;13(9):2877-80.

209. Pershing S, Enns EA, Matesic B, et al. Cost-effectiveness of treatment of diabetic macular edema. Ann Intern Med. 2014;160:18-29.

210. Regnier S, Malcolm W, Allen F, et al. Efficacy of anti-VEGF and laser photocoagulation in the treatment of visual impairment due to diabetic macular edema: a systematic review and network meta-analysis. PloS One. 2014;9:e102309.

211. Kang-Mieler JJ, Osswald CR, Mieler WF. Advances in ocular drug delivery: emphasis on the posterior segment. Expert Opin Drug Deliv 2014;11:1647-60.

212. Gamache DA, Graff G, Brady MT, et al. Nepafenac, a unique nonsteroidal prodrug with potential utility in the treatment of trauma-induced ocular inflammation: I. Assessment of anti-inflammatory efficacy. Inflammation. 2000;24:357-70.

213. Ke TL, Graff G, Spellman JM, et al. Nepafenac, a unique nonsteroidal prodrug with potential utility in the treatment of trauma-induced ocular inflammation: II. In vitro bioactivation and permeation of external ocular barriers. Inflammation. 2000;24:371-84.

214. Chastain JE, Sanders ME, Curtis MA, et al. Distribution of topical ocular nepafenac and its active metabolite amfenac to the posterior segment of the eye. Exp Eye Res 2015;145:58-67.

215. Kapin MA, Yanni JM, Brady MT, et al. Inflammation-mediated retinal edema in the rabbit is inhibited by topical nepafenac. Inflammation. 2003;27:281-91.

216. Heier JS, Awh CC, Busbee BG, et al. Vitreous nonsteroidal anti-inflammatory drug concentrations and prostaglandin E2 levels in vitrectomy patients treated with ketorolac 0.4%, bromfenac 0.09%, and nepafenac 0.1%. Retina. 2009;29:1310-3.

217. Callanan D, Williams P. Topical nepafenac in the treatment of diabetic macular edema. Clin Ophthalmology. 2008;2:689-92.

218. Hariprasad SM, Callanan D, Gainey S, et al. Cystoid and diabetic macular edema treated with nepafenac 0.1%. J Ocul Pharmacol Ther. 2007;23:585-90.

219. Singh R, Alpern L, Jaffe GJ, et al. Evaluation of nepafenac in prevention of macular edema following cataract surgery in patients with diabetic retinopathy. Clin Ophthalmology. 2012;6:1259-69.

220. Kim SJ, Flach AJ, Jampol LM. Nonsteroidal anti-inflammatory drugs in ophthalmology. Surv Ophthalmology. 2010;55:108-33.

221. Friedman SM, Almukhtar TH, Baker CW, et al. Topical nepafenec in eyes with noncentral diabetic macular edema. Retina. 2015;35:944-56.

222. Wittpenn JR, Silverstein S, Heier J, et al. A randomized, masked comparison of topical ketorolac 0.4% plus steroid vs steroid alone in low-risk cataract surgery patients. Am J Ophthalmology. 2008;146:554-60.

223. Elsawy MF, Badawi N, Khairy HA. Prophylactic postoperative ketorolac improves outcomes in diabetic patients assigned for cataract surgery. Clin Ophthalmology. 2013;7:1245-9.

224. Terada Y, Masuda A, Nejima R, et al. The anti-inflammatory effect of 0.1% bromfenac and 0.1% betamethasone combination in post-cataract surgery patients with diabetes mellitus. Nippon Ganka Gakkai Zasshi. 2014;118:645-51.

225. Sahoo S, Barua A, Myint KT, et al. Topical non-steroidal anti-inflammatory agents for diabetic cystoid macular oedema. Cochrane Database Syst Rev. 2015;2:CD010009.

226. Prausnitz MR, Noonan JS. Permeability of cornea, sclera, and conjunctiva: a literature analysis for drug delivery to the eye. J Pharm Sci. 1998;87:1479-88.

227. Loftssona T, Jarvinen T. Cyclodextrins in ophthalmic drug delivery. Adv Drug Deliv Rev. 1999;36:59-79.

228. Loftsson T, Hreinsdottir D, Stefansson E. Cyclodextrin micro-particles for drug delivery to the posterior segment of the eye: aqueous dexamethasone eye drops. J Pharm Pharmacol. 2007;59:629-35.

229. Tanito M, Hara K, Takai Y, et al. Topical dexamethasone-cyclodextrin microparticle eye drops for diabetic macular edema. Invest Ophthalmology Vis Sci. 2011;52:7944-8.

230. Kaur S, Yangzes S, Singh S, et al. Efficacy and safety of topical difluprednate in persistent diabetic macular edema. Int Ophthalmology. 2016;36(3):335-40.

231. Nakano Goto S, Yamamoto T, Kirii E, et al. Treatment of diffuse diabetic macular oedema using steroid eye drops. Acta Ophthalmologica. 2012;90:628-32.

232. Russo A, Costagliola C, Delcassi L, et al. Topical nonsteroidal anti-inflammatory drugs for macular edema. Mediators Inflamm. 2013;2013:476-525.

233. Das A, McGuire PG, Rangasamy S. Diabetic macular edema: pathophysiology and novel therapeutic targets. Ophthalmology. 2015;122:1375-94.

234. Villablanca AC. Nicotine stimulates DNA synthesis and proliferation in vascular endothelial cells in vitro. J Appl Physiol (1985). 1998;84:2089-98.

235. Heeschen C, Jang JJ, Weis M, et al. Nicotine stimulates angiogenesis and promotes tumor growth and atherosclerosis. Nat Med. 2001;7:833-9.

236. Suner IJ, Espinosa-Heidmann DG, Marin-Castano ME, et al. Nicotine increases size and severity of experimental choroidal neovascularization. Invest Ophthalmology Vis Sci. 2004;45:311-7.

237. Campochiaro PA, Shah SM, Hafiz G, et al. Topical mecamylamine for diabetic macular edema. Am J Ophthalmology. 2010;149:839-51e1.

238. McLeod DS, Lefer DJ, Merges C, et al. Enhanced expression of intracellular adhesion molecule-1 and P-selectin in the diabetic human retina and choroid. Am J Pathol. 1995;147:642-53.

239. Hogg N, Patzak I, Willenbrock F. The insider's guide to leukocyte integrin signalling and function. Nat Rev Immunol. 2011;11:416-26.

240. Gadek TR, Burdick DJ, McDowell RS, et al. Generation of an LFA-1 antagonist by the transfer of the ICAM-1 immunoregulatory epitope to a small molecule. Science. 2002;295:1086-9.

241. Rao VR, Prescott E, Shelke NB, et al. Delivery of SAR 1118 to the retina via ophthalmic drops and its effectiveness in a rat streptozotocin (STZ) model of diabetic retinopathy (DR). Invest Ophthalmology Vis Sci. 2010;51:5198-204.

242. Paskowitz DM, Nguyen QD, Gehlbach P, et al. Safety, tolerability, and bioavailability of topical SAR 1118, a novel antagonist of lymphocyte function-associated antigen-1: a phase 1b study. Eye. 2012;26:944-9.

243. Perez VL, Pflugfelder SC, Zhang S, et al. Lifitegrast, a Novel Integrin Antagonist for Treatment of Dry Eye Disease. Ocul Surf. 2016;14(2):207-15.

244. Yamada N, Olsen TW. Routes for drug delivery to the retina: topical, transscleral, suprachoroidal and intravitreal gas phase delivery. Dev Ophthalmology. 2016;55:71-83.

245. Shikamura Y, Yamazaki Y, Matsunaga T, et al. Hydrogel ring for topical drug delivery to the ocular posterior segment. Curr Eye Res. 2015:1-9.

246. Boddu SH, Gupta H, Patel S. Drug delivery to the back of the eye following topical administration: an update on research and patenting activity. Recent Pat Drug Deliv Formul. 2014;8:27-36.

247. Schopf LR, Popov AM, Enlow EM, et al. Topical Ocular Drug Delivery to the Back of the Eye by Mucus-Penetrating Particles. Transl Vis Sci Technol. 2015;4:11.

248. Bressler SB, Ayala AR, Bressler NM, et al. Persistent macular thickening after ranibizumab treatment for diabetic macular edema with vision impairment. JAMA Ophthalmology. 2016:1-8.

249. Apte RS. What Is Chronic or Persistent Diabetic Macular Edema and How Should It Be Treated? JAMA Ophthalmology. 2016:1-2.

250. Kang SW, Park SC, Cho HY, et al. Triple therapy of vitrectomy, intravitreal triamcinolone, and macular laser photocoagulation for intractable diabetic macular edema. Am J Ophthalmology. 2007;144:878-85.

251. Kim JH, Kang SW, Ha HS, et al. Vitrectomy combined with intravitreal triamcinolone acetonide injection and macular laser photocoagulation for nontractional diabetic macular edema. Korean J Ophthalmology. 2013;27:186-93.

252. Kim YT, Kang SW, Kim SJ, et al. Combination of vitrectomy, IVTA, and laser photocoagulation for diabetic macular edema unresponsive to prior treatments; 3-year results. Graefes Arch Clin Exp Ophthalmology. 2012;250:679-84.

253. Haller JA, Qin H, Apte RS, et al. Vitrectomy outcomes in eyes with diabetic macular edema and vitreomacular traction. Ophthalmology. 2010;117:1087-93e3.

254. Bonnin S, Sandali O, Bonnel S, et al. Vitrectomy with internal limiting membrane peeling for tractional and nontractional diabetic macular edema: long-term results of a comparative study. Retina. 2015;35:921-8.

255. Stefansson E. Ocular oxygenation and the treatment of diabetic retinopathy. Surv Ophthalmology. 2006;51:364-80.

256. Stefansson E. Physiology of vitreous surgery. Graefes Arch Clin Exp Ophthalmology. 2009;247:147-63.

257. Laidlaw DA. Vitrectomy for diabetic macular oedema. Eye. 2008;22:1337-41.

Chapter 29

Proliferative Diabetic Retinopathy

Pramod S Bhende, Nagesha CK, Jaya Prakash V

 INTRODUCTION

Diabetes is a global epidemic as approximately 415 million people are suffering from diabetes in the world as of 2015 and there will be an estimated 642 million people with diabetes by 2040.[1] Diabetic retinopathy occurs due to changes in the retina due to elevated blood sugars over a period of time. Initially nonproliferative changes set in and gradually progress to proliferative stage proliferative diabetic retinopathy (PDR) which is characterized by new vessels at the disc or elsewhere eventually leading to serious vision threatening complications such as traction and combined retinal detachment and anterior segment neovascularization, if left untreated.

RISK FACTORS AND PROGRESSION OF DIABETIC RETINOPATHY (DR)

As emphasized by Caird[2] et al. visual deterioration is more rapid and relentless in untreated PDR when compared to background retinopathy. Beetham et al.[3] in his series of 1149 PDR patients, followed up for 20 years, noted that 33% of patients were blind (20/200 or less) at the time of presentation and additional 25% of type 1 and 40% of type 2 diabetics deteriorated to 20/200 or worse vision over 11 years follow-up.

In eyes with PDR, prevalence of preretinal hemorrhage or vitreous hemorrhage and new vessels on or near the optic disc were noted to be important risk factors for severe vision loss. The strongest association of severe vision loss and severity of retinopathy was with the extent of new vessels over the disc.[4,5]

As noted in Early Treatment Diabetic Retinopathy Study (ETDRS), severity of intraretinal microvascular abnormalities (IRMA), retinal hemorrhages and/or microaneurysms and venous beading were found to be independent risk factors for progression of retinopathy.[6] On fluorescein angiography, fluorescein leakage (particularly diffuse), capillary loss with dilatation and various arteriolar abnormalities were associated with progression to proliferative retinopathy.[7]

The WESDR found progression to PDR[8,9] of 11% (71 of 713), 7% (31 of 418), and 2% (11 of 486), respectively in the three age group studies (younger than 30 years on insulin, those 30 years or older on insulin and 30 years or older but not on insulin at diagnosis) over 4 years. The 10 years rate of progression was 30%, 24% and 10%, respectively in these three groups.[10] After 20 years of diabetes, PDR was present in about 50%, 25% and 5% of the three groups, respectively.[11] Increased risk of PDR was associated with more severe retinopathy at baseline.

The prevalence of severe NPDR or PDR has been found to be more with increasing duration of diabetes in many studies. Also better glycemic control inhibits retinopathy across all stages and ages.[12]

A modest association was found for higher levels of high-density lipoprotein cholesterol and decreased prevalence of PDR, but no associations was found either with serum total or high-density lipoprotein cholesterol and incidence of PDR or of statin use with decreased incidence of PDR.[13]

PATHOGENESIS OF PROLIFERATIVE DIABETIC RETINOPATHY

Ashton and coworkers[14] postulated the liberation of a 'vasoformative factor' from hypoxic retina (called as factor X by Wise[15]) which stimulates secondary retinal neovascularization. It was noted that the severe degree of retinal ischemia was accompanied by optic disc pallor and neovascularization and a high incidence of rubeosis iridis with neovascular glaucoma.[16]

Aiello et al.[17] has noted potential role of Vascular Endothelial Growth Factor (VEGF) in patients with ischemic retinal diseases such as diabetic retinopathy and vascular occlusion. Further studies have shown increased concentration of VEGF in vitreous in eyes with PDR than in eyes without PDR and its inhibition is a new potential therapeutic strategy for the treatment of ocular neovascularization.[18,19] But the variable response to anti-VEGF treatment in diabetic retinopathy has led to search for alternative pathological pathways which could be contributing to development and progression of diabetic retinopathy.

Investigations are under way for the role of angiopoietin/Tie2 system in ischemia-induced angiogenesis.[20] Activation of Protein kinase C delta (PKCδ) and SRC Homology Protein 1 (SHP1) by hyperglycemia has been found to cause vascular cell apoptosis and diabetic retinopathy[21] and erythropoietin, a potent ischemia-induced angiogenic factor that acts independently of VEGF during retinal angiogenesis in proliferative diabetic retinopathy have been recently studied.[22] The clinical applications of these novel molecules as targeted therapy are still under investigation in halting progression of retinopathy as shown in recent studies.[23,24]

Role of Vitreous in PDR

The vitreoretinal relationship especially status of posterior vitreous detachment is important in the development and progression of proliferative changes in eyes with PDR. In eyes with preexisting posterior vitreous detachment (PVD), there is no support of posterior hyaloid as a scaffold, hence new vessels remain flat and do not progress to other complications. Vitreoretinal and vitreopapillary traction (generally due to incomplete PVD) can stimulate severe neovascularization and often other irreversible changes in the retina and optic nervehead.[25]

Clinically, such vitreoretinal attachments are responsible for tangential or anteroposterior or both types of traction causing varied spectrum of structural alterations ranging from surface wrinkling in early stages to extensive detachment of retina, macular edema and vitreous hemorrhage.[26-29]

Events in Tractional Retinal Detachment (TRD) Development

- Retinal ischemia is the primary insult which stimulates production of angiogenic factors notably VEGF and others like insulin-like growth factor 1, basic fibroblast growth factor.
- These growth factors lead to the development of neovascular buds (known as vascular epicenters) from retinal blood vessels and cause angiogenesis.
- Proliferation of new vessels occurs in the potential space between the retina and the posterior hyaloid (flat NVE) from the neovascular buds which later invade the posterior lamellae of the cortical vitreous producing firm adhesions.
- Leakage from these premature vessels within retrohyaloid space and presence of growth factors causes contraction and collapse of vitreous body inducing posterior hyaloid separation (PVD) from the retina.
- PVD generally starts along superotemporal arcade, temporal to macula, above and below the disc but is limited by firm vitreoretinal adhesions at the sites of vascular epicenters.
- Progressive traction on the VR attachments due to PVD further acts as stimulus for neovascular proliferation.
- The vessels proliferate continuously with an increase in the fibrous component. When these fibrous tissue

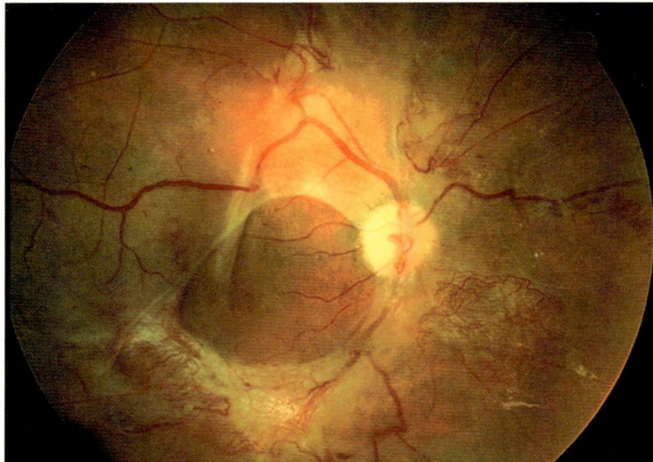

Fig. 29.1: Color image showing PDR with TRD and fibrovascular proliferation.

contracts traction is exerted on the vitreous, friable neovascular tissues and retina and leading to TRD and/or vitreous hemorrhage.
- Vitreous hemorrhage leads to more fibrosis and vitreous contraction which eventually leads to formation or further worsening of TRD.
- TRD typically appear as tented up, immobile, and concave retina with overlying contracted vitreous and/or FVP.
- TRD may involve the macula (Fig. 29.1) or it can be juxta or extra macular and may remain stationary or progress towards the macula over a period of time.

Conversion of Tractional to Combined Retinal Detachment (CRD)

- Active fibrovascular proliferation (FVP) with TRD undergoes further contraction and worsening of traction to induce break formation.
- The fibrotic tissue and the vitreous exert traction on the atrophic retina in a chronic PDR with/without TRD causing break formation.
- Anteroposteriorly directed vitreous traction on the adherent flat FVP tissue induces flap tear formation.
- Traction induced by contracting laser burn at the edge of TRD or FVP.
- Retinal break formation due to induced contraction of FVP and increased traction on the attached or detached retina following intravitreal injection of anti-VEGF agent/s.

In a combined traction/rhegmatogenous retinal detachment (Figs. 29.2A and B), generally there is a single causative retinal break often located near or at the base of FVP epicenters.

CLINICAL FEATURES OF PDR

Presence of new vessels is a hallmark of PDR which can be usually seen at the interface of perfused and nonperfused

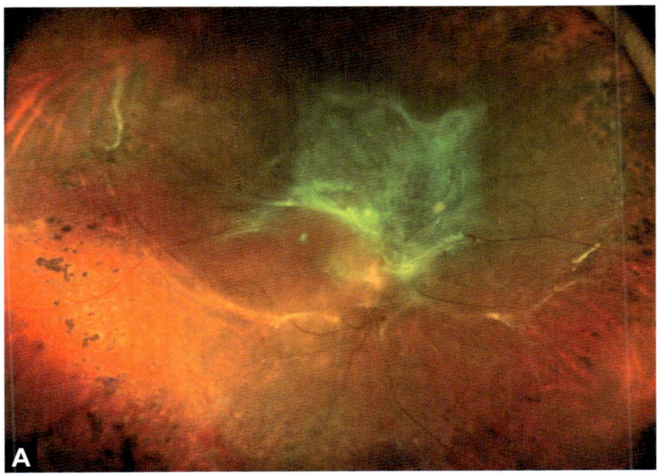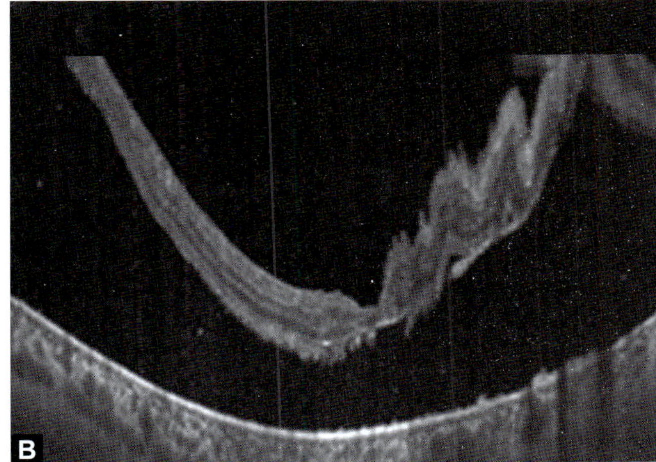

Figs. 29.2A and B: Fundus picture showing extensive fibrovascular proliferation with combined retinal detachment (Rhegmatogenous plus tractional). Ultrasonography shows detached retina.

retina and depending on their location they are described as new vessels elsewhere (NVE) or new vessels on the disc (NVD; Figs. 29.3A to C).

New vessels at the disc usually arise from the venous circulation on the disc or within 1 disc diameter of the disc and is a consequence of generalized retinal ischemia(Figs. 29.4A to D). NVD may grow directly in the vitreous cavity or can be flat along the retina.

New vessels elsewhere are flat initially as they grow between the inner surface of the retina and the posterior hyaloid face of the vitreous gel. They are seen at the junction of perfused and ischemic retina. They may look similar to IRMA on appearance.

Fibrous proliferation along NVE causes contraction and collapse of vitreous leading to separation of posterior hyaloid face and elevation of these new vessels off the retina. This traction can rupture friable new vessels leading to intraocular hemorrhage. This hemorrhage may confine to the potential space between the retina and vitreous (preretinal or subhyaloid hemorrhage Figs. 29.5A and B) or may involve vitreous gel itself (intra-gel vitreous hemorrhage) to the variable extent depending severity of the hemorrhage.

New vessel on the iris (NVI – Fig. 29.6) represents more advanced ischemic changes and sometimes occurs in association with ocular ischemia or with central retinal artery/vein occlusion. Gonioscopy should be done in all eyes to look for new vessels in the anterior chamber angle (NVA) which can lead to neovascular glaucoma, if left untreated.

PDR CLASSIFICATION

Preproliferative Retinopathy

Fundus features such as multiple large dark blot hemorrhages, presence of multiple (more than 5) cotton wool spots, and venous beading, looping and duplication, and/or IRMA are suggestive of preproliferative diabetic retinopathy. These clini-cal features are suggestive of worsening retinal ischemia which may eventually lead to the formation of the new retinal vessels.

Early PDR

There are new vessels on the retina but they do not meet the criteria for high-risk PDR.

High-Risk PDR

The Diabetic Retinopathy Study (DRS, 1972-1979),[30,31] a National Eye Institute sponsored trial has defined high-risk characteristics (HRCs) in a diabetic eye (Fig. 29.7). They are:
1. Neovascularization at or within 1 disc diameter of the optic disc (NVD) about 1/4th to 1/3rd disc area in extent, with/without vitreous or preretinal hemorrhage
2. Any NVD with vitreous hemorrhage
3. New vessels elsewhere at least 1/2th disc area in extent with vitreous hemorrhage.

High-risk PDR was defined as presence of three or more of the following high-risk characteristics:
1. Presence of preretinal or vitreous hemorrhage
2. Presence of any active neovascularization
3. Neovascularization on or within 1 disc diameter of the optic disc (NVD)
4. Severe new vessels (NVD > 1/3 disc area or NVE > ½ disc area).

In high-risk PDR, 2-year risk of severe visual loss (SVL) is decreased by 50% or more by prompt treatment with scatter laser photocoagulation (PRP).

DRS also showed that in non-high-risk PDR eyes, the probability of progression to high-risk features was 7% over 2 years and 20% over 4 years, if left untreated, in comparison to those who were treated with photocoagulation (3.2% at 2 years and 7.4% at 4 years) (Figs. 29.8A and B).

Other clinical features in PDR are:
- Preretinal, Subhyaloid and/or Vitreous hemorrhage
- Tractional retinal detachment

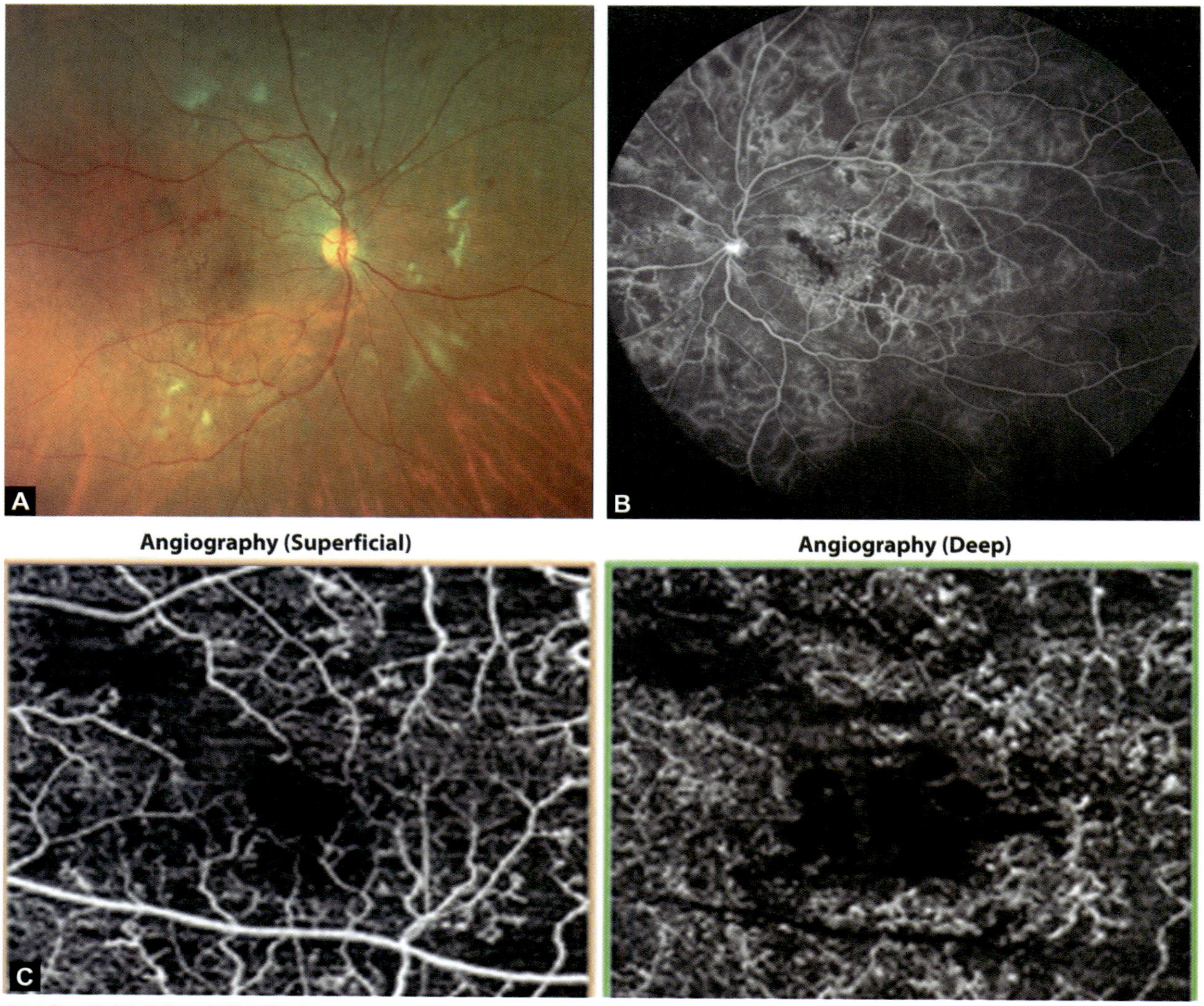

Angiography (Superficial)

Angiography (Deep)

Figs. 29.3A to C: (A) Colored UWF fundus picture showing with numerous soft exudates suggesting mixed retinopathy; (B) FFA picture showing early NVD; (C) OCTA shows macular ischemia with enlarged ,broken FAZ in superficial inner retinal vascular plexuses while deep capillary plexus reveals DME.

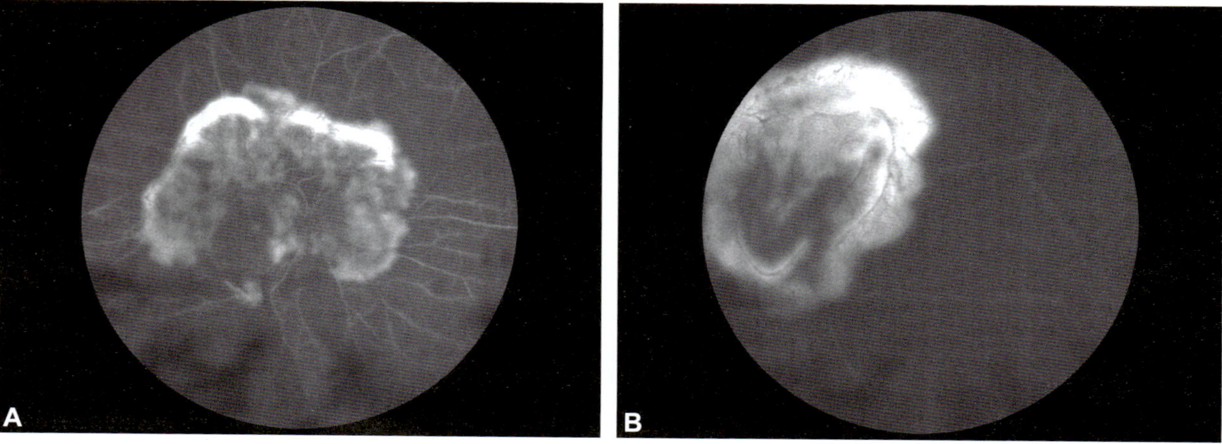

Figs. 29.4A and B

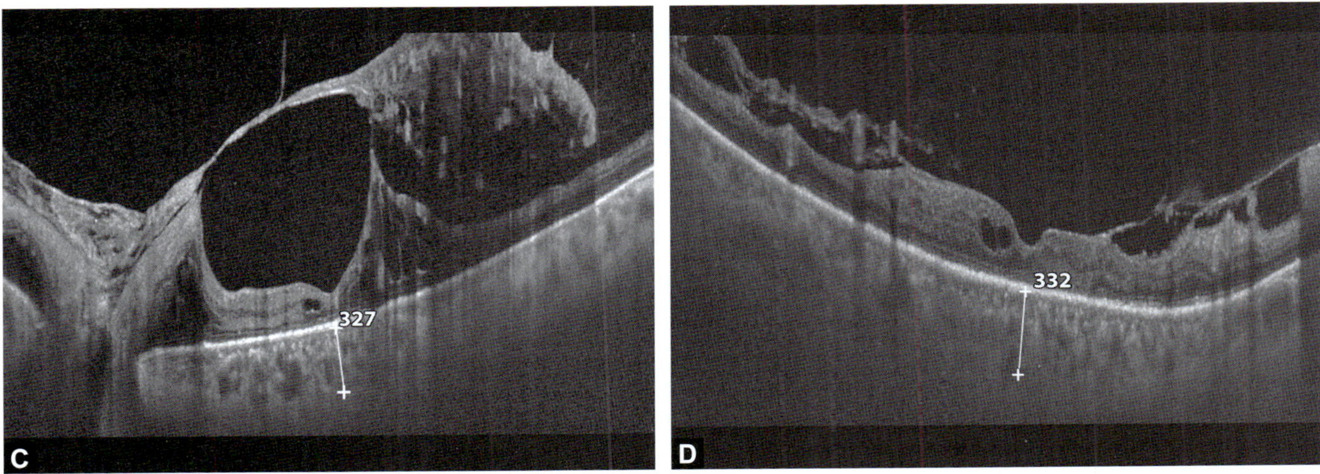

Figs. 29.4A to D: 13 year duration diabetes, poorly controlled, HbA1c-12g%; with diabetic foot was referred for eye exam first time. Showed PDR with gross ischemia on FA and atrophic macula OU.

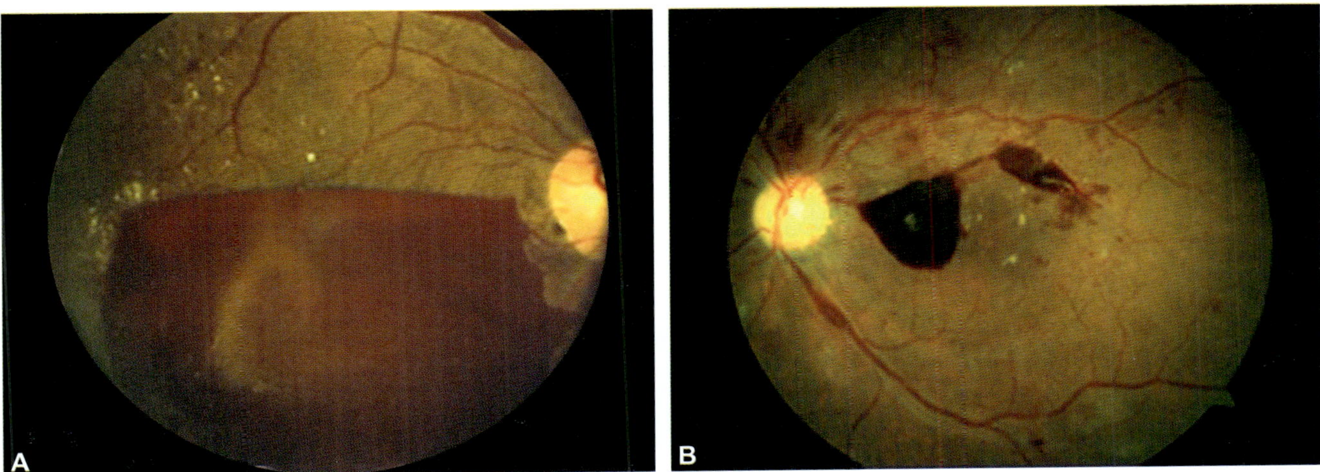

Figs. 29.5A and B: Colored fundus pictures showing premacular/subhyaloid hemorrhage.

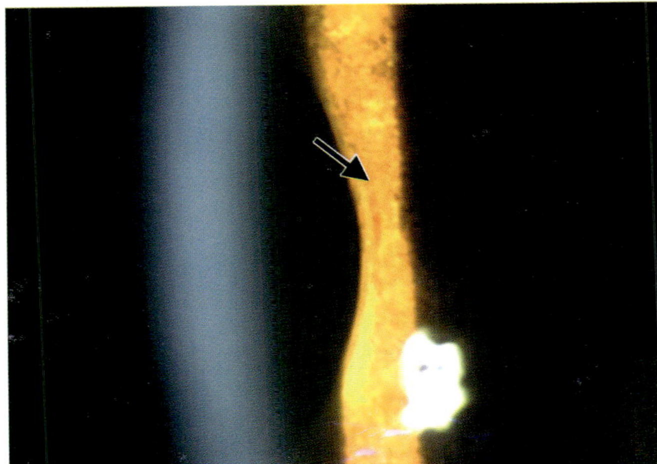

Fig. 29.6: NVI at the pupillary margin (Black arrow).

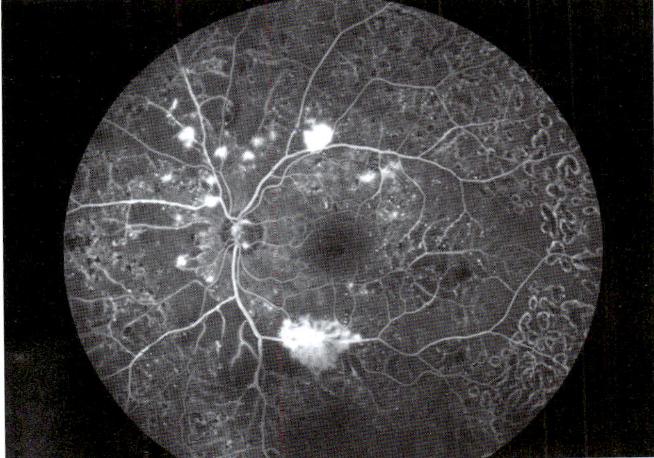

Fig. 29.7: Eye with PDR-HRC showing NVD and large (greater than 1DD NVE). NVE eyes with these HRCs have 50% risk of severe vision loss (vision ≤ 5/200), if left untreated.

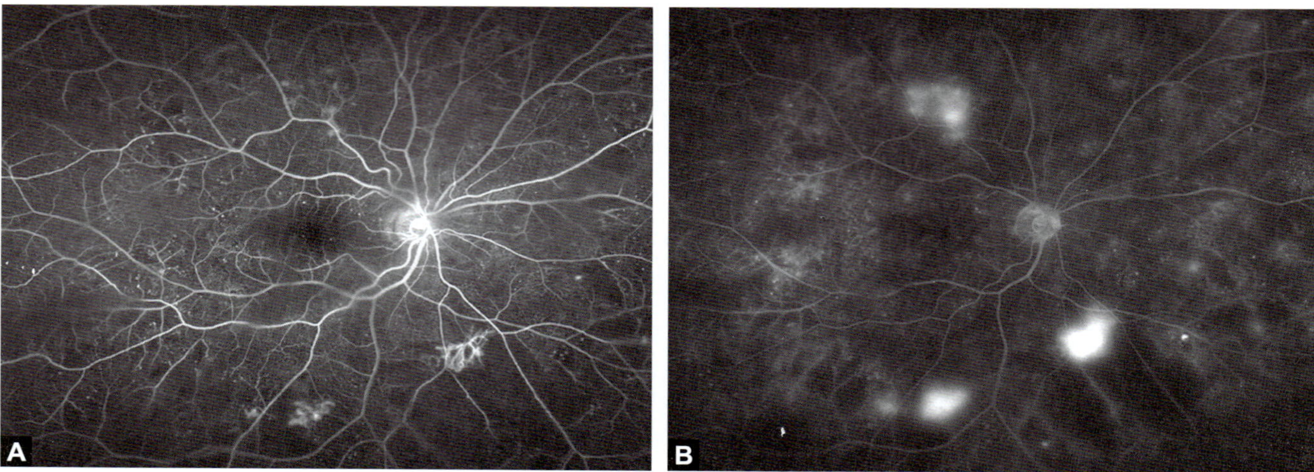

Figs. 29.8A and B: Early and late phase FA of PDR eye showing 4 quadrants of MCA's and multiple NVE ,besides vascular leakage which is also an important sign of retinopathy progression.

- Combined tractional and rhegmatogenous retinal detachment (CRD)
- Iris/Anterior chamber angle neovascularization (NVI, NVA)

PDR can be associated with macular edema of variable severity.

Visual loss in eyes with PDR could be due to vitreous or premacular hemorrhage, retinal detachment involving macula (TRD/CRD), FVP growing in front of the macula, tractional maculopathy or papillopathy and macular edema and /or ischemia.

Burned Out Retinopathy

With completion of vitreous contraction, proliferative retinopathy may enter a 'burned out stage' or 'involutional stage' which is characterized by severe retinal ischemia, reduced caliber and number of NV, thinning of fibrous tissue, reduced number of intraretinal lesions, reduced caliber of major retinal vessels and chronic macular edema.

MANAGEMENT OF PROLIFERATIVE DIABETIC RETINOPATHY

Management of Systemic Risk Factors

The Diabetes Control and Complications Trial (DCCT)[32] studying known Type 1 diabetics and the UK Prospective Diabetes Study (UKPDS)[33] involving newly diagnosed type 2 diabetics have provided good evidence on the importance of glycemic control on the development of retinopathy and its progression. It was further confirmed by ACCORD study.[34] In the DCCT/EDIC,[35] on ten years follow-up, the group which received intensive treatment previously showed 24% reduction in progression of retinopathy.

The UKPDS[36] showed that a tight control of blood pressure was associated with less need for photocoagulation and less deterioration of 2-step or more on the ETDRS retinopathy scale but ACCORD study showed no significant effect of intensive blood pressure control on retinopathy progression. EUCLID study[37] tried 10 mg of Lisinopril (Angiotensin converting enzyme blocker), and Diabetic Retinopathy Candesartan Trials (DIRECT)[38] and DIRECT-Protect 2[39] have tried oral candesartan (32 mg daily), an angiotensin-receptor blocker on the incidence and progression of diabetic retinopathy and found an overall significant change towards less severe DR in all the three trials.

In Fenofibrate Intervention and Event Lowering in Diabetes (FIELD) study[40], fenofibrate (200 mg/day) reduced the requirements for laser therapy (both macular and panretinal scatter laser) and prevented disease progression in patients with pre-existing diabetic retinopathy. The ACCORD study[34] showed a 40% reduction in the odds of having progression of retinopathy over 4 years in patients allocated to fenofibrate (160 mg/day) in combination with simvastatin, compared to simvastatin alone. It was seen that the effect exerted by fenofibrate was independent of effect on gylcemic control. Recently ACCORDION (2016, extension of ACCORD study) added that over a period of 10 years intensive control of blood sugar is beneficial, effect of fenofibrate fades and control of blood pressure does not help.[41]

Laser Therapy

Over last 35 years 'Panretinal Laser Photocoagulation' (PRP) —Figure 29.9 is the first line treatment for PDR. Reports from DRS on effect of laser photocoagulation of proliferative retina were shown to be of sustained benefit in reducing the risk of SVL.[42] The evidence of beneficial treatment effect in patients with high-risk criteria in DRS became more convincing with additional follow-up.[42-44] However, whether it is better to advise treatment at earlier stages or to defer it until high-risk characteristics develop was not firmly established from DRS data and the question was subsequently answered by ETDRS.

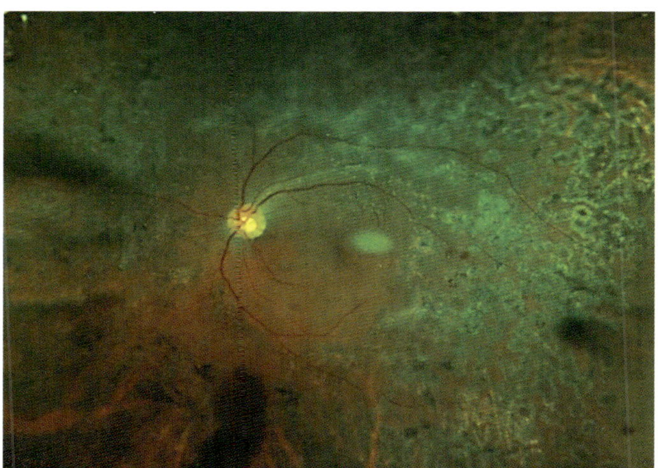

Fig. 29.9: Ultra-wide field fundus picture with panretinal photocoagulation (PRP).

The Early Treatment Diabetic Retinopathy Study (ETDRS, 1979–1987)[45], a multicenter, collaborative, clinical trial addressed three clinical questions:

a. When is it most effective to initiate photocoagulation therapy during the course of diabetic retinopathy?

b. Is photocoagulation effective in treatment of macular edema?

c. Does aspirin alter the course of diabetic retinopathy?

This study recruited patients with severe non-proliferative retinopathy and proliferative retinopathy without high-risk characteristics to determine the stage at which PRP using argon laser is most effective. Overall, the 5-year risk of SVL or need for vitrectomy was 2-6% in eyes which underwent early photocoagulation and 4-10% where photocoagulation was deferred. The conclusion was that laser PRP could be deferred until eyes approached the high-risk stage provided patient maintains proper follow-up schedule.

Supplemental aspirin did not show any beneficial effect on the course of diabetic retinopathy or cataract formation in these eyes. However, there are no ocular or systemic side effects in diabetics who require Aspirin for other cause.

These trials established the basis for the treatment of protocols for diabetic retinopathy that have subsequently been adopted worldwide. Apart from DRS high-risk characteristics, additional indications for PRP are:

- Neovascularization of iris or anterior chamber anle with/without neovascular glaucoma
- Moderate-to-severe NVE alone particularly in juvenile diabetics
- Widespread capillary non perfusion areas on fluorescein angiography
- PDR developing in pregnancy particularly with the institution of tight metabolic control
- Preproliferative retinopathy in the second eye of a juvenile diabetics with severe PDR in the other eye.

Further on, studies have found NVD to be the most important risk factor to affect the visual outcomes after photocoagulation. The risk of SVL rises with increasing severity of NVD. Other risk factors found to affect the visual outcome are hemorrhages/microaneurysms, retinal elevation (TRD), proteinuria and hyperglycemia. The risk of SVL decreases with increasing 'treatment density' thus providing support for performing additional photocoagulation when neovascularization is not reduced or stabilized by initial treatment.[45] Moreover, laser treatment may be considered for progressive proliferative retinopathy on serial follow-up even in the absence of high-risk characteristics (*see* Figs. 29.8A and B).

Conventional laser treatment causes retinal scarring and destroys photoreceptor cells and reduces O_2 demand. It further allows better O_2 diffusion across the viable retina and also modifies varies growth stimulating /inhibiting factors.

Technique of Laser Photocoagulation (DRS)[44]

Both green and red wavelength lasers can be effectively used for 'Scatter' (Panretinal) photocoagulation (PRP). Green laser penetrates choroid less hence there is relatively less pain and less risk of choroidal effusion when compare to red wavelength. Red laser penetrates vitreous hemorrhage and yellow lens nuclei better.

PRP should extend from arcade to/beyond the vortex vein ampoules (equator) and often completed in 1 to 3 sittings. With availability of Laser Indirect Ophthalmoscope (LIO), 'indirect laser delivery' system is more commonly used for PRP than 'slit lamp delivery' system.

The suggested key features of the laser techniques are summarized in the Table 29.1.

Table 29.1: Technique of laser photocoagulation (ETDRS).[46]

Burn characteristics	Recommendations
Spot size (s it lamp or LIO)	400 to 500 microns (or with 20D, 28D, or 30D indirect lens, indirect delivery)
Exposure duration	0.050 – 0.10 seconds
Intensity	Mild white/gray burns
Spacing	500 micron (one burn apart)
Number of sessions	1 to 3
Nasal proximity to disc	No closure than 500 microns
Temporal proximity to macula center	No closure than 3,000 microns
Superior/inferior limit	No further posterior than 1 burn within temporal arcade
Extent	Arcades (approx 3,000 microns from the macula center) to at least the equator
Total number of burns	1200 to 2000
Wavelength	Green (532 nm) or red

Completing the PRP in one sitting may apear convenient but increases the risk of developing macular edema. Other potential complications include iritis, serous choroidal and /or retinal detachment and anterior rotation of ciliary body leading to angle closure glaucoma.

In ETDRS, PRP was given over 2 or more sittings usually within 4 weeks. It allows the retinal edema to subside before the next sitting of PRP and is less painful for the patient. DRCR.net results found no clinically significant difference in visual acuity or OCT thickness between PRP in 1 sitting and 4 sitting more definitive results would require a large randomized trial.[47] Better visual acuity and decreased macular edema is seen in eyes receiving focal/grid laser for DME and PRP by adding intravitreal triamcinolone or anti-VEGF injectionsby.[48]

Generally treatment is well tolerated and there is no need of anaesthesia. However, treatment of retinal periphery can be more painful for the patient. Decreasing power, duration and using green wavelength may help to minimize the pain.

Though the treatment can be initiated in any quadrant, generally inferior and peripheral retina is treated first. Direct treatment to major retinal vessels, preretinal hemorrhage and dark pigmented scars should be avoided. Also limit laser photocoagulation at least 1-2 disc area away from the TRD margin.

After completion of laser, patient can be followed up after 6-8 weeks and thereafter at 4 months interval.

Repeat laser (fill-in PRP) can be considered if retinopathy is active (fine vessels, dilated buds or tips covered with hemorrhage) or increased in size or continued development of new vessels over the retina, iris or anterior chamber angle. Skip or untreated area of the retina or gaps between existing laser scars can be filled with additional laser. In eyes with vitreous hemorrhage, unobscured retina can be treated initially and additional laser can be performed as hemorrhage keeps on clearing. Red laser can be of use in these eyes.

Laser Photocoagulation—Side Effects/Complications

Side effects of the laser photocoagulation are more common that actual complications. They are:[47]

- Loss of peripheral visual field, difficult dark adaptation and decreased contrast sensitivity
- Mydriasis and paresis of accommodation (usually transient)
- Worsening of macular edema
- Vitreous hemorrhage
- Worsening of traction leading to increased TRD or retinal break formation
- Choroidal detachment with/without exudative retinal detachment
- Choroidal neovascularization due to heavy burns causing rupture of Bruch's membrane
- Foveal burn or optic disc damage
- Iris, cornea or lens burn and posterior synechiae

Due to newer laser machines and better precision of laser techniques, severity of complications has come down significantly.

Anti-VEGF Therapy in PDR

Currently, PRP is the standard treatment for PDR (Fig. 29.9), but it also has certain adverse effects being an inherently destructive procedure. Multiple studies have implicated VEGF as a major causative factor in human eye diseases characterized by neovascularization including PDR.[49,50] Thus, inhibition of VEGF would be expected to reduce PDR. Complete resolution of angiographic leakage of NVD due to PDR was reported by Avery et al. in 19 of 26 eyes (73%) that were treated with intravitreal Bevacizumab.[51]

DRCR.net Protocol S[52] evaluated non-inferiority of intravitreal Ranibizumab compared with PRP for visual acuity outcomes in patients with PDR. Individual eyes were randomly assigned to receive PRP (in 1-3 sittings), or intravitreal injection Ranibizumab (0.5 mg) at baseline and then every 4 weeks based on the treatment protocol. Both treatment groups could receive Ranibizumab for DME. The results showed that among eyes with PDR, treatment with Ranibizumab resulted in visual acuity that was noninferior to (not worse than) PRP at 2 years.

The DRCR.net Protocol S investigated whether intravitreal Ranibizumab had a beneficial effect on the vitrectomy rates of eyes with vitreous hemorrhage from PDR preventing completion of PRP compared to intravitreal saline. There was a definite reduction in vitrectomy rates with Ranibizumab treated eyes having 4% vitrectomy rates versus 15% vitrectomy rates in those eyes who underwent PRP. There was no significant difference in safety between the two treatment groups at 52-weeks.[53]

NEWER DIAGNOSTIC AND THERAPEUTIC MODALITIES FOR PDR MANAGEMENT

Role of OCTA (Dyeless Angiography) in PDR

Dyeless angiography that is Optical Coherence Tomography Angiography (OCTA) is a remarkable development which helps in diagnosis of neovascularization, macular ischemia (regularity and size of FAZ) and decreased capillary perfusion in cases of diabetic retinopathy (Figs. 29.10A and B). Major advantage is in the cases with associated severe nephropathy which precludes use of fluorescein or even in patients found allergic to fluorescein dye. The only concern with use of OCTA is that it does not show leakage.

UWFA Guided Laser Photocoagulation

Another major advantage in this field is Ultra-Wide Field Photography and Angiography (UWFA) (Optos) (Figs. 29.11A and B) which shows peripheral capillary non perfusion areas (CNP) as well as peripheral vascular leakage (PVL) (Figs. 29.12A and B) which can be targeted and lasered rather than a complete scatter laser. Targeted laser photocoagulation

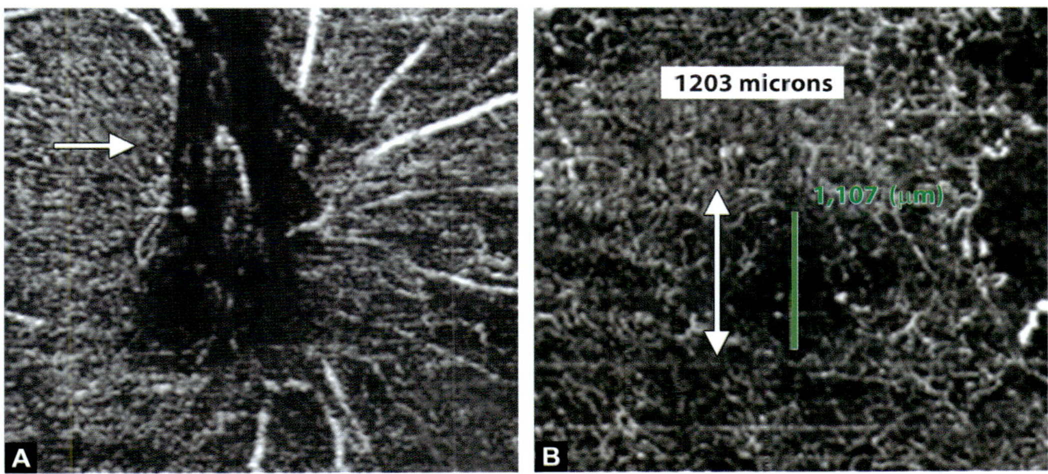

Figs. 29.10A and B: Role of OCTA in diabetic retinopathy in a case with contraindication to FFA (A) Showing NVD (white arrow); (B) Showing enlarged FAZ.

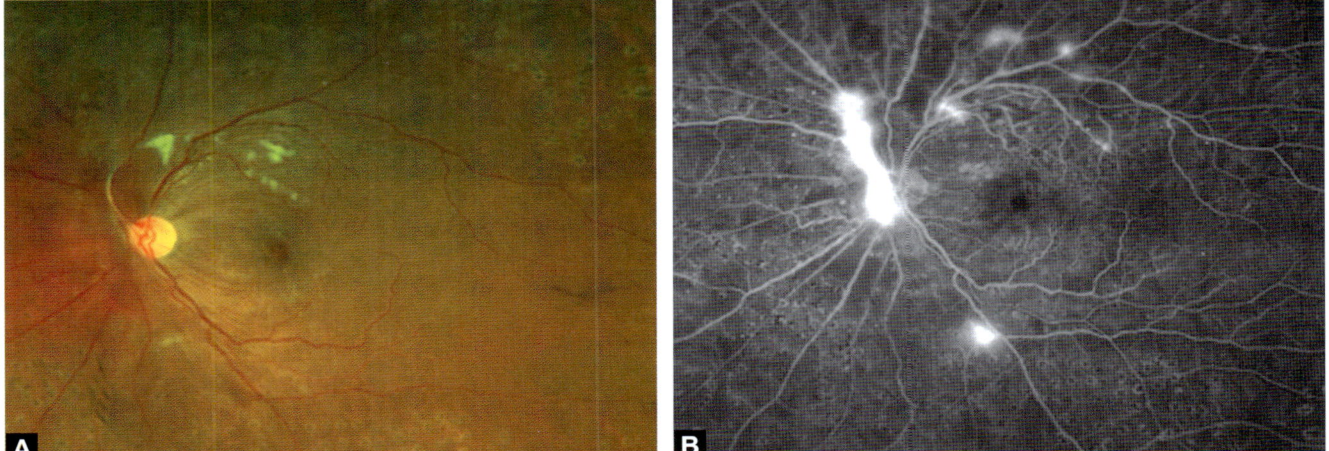

Figs. 29.11A and B: Wide field photograph showing raised NVD and NVE with laser spots with corresponding FFA showing leakage from raised NVD and multiple NVEs.

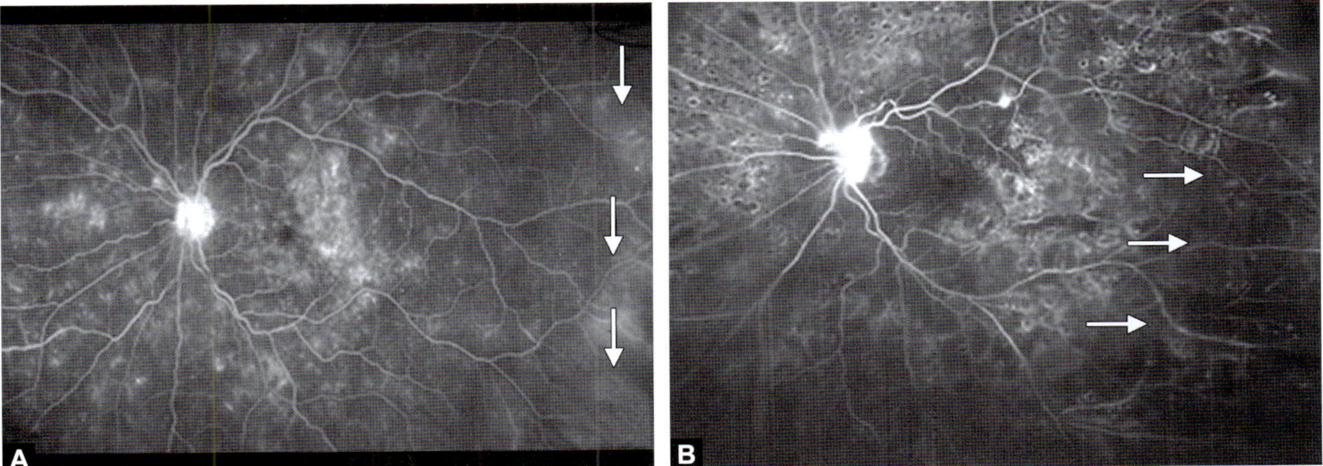

Figs. 29.12A and B: Role of ultra-wide field imaging and angiography in cases of PDR: (A) FFA showing areas of peripheral vascular leakage (PVL; white arrows); (B) FFA showing areas of capillary non perfusion areas (white arrows) causing NVD.

has been shown to be equally effective to full scatter in some studies with fewer side effects like field, accommodation loss and decreased chances of consecutive optic atrophy.

Endpoint Management

Endpoint Management is a program developed for the 577nm Pascal laser (Topcon) that allows mapping values of tissue damage based on computational modeling to a linear scale of laser energy relative to a visible titration level. The titration algorithm for Endpoint Management begins by defining the laser power required to produce a barely visible burn at a pulse duration of 20 ms. This energy is taken as 100% and all other pulse energies are expressed as a percentage of this titration threshold.

At 30% energy level only a single RPE cell in the center of the 200-µm spot is damaged. With Endpoint Management, some spots in a grid treatment pattern can be set at 100% (or above) to mark the location of the subvisible treatment with an immediately visible reference. This helps in maintaining the same ophthalmoscopic visibility throughout the fundus and provides a reproducible approach to subvisible retinal laser therapy possibly resulting in reduced dependence on injections.

Micropulse Laser

Subthreshold micropulse laser has the advantage of limiting collateral damage by delivering the laser energy in ultrashort (microseconds) pulses with adjustable on and off times. The length of these pulses must be shorter than the time required for heat to be transferred away from the irradiated tissue hence creating the rise in temperature is insufficient to cause damage to collateral retinal tissue.

This technology has mostly been tried in the treatment of DME. It minimizes scarring so much that the laser spots are usually undetectable on clinical and angiographic examination. At the same time, it has been shown to stimulate the RPE and have a beneficial effect on its activation.[23]

Nanopulse Laser

Retina Regeneration Therapy (2RT; Ellex Medical Lasers) is a subthreshold laser modality using a 532 nm laser to produce 3 ns pulses. These nanosecond pulses are purported to stimulate renewal of the RPE. 2RT combines subthreshold with micropulse laser protocols. When compared to conventional laser, the nanosecond laser using a speckle-beam profile provides a wider therapeutic range of energies over which RPE treatment can be performed without damage to the apposed retinar.[24] The use of lower energy levels is meant to cause sublethal injury to targeted RPE, rather than destroying it and leading to cytokine release by recovering RPE cells.

Targeted Retinal Photocoagulation

Targeted retinal photocoagulation (TRP) is another concept in development. Targeted or selective therapy in general is any therapy aimed to block a specific target. Examples of targeted retinal therapy include feeder vessel photocoagulation in choroidal neovascularization, focal laser photocoagulation in the treatment of DME, and selective laser to areas of nonperfusion. The idea behind TRP is to selectively treat ischemic retinal areas and adjacent intermediate areas showing leakage on angiography, while minimizing the risks and complications of conventional PRP. Muqit et al. reported that TRP for PDR using 20 ms micropulses with the Pascal laser did not produce increased macular thickness; paradoxically, it improved central retinal thickness and visual field sensitivity with reasonable regression of neovascularization.

Another major advantage of UWFA guided targeted laser (using the PASCAL or conventional single -spot laser) is it helps to reduce the retinal complications induced by heavy scatter laser. Targeted laser preferentially treats only the ischemic or leaky areas and spares the normal, healthy retina.

Micropulse Laser for PDR

By using shorter pulse duration , there is less thermal spread; PRP is less painful and creates a lighter, smaller burn with less collateral damage to the outer retina. With shorter pulse duration, there is a better stability of burn size over time and evidence of healing with less scarring, though more burns may be needed for equivalent therapeutic effect.[54] Since introduction of 577 nm yellow semi-automated pattern multispot laser delivery (PASCAL, Topcon, Capelle aan den IJssel, The Netherlands) in 2005, PRP can be delivered faster with multiple retinal laser burns being given in a set pattern with a single depression of the foot pedal. In clinical studies, good short-term control of PDR has been shown following single session pattern multispot PRP treatment. The technique shortens the procedure time, reduces total energy delivered to the eye and decreases patient pain, but top-up laser has been required with overall more laser burns delivered than with conventional laser technique.[55]

Navigated Laser Treatment (using Navilas)

A new (NAVILAS®, NAVILAS Laser System, and Irvine, CA, USA) has a retinal eye-tracking laser delivery system with integrated digital fundus imaging.

Newer Anti-VEGF Agents

Newer anti-VEGF treatments include soluble VEGF receptor analogues, Eyelea (Regeneron, Tarrytown, NY, USA), small interfering RNAs, bevasiranib (Opko Health,Miami, FL, USA) and rapamycin (Sirolimus; MacuSight, Union City, CA, USA) and also targeting a central regulator, such as Raf kinase, a mammalian target of rapamycin and the RTP 801 gene. Extended drug delivery of anti-VEGF using bioerodible implants, bioerodible microspheres and encapsulated cells are under trial. Other potential target molecules other than anti-VEGFs include angiopoietin-2, tumor necrosis factor, interleukins, proteinases, chemokines (CCL2 and CCL5) and kallikrein.[56]

CONCLUSION

Diabetic retinopathy is a microvascular complication due to progressive retinal ischemia. PDR is a potentially blinding but preventable complication of diabetes mellitus and is a major public health problem. Various multicenter trials have given clear guidelines for the management of PDR. Good metabolic control, regular examinations, early diagnosis and prompt treatment with laser photocoagulation in eyes with high-risk PDR can minimize the risk of visual loss.

REFERENCES

1. http://www.diabetesatlas.org/across-the-globe.html
2. Caird FI, Pirie A, Ramsell TG: Diabetes and the Eye. Oxford and Edinburgh: Blackwell, 1968
3. Beetham WP. Visual prognosis of proliferating diabetic retinopathy. Br J Ophthalmology. 1963;47:611-19.
4. Rand LI, Prud'homme GJ, Ederer F, Canner PL. Factors influencing the development of visual loss in advanced diabetic retinopathy. Diabetic Retinopathy Study (DRS) Report No. 10. Invest Ophthalmology Vis Sci. 1985;26:983-91.
5. Davis MD, Fisher MR, Gangnon RE, et al. Risk factors for high-risk proliferative diabetic retinopathy and severe visual loss: Early Treatment Diabetic Retinopathy Study Report #18. Invest Ophthalmology Vis Sci. 1998;39:233-52.
6. Fundus photographic risk factors for progression of diabetic retinopathy. ETDRS report number 12. Early Treatment Diabetic Retinopathy Study Research Group. Ophthalmology. 1991;98(5 Suppl):823-33.
7. Klein R, Klein BE, Moss SE, et al. The Wisconsin Epidemiologic Study of Diabetic Retinopathy. X. Four-year incidence and progression of diabetic retinopathy when age at diagnosis is 30 years or more. Arch Ophthalmology. 1989;107:244-49.
8. Klein R, Klein BE, Moss SE, Davis MD, DeMets DL. The Wisconsin Epidemiologic Study of Diabetic Retinopathy. IX. Four-year incidence and progression of diabetic retinopathy when age at diagnosis is less than 30 years. Arch Ophthalmology. 1989;107:237-43.
9. Fluorescein angiographic risk factors for progression of diabetic retinopathy. ETDRS report number 13. Early Treatment Diabetic Retinopathy Study Research Group. Ophthalmology. 1991;98(5 Suppl):834-40
10. Klein R, Klein BE, Moss SE, et al. The Wisconsin Epidemiologic Study of diabetic retinopathy. XIV. Ten-year incidence and progression of diabetic retinopathy. Arch Ophthalmology. 1994;112:1217-28.
11. Klein R, Davis MD, Moss SE, et al. The Wisconsin Epidemiologic Study of Diabetic Retinopathy. A comparison of retinopathy in younger and older onset diabetic persons. AdvExp Med Biol. 1985;189:321-35.
12. Davis MD, Fisher MR, Gangnon RE, et al. Risk factors for high-risk proliferative diabetic retinopathy and severe visual loss: Early Treatment Diabetic Retinopathy Study Report #18. Invest Ophthalmology Vis Sci. 1998;39:233-52.
13. Klein BE, Myers CE, Howard KP, et al. Serum Lipids and Proliferative Diabetic Retinopathy and Macular Edema in Persons With Long-term Type 1 Diabetes Mellitus: The Wisconsin Epidemiologic Study of Diabetic Retinopathy. JAMA Ophthalmology. 2015;133: 503-10.
14. Ashton N, Ward B, Serpell G. Effect of oxygen on developing retinal vessels with particular reference to the problem of retrolental fibroplasia. Br J Ophthalmology. 1954;38:397-432.
15. Wise GN. Retinal neovascularization. Trans Am Ophthalmology Soc. 1956;54:729-826.
16. Bresnick GH, De Venecia G, Myers FL, et al. Retinal ischemia in diabetic retinopathy. Arch Ophthalmology. 1975;93:1300-10.
17. Aiello LP, Avery RL, Arrigg PG, et al. Vascular endothelial growth factor in ocular fluid of patients with diabetic retinopathy and other retinal disorders. N Engl J Med. 1994;331:1480-87.
18. Adamis AP, Miller JW, Bernal MT, et al. Increased vascular endothelial growth factor levels in the vitreous of eyes with proliferative diabetic retinopathy. Am J Ophthalmology. 1994;118:445-50.
19. Adamis AP, Shima DT, Tolentino MJ, et al. Inhibition of vascular endothelial growth factor prevents retinal ischemia-associated iris neovascularization in a nonhuman primate. Arch Ophthalmology. 1996;114:66-71.
20. Takagi H, Koyama S, Seike H, et al. Potential role of the angiopoietin/tie2 system in ischemia-induced retinal neovascularization. Invest Ophthalmology Vis Sci. 2003;44:393-402.
21. Geraldes P, Hiraoka-Yamamoto J, Matsumoto M, et al. Activation of PKC-delta and SHP-1 by hyperglycemia causes vascular cell apoptosis and diabetic retinopathy. Nat Med. 2009;15:1298-306.
22. Watanabe D, Suzuma K, Matsui S, et al. Erythropoietin as a retinal angiogenic factor in proliferative diabetic retinopathy. N Engl J Med. 2005;353:782-92.
23. Mintz-Hittner HA. Kennedy KA, Chuang AZ; BEAT-ROP Cooperative Group. Efficacy of intravitreal bevacizumab for stage 3+ retinopathy of prematurity. N Engl J Med. 2011;364:603-15.
24. Bressler SB, Qin H, Melia M, et al. Exploratory analysis of the effect of intravitreal ranibizumab or triamcinolone on worsening of diabetic retinopathy in a randomized clinical trial. JAMA Ophthalmology. 2013;131:1033-40.
25. Takahashi M, Trempe CL, Maguire K, et al. Vitreoretinal relationship in diabetic retinopathy: a biomicroscopic evaluation. Arch Ophthalmology. 1981;99:241-45.
26. Tagawa H, McMeel JW, Furukawa H, et al. Role of the vitreous in diabetic retinopathy I. Vitreous changes in diabetic retinopathy and in physiologic aging. Ophthalmology. 1986;93:596-601.
27. Gella L, Raman R, Kulothungan V, et al. Prevalence of posterior vitreous detachment in the population with type II diabetes mellitus and its effect on diabetic retinopathy: Sankara Nethralaya Diabetic Retinopathy Epidemiology and Molecular Genetic Study SN-DREAMS report no. 23. Jpn J Ophthalmology. 2012;56:262-67.
28. Bresrick GH, Haight B, de Venecia G. Retinal wrinkling and macular heterotopia in diabetic retinopathy. Arch Ophthalmology. 1979;97:1890-95.
29. Charles S, Flinn CE. The natural history of diabetic extramacular traction retinal detachment. Arch Ophthalmology. 1981;99:66-68.
30. The Diabetic Retinopathy Study Research Group. Photocoagulation treatment of proliferative diabetic retinopathy. Clinical application of Diabetic Retinopathy Study (DRS) findings, DRS Report Number 8. Ophthalmology. 1981;88:583-600.
31. The Diabetic Retinopathy Study Research Group. Indications for photocoagulation treatment of diabetic retinopathy: Diabetic Retinopathy Study Report no. 14. Int Ophthalmology Clin. 1987;27: 239-53.
32. The relationship of glycemic exposure (HbA1c) to the risk of development and progression of retinopathy in the diabetes control and complications trial. Diabetes. 1995;44:968-83.
33. UK Prospective Diabetes Study (UKPDS) Group. Intensive blood-glucose control with sulphonylureas or insulin compared with conventional treatment and risk of complications in patients with type 2 diabetes (UKPDS 33). Lancet. 1998;352:837-53.

34. ACCORD Study Group; ACCORD Eye Study Group, Chew EY, Ambrosius WT, Davis MD, et al. Effects of medical therapies on retinopathy progression in type 2 diabetes. N Engl J Med. 2010;363:233-44.

35. White NH, Sun W, Cleary PA, et al. Prolonged effect of intensive therapy on the risk of retinopathy complications in patients with type 1 diabetes mellitus: 10 years after the diabetes control and complications trial. Arch Ophthalmology. 2008;126:1707-15.

36. Matthews DR, Stratton IM, Aldington SJ, et al. Risks of progression of retinopathy and vision loss related to tight blood pressure control in type 2 diabetes mellitus. Arch Ophthalmology. 2004;122: 1631-40.

37. Chaturvedi N, Sjolie AK, Stephenson JM, et al. Effect of lisinopril on progression of retinopathy in normotensive people with type 1 diabetes. The EUCLID Study Group. EURODIAB Controlled Trial of Lisinopril in Insulin-Dependent Diabetes Mellitus. Lancet. 1998;351:28-31.

38. Chaturvedi N, Porta M, Klein R, et al. DIRECT Programme Study Group. Effect of candesartan on prevention (DIRECT-Prevent 1) and progression (DIRECT-Protect 1) of retinopathy in type 1 diabetes: randomised, placebo-controlled trials. Lancet. 2008;372:1394-402.

39. Sjolie AK, Klein R, Porta M, et al. DIRECT Programme Study Group. Effect of candesartan on progression and regression of retinopathy in type 2 diabetes (DIRECT-Protect 2): a randomised placebo-controlled trial. Lancet. 2008;372:1385-93.

40. Keech AC, Mitchell P, Summanen PA, et al. Effect of fenofibrate on the need for laser treatment for diabetic retinopathy (FIELD study): a randomised controlled trial. Lancet. 2007;370:1687-97.

41. ACCORD Study Group; ACCORD Eye Study Group. Persistent Effects of Intensive Glycemic Control on Retinopathy in Type 2 Diabetes in the Action to Control Cardiovascular Risk in Diabetes (ACCORD) Follow-On Study. Diabetes Care. 2016 Jul;39(7):1089-100. doi: 10.2337/dc16-0024. Epub 2016 Jun 11.

42. Preliminary report on effects of photocoagulation therapy. The Diabetic. Retinopathy Study Research Group. Am J Ophthalmology. 1976;81:383-96.

43. Photocoagulation treatment of proliferative diabetic retinopathy: the second report of diabetic retinopathy study findings. Ophthalmology 1978;85:82-106.

44. Photocoagulation treatment of proliferative diabetic retinopathy. Clinical application of Diabetic Retinopathy Study (DRS) findings, DRS Report Number 8. The Diabetic Retinopathy Study Research Group. Ophthalmology 1981;88:583-600.

45. Early photocoagulation for diabetic retinopathy. ETDRS report number 9. Early Treatment Diabetic Retinopathy Study Research Group. Ophthalmology 1991;98(5 Suppl):766-85.

46. Techniques for scatter and local photocoagulation treatment of diabetic retinopathy: Early Treatment Diabetic Retinopathy Study Report no. 3. The Early Treatment Diabetic Retinopathy Study Research Group. Int Ophthalmology Clin. 1987;27:254-64.

47. Albert and Jakobiec's, Principle and Practice of Ophthalmology. Chapter 135, proliferative diabetic retinopathy. Diabetic retinopathy study and modern panretinal photocoagulation (PRP).

48. Diabetic Retinopathy Clinical Research Network, Googe J, Brucker AJ, Bressler NM, Qin H, et al. Randomized trial evaluating short-term effects of intravitreal ranibizumab or triamcinolone acetonide on macular edema after focal/grid laser for diabetic macular edema in eyes also receiving panretinal photocoagulation. Retina. 2011;31:1009-27.

49. Gonzalez VH, Giuliari GP, Banda RM, et al. Intravitreal injection of pegaptanib sodium for proliferative diabetic retinopathy. Br J Ophthalmology. 2009;93:1474-8.

50. Mason JO 3rd, Nixon PA, White MF. Intravitreal injection of bevacizumab (Avastin) as adjunctive treatment of proliferative diabetic retinopathy. Am J Ophthalmology. 2006;142:685-8.

51. Avery RL, Pearlman J, Pieramici DJ, et al. Intravitreal bevacizumab (Avastin) in the 1739 treatment of proliferative diabetic retinopathy. Ophthalmology. 2006;113:1695.e1-15.

52. Writing Committee for the Diabetic Retinopathy Clinical Research Network, Gross JG, Glassman AR, Jampol LM, et al. Panretinal photocoagulation vs intravitreous ranibizumab for proliferative diabetic retinopathy: a randomized clinical trial. JAMA. 2015; 314:2137-46.

53. Diabetic Retinopathy Clinical Research Network. Bhavser AR, Torres K, Beck RW, Bressler NM, et al. Randomized clinical trial evaluating intravitreal ranibizumab or saline for vitreous hemorrhage from proliferative diabetic retinopathy. JAMA Ophthalmology. 2013;131:283-93.

54. Muqit MM, Marcellino GR, Gray JC, et al. Pain responses of Pascal 20 ms multi-spot and 100 ms single-spot panretinal photocoagulation: Manchester Pascal Study, MAPASS report 2. Br J Ophthalmology. 2010;94:1493-8.

55. Muqit MM, Marcellino GR, Henson DB, et al. Pascal panretinal laser ablation and regression analysis in proliferative diabetic retinopathy: Manchester Pascal Study Report 4. Eye. 2011;25: 1447-56.

56. Das A, Stroud S, Mehta S, et al. New treatments for diabetic retinopathy. Diabetes, Obes Metab. 2015;17:219-30.

Chapter 30

Retinopathy in Hematological Disorders

Prateek Kakkar, Rohan Chawla, Nasiq Hasan, Amit Gadkar, Atul Kumar

LEUKEMIC RETINOPATHY

 ### INTRODUCTION

Myeloproliferative disorders like leukemia and lymphoma are systemic illnesses which may affect the eye, even before the first systemic symptom appears. In the past, ophthalmologists were relied upon for aiding in the diagnosis before bone marrow biopsy as up to 90% of patients with leukemia may have ocular involvement.[1] It may involve any ocular tissue right from the conjunctiva to the optic nerve (Fig. 30.1).[2] Retina can have direct effects due to infiltration of neoplastic cells or via associated systemic hematological abnormalities such as hyperviscosity, anemia, thrombocytopenia, or due to poor systemic immune status of the patient causing opportunistic ocular infections. Intraocular manifestations of myeloproliferative disorders are often associated with central nervous system (CNS) involvement and carry poor outcome.[3]

LEUKEMIA

Leukemia is a group of neoplastic disorders that usually begin in the bone marrow and result in high numbers of abnormal white blood cells. Leukemia may be broadly divided into B cell or T cell, or leucoid or myeloid type, according to the cell of origin. In acute stages, it presents as anemia, hemorrhage, infection, or signs and symptoms related to infiltration of organs. In chronic stages, it presents in an indolent manner with vague symptoms.

PREVALENCE AND INCIDENCE

Prevalence of intraocular leukemia has been studied both clinically and postmortem in various studies. It has been found that postmortem studies quote higher prevalence. Overall prevalence ranges from as low as 28% to as high as 90% in various studies.[1,4-6] Incidence has been noted to be slightly higher in acute leukemias than with chronic leukemias.[1]

CLINICAL MANIFESTATIONS

Only 5–10% patients with leukemia shall present with ocular symptoms while most of the patients would be referred by the physician to the ophthalmologist.[7] The manifestations are more prevalent in cases with myeloid leukemia than with lymphoid leukemia, especially more common in adults than children.[8]

The ocular manifestations of leukemia can be divided into:
- Direct manifestations (leukemic infiltrates)
- Possible direct manifestations (e.g. white-centered retinal hemorrhages) (Figs. 30.2A and B)
- Manifestations of hematological complications of leukemia like:
  - Anemia
  - Thrombocytopenia
  - Hyperviscosity states
- Opportunistic infections
- Manifestations secondary to effects of medical therapy.

It has also been seen that due to low prevalence of ocular complications or direct manifestations in the early stages of leukemia, screening may not be required, also keeping

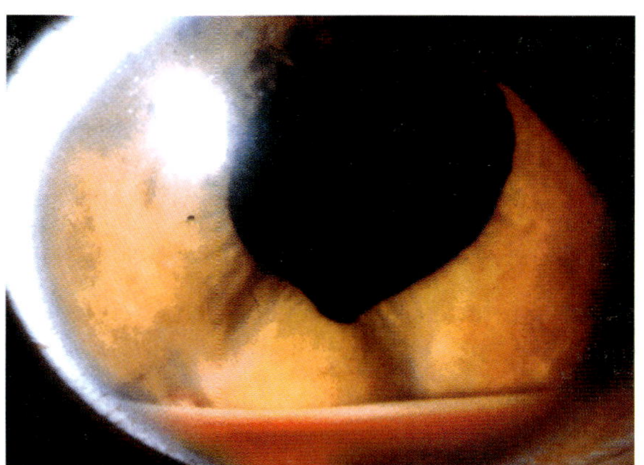

Fig. 30.1: Unusual presentation of leukemia in a child with leukemic infiltrates in anterior chamber hypopyon with hyphema.

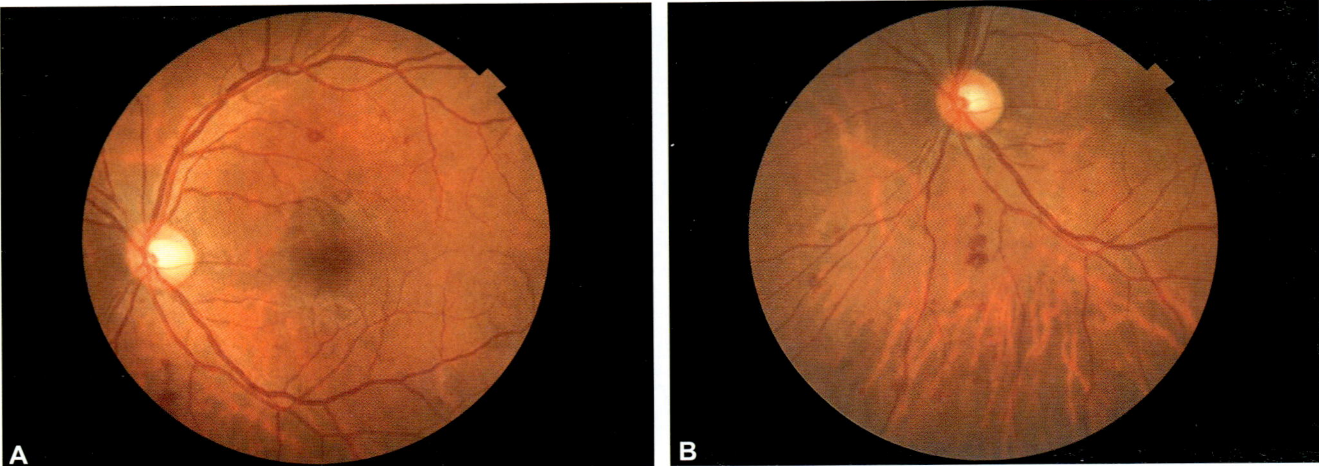

Figs. 30.2A and B: Fundus photograph of a patient with leukemia showing white-centered hemorrhages (Roth spots).

in mind the low requirement of any ocular intervention for treating ocular involvement in leukemia.

Direct Manifestations

Leukemic infiltrates are the direct manifestation due to invasion of neoplastic cells within various layers of the eye. They may be preretinal, retinal, subretinal, or choroidal (Fig. 30.3). Retinal infiltrates can range from small size to large nodules, which may be gray white in color to gray-white streaks along vessels.[9-11] These nodules are usually associated with fulminant disease and increase in size as the disease progresses.[9] Subretinal infiltrates are also seen as whitish deposits, often associated with venous vasculitis. Leukemia may also infiltrate the choroid presenting with subtle signs, unless overlying retina or retinal pigment epithelium (RPE) changes occur like depigmentation. They may be otherwise observed only when they become frank masses or have an associated serous retinal detachment.[12,13] Such patients would have shifting fluid and pinpoint fluorescein hyperfluorescence and dye leakage into the subretinal space on fundus fluorescein angiography (FFA).[14,15] As the fluid or infiltrates resolve, they leave behind coarse RPE clumping resulting in hyperpigmented regions localized to sites of serous detachment seen as black spots, especially seen at the posterior pole.[12,16,17] In worst cases it may give an appearance of *leopard spot fundus*.[12]

Vitreous opacities may range from massive collections of tumor cells in the vitreous in moribund patients to presence of few tumor cells in a patient presenting with vitreous hemorrhage. They may also present as masquerade syndrome and may give an appearance of panuveitis or chronic unilateral uveitis.[18,19] Diagnosis may be confirmed using vitreous aspiration or biopsy. Patients with vitreous infiltration are mostly associated with CNS involvement and have a positive cerebrospinal fluid tap results, especially in the blast phase of the disease.[2]

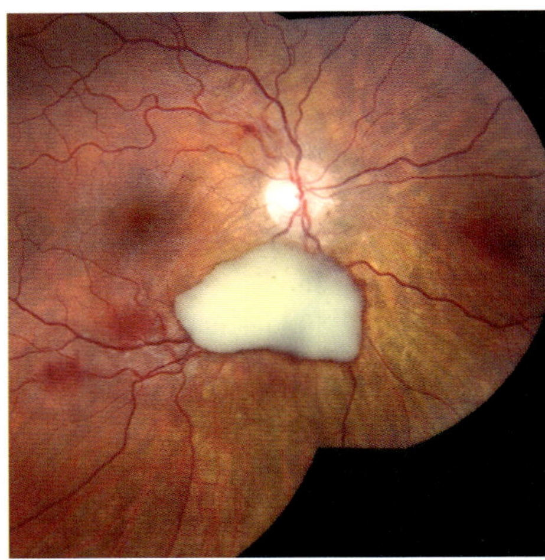

Fig. 30.3: Patient with leukemia manifesting as a single large preretinal infiltrate with multiple flame-shaped hemorrhages. Such large infiltrates are associated with poorer prognosis.

Possible Leukemic Infiltrates

White-centered retinal hemorrhages are classified as suspicious for direct intraocular manifestations of leukemia. It is due to the aggregation of leukocytes or fibrin-platelet complex in the center of white-centered hemorrhages.[20-22] The presence of perivascular infiltrates has also been counted as suspicious and not necessarily may be due to leukemia itself.

Manifestations of Complications of Leukemia—Anemia and Thrombocytopenia

Retinal hemorrhages and cotton-wool spots are the two main manifestations. Vascular tortuosity is not a sign of leukemic retinopathy. Hemorrhages may occur at any level, subretinal, deep retinal, superficial retinal, or preretinal, or even

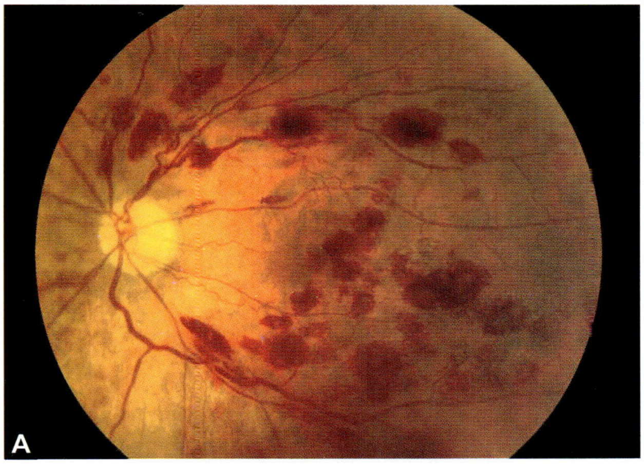

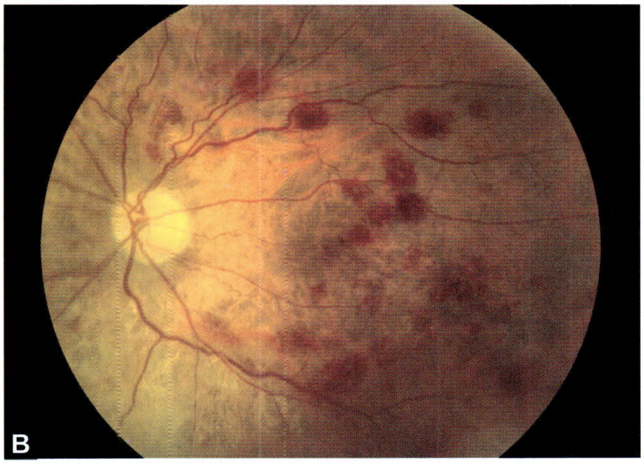

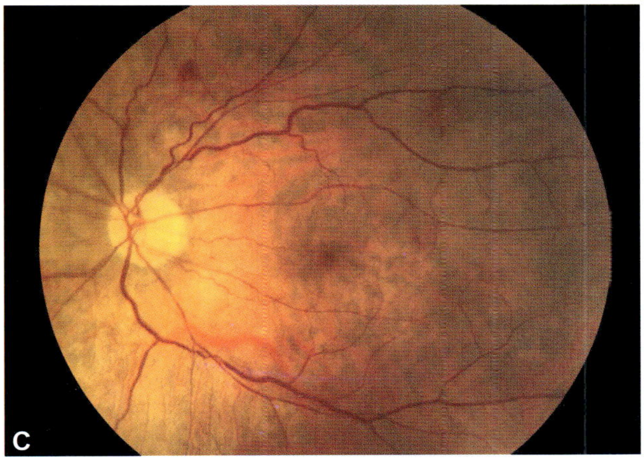

Figs. 30.4A to C: (A) Left eye of leukemic patient with many central and paracentral superficial hemorrhages, some having a white center (Roth spots); (B) Same eye after few days of chemotherapy showing resolution of hemorrhages, note the faster resolution of periphery of hemorrhages than the white center; and (C) Near complete resolution of lesions few weeks after the completion of chemotherapy.

with potential breakthrough bleeding into the vitreous cavity (Figs. 30.4 and 30.5). It is usually seen at the posterior pole.[20] Presence of hemorrhage is more in patients with lower platelet count.[23] Interestingly, it has been noted that leukemic patients presenting with macular hemorrhages are five times more prone to intracranial hemorrhages than those presenting elsewhere or without macular hemorrhages. Therefore, such patients must be closely monitored and platelet transfusions must be given to such patients.[24]

Cotton-wool spots are common and may guide one toward the diagnostic testing in suspected patients.[25] They occur due to nerve fiber layer infarcts caused either due to an abnormally large neoplastic cell or a cluster of cells. They usually do not correlate with the blood cell counts.[26]

Manifestations of Complications of Leukemia—Hyperviscosity

Hyperviscosity results due to the high blood counts, which cause especially, if white blood cell (WBC) counts reach than 50,000 cells/mm^3 and due to increase in coagulability

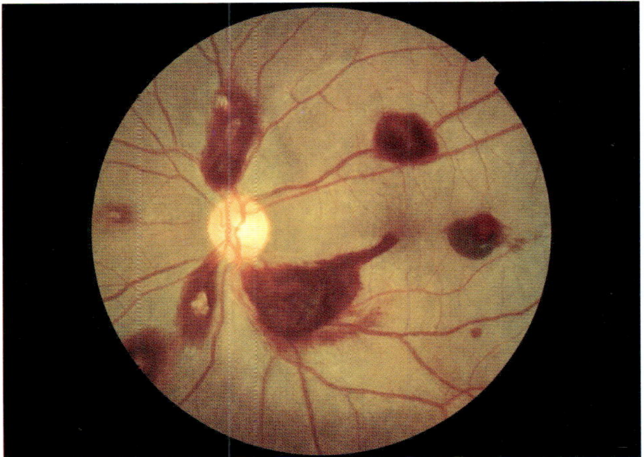

Fig. 30.5: Patient with acute leukemia showing multiple hemorrhages involving various layers of retina, ranging from: a subretinal hemorrhage temporal to macula, with superior and nasal flame-shaped hemorrhages with white centres (Roth spots), to macular subhyaloid hemorrhage.

of blood in patients with leukemia.[27] Microaneurysms are the most common presentation of the same especially in peripheral retina.[28,29] It may also present as veno-occlusive disease resulting in retinal hemorrhages, and retinal neovascularization, but most commonly manifesting as mild, or "hyperpermeable", central retinal vein occlusion.[30-33] It may also present as bilateral disc swelling similar to benign intracranial hypertension.[34] Like with proliferative sickle retinopathy (PSR), the hyperviscosity leads to nonperfusion in the peripheral areas causing retinal neovascularization.

Opportunistic Infections

Opportunistic infections are common in immunosuppressed patients like in leukemia. Cytomegalovirus (CMV) is one of the most common causes of infectious retinitis, while other common infections include herpes virus infection causing necrotizing retinal vasculitis, or progressive outer retinal necrosis (PORN), mumps uveitis, ocular toxoplasmosis, or various fungal infections.[35-39] These infections can present as retinal infiltrates with or without vitritis. A diagnostic vitreous biopsy is required in cases of diagnostic dilemma.[40,41]

MEDICAL THERAPY

Treatment of leukemia entails a cocktail of chemotherapeutic agents administered intravenously. These may lead to severe ocular side effects. Also, ocular radiation may be required which can lead to radiation retinopathy, most commonly presenting as posterior subcapsular cataract.[42] Ischemic retinopathy has also been reported in such patients, especially when they have been given higher doses of chemotherapy.[43,44]

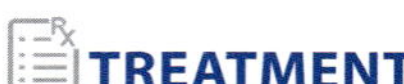 ## TREATMENT

The mainstay of leukemia therapy is systemic chemotherapy.[45,46] Ocular manifestations usually do not require direct treatment. Intrathecal chemotherapy is also done in addition to intravenous therapy for patients who have CNS involvement as well.[47] Cranial irradiation may also be done to support chemotherapy.

Chemotherapeutic agents are not known to penetrate the ocular tissues and ocular radiation may be attempted in patients, where leukemic infiltrates do not resolve.[48] General supportive measures (e.g. blood transfusions) are recommended for patients with severe anemia or thrombocytopenia. Leukapheresis may also be done to treat hyperviscosity.

A therapeutic pars plana vitrectomy (PPV) is rarely indicated in patients having associated nonresolving vitreous hemorrhage. Such patients are usually not medically fit owing to their systemic status and PPV whenever undertaken must be done under strict aseptic precautions.

PROGNOSIS

Patients with leukemic retinopathy have slightly poorer prognosis than those without it. Cotton-wool spots have been found to be associated with decreased patient survival by eight times than without it.[49] Smaller retinal infiltrates indicate worse prognosis and larger nodule-like infiltrates are usually found in moribund patients.

SICKLE CELL RETINOPATHY

 ## INTRODUCTION

Retinopathy associated with systemic disorder of sickle cell disease (SCD), which is a group of hemoglobinopathies characterized by intravascular hemolysis and defective oxygen transport by red blood cells (RBCs). Normal hemoglobin contains two α-globin subunits, two β-globin subunits, and a central heme molecule which together form the hemoglobin A (HbA). A point mutation at the sixth position on chromosome 11, leads to replacement of glutamic acid by a valine in the β-globin subunit of hemoglobin leading to abnormal hemoglobin (HbS). This leads to formation of peculiar, elongated sickle-shaped RBCs, hallmark of SCD.[50,51]

The gene transmission of SCD is autosomal recessive and therefore, one need two genes for the disease to be expressed. When both the genes are sickle cell variant the disease is denoted as SS disease. When one gene has an HbC variant the disease still manifests and is known as SC disease. This is a less severe form of the disease. When one gene is normal, the disease does not manifest and the person is known to be only carrier (SC trait). It may also be associated with β-thalassemia gene.[51]

PREVALENCE

Sickle cell disease is commonly seen in African American and Hispanic populations, approximately affecting 0.15% of the population while SC trait is seen to occur in approximately 8% of black Americans.[51,52] It is also observed in people of Mediterranean, Caribbean, South and Central American, Arab, and East Indian descent.

Patients with SS disease become symptomatic in infancy, presenting with recurrent infections and severe anemia.[53] These patients present less commonly with ocular features of SCD. Patients with SC disease have less severe systemic features though the ocular complications are more pronounced as they may have a normal life expectancy. Sickle cell trait patients may show few symptoms only in extremely hypoxic conditions.

 ### PATHOPHYSIOLOGY

Due to the genetic mutation and replacement of the polar hydrophilic amino acid glutamic acid with nonpolar hydrophobic valine, there occurs an increased tendency of the hemoglobin molecule to show polymerization and sickling of erythrocytes in conditions of hypoxia, acidosis, and dehydration. This process reverses with oxygenation of RBCs, and due to repeated cycles of oxygenation and deoxygenation, there occurs permanent sickling of the RBCs. An RBC which has undergone sickling loses the ability to conform to the shape of the vessel and leads to slowing of blood flow in capillaries. This can cause occlusion of the vessels, leading to a vaso-occlusive episode.[54] Sickling also promotes adhesion of erythrocytes to the vascular endothelium and leads to early hemolysis as well as damage to the endothelium.[55,56]

As endothelium is damaged, there is an increase in inflammatory mediators as well as a decrease in the levels of nitric oxide (NO) due to damage of NO synthase by reactive oxygen species.[57,58] This aggravates the vascular occlusion and leads to further tissue ischemia. Tissue hypoxia is therefore, a constant consequence. Due to this there is increased levels of vascular endothelial growth factor (VEGF) levels, which are found to be elevated at baseline and more so during hypoxic conditions within the serum as well as in the eyes of such patients.[59-61]

SYSTEMIC MANIFESTATIONS

Sickle cell disease affects almost all the organs of the body, from cerebrovascular accidents to painful limb as a result of vaso-occlusive crises or even death.[51] It may also lead to severe visual impairment. Systemic manifestations are more and severe with patients with SS disease than with SC disease, although the prevalence of ocular complications are more with SC disease, with as high as 33% while in SS disease is 3%.[62]

This may be attributed to shorter life span of SS disease patients, or due to the difference in hematocrit levels and lower Fetal hemoglobin (Hb F) levels. It is also proposed that patients with HbSC experience chronic hypoxia compared to HbSS patients who experience acute and anoxic conditions. This would lead to constant high levels of VEGF levels.[63,64] RBCs with HbSC retain a certain amount of flexibility and cause slower vaso-occlusion compared to the more rigid HbSS RBCs that block capillaries more commonly.[65,66]

OPHTHALMIC MANIFESTATIONS

Sickle cell may disease may affect the orbit, retina, optic nerve and other ocular structures and therefore has a variety of clinical manifestations presenting to an ophthalmologist. Vision-threatening manifestations are commonly due to retinal involvement and must be screened for in all cases.

Retrobulbar and Orbital Involvement

Orbital bone infarctions as well as orbital hematomas have been reported[67] which can lead to periorbital swelling, proptosis, restricted movements and diplopia, ultimately causing vision loss as a result of orbital compression.[68] Management is mainly conservative with antibiotic and steroid therapy, while in certain cases immediate orbital decompression may be helpful. Recurrent bilateral lacrimal gland swelling has also been reported.[69]

Anterior Segment Involvement

Conjunctiva is commonly involved with *Paton's "conjunctival sign"*, which is comma shaped or corkscrew saccular dilation of tiny conjunctival vessels.[70,71] Usually seen in inferior bulbar conjunctiva, these vessels are better seen after pharmacologically inducing vasoconstriction of normal conjunctival vessels.[72,73] The vaso-occlusive crisis causes decreased flow with vasoconstriction in these abnormal capillaries, especially seen in HbSS patients. Histopathology reports show aggregated RBCs in the distal end while dilated thinned-out proximal end with endothelial proliferation.[73]

Radial iris vessels catering to specific iris sectors have been observed to undergo ischemia. This leads to segmental iris atrophy and later neovascularization of ischemic iris stroma.[52,74-76] Rarely it may lead to neovascular glaucoma. Pupil shows sectoral changes associated with concerned iris sector.

Hyphema in SCD or sickle-cell trait patients is an ocular emergency. It can lead to increased intraocular pressures (IOPs) due to mechanical blockade of trabecular meshwork by rigid sickle cells. Even modest rise of IOP can cause central retinal artery occlusion (CRAO) or macular branch retinal artery occlusion (BRAO) and result in severe visual loss.[52,77-79] Therefore, lower IOP target must be aimed using multiple antiglaucoma medications, with caution against carbonic anhydrase inhibitors which cause systemic acidosis leading to worsening of sickling. Such patients therefore need early surgical intervention for IOP control, even at IOP of 25 mm Hg, either by paracentesis or an AC wash.[80] Role of intracameral tissue plasminogen activator (tPA) and hyperoxygenation has also been reported.[81]

Posterior Segment Involvement

Optic Nerve

Precapillary arteriolar plugging with sickled RBCs is seen at optic nerve head as small red dots, having a Y-shaped configuration. These changes are transient and not visually significant.[82,83] Rarely, optic disc neovascularization may be seen.[84-87]

NONPROLIFERATIVE SICKLE RETINOPATHY

Retinal Vasculature

In most patients, the retinal vessels may initially appear normal to increase in tortuosity, especially when affected by HbSS disease, and is thought to occur by peripheral arteriovenous (AV) anastomosis.[82,88,89] Temporal retinal vessels are narrower in the periphery and are susceptible to arterial occlusions. These occur due to sickled RBCs or due to thrombi formation after vessel wall injury.[90,91] Another abnormality observed is the AV anastomosis formation. Arterioles may appear with "silver wiring" after occlusion. These lead to peripheral retinal ischemia.

In rare cases, choroidal infarction may also be seen, occurring due to posterior ciliary artery obstruction by either impacted RBCs or thrombus formation.[92,93] Choroidal neovascularization has also been reported, spontaneously or especially after high-energy laser burns.[94,95]

Salmon-patch Hemorrhages

Salmon patch lesions are red orange to pinkish preretinal or superficial retinal hemorrhages found near the equator (Fig. 30.6). It is located between the retina and internal limiting membrane and usually resolves spontaneously without a sequelae (Fig. 30.7). These are hypothesized to arise as a result of sudden "giving way" of an occluded vessel.[96,97]

Black Sunburst

Black sunbursts are patches of RPE hypertrophy appearing clinically as flat, round areas of hyperpigmentation. It is hypothesized to occur due to localized choroidal ischemic damage of RPE, localized subretinal choroidal neovascular membrane (CNVM), or subretinal tracking of retinal hemorrhage.[98-102]

Iridescent spots may be observed when intraretinal hemorrhage clears leaving behind hemosiderin-laden macrophages in between retinal layers, appearing as glistening, refractile spots.

Vitreoretinal Interface

Most common retinal finding in sickle cell patients is peripheral retinal whitening, associated with strong vitreoretinal adhesion.[82,89,101] It appears similar to "white without pressure" areas as seen in the normal population and usually is of no pathological significance. "Dark without pressure" areas, which are brown ovoid transient lesions in the retinal periphery has also been described. These lesions are flat and show

no sequelae on disappearing. FFA and choroid are normal.[102] Only the pathologic retinal neovascularization causing vitreous hemorrhage results in sight loss.[103,104]

Macula

Macula is also affected by the ischemic pathology of the disease. Macular ischemia leads to enlarged foveal avascular zone (FAZ) and thinning of fovea especially in the outer retinal layers as seen on spectral domain optical coherence tomography (SD-OCT).[105-108] This is clinically evident, especially with red-free illumination, as dull foveal and parafoveal reflex seen as a depression in macula and hence named as "macular depression sign". Infarction of macula with associated visual loss has been reported though change in size of FAZ is not directly correlated with visual loss.[109,110] Even in asymptomatic patients with SCD, there can be areas of focal parafoveal thinning which can cause "splaying" or blunting of foveal contour. Rare complications include macular hole, epiretinal membrane (ERM) formation, foveoschisis, neovascularization at posterior pole, etc.[105-108]

Angioid streaks are found in around 1–2% of SCD patients, especially in HbSS disease patients. It is seen to increase as patient ages and is thought to occur due to hypoxic damage to the elastic Bruch's membrane.[111-115] Rarely CNVM may develop.[52]

PROLIFERATIVE SICKLE RETINOPATHY

As the disease progresses, the peripheral retinal ischemia causes the formation of abnormal new vessels, appearing as fronds in a typical shape of a sea fan. The appearance is typically of a network of vessels with an apex toward one larger vessel, having multiple side branches and branching intervening network of smaller vessels. The appearance is same as of the marine organism sea fan, or *Gorgonia flabellum*.

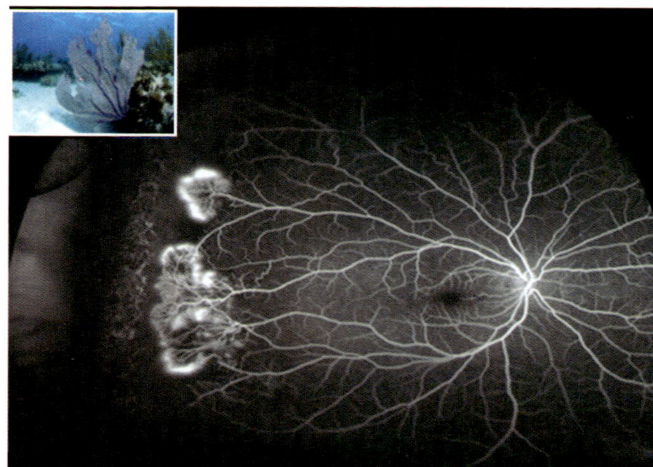

Fig. 30.6: Pinkish-red colored preretinal salmon-patch hemorrhage in a patient with nonproliferative sickle cell disease.

Fig. 30.7: Ultrawide field fundus fluorescein angiography showing sea fan neovascularization in a patient with sickle cell anemia. (Inset: Typical sea fan).

Once a sea fan neovascularization forms, it may lead to vitreous hemorrhage, or later tractional retinal detachment (TRD) formation. In certain rarer cases, combined TRD may form. This proliferative sickle cell retinopathy (SCR) may be classified into five stages (Goldberg, 1971):[116]

1. *Stage I*—Peripheral vascular occlusion with silver wiring of the arterioles, seen mostly in temporal retina.
2. *Stage II*—Arteriovenous anastomosis formation, occurring at border of perfused-nonperfused retina. It is non-leaking complex.
3. *Stage III*—Sea fan neovascularization formation, which is most common at superotemporal peripheral retina. Sea fan fronds are the hallmark of stage III PSR, and shows diffuse leakage on FFA. Chronic transudation causes vitreous degeneration and further lead to tractional component. Sea fan fronds are more commonly seen to occur from the venous component, although each complex contains a feeding artery and a draining venule.
4. *Stage IV*—Vitreous hemorrhage, without or with sudden loss, painless sight loss. It may either be localized over the site of neovascularization. It is more common with HbSC disease.[82,117] Recurrence is common with 2 or more clock hours of vitreous hemorrhage or in patients presenting with vitreous hemorrhage.[118] Chronic vitreous hemorrhage may give rise to fibroglial membranes and vitreous strands may form in cases of chronic vitreous hemorrhage which can cause TRD.[72,119]
5. *Stage V*—Presence of TRD defines Goldberg stage V. TRD is mainly in peripheral retina and less commonly needs early intervention. Chronic ischemic retinal degeneration may cause round holes or HSTs. Combined TRD and rhegmatogenous retinal detachment may also occur (Fig. 30.8).

Hemoglobin SC disease patients manifest proliferative disease more commonly than other genotypes. Also HbS-β thalassemia is more prone to developing proliferative SCD.

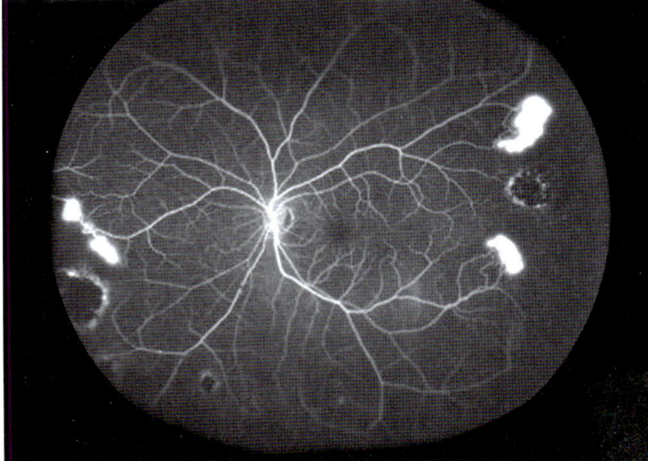

Fig. 30.8: Fluorescein angiography showing a case of proliferative sickle retinopathy with peripheral avascular zones and multiple areas of leakage indicating the presence of neovascularization.

Usually it presents by 2nd–3rd decades in men and a decade later in women. The risk of developing proliferative disease increases if there is presence of hairpin loop, high hemoglobin levels, higher mean corpuscular hemoglobin concentration (MCHC) levels, or lower HbF levels, especially in males.[120]

NATURAL HISTORY

As the disease progresses, there is a high likelihood that one-third of patients with proliferative retinopathy shall undergo spontaneous regression.[121] It is expected to occur due to occlusion of the neovascular frond. In those that do not regress develop either vitreous hemorrhage, or TRD or an ERM.[122] Patients with nonproliferative disease usually do not progress or lead to vision loss, even after a period of 10 years compared to proliferative disease.[123]

IMAGING

An ultrasonography is a must in eyes presenting with nonresolving vitreous hemorrhage. It helps to monitor the progression and rule out any TRD or choroidal detachment. The latest imaging modalities, such as ultrawide field angiography is particularly useful in early cases suspected of proliferative SCD. It helps to assess the peripheral retina for ischemic changes and record areas of neovascularization. It helps to guide in a targeted laser treatment of the patient and also to monitor the response. Conventional FFA has a limited field of evaluation and poorly assess peripheral retina.[123] Role of indocyanine green (ICG) angiography is still untapped and unclear, though it is expected to bring forward the impaired choroidal circulation abnormalities.[124]

Macular involvement has been redefined after the OCT and especially SD-OCT, with its high resolution, which provides important details about foveal anatomy. Thinning of fovea and loss of outer retinal layers have been reported and may confer poorer overall prognosis to the patent.[105-108,111]

OPHTHALMIC TREATMENTS

Normally, no ocular intervention is needed in early stages of the disease. Asymptomatic patients with peripheral nonproliferative lesions are best observed at intervals of 3–6 months, as these shall develop autoinfarctions and rarely progress further.[125,126] Proliferative disease patients may also be only observed initially as one-third may regress with autoinfarction. Only those patients that develop significant visual loss or have a disease in the contralateral eye due to proliferative disease need therapy. In cases of bilateral proliferative disease, presence of large, elevated sea fans, spontaneous hemorrhage, and rapid growth of a sea fan treatment may be needed.[100] The goal of treatment is to prevent or treat complications like vitreous hemorrhage and TRD in such eyes.

Various techniques were applied in the past for regression of sea fan neovascularization. Namely, laser photocoagulation, diathermy, or cryotherapy of the feeder vessels were attempted but were associated with higher rate of complications, such as bleeding from the vessels, retinal break formation, or development of CNVM from Bruch's membrane tear.[125,126] Currently, targeted laser therapy of the ischemic diseased areas is the mainstay of the treatment and works on the same principle of destruction of diseased retina to decrease the mediators of neovascularization and decrease the oxygen demand in the retinal tissue, and shunting oxygen supply to the healthy retinal tissue.

Complete regression of retinal neovascularization and resolution of vitreous hemorrhage has been reported following intravitreal injection of anti-VEGF agents in eyes with PSR.[127,128] No well-studied data is available and further data is needed before anti-VEGFs must be used for treatment.

For patients with vitreous hemorrhage, an ultrasonography is must to rule out associated retinal detachment. When not associated with RD, observation may be done for hemorrhage to clear up. When nonresolving, the vitrectomy may be combined with endolaser photocoagulation and a preoperative anti-VEGF injection to decrease the amount of new vessels. Such patients are prone to intraoperative anterior segment ischemia. Therefore, precaution must be taken to maintain adequate oxygenation throughout the procedure. To minimize complications from surgically-induced anterior segment ischemia presence of large, elevated sea fans, spontaneous hemorrhage have been tried.[109]

The pathological retinal tissue is friable and peeling or delamination from its surface often leads to iatrogenic retinal tear formation. Therefore, an approach toward segmentation is preferable during vitrectomy. Scleral buckling may be used with caution to counter the anterior traction on the retina, with the risk of anterior segment ischemia.[110,129]

SYSTEMIC THERAPY

Various medications to improve the overall systemic circulation and increase the oxygen carrying capacity of blood have been tried. Agents like hydroxyurea reduce inflammation and the overall load of inflammatory mediators, arginine increases NO levels in blood and leads to vasodilation decreasing the risk of occlusion. It has also been observed that agents that increase HbF levels help reduce the adverse events of SCD as it interferes with HbS polymerization, including agents like hydroxyurea, omega-3 fatty acids, and erythropoietin. Blood transfusion and hemapheresis attempt at reducing HbS levels in systemic circulation but are of temporary use. Hematopoietic stem cell transplantation is a more permanent solution but is still under investigation.[51]

REFERENCES

1. Kincaid MC, Green WR. Ocular and orbital involvement in leukemia. Surv Ophthalmology. 1983;27:211-32.
2. Swartz M, Schumann B. Acute leukemic infiltration of the vitreous diagnosed by pars plana aspiration. Am J Ophthalmology. 1980;90: 326-30.
3. Allen RA, Straatsma BR. Ocular involvement in leukemia and allied disorders. Arch Ophthalmology. 1961;66:490-508.
4. Schachat AP, Markowitz JA, Guyer DR, et al. Ophthalmic manifestations of leukemia. Arch Ophthalmology. 1989;107:697-700.
5. Nelson CC, Hertzberg BS, Klintworth GK. A histopathologic study of 716 selected eyes in patients with cancer at the time of death. Am J Ophthalmology. 1983;95:788-93.
6. Karesh JW, Goldman EJ, Reck K, et al. A prospective ophthalmic evaluation of patients with acute myeloid leukemia: correlation of ocular and hematologic findings. J Clin Oncol. 1989;7:1528-32.
7. Reddy SC, Menon BS. A prospective study of ocular manifestations in childhood acute leukemia. Acta Ophthalmology Scand. 1998;76: 700-3.
8. Reddy SC, Jackson N, Menon BS. Ocular involvement in leukemia—a study of 288 cases. Ophthalmologica. 2003;217:441-5.
9. Kuwabara T, Aiello L. Leukemic miliary nodules in the retina. Arch Ophthalmology. 1964;72:494-7.
10. Robb RM, Ervin LD, Sallan SE. A pathological study of eye involvement in acute leukemia of childhood. Trans Am Ophthalmology Soc. 1978;76:90-101.
11. Merle H, Donnio A, Gonin C, et al. Retinal vasculitis caused by adult T-cell leukemia/lymphoma. Jpn J Ophthalmology. 2005;49:41-5.
12. Clayman HM, Flynn JT, Koch K, et al. Retinal pigment epithelial abnormalities in leukemic disease. Am J Ophthalmology. 1972;74: 416-9.
13. Rosenthal AR. Ocular manifestations of leukemia: a review. Ophthalmology. 1983;90:899-905.
14. Kincaid MC, Green WR, Kelley JS. Acute ocular leukemia. Am J Ophthalmology. 1979;87:698-702.
15. Gass JD. Stereoscopic Atlas of Macular Diseases: Diagnosis and Treatment, 4th edition. St Louis: Mosby; 1997.
16. Tang RA, Vila-Coro AA, Wall S, et al. Acute leukemia presenting as a retinal pigment epithelium detachment. Arch Ophthalmology. 1988;106:21-2.
17. Jakobiec F, Behrens M. Leukemic retinal pigment epitheliopathy with report of a unilateral case. J Pediatr Ophthalmology. 1975;12:10-5.
18. Dhar-Munshi S, Alton P, Ayliffe WH. Masquerade syndrome: T-cell prolymphocytic leukemia presenting as panuveitis. Am J Ophthalmology. 2001;132:275-7.
19. Belmont JB, Michelson JB, Bordin GM. Ocular inflammation associated with chronic lymphocytic leukemia. J Ocul Ther Surg. 1985;4:125-9.
20. Duane TD, Osher RH, Green WR. White centered hemorrhages: their significance. Ophthalmology. 1980;87:66-9.
21. Holt JM, Gordon-Smith EL. Retinal abnormalities in diseases of the blood. Br J Ophthalmology. 1969;53:145-60.
22. Phelps CD. The association of pale-centered retinal hemorrhages with intracranial bleeding in infancy. Am J Ophthalmology. 1971;73:348-50.
23. Melberg NS, Grand MG, Rup D. The impact of acute lymphocytic leukemia on diabetic retinopathy. J Pediatr Hematol Oncol. 1995;17:81-4.
24. Jackson N, Reddy SC, Harun MH, et al. Macular haemorrhage in adult acute leukaemia patients at presentation and the risk of subsequent intracranial haemorrhage. Br J Haematol. 1997;98: 204-9.
25. Brown GC, Brown MM, Hiller T, et al. Cotton wool spots. Retina. 1985;5:206-14.
26. Bishop JE, Salmonsen PC. Presumed intraocular Hodgkin's disease. Ann Ophthalmology. 1985;17:589-92.

27. Stephens DJ. Relation of viscosity of blood to leukocyte count with particular reference to chronic myelogenous leukemia. Proc Soc Exp Biol Med. 1936;35:251-6.

28. Duke JR, Wilkinson CP, Sigelman S. Retinal microaneurysms in leukemia. Br J Ophthalmology. 1968;52:368-74.

29. Jampol LM, Goldberg MF, Busse B. Peripheral microaneurysms in chronic leukemia. Am J Ophthalmology. 1975;80:242-8.

30. Frank RN, Ryan SJ. Peripheral retinal neovascularization with chronic myelogenous leukemia. Arch Ophthalmology. 1972;87:585-9.

31. Levielle AS, Morse PH. Platelet-induced retinal neovascularization in leukemia. Am J Ophthalmology. 1981;91:640-3.

32. Little HL. The role of abnormal hemorrheodynamics in the pathogenesis of diabetic retinopathy. Trans Am Ophthalmology Soc. 1976;74:573-636.

33. Morse PH, McCready JL. Peripheral retinal neovascularization in chronic myelocytic leukemia. Am J Ophthalmology. 1971;72:975-8.

34. Guymer RH, Cairns JD, O'Day J. Benign intracranial hypertension in chronic myeloid leukemia. Aust NZJ Ophthalmology. 1993;21:181-5.

35. Levy-Clarke GA, Buggage RR, Shen D, et al. Human T-cell lymphocytic virus type-1 associated T-cell leukemia/lymphoma masquerading as necrotizing retinal vasculitis. Ophthalmology. 2002;109:1717-22.

36. Brody JM, Butrus SI, Ashraf MF, et al. Multiple myeloma presenting with bilateral exudative macular detachments. Acta Ophthalmology Scand. 1995;73:81-2.

37. Al-Rashid RA, Cress C. Mumps uveitis complicating the course of acute leukemia. J Pediatr Ophthalmology. 1977;14:100-2.

38. Lewis JM, Nagae Y, Tano Y. Progressive outer retinal necrosis after bone marrow transplantation. Am J Ophthalmology. 1996;122:892-5.

39. Phillips WB, Shields CL, Shields JA, et al. Nocardia choroidal abscess. Br J Ophthalmology. 1992;76:694-6.

40. Gordon KB, Rugo HS, Duncan JL, et al. Ocular manifestations of leukemia: leukemic infiltration versus infectious process. Ophthalmology. 2001:108:2293-300.

41. Palkovacs EM, Correa Z, Ausburger JJ, et al. Acquired toxoplasmic retinitis in an immunosuppressed patient: diagnosis by transvitreal fine-needle aspiration biopsy. Graefes Arch Clin Exp Ophthalmology. 2008;246:1495-7.

42. Hoover DL, Smith LE, Turner SJ, et al. Ophthalmic evaluation of survivors of acute lymphoblastic leukemia. Ophthalmology. 1988;95:151-5.

43. Lopez PF, Sternberg F, Dabbs CK, et al. Bone marrow transplant retinopathy. Am J Ophthalmology. 1991;112:635-46.

44. Webster AR, Anderson JR, Richards EM, et al. Ischemic retinopathy occurring in patients receiving bone marrow allografts and Campath-1G: a clinicopathological study. Br J Ophthalmology. 1995;79:687-91.

45. Jabbour E, Branford S, Saglio G, et al. Practical advice for determining the role of BCR-ABL mutations in guiding tyrosine kinase inhibitor therapy in patients with chronic myeloid leukemia. Cancer. 2011;117:1800-811.

46. Pollyea DA, Kohrt HE, Medeiros BC. Acute myeloid leukaemia in the elderly: a review. Br J Haematol. 2011;152:524-42.

47. Pui CH. Recent research advances in childhood acute lymphoblastic leukemia. J Formos Med Assoc. 2010;109:777-87.

48. Ellis W, Little HL. Leukemic infiltration of the optic nerve head. Am J Ophthalmology. 1983;75:867-71.

49. Abu el-Asrar AM, al-Momen AK, Kangave D, et al. Prognostic importance of retinopathy in acute leukemia. Doc Ophthalmology. 1996;91:273-81.

50. Ashley-Koch A, Yang Q, Olney RS. Sickle hemoglobin (HbS) allele and sickle cell disease: a HuGE review. Am J Epidemiol. 2000;151:839-45.

51. Elagouz M, Jyothi S, Gupta B, et al. Sickle cell disease and the eye: old and new concepts. Surv Ophthalmology. 2010;55:359-77.

52. Emerson GG, Harlan JB, Fekrat S, et al. Hemoglobinopathies. In: Ryan SJ (Ed). Retina, 4th edition. Edinburgh: Elsevier; 2006. pp. 1429-45.

53. Gill FM, Sleeper LA, Weiner SJ, et al. Clinical events in the first decade in a cohort of infants with sickle cell disease: cooperative study of sickle cell disease. Blood. 1995;86:776-83.

54. Bunn HF. Pathogenesis and treatment of sickle cell disease. N Engl J Med. 1997;337:762-9.

55. Fabry ME, Kaul DK. Sickle cell vaso-occlusion. Hematol/Oncol Clin North Am. 1991;5:375-98.

56. Hebbel RF. Adhesive interactions of sickle erythrocytes with endothelium. J Clin Invest. 1997;100:S83-6.

57. Vichinsky E. New therapies in sickle cell disease. Lancet. 2002;360:629-31.

58. Wood KC, Hsu LL, Gladwin MT. Sickle cell disease vasculopathy: a state of nitric oxide resistance. Free Radic Biol Med. 2008;44:1506-28.

59. Gurkan E, Tanriverdi K, Baslamish F. Clinical relevance of vascular endothelial growth factor levels in sickle cell disease. Ann Hematol. 2005;84:71-5.

60. Cao J, Kunz Mathews MK, McLeod DS, et al. Angiogenic factors in human proliferative sickle cell retinopathy. Br J Ophthalmology. 1999;83:838-46.

61. Kim EY, Mocanu V, McLeod DS, et al. Expression of pigment epithelium derived factor (PEDF) and vascular endothelial growth factor (VEGF) in sickle cell retina and choroid. Exp Eye Res. 2003;7:433-45.

62. Lutty GA, Goldberg MF. Ophthalmological complications. In: Embury SH, Hebbel RP, Mohandas N (Eds). Sickle Cell Disease: Basic Principles and Clinical Practice. New York: Raven Press; 1992. pp. 703-24.

63. Ballas SK, Lewis CN, Noone AM, et al. Clinical, hematological, and biochemical features of Hb SC disease. Am J Hematol. 1982;13:37-51.

64. Pauling L, Itano HA, Singer SJ, et al. Sickle cell anemia: a molecular disease. Science. 1949;110:543-8.

65. Powars D, Hiti A. Sickle cell anemia. Beta s gene cluster haplotypes as genetic markers for severe disease expression. Am J Dis Child. 1993;147:1197-202.

66. Lutty GA, Phelan A, Mcleod DS, et al. A rat model for sickle-cell mediated vaso-occlusion in retina. Microvasc Res. 1996;52:270-80.

67. Ganesh A, William RR, Mitra S, et al. Orbital involvement in sickle cell disease: a report of 5 cases and review literature. Eye. 2001;15:774-80.

68. Perlman JI, Forman S, Gonzalez ER. Retrobulbar ischemic optic neuropathy associated with sickle cell disease. J Neuro Ophthalmology. 1994;14:45-8.

69. Adewoye AH Ramsey J, McMahon L, et al. Lacrimal gland enlargement in sickle cell disease. Am J Hematol. 2006;81:888-9.

70. Condon PI, Sergeant GR. Ocular findings in elderly cases of homozygous sickle cell disease in Jamaica. Br J Ophthalmology. 1976;60:361-4.

71. Paton D. The conjunctival sign of sickle cell disease. Arch Ophthalmology. 1961;66:90-4.

72. Nagpal KC, Goldberg MF, Rabb MF. Ocular manifestations of sickle hemoglobinopathies. Surv Ophthalmology. 1977;21:391-411.

73. Funahashi T, Fink A, Robinson M, et al. Pathology of conjunctival vessels in sickle-cell disease: a preliminary report. Am J Ophthalmology. 1964;57:713-8.

74. Chambers J, Puglisi J, Kernitsky R, et al. Iris atrophy in hemoglobin SC disease. Am J Ophthalmology. 1974;77:247-9.

75. Galinos S, Rabb MF, Goldberg MF, et al. Hemoglobin SC disease and iris atrophy. Am J Ophthalmology. 1973;75:421-5.

76. Bergren RL, Brown GC. Neovascular glaucoma secondary to sickle cell retinopathy. Am J Ophthalmology. 1992;113:718-9.

77. Goldberg MF. The diagnosis and treatment of secondary glaucoma after hyphema in sickle cell patients. Am J Ophthalmology. 1979;87:43-9.

78. Goldberg MF. Sickled erythrocytes, hyphema, and secondary glaucoma: IV. The rate and percentage of sickling of erythrocytes in rabbit aqueous humor, in vitro and in vivo. Ophthalmic Surg. 1979;10:62-9.

79. Goldberg MF. Sickled erythrocytes, hyphema, and secondary glaucoma: I. The diagnosis and treatment of sickled erythrocytes in human hyphemas. Ophthalmic Surg. 1979;10:17-31.

80. Goldberg MF, Dizon R, Raichand M. Sickled erythrocytes, hyphema, and secondary glaucoma: II. Injected sickle cell erythrocytes into human, monkey, and guinea pig anterior chambers: the introduction of sickling and secondary glaucoma. Ophthalmic Surg. 1979;10:32-51.

81. Karaman K, Culić S, Erceg I, et al. Treatment of post-traumatic trabecular meshwork thrombosis and secondary glaucoma with intracameral tissue plasminogen activator in previously unrecognized sickle cell anemia. Coll Antropol. 2005;29:123-6.

82. Condon PI, Serjeant GR. Ocular findings in homozygous sickle cell anemia in Jamaica. Am J Ophthalmology. 1972;73:533-43.

83. Goldberg MF. Retinal vaso-occlusion in sickling hemo-globinopathies. Birth Defects Orig Artic Ser. 1976;12:475-515.

84. Condon PI, Serjeant GR. Behaviour of untreated proliferative sickle retinopathy. Br J Ophthalmology. 1980;64:404-11.

85. Kimmel AS, Magargal LE, Tasman WS. Proliferative sickle retinopathy and neovascularization at the disc: regression following treatment with peripheral scatter laser photocoagulation. Ophthalmic Surg. 1986;17:20-2.

86. Ober RR, Michels RG. Optic disk neovascularization in hemoglobin SC disease. Am J Ophthalmology. 1978;85:711-4.

87. Raichand M, Goldberg MF, Nagpal KC, et al. Evolution of neovascularization in sickle cell retinopathy. A prospective fluorescein angiographic study. Arch Ophthalmology. 1977;95:1543-52.

88. Welch RB, Goldberg MF. Sickle-cell hemoglobin and its relation to fundus abnormality. Arch Ophthalmology. 1966;75:353-62.

89. Condon PI, Serjeant GR. Ocular findings in hemoglobin SC disease in Jamaica. Am J Ophthalmology. 1972;74:921-31.

90. Savitt TL. Tracking down the first recorded sickle cell patient in Western medicine. J Natl Med Assoc. 2010;102:981-92.

91. Fine LC, Petrovic V, Irvine AR, et al. Spontaneous central retinal artery occlusion in hemoglobin SC disease. Am J Ophthalmology. 2000;130:680-1.

92. Lutty GA, Merges C, Crone S, et al. Immunohistochemical insights into sickle cell retinopathy. Curr Eye Res. 1994;13:1251-38.

93. McLeod DS, Goldberg MF, Lutty GA. Dual-perspective analysis of vascular formations in sickle cell retinopathy. Arch Ophthalmology. 1993;111:1234-45.

94. Liang JC, Jampol LM. Spontaneous peripheral chorioretinal neovascularization in association with sickle cell anemia. Br J Ophthalmology. 1983;67:107-10.

95. Condon PI, Jampol LM, Ford SM, et al. Choroidal neovascularization induced by photocoagulation in sickle cell disease. Br J Ophthalmology. 1981;65:192-7.

96. Romayananda N, Goldberg MF, Green WR. Histopathology of sickle cell retinopathy. Trans Am Acad Opthalmol Otol. 1973;77:652-76.

97. Gagliano DA, Goldberg MF. The evolution of salmon-patch hemorrhages in sickle cell retinopathy. Arch Ophthalmology. 1989;107:1814-5.

98. Serjeant GR, Serjeant BE. The eyes. In: Serjeant GR, Serjeant BE (Eds). Sickle cell disease, 3rd edition. Oxford: Oxford University Press; 2001. pp. 366-92.

99. Emerson GG, Lutty GA. Effects of sickle cell disease on the eye: clinical features and treatment. Hematol Oncol Clin North Am. 2005;19:957-63.

100. Lutty GA, McLeod DS, Pachinis A, et al. Retinal and choroidal neovascularization in a transgenic mouse model of sickle cell disease. Am J Pathol. 1994;145:490-7.

101. Condon PI, Serjeant GR. Ocular findings in sickle cell thalassemia in Jamaica. Am J Ophthalmology. 1972;74:1105-9.

102. Nagpal KC, Goldberg MF, Asdourian G, et al. Dark-without-pressure fundus lesions. Br J Ophthalmology. 1975;59:476-9.

103. Henry MD, Chapman AZ. Vitreous hemorrhage and retinopathy associated with sickle cell disease. Am J Ophthalmology. 1954;38:204-9.

104. Hannon JF. Vitreous hemorrhages associated with sickle cell-hemoglobin C disease. Am J Ophthalmology. 1956;42:707-12.

105. Goldbaum MH. Retinal depression sign indicating a small retinal infarct. Am J Ophthalmology. 1978;86:45-55.

106. Sanders RJ, Brown GC, Rosenstein RB, et al. Foveal avascular zone diameter and sickle cell disease. Arch Ophthalmology. 1991;109:812-5.

107. Witkin AJ, Rogers AH, Ko TH, et al. Optical coherence tomography demonstration of macular infarction in sickle cell retinopathy. Arch Ophthalmology. 2006;124:746-7.

108. Hoang QV, Chau FY, Shahidi M, et al. Central macular splaying and outer retinal thinning in asymptomatic sickle cell patients by spectral-domain optical coherence tomography. Am J Ophthalmology. 2011;151:990-4.

109. Bove JR. Transfusion-transmitted diseases: current problems and challenges. Prog Hematol. 1986;14:123-47.

110. Williamson TH, Rajput R, Laidlaw DA, et al. Vitreoretinal management of the complications of sickle cell retinopathy by observation or pars plana vitrectomy. Eye. 2009;23:1314-20.

111. Murthy RK, Grover S, Chalam K. Temporal macular thinning on spectral domain optical coherence tomography in proliferative sickle cell retinopathy. Arch Ophthalmology. 2011;129:247-9.

112. Raichland M, Dizon RV, Nagpal KC, et al. Macular holes associated with proliferative sickle cell retinopathy. Arch Ophthalmology. 1987;96:1592-6.

113. Moriarty BJ, Acheson RW, Serjeant GR. Epiretinal membranes in sickle cell disease. Br J Ophthalmology. 1987;71:466-9.

114. Schubert HD. Schisis in sickle cell retinopathy. Arch Ophthalmology. 2005;123:1607-9.

115. Frank RN, Cronin MA. Posterior pole neovascularization in a patient with hemoglobin SC disease. Am J Ophthalmology. 1979;88:680-2.

116. Goldberg MF. Natural history of untreated proliferative sickle retinopathy. Arch Ophthalmology. 1971;85:428-37.

117. Clarkson JG. The ocular manifestations of sickle cell disease: a prevalence and natural history study. Trans Am Ophthalmology Soc. 1992;90:481-504.

118. Condon PI, Whitelocke RA, Bird AC, et al. Recurrent visual loss in homozygous sickle cell disease. Br J Ophthalmology. 1985;69:700-6.

119. Goldberg MF. Retinal neovascularization in sickle cell retinopathy. Trans Sect Ophthalmology Am Acad Ophthalmology Otolaryngol. 1977;83:OP409-31.

120. Fox PD, Dunn DT, Morris JS, et al. Risk factors for proliferative sickle retinopathy. Br J Ophthalmology. 1990;74:172-6.

121. Downes SM, Hambleton IR, Chuang EL, et al. Incidence and natural history of proliferative sickle cell retinopathy: observations from a cohort study. Ophthalmology. 2005;112:1869-75.

122. Moriarty BJ, Acheson RW, Condon PI, et al. Patterns of visual loss in untreated sickle cell retinopathy. Eye. 1988;2:330-5.

123. Penman AD, Talbot JF, Chuang EL, et al. New classification of peripheral retinal vascular changes in sickle cell disease. Br J Ophthalmology. 1994;78:681-9.

124. Diallo JW, Kuhn D, Hayman-Gawrilow P, et al. Contribution of indocyanine green angiography in sickle cell retinopathy. J Fr Ophthalmology. 2009;32:430-5.

125. Condon P, Jampol LM, Farber MD, et al. A randomized clinical trial of feeder vessel photocoagulation of proliferative sickle cell retinopathy. II. Update and analysis of risk factors. Ophthalmology. 1984;91:1496-8.

126. Rednam KR, Jampol LM, Goldberg MF. Scatter retinal photocoagulation for proliferative sickle cell retinopathy. Am J Ophthalmology. 1982;93:594-9.

127. Shaikh S. Intravitreal bevacizumab (Avastin) for the treatment of proliferative sickle retinopathy. Indian J Ophthalmology. 2008;56:259.

128. Siquiera RC, Costa RA, Scott IU, et al. Intravitreal bevacizumab (Avastin) injection associated with regression of retinal neovascularization caused by sickle cell retinopathy. Acta Ophthalmology Scand. 2006;84:834-5.

129. Pulido JS, Flynn HW, Clarkson JG, et al. Pars plana vitrectomy in the management of complications of proliferative sickle retinopathy. Arch Ophthalmology. 1988;106:1553-7.

Chapter 31

Macular Telangiectasia

Atul Kumar, Pooja Shah, Rohan Chawla, Raghav Ravani

INTRODUCTION

Telangiectasia of retina has been recognized since 18th century, following the work of Carl Ferdinand Graefe.[1] A century later, Coats described congenital retinal telangiectasia with exudation and Leber described 'miliary aneurysms,'[2] which are the part of spectrum of the same disease in children or adults as proposed by Reese in 1956.[1] While retinal telangiectasia, i.e. abnormal dilatation of retinal capillaries occurs in several ocular and systemic disease, Gass in 1968 identified a distinct form of retinal telangiectasia limited to perifoveal region with no apparent cause and termed it as idiopathic juxtafoveolar retinal telangiectasia (IJRT).[3]

CLASSIFICATION

Several attempts at classification of macular telangiectasia (MacTel) have been made in past. Gass and Oyakawa, in 1982,[3,4] grouped IJRT in four groups based on clinical and fluorescein angiography (FA) characteristics which was later modified by Gass and Blodi in 1993,[5] to include three groups. However, Gass classification (Table 31.1) was too complex. Yannuzzi et al.[6] published a simplified classification of Macular Telangiectasia with indocyanine green, and FA as well as optical coherence tomography (OCT) findings. Groups 1A and 1B of Gass classification were merged into one group called aneurysmal telangiectasia or idiopathic macular telangiectasia type 1 or MacTel type 1. In fact, Gass et al. believed that this group of idiopathic juxtafoveal telangiectasia may be a part of the spectrum of congenital retinal telangiectasis or Coats' disease similar to the miliary retinal aneurysms as described previously by Leber.[2] Group 2A was renamed as idiopathic perifoveal telangiectasia or MacTel type 2, whereas rare entities like group 2B and 3 were removed. This is the most common type of IJFT, and differs completely from IJFT I. It is congenital. MacTel type 2 with has a nonproliferative stage with presence of telangiectasia and foveal atrophy and a proliferative stage characterized by the presence of subretinal neovascularization (SRNV). The focus of this chapter is MacTel type 2, most common form of MacTel.

Table 31.1: Classification of IJRT by Gass and Blodi, 1993.[5]

Group	Description
1	Congenital unilateral telangiectasia with male preponderance, uncommon
1A	Visible and exudative IJRT
1B	Visible, exudative, and focal IJRT
2	Acquired bilateral telangiectasia. Usually found in middle-aged or older patients
2A	Occult nonexudative IJRT. Most common form of IJRT (MacTel)
2B	Juvenile occult familial IJRT
3	Rare and poorly understood primarily occlusive phenomenon
3A	Occlusive IJRT
3B	Occlusive IJRT associated with CNS vasculopathy

(IJRT: Idiopathic juxtafoveolar retinal telangiectasia; CNS: Central nervous system)

It is likely that MacTel 2 is under diagnosed due to difficulty in diagnosis of its early stage, while in late stages it simulates age-related macular degeneration.[7] Hence, there is limited information on incidence and prevalence of MacTel type 2. The prevalence estimates of existing population-based studies using fundus photography report significant discrepancy. The Beaver Dam Study[8] reported a prevalence of 0.1% in white Americans over the age of 43 which is much higher than study of white Australians over 47 years of age, where the prevalence was found to be 0.0045–0.022%.[9] This discrepancy is perhaps due to differences in the methodology of the study or genetic variances amongst two races.[10]

Usual presentation of this acquired disease is during the 5th and 6th decades of life with a mean age of 55 years and no predilection for gender or race. Although typically it presents as bilateral symmetric disease, some may have an asymmetric disease and appear as unilateral in its initial stages.[5,6] Patients may be asymptomatic or have vague complaints of mild blurring of vision, difficulty in reading, and metamorphopsia especially in nasal quadrant of central visual field,[11] paracentral, or central scotoma. Visual impairment is usually mild and progresses very slowly over years.[10] 50% of patients in MacTel project had visual acuity, of 20/32 or better. However, despite good visual acuity performance on the National Eye Institute Visual Function Questionnaire was poor in MacTel project highlighting the fact that central visual acuity is a poor indicator of visual dysfunction in MacTel 2.[12] Microperimetry may be useful to detect and quantify functional changes and correlate it with structural lesions in such patients. Risk factors for drop in visual acuity to less than equal to 20/80 include subretinal neovascular membrane or central photoreceptor atrophy.[10]

Earliest fundus change seen on slit lamp biomicroscopy is the loss of transparency of temporal perifoveal retina eventually progressing all around in an oval configuration.[5,6,14] It is visualized as mild graying of retina caused by low-grade edema due to middle retinal layer ischemia. Retinal capillary telangiectasis is barely evident clinically, readily demonstrated on FA, and typically not associated with lipid exudates or hemorrhages.[6] Dilated and blunted retinal venule running at right angle may be visualized. Abnormal parafoveal capillary network is best visualized on FA. Multiple small, yellow, and refractile deposits may be seen at vitreoretinal interface close to the telangiectatic vessels, but they do not correlate with severity of disease.[5] Various hypotheses like byproduct of degenerating Müller cells, lipofuscin containing cells, and retinoids of visual cycle have been proposed to explain the origin of crystals but the exact cause is largely elusive.[10]

A few patients may have intraretinal yellow spot without significant loss of foveal contour. The spot size is usually between 100 μ to 300 μ and may be confused with adult vitelliform foveomacular dystrophy or Best disease. Intraretinal yellow spot can be seen in 5% of patients with MacTel 2.[10] Other foveal lesions seen include focal atrophy, lamellar macular hole, and full thickness macular hole occur probably secondary to Müller cell dysfunction. Lamellar macular holes have a distinct circular or irregular margin and associated focal foveolar retinal atrophy is present within the foveal avascular zone. The cause of full-thickness macular hole is postulated as Müller cell loss and dysfunction. Some may develop intraretinal black pigmented plaques due to migration of hyperplastic retinal pigment epithelium (RPE) along right angle venule[5] (Figs. 31.1A to F). Subretinal neovascular membrane frequently occurs near such pigmented plaques and may lead to profound visual loss due to lipid exudation, intra and subretinal hemorrhages, cystoid macular edema, and disciform scar when it resembles age related macular degeneration. However, SRNV in MacTel 2 is not associated with pigment epithelial detachment versus age-related macular degeneration (AMD).

FUNDUS AUTOFLUORESCENCE

Fundus autofluorescence (FAF) shows decreased foveal hypofluorescence, which is the earliest sign on imaging. This increased signal on shortwave autofluorescence is due to loss of foveal luteal pigments because of Müller cell degeneration, which also results in increased confocal blue reflectance. Areas of RPE hyperplasia will appear as hyperfluorescent spots on FAF.

FLUORESCEIN ANGIOGRAPHY

Fluorescein angiography appearance varies from mild late retinal staining of the outer juxtafoveolar retina to features similar to classic neovascularization[6] (Figs. 31.2A to D). Dilated right-angle vessels may be of arteriolar or venular origin.[10] CNVM is of retinal origin, as FA shows a feeding arteriole and a draining venule. Size of foveal avascular zone is reduced as compared to normal subjects.[10] Abnormal vasculature, which is difficult to visualize on FA due to leakage, is better seen on OCT angiography (Figs. 31.3A and B).

Optical coherence tomography shows enlargement of temporal foveal pit due to outer nuclear layer and ellipsoid zone loss that can progress into large cysts (often called 'cavitation') seen as a hyporeflective space encompassing all retinal layers.[15-17] Often, only the internal limiting membrane is left in place over these areas described as 'ILM drape' sign seen as superficial hyporeflective void[18,19] (Fig. 31.4). Hyperreflective areas on OCT correlate with areas of RPE hyperplasia and migration. Retinal thinning at fovea with low-grade edema may be seen. Parafoveal retinal thickness correlates with visual acuity. Ellipsoid layer disruption suggests photoreceptor atrophy.[20]

OPTICAL COHERENCE TOMOGRAPHY ANGIOGRAPHY OF MACULAR TELANGIECTASIA TYPE 2

Macular telangiectasia type 2 is a macular disease affecting all the layers of the macula and can lead to neovascularization from retinal as well as choroidal circulation. The earliest changes in the retinal microvasculature involve the temporal aspect of the parafoveal deep capillary plexus is involved early in the disease and can be seen on OCT angiography (OCTA) (Figs. 31.5A to D). With progression of disease, dilated anastomoses form between the superficial and deep capillary plexuses and cyst formation occurs with loss of photoreceptor outer segments and the retina becomes more atrophic. OCTA is advantageous because it is safer, more comfortable for the patient, and more easily repeatable, it can be performed during follow-up visits, and it produces both intensity-based OCT images and flow-based images which allow for visualization of the macular microvasculature. OCTA can be used as the primary modality of imaging for diagnosing and monitoring MacTel 2.

ADAPTIVE OPTICS

Adaptive optics (AO) allows high resolution imaging of photoreceptors by correcting ocular aberrations. Reduced cone density, ring like or patchy dark areas suggesting disruption

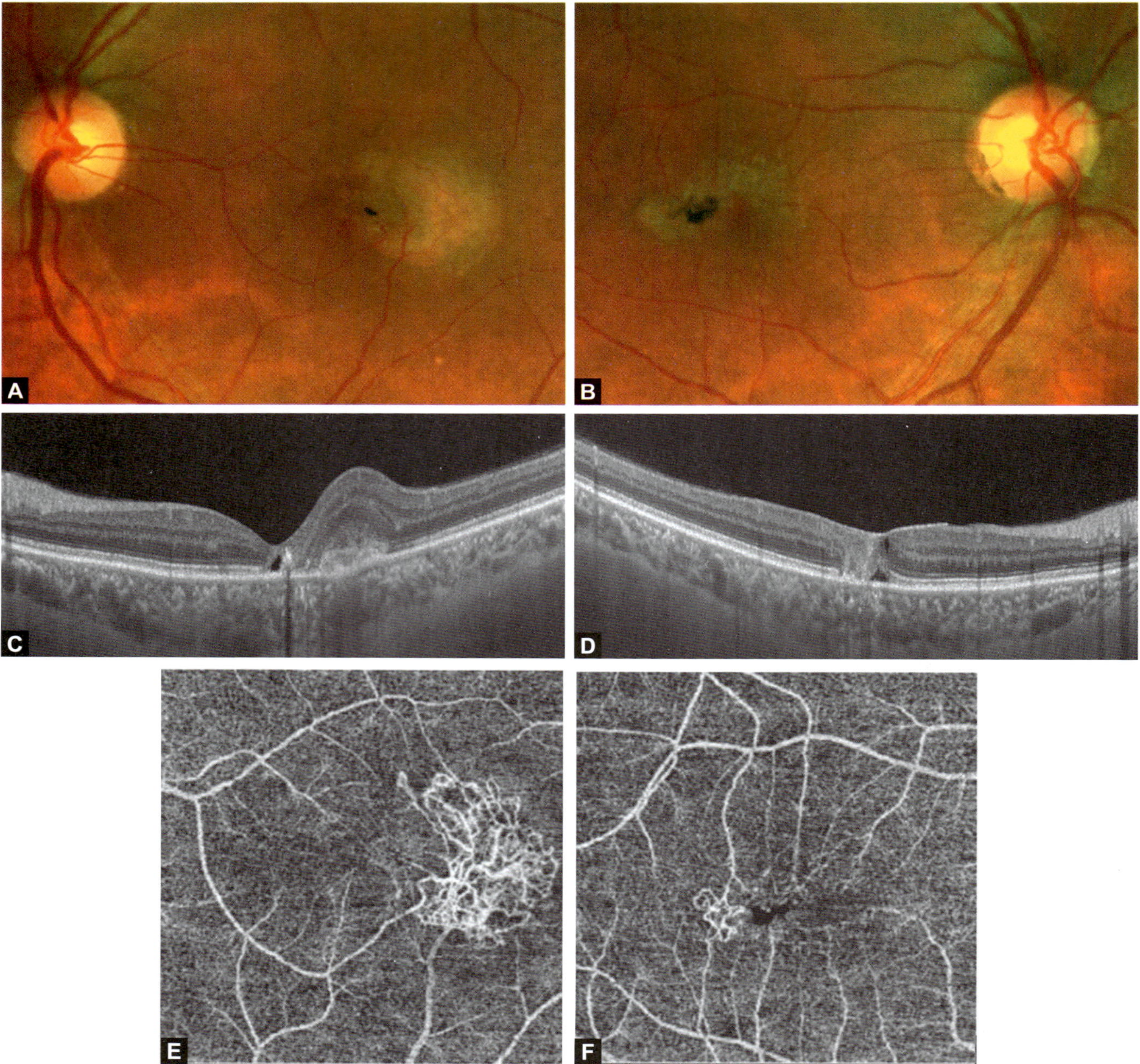

Figs. 31.1A to F: Fundus photograph showing macular telangiectasia type 2 (MacTel) with parafoveal metallic sheen with pigmentation. Evidence of secondary CNV OU is visible on OCTA.
(CNV: Choroidal neovascularization; OCTA: Optical coherence tomography angiography).

of cone mosaic are reported on AO imaging in areas with normal and abnormal vasculature supporting the hypothesis that neurodegeneration precedes vascular abnormalities.[21]

HISTOPATHOLOGY

The histopathological features of IJFT IIA have been described by Green et al.[12] who found thickening of retinal capillaries caused by multilayered basement membrane proliferation associated with narrowing of lumen. They did not actually find any telangiectasis of the retinal vessels. Degeneration of pericytes was also seen primarily in juxtafoveal area. These histopathological features support postulate of Gass that capillary dilation and "telangiectasis" does not occur until later in the process.[13]

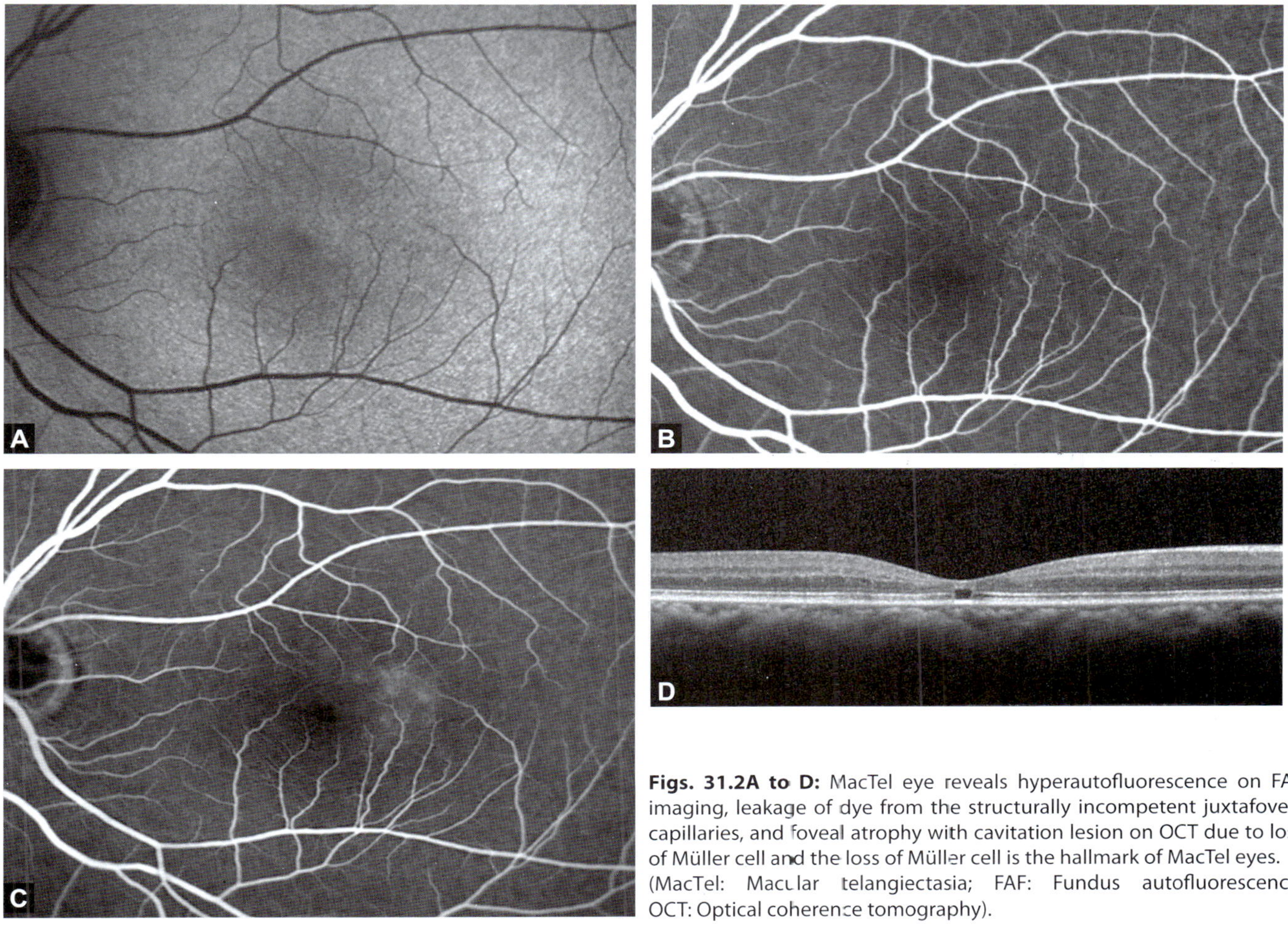

Figs. 31.2A to D: MacTel eye reveals hyperautofluorescence on FAF imaging, leakage of dye from the structurally incompetent juxtafoveal capillaries, and foveal atrophy with cavitation lesion on OCT due to loss of Müller cell and the loss of Müller cell is the hallmark of MacTel eyes. (MacTel: Macular telangiectasia; FAF: Fundus autofluorescence: OCT: Optical coherence tomography).

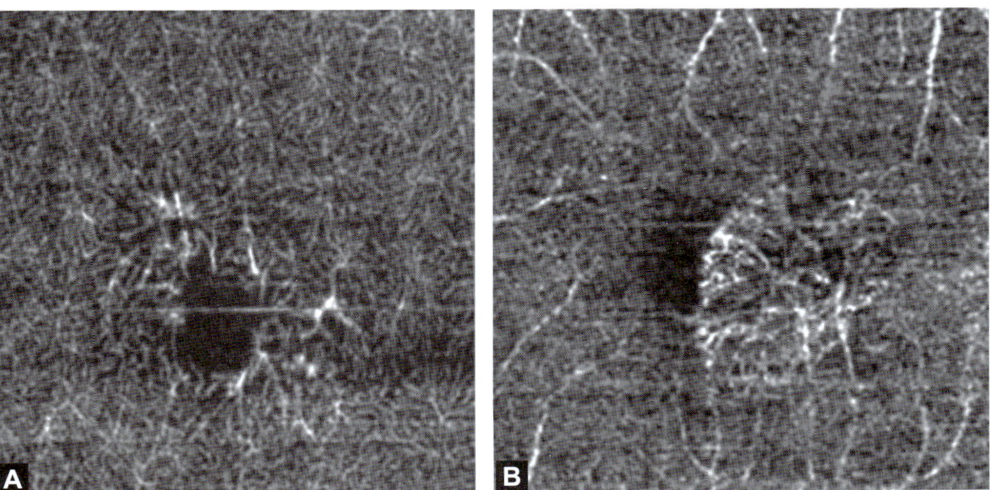

Figs. 31.3A and B: OCT angiography showing abnormal capillary network in retinal layers in the first two frames and a type 2 neovascularization in the last frame.
(OCT: Optical coherence tomography).

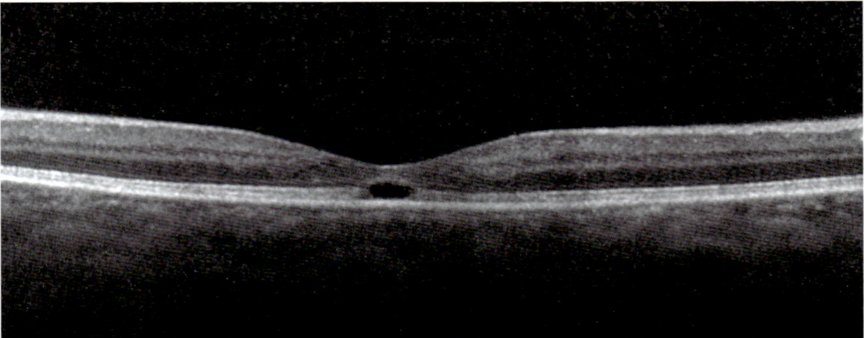

Fig. 31.4: Cavitation lesion at fovea with foveal atrophy in macular telangiectasia on OCT. (OCT: Optical coherence tomography).

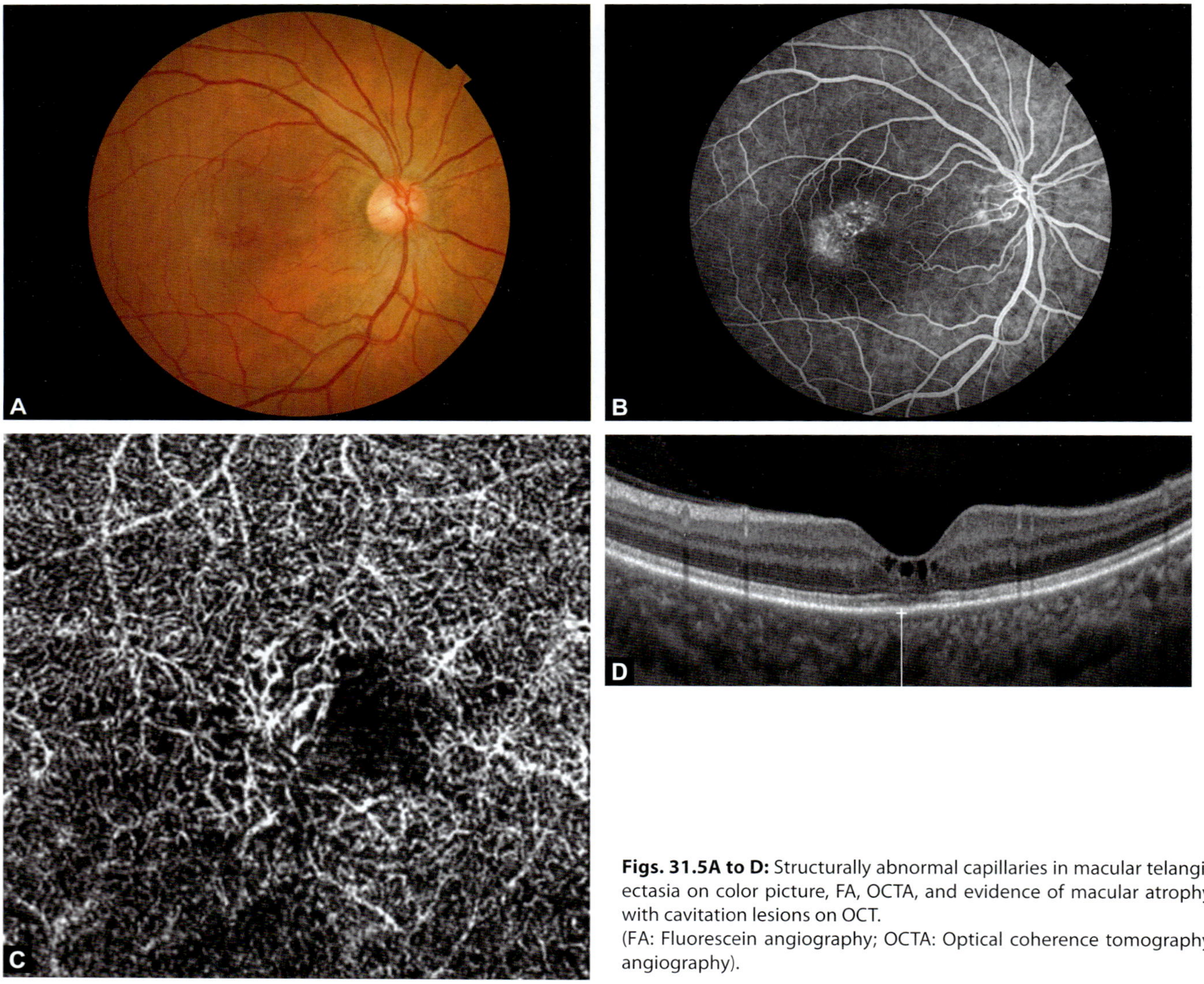

Figs. 31.5A to D: Structurally abnormal capillaries in macular telangiectasia on color picture, FA, OCTA, and evidence of macular atrophy with cavitation lesions on OCT.
(FA: Fluorescein angiography; OCTA: Optical coherence tomography angiography).

PATHOPHYSIOLOGY

There are controversies regarding the exact pathogenesis of IJFT IIA. Initially a primary role of the retinal capillaries was proposed by Gass and associates.[3] Alteration in the capillary wall along with increased endothelial permeability and metabolic alterations leads to chronic nutritional damage to the retina especially the Müller cells.[14]

Gass commented that IJFT IIA 'is not primarily a leaky retinal blood vessel disease', but rather 'the primary abnormality may reside in one or both of the parafoveal retinal neural or Müller cells' as he observed central vision is lost due to atrophy of photoreceptors without any macular edema and telangiectatic capillary dilation does not occur until late in the course of disease. A common finding is superficial crystalline deposits located near the ILM, which are thought to represent the remnants of degenerated Müller cells.[5]

Recent advances like AO imaging, short-wavelength autofluorescence, confocal blue reflectance and few histopathological studies suggest macular pigment depletion and Müller cell degeneration as central in pathogenesis of MacTel type 2 supporting that it is a primary neurodegenerative disorder.[10,22]

DIFFERENTIAL DIAGNOSIS

Differential diagnosis of retinal capillary telangiectasia includes several inflammatory and vaso-occlusive diseases. Branch retinal vein occlusion causes segmental capillary changes distal to arteriovenous crossing. Diabetic retinopathy has widespread involvement, prominent exudates, and neo-vascularization at vitreoretinal interface. Radiation retinopathy involves larger area, cotton wool spots, and preretinal neovascularization apart from history of prior radiotherapy. In cases of neovascularization, AMD should be ruled out.[17]

SYSTEMIC ASSOCIATIONS

Up to 45% of patients with MacTel type 2 may have an associated systemic disorder.[7] Several studies support an association between diabetes mellitus and MacTel type 2,[10] while some do not[5,6] and current evidence is insufficient to establish the true relationship between the two.[10] Other reported systemic associations include hypertension, coronary artery disease, celiac sprue, polycythemia vera, calcinosis, Raynaud phenomenon, esophageal dysmotility, sclerodactyly, and telangiectasia (CREST) syndrome, Alport disease, and pseudoxanthoma elasticum, while ocular associations include epiretinal membranes, microhemangiomas of the pupillary margin, soft confluent drusen and wider retinal arteriolar, and venular calibers beyond fovea with probable explanation being generalized dysfunction in retinal vascular pericytes or glial cells or a consequence of venous congestion.[10] The Beaver Dam Study supports an association between cigarette smoking and MacTel type 2.[8]

Gass and Blodi observed the orderly appearance of various lesions of MacTel type 2 and proposed a clinical staging system (Table 31.2).[5] This system was proposed before the availability of current advanced imaging techniques and has limited value at present.[10,17]

Macular telangiectasia type 1 or aneurysmal telangiectasia or group 1 or visible and exudative idiopathic

Table 31.2: Various lesions of MacTel type 2 and proposed a clinical staging system.

Stage Yannuzzi et al.	Gass and Blodi	Prominent features	Visual symptoms	Biomicroscopy	Fluorescein angiography
Nonproliferative perifoveal telangiectasia	1	Occult vascular abnormalities	Asymptomatic	Slight parafoveal graying (may be difficult to detect)	Minimal or no evidence of capillary dilation and late retinal staining
	2	No clinically visible telangiectasis	Asymptomatic or mild visual disturbances	Mild loss of parafoveolar retinal transparency or no visible telangiectatic vessels or superficial refractile crystals possible	Early staining of capillary walls in outer retinal network or diffuse late staining
	3	Prominent dilated right-angled retinal venules	Metamorphopsia, mild scotoma	Parafoveal right-angled venules, draining telangiectasis or visible capillary dilation	Capillary dilation and leakage beneath right-angled venules causing late retinal staining or no pooling of fluid

Contd...

Contd...

Stage					
Yannuzzi et al.	*Gass and Blodi*	*Prominent features*	*Visual symptoms*	*Biomicroscopy*	*Fluorescein angiography*
	4	Retinal pigment hyperplasia extending into the retina	Progressive visual decline	Retinal pigment epithelial hyperplasia or clumps around right-angled venules	Capillary dilation and leakage beneath right-angled venules causing late retinal staining or no pooling of fluid or blocked fluorescence in areas of pigment
Proliferative perifoveal telangiectasia	5	Subretinal neovascularization	Rapid and severe visual loss	Subretinal exudation and hemorrhage or retinochoroidal anastomosis	Like classic neovascularization with features of stages 3–4

(MacTel type: Macular telangiectasia)

juxtafoveal telangiectasia is commonly found in middle-aged male patients. They present with blurring of vision in central field, often mild and unilateral. On slit lamp biomicroscopy, prominently visible telangiectatic retinal capillaries with variable-sized aneurysmal dilations are a hallmark[5] involving up to two disc diameter or greater area temporal to the fovea.[8] This type of IJFT is not associated with blunted right-angled venules, superficial vitreoretinal interface crystalline deposits, plaques of pigment epithelial hyperplasia, intraretinal pigment migration, or SRNV.[5] Lipid deposition and macular edema are characteristically seen.

MANAGEMENT

Over the years, researchers have studied many MacTel treatments. None have proven to significantly improve vision. Since the disease has a relatively good prognosis, most patients may not need treatment.

Therapy is largely directed towards neovascular complications of MacTel type 2. Laser photocoagulation and photodynamic therapy of leaking lesions in nonproliferative MacTel type 2 have been attempted with no stabilization of disease process.[10] Intravitreal antivascular endothelial growth factor (VEGF) agents, photodynamic therapy and transpupillary thermotherapy have been tried for the treatment of SRNV. Submacular surgery for SRNV was attempted in the past with poor success. A decrease in retinal thickness, reduction in angiographic leakage, and an improvement in visual acuity have been reported with single and multiple intravitreal anti-VEGF injections but no change in progression of disease. But despite few encouraging results, anti-VEGF therapy should be used cautiously as VEGF has several functions in eye including role in neuroprotection and cell survival.[10] Pars plana vitrectomy surgery, membrane peeling and gas

tamponade for full thickness macular hole associated with MacTel type 2 is associated with poor success than idiopathic macular hole possibly due to neurodegeneration involved in MacTel type 2.[10] Further studies evaluating role of neuroprotective agents and randomized controlled trials evaluating anti-VEGF agents may be considered.

REFERENCES

1. F P Campbell. Coats' disease and congenital vascular retinopathy. Trans Am Ophthalmology Soc. 1976;74:365-424.
2. Leber T. Ueber Vorkommen durch eine multipler Miliaraneurysmen charakterisierte Form von Retinal Degeneration. F Arch Ophthalmology. 1912;81(81):1-14.
3. Gass JD, Oyakawa RT. Idiopathic juxtafoveolar retinal telangiectasis. Arch Ophthalmology. 1982;100(5):769-80.
4. Cahill M, O'Keefe M, Acheson R, et al. Classification of the spectrum of Coats' disease as subtypes of idiopathic retinal telangiectasis with exudation. Acta Ophthalmology Scand. 2001;79(6):596-602.
5. Gass JD, Blodi BA. Idiopathic juxtafoveolar retinal telangiectasis. Update of classification and follow-up study. Ophthalmology. 1993;100(10):1536-46.
6. Yannuzzi LA, Bardal AMC, Freund KB, et al. Idiopathic macular telangiectasia. Arch Ophthalmology. 2006;124(4):450-60.
7. Clemons TE, Gillies MC, Chew EY, et al. Baseline characteristics of participants in the natural history study of macular telangiectasia (MacTel) MacTel Project Report No. 2. Ophthalmic Epidemiol. 2010;17(1):66-73.
8. Klein R, Blodi BA, Meuer SM, et al. The Prevalence of Macular Telangiectasia Type 2 (MT2) in the Beaver Dam Eye Study. Am J Ophthalmology. 2010;150(1):55-62.e2.
9. Aung KZ, Wickremasinghe SS, Makeyeva G, et al. The prevalence estimates of macular telangiectasia type 2: the Melbourne Collaborative Cohort Study. Retina. 2010;30(3):473-8.
10. Wu L, Evans T, Arevalo JF. Idiopathic macular telangiectasia type 2 (idiopathic juxtafoveolar retinal telangiectasis type 2A, MacTel 2). Surv Ophthalmology. 2013;58(6):536-59.

11. Charbel Issa P, Holz FG, Scholl HP. Metamorphopsia in patients with macular telangiectasia type 2. Doc Ophthalmology. 2009; 119(2):133-40.
12. Green WR, Quigley HA, De la Cruz Z, et al. Parafoveal retinal telangiectasis: light and electron microscopy studies. Trans Ophthalmology Soc UK. 1980;100(Pt 1):162-70.
13. Gass JD. Histopathologic study of presumed parafoveal telangiectasis. Retina. 2000;20(2):226-7.
14. Gass JD. Diagnosis and Treatment. In: Gass JD (Ed). Stereoscopic Atlas of Macular Diseases, 4th edition. St Louis: Mosby; 1997.pp. 505-11.
15. Clemons TE, Gillies MC, Chew EY, et al. Medical characteristics of patients with macular telangiectasia type 2 (MacTel Type 2) MacTel project report no. 3. Ophthalmic Epidemiol. 2013;20(2): 109-13.
16. Surguch V, Gamulescu MA, Gabel VP. Optical coherence tomography findings in idiopathic juxtafoveal retinal telangiectasis. Graefes Arch Clin Exp Ophthalmology. 2007;245(6):783-8.
17. Cohen SM, Cohen ML, El-Jabali F, et al. Optical coherence tomography findings in nonproliferative group 2a idiopathic juxtafoveal retinal telangiectasis. Retina. 2007;27(1):59-66.
18. Schmitz-Valckenberg S, Ong EEL, Rubin GS, et al. Structural and functional changes over time in MacTel patients. Retina. 2009;29(9):1314-20.
19. Abujamra S, Bonanomi MT, Cresta FB, et al. Idiopathic juxta-foveolar retinal telangiectasis: clinical pattern in 19 cases. Ophthalmologica. 2000;214(6):406-11.
20. Paurescu LA, Ko TH, Duker JS, et al. Idiopathic juxtafoveal retinal telangiectasis: new findings by ultrahigh-resolution optical coherence tomography. Ophthalmology. 2006;113(1):48-57.
21. Ooto S, Hangai M, Takayama K, et al. High-resolution photo-receptor imaging in idiopathic macular telangiectasia type 2 using adaptive optics scanning laser ophthalmoscopy. Invest Ophthalmology Vis Sci. 20111;52(8):5541-50.
22. Wu L. Multimodality imaging in macular telangiectasia 2: A clue to its pathogenesis. Indian J Ophthalmology. 2015;63(5):394-8.

Chapter 32

Miscellaneous Retinal Vascular Diseases

Prateek Kakkar, Nawazish Shaikh, Farin Shaikh, Atul Kumar

VALSALVA RETINOPATHY

Thomas Duane in 1972 was the first to describe Valsalva retinopathy as a hemorrhagic retinal pathology secondary to sudden increase in intrathoracic pressure.[1] It is usually reported in otherwise healthy eyes and is known to resolve spontaneously.

 PATHOPHYSIOLOGY

Valsalva maneuver is the forceful expiration against closed glottis leading to raised intrathoracic pressure and thus reduced venous return to right side of heart. This culminates into reduced cardiac stroke volume and raised systemic venous system pressure.[2] Sudden rise in intraocular venous pressure leads to rupture of superficial retinal capillaries presenting as preretinal or subhyaloid bleed.[2] Table 32.1 represents the phases of Valsalva maneuver.

Valsalva retinopathy is characteristically observed after sudden increase in intrathoracic or intra-abdominal pressure. Common conditions causing this are coughing, vomiting, heavy weight lifting, choking, Heimlich maneuver, sexual intercourse, labor, straining and blowing musical instruments. Valsalva retinopathy is also observed in patients of compressive injuries.

Incompetent valves in head and neck veins can also cause direct transmission of intrathoracic or intra-abdominal pressure into head and neck venous circulatory system. This raised pressure can lead to decompensation of retinal capillary bed causing retinal hemorrhages. Hemorrhages are seen below the internal limiting membrane (ILM), which can sometimes breakthrough in the subhyaloid or vitreous.[3]

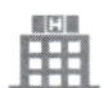 RISK FACTORS

It usually occurs in otherwise healthy eyes but may be associated with congenital conditions like retinal telangiectasia and congenital retinal artery tortuosity or acquired retinal vascular abnormalities like diabetic or hypertensive retinopathy.[2,4]

 CLINICAL PRESENTATION

Patient usually complains of either unilateral or bilateral sudden painless loss of vision or central scotoma with a typical history suggestive of Valsalva maneuver. Unilateral form is seen more commonly than the bilateral form.

Anterior segment evaluation may reveal associations like subconjunctival hemorrhage and occasional presence of retrolental cells. Fundus examination reveals round or bi-lobed (dumb-bell shaped), well-circumscribed red elevation causing hemorrhagic detachment of the ILM (Figs. 32.1A and B). It is typically located in premacular region and below the ILM (Fig. 32.2). Although it may occasionally break through into the subhyaloid or intravitreal space. Rarely associated choroidal hemorrhage may be seen.

Blood initially appears bright red (Fig. 32.3A) but turns yellow with associated fluid level after several days to weeks (Fig. 32.3B). Serous detachment may persist up to weeks.[5] Visual acuity almost always returns to the baseline after resolution of the hemorrhage.

Table 32.1: Phases of Valsalva maneuver.

Phase I	Sudden increase in intrathoracic pressure decreasing cardiac venous return
Phase II	Decreased cardiac filling causes lowering of the mean arterial pressure leading to reflex tachycardia and peripheral vasoconstriction
Phase III	When the strain is released, a sudden decrease in intrathoracic pressure causes further decrease in blood pressure and increased cardiac pressure
Phase IV	Sudden increase in blood pressure as venous blood goes back to the heart causing reflex bradycardia

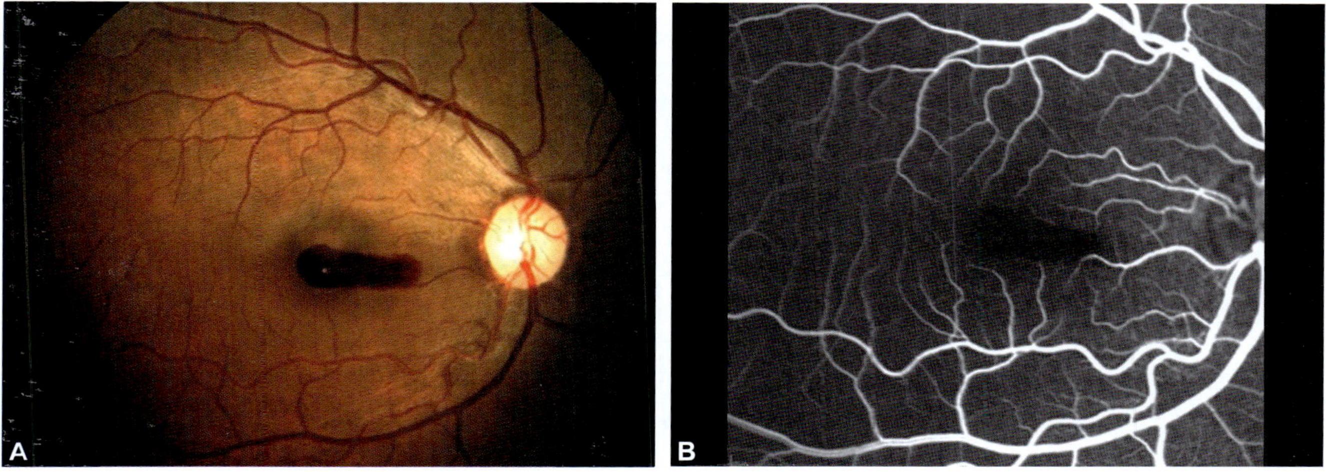

Figs. 32.1A and B: Clinical photograph and fluorescein angiography of Valsalva retinopathy showing blocked fluorescence due to preretinal blood.

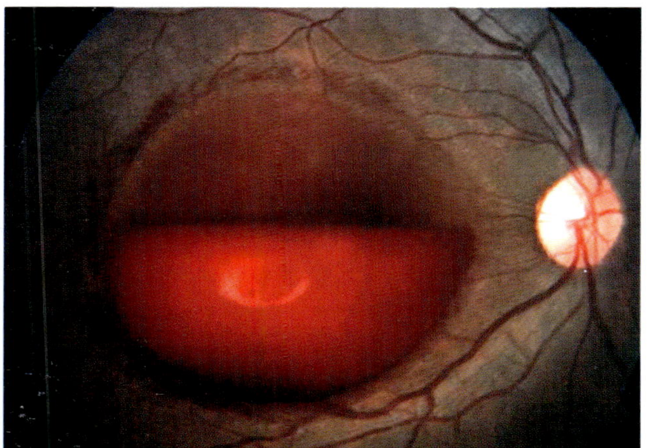

Fig. 32.2: Clinical photograph showing premacular bleed secondary to Valsalva retinopathy, associated with fluid level.

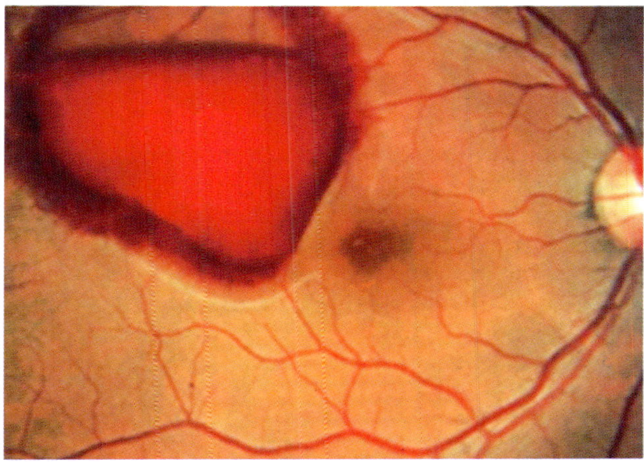

Fig. 32.3A: Clinical photograph showing subhyaloid hemorrhage seen superotemporal to the fovea.

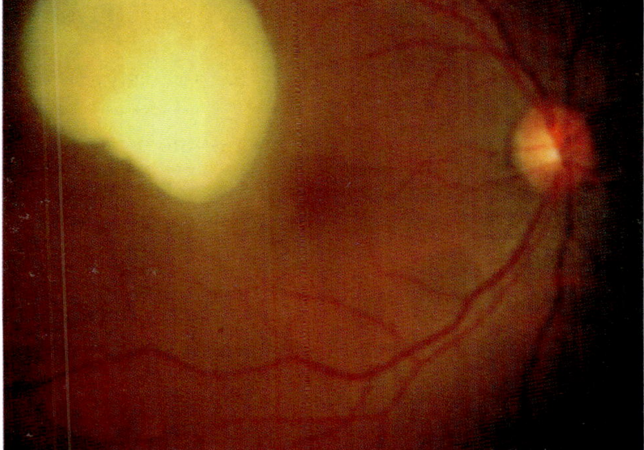

Fig. 32.3B: Clinical fundus picture showing change in the hemorrhage color at 3 weeks with some of it entering the vitreous cavity.

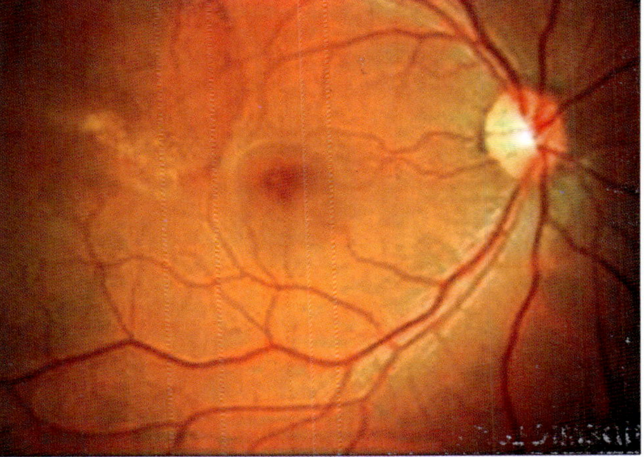

Fig. 32.3C: Clinical picture showing spontaneous resolution of the hemorrhage by around 6 weeks.

MANAGEMENT

Valsalva retinopathy is a diagnosis of exclusion. Laboratory studies like complete blood count, fasting blood sugar, glucose tolerance test, prothrombin time, activated partial thromboplastin time, sickle-cell preparation, hemoglobin electrophoresis, antiphospholipid antibodies and urinalysis can be used to rule out predisposing risk factors like diabetes, sickle cell disease, anemia, idiopathic thrombocytopenic purpura and other blood dyscrasias.

Serial monitoring on follow-up for progression and resolution of hemorrhages can be done with the help of fundus photographs. Optical coherence tomography (OCT) can be used to find the level of bleed whether sub-ILM or subhyaloid.[6] Fundus fluorescein angiography (FFA) may be done to rule out any neovascularization or other etiological diagnosis.

Treatment for Valsalva retinopathy is usually observation and propped up positioning. Propped up position helps in settling of blood and may improve visual acuity. Preretinal hemorrhages usually resolve over few weeks (Fig. 32.3C). Whereas, vitreous hemorrhage can take around 3–6 months to resolve.[7]

Counseling of patient should be done with respect to avoiding predisposing factors like strenuous activities and anticoagulants to prevent rebleed. Stool softeners may be advised to avoid straining.

Neodymium-doped yttrium aluminum garnet (Nd:YAG) laser or argon laser membranotomy can be used in patients with large hemorrhage, more so, in one eyed patients (Figs. 32.4A to C). It is usually preferred in macular subhyaloid hemorrhage of less than 3 weeks in duration and more than 3-disc diameter in size. Occasionally, vitrectomy may be required to clear nonresolving subhyaloid or vitreous hemorrhage.

PROGNOSIS

Prognosis is usually good with observation alone leading to resolution of hemorrhages.

TERSON'S SYNDROME

Terson's syndrome (TS) is named after the French ophthalmologist Albert Terson who described the disease in 1900 as vitreous bleeding observed in association with subarachnoid hemorrhage (SAH).[8] Although history of this clinical entity dates back to 1881, when the similar condition was described by Litten.[9]

Terson's syndrome is known as intraocular hemorrhage of any type (intraretinal, subhyaloid or intravitreal) associated with SAH, intracerebral bleed or cerebral trauma.

EPIDEMIOLOGY

Terson's syndrome has been reported in 10–40% of individuals with subarachnoid hemorrhage.[10-15] Whereas, incidence

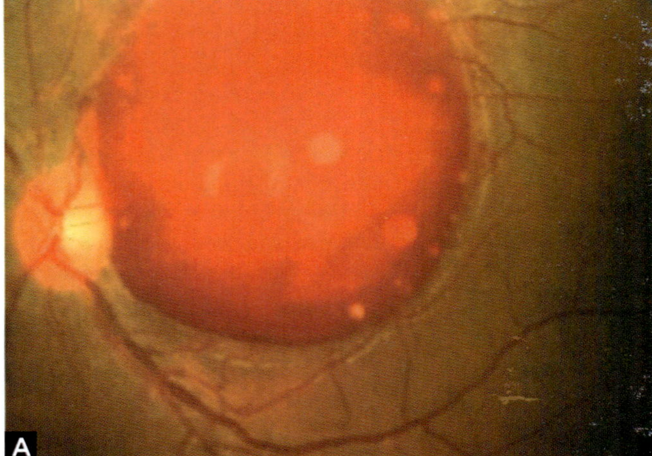

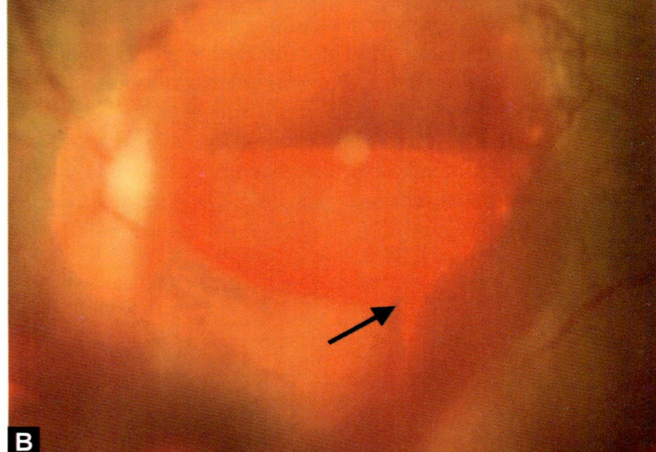

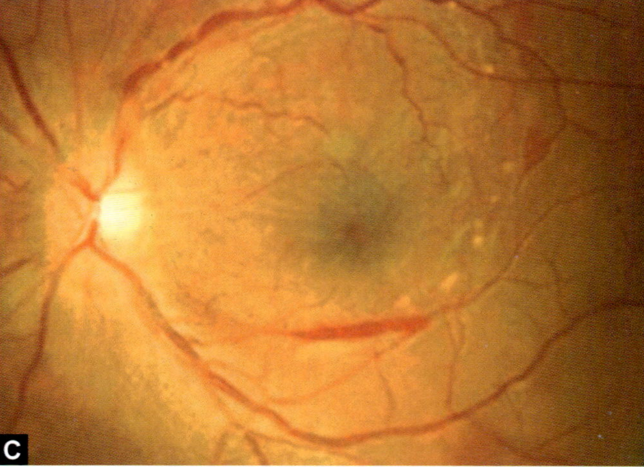

Figs. 32.4A to C: Clinical fundus image showing (A) A large premacular hemorrhage obscuring the fovea due to Valsalva retinopathy; (B) Yttrium aluminum garnet (YAG) hyaloidotomy is performed for early visual rehabilitation. Black arrow shows blood escaping through opening made by the YAG laser: (C) 1 week following laser the vitreous and subhyaloid space is mostly free of blood with the patient recovering 6/6 visual acuity.

of vitreous hemorrhage[16] seen in cases of TS is 3–13%. TS can be unilateral or bilateral. It has been suggested by Manschot et al. that patients with bilateral hemorrhage have more pronounced intracranial hemorrhage than patients with unilateral involvement.[17]

Mean age is 47.3 years in patients reported to have TS, 28.3 years in cases associated with trauma, and 56.1 years in cases with vasculogenic cause of intracranial hemorrhage. Male : female ratio in TS is 2:1 and is consistent with the sex difference in incidence of aneurysmal subarachnoid hemorrhage. No difference in the sex ratio is seen between those with and without vitreous hemorrhage.[18] Terson's syndrome in patients with subarachnoid hemorrhage is also associated with increased mortality.[19]

PATHOPHYSIOLOGY

Pathophysiological mechanism of TS has been a matter debated for many years with two distinct schools of thoughts. Manschot[17] et al. suggested that sudden increase in intracranial pressure occurs following subarachnoid bleed, which forces blood into the subarachnoid space of the optic nerve. Whereas, Hedges and Walsh[20] suggested that pressure leads to rapid effusion of cerebrospinal fluid (CSF) into the optic nerve sheath space and decrease in venous return to the cavernous sinus or obstruction of the retinochoroidal anastomoses and central retinal vein, culminating in venous stasis and hemorrhage.

Michalewska et al. using spectral domain OCT suggested that blood enters the vitreous cavity around the peripapillary vessels and may spread intraretinal, below the ILM or along retinal vessels. It is now generally accepted that vitreous hemorrhage results from ocular blood.[21-23]

Magnetic resonance imaging (MRI) findings also suggest that subarachnoid hemorrhage within the optic nerve sheath can enter into the space beneath the ILM and subsequently beneath the vitreous. ILM breakdown can cause glial cell proliferation and epiretinal membrane formation.

Subhyaloid hemorrhages are diffuse, irregularly edged, and have variable density; whereas sub-ILM hematomas are well-demarcated and dome-shaped.[18] The "double ring" sign is seen when subhyaloid hemorrhage and sub-ILM hemorrhage are present concurrently.[24] Hemorrhage beneath the ILM causes elevation of the ILM known as "macular ring" reported by Sadeh et al.[15] As the hematoma contracts and serum is absorbed, wrinkling of the ILM occurs appearing as a folded reflective surface. Glatt and Machemer demonstrated toxic effects of blood on the photoreceptors, especially in the first 7 days after the hemorrhage. The iron from hemoglobin catalyzes the conversion of hydrogen peroxide into hydroxyl radical leading to oxidative damage. Since, the main function of the retinal pigment epithelium (RPE) is to phagocyte the lipid-rich photoreceptors external segments, retina and the RPE are more prone to this oxidative damage.[25]

ETIOLOGY

Subarachnoid or intracranial hemorrhage, head trauma, raised intracranial pressure and tumor. Ruptured cerebral vessel aneurysms, mainly in the internal carotid artery, middle cerebral artery bifurcation and upper part of the basal artery are associated with TS. There is also no relationship between the location of the aneurysm and which eye is affected by TS.

Other causes of TS include carotid artery occlusion, cortical venous sinus thrombosis, moyamoya disease, lumbosacral myelomeningocele, and intraoperative bleeding during endoscopic third ventriculostomy.

CLINICAL PRESENTATION

Terson's syndrome usually presents with dome-shaped hemorrhages at the macula. Classic macular double-ring sign can be seen. Preretinal hemorrhage often precedes the vitreous hemorrhage.[10,19]

Funduscopic examination is the gold standard for diagnosis of TS. Loss of red reflex is seen in 20% of the cases. Median time from visual symptoms to referral to an ophthalmologist is 4–5 months due to systemic condition of the patient. Although, CT scan may be useful to identify possible TS.

Approximately, 12–16% of patients with subarachnoid hemorrhage do not reach hospital to be clinically assessed.[26,27] Fahmy et al. suggested that aneurysmal rupture can occur in about one-third of cases of subarachnoid hemorrhage and should be suspected in any patient with retinal hemorrhage who has temporarily lost consciousness. Although there is no correlation between the side of retinal hemorrhage and the site of aneurysm.[14,28]

COMPLICATIONS

Epiretinal membrane formation is one of the most common complications, which can occur in Terson's, with an incidence of up to 78%. Complications are usually secondary to proliferation of glial and retinal pigment epithelial elements capable of causing retinal distortion and fibrotic adhesions.[29] Other complications include visual loss, macular holes, retinal folds, proliferative vitreoretinopathy and retinal detachment.[15,29-34]

Hemorrhage of the optic nerve sheath within the dural sheath, subdural space, subarachnoid space or pia mater is also reported as one of the complications of TS. These optic nerve hemorrhages of TS were noted to be locally multifocal and not an extension of intracranial blood.[22]

Other reported long-term complications include RPE mottling, optic atrophy, cystoid retinal changes and cataract formation.

 ## MANAGEMENT

Terson's syndrome is a frequent cause of visual loss following subarachnoid hemorrhage.[35] Earlier definition of the extent and location of bleeding before 3 months can optimize clinical management. Vitrectomy with or without membrane peeling and ILM peeling can be performed to remove the VH, epiretinal gliosis and the sub-ILM bleeding in cases with non-resolving vitreous hemorrhage.[36] Current recommendation in literature is to observe for 3–6 months after the acute event, later on, vitrectomy can be done if visual acuity does not improve.[13,37,38] Improvement in visual acuity is usually seen after vitrectomy.[15,39,40] New instruments and dyes available for microsurgery facilitate peeling resulting in better results.[41] Daus et al. suggested early vitrectomy in patients with bilateral hemorrhage.[42] High incidence of development of intraoperative breaks requiring supplementary treatment with laser therapy, cryotherapy and gas tamponade has also been reported in TS eyes undergoing vitrectomy.[39] Ultrasound, MRI and ocular coherence tomography can be a useful aid in clinicopathological correlation.

In 1991, Lewis introduced tissue plasminogen activator (tPA) in management of TS, which helps in breaking down of the blood clot in cases of submacular hemorrhages.[43] The tPA is a protease that transforms plasminogen into plasmin, which subsequently breaks the fibrin clot. It can be used as a subretinal injection during vitrectomy or intravitreal injection along with the pneumatic displacement of the clot.[44]

In cases with premacular subhyaloid hemorrhages long-standing visual impairment may occur due to poor resorption of the blood. Ulbig et al. concluded that puncturing the posterior hyaloid face or the ILM using a pulsed Nd:YAG laser is a viable alternative treatment to vitrectomy.[45]

PROGNOSIS

Patients diagnosed with TS have a 40–60% mortality rate, 3–9 times higher comparative to the patients who only present with subarachnoid hemorrhage unaccompanied by ocular manifestations.[46] The amount of intraocular hemorrhage is influenced by the speed of accumulation and magnitude of the intracranial pressure elevation.[15] Degree of vision loss is usually related to the extent of the intraocular hemorrhage. It can vary from 20/20 to light perception. Final visual prognosis is influenced by factors like the age of the patient, the rate of pre- and postoperative complications like epiretinal membrane formation and cataract.

PURTSCHER AND PURTSCHER-LIKE RETINOPATHY

Dr Otmar Purtscher, an Austrian ophthalmologist, first described Purtscher's retinopathy or *angiopathia retinae traumatica* in the year 1910 when he noted fundus abnormalities like multiple retinal hemorrhages and retinal whitening confined to posterior pole, in a middle-aged man who complained of bilateral visual loss after few hours of head trauma due to fall from tree. Despite the grave visual loss, the patient recovered without any specific treatment.[47]

Purtscher retinopathy is a chorioretinopathy associated with indirect trauma, with typical retinal findings including retinal hemorrhages, cotton–wool spots, optic disc edema and Purtscher flecken (polygonal areas of inner retinal whitening due to larger capillary bed infarcts). It is typically associated with compression trauma.

The term Purtscher-like retinopathy is used when these retinal signs are present without the history of trauma. In 1975, Inkeles and Walsh first described it in a patient with acute pancreatitis.[48]

CAUSES

Purtscher and Purtscher-like retinopathy are collectively referred to as "Purtscher retinopathy" because they share a common pathophysiological mechanism, clinical presentation and treatment.

The causes of Purtscher retinopathy can be broadly classified as traumatic and nontraumatic. The traumatic causes include head trauma,[47] chest compression, long bone fracture,[49] crush injury, orthopedic surgery, weight lifting,[50] barotrauma,[51] and battered baby syndrome.[52] Nontraumatic causes described are acute pancreatitis,[48,53] pancreatic adenocarcinoma,[54] chronic renal failure,[55] preeclampsia, HELLP syndrome and childbirth,[56] connective tissue disorders (like systemic lupus erythematosus, dermatomyositis,[57] scleroderma, etc.), fat embolism syndrome, amniotic fluid embolism,[58,59] Valsalva maneuver, lymphoproliferative disorders (like Hodgkin lymphoma) and bone marrow transplantation,[60] steroid injections in and around the orbit and nasal passages,[61] retrobulbar anesthesia,[62] hemolytic uremic syndrome,[63,64] and cryoglobulinemia.[65]

The most common cause is trauma followed by acute pancreatitis.[66]

SYMPTOMS

Most important symptom is diminution of vision and visual field loss in the form of scotoma. Peripheral visual field is usually preserved.[67] 60% of patients present bilaterally and mostly associated with acute pancreatitis.[68,69]

SIGNS

Majority of the cases are bilateral but unilateral cases are also reported.[50,58,62] The most common fundus abnormalities are cotton–wool spots (93%). Other signs commonly seen are retinal hemorrhages (65%) and Purtscher flecken (63%)[66] (Fig. 32.5). Purtscher flecken, the pathognomonic finding, are defined as polygonal areas of whitening in the inner nuclear layers with a characteristic clear demarcating zone (within

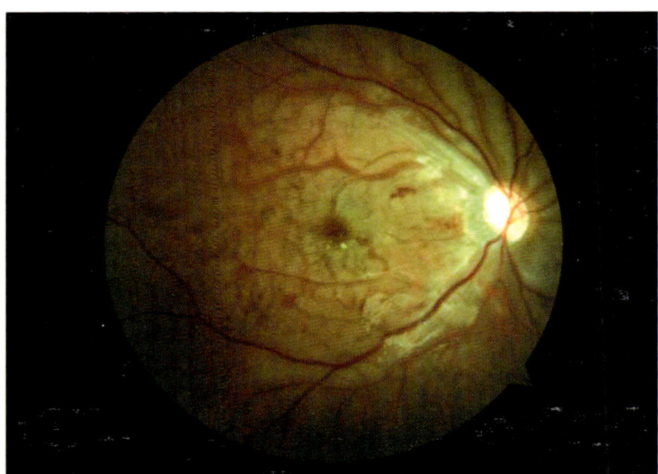

Fig. 32.5: Clinical fundus image of right eye showing peripapillary retinal whitening with macular involvement, dilated retinal venous system, Purtscher flecken and multiple hemorrhages.

50 µm, corresponding to capillary-free area) between the affected retina and adjoining normal retinal vessels.

In more than 50% cases, perivascular retina is spared classically.[69] The lesions, usually affecting the superficial aspect of inner retina, may be isolated, multiple and of variable size. They classically affect the posterior pole, i.e. around the disc and macular area. This may be postulated to be due to fewer arteriolar feeders and anastomoses in this area making the arterioles and capillaries in this area more susceptible to embolic occlusion.[67,70] When this whitening occurs around the fovea, it may give rise to pseudo-cherry red spot. Usually, there are minimal retinal hemorrhages that are typically flame-shaped but dot and blot hemorrhages may also occur.

The retina may remain normal initially for 1–2 days after the systemic illness. In 40% of the patients, the lesions resolved without any treatment but optic atrophy (usually temporal disc pallor) was reported in around two-thirds of cases. The other changes seen were RPE mottling, retinal thinning, and arterial narrowing or sheathing.[66]

DIAGNOSIS

Diagnosis is mainly clinical for Purtscher retinopathy. Miguel et al.[66] proposed the following diagnostic criteria:
- Purtscher flecken
- Retinal hemorrhages, in low-to-moderate number
- Cotton–wool spots (confined to the posterior pole)
- Probable explanatory etiology
- Complementary investigation compatible with diagnosis.

Presence of at least three out of the above five criteria is essential for the diagnosis of Purtscher retinopathy.

INVESTIGATIONS

Optical Coherence Tomography

Initially, there will be hyper-reflectivity in the inner retinal layers due to cotton–wool spots. Macular edema may or may not be present. In chronic cases, there will be evidence of variable atrophy of outer layers of retina and loss of photoreceptors, which is of prognostic significance.[71-73]

Fundus Fluorescein Angiography

Presence of retinal whitening and/or blood at the posterior pole gives area of blocked choroidal fluorescence, especially in the acute phase (within 2 hours). Other findings include arteriolar occlusion, areas of capillary nonperfusion, delayed leakage from the retinal vasculature and optic disc edema.[74,75]

Indocyanine Angiography

It shows areas of hypofluorescence inferring that the choroidal vasculature is also involved.[76]

Electroretinography

Multifocal electroretinography (ERG) reveals depression in both a-wave and b-wave in the affected part, suggesting involvement of both the outer and inner retina.[77]

PATHOGENESIS

The pathogenesis has been controversial in the past times. In the original report titled *angiopathia retinae traumatica*, Purtscher postulated that the lesions were a due extravasation of lymph from the vessels after a sudden rise in intracranial tension.

Presently, the most accepted hypothesis emphasizes on microembolization, leading to precapillary arteriolar occlusion and infarction of retinal nerve fiber layer.[67,78] Sources of embolism described are fat emboli (e.g. long bone fractures), disseminated pancreatic proteases and free-fatty acids in the systemic circulation (acute pancreatitis) and leukoembolization (leukocyte aggregation and C5 complement activation resulting in secondary lymph extravasation).[79,80] In cases secondary to chest compression, battered baby syndrome, weight lifting or asphyxia, there is decreased venous return with sudden expansion of retinal veins leading to retinal hemorrhages, cotton–wool spots and sometimes Purtscher flecken.[51]

The primary pathogenic process lies in the precapillary arterioles,[81] and is further supported by the existence of the demarcation line in Purtscher flecken because if the size of emboli was small, it would lodge in the distal end of capillaries and cause cotton–wool spots.

HISTOPATHOLOGY

Purtscher retinopathy has a benign course and hence there is relatively less data from the histopathology studies.

Holló et al. described these changes in a patient with necrotizing pancreatitis who died after a 6-day interval.[81,82] They observed cotton–wool spots similar in appearance to other pathologies and that the entire retinal vasculature, including the vessels in and around the cotton-wool spots were not obstructed. Hence, they concluded that microembolization with resulting vascular obstruction and endothelial injury is not a prerequisite for the development of these cotton wool spots in cases of acute pancreatitis. Kincaid et al. also published the histopathological changes in a patient with acute pancreatitis but the interval between onset and examination was 23 days.[78] They noticed focal discrete areas of edema, with cystoid spaces, within the inner retinal layers and disruption of the normal architecture. Abrupt transition was present between the normal and affected retina. In the affected areas, there were more obvious changes in the outer retina as compared to inner retina, but the RPE and choroid were still within the normal limits. The emboli occluding retinal vessels were positive for periodic acid-Schiff and also stained positive for fibrin. Electron microscopy revealed that small arterioles with narrowed lumen contained protein like material placed centrally, which was considered to be in accordance with recanalized thrombi.

⊕ DIFFERENTIAL DIAGNOSIS

Important conditions to be ruled out include branch or central retinal artery occlusion and commotio retinae. History, thorough examination and diagnostic tests help in accurate diagnosis.

▤ TREATMENT

Owing to the benign course of disease, observation is the most recommended strategy. First step includes treating the underlying cause wherever known. Numerous authors[47,66,69,78] have reported no statistically significant difference in visual acuity gain between patients receiving no treatment and those getting high-dose corticosteroids. The conclusion held true even for longer studies regardless of the cause.[83,84]

Wang et al.[74] and Atabay et al.[83] have published successful results with the use of high-dose intravenous corticosteroids. They postulated that the high-dose corticosteroids stabilized damaged neuronal membrane and vessels, which resulted in partial recovery of neurons that have not yet been damaged irreversibly. Steroids also hinder activation of complement and granulocyte aggregation.[85,86]

Newer treatment modalities like Papaverine hydrochloride[84] and hyperbaric oxygen[87-89] have been suggested, but there is limited data.

PROGNOSIS

Visual recovery is variable and heterogeneous. Prognosis depends on the presenting visual acuity and it is noted that patients with a worse visual acuity at presentation are more likely to have persistent fundus changes at 1 month follow-up.[69] Other possible prognostic factors associated with a poor visual outcome include optic disc edema, leakage on FFA, choroidal hypoperfusion, outer retinal layers involvement and capillary nonperfusion areas.[67] The absence of development of macular edema is associated with better prognosis at 6 months. Duration of acute fundus changes, alone, is the main factor affecting the late prognosis.[71] In patients with severe necrotizing pancreatitis, development of Purtscher retinopathy indicates multiple-organ failure and poor clinical prognosis.[89]

HELLP SYNDROME

HELLP syndrome, associated with toxemia of pregnancy, is characterized by consumptive coagulopathy, specifically having the major symptoms of hemolysis (H), elevated liver enzymes (EL) and low-platelet count (LP). The incidence of the HELLP syndrome is reported to be between 0.2% and 0.6% of all pregnancies and in 4–12% of patients with pre-eclampsia. It typically occurs after 27th week of gestation or delivery or immediately postpartum in 15–30% of cases.[90-94] It is a microangiopathy like thrombotic thrombocytopenic purpura (TTP), although it may progress to disseminated intravascular coagulation (DIC) in about 20% patients. Other causes of morbidity include abruptio placentae (16%), acute renal failure (7%) or pulmonary edema (6%).[95] Death rate can be decreased to about 1% when adequately managed.

⚚ PATHOPHYSIOLOGY AND CLINICAL FEATURES

There are hemorrhages at all levels within the eye, including subconjunctival and also subcutaneous due to anemia and thrombocytopenia, which is usually severe. The hypercoagulable state typically leads to occlusion of choriocapillaris by fibrin–platelet clots.[96-99] Microthrombi in the choriocapillaris result in localized ischemic damage to the RPE, resulting in a dysfunction of the outer blood–retinal barrier and decreased ability of the RPE to transport fluid out of the subretinal space.[100] Fluid exudating from choroidal vessels passes through small defects in the RPE further extending into the subretinal space causing serous retinal detachments and choroidal thickening (Figs. 32.6A and B). Compression of choroidal vessels, due to extravasation in choroidal stroma, leads to ground glass appearance of the choroid.[101]

The visual loss from fluid accumulation and hemorrhage may recover following resolution as resorption occurs. There may be coexistent signs of hypertensive retinopathy like arteriovenous crossing, optic disc edema, hemorrhages, cotton–wool spots and Elschnig spots. The presence of serous retinal detachments is not a specific sign of any coagulopathy but may also be seen in pregnancy itself.

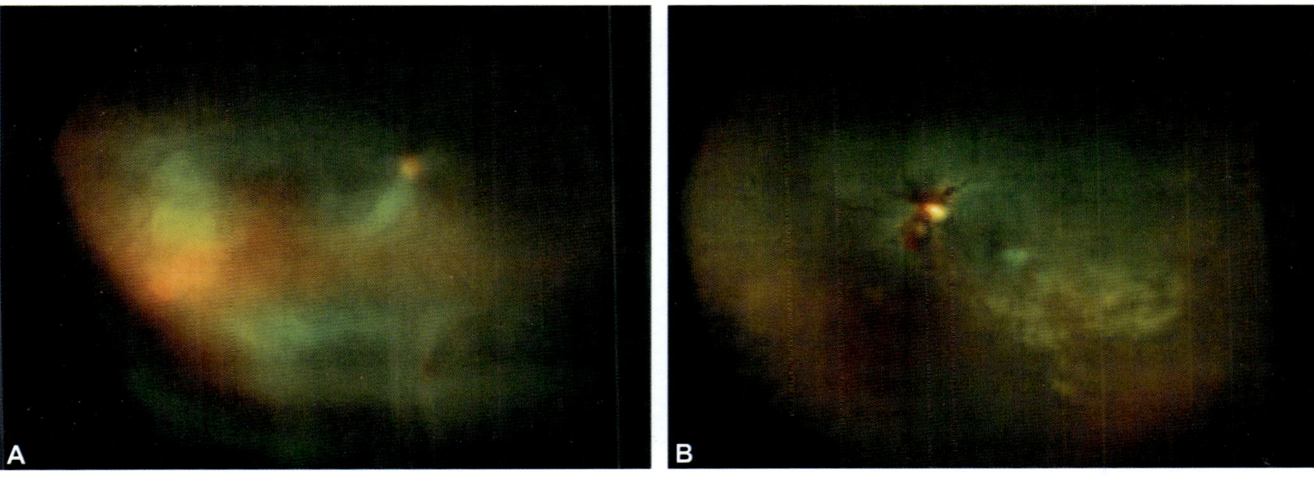

Figs. 32.6A and B: Clinical fundus image (A) Right eye showing massive exudative retinal detachment with characteristic hemorrhage; (B) Left eye of the same patient showing localized areas of early exudative retinal detachment.

REFERENCES

1. Duane TD. Valsalva hemorrhagic retinopathy. Trans Am Ophthalmology Soc. 1972;70:298-313.
2. Chandra P, Azad R, Pal N. Valsalva and Purtscher's retinopathy with optic neuropathy in compressive thoracic injury. Eye. 2005;19(8):914-5.
3. Tildsley J, Srinivasan S. Valsalva retinopathy. Postgrad Med J. 2009;85:110.
4. Choi SW, Lee SJ, Rah SH. Valsalva retinopathy associated with fiber optic gastroenteroscopy. Can J Ophthalmology. 2006;41(4):491-3.
5. Saricaoglu MS, Kalayci D, Guven D, et al. Decompression retinopathy and possible risk factors. Acta Ophthalmology. 2009;87(1):94-5.
6. Shukla D, Naresh KB, Kim R. Optical coherence tomography findings in Valsalva retinopathy. Am J Ophthalmology. 2005;140:134-6.
7. Khan MT, Saeed MU, Shehzad MS, et al. Nd:YAG laser treatment for Valsalva premacular hemorrhages: 6 month follow up: alternative management options for preretinal premacular hemorrhages in Valsalva retinopathy. Int Ophthalmology. 2008;28(5):325-7.
8. Terson A. De l'he´morrhagie dans le corps vitre au cours de l'he´morrhagie cerebrale. Clin Ophthalmology. 1900;6:309-12.
9. Litten M. Ueber Einige vom Allgemein-Klinischen Standpunkt aus Interessante Augenvera¨nderungen. Berl Klin Wochenschr. 1881;18:23-7.
10. Fahmy JA. Fundal haemorrhages in ruptured intracranial aneurysms. I. Material, frequency and morphology. Acta Ophthalmology. 1973;51:289-98.
11. Ness T, Janknecht P, Berghorn C. Frequency of ocular hemorrhages in patients with subarachnoidal hemorrhage. Graefes Arch Clin Exp Ophthalmology. 2005;243:859-62.
12. Medele RJ, Stummer W, Mueller AJ, et al. Terson's syndrome in subarachnoid hemorrhage and severe brain injury accompanied by acutely raised intracranial pressure. J Neurosurg. 1998;88:851-4.
13. Fountas KN, Kapsalaki EZ, Lee GP, et al. Terson hemorrhage in individuals suffering aneurysmal subarachnoid hemorrhage: predisposing factors and prognostic significance. J Neurosurg. 2008;109:439-44.
14. Pfausler B, Belcl R, Metzler R, et al. Terson's syndrome in spontaneous subarachnoid hemorrhage: a prospective study in 60 consecutive patients. J Neurosurg. 1996;85:392-4.
15. Kuhn F, Morris R, Witherspoon CD, et al. Terson syndrome. Results of vitrectomy and the significance of vitreous hemorrhage in patients with subarachnoid hemorrhage. Ophthalmology. 1998;105:472-7.
16. Middleton K, Esselman P, Lim PC. Terson syndrome: an underrecognized cause of reversible vision loss in patients with subarachnoid hemorrhage. Am J Phys Med Rehabil. 2012;91(3):271-4.
17. Manschot WA. The fundus oculi in subarachnoid haemorrhage. Acta Ophthalmology. 1944;22:281-99.
18. Ko F, Knox DL. The ocular pathology of Terson's syndrome. Ophthalmology. 2010;117(7):1423-9.e2
19. Shaw HEJ, Landers MB, Sydnor CF. The significance of intraocular hemorrhages due to subarachnoid hemorrhage. Ann Ophthalmology. 1977;9:1403-5.
20. Hedges TR Jr, Walsh FE. Optic nerve sheath and subhyaloid hemorrhage as a complication of angiocardiography. AMA Arch Ophthalmology. 1955;54:425-7.
21. Castren JA. Pathogenesis and treatment of Terson syndrome. Acta Ophthalmology. 1963;41:430-4.
22. Ballantyne AJ. The ocular manifestations of spontaneous subarachnoid haemorrhage. Br J Ophthalmology. 1943;27:383-414.
23. Ogawa T, Kitaoka T, Dake Y, et al. Terson syndrome: a case report suggesting the mechanism of vitreous hemorrhage. Ophthalmology. 2001;108:1654-6.
24. Srinivasan S, Kyle G. Subinternal limiting membrane and subhyaloid haemorrhage in Terson syndrome: the macular 'double ring' sign [letter]. Eye. 2006;20:1099-101.
25. Song D, Dunaief JL. Retinal iron homeostasis in health and disease. Front Aging Neurosci. 2013;5:24.
26. Pobereskin LH. Incidence and outcome of subarachnoid haemorrhage: a retrospective population based study. J Neurol Neurosurg Psychiatry. 2001;70:340-3.
27. Bamford J, Dennis M, Sandercock P, et al. The frequency, causes and timing of death within 30 days of a first stroke: the Oxfordshire Community Stroke Project. J Neurol Neurosurg Psychiatry. 1990;53:824-9.

28. Fahmy JA. Symptoms and signs of intracranial aneurysms with particular reference to retinal haemorrhage. Acta Ophthalmology. 1972;50:129-36.

29. Rubowitz A, Desai U. Nontraumatic macular holes associated with Terson syndrome. Retina. 2006;26:230-2.

30. Yokoi M, Kase M, Hyodo T, et al. Epiretinal membrane formation in Terson syndrome. Jpn J Ophthalmology. 1997;41:168-73.

31. Sharma T, Gopal L, Biswas J, et al. Results of vitrectomy in Terson syndrome. Ophthalmic Surg Lasers. 2002;33:195-9.

32. Keithahn MA, Bennett SR, Cameron D, et al. Retinal folds in Terson syndrome. Ophthalmology. 1993;100:1187-90.

33. Ritland JS, Syrdalen P, Eide N, et al. Outcome of vitrectomy in patients with Terson syndrome. Acta Ophthalmology Scand. 2002;80:172-5.

34. Velikay M, Datlinger P, Stolba U, et al. Retinal detachment with severe proliferative vitreoretinopathy in Terson syndrome. Ophthalmology. 1994;101:35-7.

35. McCarron MO, Alberts MJ, McCarron P. A systematic review of Terson's syndrome: frequency and prognosis after subarachnoid haemorrhage. J Neurol Neurosurg Psychiatry. 2004;75(3):491-3.

36. Murjaneh S, Hale JE, Mishra S, et al. Terson's syndrome: surgical outcome in relation to entry site pathology. Br J Ophthalmology. 2006;90(4):512-3.

37. Garfinkle AM, Danys IR, Nicolle DA, et al. Terson's syndrome: a reversible cause of blindness following subarachnoid hemorrhage. J Neurosurg. 1992;76:766-71.

38. Biousse V, Mendicino ME, Simon DJ, et al. The ophthalmology of intracranial vascular abnormalities. Am J Ophthalmology. 1998;125:527-44.

39. Spraul CW, Grossniklaus HE. Major review, vitreous haemorrhage. Surv Ophthalmology. 1997;42:3-39.

40. Gnanaraj L, Tyagi AK, Cottrell DG, et al. Referral delay and ocular surgical outcome in Terson syndrome. Retina. 2000;20:374-7.

41. Abdelkader E, Lois N. Internal limiting membrane peeling in vitreo-retinal surgery. Surv Ophthalmology. 2008;53:368-96.

42. Daus W, Kasmann B, Alexandridis E. Terson syndrome. Complicated clinical course [in German]. Ophthalmologe. 1992;89:77-81.

43. Lewis H, Resnick SC, Flannery JG, et al. Tissue plasminogen activator treatment of experimental subretinal hemorrhage. Am J Ophthalmology. 1991;111:197-204.

44. Hillenkamp J, Surguch V, Framme C, et al. Management of submacular hemorrhage with intravitreal versus subretinal injection of recombinant tissue plasminogen activator. Graefes Arch Clin Exp Ophthalmology. 2010;248:5-11.

45. Ulbig MW, Mangouritsas G, Rothbacher HH, et al. Long-term results after drainage of premacular subhyaloid hemorrhage into the vitreous with a pulsed Nd:YAG laser. Arch Ophthalmology. 1998;116:1465-9.

46. Skevas C, Czorlich P, Knospe V, et al. Terson's syndrome-rate and surgical approach in patients with subarachnoid hemorrhage: a prospective interdisciplinary study. Ophthalmology. 2014;121(8):1628-33.

47. Purtscher O. Noch unbekannte befunde nach schadel trauma. Ber Dtsch Ophthalmology Ges. 1910;36:294-301.

48. Inkeles DM, Walsh JB. Retinal fat emboli as sequela to acute pancreatitis. Am J Ophthalmology. 1975;80(5):935-8.

49. Chuang EL, Miller FS, Kalina RE. Retinal lesions following long bone fractures. Ophthalmology. 1985;92:370-4.

50. Kocak N, Kaynak S, Kaynak T, et al. Unilateral Purtscher-like retinopathy after weight-lifting. Eur J Ophthalmology. 2003;13:395-7.

51. Marr WG, Marr EG. Some observations on Purtscher's disease: traumatic retinal angiopathy. Am J Ophthalmology. 1962;54:693-705.

52. Tomasi LG, Rosman NP. Purtscher's retinopathy in the battered child syndrome. Am J Dis Child. 1975;129(11):1335-7.

53. Carrera CRL, Pierre LM, Medina FMC, et al. Purtscher-like retinopathy associated with acute pancreatitis. Sao Paulo Med J. 2005;123(6):289-91.

54. Tabandeh H, Rosenfeld PJ, Alexandrakis G, et al. Purtscher-like retinopathy associated with pancreatic adenocarcinoma. Am J Ophthalmology. 1999;128:650-2.

55. Stoumbos VD, Klein ML, Goodman S. Purtscher-like retinopathy in chronic renal failure. Ophthalmology. 1992;99:1833-9.

56. Blodi BA, Johnson MW, Gass JD, et al. Purtscher's-like retinopathy after childbirth. Ophthalmology. 1990;97:1654-9.

57. Bader-Meunier B, Monnet D, Barnerias C, et al. Thrombotic microangiopathy and Purtscher-like retinopathy as a rare presentation of juvenile dermatomyositis. Pediatrics. 2012;129(3):e821-4.

58. Roden D, Fitzpatrick G, O'Donoghue H, et al. Purtscher's retinopathy and fat embolism. Br J Ophthalmology. 1989;73:677-9.

59. Scotton WJ, Kohler K, Babar J, et al. Fat embolism syndrome with Purtscher's retinopathy. Am J Respir Crit Care Med. 2013;187(1):106.

60. Parc C. Purtscher-like retinopathy as an initial presentation of a thrombotic microangiopathy associated with antineoplastic therapy. Am J Hematol. 2007;82:486-8.

61. Wilkinson WS, Morgan CM, Baruh E, et al. Retinal and choroidal vascular occlusion secondary to corticosteroid embolisation. Br J Ophthalmology. 1989;73:32-4.

62. Lemagne JM, Michiels X, Van Causenbroeck S, et al. Purtscher-like retinopathy after retrobulbar anesthesia. Ophthalmology. 1990;97:859-61.

63. Lauer AK, Klein ML, Kovarik WD, et al. Hemolytic uremic syndrome associated with Purtscher-like retinopathy. Arch Ophthalmology. 1998;116:1119-20.

64. Patel MR, Bains AK, O'Hara JP, et al. Purtscher's retinopathy as the initial sign of thrombotic thrombocytopenic purpura/hemolytic uremic syndrome. Arch Ophthalmology. 2001;119:1388-9.

65. Myers JP, Di Bisceglie AM, Mann ES. Cryoglobulinemia associated with Purtscher-like retinopathy. Am J Ophthalmology. 2001;131:802-4.

66. Miguel IM, Henriques F, Azevedo LFR, et al. Systematic review of Purtscher's and Purtscher-like retinopathies. Eye (Lond). 2013;27(1):1-13.

67. Michaelson IC, Campbell ACP. The anatomy of the finer retinal vessels. Trans Ophthalmology Soc UK. 1940;60:71-111.

68. Agrawal A, McKibbin MA. Purtscher's and Purtscher-like retinopathies: a review. Surv Ophthalmology. 2006;51(2):129-36.

69. Agrawal A, McKibbin M. Purtscher's retinopathy: epidemiology, clinical features and outcome. Br J Ophthalmology. 2007;91(11):1456-9.

70. Holak HM, Holak S. Prognostic factors for visual outcome in Purtscher retinopathy. Surv Ophthalmology. 2007;52(1):117-8; author reply page 118-9.

71. Giani A, Deiro AP, Sabella P, et al. Spectral domain-optical coherence tomography and fundus autofluorescence findings in a case of Purtscher-Like retinopathy. Retin Cases Brief Rep. 2010;5(2):167-70.

72. Soliman W, Zibrandtsen N, Jørgensen T, et al. Sequels of Purtscher's retinopathy imaged by enhanced optical coherence tomography. Acta Ophthalmology Scand. 2007;85(4):450-3.

73. Kincaid MC, Green WR, Knox DL, et al. A clinicopathological case report of retinopathy of pancreatitis. Br J Ophthalmology. 1982;66(4):219-26. [online] Available from: http://www.

pubmedcentral.nih.gov/articlerender.fcgi?artid = 1039760&tool = pmcentrez&rendertype = abstract. [Accessed December, 2017].

74. Wang A, Yen M, Liu J. Pathogenesis and neuroprotective treatment in Purtscher's retinopathy. Japanese J Ophtalmol. 1998;42:318-22.

75. Gomez-Ulla, Ferte B, Torreiro MG, et al. Choroidal vascular abnormality in Purtscher's retinopathy shown by indocyanine green angiography. Am J Ophthalmology. 1996;122(2):261-3.

76. Haq F, Vajaranant T, Szlyk J, et al. Sequential multifocal electroretinogram findings in a case of Purtscher-like Retinopathy. Am J Ophthalmology. 2002;134(1):125-8.

77. Sellami D, Ben-Zina B, Jelliti B, et al. Purtscher-like retinopathy in systemic lupus erythematosus. Two cases. J Fr Ophtalmol. 2002;25(1):52-5.

78. Beckingsale AB, Rosenthal AR. Early fundus fluorescein angiographic findings and sequelae in traumatic retinopathy: case report. Br J Ophthalmology. 1983;67(2):119-23. [online] Available from: http://www.pubmedcentral.nih.gov/articlerender. fcgi?artid=1039979&tool=pmcentrez&rendertype=abstract. [Accessed December, 2017].

79. Craddock PR, Hammerschmidt D, White JG, et al. Complement (C5a)-Induced Granulocyte Aggregation in Vitro. J Clin Invest. 1977;60(1):260-4.

80. Shapiro I, Jacob H. Leukoembolization in ocular vascular occlusion. Ann Ophtalmol. 1982;14:60-2.

81. Holló G, Popik E. Is retinopathy in pancreatitis caused by leukocyte emboli? Acta Ophthalmology. 1992;70(6):820-3.

82. Holló G, Bobek I. Clinicopathology of a case with retinopathy of pancreatitis. Acta Ophthalmology Scand. 1993;71(3):422-5.

83. Atabay C, Kansu T, Nurlu G. Late visual recovery after intravenous methylprednisolone treatment of Purtscher's retinopathy. Ann Ophthalmology. 1993;25(9):330-3.

84. Weinberger AW, Siekmann UP, Wolf S, et al. Treatment of Acute Central Retinal Artery Occlusion (CRAO) by Hyperbaric Oxygenation Therapy (HBO)—Pilot study with 21 patients. Klin Monbl Augenheilkd. 2002;219(10):728-34.

85. Hammerschmidt DE, White JG, Craddock PR, et al. Corticosteroids inhibit complement-induced granulocyte aggregation. A possible mechanism for their efficacy in shock states. J Clin Invest. 1979;63(4):798-803.

86. Frayser R, Hickam JB. Effect of vasodilator drugs on the retinal blood flow in man. Arch Ophthalmology. 1965;73(5):640-2.

87. Bojić L, Ivanisević M, Gosović G. Hyperbaric oxygen therapy in two patients with non-arteritic anterior optic neuropathy who did not respond to prednisone. Undersea Hyperb Med. 2002;29(2):86-92.

88. Kiryu J, Ogura Y. Hyperbaric oxygen treatment for macular edema in retinal vein occlusion: relation to severity of retinal leakage. Ophthalmologica. 1996;210:168-70.

89. Holló G, Tarjányi M, Varga M, et al. Retinopathy of pancreatitis indicates multiple-organ failure and poor prognosis in severe acute pancreatitis. Acta Ophthalmology. 1994;72(1):114-7.

90. Stella C, Malik K, Sibai B. HELLP syndrome: an atypical presentation. Am J Obstet Gynecol. 2008;198:e6-e8.

91. Martin JN Jr, Magann EF, Blake PG. Analysis of 454 pregnancies with severe preeclampsia/eclampsia/ HELLP syndrome using the 3-class system of classification. Am J Obstret Gynecol. 1993;68:386.

92. Martin JN Jr, Magann EF. HELLP syndrome current principles and recommended practice. Curr Obstet Med. 1996;4:129-75.

93. Sibai BM, Ramamdan MK, Usta I, et al. Maternal morbidity and mortality in 442 pregnancies with HELLP syndrome. Am J Obstet Gynecol. 1993;169 1000-6.

94. Ukomadu C, Greenberger N, Blumberg R, et al. Chapter 8: Hepatic complications of Pregnancy. Current Diagnosis and treatment: Gastroenterology, Hepatology and Endoscopy. New York: McGraw Hills and Company; 2009. p 98.

95. Barton JR, Sibai BM. Diagnosis and management of hemolysis, elevated liver enzymes, and low platelets syndrome. Clin Perinatol. 2004;31:807-33.

96. Majji A, Bhatia K, Mathai A. Spontaneous bilateral peripapillay, subhyalid and vitreous hemorrhage with severe anemia secondary to idiopathic thrombocytopenic purpura. Ind J Ophthalmology. 2010;58:234-6.

97. Karagiannis D, Gregor Z. Valsalva retinopathy associated with idiopathic thrombocytopenic purpura and positive anti-phospholipid antibodies. Eye. 2006;20:1447-9.

98. Sodhi PK, Jose R. Subconjunctival hemorrhage: the first presenting clinical feature of idiopathic thrombocytopenic purpura. Jpn J Ophthalmology. 2003;47:316-18.

99. Okuda A, Inoue M, Shinoda K, et al. Massive bilateral vitreoretinal hemorrhage in patient with chronic refractory idiopathic thrombocytopenic purpura. Graefes Arch Clin Exp Ophthalmology. 2005;243:1190-3.

100. Narayakkara P, Gans RO, Reichert-Thoen J, et al. Serous retinal detachment as an early presentation of thrombotic thrombocytopenic purpura. Eur J Intern Med 2000;11:286-8.

101. Kasai A, Sugano Y, Maruko I, et al. Choroidal morphology in a patient with HELLP syndrome. Retin Cases Brief Rep. 2016; 10(3):273-277.

Pediatric Retinal Disease

Chapter 33

Etiopathogenesis, Clinical Features and Screening of Retinopathy of Prematurity

Parijat Chandra, Nitesh Salunkhe

INTRODUCTION

Retinopathy of prematurity (ROP) is a retinal vasoproliferative disorder affecting preterm and low-birth-weight babies. Over the years, it has emerged as a major cause of childhood blindness across the world and is now emerging in epidemic proportions in developing countries due to mushrooming of neonatal intensive care units (NICU) and survival of more preterm babies. Lack of proper training and poor NICU practices is leading to the development of ROP in bigger babies as well.[1] Lack of awareness amongst pediatricians and ophthalmologists is causing poor coverage of ROP screening programs, leading to advanced ROP and a large proportion of ROP-related blindness.[2]

It is estimated that globally at least 50,000 children suffer from blindness due to ROP, and ROP is a major cause of blindness not only in developed countries but is also a significantly cause of visual handicap in many middle-income countries.[3] An assessment of the ROP burden at the global and regional levels suggests that in the year 2010, 184,700 preterm babies developed any stage of ROP, 20,000 of these became blind from ROP, and 12,300 developed mild/moderate visual impairment.[4] An alarming sign is that 65% of these were born in middle-income countries. The South Asia region is reported to have the highest number of live births (37.1 million, 28%) and largest number of preterm births (4.95 million, 33%) are reported, which predisposes an estimated 79,600 babies to have high risk of developing ROP annually.[4]

EPIDEMIOLOGY

Retinopathy of prematurity is a growing concern for childhood blindness and the incidence is growing worldwide as more preterm babies continue to survive. However, ROP occurrence is exceptionally low in countries like Sub-Saharan Africa with high infant mortality rates, where survival of premature babies is less.

The first epidemic of ROP occurred in the 1940s and 1950s when unmonitored oxygen therapy was used for treatment of respiratory ailments in premature infants. Though it improved survival, it led to an uncontrolled rise of ROP and it emerged as an important cause of childhood blindness during that time in the developed world.[5]

Since high O_2 supplementation increased the risk of retinopathy of prematurity, NICUs dramatically decreased the use of high oxygen concentration, and though this decreased ROP blindness, it led to an increase in mortality and morbidity in the following decades. With the emergence of advanced NICUs in the early 1970s, a second epidemic followed by improved survival in high-income countries.[6] This was controlled following improvements in NICU facilities and the introduction of retinal ablative therapy using cryotherapy and laser.

Now with improvement in NICU care in middle-income countries, more preterm babies continue to survive, but poor NICU practices have led to larger babies also developing ROP. Therefore, in these last two decades, a third epidemic of ROP has ensued in many countries.[7-9]

PATHOGENESIS

During the course of normal retinal vascularization, the retinal vessels start to develop and grow outwards from the optic disc at 16 weeks gestation and proceed towards the retinal periphery anteriorly. The retinal vessels reach the edge of the nasal ora serrata by 36 weeks gestation age and the temporal ora serrata by 40 weeks gestation age.

Some popular theories to explain the pathogenesis of ROP are as follows:

- *The classical theory:* This theory was proposed by Ashton and Patz. They suggested that high concentrations of oxygen over a sustained period causes severe vasoconstriction of immature vessels and often leads to permanent vascular occlusion. Even if partial vessel reopening occurs, it continues to incite the development of neovascularization and abnormal fibrovascular proliferation which can lead to retinal hemorrhages and tractional retinal detachment.[10-12]

- *Spindle cell theory:* According to this theory proposed by Kretzer, hyperoxia leads to free oxygen diffusion across the retina from the choroidal vasculature, which causes free radical damage of the spindle cells in the avascular retina. The damaged spindle cells stop forming inner retinal vessels by canalization, stop migrating peripherally and start secreting angiogenic factors. Thereafter, myofibroblasts begin to differentiate from stem cells and form contractile sheets which invaded the vitreous and cause tractional retinal detachment.[13,14]

The development of ROP is attributed to multiple factors in the antenatal, natal, and postnatal period of the preterm neonate. It is suggested that the disease progresses in two phases[15] as follows:

1. *Phase I:* Occurs around 22–30 weeks of postmenstrual age, wherein relative hyperoxia exacerbated by supplemental oxygen leads to vasoconstriction, and continuous exposure can lead to permanent vascular closure, which leads to stoppage of peripheral retinal vascular growth. This phase is typically characterized by low vascular endothelial growth factor (VEGF) levels.
2. *Phase II:* This phase occurs around 31–44 weeks of postmenstrual age. There is relative hypoxia which induces a rapid increase in VEGF and other angiogenic factors which were suppressed in phase I. This leads to rapid neovascularization, which can lead to vitreous hemorrhage and tractional retinal detachment.

The understanding of these phases of ROP has allowed targeting of VEGF levels for ROP treatment using various pharmacological drugs like bevacizumab.

RISK FACTORS AND PREVENTION

It is well known that ROP occurs in low-birth-weight and low-gestation-age babies; the lower the gestation age or birth weight, higher is the risk for development of ROP. Besides these two most important risk factors, there are many other risk factors which predispose preterm babies to the development of ROP. Several risk factors have been reported in literature[16,17] like prolonged oxygen therapy, low Apgar score, sepsis, anemia, necrotizing enterocolitis, intraventricular hemorrhage, respiratory distress syndrome, bronchopulmonary dysplasia, multiple gestations, multiple blood transfusions, hypotension, hypothermia, assisted conception, etc.

It is also well known that ROP can be prevented. The NICUs which follow best neonatal practices have very low incidence of ROP, and even if ROP does occur, it is of very low severity and rarely needs treatment. The most important NICU practice which helps to reduce the occurrence of ROP is judicious oxygen therapy.[18,19] Oxygen should be considered as a drug and only used when it is absolutely necessary. It is essential to maintain tight recommended oxygen saturation levels while preventing fluctuations with episodes of hyperoxia or hypoxia. Every NICU should maintain written policies and train their staff for same. It is important to use blenders to ensure proper control of oxygen delivered. Judicious use of blood transfusion is necessary. Some other useful options[4] are delayed cord clamping, preventing hypothermia, avoiding 100% oxygen, vitamin E supplementation, and breastfeeding. Antenatal administration of steroids[20] helps in accelerated fetal lung maturation and might help to prevent respiratory distress and intraventricular hemorrhage, both of which are considered as high-risk factors for the development of ROP.

 CLINICAL FEATURES AND CLASSIFICATION

There was a need to create a universal classification of ROP to facilitate communication between ROP teams and to develop standardized criteria which could be followed across the world. It had to be modern, universally acceptable, and easy to understand and implement. Therefore, the International Classification of Retinopathy of Prematurity (ICROP) group suggested a classification which was first published in 1984[21] and later expanded in 1987.[22] It was subsequently updated in 2005[23] with new terminology as well.

Retinopathy of Prematurity Zones

Since the normal vascularization develops from the optic disc and proceeds outwards towards the retinal periphery, the group described ROP as occurring in three concentric zones (Fig. 33.1):

1. *Zone I:* This is the innermost zone and the circle extends from the center of the disc with a radius of twice the distance from disc to macula. The most severe disease occurs in this zone.
2. *Zone II:* This zone is outside zone I. It extends from the nasal edge of zone I to ora serrata nasally and up to the retinal equator temporally. This is the commonest zone where ROP appears.
3. *Zone III:* This is the outermost zone, outside zone II. It includes the temporal crescent of retina anterior to zone II and has the least severe disease.

Retinopathy of Prematurity Stages

The ICROP group described five stages depending on the severity and progression. If the child is examined early enough, then probably the examiner will observe normal retinal vessels proceeding from the disc towards the retinal periphery, and this is termed as immature retina. However, when ROP develops, following stages are described (Figs. 33.2 to 33.6):

- *Stage 1 (demarcation line):* This is the earliest sign signifying the appearance of ROP. It is characterized by the development of a flat white line at the junction of vascularized and avascular retina. The demarcation line can develop in any zone depending upon the level of prematurity.

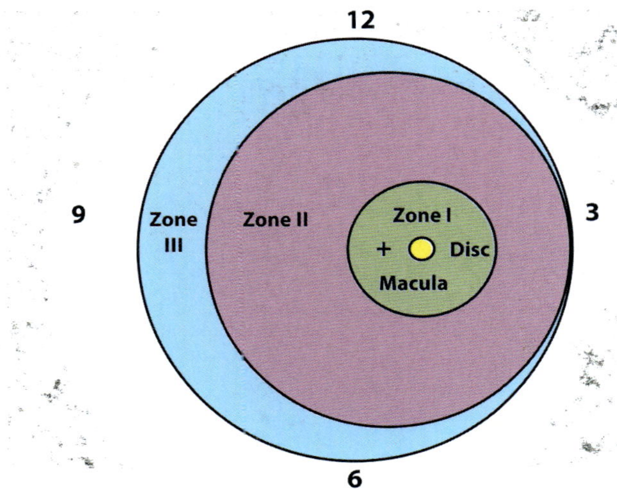

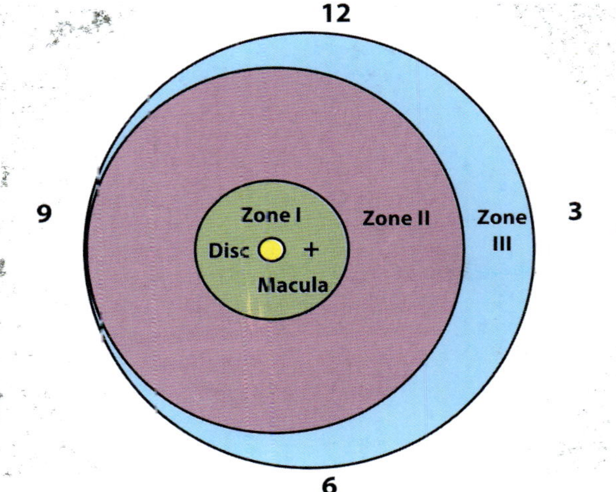

Fig. 33.1: Zones in retinopathy of prematurity classification.

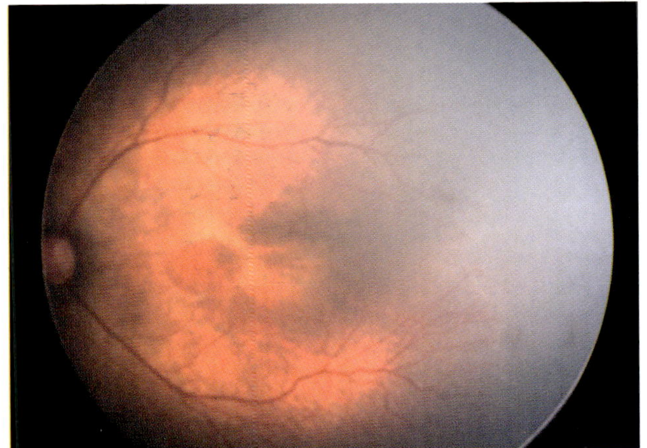

Fig. 33.2: Stage 1 retinopathy of prematurity (ROP) with demarcation line.

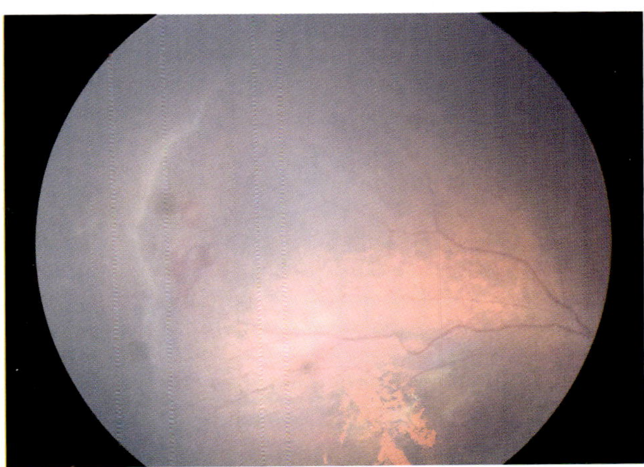

Fig. 33.3: Stage 2 retinopathy of prematurity (ROP)—demarcation ridge.

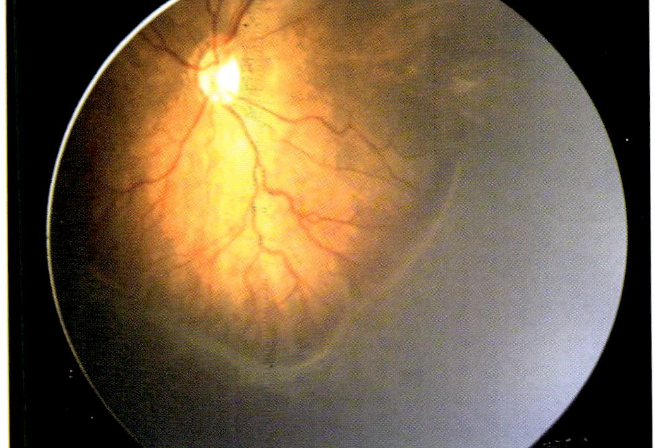

Fig. 33.4: Stage 3 retinopathy of prematurity (ROP)—extraretinal fibrovascular neovascularization.

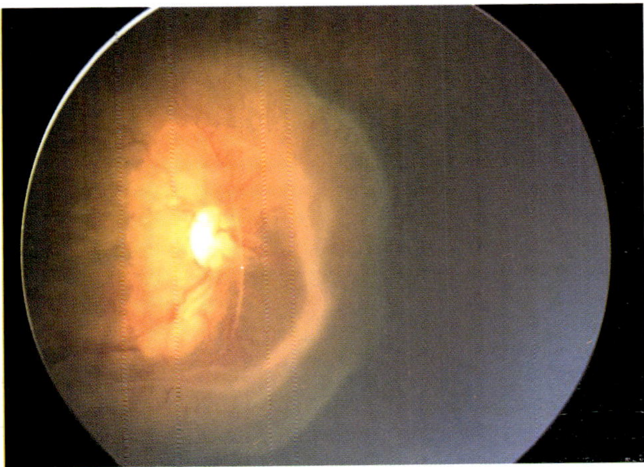

Fig. 33.5: Stage 4 retinopathy of prematurity (ROP)—subtotal retinal detachment.

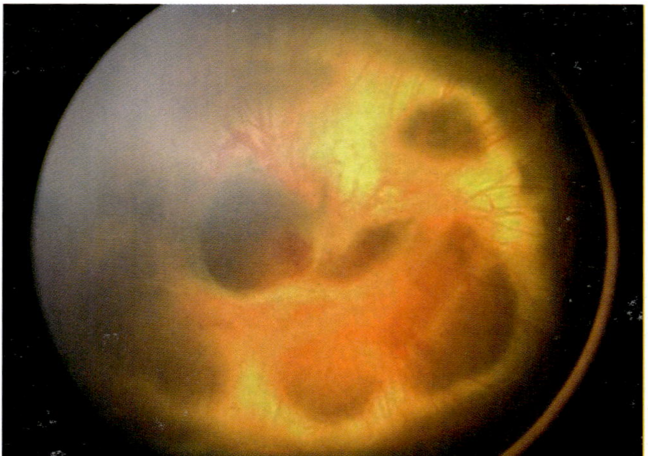

Fig. 33.6: Stage 5 retinopathy of prematurity (ROP)—total retinal detachment.

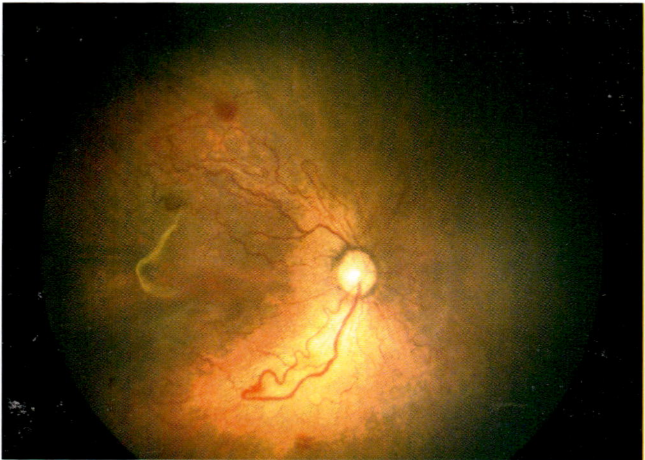

Fig. 33.7: Aggressive posterior retinopathy of prematurity (ROP) in the right eye with severe plus disease in zone I. Note unclear demarcation between vascular and avascular retina.

- *Stage 2 (demarcation ridge):* In this next stage, the demarcation line gains height and width and progresses to become a ridge which is a pink or white elevation of the thickened tissue. Some neovascular tufts can sometimes be seen posterior to this ridge.
- *Stage 3 (extraretinal fibrovascular proliferation):* The highlight of this stage is the development of neovascular tissue into and above the ridge. The vessels can also grow into the vitreous and can lead to patches of vitreous hemorrhage.
- *Stage 4 (partial retinal detachment):* As fibrovascular proliferation into the vitreous cavity pulls on the retina, it causes a tractional retinal detachment. It can be partial retinal detachment without foveal involvement (stage 4a) or with foveal involvement (stage 4b).
- *Stage 5 (total retinal detachment):* The configuration of such detachments are usually funnel-shaped, which may be classified on the basis of ultrasonography as open or closed anteriorly and open or closed posteriorly.

Some other important terminologies associated with ROP are given below.

Plus Disease

It is defined as venous dilation and arterial tortuosity of the posterior pole retinal vessels, which is comparable or more than the standard plus photograph.[21] The Early Treatment for Retinopathy of Prematurity (ETROP) group[24] defined plus disease as at least two quadrants of dilation and tortuosity of the posterior retinal blood vessels.

It is often associated with iris congestion, pupillary rigidity, and vitreous haze. When pupils do not dilate during screening, despite adequate instillation of dilating drops, then plus disease must always be considered and it is essential to look at the posterior pole in all these cases to rule out severe variants like aggressive posterior retinopathy of prematurity (APROP). It indicates severity of ROP and is often used on follow-up to track progression/regression of the disease (Fig. 33.7).

Preplus Disease

This is indicative of vascular abnormality at the posterior pole that is not sufficient for being diagnosed under plus disease, but there is more tortuosity of arteries and dilatation of veins than what is normally observed. Preplus disease can progress later to become plus disease which is an indication of increased severity and activity of ROP.

Aggressive Posterior Retinopathy of Prematurity (APROP)

APROP was a new terminology suggested in the last update by ICROP group.[23] It is typically seen in very small babies with high-risk factors. It was meant to replace various confusing terminologies earlier being used in literature like fulminate ROP or rush disease, which basically signified a very severe disease which progressed despite laser treatment and had a poor prognosis, if not treated in time.

APROP is a severe form of ROP that characteristically occurs in posterior zone II or zone I. Typically, because the retina is vascularized in a very small area, severe neovascularization occurs quickly. The junction between the vascular and avascular retina is featureless, and there is presence of avascular loops and shunts instead of a well-defined ridge. However plus disease is very significant and contrasts with the quiet junction. The disease quickly develops flat neovascularization and rapidly progresses to advanced stages of ROP. Severe plus disease leads to poorly dilating pupils and a high index of suspicion for APROP should always be considered (Fig. 33.7).

Type 1 and 2 Retinopathy of Prematurity

The ETROP group[24] classified ROP into 2 types based on the ROP findings. Type 1 ROP needs treatment and includes eyes with zone I, any stage with plus; zone I, stage 3 without plus; and zone II, stage 2–3 with plus. Type 2 ROP needs close follow-up and includes eyes with zone I, stage 1–2 without plus; and zone II stage 3 without plus.

Threshold Retinopathy of Prematurity

It is defined as stage 3 + ROP in zone I-II, occupying at least 5 contiguous clock hours or 8 noncontiguous clock hours of the retina, with the presence of plus disease. This was considered the treatment indication in several earlier studies but led to suboptimal outcomes, but now laser treatment is done earlier at prethreshold stage as per the ETROP treatment criteria.[24]

Prethreshold Retinopathy of Prematurity

It is defined as any stage of ROP in zone I with plus disease and ROP stage 3+ with 3 contiguous or 5 noncontiguous clock hours of involvement of retina in zone II, but less than threshold stage. The ETROP group considered a variant of this for the new treatment indications which are now being followed worldwide.

Thus, it is essential to be aware of the epidemiology and pathogenesis of ROP to better understand the ROP disease process. Every ROP specialist must be well-versed with universally standardized classification and terminologies to perform optimal ROP screening, ensure proper documentation, and advise timely ROP treatment, if needed.

SCREENING OF RETINOPATHY OF PREMATURITY

Timely screening of premature infants at risk of developing ROP is important as early detection and treatment can result in improved visual outcomes. India has the highest number of preterm births in the world, but very few NICUs in our country have effective ROP screening programs.

This is mainly due to a lack of awareness and collaboration among ophthalmologists and pediatricians to run ROP screening programs at their facilities. Therefore, a large number of premature babies continue to survive but fail to undergo ROP screening or treatment in time, which is leading to a large number of these babies with advanced ROP presenting to tertiary eye care facilities. Advanced stage 5 ROP has a poor prognosis, and there are very few advanced vitreoretinal surgical setups and trained ROP surgeons in the country to manage these babies.

The only way to detect and treat ROP in time is to run an ROP screening program in every NICU. As a large number of NICUs continue to mushroom across the country, with poor neonatal care practices—ROP is reaching epidemic proportions and has emerged as an important public health problem. There is an urgent need to develop ROP screening centers across the country to prevent this important cause of childhood blindness.

Whom to Screen?

It is very important to establish which babies need to be screened for ROP. Screening guidelines for ROP vary throughout the world with different cutoffs for birth weight and gestational age. This is because in developed countries ROP appears in very low-birth-weight babies, but in developing countries, while very small babies continue to develop ROP, even larger heavier birth weight babies develop ROP because of poor NICU practices.[1] This poses a unique challenge because it brings many more babies into the screening program.

The aim of every ROP screening program is to include all babies at risk for developing ROP, therefore the same guidelines cannot be used in developing and developed countries. In countries where detailed statistics about ROP profile are available, they devise their own ROP screening guidelines based on their own data. Thus, there is a wide variation of ROP screening guidelines observed across the world.

The American guidelines[25] recommend screening for infants with less than and equal to 1,500 g birth weight and/or gestation age of 30 weeks or less; though bigger babies can also be screened with a birth weight between 1,500 g and 2,000 g or gestational age of more than 30 weeks with an unstable clinical course, including those requiring cardiorespiratory support and who are believed by their attending pediatrician or neonatologist to be at high risk for ROP.

In India, most eye care facilities usually follow the National Neonatology Forum (NNF) guidelines[26] which state that ROP screening should be performed in all preterm neonates who are less than 34 weeks gestation age and/or less than 1,750 g birth weight. Larger babies between 34 weeks and 36 weeks gestational age or birth weight between 1,750 g and 2,000 g can also be screened, if they have risk factors for ROP.

Recently, the Government of India ROP expert groups have recommended that all babies born less than 34 weeks gestation age or less than 2,000 g birth weight should be screened; while those more than 34 weeks can also be screened, if associated ROP risk factors are present. The risk factors to consider are poor postnatal weight gain, cardiorespiratory support, prolonged oxygen requirement, respiratory distress syndrome, chronic lung disease, blood transfusion, fetal hemorrhage, sepsis, exchange transfusion, intraventricular hemorrhage, and apnea.

When to Screen?

It is very important to decide when to start screening the babies which have been identified to undergo ROP screening. The guidelines again differ across developing and developed countries to screen babies depending on the ROP profile of the region.

The American screening guidelines[25] suggest that we should screen all babies at 31 weeks of postconceptional age or 4 weeks after birth whichever is later. The Indian guidelines proposed by the NNF[26] suggest that the first screening should be performed not later than 4 weeks of age. However, in very small infants born less than 28 weeks or less than 1,200 g birth weight, they can be screened as early as 2–3 weeks of age, to enable early identification of severe variants like APROP.

Recently, the Government of India ROP expert groups have recommended first screening of all preterm babies eligible for ROP screening be performed within thirty days of birth.

Where to Screen?

Screening should be performed preferably in a NICU setting, under the supervision of a pediatrician or neonatologist. The NICU team identifies the babies to be screened and keeps them ready for examination on a particular day and time of the week. The pediatric nurse coordinates all ROP activities and ensures all ROP screening forms are properly filled and signed by the visiting teams.

For discharged babies, at every visit, the pediatrician should assess the health of the infant and ROP screening is incorporated into the routine follow-up visits of the baby to the NICU. The NICU setting helps the pediatricians or the pediatrics nurse to monitor the baby during ROP screening and deal with any emergency during the screening procedure.

How to Follow-up?

It is very important that babies in the ROP screening program continue to follow-up on a regular basis, so as to detect progressive changes in the disease in a timely manner. A large number of babies will undergo spontaneous regression characterized by clearance of tunica vasculosa lentis, improved pupillary dilation, reduction in ridge width/height, and resolution of plus disease.

The ROP screening program is designed to pick up treatable disease at an early stage, so that, if laser treatment is needed as per ETROP[24] protocol guidelines[24], the outcomes are very good. ETROP classified ROP into two types based on the findings. Type 1 ROP needs treatment and includes eyes with zone I, any stage with plus; zone I, stage 3 without plus; and zone II, stage 2–3 with plus. Type 2 ROP needs close follow-up and includes eyes with zone I, stage 1–2 without plus; zone II, and stage 3 without plus.

It is essential that parents realize the need for follow-up and proper counseling is mandatory after examination. Proper parent counseling is highly essential as many times babies are lost to follow-up and continue to develop advanced disease with poor visual outcomes.

The time and interval for revisit and re-examination depend upon the age at examination and the observed retinal findings and usually, it is advised to screen at every 1–2 weeks. If laser treatment is recommended, it is usually performed within 48 hours. The screening is stopped when the retina vascularization is complete (retina is mature) or vessels reach till one disc diameter of the temporal ora serrata. Usually, ROP screening is completed by 45–50 weeks of postconceptional age.

Since ROP has a significant impact on ocular development, more so in cases with severe ROP, a large number of these babies develop myopia, astigmatism, and strabismus.[27,28] Thus, it becomes very important that after the intensive ROP screening is completed and disease has regressed, the baby continues to maintain long-term follow-up every 3–6 months so that they can be adequately evaluated for retinal status, refractive errors and proper spectacles correction can be provided in case it is required.

How to Screen?

Retinal examinations of preterm babies should be performed by a trained ophthalmologist experienced in screening ROP. He must be adequately trained and be able to identify and classify ROP based on its location and extent and experienced enough to diagnose and document sequential changes of ROP.

Pupils Dilation

This step is very important for proper ROP screening. Often pupils do not dilate, due to plus disease which leads to pupillary rigidity. It is important that ROP screening still be performed in these babies even through a smaller pupil because of the high risk of severe ROP in these cases. It is almost always possible to examine the posterior pole for plus disease even through a small pupil. Never delay ROP screening because of poorly dilating pupils, as it is mostly a manifestation of plus disease indicating severe disease.

The eye drops used for pupillary dilation are a combination of phenylephrine (2.5%) and tropicamide (0.5%). This is half the strength of similar commercially available combinations and can readily be prepared by diluting 1:1 with tear supplements. The eye drops are instilled twice at 15-minute intervals half an hour prior to the procedure. It is important to ensure that the eye drops properly enter the eye, and are associated with punctal occlusion to prevent systemic absorption of the drug. The excess drug should be wiped from the facial skin. It is essential to advise that over medication should not be done.

Procedure

ROP screening is a very cost-effective strategy and is performed using a good quality indirect ophthalmoscope (IO) accompanied by a 28D/30D lens. The advantage of the 28D/30D lens is that it provides a wide-field view which is very helpful while examining the retinal periphery, with lesser need for scleral indentation. Moreover, it also helps in retinal examination through a small pupil, which commonly occurs in severe ROP with plus disease. A 20D lens is useful sometimes as it provides better magnification and better assessment of retinal details, if needed (Fig. 33.8).

It is essential that the baby is comfortable during ROP screening examination. The baby is kept fasting for 1 hour prior to the procedure. Proparacaine 0.5% eye drops are instilled to provide topical anesthesia. A pediatric wire specu-

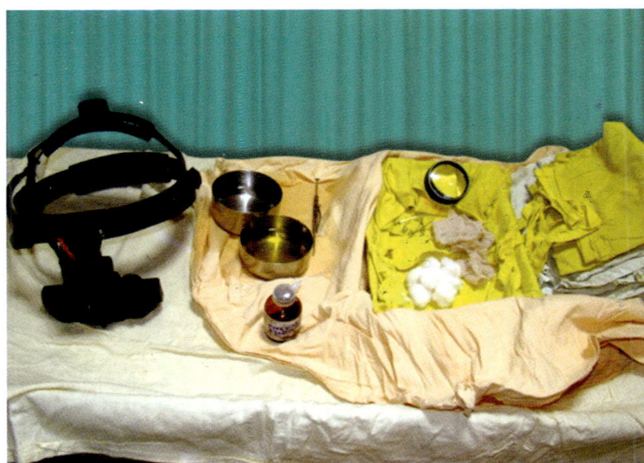

Fig. 33.8: Equipment needed for retinopathy of prematurity (ROP) screening.

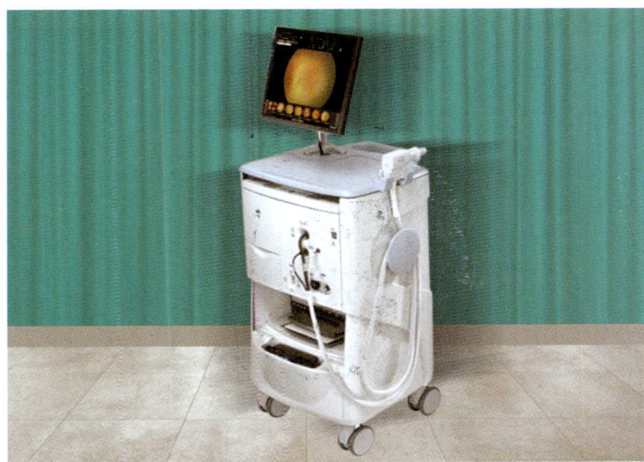

Fig. 33.9: RetCam 3 wide view imaging system for retinopathy of prematurity (ROP) screening.

lum may be used during examination. Sometimes experts like to examine even without the wire speculum as they believe it is more comfortable for the baby.

Initial examination includes that of anterior segment. This includes examination for extent of dilation of pupil, lens/media clarity and tunica vasculosa lentis. This is then followed by the detailed examination of posterior pole for plus disease followed by a detailed and thorough examination of retinal periphery in every clock hours. The examination of the nasal and temporal periphery is essential to look for vascularization in zone II-III.

Scleral depression is an important component of ROP screening. It helps the expert to examine peripheral retinal areas, and rotate/stabilize the constantly moving eye. It helps to detect disease in the retinal periphery which might not be seen otherwise. The pediatric scleral depressor needs to be gently used with care or it may lead to complications like conjunctival hemorrhage or rarely even conjunctival laceration. Always ensure there is not much pressure from the speculum or sclera depressor as it might alter the appearance of plus disease.

Documentation

The proper documentation of an ROP examination is highly essential on a well-structured proforma. It should include accurate details (as per ICROP classification[23]) of ROP zone, stage, clock hours of disease, the presence of preplus or plus disease, and change since the last follow-up. The next follow-up and the disease status of the baby should be discussed with the parents and clearly put in the medical records.

Proper documentation is essential because many of these babies are on regular follow-up and it helps to clearly establish the course of the disease over different examinations. It also helps to avoid interobserver variation among various examiners and is useful when referring patients to other experts. With the growing number of medicolegal cases, it is very important that proper documentation is maintained.

DIGITAL RETINOPATHY OF PREMATURITY SCREENING

Digital screening is emerging as a popular way to screen ROP. RetCam is a useful tool in screening and management of ROP. RetCam stands for the retinal camera and is basically a wide field pediatric digital imaging system (Clarity Medical Systems Inc., USA). It is a mobile complete unit which can be easily transported for use in the NICU, operation theatres or moved across in a mobile van. It allows trained nurses and technicians to capture images without needing expertise for indirect ophthalmoscopy or scleral indentation. It serves as a useful tool not only for teaching residents, but also to explain to the parents about the disease status of their child. With the rising number of medicolegal cases, it has the advantage of storing and retrieving long-term follow-up images when required.

Currently, RetCam 3 and RetCam Shuttle are the two models in use (Figs. 33.9 and 33.10). The RetCam 3 is the more expensive and comprehensive equipment which also allows the user to perform fluorescein angiography. The RetCam Shuttle is the cheaper and portable model, as most components are incorporated into a laptop.

Procedure

The patient and ocular preparation are similar to that for NICU based ROP screening described earlier. Since this is a contact procedure, a coupling gel-like methylcellulose is instilled over the cornea after topical anesthesia. The hand-held camera is then placed over the eye, and adjustments are made to brightness and focusing, and suitable images are

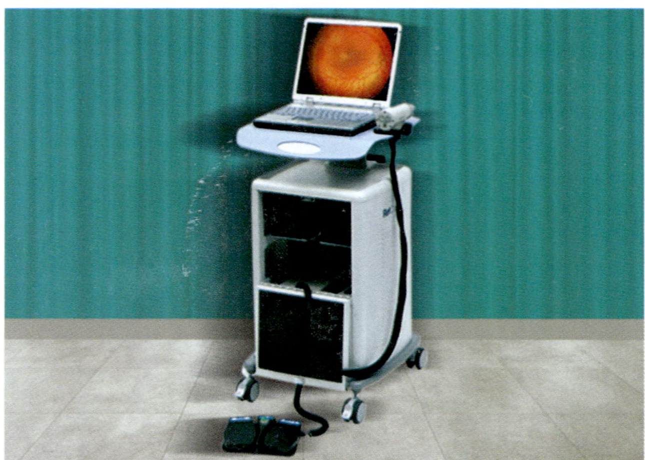

Fig. 33.10: RetCam Shuttle wide view imaging system for retinopathy of prematurity (ROP) screening.

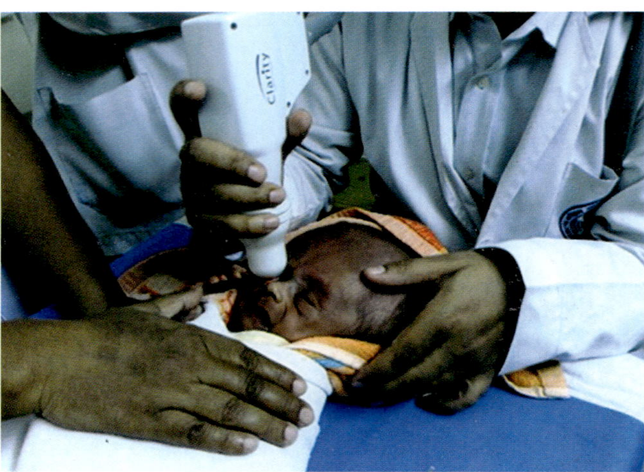

Fig. 33.11: A preterm baby with hydrocephalus undergoing retinopathy of prematurity (ROP) screening using RetCam.

captured in all quadrants. The wide-field 130° lens allows the entire retinal imaging to be done in as few as five images. Multiple interchangeable lenses are available for different views and magnifications. The foot pedal-assisted controls allow focused image capture to be done easily. The facility for video capture is sometimes useful to extract suitable images in an uncooperative child (Fig. 33.11).

Retinopathy of Prematurity Fluorescein Angiography

An added advantage of the RetCam 3 model is that it allows users to perform fluorescein angiography in ROP eyes where needed.[29,30] A special yellow filter is placed inside the hand-held camera and the light source is switched to blue light. The procedure involves intravenous injection of dye (0.04 mL/kg of 20% sodium fluorescein) and the images are documented in the RetCam. It is essential to perform this procedure in the presence of a pediatrician and informed consent of the parents is necessary (Fig. 33.12).

The fluorescein angiography is very helpful in identifying demarcation junctions, avascular areas as well as flat neovascularization patches which are difficult to visualize by routine fundus imaging. It serves especially useful in cases of APROP as it helps in better assessment of avascular retina with the area's needed to be treated and is particularly useful for new trainees when they start managing such complex cases.

RETINOPATHY OF PREMATURITY TELESCREENING

Tele screening is an important novel addition in the screening of ROP. As part of ROP telescreening programs, ROP screening is performed by trained technicians in mobile vans, wherein they can capture images and send across to reading centers or ROP experts who can opine about the case using mobile apps

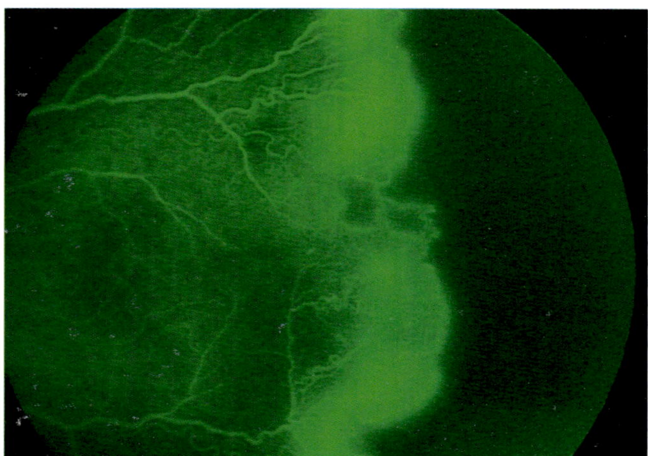

Fig. 33.12: RetCam assisted Fluorescein angiography of left eye showing extensive leakage of dye at ridge suggestive of neovascularization at ridge.

on their smartphones. This allows a larger population to be screened without the need for ophthalmologists to physically visit these areas. Moreover, these small and often sick babies do not need to travel across to major eye care facilities for routine screening every week.

Several large telescreening studies like Stanford University Network for Diagnosis of Retinopathy of Prematurity (SUNDROP)[31] telemedicine initiative have clearly established high sensitivity and specificity of digital screening for detecting treatment warranted ROP. The notable example in India is the Karnataka Internet Assisted Diagnosis of Retinopathy of Prematurity (KIDROP) program,[32] a public-private partnership which has helped to establish an ROP network in urban and semi-urban population across the State of Karnataka. It follows the triple T philosophy—tele-ROP, training of peripheral ophthalmologists and ophthalmic assistants, and talking to neonatologists, pediatricians and gynecologists.

With the rising number of ROP cases in the community and lack of trained personnel to screen them on a routine basis, digital telescreening is emerging as a popular option for establishing ROP services in the community. In fact, for wider implementation of ROP services, there is a new push for neonatology-led screening programs where trained technicians in NICU will digitally screen babies and only refer babies which need urgent ophthalmic opinion.[33]

The only hindrance currently is the very expensive cost of the RetCam. Newer hand-held cameras are on the horizon, which are indigenously made at low cost and will give a huge boost to the spread of digital ROP screening across the country. They will make ROP screening facilities accessible to a larger population which will go a long way to prevent ROP-related blindness. ROP screening is the right of every premature baby, and we must ensure every preterm child undergoes ROP screening.

REFERENCES

1. Vinekar A, Dogra MR, Sangtam T, et al. Retinopathy of prematurity in Asian Indian babies weighing greater than 1250 grams at birth: ten year data from a tertiary care center in a developing country. Indian J Ophthalmology. 2007;55(5):331-6.
2. Sanghi G, Dogra MR, Katoch D, et al. Demographic profile of infants with stage 5 retinopathy of prematurity in North India: implications for screening. Ophthalmic Epidemiol. 2011;18(2): 72-4.
3. Gilbert C. Retinopathy of prematurity: a global perspective of the epidemics, population of babies at risk and implications for control. Early Hum Dev. 2008;84(2):77-82.
4. Blencowe H, Lawn JE, Vazquez T, et al. Preterm-associated visual impairment and estimates of retinopathy of prematurity at regional and global levels for 2010. Pediatr Res. 2013;74 Suppl 1:35-49.
5. Campbell K. Intensive oxygen therapy as a possible cause of retrolental fibroplasia; a clinical approach. Med J Aust. 1951;2(2): 48-50.
6. Flynn JT, Bancalari E, Snyder ES, et al. A cohort study of transcutaneous oxygen tension and the incidence and severity of retinopathy of prematurity. N Engl J Med. 1992;326(16):1050-4.
7. Gilbert CE, Anderton L, Dandona L, et al. Prevalence of visual impairment in children a review of available data. Ophthalmic Epidemiol. 1999;6(1):73-82.
8. Gilbert C, Fielder A, Gordillo L, et al. Characteristics of infants with severe retinopathy of prematurity in countries with low, moderate, and high levels of development: implications for screening programs. Pediatrics. 2005;115(5):e518-25.
9. Gilbert C, Rahi J, Eckstein M, et al. Retinopathy of prematurity in middle-income countries. Lancet Lond Engl. 1997;350(9070):12-4.
10. Ashton N, Pedler C. Studies on developing retinal vessels: IX. Reaction of endothelial cells to oxygen. Br J Ophthalmology. 1962; 46(5):257-76.
11. Patz A. Current concepts of the effect of oxygen on the developing retina. Curr Eye Res. 1984;3(1):159-63.
12. Ashton N, Ward B, Serpell G. Effect of oxygen on developing retinal vessels with particular reference to the problem of retrolental fibroplasia. Br J Ophthalmology. 1954;38(7):397-432.
13. Kretzer FL, Hittner HM. Retinopathy of prematurity: clinical implications of retinal development. Arch Dis Child. 1988;63(10 Spec No):1151-67.
14. Kretzer FL, Hittner HM. Spindle cells and retinopathy of prematurity: interpretations and predictions. Birth Defects Orig Artic Ser. 1988;24(1):147-68.
15. Smith LEH. Through the eyes of a child: understanding retinopathy through ROP the Friedenwald lecture. Invest Ophthalmology Vis Sci. 2008;49(12):5177-82.
16. Port AD, Chan RVP, Ostmo S, et al. Risk factors for retinopathy of prematurity: insights from outlier infants. Graefes Arch Clin Exp Ophthalmology. 2014;252(10):1669-77.
17. Chaudhari S, Patwardhan V, Vaidya U, et al. Retinopathy of prematurity in a tertiary care center--incidence, risk factors and outcome. Indian Pediatr. 2009;46(3):219-24.
18. 18.Carlo WA. Finer NN, Walsh MC, et al. Target ranges of oxygen saturation in extremely preterm infants. N Engl J Med. 2010; 362(21):1959-69.
19. Stenson BJ, Tarnow-Mordi WO, Darlow BA, et al. Oxygen saturation and outcomes in preterm infants. N Engl J Med. 2013;368(22): 2094-104.
20. Roberts D, Dalziel S. Antenatal corticosteroids for accelerating fetal lung maturation for women at risk of preterm birth. Cochrane Database Syst Rev. 2006;(3):CD004454.
21. An international classification of retinopathy of prematurity. The Committee for the Classification of Retinopathy of Prematurity. Arch Ophthalmology. 1984;102(8):1130-4.
22. An international classification of retinopathy of prematurity. II. The classification of retinal detachment. The International Committee for the Classification of the Late Stages of Retinopathy of Prematurity. Arch Ophthalmology. 1987;105(7):906-12.
23. International Committee for the Classification of Retinopathy of Prematurity. The International Classification of Retinopathy of Prematurity revisited. Arch Ophthalmology. 2005;123(7):991-9.
24. Good WV. Final results of the Early Treatment for Retinopathy of Prematurity (ETROP) randomized trial. Trans Am Ophthalmology Soc. 2004;102:233-50.
25. Fierson WM, American Academy of Pediatrics Section on Ophthalmology, American Academy of Ophthalmology, et al. Screening examination of premature infants for retinopathy of prematurity. Pediatrics. 2013;131(1):189-95.
26. Pejaver RK, Vinekar A, Bilagi AP, et al. NNF Clinical Practice Guidelines for Retinopathy of Prematurity. [online] Available from: http://v2020eresource.org/content/files/NNF.html [Accessed December 2017].
27. Ouyang L-J, Yin Z-Q, Ke N, et al. Refractive status and optical components of premature babies with or without retinopathy of prematurity at 3–4 years old. Int J Clin Exp Med. 2015;8(7): 11854-61.
28. Shah PK, Ramakrishnan M, Sadat B, et al. Long-term refractive and structural outcome following laser treatment for zone 1 aggressive posterior retinopathy of prematurity. Oman J Ophthalmology. 2014; 7(3):116-9.
29. Azad R, Chandra P, Khan MA, et al. Role of intravenous fluorescein angiography in early detection and regression of retinopathy of prematurity. J Pediatr Ophthalmology Strabismus. 2008;45(1):36-9.
30. Lepore D, Molle F, Pagliara MM, et al. Atlas of fluorescein angiographic findings in eyes undergoing laser for retinopathy of prematurity. Ophthalmology. 2011;118(1):168-75.
31. Wang SK, Callaway NF, Wallenstein MB, et al. SUNDROP: six years of screening for retinopathy of prematurity with telemedicine. Can J Ophthalmology. 2015;50(2) 101-6.
32. Vinekar A. Gilbert C, Dogra M, et al. The KIDROP model of combining strategies for providing retinopathy of prematurity screening in underserved areas in India using wide-field imaging, telemedicine, nonphysician graders and smart phone reporting. Indian J Ophthalmology. 2014;62(1):41-9.
33. Gilbert C, Wormald R, Fielder A, et al. Potential for a paradigm change in the detection of retinopathy of prematurity requiring treatment. Arch Dis Child Fetal Neonatal Ed. 2016;101(1):6-9.

Laser Treatment for Retinopathy of Prematurity

Mangat R Dogra, Deeksha Katoch

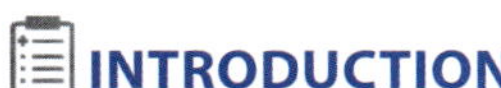 INTRODUCTION

Retinopathy of prematurity (ROP) is a proliferative vitreoretinopathy affecting preterm infants and is now a leading cause of blindness in children across the globe. The advancement and wider availability of neonatal care has led to increasing survival of preterm infants. However, the quality of neonatal care being provided is highly variable. Delayed or absent screening for ROP has led to developing countries like India witnessing the "third epidemic" of ROP blindness.[1]

Blindness from ROP is potentially preventable as highly effective therapy is available in the form of laser photocoagulation. Timely screening and laser treatment of ROP offers the best opportunity for a better visual outcome in the long-term.

RATIONALE FOR THERAPY

The underlying pathological change in ROP is hypoxia of the peripheral avascular retina. This hypoxia increases vascular endothelial growth factor (VEGF) expression which stimulates abnormal retinal neovascularization. The success of therapy depends on the destruction of the hypoxic retinal areas due to nonperfusion thereby leading to decrease in production of angiogenic factors like VEGF. This can be achieved by either cryotherapy or laser photocoagulation.

INDICATIONS FOR TREATMENT

Cryotherapy was the earliest established treatment for sight threatening ROP. The efficacy of cryotherapy for ROP was proven by the multicenter CRYO-ROP study. This study showed that the rates of unfavorable structural outcome were reduced from 43% to 22% at 3 months when cryotherapy was performed in eyes with "threshold ROP", i.e. at least 5 contiguous or 8 cumulative clock hours of stage 3 ROP in zone I or II in the presence of plus disease (defined as a degree of dilation and tortuosity of the posterior retinal blood vessels meeting or exceeding that of a standard photograph).[2]

However, this treatment modality is technically challenging. It requires general anesthesia, an operating room and equipment which may not be portable. Cryotherapy is also associated with more postoperative complications such as eyelid edema and conjunctival chemosis. In addition, cryotherapy is particularly difficult in the treatment of the posterior retina which may require a conjunctival peritomy. Long-term retinal complications such as disc drag, macular drag, narrow arcades and temporal crescent have also been reported following cryotherapy for threshold ROP which may affect long-term visual acuity outcomes.[3]

Laser photocoagulation is now the preferred modality (gold standard) for treatment of retinopathy of prematurity replacing cryotherapy ever since findings of the "Early Treatment for Retinopathy of Prematurity" (ETROP) study were published.[4] The ETROP study was a multicenter, randomized trial designed to determine whether early treatment using ablation of the avascular retina in high-risk (high likelihood of progression to unfavorable outcome) prethreshold ROP results in improved grating visual acuity and retinal structural outcomes compared with conventional treatment. The study showed that early treatment of high-risk prethreshold ROP significantly reduced unfavorable visual outcomes from 19.8% to 14.3% and unfavorable structural outcomes from 15.6% to 9%.[5]

The ETROP study developed an algorithm based on the International Classification of ROP (ICROP) identifying infants who will benefit from early treatment (Type I ROP) (Figs. 34.1A and B) versus those who are not likely to benefit from treatment (Type II ROP).

Box 34.1 summarizes the recommended categories for treatment with laser photocoagulation as per the ETROP study. These criteria are universally followed and are standard treatment guidelines now.

In addition to the ETROP recommendations, early treatment is warranted in aggressive posterior ROP (APROP). APROP is a distinct clinical entity recognized in 2005[6] by the revised ICROP classification. It is characterized by disturbed vasculogenesis resulting in severe plus disease and flat neovascularization in the absence of a definite demarcation line or ridge. APROP is most often encountered in zone I or posterior zone II and can rapidly progress to stage 5 without passing through the intervening stages.

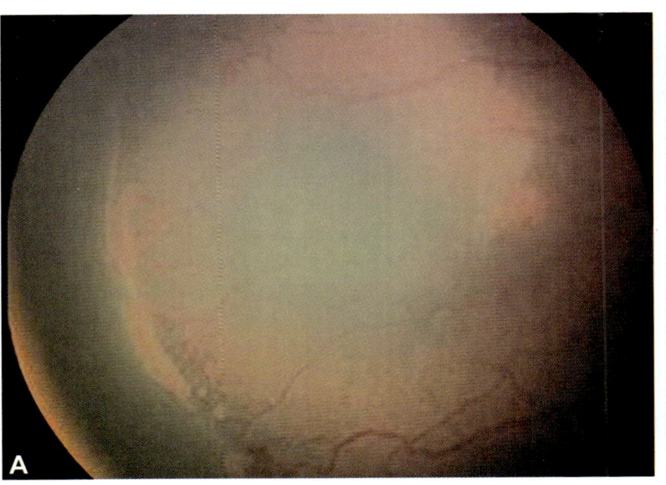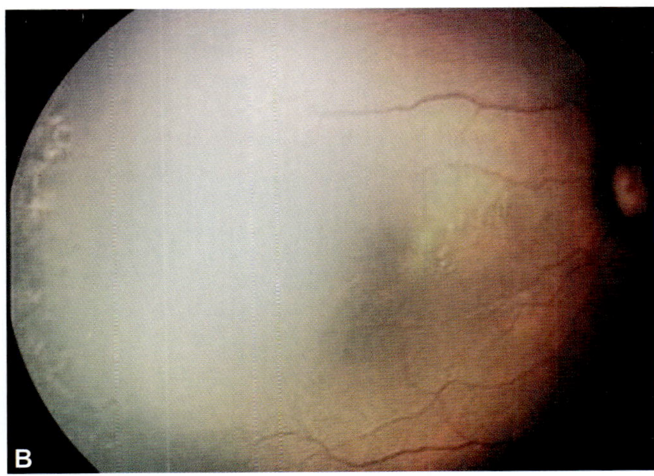

Figs. 34.1A and B: RetCam images showing stage 3 retinopathy of prematurity (ROP) and regression following confluent laser photocoagulation.

Box 34.1: Recommendations for treatment.

Early treatment for retinopathy of prematurity (ETROP) recommendations for laser treatment

Type 1 retinopathy of prematurity (ROP)—Laser treatment indicated

Zone I: Any stage of ROP with plus

Zone I: Stage 3 ROP without plus

Zone II: Stage 2 or 3 ROP with plus

Type 2 ROP: Observe

Zone I: Stage 1 or 2 ROP without plus

Zone II: Stage 3 ROP without plus

"PLUS" DISEASE

The presence of plus disease has now become the sine qua non for the requirement of laser treatment for ROP. It is probably more relevant that either the stage of ROP or the zone of the disease. Dilatation of the retinal arteries and veins in the course of development of ROP was first described by Owens and Owens. This dilatation was more marked in the veins and tortuosity was particularly seen in the arterioles.[7] In 1982, Quinn et al. used the term "retinopathy of prematurity plus" to classify the virulent form of ROP characterized by rapid progression and posterior pole vascular tortuosity and dilation.[8]

The ICROP, in 1984, recognized the importance of these vascular changes and originally defined "plus" as being present when "the vascular changes are so marked that the posterior veins are enlarged and the arterioles tortuous."[9] CRYO-ROP trial then introduced a standard photograph to allow comparison as the minimum abnormality necessary for diagnosing plus disease.[10] Plus disease in the ETROP study[4] was defined as at least two quadrants (6 or more clock hours) of dilation and tortuosity of the posterior retinal blood vessels.

In 2005, the ICROP[6] published a revised version of the existing classification (ICROP revisited) which provided additional standard photographs for comparison and in addition described "preplus" disease. The committee defined pre-plus disease as "vascular abnormalities of the posterior pole that are insufficient for the diagnosis of plus disease but demonstrate more arterial tortuosity and more venous dilatation than normal."[6]

These may be due to decreased resistance of capillaries and increase of blood flow to retina in response to ischemia.[11,12]

In a kitten model of ROP, it was shown that during the hypoxic phase there is impaired smooth muscle cell differentiation suggesting a decreased ability to regulate blood flow.[13] Retinal veins are more distensible compared to the arterioles and thus veins dilate in response to increased blood flow, while the arterioles become tortuous. Another mechanism[14] for plus disease is local production of VEGF due to ischemia that acts on central retinal vessels leading to dilation and tortuosity.

The major challenge in the diagnosis of plus disease is its subjectivity and high interobserver variability[15] even among the ROP experts. Most experts now recognize that there exists a spectrum of posterior retinal vascular changes and plus disease is on the extreme end of the spectrum. This suggests that less severe forms of the retinal vascular changes are probably as important and also require early recognition. With advent and accessibility of newer objective diagnostics tools, the early identification of these changes is possible. The RetCam allows objective documentation and comparison of these changes from the wide-field fundus photographs. A few computer-assisted quantification tools[16,17] are available that help in measuring these vascular changes in retinal images. These include the "ROP tool" (a semi-automated computer program that helps quick and easy tracing and measurement of retinal blood vessels from high-quality RetCam images), computer-aided image analysis of the retina (CAIAR) and the retinal image multiscale analysis (RISA). Most of such software available as of now are semi-automated and development of a fully-automated software may help in providing consistency and accuracy in the diagnosis of plus in the future.

ANESTHESIA

Various modalities for anesthesia have been used for laser treatment. These include general anesthesia, intravenous sedation, subtenon anesthesia and topical anesthesia. The choice of anesthesia largely depends upon the facilities and manpower available, preference of the surgeon and the infant's systemic condition.

In most centers in our country laser treatment is done under topical anesthesia using 0.5% proparacaine eye drops. It is critical that all treatments are performed under strict monitoring by a neonatologist or an anesthesiologist. Comfort care techniques (e.g. administering oral sucrose solution on a gauze as a pacifier, nesting, swaddling) may be considered while doing the laser procedure under topical anesthesia. It is done either in the neonatal intensive care unit (NICU) or in an operating room equipped with drugs and instruments required for resuscitation in the rare event of apnea or cardiac arrest. The neonatologist/anesthesiologist must monitor the baby after treatment until he or she is fed and stable. Babies who are unstable and cannot be brought out of the incubator can be safely treated within the incubator itself through its sloping wall.[18]

LASER EQUIPMENT

A portable laser indirect ophthalmoscope (LIO) delivery system and a 20- or 28-diopter aspheric condensing lens are used for the treatment of ROP. Laser wavelengths which can be used for laser ablation include either a diode (810 nm), argon-green (514 nm) or green (532 nm) laser. The diode laser had been the preferred modality in most studies due to its deeper penetration, even in eyes with tunica vasculosa lentis and vitreous hemorrhage and a lower risk of cataract formation. However, the neodymium-doped yttrium aluminum garnet (Nd:YAG) (532 nm) green laser has been reported to be equally safe as compared to the diode laser[19] even in eyes with tunica vasculosa lentis and is routinely being used in many centers. The power is usually kept at 300–400 mW, duration 300–400 milliseconds for diode laser and 150–200 mW with a duration of 0.1–0.2 seconds for green laser titrated to achieve a grayish-white burn.

Transscleral diode lasers (TSDL) are also available for the treatment of ROP.[20] The transscleral probe is applied to the external surface of the sclera and has a diode aiming beam that allows the targeted retina to be visualized using an indi-rect ophthalmoscope. Potential advantages of transscleral treatment compared to transpupillary treatment include the reduced risk of thermal injury to the iris and lens. Another advantage is the ability to treat through media opacities such as vitreous hemorrhage and a nondilating pupil. The disadvantage of transscleral therapy is the technical difficulty in treating posterior disease such as in zone 1 requiring conjunctival incisions to allow laser delivery.

TREATMENT PROCEDURE

Once the decision to treat an infant is made, a written informed consent explaining the severity of disease, nature of the treatment and potential complications should be obtained from the parents or the legal guardian. The possibility of retreatment, further surgical intervention and the need for long-term follow-up for refractive errors and other sequelae should be explained. Pupils can be dilated with 2.5% phenylephrine hydrochloride and 0.5% cyclopentolate or 0.5–1% tropicamide taking care to wipe off the excess drops from the medial canthus and/or cheek area to avoid absorption and systemic toxicity. Feeding should be withheld at least half an hour prior to treatment to avoid regurgitation during the procedure. Both eyes can be safely treated in the same session in most situations unless a systemic adverse event occurs during the procedure.

Treatment is done to the entire avascular retina up to the ora-serrata getting as close to the ridge as possible. The density of treatment can have a profound impact on the progression of the disease. Banach et al.[21] have addressed this question in their randomized trial comparing near confluent laser pattern versus burns spaced 1–1.5 burns apart. In this study, two cohorts treated with either a near-confluent (0.25 burn width apart) or laser burns 1–1.5 burn width apart were compared for progression to stage 4A, 4B or stage 5. The progression rate of eyes treated in a near confluent pattern was 3.6% whereas those treated with burns 1–1.5 width apart was 29.4% which was statistically significant. In addition, prompt retreatment in the presence of plus disease was also associated with reduced progression rates in this study. Adequate laser treatment is imperative as any avascular retina acts as a reservoir of VEGF production and can lead to progression of the disease. Near confluent pattern of treatment as well as prompt retreatment when indicated are the cornerstones of obtaining a favorable outcome and preventing progression to stage 4 in ROP. The consensus guidelines[22] of the leading ROP experts in our country regarding the technical aspects of laser treatment of ROP have been published and are available to serve as a guide.

At the end of the procedure, both the eyes should be reexamined 360° to identify any areas missed (skip areas) initially; these areas need fill-in laser so that no avascular retina is left untreated. In cases with severe plus disease or tunica vasculosa lentis, pupils may not dilate with dilator eye drops. The treating ophthalmologist should be aware of such a situation

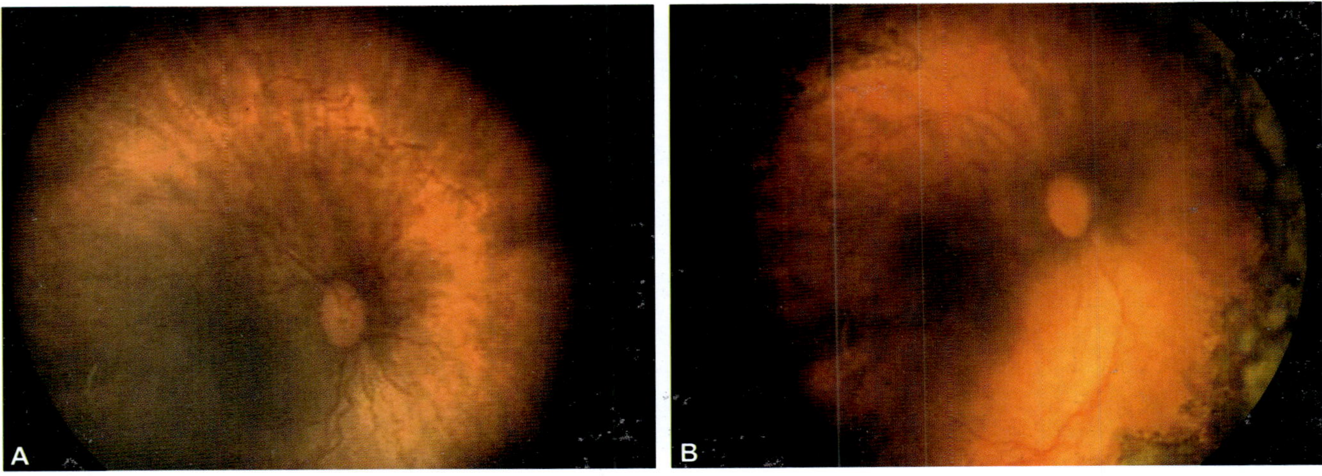

Figs. 34.2A and B: RetCam images showing APROP and regression following confluent laser photocoagulation. (APROP: Aggressive posterior retinopathy of prematurity).

and refrain from instilling more and more dilators in such a "bowed-down" pupil as it will only result in systemic toxicity. In these situations, pupils may dilate during the course of treatment as a result of mechanical pupillary stretching by scleral indentation. There is a role of anti-VEGF therapy in such situations. Anti-VEGF therapy will help in the resolution of the tunica vasculosa lentis and regression of the "plus disease" allowing dilatation of the pupil and facilitating laser treatment which can be scheduled 1–2 weeks later.

Aggressive posterior ROP poses a therapeutic challenge (Figs. 34.2A and B). The disease is most commonly present in Zone 1 or posterior Zone II and the fovea itself may be avascular. In this situation, the entire peripheral avascular retina is ablated getting as close as possible to the edge of the vascularization. It is important to first delineate the posterior pole area with laser to prevent inadvertent laser application to the fovea. Treatment of the flat neovascular fronds can be done in two ways as suggested by the PHOTO-ROP study.[23] The first option is to treat these areas in the first sitting itself. Alternatively, a second session 5–10 days later may be performed in the area where the flat neovascular frond has involuted, exposing the underlying avascular retina. The study also indicates that even in eyes adequately treated for APROP, retreatment may be required for the avascular retina which gets exposed after the flat neovascularization regresses.

POSTOPERATIVE CARE

Antibiotic and steroid drops are advised three to four times a day for a week after laser treatment. Follow-up examinations are scheduled every week initially. At each visit examination should be done to evaluate the response to treatment by looking at the following parameters:

- Persistence/regression of tunica vasculosa lentis
- Persistence/regression of plus disease
- Status of the ridge or preexisting fibrovascular proliferation

- New onset vitreous hemorrhage/fibrovascular proliferation.

At 1–2 weeks, if plus disease persists or there appear any "skip" areas it is advisable to perform additional laser to these areas. Weekly follow-ups should be continued until the plus disease regresses. Thereafter 2 weekly follow-ups are recommended until regression of ROP, defined as the absence of plus disease and complete disappearance of any active neovascular tissue, i.e. ridge or fibrovascular proliferation. This may take 6–12 weeks following laser. At this time if there is no fibrovascular organization in the vitreous, the infant can be next seen at 6 months of age. However, if there is fibrovascular proliferation the infant is followed up at weekly intervals for the development of any retinal detachment. New onset fibrovascular organization is a significant risk factor for the development of retinal detachment after laser for acute ROP.[24,25]

Less than 3 clock hours of extramacular detachment (localized stage 4a) may be observed till the fibrovascular membrane separates into the vitreous cavity, leading to spontaneous regression or there is progression. More than 4 clock hours of stage 4a or 4b (macular detachment) requires surgical intervention (lens sparing vitrectomy) (Figs. 34.3A to E).

According to the CRYO-ROP study, the unfavorable outcome is defined as any of the following:

- A posterior retinal fold (falciform) involving the macula
- A retinal detachment involving the macula
- Retrolental tissue or mass obscuring the view of the posterior pole.

COMPLICATIONS AND SEQUELAE

Retinopathy of prematurity treatment may be associated with significant systemic stress and potentially life-threatening cardiorespiratory events. Babies undergoing treatment for ROP are frequently unwell and may be suffering from other complications of preterm delivery. The strong light stimulus

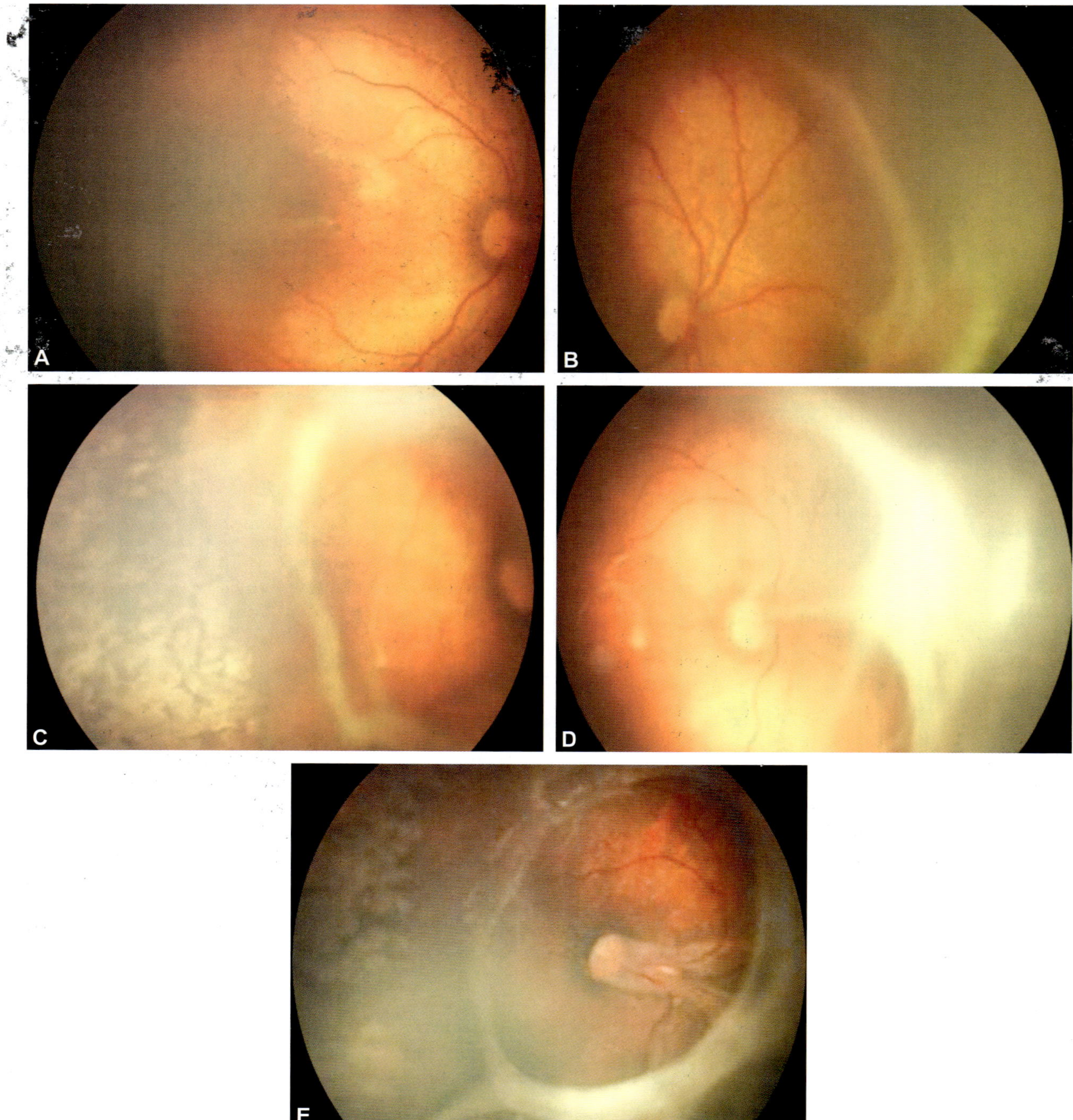

Figs. 34.3A to E: (A and B) RetCam images of the right eye showing avascular retina in posterior zone II along with extensive (>3 clock hours) stage 4A retinopathy of prematurity (ROP). (C and D) Showing progression to Stage 4B despite confluent laser photocoagulation. (E) Shows the same eye following lens sparing vitrectomy.

from the indirect ophthalmoscope, manipulation of the globe with scleral indentation and the laser itself may contribute to neonatal stress and pain. Bradycardia, apnea, oxygen desatu- ration and hypothermia can occur during treatment. There may be infants who may require resuscitation and ventilator support. Hence, all laser treatments for ROP should only be

Role of Antivascular Endothelial Growth Factor Drugs and Surgical Management of Retinopathy of Prematurity

Parijat Chandra, Ruchir Tewari

INTRODUCTION: ANTIVASCULAR ENDOTHELIAL GROWTH FACTOR DRUGS

It is well known that retinopathy of prematurity (ROP) is a vasoproliferative retinopathy and early exposure of an immature and poorly vascularized retina to hyperoxic environment leads to the development of ROP. Laser ablation of peripheral avascular retina with laser photocoagulation is the mainstay for treatment.

However, zone I or zone II posterior disease and the severe variant of aggressive posterior ROP (APROP)[1] pose a unique challenge to the ROP experts as it sometimes leads to a severe disease, which might progress to advanced stages despite timely and complete laser treatment. The large zone of avascular retina stimulates rapid production of angiogenic factors, leading to extensive neovascularization. Many times the cases of severe ROP present late due to lack of screening and referral with extensive neovascular disease, which might not be controlled by laser treatment alone. In these scenarios, laser treatment is late or partially effective and there is a need for an adjuvant agent that can help to control the disease in these cases.

With advances in our understanding of the disease process, newer interventions are being explored and antivascular endothelial growth factor (VEGF) agents have shown great promise.

RATIONAL OF USE OF ANTIVASCULAR ENDOTHELIAL GROWTH FACTOR DRUGS IN RETINOPATHY OF PREMATURITY

It is important to understand the mechanism by which ROP occurs. The development of ROP occurs in two distinct phases[2]—the first phase of hyperoxia-induced vaso-obliteration that occurs from 22 weeks to 30 weeks postmenstrual age and the second phase of ischemia induced vasoproliferation from 31 weeks to 44 weeks. Alon et al.[3] showed that the first phase is marked by a sudden hyperoxia induced decline in VEGF levels with the destruction of endothelial cells leading to vasoconstriction and vaso-obliteration; proposing the role of VEGF in stimulation as well as maintenance of newly developing normal capillary network. The second phase[2] involves ischemia associated rise in VEGF with the development of abnormal vessels at the junction of the avascular and vascular retina. Thus, VEGF has a key role in different phases of development of ROP, and inhibition of VEGF in the second phase could potentially change the course of the disease. Anti-VEGF agents bind to either VEGF molecules or to VEGF receptors and inhibit the action of VEGF in the desired tissue.

ROLE OF ANTIVASCULAR ENDOTHELIAL GROWTH FACTOR DRUGS IN RETINOPATHY OF PREMATURITY

With the revelation of increased levels of VEGF in vitreous cavity of babies with ROP, it was only natural that researchers started experimenting with these drugs for ROP treatment. Initial efforts of its use with laser therapy for aggressive zone 1 disease resulted in good outcomes.[4] This was followed by several reports of successful use of anti-VEGF agents for ROP.[5,6]

To better understand the efficacy of these drugs in ROP, the first randomized clinical trial was conducted. The Bevacizumab Eliminates Angiogenic Threat for ROP (BEAT-ROP)[7] trial compared the efficacy of intravitreal bevacizumab monotherapy (0.625 mg) with conventional laser therapy bilaterally in zone 1 or zone 2 posterior stage 3 + ROP. The results suggested significant benefit in zone 1 ROP with decreased recurrences. Another advantage was that revascularization of avascular retina continued to occur with bevacizumab, while on the other hand, the laser therapy destroyed large parts of the retina, thereby restricting visual fields. However, the trial was too small to assess safety.

This has led to several usage options of anti-VEGF drugs—many use it for a primary treatment instead of laser,[7] some use it as combination or rescue therapy with laser treatment,[8] while others find it useful prior to vitreous surgery to reduce the vascularization[9] (Figs. 35.1 and 35.2).

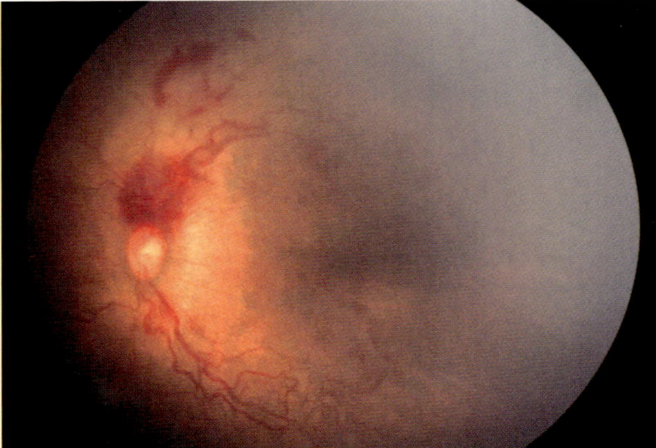

Fig. 35.1: A case with zone I aggressive posterior ROP in the left eye with preretinal hemorrhages, plus disease, and unclear demarcation between vascular and avascular retina.

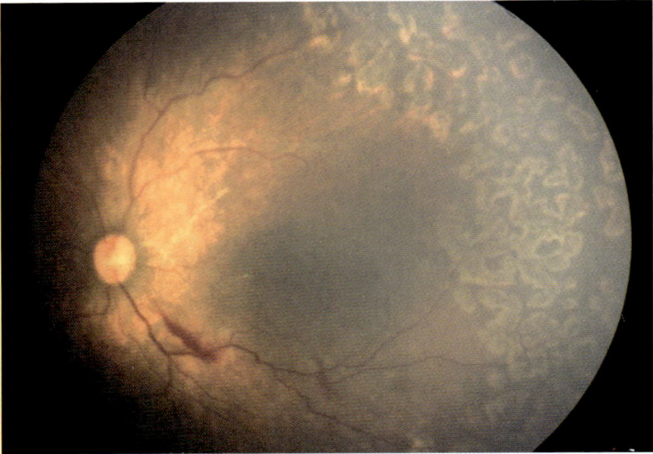

Fig. 35.2: The same case of zone 1 AP ROP showing disease regression at 3 weeks following single intravitreal injection of bevacizumab and laser treatment.
(AP ROP: Aggressive posterior retinopathy of prematurity)

There are several anti-VEGF agents which have used in the management, which of ROP, though all have been "off-label" uses. Bevacizumab is a humanized monoclonal antibody that binds human VEGF-A, is among the first drugs to be used and has been used most extensively for management of ROP.[4] Ranibizumab is a humanized anti-VEGF-A recombinant Fab fragment and is showing promise in varying doses with good outcomes.[10,11] Recently, VEGF-Trap (Aflibercept) has been introduced which is a fusion protein that inhibits VEGF by acting as a decoy receptor for the ligand binding regions of VEGF, has much higher affinity for VEGF and also binds with VEGF-B and placental growth factor (PlGF). Few case reports have described successful use of aflibercept in ROP.[12]

INTRAVITREAL ANTIVASCULAR ENDOTHELIAL GROWTH FACTOR INJECTION

The procedure for intravitreal injection of anti-VEGF drugs is almost similar to that in adults. It is preferable to give these injections under sedation or general anesthesia, as the injection is more controlled and easier to perform at the correct site with lower complications. Many surgeons prefer to give an intravitreal injection under topical anesthesia as it minimizes the risk of anesthesia-related complications—but then the child's eye is constantly moving and there is more risk of complications like wrong site of injection, needle induced injuries leading to cataract, etc.

Strict aseptic measures should be followed. Clean the eye using povidone-iodine, use sterile drapes, and clearly mark site of injection, which is usually 1.5–2 mm from the limbus, depending on the age of the baby. The drug is loaded in a tuberculin syringe with attached 30G needle. For bevacizumab, 0.625 mg in 0.025 mL can be used as suggested by BEAT-ROP study.[7] Some surgeons prefer to use lesser doses.

The eye is fixated with fixation forceps, the needle is slid on the conjunctiva and inserted using a multistep technique such that a self-sealing wound is created. Once the needle is inside, it is perpendicularly oriented to inject the drug into the mid-vitreous. After completion of the injection, the needle is quickly removed with pressure on the site with a swab such that the drug does not escape out. This is followed by instillation of antibiotic eye drops.

CHALLENGES AND CONCERNS OF ANTIVASCULAR ENDOTHELIAL GROWTH FACTOR DRUG USAGE

A recent meta-analysis[13] studied 24 original reports including 1,457 eyes on VEGF inhibitor treatment for ROP over the last few years. They observed that there were significant benefits with the use of anti-VEGF agents in zone 1 ROP, not only in terms of disease regression but also fewer recurrences, preservation of visual field, and less induction of myopia.

The study highlighted another major concern about the lack of long-term safety data to establish the systemic safety of these drugs. While half the adult dose is being commonly used, many consider the dosage is still high, and lowest sufficient dose data is still not available. While no systemic complications are reported, better documentation and long-term observational data is needed, which is difficult to obtain in small preterm babies.

Vascular endothelial growth factor is an important mediator of physiological angiogenesis, as well as acts as a neuroprotective agent and its systemic suppression in preterm infants, may lead to potential developmental defects in other growing organs of the body. Considering the larger molecular size of bevacizumab, it was earlier thought it would be unable to penetrate retinal layers and would lead to minimal systemic absorption. Kong et al.[14] measured serum levels of bevacizumab, VEGF, and insulin-like growth factor 1 (IGF-1) levels after treatment with 0.625 mg and 0.25 mg doses of bevacizumab and laser treatment in ROP. They found that serum clearance of bevacizumab takes at least 2 months. They noted that serum-free VEGF levels decreased significantly with bevacizumab treatment compared to laser, and they suggested that potential long-term effects need to be studied further. But a much larger sample size is needed to study mortality and morbidity associated with anti-VEGF use.

Rarely, Bevacizumab use in advanced stages of disease has been noted to cause severe contraction of proliferative membranes and development of tractional retinal detachment (TRD).[15-17] Another important concern is delayed recurrence and late reactivation of disease after anti-VEGF treatment, which can occur several weeks after injection.[18,19] This necessitates a prolonged and frequent follow-up even after "apparent" regression of disease.

Summary

Currently, anti-VEGF drugs are being used by many ROP experts in select cases of zone 1 ROP or APROP, with severe progressive neovascular disease with or without additional laser treatment. In very small zone I disease, where even macula is avascular, they have the added benefit of allowing retinal vascular growth, aiding in the development of macular region. They are especially useful in cases of nondilating pupils with dense iris neovascularization in APROP with severe plus disease, as they can help in faster regression of iris new vessels and reduce plus disease, thereby allowing early pupillary dilation facilitating laser treatment. But we need to remember that the usage is currently off label and parents need to be counseled well, and detailed informed consent is essential.

There is hope that pharmacological approaches to the treatment of ROP might become the treatment of choice in the future. It will avoid the permanent destruction of retinal tissue and visual field loss caused by laser therapy, as well as bypass the expertise needed for laser treatment and alleviate the prolonged pain experienced by babies during laser treatment. Systemic safety and long-term results through new multicentric trials will give clarity about the definitive role of anti-VEGF drugs in ROP. Till then laser treatment remains the gold standard for treatment of ROP, supported by validated long-term results. With further research, anti-VEGF agents or other emerging newer drugs have the potential to change our perspective towards managing ROP.

SURGICAL MANAGEMENT OF RETINOPATHY OF PREMATURITY

Laser is the gold standard for treatment, and ROP treated in time most often regresses uneventfully. However, in developing countries like India, there is a lack of awareness among ophthalmologists and pediatricians, which leads to the absence of effective ROP screening programs. This leads to a large number of babies presenting to tertiary eye care facilities with advanced stages of ROP.[20]

Based on the international ROP classification by the International Classification of ROP (ICROP) group, advanced stage ROP includes stages 4–5 ROP. Stage 4 ROP means subtotal retinal detachment which can be stage 4A with subtotal retinal detachment without foveal involvement, and stage 4B with subtotal retinal detachment and foveal detachment.

Advanced stages of ROP often occur in severe variants like zone 1 APROP, which can progress despite laser treatment. However, many cases are referred for advanced ROP because of lack of screening or treatment, leading to worsening of ROP.

Advanced ROP needs surgical intervention. ROP surgery involves complex vitreoretinal surgery performed by experienced ROP surgeons with high-tech vitreoretinal surgical setups. The availability of such surgical setups and experienced surgeons are limited, therefore a large number of such babies continue to go blind due to lack of access to care. However surgery for stage 4 ROP has a better prognosis if performed early, while the surgical outcomes in stage 5 ROP are poor.

INDICATIONS FOR RETINOPATHY OF PREMATURITY SURGERY

Stage IV: Surgery is indicated in most cases in stage IV ROP, though not all eyes with detachment require or benefit from surgery. Early stage IVA with small peripheral detachments presenting late may be treated with laser and observed for subsequent regression. If traction persists, then posterior barrage laser can prove useful, as it helps to anchor the retinal posterior to the ridge, eliminates the posterior avascular areas behind the ridge, and sometimes helps in faster and more complete regression.[21]

However, when traction increases in height, extends across many clock hours with posterior extension (which can threaten the macula), surgery is warranted. When multiple areas of TRD join together, the traction progresses at a much faster rate and early surgery is recommended. Delayed surgery can cause fibrovascular proliferation to extend behind the lens, making lens sparing surgery difficult. More neovascular component predisposes to high-risk of bleeding intraoperatively as well as postoperatively.

Zone 1 disease or APROP is particularly tricky as retinal detachment progresses very fast, is more vascular in nature and can cause early macular detachment. Moreover, these small babies are usually sick and anesthesia clearance for surgery might also be difficult.

Stage V: Surgery in stage 5 ROP is particularly challenging, and not all cases are suitable for surgical intervention. Many of these cases have associated posterior synechiae, cataract, shallow anterior chamber, corneal opacities, secondary glaucoma, dense retrolental plaques, hypotony, etc.—which contribute to poor surgical prognosis.

Since the retinal status is not visible, ultrasonography is useful to determine the retinal funnel status.[22] Based on ultrasonography findings, the retinal funnel is divided into anterior and posterior parts, which can be an open or closed funnel. Thus, an open-closed funnel would mean the retinal funnel is open anteriorly and closed posteriorly. Most ROP surgeons will operate cases with open-open funnel configuration as they have better surgical outcomes. Closed-closed funnel configuration has worse prognosis. Ultrasonic biomicroscopy is also a useful tool to assess prognosis and determine anterior surgical space for allowing safe instruments entry.[23]

Early stage 5 ROP as seen in cases of progressing stage 4 may have better anatomic and functional outcomes. Bilateral stage V cases can be offered surgery with the hope that even minimal surgical benefit can help to provide navigable vision to the child. Resurgery might be indicated following postoperative bleeding, persistent traction, or improved retinal configuration, which can be operated further to relieve traction.

With advancement in surgical techniques and availability of better instrumentation, surgery has become safer than before, leading to the adoption of an aggressive approach and expansion of indications.

PREOPERATIVE PREPARATION

Proper preoperative evaluation and planning are imperative in all cases. As surgery is performed under general anesthesia, systemic evaluation and neonatal intensive care support are essential. It is a challenging situation for the parents as they have to give high-risk informed consent for surgery. An experienced anesthesia team is needed to safely administer general anesthesia to a preterm baby. A robust neonatal intensive care unit (NICU) support is required to monitor the baby postoperatively and manage any related complications.

Since advanced ROP has a potential for medicolegal implications, it is imperative that the parents should be clearly explained the advanced nature of the disease, the surgical procedure, the guarded or poor surgical prognosis, and have realistic expectations from the surgical intervention.

ROLE OF SCLERAL BUCKLING

Scleral buckling was first described for both stages 4 and 5 disease although it was found to be more beneficial for stage 4.[24] Although no large scale comparative studies have been performed, different case series have reported variable limited success rates of scleral buckling for both stages 4A and 4B ROP.[24-26]

Scleral buckling involves placement of an encircling band with or without a scleral buckle in the clock hours of traction. Drainage of subretinal fluid is not mandatory and a nondrainage procedure requires an anterior chamber paracentesis to check the rise in intraocular pressure. Once the traction is relieved, the fluid absorbs and the retina settles back. It is essential to cut the encircling band after 3 months to allow growth of the eyeball and decrease the amount of anisometropia, which can lead to anisometropic amblyopia.[27,28]

However, with improvements in instrumentation and development of small gauge vitrectomy systems and more experienced surgeons, the safety and outcome of primary vitreous surgery has improved immensely leading to its global adoption as the preferred modality for treating ROP detachments and buckling surgery for ROP is now rarely done.[22]

VITREORETINAL SURGERY FOR STAGE 4 RETINOPATHY OF PREMATURITY

Lens sparing vitrectomy (LSV) has become the procedure of choice for stages 4A and 4B ROP. Increasing vitreoretinal traction from the vertically growing neovascular ridge leads to TRD and primary vitrectomy helps by directly relieving this traction. It also removes the vitreous rich in angiogenic factors and decreases the angiogenic stimulus. The dissection and removal of fibrous membranes helps the retina fall back and releases the circumferential fibrous tissue, thereby preventing the closure of the retinal funnel.

Most surgeons prefer to use 25/27 G vitrectomy systems as the fine instruments allow easy manoeuvrability and dissection, cause less retinal damage, ensure better chamber stability, and allow sutureless closure. The surgical steps include the creation of standard three ports at pars plicata usually at 1.5–2 mm from the limbus (depending on age) as these surgeries are lens sparing.[29] The site of the ports is assessed prior to surgery by indirect ophthalmoscopy and scleral indentation to avoid areas of traction, to prevent subretinal entry of instruments. This is followed by core vitrectomy, relief of traction over the TRD, dissection of membranes, induction of posterior vitreous detachment, diathermy of bleeding vessels, and relief of circumferential traction. No attempt is made to create a retinotomy or drain subretinal fluid. After successful vitrectomy, a partial air-fluid exchange is done, and ports are left sutureless or closed with 8–0 Vicryl sutures. Care should be taken to avoid intraoperative bleeding, prevent retinal breaks, and gently perform surgery, so as to avoid iatrogenic complications. No long-term tamponade is required as after the traction is relieved, the fibrovascular tissue regresses and the traction retinal detachment settles down over the next few weeks (Figs. 35.3 and 35.4).

Postoperative bleeding is a common complication and can be minimized by minimal intervention of fibrovascular tissue, and ensuring there are no bleeders at the end of surgery. Lens touch is another complication, which can be avoided by ensuring proper entry of instruments at the correct site and distance from the limbus and avoiding close retrolental dissection of TRD. Most reports indicate good long-term lens clarity after LSV for stage 4 ROP.[30] Sometimes, persistent rise in intraocular pressure has been reported after ROP surgery.[31]

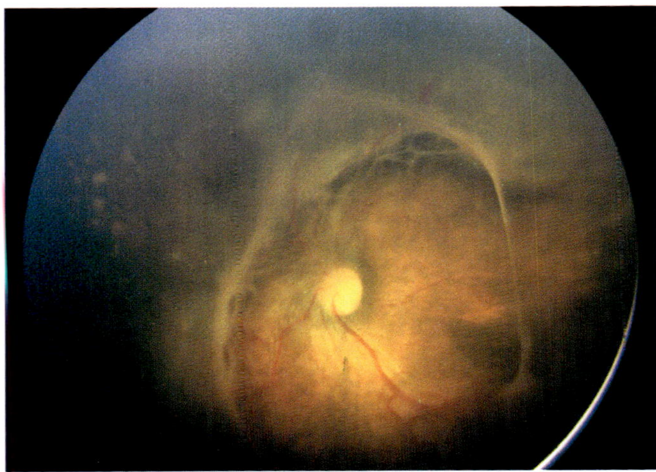

Fig. 35.3: Advanced stage 4a ROP in the left eye showing anterior and circumferential traction with subtotal retinal detachment.
(ROP: Retinopathy of prematurity)

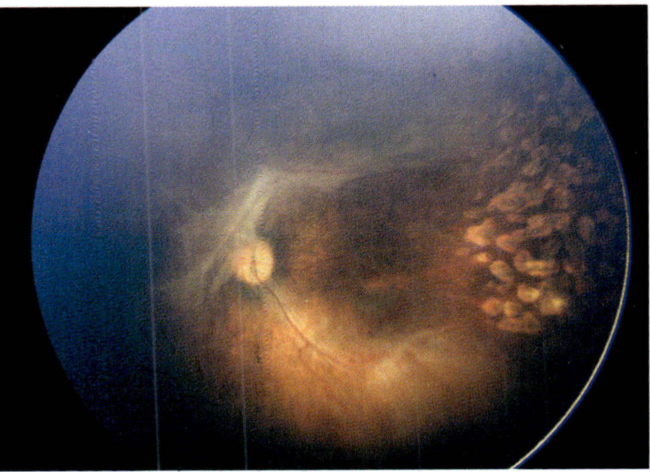

Fig. 35.4: Operated case of stage 4A ROP showing resolution of retinal detachment and disease regression at 3 weeks.
(ROP: Retinopathy of prematurity)

Multiple case series have reported good outcome with primary vitrectomy for stage 4ROP. Bhende et al.[32] studied outcomes of lens sparing surgery for stage 4ROP in 39 eyes and reported 74% anatomic success and 63% favorable functional outcome on a mean follow-up of 15 months. Singh et al.[33] reported the long-term functional outcome of LSV for stage 4ROP and found that 63% of cases had measurable visual acuity (VA) (mean logMAR 0.92 for stage 4A and 1.63 for stage 4B) and 19% had form vision, and remaining 18% had only light perception or less. A similar outcome was reported by Choi et al.[34] in stage 4B ROP, wherein with a mean follow-up of 5.6 years they reported 62% anatomic success and 78% with vision more than form sense. In another large series of 496 eyes, they found that the attachment rate after a single LSV surgery was 82.1% for stage 4a, and 69.5% for stage 4B.[30]

Some surgeons now advocate bilateral eye surgery for stage 4ROP in the same sitting.[35] They found it very effective and safe with no increased rates of infection, though strict aseptic precautions are necessary. Their anatomic success was 100% for stage 4A (11 eyes) and 89% for stage 4B (9 eyes). This approach is useful as it provides surgical benefit for both eyes together in a single general anesthesia sitting and prevents delay.

VITREORETINAL SURGERY FOR STAGE 5 RETINOPATHY OF PREMATURITY

Stage 5ROP involves total retinal detachment and is usually the culmination of a progressive untreated disease. Early stage 5 disease where shallow total detachment has occurred but fibrous membranes have not yet formed behind the lens (as in cases which are progressing from stage 4), may be amenable to LSV with better outcomes than seen in end-stage 5ROP. The cases which present with end-stage 5ROP have retrolental membranes, total TRD, dense fibrovascular proliferation, and subretinal exudation with no view of the fundus.

Ultrasonography plays an important role in surgical planning and prognostication of stage 5ROP.[22] It helps in determination of true configuration of retinal detachment where visualization is hampered. Typically, open-open retinal funnel configurations have better prognosis and surgery is attempted. The closed-closed retinal configuration has a poor prognosis and most surgical attempts lead to failure.

Different surgical techniques have been described for stage 5ROP. Open sky vitrectomy is the first described method for operating stage 5ROP.[36] It is rarely done now and reserved only for cases with associated corneal clouding that hampers visualization. Closed lensectomy, vitrectomy, and membrane peeling are the procedures of choice in established stage 5 disease with fibrous membranes reaching up to the lens.

The surgical steps we practice involve making three clear corneal incisions near limbus with the 20G/23G MVR blade. The 23G/25G instruments can easily pass through these incisions. Partial iridectomy becomes necessary when pupillary dilation is poor, to gain surgical space. Once lensectomy is completed, the entire capsular bag complex can sometimes be pinched out using a fine forceps, to prevent the postoperative inflammatory closure of the pupil. This step also relieves the traction on the retrolental tissue and provides access for further dissection. Two bent 26G needles or Sinskey hooks can be used for the further opening of the central funnel in the retrolental tissue. A close dissection of membranes is then performed with different instruments such as vitreous cutter, intravitreal scissors, and forceps. As the dissection proceeds more posteriorly into the funnel, viscoelastics can also be used to safely open up the funnel further. No attempt is made to create a retinotomy or drain the subretinal fluid. Once the

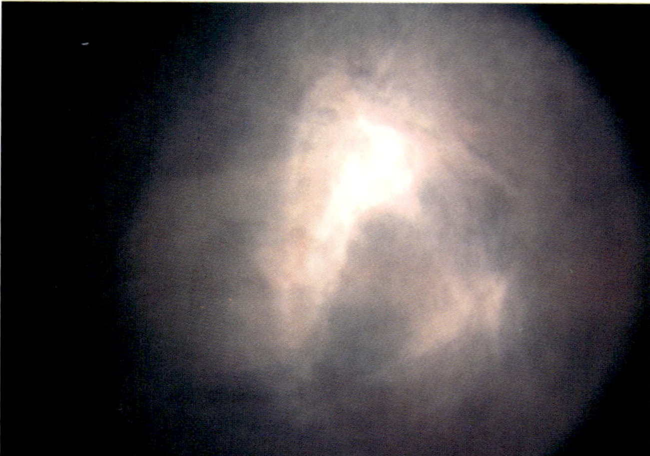

Fig. 35.5: Stage 5ROP showing retrolental membrane with poor retinal visibility and underlying total retinal detachment. (ROP: Retinopathy of prematurity)

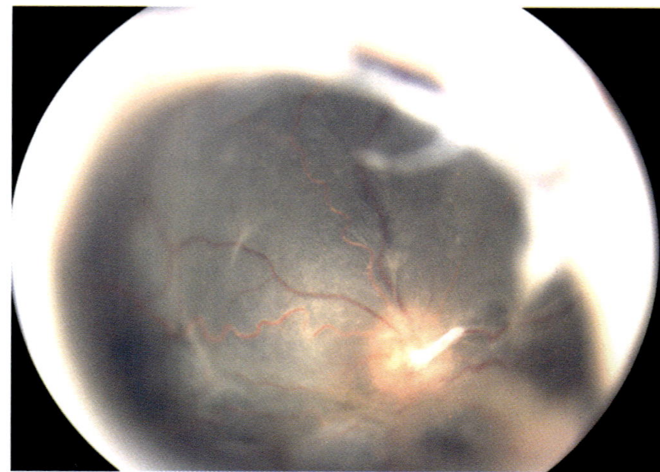

Fig. 35.6: Operated case of stage 5ROP showing centrally open retinal funnel with visible posterior pole at 8 weeks. (ROP: Retinopathy of prematurity)

traction is relieved, the fluid absorbs gradually over months and the retinal settles as much as possible. Since there is a dense meshwork of vessels, care should be taken to not traumatize them as profuse bleeding might occur. At the end of the surgery, air can be filled in the anterior chamber and ports can be hydrated for sutureless closure or sutured with 10-0 monofilament nylon sutures. Sutures can be later removed after a few weeks on subsequent examination under general anesthesia (Figs. 35.5 and 35.6).

Usually, results after stage 5ROP surgery are not encouraging. Even after removing traction maximally, the retina is often contracted irreversibly and an attached posterior retina is difficult to achieve. Most literature reports that anatomic success is very poor.[32,34,37,38] Often the postoperative outcomes are further complicated by secondary glaucoma, corneal edema, recurrent uveitis, chronic hypotony, etc. Long-term functional success is also limited with most children achieving only light perception vision, while few others might obtain suboptimal vision.[39,40] Visual rehabilitation remains a big challenge due to primary poor visual recovery, aphakia, and fibrous reproliferation reversing the results of surgery. In the few cases where the posterior retina does attach, early refractive correction is essential to prevent amblyopia.

LATE RETINAL DETACHMENTS IN RETINOPATHY OF PREMATURITY

Retinal detachment can sometimes occur in eyes with regressed ROP, later in life (Figs. 35.7A to D). Following the acute phase of ROP, vascular activity diminishes and ROP may regress. Once regressed, retinal changes may occur includ-

ing peripheral vascular abnormalities, pigmentary changes of the retina, cicatricial vitreoretinal interface abnormalities, peripheral retinal folds, lattice-like degeneration, dragging of the retina, retinal breaks, and tractional and rhegmatogenous retinal detachment. Several other authors have reported their experience with late-onset retinal detachments after ROP in adults.[41-46] They found that regressed ROP-associated retinal detachments can occur at any time during the life of the patient.

Repair of late retinal detachments in children (aged 2–15 years) offer a difficult surgical challenge with limited visual outcomes and decreased primary success rates. In a study, anatomical success following single surgery was 43.6%.[42] VA better than 20/200 was achieved in only 2 of 16 eyes studied, possibly due to delayed detection and abnormal development of visual function.

SUMMARY

Surgery for ROP has good results in early cases of stage 4A ROP. As the ROP continues to worsen and reaches stage 4B and stage 5 the prognosis continues to worsen. There are very few surgical centers as well as trained surgeons to manage these babies, and therefore most of these babies go blind, thereby causing a huge economic and social burden on the society.[47]

The best way to prevent these surgical challenges is to establish effective ROP screening programs which can screen, refer, and treat ROP in time so that babies do not develop advanced ROP. There is a need for creating awareness amongst ophthalmologists, pediatricians, and parents about the blinding outcomes of ROP and ensure that no baby goes blind.

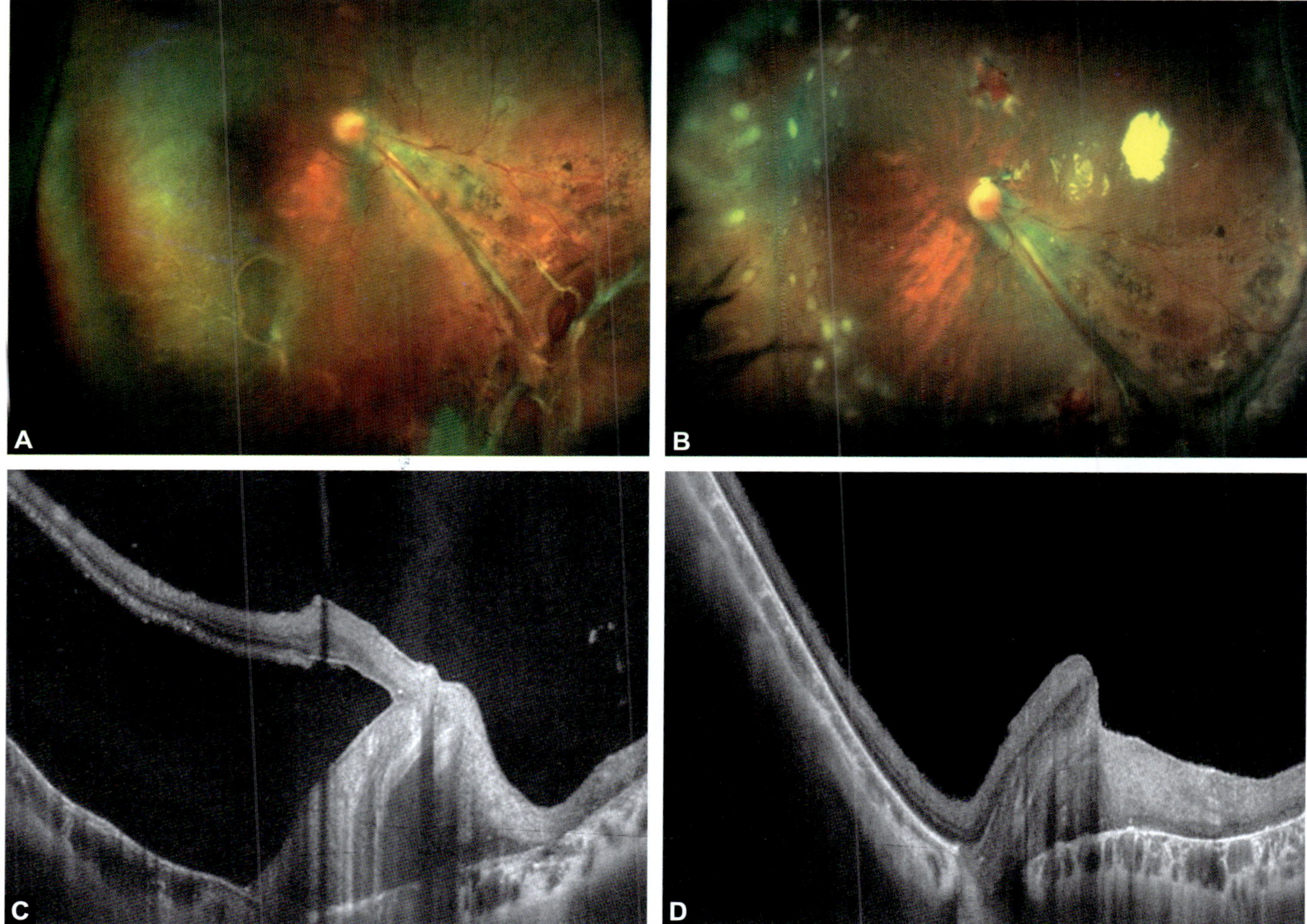

Figs. 35.7A to D: (A) Retinal detachment with dragged retina and break(s) in an eye with regressed ROP (BCVA - HMCF). (B) Postoperatively the retina is well settled (BCVA - 6/60), with visible laser marks. (C) OCT shows preoperative detachment with elevated retinal fold visible and (D) postoperatively attached retina draped around the fold.
(ROP: Retinopathy of prematurity; BCVA: Best Corrected Visual Acuity, HMCF: Hand movement close to face; OCT: Optical coherence tomography)

REFERENCES

1. International Committee for the Classification of Retinopathy of Prematurity. The International Classification of Retinopathy of Prematurity revisited. Arch Ophthalmology. 2005;123(7):991-9.
2. Smith LEH. Through the eyes of a child: understanding retinopathy through ROP the Friedenwald lecture. Invest Ophthalmology Vis Sci. 2008;49(12):5177-82.
3. Alon T, Hemo I, Itin A, et al. Vascular endothelial growth factor acts as a survival factor for newly formed retinal vessels and has implications for retinopathy of prematurity. Nat Med. 1995;1(10):1024-8.
4. Chung EJ, Kim JH, Ahn HS, et al. Combination of laser photocoagulation and intravitreal bevacizumab (Avastin) for aggressive zone I retinopathy of prematurity. Graefes Arch Clin Exp Ophthalmology. 2007;245(11):1727-30.
5. Quiroz-Mercado H, Martinez-Castellanos MA, Hernandez-Rojas ML, et al. Antiangiogenic therapy with intravitreal bevacizumab for retinopathy of prematurity. Retina. 2008;28(3 Suppl):S19-25.
6. Kusaka S, Shima C, Wada K, et al. Efficacy of intravitreal injection of bevacizumab for severe retinopathy of prematurity: a pilot study. Br J Ophthalmology. 2008;92(11):1450-5.
7. Mintz-Hittner HA, Kennedy KA, Chuang AZ; BEAT-ROP Cooperative Group. Efficacy of intravitreal bevacizumab for stage 3+ retinopathy of prematurity. N Engl J Med. 2011;364(7):603-15.
8. Lee JY, Chae JB, Yang SJ, et al. Effects of intravitreal bevacizumab and laser in retinopathy of prematurity therapy on the development of peripheral retinal vessels. Graefes Arch Clin Exp Ophthalmology. 2010;248(9):1257-62
9. Xu Y, Zhang Q, Kang X, et al. Early vitreoretinal surgery on vascularly active stage 4 retinopathy of prematurity through the preoperative intravitreal bevacizumab injection. Acta Ophthalmology. 2013;91(4):e304-10.
10. Baumal CR, Goldberg RA, Fein JG. Primary intravitreal ranibizumab for high-risk retinopathy of prematurity. Ophthalmic Surg Lasers Imaging Retina. 2015;46(4):432-8.
11. Yi Z, Su Y, Zhou Y, et al. Effects of Intravitreal Ranibizumab in the Treatment of Retinopathy of Prematurity in Chinese Infants. Curr Eye Res. 2016 41(8):1092-97.

12. Salman AG, Said AM. Structural, visual and refractive outcomes of intravitreal aflibercept injection in high-risk prethreshold type 1 retinopathy of prematurity. Ophthalmic Res. 2015;53(1):15-20

13. Pertl L, Steinwender G, Mayer C, et al. A Systematic Review and Meta-Analysis on the Safety of Vascular Endothelial Growth Factor (VEGF) Inhibitors for the Treatment of Retinopathy of Prematurity. PloS One. 2015;10(6):e0129383.

14. Kong L, Bhatt AR, Demny AB, et al. Pharmacokinetics of bevacizumab and its effects on serum VEGF and IGF-1 in infants with retinopathy of prematurity. Invest Ophthalmology Vis Sci. 2015; 56(2):956-61.

15. Lee BJ, Kim JH, Heo H, et al. Delayed onset atypical vitreoretinal traction band formation after an intravitreal injection of bevacizumab in stage 3 retinopathy of prematurity. Eye (Lond). 2012;26(7):903-10.

16. Honda S, Hirabayashi H, Tsukahara Y, et al. Acute contraction of the proliferative membrane after an intravitreal injection of bevacizumab for advanced retinopathy of prematurity. Graefes Arch Clin Exp Ophthalmology. 2008;246(7):1061-3.

17. Jalali S, Balakrishnan D, Zeynalova Z, et al. Serious adverse events and visual outcomes of rescue therapy using adjunct bevacizumab to laser and surgery for retinopathy of prematurity. The Indian Twin Cities Retinopathy of Prematurity Screening database Report number 5. Arch Dis Child Fetal Neonatal Ed. 2013;98(4):F327-33.

18. Hu J, Blair MP, Shapiro MJ, et al. Reactivation of retinopathy of prematurity after bevacizumab injection. Arch Ophthalmology. 2012;130(8):1000-6.

19. Wong RK, Hubschman S, Tsui I. Reactivation of retinopathy of prematurity after ranibizumab treatment. Retina. 2015;35(4):675-80.

20. Sanghi G, Dogra MR, Katoch D, et al. Demographic profile of infants with stage 5 retinopathy of prematurity in North India: implications for screening. Ophthalmic Epidemiol. 2011;18(2):72-4.

21. Ells AL, Gole GA, Lloyd Hildebrand P, et al. Posterior to the ridge laser treatment for severe stage 3 retinopathy of prematurity. Eye (Lond). 2013;27(4):525-30.

22. Muslubas IS, Karacorlu M, Hocaoglu M, et al. Ultrasonography Findings in Eyes With Stage 5 Retinopathy of Prematurity. Ophthalmic Surg Lasers Imaging Retina. 2015;46(10):1035-40.

23. Azad R, Mannan R, Chandra P. Role of ultrasound biomicroscopy in management of eyes with stage 5 retinopathy of prematurity. Ophthalmic Surg Lasers Imaging. 2010;41(2):196-200.

24. Greven C, Tasman W. Scleral buckling in stages 4B and 5 retinopathy of prematurity. Ophthalmology. 1990;97(6):817-20

25. Beyrau K, Danis R. Outcomes of primary scleral buckling for stage 4 retinopathy of prematurity. Can J Ophthalmology. 2003;38(4):267-71.

26. Chuang YC, Yang CM. Scleral buckling for stage 4 retinopathy of prematurity. Ophthalmic Surg Lasers. 2000;31(5):374-9.

27. Choi MY, Yu YS. Efficacy of removal of buckle after scleral buckling surgery for retinopathy of prematurity. J AAPOS. 2000;4(6):362-5.

28. Chow DR, Ferrone PJ, Trese MT. Refractive changes associated with scleral buckling and division in retinopathy of prematurity. Arch Ophthalmology. 1998;116(11):1446-8.

29. Hairston RJ, Maguire AM, Vitale S, et al. Morphometric analysis of pars plana development in humans. Retina. 1997;17(2):135-8.

30. Nudleman E, Robinson J, Rao P, et al. Long-term outcomes on lens clarity after lens-sparing vitrectomy for retinopathy of prematurity. Ophthalmology. 2015;122(4):755-9.

31. Iwahashi-Shima C, Miki A, Hamasaki T, et al. Intraocular pressure elevation is a delayed-onset complication after successful vitrectomy for stages 4 and 5 retinopathy of prematurity. Retina. 2012; 32(8):1636-42.

32. Bhende P, Gopal L, Sharma T, et al. Functional and anatomical outcomes after primary lens-sparing pars plana vitrectomy for Stage 4 retinopathy of prematurity. Indian J Ophthalmology. 2009;57(4):267-71.

33. Singh R, Reddy DM, Barkmeier AJ, et al. Long-term visual outcomes following lens-sparing vitrectomy for retinopathy of prematurity. Br J Ophthalmology. 2012;96(11):1395-8.

34. Choi J, Kim JH, Kim SJ, et al. Long-term results of lens-sparing vitrectomy for stages 4B and 5 retinopathy of prematurity. Korean J Ophthalmology. 2011;25(5):305-10.

35. Yonekawa Y, Wu WC, Kusaka S, et al. Immediate Sequential Bilateral Pediatric Vitreoretinal Surgery. Ophthalmology. 20161;123(8):1802-8.

36. Tasman W, Borrone RN, Bolling J. Open sky vitrectomy for total retinal detachment in retinopathy of prematurity. Ophthalmology. 1987;94(4):449-52.

37. Gopal L, Sharma T, Shanmugam M, et al. Surgery for stage 5 retinopathy of prematurity: the learning curve and evolving technique. Indian J Ophthalmology. 2000;48(2):101-6.

38. Trese MT, Droste PJ. Long-term postoperative results of a consecutive series of stages 4 and 5 retinopathy of prematurity. Ophthalmology. 1998;105(6):992-7.

39. Cusick M, Charles MK, Agrón E, et al. Anatomical and visual results of vitreoretinal surgery for stage 5 retinopathy of prematurity. Retina. 2006;26(7):729-35.

40. Mintz-Hittner HA, O'Malley RE, Kretzer FL. Long-term form identification vision after early, closed, lensectomy-vitrectomy for stage 5 retinopathy of prematurity. Ophthalmology. 1997;104(3):454-9.

41. Tasman W, Brown GC. Progressive visual loss in adults with retinopathy of prematurity (ROP). Tr Am Opth Soc. 1988;86:357-79.

42. Park KH, Hwang JM, Choi MY, et al. Retinal detachment of regressed retinopathy of prematurity in children aged 2 to 15 years. Retina. 2004;24(3):368-75.

43. Tufail A, Singh AJ, Haynes RJ, et al. Late onset vitreoretinal complications of regressed retinopathy of prematurity. Br J Ophthalmology. 2004;88(2):243-6.

44. Terasaki H, Hirose T. Late onset retinal detachment associated with regressed retinopathy of prematurity. Jap J Ophthamol. 2003;47(5):492-7.

45. Ferrone PJ, Trese MT, Williams GA, et al. Good visual acuity in an adult population with marked posterior segment changes secondary to retinopathy of prematurity. Retina. 1998;18:335-8.

46. Machemer R. Late traction detachment in retinopathy or ROP like cases. Graefes Arch Clin Exp Ophthalmology. 1993;231(7):389-94.

47. Azad R. Retinopathy of prematurity a giant in the developing world. Indian Pediatr. 2009;46(3):211-2.

Chapter 36

Familial Exudative Vitreoretinopathy

Atul Kumar, Dheepak Sundar, Rohan Chawla

 ## INTRODUCTION

Familial exudative vitreoretinopathy (FEVR) is a rare hereditary disorder characterized by incomplete and aberrant retinal angiogenesis. Criswick and Schepens first described FEVR in 1969.[1] In 1972, Canny and Oliver further outlined the vascular features with the help of fluorescein angiography.[2] The disease closely resembles retinopathy of prematurity (ROP) and shows marked phenotypic variability. The clinical features may range from asymptomatic avascular peripheral retina to total retinal detachment causing severe vision loss.[3,4]

 ## PATHOPHYSIOLOGY AND INHERITANCE

Retinal vascularization starts at about 18 weeks of gestation and gets completed by 38–40 weeks. The organization of vascular plexus involves two critical steps: vasculogenesis and angiogenesis. Vasculogenesis is the de novo formation of vessels from the endothelial precursor cells. The endothelial cells unite together to form cords, which later develop lumen. Angiogenesis involves the development of newer vessels from the existing vascular network. It is believed that the primary vascular plexus of the retina is formed by the process of vasculogenesis whereas the remaining capillary layers in the deeper and peripheral retina develop by angiogenesis.[5] FEVR is a disorder of retinal angiogenesis.[6]

At the molecular level, Wnt and the Norrin-signaling pathways are vital for organogenesis and angiogenesis in the eye. Typical mutations in FEVR are as shown in Table 36.1. The products of these genes are involved in the Wnt pathway. Norrin coded by Norrie disease protein gene (*NDP*) has a strong affinity and binds to Frizzled-4 (FZD4) receptor. Low-density lipoprotein receptor-related protein 5 (LRP5) acts like a coreceptor. The ligand receptor complex is mediated by Tetraspanin-12 (TSPAN12), an auxiliary transmembrane protein. The Norrin receptor complex thereby activates the Wnt signaling. Thus, mutation in any of these factors leads to defective Wnt signaling and hence affects retinal angiogenesis.[7-11]

A positive family history can be identified in 20–40% of the cases. Currently, three different inheritance patterns have been described: autosomal dominant (AD), autosomal recessive (AR) and X-linked recessive; with the AD form being the most common. The disease shows variable expressivity, explaining the wide spectrum of clinical presentation even among members of the same family.[4,7]

Phenotypic Variability

The severity of the disease depends on the phenotypic variability. The members of the same family with a mutation at the same genetic loci may have different clinical presentations.[12] The phenotypic variability is believed to be a consequence of genetic modifiers and environmental influences. The genetic modifiers that vary among individuals may either protect the individual from the effects of mutation or aggravate it. The environmental factors may be systemic or local. For example,

Table 36.1: Mutations related to familial exudative vitreoretinopathy (FEVR).[6]

S. No	Gene	Protein	Inheritance	Chromosome
1	NDP	Norrin disease protein	X-linked recessive	X
2	FZD 4	Frizzled-4	Autosomal dominant (AD)	11
3	LRP 5	Low density lipoprotein receptor protein-5	AD and Autosomal recessive (AR)	11
4	TSPAN 12	Tetraspanin-12	AD	7
Others	ZNF408 (AD)			

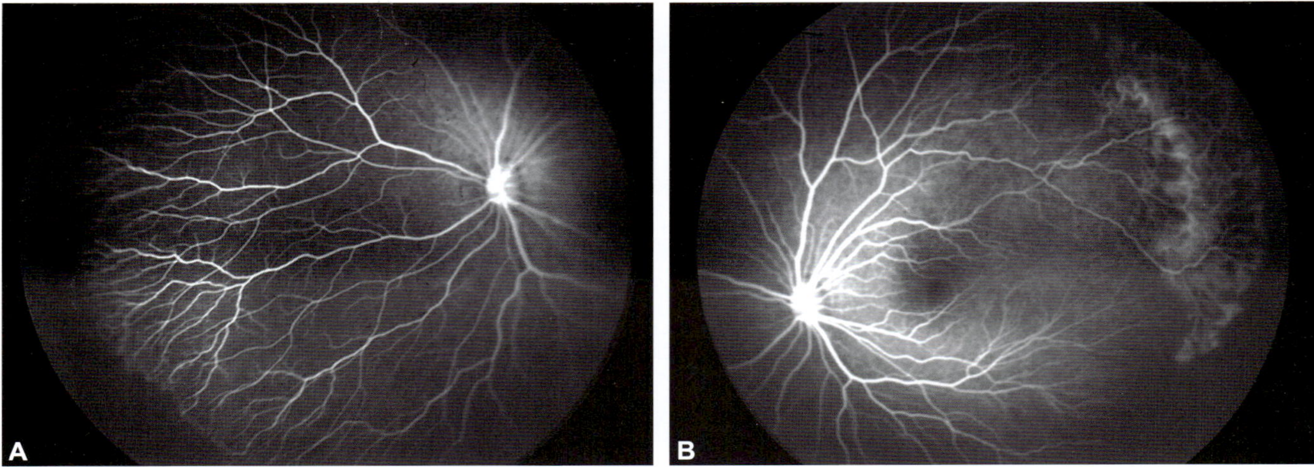

Figs. 36.1A and B: Fluorescein angiography of a child with familial exudative vitreoretinopathy (FEVR) showing (A) peripheral avascularity, (B) avascularity, venous-venous anastomosis and neovascularization with leakage.

minimal changes in the partial pressure of oxygen (PaO_2) or exposure to certain drugs during intra uterine development may alter the phenotypic presentation. Another interesting feature is the asymmetric nature of the disease. That is, one eye of the patient may present with retinal detachment (RD) and the other may exhibit subtle vascular changes only. The asymmetry is again believed to be a result of local environmental differences during ocular development.[6,13]

CLINICAL PRESENTATION, DIAGNOSIS AND STAGING

The most prominent feature of FEVR is the peripheral retinal avascularity as explained previously by the defective retinal angiogenesis.[14] The severity of the disease due to the phenotypic variability may be mild to advance. The age of presentation in turn depends on the severity. In mild cases, the patient is asymptomatic with subtle peripheral vascular changes. Vitreoretinal adhesions, venous-venous anastomoses, supernumerous vascular branching and V-shaped retinochoroidal degenerations are some of the prominent features. In moderate to severe cases, neovascularization is seen. The pre-retinal new vessels are visible at the junction of vascular and avascular retina similar to ROP (Figs. 36.1 and 36.2). The fibrosis associated with these vessels causes traction of the macula and the blood vessels. They can lead to macular ectopia and the patients show a drop in visual acuity. Radial folds spanning the macula may develop which is another hallmark feature of severe FEVR. They are termed as falciform folds or knife-like folds based on their clinical appearance (Figs. 36.3A and B). Vitreous hemorrhage from the new vessels is also a common presenting feature.

Retinal detachments are seen in 21–64% of the cases. They can be serous, tractional or rhegmatogenous (Figs. 36.4A

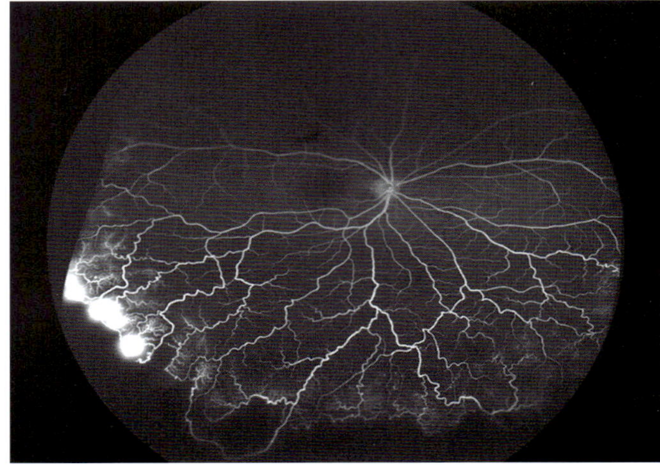

Fig. 36.2: Ultra-wide-field fundus fluorescein angiography of a 17-year-old familial exudative vitreoretinopathy (FEVR) patient revealing inferior combined retinal detachment with peripheral neovascularization.

and B). Other common findings include retinal exudation, secondary epiretinal membrane, vitreoretinal adhesion, hyaloid vascular remnants, capillary angioma, peripheral schisis and secondary glaucoma.[6,11]

Examination of the retinal periphery with UWF color picture and FA is paramount at diagnosis and for follow-up. This being a lifelong disease with exacerbations, hence requiring careful peripheral retina imaging.

Recently spectral domain optical coherence tomography (OCT) characteristics of FEVR were reported. Posterior hyaloidal organization, cystoid macular edema and ellipsoid zone disruption are a few OCT findings indicating the cause of vision loss.[15] Fundus fluorescein angiography (FFA) on a

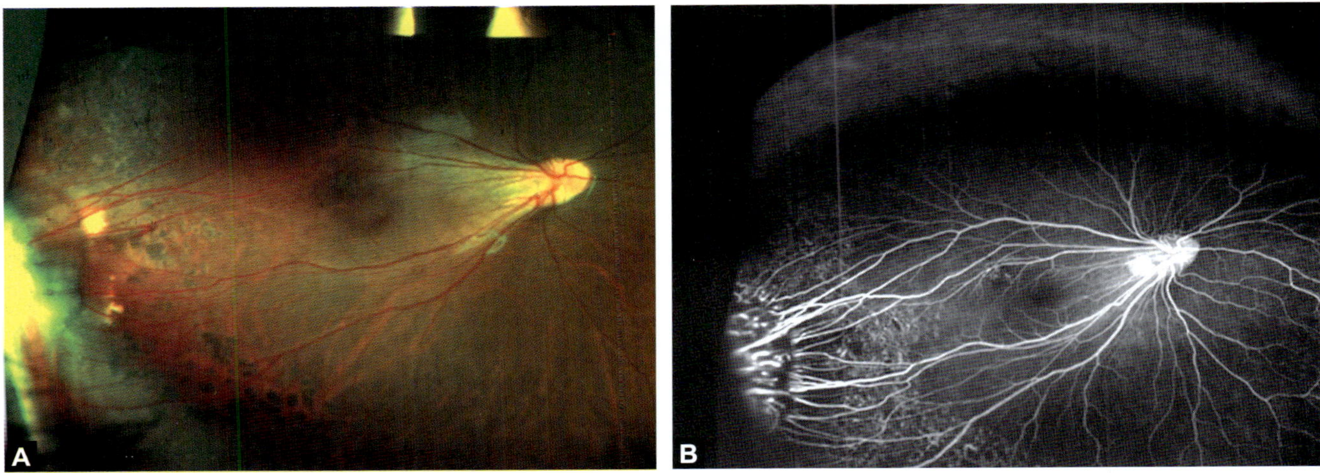

Figs. 36.3A and B: Ultra-wide-field imaging (A) falciform folds originating from the disc (B) abnormal straightening of the vessels at the posterior pole with peripheral laser mark.

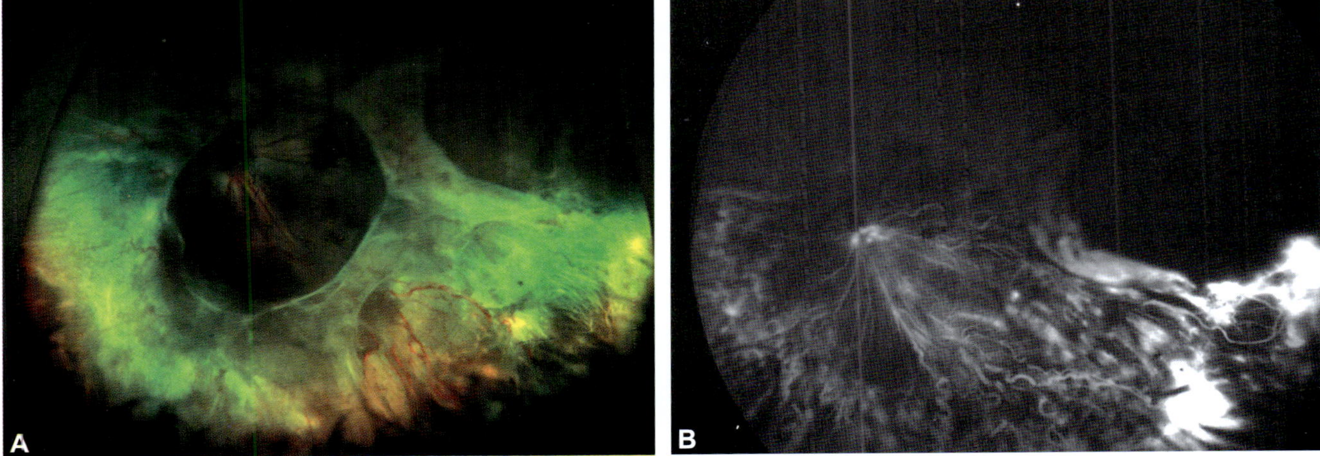

Figs. 36.4A and B: (A) Advanced stage of familial exudative vitreoretinopathy (FEVR) showing combined retinal detachment with severe proliferative vitreoretinopathy (PVR) with peripheral leakage on ultrawide field FA (B).

yearly basis helps in detecting leakage and ischemic zones in mild cases.[11]

Though there are no established criteria, the diagnosis of FEVR can be made considering the following:

- Presence of avascular areas in the peripheral retina in at least one eye
- Lack of a history of prematurity and any other features suggestive of ROP
- Other clinical manifestations representing the sequelae of retinal avascularity as explained before.[16]

A positive family history may further help in confirming the diagnosis, whereas a negative history does not necessarily rule out FEVR.[11]

Various staging and classification systems have been devised for prognostication and treatment purposes. The staging system proposed by Pendergast and Trese.[17] that was recently updated is the most comprehensive of all (Table 36.2). It is to be noted that the staging systems are based on the clinical presentation and do not represent the course of disease advancement.

DIFFERENTIAL DIAGNOSIS

Norries disease is one of the differential diagnoses of FEVR. It is considered as a severe form of FEVR and may be associated with systemic features. Deletion mutation of NDP gene exclusively leads to this X-linked retinal dysplasia. Missense mutation can cause either X-linked recessive FEVR or Norries disease. Cases of Norries disease present with a classic glistening whitish retinal mass with almost total loss of vision.

Table 36.2: Updated clinical classification of familial exudative vitreoretinopathy.[4,21]

Stage	Exudate*		Clinical features
	Without	*With*	
1	A	B	Avascular retinal periphery
2	A	B	Extraretinal neovascularization
3	A	B	Retinal detachment not involving macula
4	A	B	Retinal detachment involving macula
5	A (open funnel)	B (closed funnel)	Total retinal detachment

*: For stages 1–4.

Associated systemic features include progressive hearing loss and mental retardation. It can be differentiated from FEVR by its rapidly progressive course and absence of preretinal new vessels. The disease is as such nontreatable. Management is mainly concerned with preventing secondary complication to maintain the organization of the globe.[6,11,18]

Osteoporosis pseudoglioma (OPPG) is caused by mutation in *LRP 5* gene. Ocular features resemble the presentation of severe FEVR. The patient has associated with osteoporosis. A congenitally blind patient with frequent history of childhood fractures draws the diagnosis toward OPPG. The visual prognosis is poor with the systemic disease requiring bisphosphonate therapy.[19,20]

Retinopathy of prematurity has a similar clinical picture but there is a definite history of prematurity. Bilateral presentation at an earlier age is more common with early regression and absence of late recurrences.[21]

LONG-TERM OUTCOMES

Most patients with mild-to-moderate FEVR have stable vision if properly monitored and treated with 64–74% of affected patients maintaining a vision of 6/12 or better.[22,23] FEVR is a life-long disease requiring regular examinations, follow-up and prompt treatment.

 MANAGEMENT

Treatment is strategized based on the stage of FEVR. Stage 1 requires regular monitoring and follow-up. In stage 2 (neovascularization), after confirming the leakage with fluorescein angiography (FA), laser photocoagulation of the capillary nonperfusion areas is done. Cryotherapy is useful in treating neovascularization, when the media is hazy or in cases with non-dilating pupil.[11,23] Few studies have quoted the role of antivascular endothelial growth factor (VEGF) in treating neovascularization based on the finding that the dysregulation of Wnt pathway was associated with elevated levels of VEGF in FEVR patients. Regression of new vessels was observed following the administration of anti-VEGFs.[24]

Advanced stages require surgical treatment. Scleral buckling and pars plana vitrectomy or a combination of both can be considered based on the configuration of the detachment (Figs. 36.5 to 36.8). Final reattachment rate reported in various studies range from 50% to 85%.[11,17] Role of intravitreal plasmin

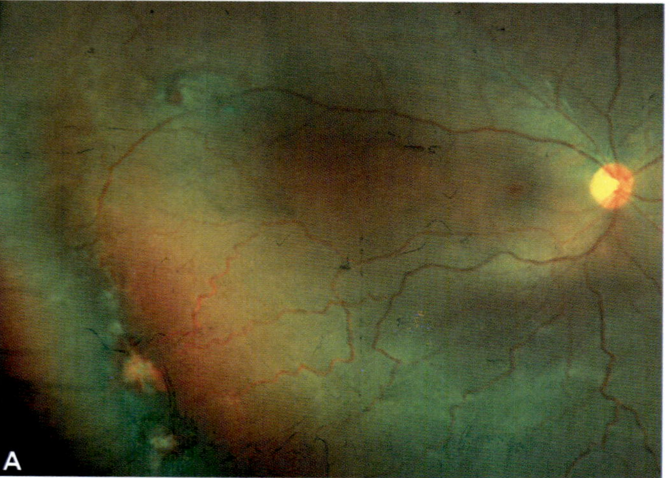
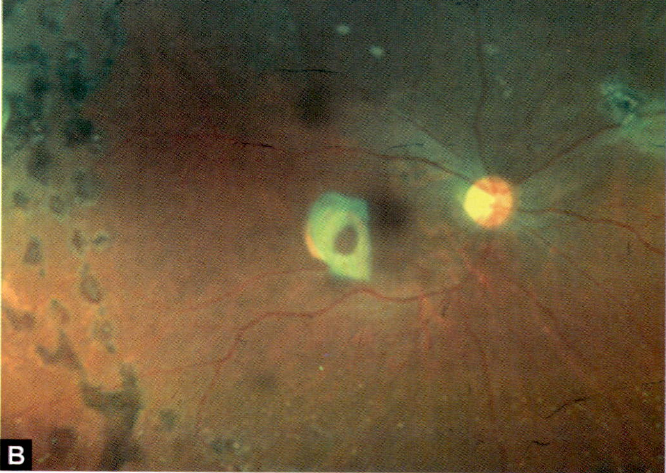

Figs. 36.5A and B: Preoperative familial exudative vitreoretinopathy (FEVR) with retinal detachment. Note the peripheral vascular abnormalities, and postoperatively the retina on with laser marks.

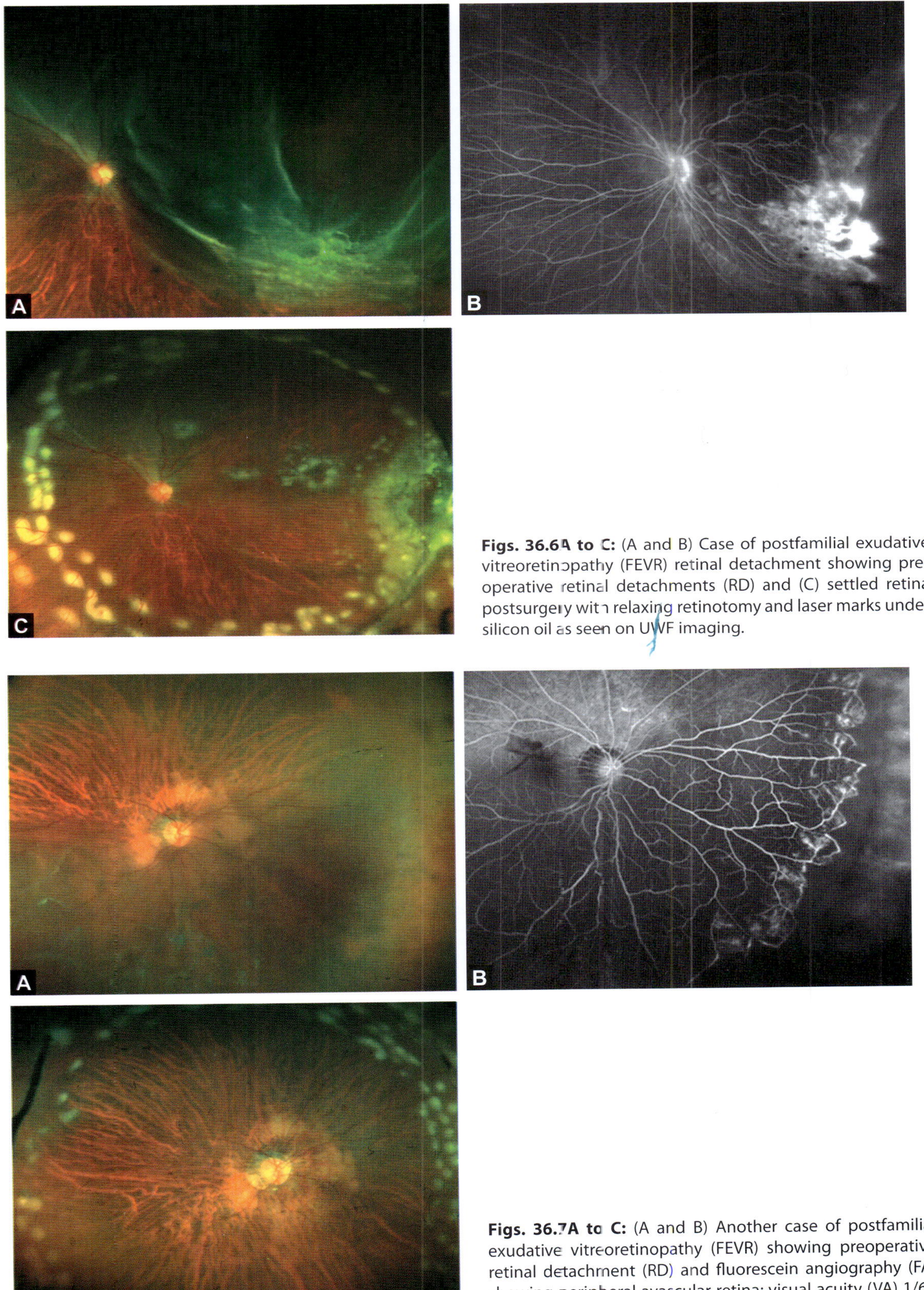

Figs. 36.6A to C: (A and B) Case of postfamilial exudative vitreoretinopathy (FEVR) retinal detachment showing preoperative retinal detachments (RD) and (C) settled retina postsurgery with relaxing retinotomy and laser marks under silicon oil as seen on UWF imaging.

Figs. 36.7A to C: (A and B) Another case of postfamilial exudative vitreoretinopathy (FEVR) showing preoperative retinal detachment (RD) and fluorescein angiography (FA) showing peripheral avascular retina; visual acuity (VA) 1/60 and (C) settled retina postsurgery; VA 6/24.

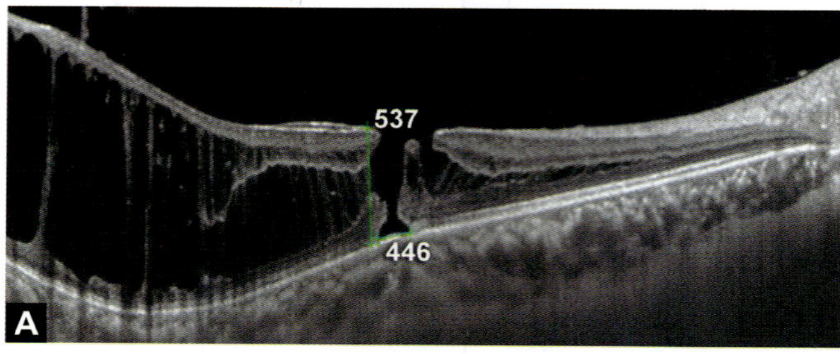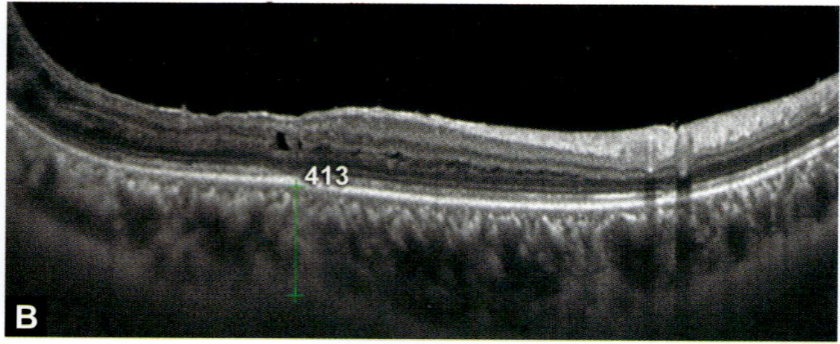

Figs. 36.8A and B: A young lady of 18 years presented with familial exudative vitreoretinopathy (FEVR) (Visual acuity (VA) - 3/60; FEVR was also evident in the mother on indirect ophthalmoscopy (IO) examination, optical coherence tomography (OCT) revealed marked retinoschisis with macular hole, which after surgery subsided and hole closed (final vision VA at 6 weeks 6/36).

to create a smooth surgical plane of dissection counteracting the traction due to the taut posterior hyaloid has also been studied.

Systemic investigation is mandatory when the clinical features indicate Norries disease or OPPG. Dexa scan to rule out osteoporosis and a thorough pediatric examination to evaluate hearing loss and mental retardation are required.[25]

Screening of asymptomatic family members helps in early detection and to provide genetic counseling. The ultra-wide-field fluorescein angiography is a fast growing screening tool, which guides in identifying peripheral vascular changes at an earlier stage.[26]

REFERENCES

1. Criswick VG, Schepens CL. Familial exudative vitreoretinopathy. Am J Ophthalmology. 1969;68:578-94.
2. Canny CL, Oliver GL. Fluorescein angiographic findings in familial exudative vitreoretinopathy. Arch Ophthalmology. 1976;94:1114-20.
3. Quiram PA, Drenser KA, Lai MM, et al. Treatment of vascularly active familial exudative vitreoretinopathy with pegaptanib sodium (Macugen). Retina. 2008;28:S8-12.
4. Kashani AH, Learned D, Nudleman E, et al. High prevalence of peripheral retinal vascular anomalies in family members of patients with familial exudative vitreoretinopathy. Ophthalmology. 2014;121:262-8.
5. Hughes S, Yang H, Chan-Ling T. Vascularization of the human fetal retina: roles of vasculogenesis and angiogenesis. Invest Ophthalmology Vis Sci. 2000;41:1217-28.
6. Gilmour DF. Familial exudative vitreoretinopathy and related retinopathies. Eye (Lond). 2015;29:1-4.
7. Jia LY, Li XX, Yu WZ, et al. Novel frizzled-4 gene mutations in Chinese patients with familial exudative vitreoretinopathy. Arch Ophthalmology. 2010;128:1341-9.
8. Robitaille JM, Zheng B, Wallace K, et al. The role of Frizzled-4 mutations in familial exudative vitreoretinopathy and Coats disease. Br J Ophthalmology. 2011;95:574-9.
9. Nikopoulos K, Venselaar H, Collin RW, et al. Overview of the mutation spectrum in familial exudative vitreoretinopathy and Norrie disease with identification of 21 novel variants in FZD4, LRP5, and NDP. Hum Mutat. 2010;31:656-66.
10. Poulter JA, Davidson AE, Ali M, et al. Recessive mutations in TSPAN12 cause retinal dysplasia and severe familial exudative vitreoretinopathy (FEVR). Invest Ophthalmology Vis Sci. 2012;53:2873-9.
11. Sızmaz S, Yonekawa Y, Trese MT. Familial exudative vitreoretinopathy. Turk J Ophthalmology. 2015;45:164-8.
12. Toomes C, Bottomley HM, Scott S, et al. Spectrum and frequency of FZD4 mutations in familial exudative vitreoretinopathy. Invest Ophthalmology Vis Sci. 2004;45:2083-90.
13. Sylvester CL. Retinopathy of prematurity. Semin Ophthalmology. 2008;23:318-23.
14. Boonstra FN, van Nouhuys CE, Schuil J, et al. Clinical and molecular evaluation of probands and family members with familial exudative vitreoretinopathy. Invest Ophthalmology Vis Sci. 2009;50:4379-85.
15. Yonekawa Y, Thomas BJ, Drenser KA, et al. Familial exudative vitreoretinopathy: spectral-domain optical coherence tomography of the vitreoretinal interface, retina, and choroid. Ophthalmology. 2015;122:2270-7.
16. Ranchod TM, Ho LY, Drenser KA, et al. Clinical presentation of familial exudative vitreoretinopathy. Ophthalmology. 2011;118:2070-5.
17. Pendergast SD, Trese MT. Familial exudative vitreoretinopathy. Results of surgical management. Ophthalmology. 1998;105:1015-23.
18. Sims KB. NDP-Related Retinopathies. In: Pagon RA, Adam MP, Ardinger HH, Wallace SE (Eds). GeneReviews®. Seattle (WA): University of Washington, Seattle; 1993–2017. [online] Available from: https://www.ncbi.nlm.nih.gov/books/NBK1331/ [Accessed December, 2017].
19. Ai M, Heeger S, Bartels CF, et al. Clinical and molecular findings in osteoporosis-pseudoglioma syndrome. Am J Hum Genet. 2005;77:741-53.
20. Streeten EA, McBride D, Puffenberger E, et al. Osteoporosis-pseudoglioma syndrome: description of 9 new cases and beneficial response to bisphosphonates. Bone. 2008;43:584-90.
21. Ranchod TM, Ho LY, Drenser KA, et al. Clinical presentation of familial exudative vitreoretinopathy. Ophthalmology. 2011;118:2070-5.
22. van Nouhuys CE. Signs, complications, and platelet aggregation in familial exudative vitreoretinopathy. Am J Ophthalmology. 1991;111:34-41.
23. Shukla D, Singh J, Sudheer G, et al. Familial exudative vitreoretinopathy (FEVR). Clinical profile and management. Indian J Ophthalmology. 2003;51:323-8.
24. Tagami M, Kusuhara S, Honda S, et al. Rapid regression of retinal hemorrhage and neovascularization in a case of familial exudative vitreoretinopathy treated with intravitreal bevacizumab. Graefes Arch Clin Exp Ophthalmology. 2008;246:1787-9.
25. Joshi MM, Ciaccia S, Trese MT, et al. Posterior hyaloid contracture in pediatric vitreoretinopathies. Retina. 2006;26:38-41.
26. Lyu J, Zhang Q, Wang SY, et al. Ultra-wide-field scanning laser ophthalmoscopy assists in the clinical detection and evaluation of asymptomatic early-stage familial exudative vitreoretinopathy. Graefes Arch Clin Exp Ophthalmology. 2017;255:39-47.

Chapter 37

Coats' Disease

Rohan Chawla, Shreyans Jain, Ruchir Tewari

INTRODUCTION

Coats' disease was first described by a Scottish ophthalmologist George Coats in 1908.[1] it is an idiopathic disorder characterised by aneurysmal and telangiectatic retinal vessels with intraretinal and subretinal exudation and fluid.[2] Exudative retinal detachment is a common feature present in this disease. Generally, the onset is in early childhood and a male preponderance with a male:female (M:F) ratio of 3:1 is seen. It is unilateral in 80–95% of cases.[3-5]

ETIOPATHOGENESIS AND HISTOLOGY

A genetic predisposition has been proposed as the etiology. Norrie disease pseudoglioma (NDP) gene mutation on chromosome Xp11.2 is seen in some patients. Norrin (a retinal protein) has been found to be deficient pointing towards pathogenesis of this disease.[6,7]

Coats' disease is a part of a spectrum of related genetic disorders known as "retinal hypovasculopathies"[8,9] which consists of Norrie disease, familial exudative vitreoretinopathy (FEVR), fascioscapulohumeral muscular dystrophy (FSHD), and the osteoporosis pseudoglioma syndrome.[10-13] All the above-mentioned diseases have a similar phenotypic feature which is failure of peripheral retinal vascularization and associated telangiectatic, incompetent remnant vasculature.

Fundus examination typically shows a bullous retinal detachment. The subretinal fluid is a viscous, lipid-rich, yellow fluid with glistening crystals. On microscopic examination of subretinal fluid, the exudation consists of collection of histiocytes and cholesterol clefts (Fig. 37.1). These exudates cause thickening of the outer retinal layer and inner retinal layer to some extent. Areas of the inner retina also contain numerous large, dilated, and telangiectatic vessels.[14]

CLINICAL PRESENTATION

The patient usually presents in the first decade of life (average 5 years). The patient may present with unilateral loss of

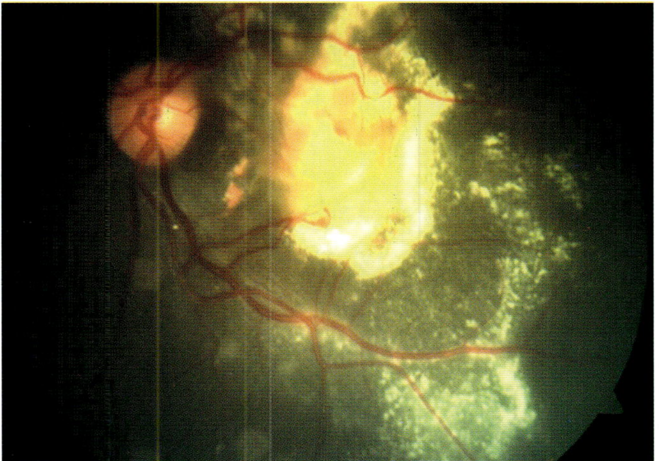

Fig. 37.1: Left eye fundus image shows extensive subretinal exudation in the macular region.

vision, strabismus and leukocoria.[4] Rarely, the patient may remain asymptomatic. Bilateral presumed Coats is very rare and other conditions like retinitis pigmentosa, pars planitis, FSHD, FEVR, Lebers congenital amaurosis (LCA) or other diseases that mimic Coats' like exudative retinopathy should be evaluated.[15-17] Anterior segment is usually normal in nearly 90% of eyes with the rest presenting with cataract, iris neovascularization, shallow anterior chamber or corneal edema.[18,19] Retinal findings include peripheral telangiectatic vessels, usually in the inferior and temporal quadrants beyond the equator with intraretinal and subretinal exudation (Figs. 37.2A and B). This progresses to an exudative retinal detachment, associated with retinal hemorrhages, retinal macrocyst, vasoproliferative tumor formation and optic disc neovascularization.[20] As the disease progresses it can lead to secondary complications like iridocyclitis, cataract, and secondary neovascular glaucoma which can further progress to phthisis bulbi in severe cases.[21,22]

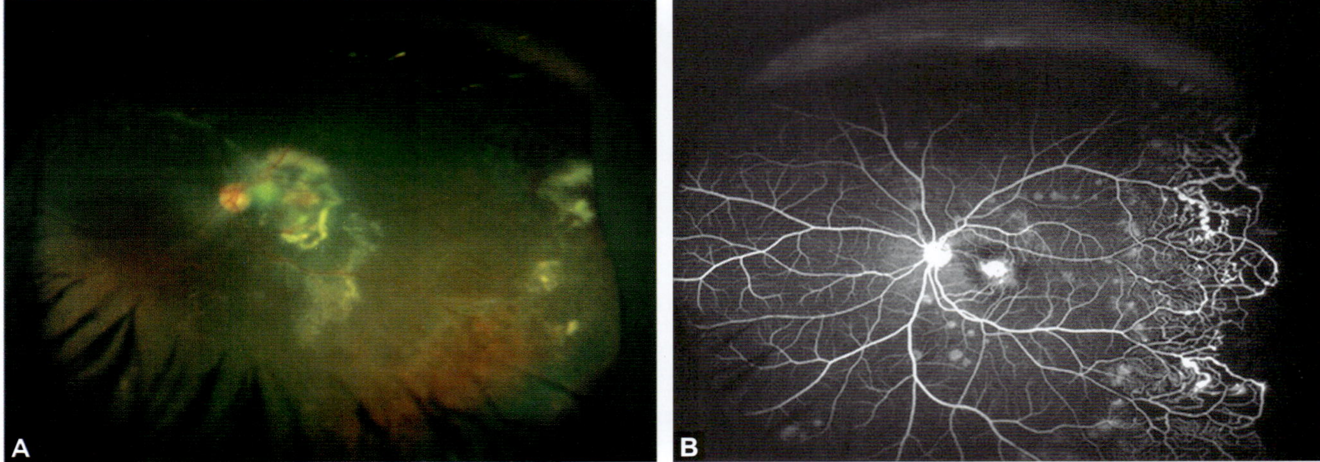

Figs. 37.2A and B: Coats' disease showing leaking angioma at the macula with peripheral telangiectatic vessels with some leakage and peripheral retinal ischemia.

STAGING

Initially divided by George Coats into three stages, it has been variously classified, and the most commonly followed staging system as given by Shields et al.:[23]

- Stage 1: Retinal telangiectasia only
- Stage 2A: Retinal telangiectasia and extrafoveal intraretinal exudation
- Stage 2B: Retinal telangiectasia and foveal intraretinal exudation
- Stage 3A$_1$: Subtotal extrafoveal exudative detachment
- Stage 3A$_2$: Subtotal foveal exudative detachment
- Stage 3B: Total exudative retinal detachment
- Stage 4: Total retinal detachment with elevated intraocular pressure
- Stage 5: Phthisis bulbi

The staging system also helps in prognosticating as visual acuity and final anatomic outcome have been found to be highly correlated with the disease stage.[24]

DIAGNOSIS

Usual ophthalmoscopic evaluation is enough for the diagnosis of Coats' retinopathy, but other disorders need to be ruled out, especially retinoblastoma.

Fundus fluorescein angiography (FFA) in mild cases shows early hyperfluorescence from the telangiectatic vessels. Other findings better defined on angiography are aneurysmal dilatation, vessel wall beading, and multiple communicating channels with larger vessels (Figs. 37.3A and B). These vessels display early and persistent leakage, representing breakdown of blood-retinal barrier (BRB). Capillary nonperfusion areas denote areas of microvascular involvement.

Newer modalities such as ultra-widefield angiography (UWFA) are useful to document and follow up patients,

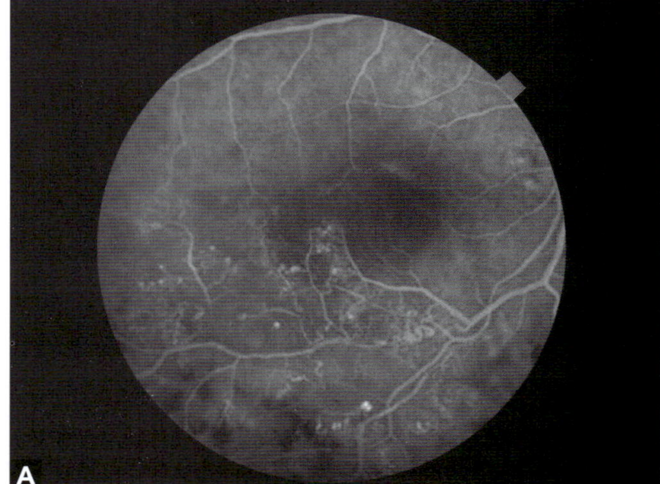

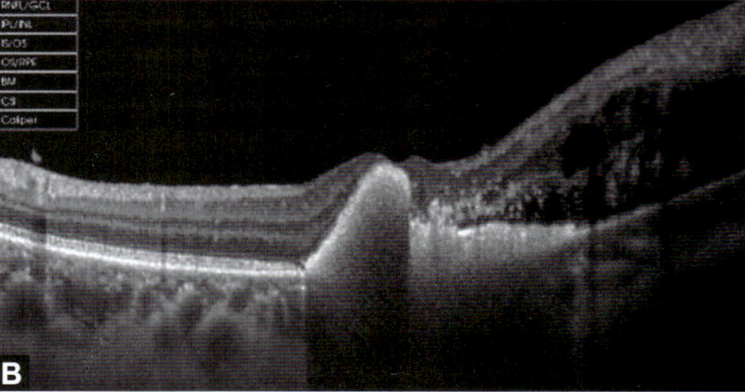

Figs. 37.3A and B: (A) Fundus fluorescein angiography (FFA) picture showing telangiectatic vessels with bulb like endings. (B) Optical Coherence Tomography (OCT) showing hyperreflective shadow corresponding to subretinal exudates with intraretinal edema.

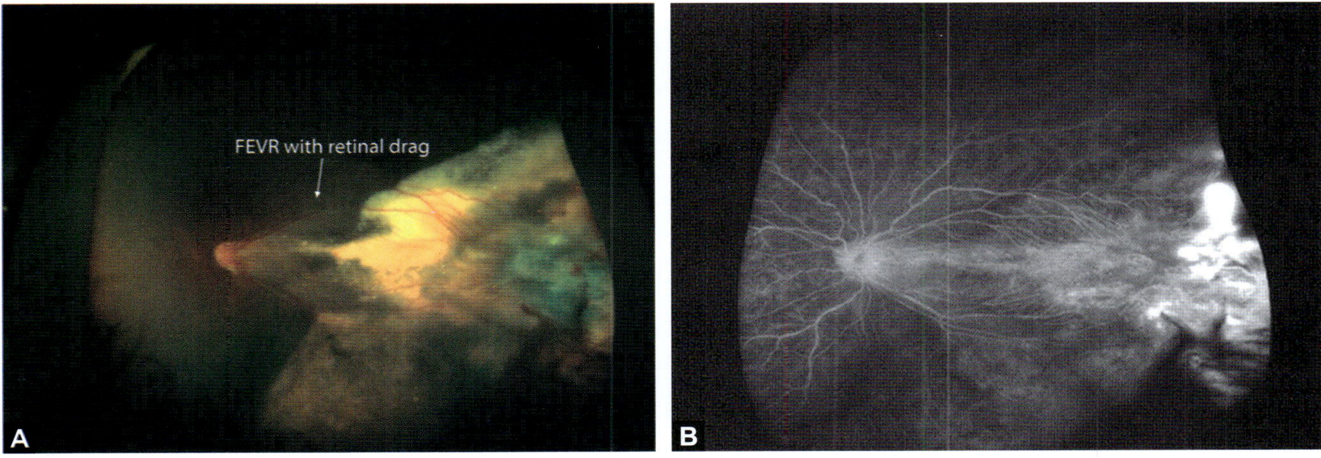

Figs. 37.4A and B: (A) Ultra-widefield (UWF) pseudocolor image of the left eye of a patient with familial exudative vitreoretinopathy (FEVR) shows straightening of retinal vessels and massive subretinal exudation along with abnormal peripheral vascular endings. (B) ultra-widefield (UWF) angiography picture shows extensive leakage from the peripheral vascular endings.

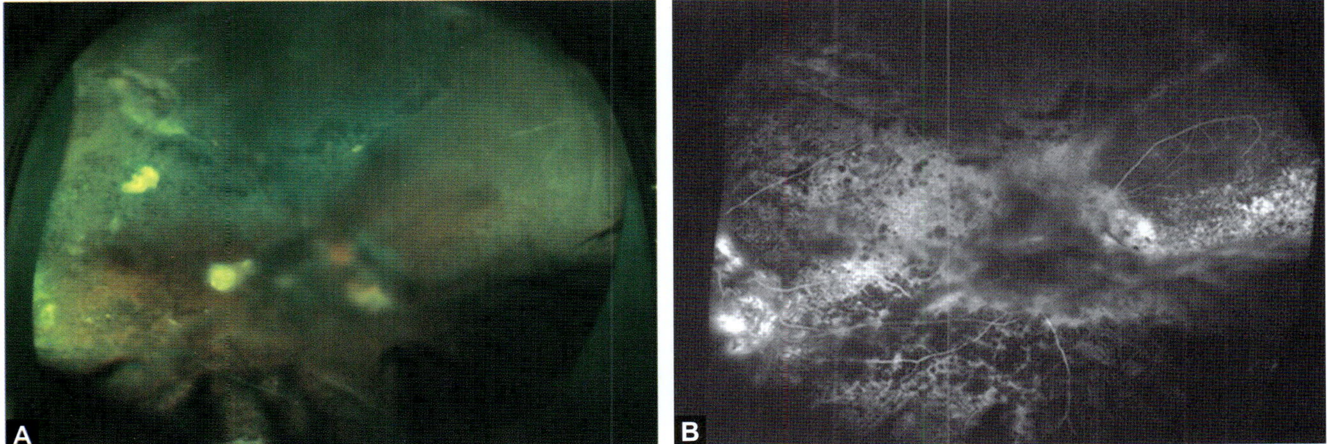

Figs. 37.5A and B: (A) Ultra-widefield (UWF) image showing lasered Coats' with scarring and exudation. (B) Peripheral leakage is noted in the UWF angiogram of the same eye.

especially in early stages of the disease (Figs. 37.4A and B). Detection and documentation of peripheral capillary nonperfusion (CNP) areas and from the peripheral telangiectatic vessels helps in early initiation of targeted treatment.

Ultrasonographic examination may help to differentiate retinoblastoma and Coats' disease as intraocular calcification is not usually seen in Coats' disease unlike retinoblastoma.

CT scan is helpful in characterizing the morphology, measuring subretinal opacities, determining vascularity in the subretinal space by contrast enhancement and indentifying other associated abnormalities in the orbital or intracranial space.

Optical coherence tomography (OCT) may be useful in cooperative children to rule out macular involvement and planning of treatment.

Histological examination of subretinal fluid can be done to confirm the diagnosis but it is rarely used. It reveals cholesterol crystals and pigment-laden macrophages without tumor cells.[25] FEVR can present as an exudative vitreoretinopathy with disc and retinal dragging and can be a differential diagnosis for Coats' disease.

MANAGEMENT

Observation and regular follow-up is advised in patients with mild, nonvision threatening disease (stage 1) in which the patient has no symptoms and in those who have end-stage disease with retinal detachment in which visual prognosis is nil. Laser photocoagulation to areas of telangiectasia and CNP should be considered if progressive exudation is documented (Figs. 37.5A and B). Direct laser of leaking vessels can be done under fluorescein guidance. Frequently more than one treatment session is required to obliterate the peripheral telangiectasia and induce resolution of remote exudation at the macula.[26-28] Cryotherapy, with a double freeze-thaw method, is useful in eyes with marked peripheral exudation or subtotal retinal detachment, although, this may result in marked reaction with increased leakage. Therefore, laser photocoagulation is still the preferred option wherever possible.

Intravitreal triamcinolone acetonide (IVTA) is used to decrease macular edema and subretinal exudation.[29,30] Anti-vascular endothelial growth factor (VEGF) therapy use is limited as only few studies of anti-VEGF therapy for Coats' have been carried out to date, but initial results as an adjunctive treatment to laser, cryo, or IVTA are promising.[31-33] Long-term safety in children remains unknown. Vitreoretinal surgery may be considered in eyes with total retinal detachment. The visual prognosis in such cases is usually poor though a successful retinal reattachment often prevents the subsequent development of neovascular glaucoma. Enucleation may be required in painful eyes with neovascular glaucoma. Transscleral diode laser cyclophotocoagulation (DLCP) is an alternative in cases with neovascular glaucoma.[34,35]

PROGNOSIS

The prognosis depends on the severity of involvement and stage of the disease at presentation. Young children, particularly those under 3 years of age, frequently have a hostile progression and already have extensive retinal detachment at presentation. However, older children and young adults have a more benign disease with decreased rate of progression to exudation or retinal detachment. Rarely, spontaneous regression is known to occur in older children with mild disease.

REFERENCES

1. Coats G. Forms of retinal disease with massive exudation. R Lond Ophthalmology Hosp Rep. 1908;525:440-525.
2. Egbert PR, Chan CC, Winter FC. Flat preparations of the retinal vessels in Coats' disease. J Pediatr Ophthalmology. 1976;13:336-9.
3. Egerer I, Tasman W, Tomer T. Coats' disease. Arch Ophthalmology. 1974;92:109-12.
4. Shields JA, Shields CL, Honavar SG, et al. Clinical variations and complications of Coats disease in 150 cases: the 2000 Sanford Gifford Memorial Lecture. Am J Ophthalmology. 2001;131:561-71.
5. Shields JA, Shields CL. Differentiation of Coats' disease and retinoblastoma. J Pediatr Ophthalmology Strabismus. 2001;38:262-
6. Black GC, Perveen R, Bonshek R, et al. Coats' disease of the retina (unilateral retinal telangiectasis) caused by somatic mutation in the NDP gene: a role for norrin in retinal angiogenesis. Hum Mol Genet. 1999;8:2031-5.
7. Shastry BS, Trese MT. Overproduction and partial purification of the Norrie disease gene product, norrin, from a recombinant baculovirus. Biochem Biophys Res Commun. 2003;312:229-34.
8. Ye X, Wang Y, Cahill H, et al. Norrin, frizzled-4, and Lrp5 signaling in endothelial cells controls a genetic program for retinal vascularization. Cell. 2009;139:285-98.
9. Clevers H. Eyeing up new Wnt pathway players. Cell. 2009;139: 227-9.
10. Lin P, Shankar SP, Duncan J, et al. Retinal vascular abnormalities and dragged maculae in a carrier with a new NDP mutation (c. 268delC) that caused severe Norrie disease in the proband. J AAPOS. 2010;14:93-6.
11. Dickinson JL, Sale MM, Passmore A, et al. Mutations in the NDP gene: contribution to Norrie disease, familial exudative vitreoretinopathy and retinopathy of prematurity. Clin Exp Ophthalmology. 2006;34:682-8.
12. Warden SM, Andreoli CM, Mukai S. The Wnt signaling pathway in familial exudative vitreoretinopathy and Norrie disease. Semin Ophthalmology. 2007;22:211-7.
13. Qin M, Hayashi H, Oshima K, et al. Complexity of the genotype–phenotype correlation in familial exudative vitreoretinopathy with mutations in the LRP5 and/or FZD4 genes. Hum Mutat. 2005;26:104-12.
14. Woods AC, Duke JR. Coats's disease. I. Review of the literature, diagnostic criteria, clinical findings, and plasma lipid studies. Br J Ophthalmology. 1963;47:385-412.
15. Vance SK, Wald KJ, Sherman J, et al. Subclinical facioscapulohumeral muscular dystrophy masquerading as bilateral Coats disease in a woman. Arch Ophthalmology. 2011;129:807-9.
16. Kan E, Yilmaz T, Aydemir O, et al. Coats-like retinitis pigmentosa: Reports of three cases. Clin Ophthalmology. 2007;1:193-8.
17. Kumar V, Tewari R, Chandra P, et al. Ultra wide field imaging of Coats like response in Leber's congenital amaurosis. Saudi J Ophthalmology. 2017;31:122-3.
18. Gupta N, Beri S, D'Souza P. Cholesterolosis bulbi of the anterior chamber in Coats disease. J Pediatr Ophthalmology Strabismus. 2009;doi: 10.3928/01913913-20090616-04.
19. Shields JA, Eagle RC Jr, Fammartino J, et al. Coats' disease as a cause of anterior chamber cholesterolosis. Arch Ophthalmology. 1995;113:975-7.
20. Jumper JM, Pomerleau D, McDonald HR, et al. Macular fibrosis in Coats disease. Retina. 2010;30:S9-14.
21. Naumann GD, Portwich E. Etiology and final clinical cause for 1000 enucleations. (A clinico-pathologic study) (author's transl.). Klin Monbl Augenheilkd. 1976;168:622-30.
22. Friedenwald H, Friedenwald JS. Terminal stage in a case of retinitis with massive exudation. Trans Am Ophthalmology Soc. 1929;27: 188-94.
23. Shields JA, Shields CL, Honavar SG, et al. Classification and management of Coats disease: the 2000 Proctor Lecture. Am J Ophthalmology. 2001;131:572-83.
24. Lai CH, Kuo HK, Wu PC, et al. Manifestation of Coats' disease by age in Taiwan. Clin Exp Ophthalmology. 2007;35:361-5.
25. Haik BG. Advanced Coats' disease. Trans Am Ophthalmology Soc. 1991;89:371-476.
26. Schefler AC, Berrocal AM, Murray TG. Advanced Coats' disease. Management with repetitive aggressive laser ablation therapy. Retina. 2008;28(Suppl):S38-41.
27. Spitznas M, Joussen F, Wessing A. Treatment of Coats' disease with photocoagulation. Albrecht Von Graefes Arch Klin Exp Ophthalmology. 1976;199:31-7.
28. Shapiro MJ, Chow CC, Karth PA, et al. Effects of green diode laser in the treatment of pediatric Coats disease. Am J Ophthalmology. 2011;151:725-31. e722.
29. Othman IS, Moussa M, Bouhaimed M. Management of lipid exudates in Coats disease by adjuvant intravitreal triamcinolone: effects and complications. Br J Ophthalmology. 2010;94:606-10.
30. Jarin RR, Teoh SC, Lim TH. Resolution of severe macular oedema in adult Coat's syndrome with high-dose intravitreal triamcinolone acetonide. Eye (Lond). 2006;20:163-5.

31. Kaul S, Uparkar M, Mody K, et al. Intravitreal anti-vascular endothelial growth factor agents as an adjunct in the management of coats' disease in children. Indian J Ophthalmology. 2010;58(1):76-8.

32. Sun Y, Jain A, Moshfeghi DM. Elevated vascular endothelial growth factor levels in Coats disease: Rapid response to pegaptanib sodium. Graefes Arch Clin Exp Ophthalmology. 2007;245: 1387-8.

33. Venkatesh P, Mandal S, Garg S. Management of Coats disease with bevacizumab in 2 patients. Can J Ophthalmology. 2008;43:245-6.

34. Egerer I, Tasman W, Tomer TT. Coats disease. Arch Ophthalmology. 1974;92:109-12.

35. Matsuzaka T, Sakuragawa N, Terasawa K, et al. Facioscapulohumeral dystrophy associated with mental retardation, hearing loss, and tortuosity of retinal arterioles. J Child Neurol. 1986;1:218-23.

Chapter 38

Fundus Coloboma

Vineet Mutha, Anin Sethi, Atul Kumar

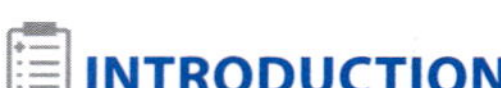 INTRODUCTION

The word coloboma is derived from a Greek word "koloboma" which means defect. "Coloboma" term was first used by Walther,[1] while the first clinical description of choroidal coloboma was given by Von Ammon in 1830. Coloboma is a defect in ocular tissue which may involve lid, lens, iris or choroid with each having different embryological mechanisms. Fundus coloboma is a relatively rare disease and occurs in 0.14% of the general population.[2] Still it is important to understand this condition because it may lead to a retinal detachment in as high as 40% cases.[2,3]

EMBRYOLOGY

Various theories have been suggested in the past to explain the development of a coloboma such as vascular abnormality, inflammatory mechanisms and chorioretinal scarring. Present knowledge suggests that *fundus coloboma occurs due to defective closure of the embryonic fissure.* At 4th week (7.5 mm stage) of gestation, an invagination occurs in the inferonasal part of the optic cup and stalk from where mesenchyme and axons of ganglion cells get incorporated in the optic nerve. This fissure gets completely closed bilaterally at 6th week of gestation in a zipper like fashion (Figs. 38.1A and B). The central portion fuses first while the proximal and distal portions fuse last. Thus, the area of coloboma has defective neuroectodermal elements with absence of outer retina and choroid. Inner retinal layers form a thinned out intercalary membrane over the coloboma and the outer retinal layers get curled up at the margin of coloboma forming the *Locus minoris resistentiae.* The sclera in the area of coloboma gets thinned out and ectatic.[4,5]

GENETICS AND SYNDROMIC ASSOCIATIONS

More than 30 genetic loci have been linked with coloboma and associated syndromes. Recently coloboma gene network (CGN) has been proposed for simplifying the genetic abnormality. According to this, *Sonic HedgeHog (SHH)* and *PAX6* genes are the most important genes involved in the development of coloboma. Various multisystem abnormalities such as CHARGE (coloboma, heart defects, atresia choanae, growth retardation, genital abnormalities, and ear abnormalities) syndrome have iris/choroidal coloboma in about 80% cases but the underlying mechanism is unknown. Genetic associations have been enumerated in Table 38.1.[6]

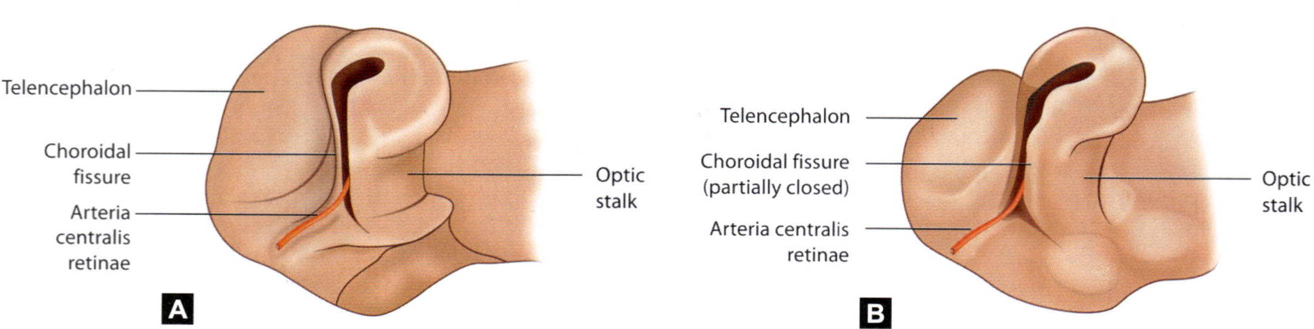

Figs. 38.1A and B: Schematic diagram showing the closure of embryonic fissure. (A) Open choroidal fissure. (B) Partially closed choroidal fissure. *Source*: Dr Anin Sethi.

Table 38.1: Genetic associations with fundal coloboma.

Genetic loci	Disease/Syndrome
7q36; Autosomal dominant; *SHH* gene	Uveoretinal coloboma syndrome
9q34.3; Autosomal Recessive	Joubert syndrome
11p13; Autosomal Dominant; *PAX6* gene	Ocular coloboma
10q24; Autosomal Dominant; *PAX2* gene	Renal coloboma
12q24; Autosomal Dominant; *PTPN11* gene	Noonan syndrome
14q/15q; AD/AR; *CHX10* gene	Microphthalmia syndromes
2q24-2q31	Craniosynostosis
8q21.1 del; *CHD7* gene	CHARGE association
22q11	Cat eye syndrome
22q11	Di George syndrome

ENVIRONMENTAL CAUSES

Literature suggests that coloboma may be a result of teratogenic effects of various drugs used during pregnancy. Drugs such as thalidomide and alcohol have been linked with a number of ocular abnormalities including coloboma. Lysergic acid diethylamide (LSD) and carbamazepine consumption during pregnancy have also been linked with the same. Maternal vitamin A and E deficiency, exposure to ionizing radiation and hyperthermia have also been found to be associated with coloboma. Among infectious causes, cytomegalovirus and toxoplasmosis were seen to be associated with coloboma.[6]

CLINICAL FEATURES

Fundus coloboma usually presents as a bilateral (80%) asymmetric condition in the first decade of life with more than 85% cases with associated iris involvement which appears as a keyhole like defect on gross examination (Fig. 38.2). It is first recognized by parents when they notice that the child is unable to follow objects. Other manifestations which may lead to the diagnosis are nystagmus or nystagmoid movements with squint and rarely a white/yellow reflex—"leukocoria". Nystagmoid movements are present in more than 50% of coloboma cases. In cases with macular involvement visual acuity is markedly reduced. However, many cases may go unnoticed and present in later life (2nd or 3rd decade) with retinal detachment (40%) or rarely choroidal neovascular membrane. Microphthalmia (40%) and high myopia (20%) are among other frequent associations. Developmental cataract, complicated cataract and glaucoma may also lead to decreased visual acuity apart from coloboma alone.[4]

Most commonly fundus colobomas are located in the inferonasal quadrant and thus these are labeled "typical". However, rarely they can be seen in other quadrants as well which are referred to as "atypical colobomas".[7] We have seen one such case with a superotemporal fundus coloboma (Fig. 38.3).

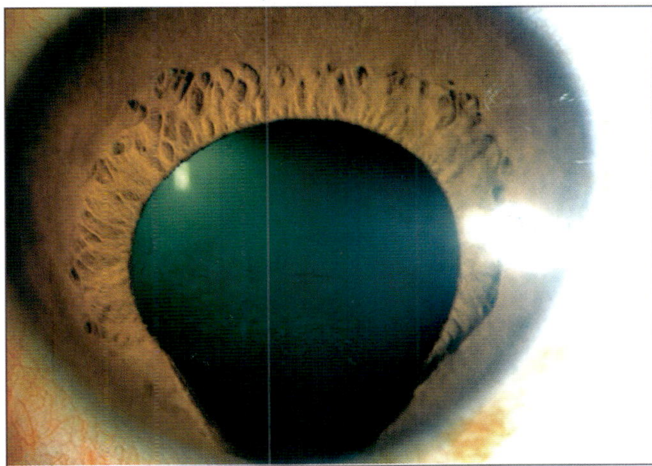

Fig. 38.2: Anterior segment photograph showing iris coloboma.

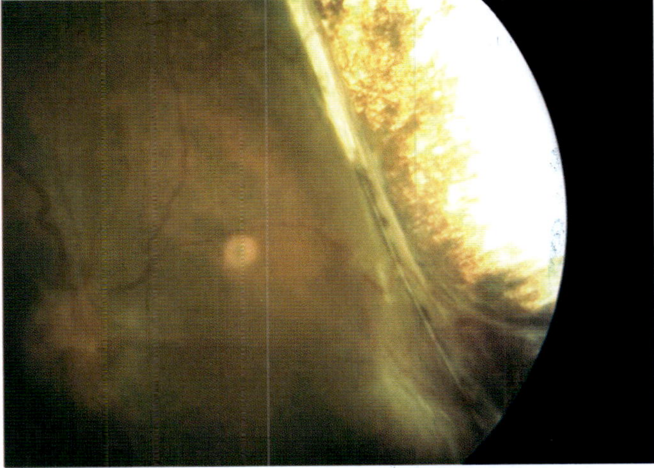

Fig. 38.3: Fundus photograph of atypical choroidal coloboma located superotemporally.

Investigations like visual fields, optical coherence tomography, fluorescein angiography and ultrasonography may be performed depending upon case profile and are not required in all cases as the diagnosis is mostly made on clinical examination.

CLASSIFICATION OF CHOROIDAL COLOBOMA

Prof Ida Mann published a classification of choroidal coloboma in 1937 in her book "Developemental abnormalities of eye". The classification is based on anatomical area of globe involved by coloboma. In 1996 Prof. Lingam Gopal published another classification based on involvement of optic nerve and emergence of blood vessels from disc area in an attempt to understand factors predicting visual acuity in these patients (Table 38.2 and Figs 38.4 to 38.7).

DIFFERENTIAL DIAGNOSIS

- *Posterior staphyloma (Fig. 38.8)*: It is an outpouching of the ocular coats (retina, choroid and sclera) at the posterior pole usually seen in pathological myopia. It can be easily differentiated from coloboma as it is on the posterior pole (cf. colobomas are inferonasal) and all layers of ocular coats are intact unlike coloboma with deficient choroid and outer retinal layers.
- *Macular coloboma (Fig. 38.9)*: Macular coloboma is a fundus coloboma but is not due to faulty closure of embryonic fissure rather due to incomplete differentiation of arcuate bundles along the horizontal raphe. These are also bilateral which differentiates them from a more common condition with similar appearance—toxoplasmosis scar.
- *Rarely large confluent cryo spots*: Primarily these can be differentiated on the basis of history as patient will give a definite history of previous therapeutic procedure.

Clinically the margins of cryo spot are not sharp as of coloboma and the base is not excavated and multiple cryo spots form a club-shaped structure contrasting to pear-shaped coloboma.

ROLE OF PROPHYLACTIC LASER BARRAGE

This is a matter of debate but according to a study by Uhumwangho and Jalali, only 2.9% of those who underwent prophylactic laser barrage of fundus coloboma developed retinal detachment while this percentage went as high as 24% in unlasered cases.[10] In a retrospective study from our center by Koushik et al., only 0.6% of lasered cases developed rhegmatogenous retinal detachment (RRD).[11]

Laser (Fig. 38.10) is usually done on a slit-lamp delivery system or laser indirect ophthalmoscopy (LIO). Laser settings on a slit-lamp delivery system are spot size of about 300–500 microns, burn duration of 0.2–0.3 seconds and interspot duration of about 0.1–0.2 second. Three rows of laser burns at margins of coloboma with moderate retinal whitening and interspot distance of about 0.25 spot size are sufficient. Laser should be done at first presentation considering the high risk of retinal detachment. In children laser can be done with LIO under general anesthesia with power settings of about 100 mW and aforementioned burn and interspot duration. In eyes with nystagmus, laser can be done under peribulbar infiltrative block with LIO keeping similar settings. LIO is also useful if anterior margin of coloboma is uncovered using conventional slit-lamp delivery.

Laser acts by creating strong chorioretinal adhesions at margin of coloboma thus decreasing chances of retinal detachment as described by Uhumwangho and Jalali.[9] Extensive white burn may itself lead to retinal breaks and detachment while widely spaced mild burns may not be able to prevent retinal detachment.

Table 38.2: Classifications of choroidal coloboma.

Classification by Lingam Gopal (1996)[5]		Classification by Ida Mann (1937)[9]	
Normal disc outside coloboma	Type I	Upper edge of coloboma passing above the optic disc (Fig. 38.5)	Type 1
Abnormal but noncolobomatous disc outside coloboma (Fig. 38.7)	Type II	Upper edge of coloboma passing at the level of optic disc or at its inferior border (Fig. 38.6)	Type 2
Colobomatous disc outside coloboma	Type III	Optic disc and upper edge of coloboma separated by retina (Fig. 38.7)	Type 3
Near normal disc inside coloboma (Fig. 38.5)	Type IV	Inferior crescent at the lower margin of disc	Type 4
Colobomatous disc inside coloboma (Fig. 38.6)	Type V	Isolated fundus coloboma that is isolated defect in the line of closure of embryonic fissure	Type 5
Disc not identifiable as it completely merges with colobomatous area	Type VI	Inferior zone/area of abnormal pigmentation	Type 6
		Coloboma located in far periphery	Type 7

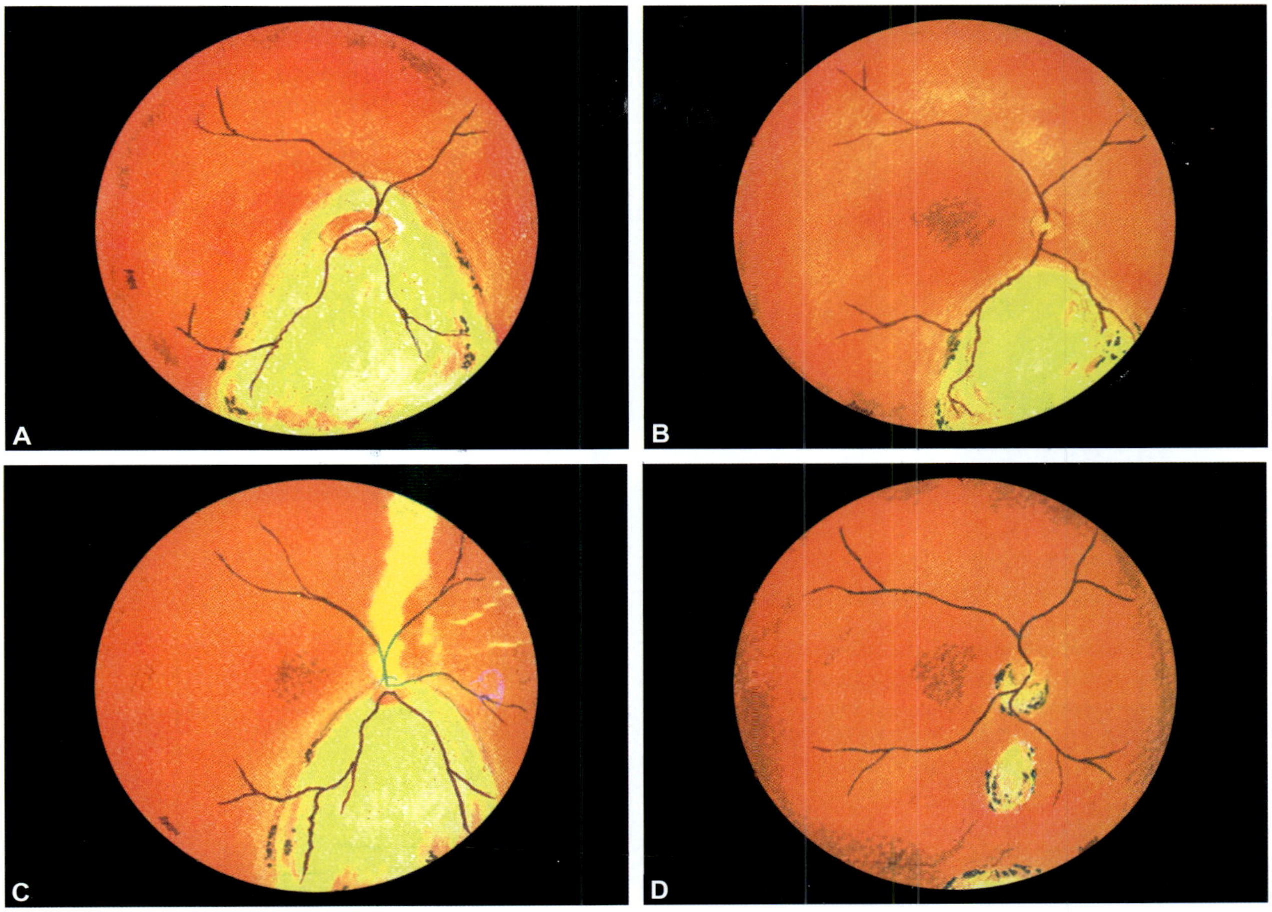

Figs. 38.4A to D: Color diagrams showing Ida Mann (A) type 1, (C) type 2, (B) type 3 and (D) type 4, 5 and 7.
Source: Dr Anin.

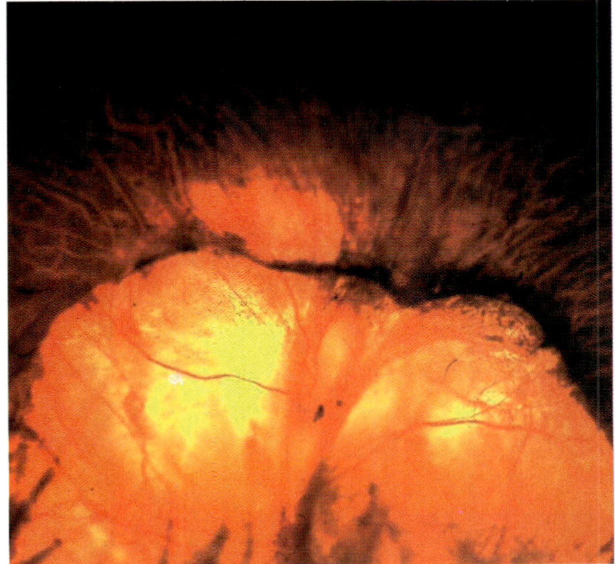

Fig. 38.5: Ida Mann type 1 and Gopal Lingam type IV.

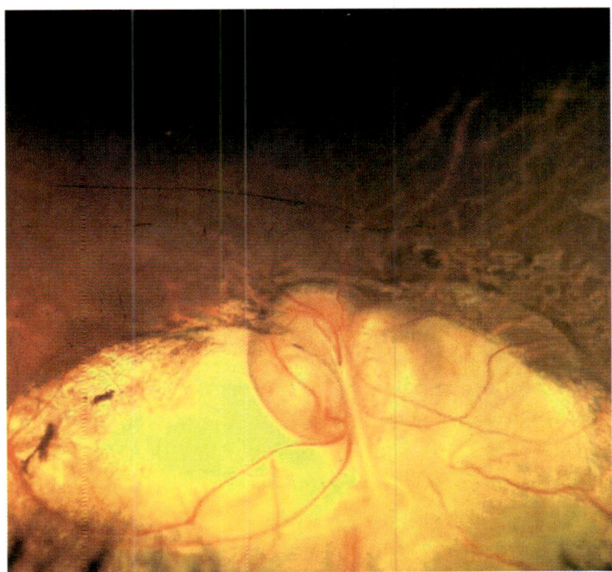

Fig. 38.6: Ida Mann type 2 and Gopal Lingam type V coloboma.

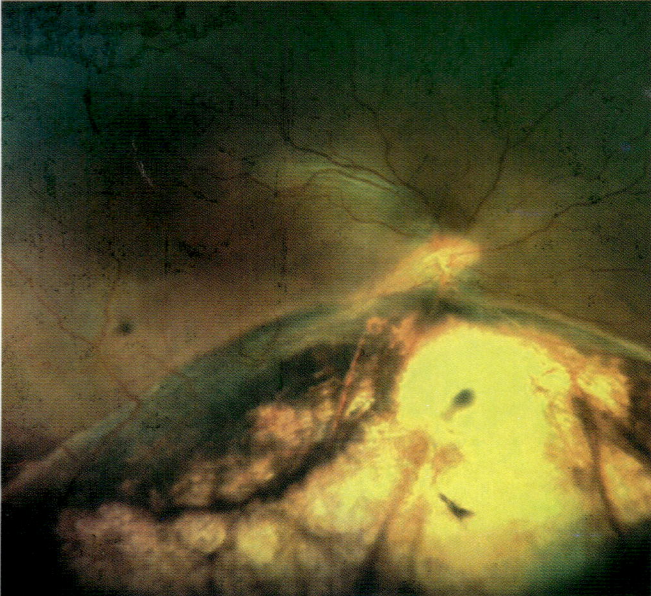

Fig. 38.7: Ida Mann type 3 and Gopal Lingam type II coloboma.

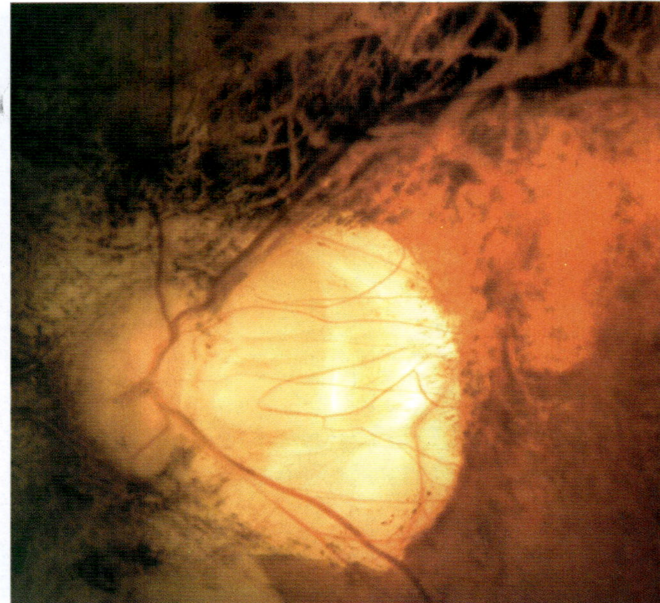

Fig. 38.8: Clinical fundus picture of posterior staphyloma in a patient with pathological myopia.

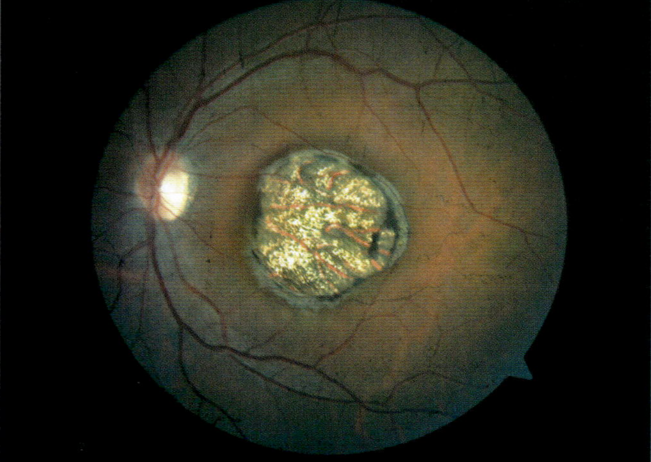

Fig. 38.9: Clinical fundus picture showing macular coloboma.

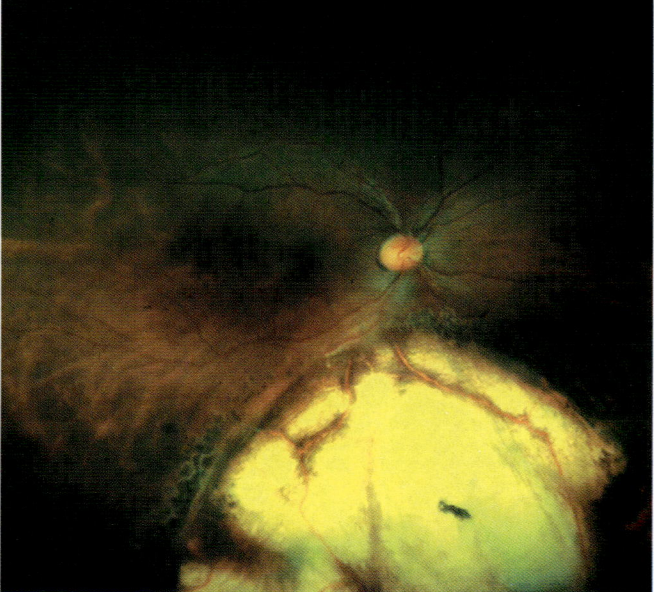

Fig. 38.10: Laser barraged coloboma with minimal burns just outside the inferior arcade.

COLOBOMA AND RETINAL DETACHMENT[11-14]

The complexity of retinal detachment increases in eyes with coloboma. As already mentioned, fundus coloboma may lead to a rhegmatogenous retinal detachment in 30–40% cases. Most commonly the break is found in the intercalary membrane (60% cases) and is usually difficult to find as there is absence of choroid underneath. These breaks are commonly round atrophic holes which first lead to detachment of intercalary membrane and then may progress to complete retinal detachment. Here comes the role of prophylactic barrage laser which prevents this progression. Severe prolifera-tive vitreoretinopathy (PVR) occurs in around 8% cases as younger age group is involved.

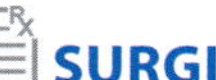

SURGICAL MANAGEMENT

Surgery for retinal detachment associated with coloboma is challenging. Patient and his/her family should be explained about higher risk of redetachment and a written informed consent should be taken prior. If cataract is present then it can be removed in a single stage surgery or sequential surgeries depending upon its grade. After a complete peritomy and an encircling band, three standard pars plana ports (23G/25G/27G) are made followed by tricot assisted posterior vitreous detachment induction. Then vitrectomy along with vitreous base shaving is done. Subretinal fluid is drained after making a small retinotomy usually superonasal followed by 360° endolaser along with laser around breaks and around coloboma margins. Silicone oil should be injected in view of high risk of redetachment.

Placement of an encirclage helps in peripheral vitreous shaving and relieving traction. Yet redetachment rate with or without encirclage is around 12%. Difficulty in inducing posterior vitreous detachment due to tight adhesions of the posterior vitreous to the retina further increases the intricacy of the procedure. Perfluorocarbon liquid (PFCL) use is another area of debate as it may collect in the colobomatous area making it difficult to remove the same and also there is a risk of subintercalary migration of PFCL which is almost impossible to extract in coloboma eyes. Similar is the chance of migration of silicone oil beneath the intercalary membrane but here benefits outweigh risk as silicone oil is a must for tamponade in coloboma associated detachments (Fig. 38.11).

According to a recent (2017) multicentric study, an anatomical success of about 88% is achieved in coloboma related detachments with better results with a long-acting tamponade. Cryotherapy was associated with worse outcomes while encircling band had no effect on final success in coloboma related retinal detachments. Another study from our center by Pal et al. in 2006 reported a similar success rate with redetachment rates of around 10% and as already mentioned, severe proliferative vitreoretinopathy (PVR) was found in up to 8% cases.

Fundus visualization can be tough in the postoperative period due to nystagmus and poor pupillary dilation.

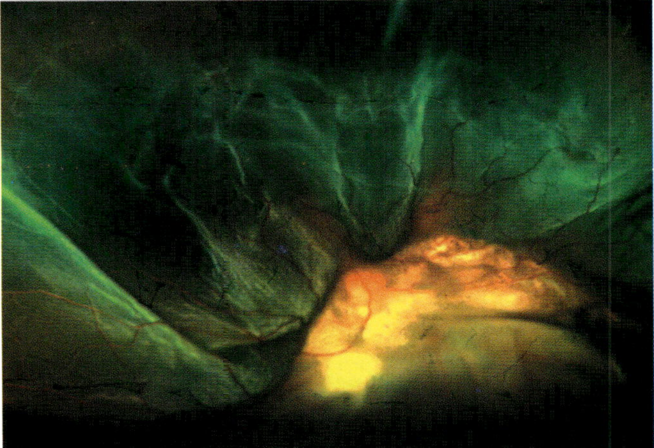

Fig. 38.11: Retinal detachment associated with fundus coloboma.

Patient may require frequent examinations under anesthesia for fundus assessment along with refraction. Apart from this, the chances of secondary glaucoma (46%) and cataract (100%) are higher in coloboma eyes postvitreoretinal surgery. Silicone oil removal (SOR) should be performed between 3 months and 8 months though it can be left in situ in one-eyed patients till significant emulsification in those with complex retinal detachments with extensive PVR as there is a high risk of redetachment post-SOR. Use of 5,000 centistokes oil which does not emulsify early is recommended in such eyes.[13]

PROGNOSIS

The prognosis depends on the type of coloboma, macular involvement, presence of microphthalmos and retinal detachment. Visual acuity is worse than LogMAR 1 (20/200) in eyes with type 1 and type 2 colobomas which frequently involve macula. Postoperative visual acuity in eyes with retinal detachment can range from LogMAR 0.9 to 3 but a median acuity is reported as finger counting at 2 meters even though the anatomical success rates approach 90%. Eyes with type 3–7 have a very good prognosis as macula is spared. Retinal detachment surgeries in these eyes also have a much better outcome than those in type 1 and type 2.[12]

OPTIC DISC COLOBOMA AND OTHER DISC ANOMALIES

Optic Nerve Coloboma

Optic nerve coloboma is commonly inherited as an autosomal dominant trait and are bilateral in more than 60% cases.[14] It can be an isolated finding or can be associated with syndromes of known or unknown etiology. The structure of a colobomatous optic nerve can vary from slightly increased physiological cupping to marked excavation. Most common ocular associations are microphthalmia and retinal detachment. They may also be associated with central nervous system abnormalities like olfactory dysplasia, transsphenoidal encephalocoele. Craniocerebrofacial clefts, agenesis of the corpus callosum, arachnoid cysts, hydrocephalus, epilepsy and mental retardation.[16]

There have been reported cases of retinoschisis and nonrhegmatogenous retinal detachment associated with optic disc coloboma which showed signs similar to that of optic disc pit maculopathy but the pathophysiology has not been identified.[17]

Morning Glory Syndrome

Morning glory syndrome (Fig. 38.12) is another optic disc anomaly which looks similar to optic disc coloboma. It is named as it resembles a morning glory flower. The differentiating features are the presence of a larger optic disc surrounded by an annular zone of retinal depigmentation with an elevated glial tuft overlying the center of the disc and anomalous vessels arising from the periphery of the disc compared to a large white, glistening excavation within an enlarged optic disc.[18] Morning glory syndrome can be associated with transsphenoidal basal encephalocele, which is the outpouching of the meninges often containing optic chiasm and hypothalamus through a defect in the sphenoid bone.

Occurrence of serous detachment, rhegmatogenous retinal detachment and combined traction-rhegmatogenous retinal detachment has been reported with morning glory syndrome.[19,20] Rhegmatogenous retinal detachment in morning glory syndrome may be due to a small slit-like break at the edge of anomalous disc (peripapillary break) leading to total retinal detachment which requires vitreoretinal surgery achieve anatomical reattachment and some functional vision (Fig. 38.11).[19] Serous detachment is postulated to be due to anomalous communication between the intraocular and extraocular compartments leading movement of vitreous humor or cerebrospinal fluid within and under the retina because of dynamic fluctuations in the gradient between intraocular and intracranial pressures.[21] Serous detachment may respond to peripapillary laser, vitrectomy with gas tamponade or oral acetazolamide.[21,22]

Optic Nerve Hypoplasia

Optic nerve hypoplasia (Fig. 38.12) occurs due to the underdevelopment of optic nerve characterized by decreased number of optic nerve axons. It is usually congenital and has been associated with many prenatal risk factors like young maternal age, maternal drug abuse, viral infections and fetal alcohol syndrome. Double ring sign is classical in these patients. De Morsier syndrome or septo-optic dysplasia is congenital malformation featuring optic nerve hypoplasia, absence of septum pellucidum and pituitary gland dysfunction.[23] Valproate toxicity in utero is a possible etiology of this condition.[24]

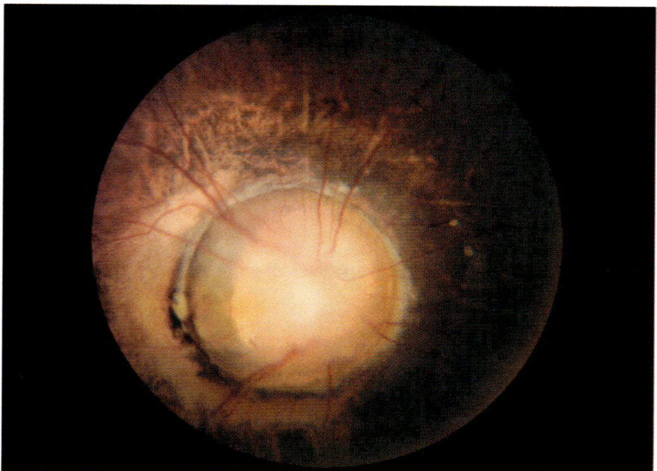

Fig. 38.12: Optic nerve head with morning glory syndrome.

SUMMARY

- Fundus coloboma is formed due to improper closure of embryonic fissure and is usually associated with iris coloboma (about 90%)
- May be associated with microphthalmia, nystagmus, squint and poor visual acuity
- Risk of retinal detachment is around 40% with breaks most commonly found in the intercalary membrane (60%)
- Prognosis is poor in type 1 and type 2 coloboma
- Early diagnosis and prophylactic laser delimitation may prevent retinal detachments associated with coloboma.

REFERENCES

1. Walther J Chir. Augenheilk 2:598, 1821; quoted by Duke-Elder, System of Ophthalmology. Vol. III, Part 2, St. Louis, C. V. Mosby Co., 1963. p. 456.
2. Jesberg D, Schepens C. Retinal detachment associated with coloboma of the choroid. Arch Ophthalmology. 1961;65:163-73.
3. Von Ammon. Anatomische Untersuchung von Coloboma bulbi. Z Ophthalmology. 1830:I.
4. Schepens CL. Retinal Detachment and Allied Diseases, Vol 2. Philadelphia: WB Saunders; 1983. pp. 615-7.
5. Gopal L, Badrinath SS, Kumar KS, et al. Optic disc in fundus coloboma. Ophthalmology. 1996;103(12):2120-7.
6. Schubert HD. Structural organization of choroidal colobomas of young and adult patients and mechanism of retinal detachment. Trans Am Ophthalmology Soc. 2005;103:457-72.
7. Gregory-Evans CY, Williams MJ, Halford S, et al. Ocular coloboma: a reassessment in the age of molecular neuroscience. J Med Genet. 2004;41(12):881-91.
8. Gopal L, Khan B, Jain S, et al. A clinical and optical coherence tomography study of the margins of choroidal colobomas. Ophthalmology. 2007;114(3):571-80.
9. Mann I. Developmental Abnormalities of the Eye. London: Cambridge University Press; 1937. pp. 65–103.
10. Uhumwangho OM, Jalali S. Chorioretinal coloboma in a paediatric population. Eye (Lond). 2014;28(6):728-33.
11. Tripathy K, Chawla R, Sharma YR, et al. Prophylactic laser photocoagulation of fundal coloboma: does it really help? Acta Ophthalmology. 2016;94(8):e809-10.
12. Pal N, Azad RV, Sharma YR. Long-term anatomical and visual outcome of vitreous surgery for retinal detachment with choroidal coloboma. Indian J Ophthalmology. 2006;54(2):85-8.
13. Ramezani A, Dehghan M-H, Rostami A, et al. Outcomes of retinal detachment surgery in eyes with chorioretinal coloboma. J Ophthalmic Vis Res. 2010;5(4):240-5.
14. Abouammoh MA, Alsulaiman SM, Gupta VS, et al. Surgical outcomes and complications of rhegmatogenous retinal detachment in eyes with chorioretinal coloboma: the results of the KKESH International Collaborative Retina Study Group. Retina. 2017;37:1942-7.
15. Pyhtinen J, Lindholm EL. Imaging in optic nerve coloboma. Neuroradiology. 1996; 38:171-4.
16. Hittner HM, Hirsch NJ, Kreh GM, et al. Colobomatous microphthalmia, heart disease, hearing loss and mental retardation: a syndrome. J Pediatr Ophthalmology Strabismus. 1979;16:122-8.
17. Hotta K, Hirakata A, Hida T. Retinoschisis associated with disc coloboma. Br J Ophthalmology. 1999;83:124.
18. Brodsky MC. Morning glory disc anomaly or optic disc coloboma? Arch Ophthalmology. 1994;112:153.

19. Ho CL, Wei LC. Rhegmatogenous retinal detachment in morning glory syndrome pathogenesis and treatment. Int Ophthalmology. 2001;24:21-4.

20. Harris MJ, de Bustros S, Michels RG, et al. Treatment of combined traction-rhegmatogenous retinal detachment in the morning glory syndrome. Retina. 1984;4(4):249-52.

21. Jain N, Johnson MW. Pathogenesis and treatment of maculopathy associated with cavitary optic disc anomalies. Am J Ophthalmology. 2014;158(3):423-35.

22. Prakash P, De Salvo G, Lotery AJ. Morning glory with serous macular detachment responds to oral acetazolamide. Eye (Lond). 2010;24(11):1732-3.

23. Gleason CA, Devascar S. Congenitalmalformations of the central nervous system. In: Avery's Diseases of the Newborn, 9th edition. Saunders; 2011. p. 857.

24. Strauss JF, Barbieri RL (eds). Yen and Jaffe's Reproductive Endocrinology: Physiology, Pathophysiology and Clinical Management. 6th Edition Elsevier Saunders, Philadelphia. 2009. pp. 421.

Choroidal and Retinal Inflammations

Chapter 39

Noninfectious Inflammations

Reema Bansal, Amod Gupta, Vishali Gupta

WHITE DOT SYNDROMES

White dot syndromes (WDSs) are a wide spectrum of inflammatory disease involving the choroid and retina of unknown etiology primarily involving the choriocapillaris. Typically, young healthy adults are affected with discrete, whitish lesions at various levels of the retina, retinal pigment epithelium (RPE) and the choroid.[1] While an infectious trigger or a viral prodrome has been hypothesized in some, an autoimmune etiology has been associated with others.[2] Some of the entities are self-limiting and have a good visual prognosis, and others have relapsing and remitting course with significant visual morbidity. Although there is a great resemblance of lesions among different entities, the differentiation and their diagnosis is mostly clinical, depending on morphology of the lesions, their natural course and pattern on fluorescein angiography (FA).[3,4] Here we discuss acute posterior multifocal placoid pigment epitheliopathy (APMPPE), multiple evanescent white dot syndrome (MEWDS), acute retinal pigment epitheliitis (ARPE), acute zonal occult outer retinopathy (AZOOR), birdshot chorioretinopathy, punctate inner choroidopathy (PIC), multifocal choroiditis with panuveitis (MCP), and serpiginous choroiditis (SC).

Acute Posterior Multifocal Placoid Pigment Epitheliopathy

Acute posterior multifocal placoid pigment epitheliopathy affects young healthy adults (20–40 years) with a slight female preponderance.[5] It is usually bilateral (one eye followed by the fellow eye), and may follow a flu-like illness. While an autoimmune etiology has been speculated for APMPPE, an infectious trigger is also associated with mumps, tuberculosis, syphilis, and Lyme disease. A morphological presentation of APMPPE-like lesions has also been described in sarcoidosis, ulcerative colitis and Wegener's granulomatosis.[6] The anterior chamber is often quiet with cells in the vitreous. Funduscopic examination reveals multiple, discrete, well-defined, creamish-yellow placoid lesions (less than one disc diameter in size), primarily involving the posterior pole. FA reveals hypofluorescence in the early phase, and staining of the lesions in the late phase[7] (Figs. 39.1A and B). Hypofluorescence of active as well as healed lesions is seen on indocyanine green

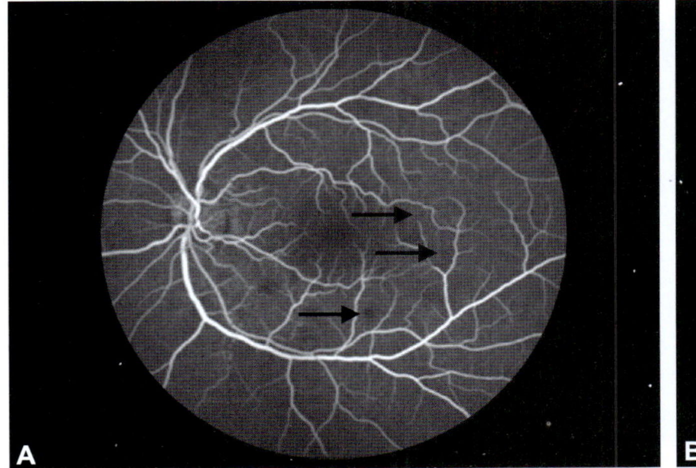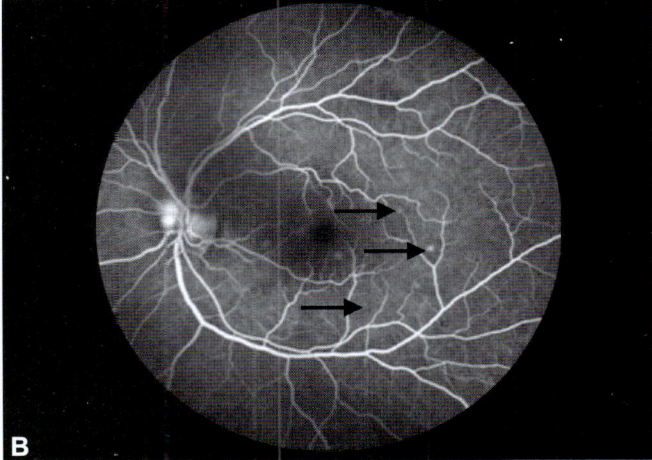

Figs. 39.1A and B: Fluorescein angiography of an APMPPE patient showing early hypofluorescence and late hyperfluorescence (black arrows).

angiography (ICGA), suggesting choroidal nonperfusion or choroidal infarction.[8] Autofluorescence (AF) imaging shows hypoautofluorescence in active lesions. A delay in 30-Hz flicker cone response is seen on electroretinogram (ERG). An alternate mechanism of precapillary arteriolar obstruction due to choroidal vasculitis has also been suggested.[6] The lesions start disappearing within 1–2 weeks, leaving mild pigmentation of the RPE.

Although the cause of APMPPE remains unknown, infectious etiologies need to be ruled out in these patients.[9] While the disease is usually self-limiting, some physicians do recommend systemic corticosteroids, particularly in cases of foveal involvement or cerebral vasculitis. The visual prognosis is good. Rare complications include recurrences and choroidal neovascular membranes (CNVMs).[10]

Multiple Evanescent White Dot Syndrome

Multiple evanescent white dot syndrome is usually unilateral, affecting healthy females with a moderate myopia in third to fifth decades. Bilateral involvement is very rare.[11] About half of them complain of a viral prodrome. Ocular symptoms include blurred vision, scotomas and photopsias usually in the temporal field. The anterior segment is quiet, and vitritis is often mild. The white dots are multiple, small, and at the outer retina or RPE and affect the posterior pole. Fovea shows a classical granular appearance, which persists even after the active inflammation subsides (Fig. 39.2). Macular edema, vasculitis and optic neuritis may be rarely associated.

Fluorescein angiography shows punctate hyperfluorescence in both early and late phases in a wreath-like pattern, with optic disc hyperfluorescence. These lesions appear as hypofluorescent discrete dots on ICGA, which reveals much more number of lesions than seen clinically or on FA, suggesting concomitant choroidal involvement.[12] ERGs and electro-oculograms (EOGs) show changes in acute stages, suggesting a primary involvement of the photoreceptors that resolve after resolution of inflammation.[13] The angiographic and ERG findings corroborate the outer level of involvement (photoreceptors, RPE and choroid). The lesions resolve spontaneously over few weeks, and visual prognosis is extremely good. However, scotomas and photopsias may persist. Recurrences and CNVM may occur rarely.

Acute retinal Pigment Epitheliitis

Also known as Krill's disease, ARPE is a benign, unilateral condition of unknown etiology. It has no sex predilection and affects young, healthy adults in the second to fourth decades.[14] It was first described by Krill and Deutman.[14] Ocular symptoms include mild visual blurring and central metamorphopsia. Initial lesions may be subtle, but they appear as hyperpigmented fine spots surrounded by a halo of yellowish-white hypopigmentation in the macular region about 1–2 weeks after their onset. AF reveals hyperautofluorescence of the lesions. An early hyperfluorescence in a halo configuration is seen on FA with staining (without any leakage) in the late phase. Spectral-domain optical coherence tomography (SD-OCT) reveals disruption of the photoreceptors inner segment-outer segment (IS-OS) band along with a wider RPE band disruption.[15] A normal ERG and an abnormal EOG suggest that the disease primarily affects the RPE. A higher concentration of the photoreceptors in the macula and an increased metabolic demand of the RPE cells in the macula as compared to the peripheral retina may predispose this region to develop ARPE. The lesions are self-limiting, and resolve without any pigmentation.[16] The visual acuity returns to normal without needing any treatment. CNVM is not seen.

Acute Zonal Occult Outer Retinopathy

Acute zonal occult outer retinopathy has been described by Gass as representing various retinal disorders within the spectrum of "AZOOR complex" that includes a heterogenous group of disorders.[17] It typically affects young, myopic, healthy females and may be unilateral or bilateral. Although not clear, various etiologies may include a viral cause,[18] toxic or an immune-mediated retinopathy[2,19] or fungal infections.[20,21] The patient may have photopsia and a rapid loss of peripheral visual field (zonal field loss), which is not consistent with the near normal fundus findings at the onset of the disease.[22] Vitreous inflammation is usually mild. The clinical spectrum ranges from a normal fundus to an extensive retinal damage. Progressive development of zonal areas of retinal atrophy and pigmentary degeneration denote a widespread disease. Electrophysiologic findings show characteristic abnormalities suggesting significant retinal dysfunction, even in the presence of a normal looking fundus.[23]

Abrupt episodes and recurrences are common. Unilateral and asymmetric presentation may be seen in AZOOR that may help to differentiate it from hereditary, autoimmune and toxic chorioretinopathies. While Gass proposed the hypothesis of outer retinal involvement many years ago, modern multimodal imaging reveals these characteristic findings that

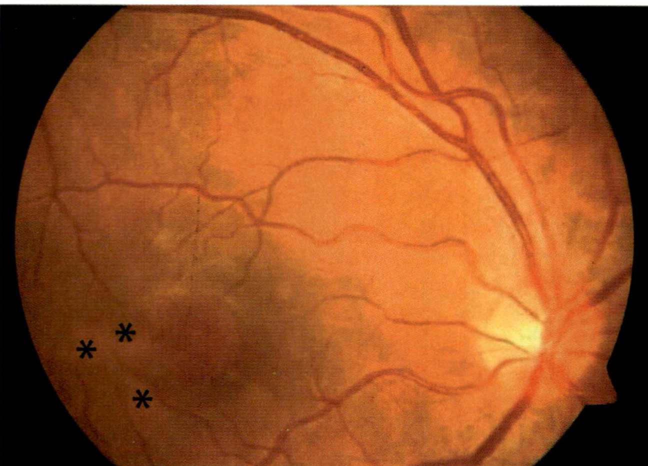

Fig. 39.2: Clinical picture of a patient showing characteristic evanescent lesions at macula [black asterix (*)].

help to differentiate AZOOR from other WDSs.[24] A trizonal pattern is seen on fundus autofluorescence (FAF), ICGA and SD-OCT. A hyperautofluorescent line demarcates the AZOOR lesion from normal retina on FAF imaging (which may be seen clinically as a white or gray line), unlike any other simulating disease. The trizonal pattern of chorioretinal degeneration involves outer retina, RPE and choroidal zonal lesions. SD-OCT reveals disruption of ellipsoid and interdigitation lines.

Birdshot Chorioretinopathy

Birdshot chorioretinopathy is characterized by hypopigmented, cream-colored, small ovoid postequatorial lesions, affecting the posterior pole and mid-periphery.[25,26] In 1980, Ryan and Maumenee described the fundus in this disease as resembling the scatter of a shotgun blast (birdshot), with the yellowish lesions radiating out from the optic nerve. The lesions are lower than one disc diameter in area. It is a bilateral chronic inflammation, affecting females more commonly than males in the fourth to sixth decades. The nasal retina is usually involved and the pattern is symmetrical in both eyes. Vitritis and retinal vasculitis are typically present with no anterior segment involvement. Typically, lesions heal without causing pigmentation around them.

All patients are human leukocyte antigen (HLA)-A29 positive, although the cause is not clearly known.[27] Vasculitis, optic disc staining and cystoid macular edema (CME) are typically seen on FA, but the birdshot lesions are seen better on ICGA than on FA as hypofluorescent lesions, radiating along the large choroidal veins.[28,29] Diffuse retinal atrophy can be well appreciated on FAF, and electroretinography as significant rod and cone dysfunction, differentiating it from other WDSs that have focal retinal dysfunction.[30] Chronic hypoperfusion may lead to global RPE and choroid involvement. The disease is usually recurrent with multiple exacerbations and remissions.[31] Chronic CME, optic atrophy and rarely, CNVM, cause visual loss.[26,32] Besides systemic corticosteroids, immunosuppressive agents are needed for long-term suppression of choroidal inflammation. Periocular or intravitreal steroids may be used for recalcitrant CME.[33,34]

Punctate Inner Choroidopathy

Punctate inner choroidopathy is an uncommon, bilateral disorder affecting healthy, myopic, young women.[35,36] Patients complains of floaters, blurring of vision, central or paracentral scotomas, or photopsias. Fundus examination reveals small, well-defined, yellowish-white lesions, 100–300 µm in size, involving the posterior pole or mid-periphery, at the level of RPE and choroid. There may be a serous retinal detachment (RD) overlying these lesions. Peripheral retina is usually not involved. The anterior chamber or the vitreous does not show any cells. The lesions show an early hyperfluorescence on FA that increases in the late phases, and hypofluorescence on ICGA.[34] The lesions are often benign, do not require treatment, and resolve within few weeks into atrophic chorioretinal scars.[37] Visual prognosis is usually favorable, unless complicated by CNVM or subretinal fibrosis. Rates of CNVM have been reported in 25–75% of PIC cases.[38,39] Cases with CNVM require treatment in the form of systemic corticosteroids, immunosuppressive agents, laser photocoagulation, photodynamic therapy (PDT), intravitreal anti-vascular endothelial growth factor (VEGF) agents and submacular surgery.[37]

Multifocal Choroiditis with Panuveitis

Multifocal choroiditis with panuveitis is a bilateral panuveitis of unknown cause, affecting females in the second to sixth decades.[38] Patients present with decreased vision and photopsias. Presence of cells in the anterior chamber and vitreous differentiate it from other WDSs, particularly PIC.[40] Fundus examination reveals acute lesions as yellow or gray lesions (100–300 µm) in the posterior pole and/or periphery at the level of RPE or choroid. The lesions may be solitary or in clumps. As the lesions heal, they become atrophic, attain a "punched out" appearance and acquire varying amounts of pigmentation.[41,42] Early hypofluorescence and late hyperfluorescence of the acute lesions are seen on FA, and persisting hypofluorescence is seen on ICGA. Visual loss commonly occurs due to CME (Figs. 39.3A and B). The other secondary causes of visual loss include CNVM, subretinal fibrosis and RPE metaplasia.[43] CNVM may be juxtafoveal, extrafoveal or peripapillary.

Corticosteroids control the disease in initial stages (Fig. 39.4), but recurrences are common. Immunosuppressive agents are required in cases complicated with CNVM or subretinal fibrosis.

Serpiginous Choroiditis

Serpiginous choroiditis is a bilateral, chronic recurrent inflammation mainly involving the inner choroid and RPE (Figs. 39.5A to C).[44,45] Clinically, it manifests as grayish-yellow subretinal lesions, typically beginning in the peripapillary region, contiguous to the optic disc, and spreading centrifugally in a serpentine manner.[46] It was earlier called helicoid peripapillary chorioretinal degeneration or geographic choroidopathy due to its morphological pattern.[47,48] Chronic and recurrent course leads to severe visual loss due to foveal involvement.[46] The etiology is unclear, but an autoimmune mechanism has been believed to be the main cause.[49,50] Systemic diseases such as sarcoidosis, systemic lupus erythematosus (SLE), celiac disease, Crohn's disease and non-Hodgkin's lymphoma (NHL) have been rarely associated with SC. Infective agents (tuberculosis, herpes virus) have also been proposed in the pathogenesis of SC.[51,52]

Classically, vitreous and anterior chamber are not involved, and the fundus lesions are solitary. In case of a recurrence, the new active lesion arises from the peripapillary scar. The active lesions are hypofluorescent in early and hyperfluorescent in late phases of FA. The early and intermediate phases of ICGA reveal hypofluorescence, which remains

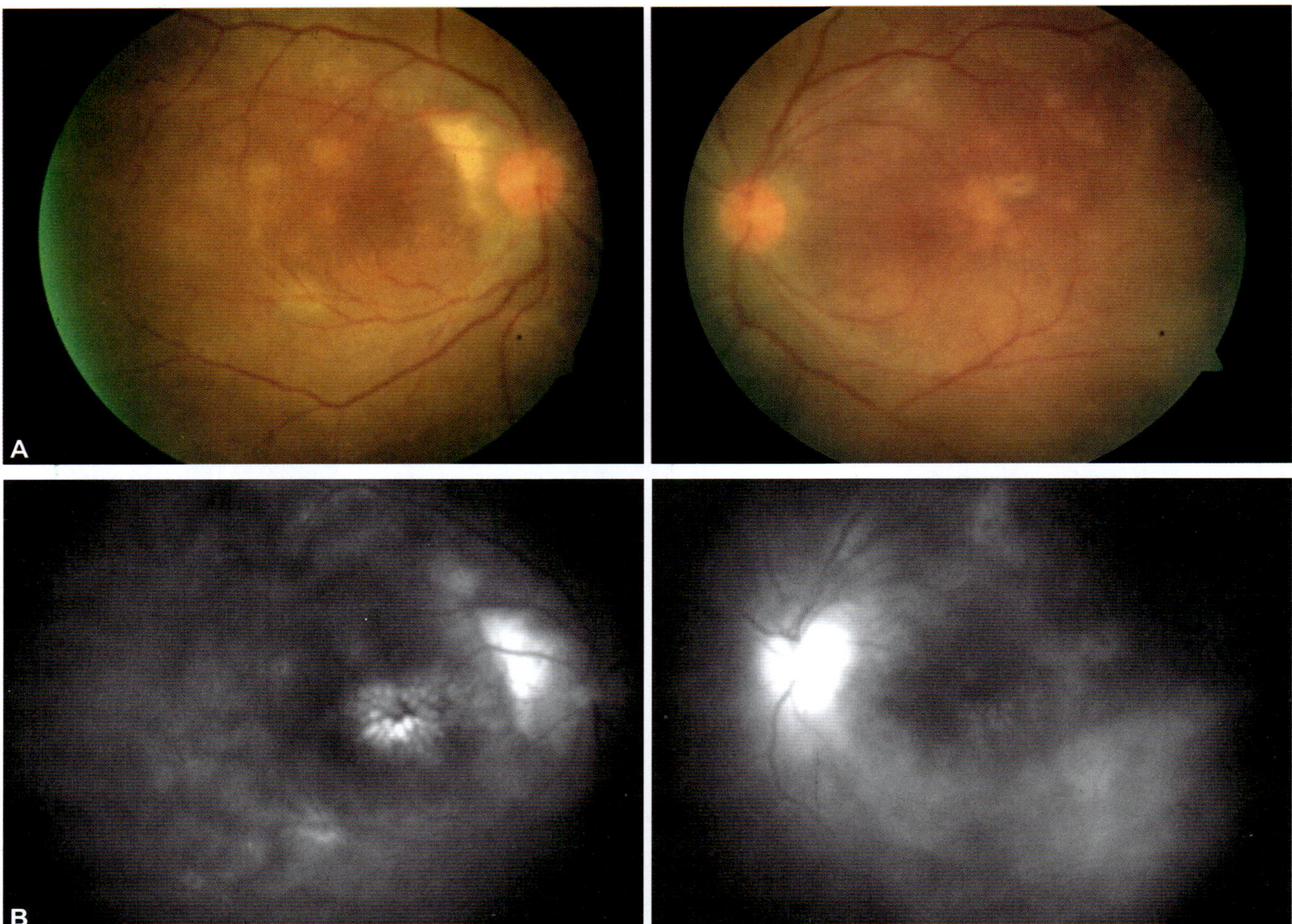

Figs. 39.3A and B: (A) Bilateral multifocal choroiditis with panuveitis, showing yellowish-gray lesions in posterior pole; (B) The right eye has a juxtapapillary CNVM. Fluorescein angiography shows cystoid macular edema (CME), with leakage from CNVM and optic discs.

hypofluorescent or becomes isofluorescent in late phase. FAF helps in a quick clinical assessment of the lesions as they evolve. The course is chronic, with multiple recurrences and relentless progression.[53] Corticosteroids and immunosuppressive agents are administered over long periods. The most frequent complication is CNVM, reported in 13–35% of cases.[54-56]

Tubercular Serpiginous-Like Choroiditis

Bansal R and Gupta A et al. described a variant of the classical serpiginous choroiditis which they concluded that it presented as a multifocal serpiginoid choroiditis affecting predominantly young to middle-aged men. It was frequently bilateral with overlying vitreous inflammation and multifocal lesions that were noncontiguous to the optic disc and showed a serpiginoid spread. Antitubercular therapy significantly reduced recurrences. These lesions responded dramatically to combined antitubercular and steroid therapy. An as they also tended to spare the fovea, they had a satisfactory final visual acuity.[57]

INFLAMMATORY VASCULITIS

Retinal vasculitis often presents as an isolated ocular disease, and is less commonly associated with a systemic etiology, infectious or inflammatory.[58] Diagnosis is usually clinical, and FA plays a significant role in demonstrating the extent and severity of vasculitis. Infectious causes of retinal vasculitis include tuberculosis, viral infections, toxoplasmosis, syphilis, Lyme disease, cat-scratch disease, brucellosis, West Nile virus fever, etc. Isolated ocular vasculitis may present as frosted branch angiitis (Fig. 39.6), idiopathic retinal vasculitis, aneurysms and neuroretinitis (IRVAN), idiopathic recurrent branch retinal vein occlusion, birdshot chorioretinopathy or acute multifocal hemorrhagic retinal vasculitis. It may occur in association with neurological disorders such as multiple sclerosis or Susac's syndrome, or may occur as an ocular manifestation of masquerade syndromes like lymphoma, or

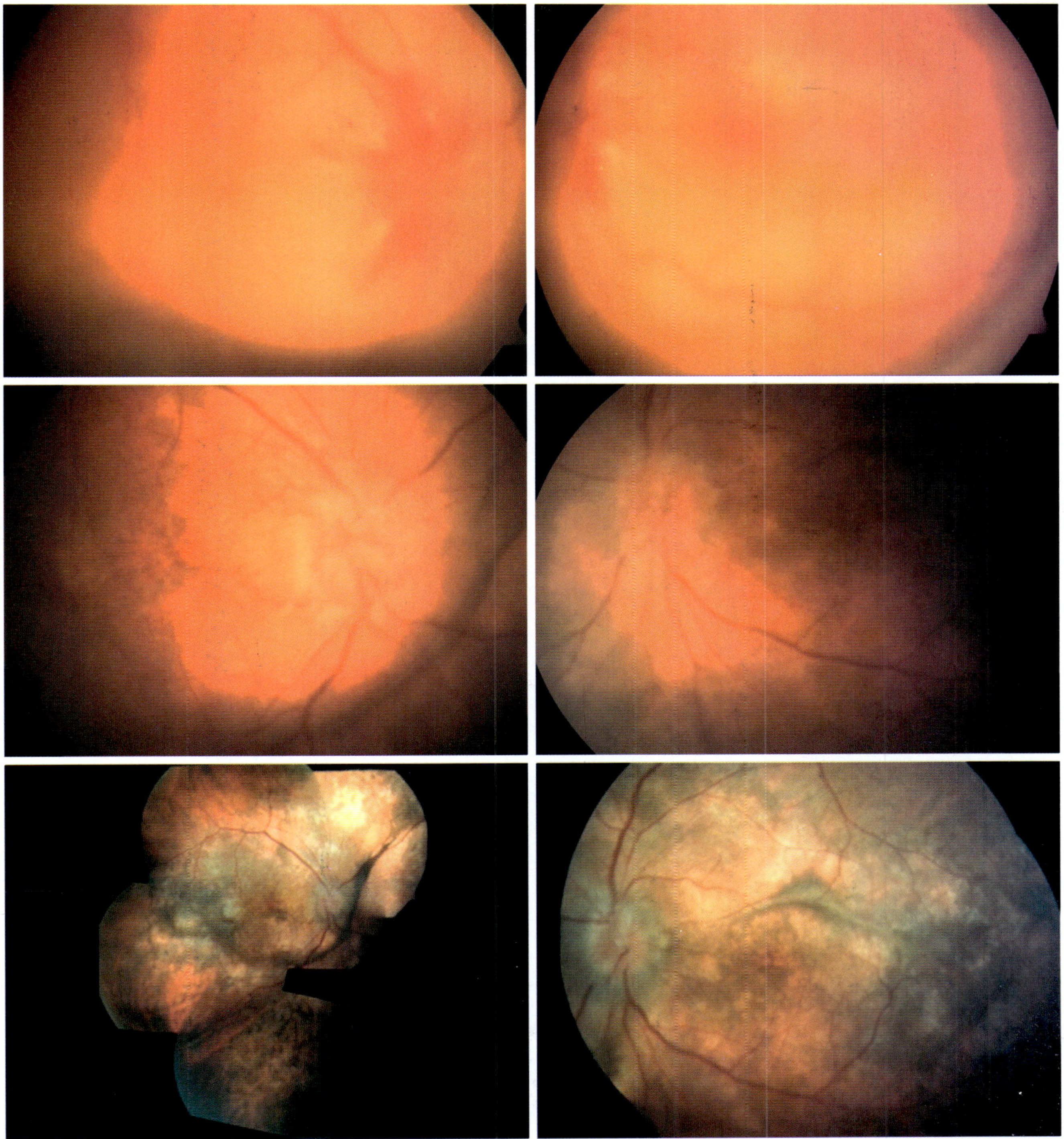

Fig. 39.4: Severe panuveitis responding to steroids with development of subretinal fibrosis.

paraneoplastic syndromes. Inflammatory causes of retinal vasculitis include sarcoidosis (Figs. 39.7A and B), Behçet's disease, SLE, Wegener's granulomatosis, polyarteritis nodosa (PAN), relapsing polychondritis, rheumatoid arthritis, Crohn's disease, polymyositis, Takayasu's disease, Buerger's disease, and Churg-Strauss syndrome.

Retinal vasculitis in sarcoidosis is nonocclusive, and usually manifests as "candle wax drippings", characterized

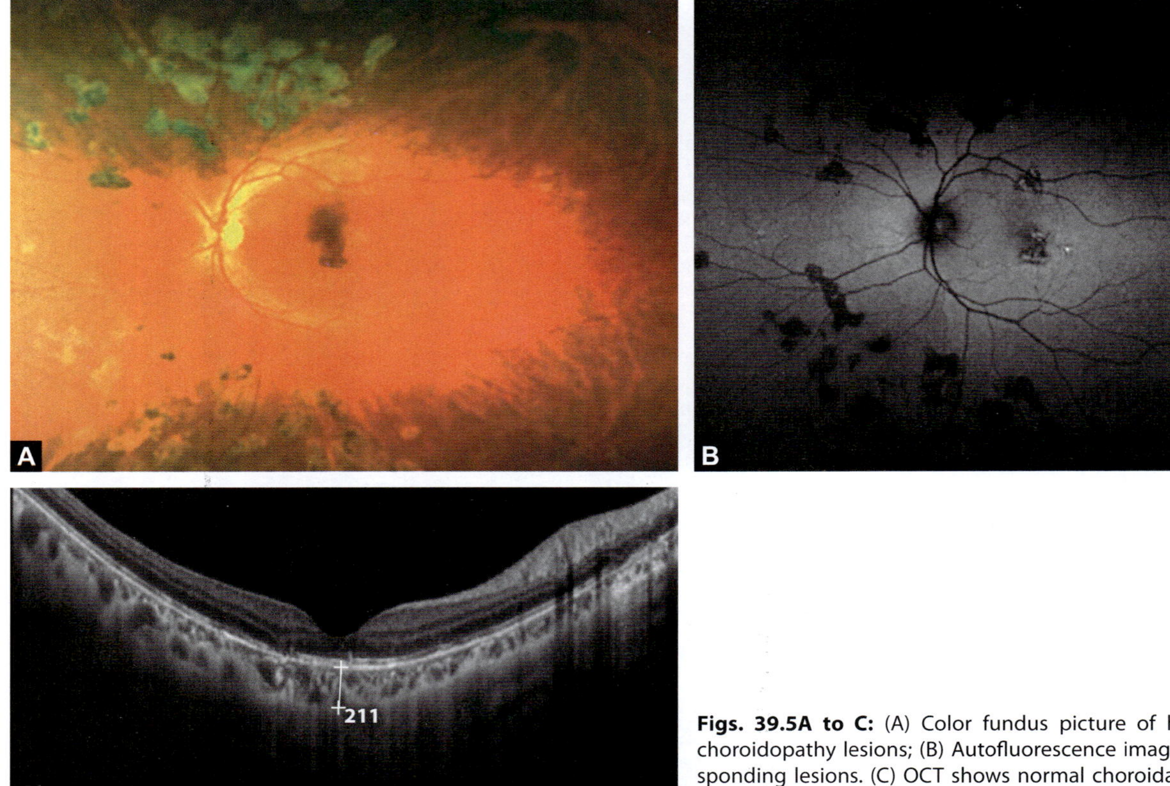

Figs. 39.5A to C: (A) Color fundus picture of healed serpiginous choroidopathy lesions; (B) Autofluorescence imaging showing corresponding lesions. (C) OCT shows normal choroidal thickness and no retinal pathology.

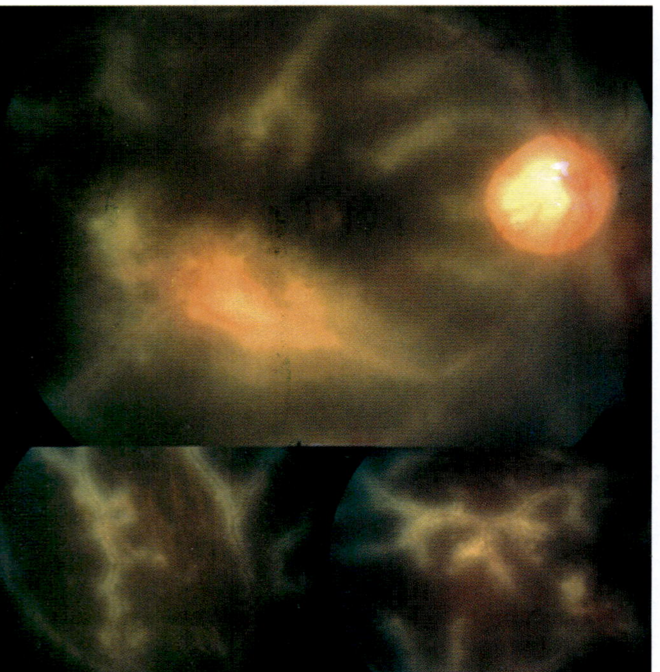

Fig. 39.6: Fundus color photograph of a patient with frosted branch angiitis.

by segmental cuffing, perivascular exudates, and sheathing of vessels. Other posterior segment manifestations include peripheral multifocal chorioretinitis, optic disc edema with/without neovascularization, choroidal granuloma(s)/optic disc granuloma (Fig. 39.8), or arterial macroaneurysms.[59-62] Other features of sarcoid uveitis include anterior uveitis (the most common presentation), mutton-fat keratic precipitates, granulomas on iris surface or angle, iris neovascularization, intermediate uveitis and neuroretinitis.[59-62] Response to systemic steroids is quite favorable. Anergy test, pulmonary imaging and biopsy play an important role in diagnosing systemic sarcoidosis.

Retinal vasculitis in Behçet's disease (Figs. 39.9A and B) is usually occlusive, and is accompanied by recurrent episodes of nongranulomatous (often bilateral) panuveitis with or without hypopyon, vitritis, retinitis, and/or optic disc edema.[63-66] FA reveals extensive vasculitis, demonstrating periphlebitis as well as capillaritis.

Vascular sheathing is not a feature during acute episodes, but gliotic sheathing may be seen once active inflammation is controlled. Extensive venous occlusion may simulate frosted branch angiitis. Retinal neovascularization may develop secondary to retinal ischemia (Fig. 39.10). Recurrences are common and immunosuppressive agents are needed as steroid-sparing therapy.[66] Other complications include cataract, glaucoma, CME, and optic atrophy.

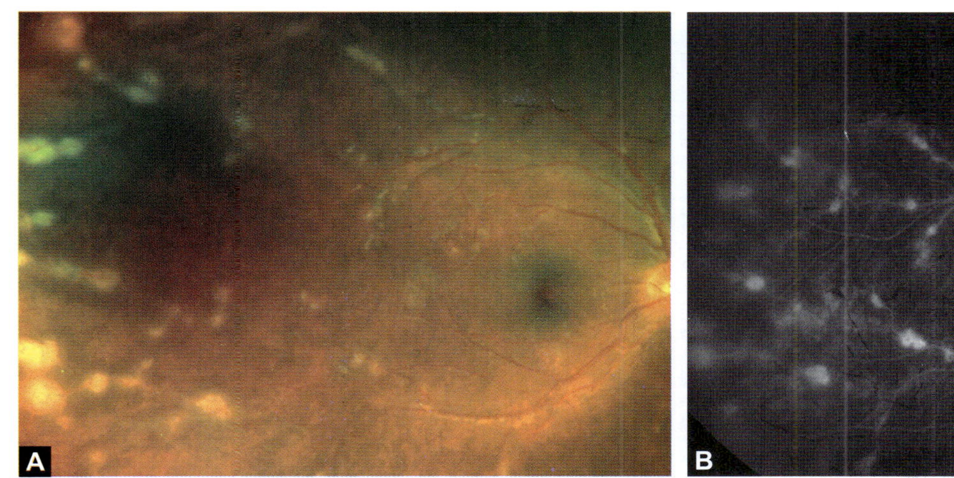

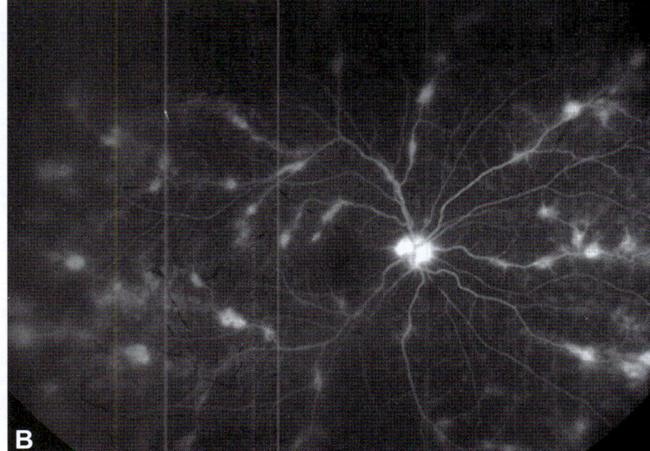

Figs. 39.7A and B: Segmental vasculitis in an eye with systemic sarcoidosis.

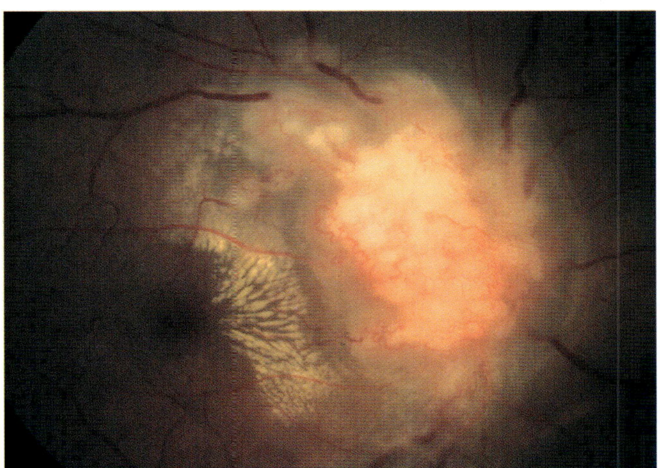

Fig. 39.8: Optic disc granuloma in a patient with sarcoidosis.

Retinal vasculitis may be seen in Wegener's granulomatosis besides other ocular manifestations of scleritis, episcleritis, orbital involvement, corneal ulcer, retinal/choroidal artery occlusion and optic nerve vasculitis.[67-70] Wegener's granulomatosis is characterized by necrotizing, granulomatous inflammation of the small vessels (sometimes medium vessels), chiefly of the airways and kidneys. The diagnosis is supported by presence of specific markers such as antineutrophil cytoplasmic antibodies (ANCAs) and histological findings. In SLE, retinal vascular occlusion occurs as a result of immune complex deposition in the vessel wall of arterioles of the retina and choroid. The various ocular manifestations are cotton wool spots, retinal hemorrhages, extensive capillary nonperfusion, frosted branch periphlebitis and rarely, exudative maculopathy and cilioretinal artery occlusion.[71-74] Arterial occlusion is also a feature of retinal vasculitis in PAN and Churg-Strauss syndrome.[75-78]

EALES DISEASE

Eales disease is an idiopathic disease which obliterates vessels usually involving the peripheral retina of young healthy adults. It was first described in 1880 by Henry Eales in young healthy males with abnormal retinal veins and recurrent vitreous hemorrhages. Signs of vascular sheathing with adjacent nerve fiber layer hemorrhages can be seen (Figs. 39.11A and B). It usually affects the retinal veins, but arteriolar involvement has also been noted. Peripheral nonperfusion areas are classically seen in Eales disease.

Confluent areas of temporal retina are affected more commonly. Signs of vascular tortuosity, and microvascular abnormalities like microaneurysms, arteriovenous (AV) shunts, venous beading, hard exudates and cotton wool spots can be seen. Neovascularization is a common phenomenon of which neovascularization of the disc (NVD) or neovascularization elsewhere (NVE) can be seen in up to 80% of the patients (Fig. 39.12). The NVE usually is located peripherally, at the junction of perfused and nonperfused retina and it may cause vitreous hemorrhage leading to diminution of vision. It may further lead to rubeosis iridis or formation of neovascularization of the iris (NVI) resulting in neovascular glaucoma. Other common complication is the formation of fibrovascular proliferation leading to tractional RD in these eyes.

Cystoid macular edema can occur in patients leading to significant vision loss. Vestibuloauditory dysfunction has been reported in patients with Eales disease. It is presumed that a similar mechanism of vascular occlusion and hypoxia leads to these systemic findings.

Eales disease is an idiopathic phenomenon and the cause is unknown. It is usually a diagnosis of exclusion. Hypersensitivity reaction to tuberculin protein has been reported but is not conclusive. Few reports have shown elevated erythrocyte sedimentation rate (ESR), high tuberculin skin test (TST) result, and vitreous polymerase chain reaction (PCR) positive

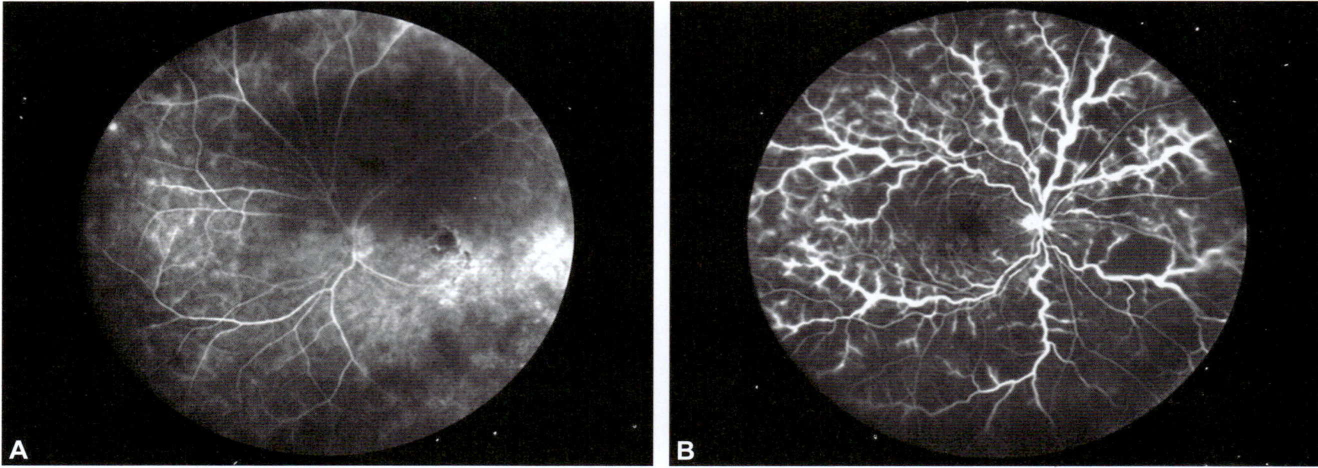

Figs. 39.9A and B: Capillaritis seen in both eyes of a female with HLA-B5 positive Behçet's disease.

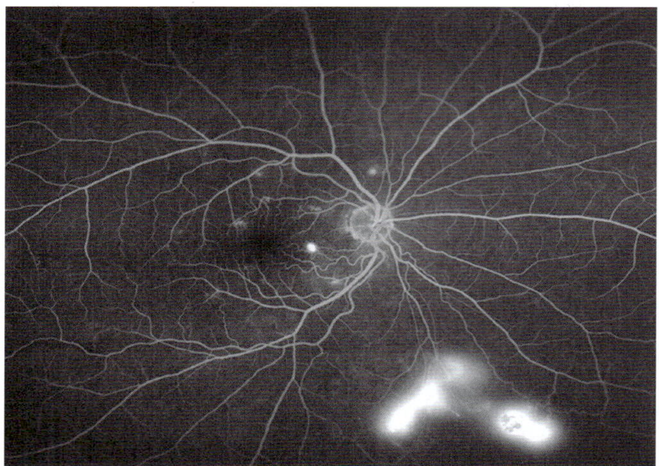

Fig. 39.10: Eye with postidiopathic healed vasculitis and sea-fan neovascularization. The patient on the recent visit had also developed a central serous chorioretinopathy (CSC) leak visible on this FA frame.

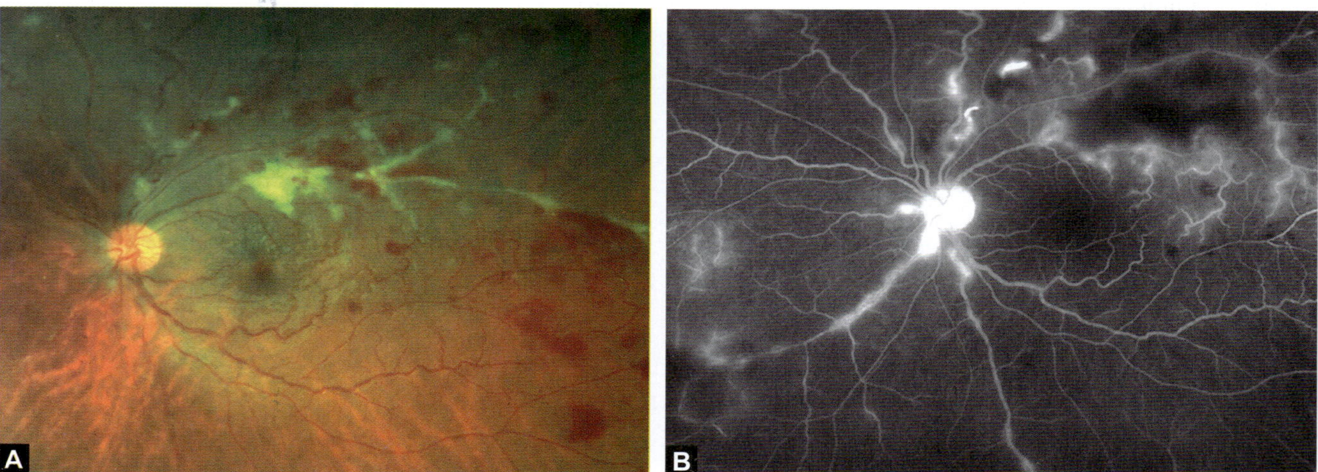

Figs. 39.11A and B: Color picture and FA of patient with idiopathic vasculitis (presumed Eales) showing intense sheathing and exudation from venules.

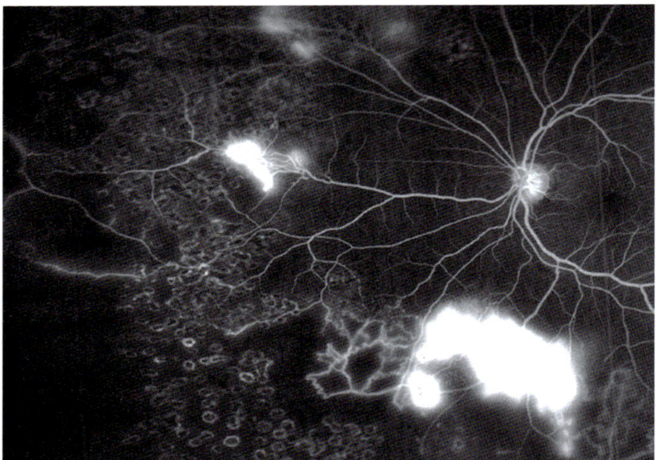

Fig. 39.12: Eye with long-standing partially lasered idiopathic Eales disease shows sea-fan NVE and areas of capillary nonperfusion.

for Mycobacterium tuberculosis indicating a more likely diagnosis of Eales disease.[78,79]

VOGT-KOYANAGI-HARADA DISEASE

Choroid is the primary site of inflammation in Vogt-Koyanagi-Harada (VKH) disease.[79] Conventionally, FA and ICGA have been used for its diagnosis and management.[80] However, persisting subclinical inflammation within the choroid is difficult to diagnose clinically. The recent enhanced-depth imaging OCT (EDI-OCT) has provided a new insight into the ultrastructural changes taking place within the choroid during acute as well as convalescent stages.[81-83] The four clinical stages of VKH disease (prodromal, acute, chronic convalescent and chronic recurrent stages) reveal specific manifestations. The ocular signs of acute stage typically follow the prodromal stage of neurologic and auditory disturbances, and include bilateral posterior uveitis with diffuse granulomatous choroiditis.[84,85] Vitritis, optic disc edema and exudative RD occur with/without anterior segment inflammation (Fig. 39.13A). Exudative RD begins as multifocal, shallow detachments of neurosensory retina in the posterior pole, which may become bullous in extreme cases. Sometimes, optic disc edema and vitritis along with multifocal choroiditis may be seen preceding exudative RD. Retinal and/or choroidal folds may also be seen.[86] FA reveals patchy hypofluorescence due to delayed choroidal filling and multiple punctate hyperfluorescent dots at the level of RPE in early frames.[86,88] In late frames, these hyperfluorescent dots enlarge, and the dye stains the surrounding subretinal fluid, revealing the extent of neurosensory detachments (Fig. 39.13B). Optic disc hyperfluorescence is a common finding in late frames. Alternate hypofluorescent and hyperfluorescent bands on FA indicate choroidal folds.[89] International classification (American Uveitis Society classification revised by International Nomenclature Committee) for VKH is as follows:

- No history of penetrating ocular trauma or surgery preceding the initial onset of uveitis
- No clinical or laboratory evidence suggestive of other ocular disease entities
- Bilateral ocular involvement (a or b must be met, depending on the stage of disease when the patient is examined)
  - Early manifestations of disease
    - Evidence of diffuse choroiditis (with or without anterior uveitis, vitreous inflammatory reaction or optic disc hyperemia) which may manifest as (a)focal areas of subretinal fluid or (b) bullous exudative RDs
  - Late manifestations of disease
    1. History suggestive of prior presence of early findings noted in 3a and either (2) or (3) below, or multiple signs from (3)
    2. Ocular depigmentation; either (a) sunset glow fundus or (b) Sugiura' sign
    3. Other ocular signs including (a nummular chorioretinal depigmented scars, or (b) retinal pigment epithelium clumping and/or migration or (c) recurrent or chronic anterior uveitis
- Neurological/auditory findings (may resolve by time of evaluation)
  - Meningismus (malaise, fever, headache, nausea, abdominal pain, stiffness of the neck and back, or a combination of these factors); note that headache alone is not sufficient to meet the definition of meningismus
  - Tinnitus
  - Cerebrospinal fluid pleocytosis
- Integumentary finding (not preceding onset of central nervous system (CNS) or ocular disease)
  - Alopecia, or
  - Poliosis, or
  - Vitiligo

Complete VKH: criteria 1–5 must be present.
Incomplete VKH: criteria 1–3 and either 4 or 5 must be present
Probable VKH (isolated ocular disease): criteria 1–3 must be present
VKH: Vogt-Koyanagi-Harada.

Ultrasound B-scan reveals peripapillary retinochoroidal thickening. On ICGA, the acute phase reveals patchy filling delay of choriocapillaris as well as those of large choroidal arteries.[80,90,91] The intermediate phase reveals diffuse leaking fuzzy vessels with persisting hypofluorescent dark dots. In the late phase, the hypofluorescent dark dots either become isofluorescent or remain hypofluorescent against a background of diffuse choroidal hyperfluorescence, suggesting partial or full-thickness granulomas, respectively.

Several weeks/months later after the acute inflammation subsides, chronic convalescent phase follows with variable degrees of choroidal and integumentary depigmentation. Sunset glow fundus (Fig. 39.14) that develops as a result of loss of choroidal melanocytes, is highly specific to chronic phase of VKH disease.[92] Nummular, depigmented, round, well-defined chorioretinal scars develop in the mid-peripheral fundus, which are suggestive of focal RPE atrophy (Fig. 39.14).

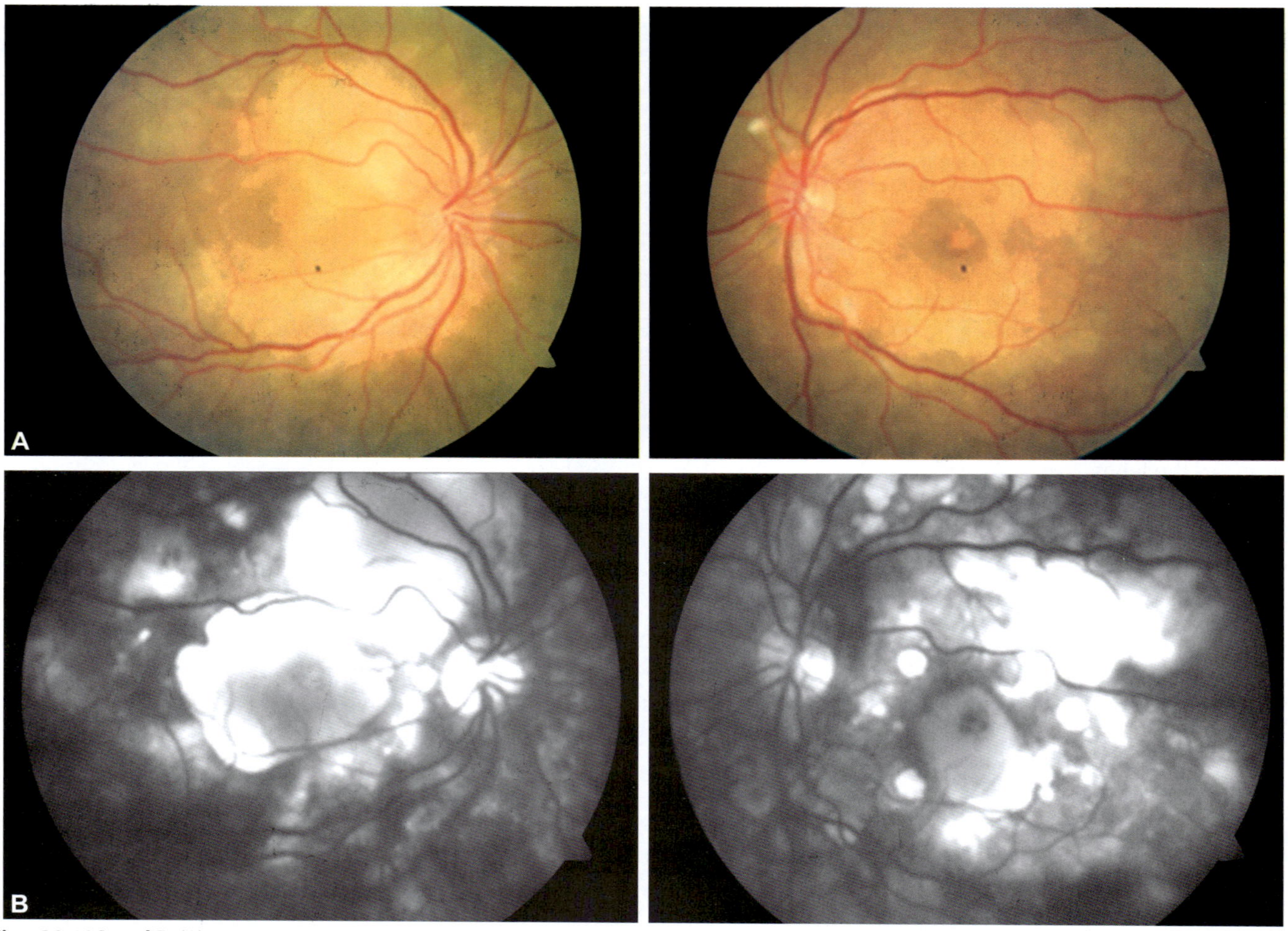

Figs. 39.13A and B: (A) Acute Vogt-Koyanagi-Harada disease showing exudative retinal detachment (RD) in posterior pole; (B) Fluorescein angiography reveals pooling of dye into the subretinal space in late phase.

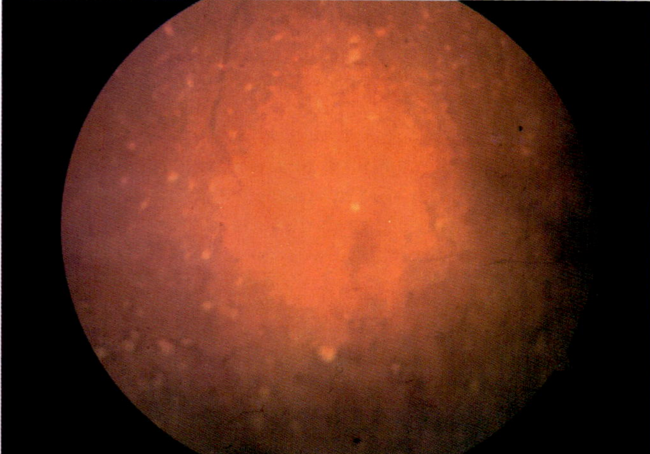

Fig. 39.14: Sunset glow fundus with nummular hypopigmented scars in chronic VKH disease.

Hyperpigmented linear focal lesions develop as a result of RPE migration/clumping.[84] Other signs of ocular depigmentation are rare, which include perilimbal vitiligo (Sugiura's sign) and peripheral iris depigmentation.[84,85] Cutaneous manifestations during this phase include vitiligo, alopecia and poliosis of eyelashes or eyebrows. Chronic recurrent phase is characterized by recurrent/chronic anterior uveitis leading to sight-threatening complications.[84] The anterior segment inflammation is typically granulomatous with mutton-fat keratic precipitates with/without iris nodules. The posterior segment examination reveals sunset glow fundus and depigmented chorioretinal scars. Active lesions of acute phase such as choroidal granulomas and exudative RD are highly unlikely during this phase.

Spectral-domain OCT aids in monitoring response to therapy, particularly in acute phase as it shows resolution of subretinal fluid/fibrin, and RPE undulations.[93,94] Prompt administration of systemic corticosteroids is the mainstay of therapy, with gradual tapering. Immunosuppressive agents are used as steroid-sparing agents, or in cases showing poor response/adverse effects to corticosteroids, or recurrence.[95,96] While diffuse choroidal thickening and loss of focal hyper-reflectivity in the inner choroid on EDI-OCT is a known feature of acute and convalescent VKH disease,[81-83] a transient, localized thickening of the choroid (choroidal bulging) has been more recently shown in eyes with uveitis in nonacute stage suggesting subclinical choroidal inflammation.[97] The most common complications include cataract, glaucoma, CNVM and subretinal fibrosis.[98-100]

SYMPATHETIC OPHTHALMIA

Sympathetic ophthalmia (SO) is a bilateral, diffuse granulomatous uveitis that occurs following surgery or penetrating trauma to the fellow eye.[101-104] Its onset is variable, occurring within days or months (majority of cases occurring within 1 year), or even decades later. Its incidence ranges from 0.01% to 0.5%.[104] The classical presentation includes bilateral anterior uveitis associated with mutton-fat keratic precipitates, vitritis, choroiditis, and papillitis. Optic nerve swelling and exudative RD are usually the presenting features of an acute disease (posterior SO) (Fig. 39.15A).[104] Granulomatous anterior uveitis can be visualized in severe and/or chronic recurrent cases. Yellowish-white subretinal nodular lesions on fundus examination correspond to the histopathologic Dalen-Fuchs nodules.

The diagnosis is essentially clinical, and does not require any laboratory or serological tests. Other causes such as VKH disease or sarcoidosis must be ruled out in the absence of history of ocular injury. Another way to differentiate it from VKH is the involvement of choriocapillaris in VKH but not in SO. FA and ICGA provide diagnostic clues. Multiple hyperfluorescent pinpoint leaks are seen in early frames of FA that leak the dye in late phases causing dye pooling in pockets of neurosensory detachments (Figs. 39.15B and C). The other presentation on FA may manifest as early hypofluorescent choroiditis lesions that become hyperfluorescent in late phase like other multifocal choroidopathies. Optic disc staining suggests disc swelling. Early hypofluorescent lesions on ICGA remain hypofluorescent in late phases suggesting choroidal hypoperfusion. B-scan ultrasonography demonstrates peripapillary choroidal thickening due to cellular infiltrates. Recently, OCT

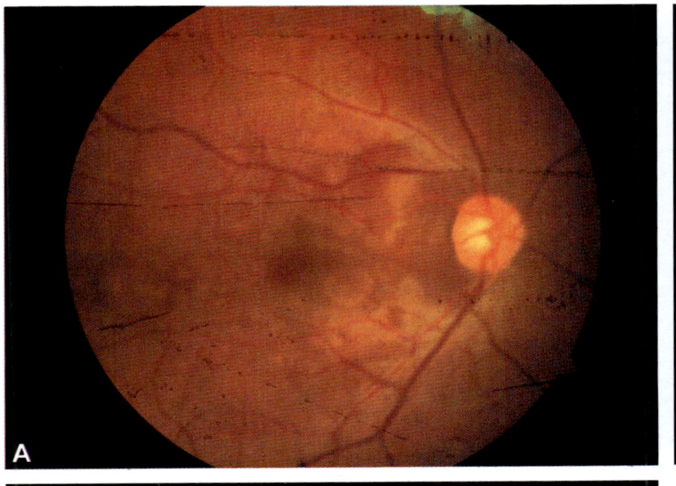

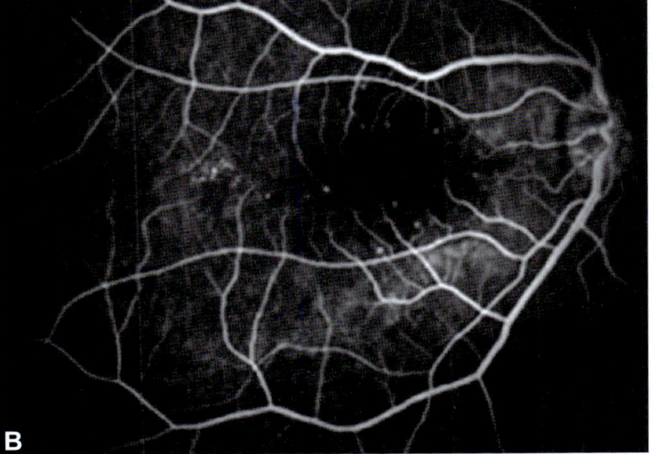

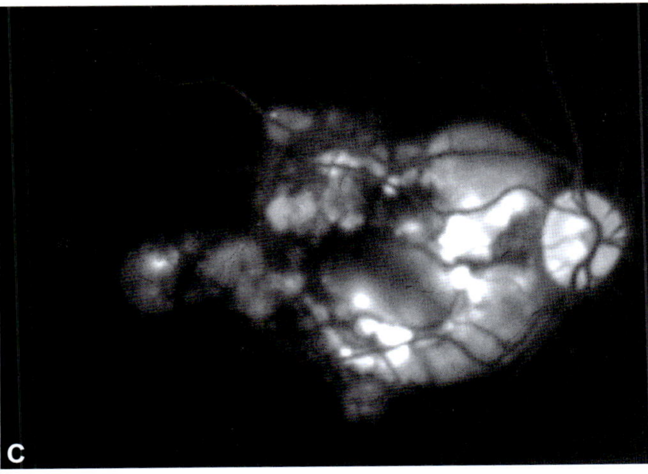

Figs. 39.15A to C: Acute exudative retinal detachment in the right eye (A) in a patient with left eye phthisis (following penetrating eye injury), with punctate hyperfluorescent leaks in early phase of fluorescein angiography (B) that leak profusely in late phase (C), suggesting sympathetic ophthalmia.

has been used as a regular tool for documenting and monitoring subretinal fluid and choroidal thickening before and after treatment.[105] Chronic, recurrent uveitis produces sight-threatening complications like cataract, glaucoma and maculopathy.[106]

Histopathologic studies reveal uveal infiltration by granulomas consisting primarily of lymphocytes, macrophages, and multinucleated giant cells.[107,108] Retinal and choriocapillaris involvement is rare. Autoimmunity and cell-mediated immunity play a key role in the pathogenesis of SO.[109,110]

High-dose systemic corticosteroids are the mainstay of therapy. In acute cases, intravenous pulse steroid therapy is given (methylprednisolone 1.0 g/day for 3–5 days), followed by oral prednisone (1.0–2.0 mg/kg/day), which is tapered slowly over 3–4 months. Adjunctive topical corticosteroids and cycloplegics are indicated in anterior uveitis to prevent posterior synechia formation. Immunomodulatory therapy is started as a steroid-sparing therapy, or in cases with inadequate response to corticosteroids.[111,112] Azathioprine, cyclosporine, chlorambucil, cyclophosphamide, etc. may be used in consultation with the internist with regular systemic monitoring.

INTRAOCULAR LYMPHOMA

Primary intraocular lymphoma (PIOL), or primary vitreoretinal lymphoma (PVRL), is predominantly a NHL and a subtype of primary central nervous system lymphoma (PCNSL) that originates in the eye, or is detected first in the eye.[113-115] About 80% of PVRL eventually develop CNS involvement, while 20% of PCNSL develop intraocular disease.[116,117] Patients with PIOL present with floaters and blurred vision, which is usually unilateral to begin with. While the anterior segment examination reveals mild inflammation (aqueous cells and few keratic precipitates), vitritis is significant. The typical fundus lesions are yellowish-white or cream-colored sub-RPE infiltrates which may or may not be confluent and can be seen in any part of the fundus (Figs. 39.16A to C).

Fundus autofluorescence plays a crucial role in demonstrating RPE abnormalities in the form of granular, mixed fluorescence, and mottling. Patchy window defects and late staining patterns are seen on FA, besides other features like diffuse retinal vasculitis, or sometimes CME.[118] SD-OCT typically reveals sub-RPE elevations. In patients with suspected

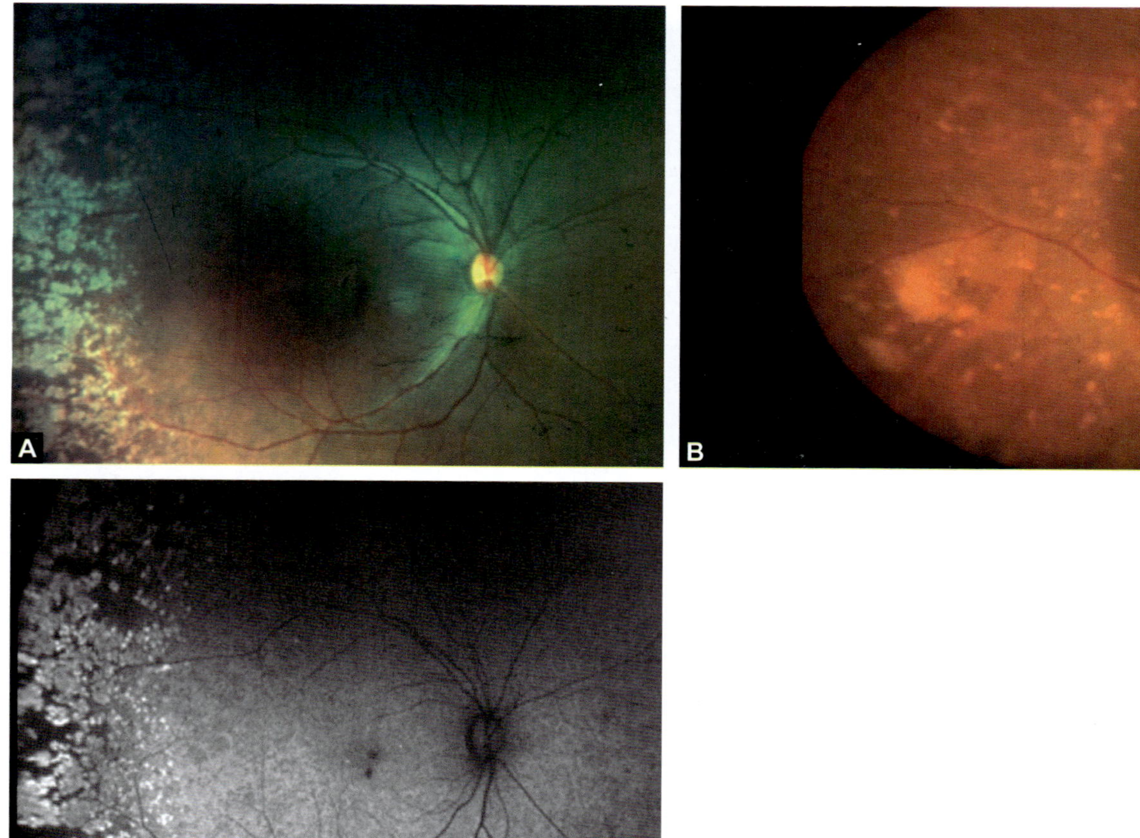

Figs. 39.16A to C: (A and B) Cream-colored sub-RPE infiltrates in a patient with primary vitreoretinal lymphoma; (C) A corresponding red free fundus picture showing the lesions.

PVRL, magnetic resonance imaging (MRI) of the brain should be done to evaluate CNS involvement. Cytological or histopathological demonstration of PIOL cells from the eye (vitreous or retinal/choroidal biopsy) forms the gold standard for diagnosing PVRL. As lymphoma cells are scarce in vitreous samples and highly susceptible to necrosis, the processing of sample and availability of an experienced cytopathologist are the most crucial steps in facilitating its cytological diagnosis. PVRL samples display several large, atypical cells with large nuclei, scanty basophilic cytoplasm, and prominent nucleoli.[119,120]

The yield of vitreous biopsy is low in PVRL in most of the cases. A transvitreal retinochoroidal biopsy or an external chorioretinal biopsy of the subretinal, yellowish deposits is performed in these cases for histopathologic analysis. Lymphoma cells are seen infiltrating the sub-RPE, subretinal and retinal layers.[121] Analysis of interleukin-10 (IL-10) in the vitreous fluid provides an additional method for diagnosing PVRL if the IL-10:IL-6 ratio is greater than 1.0.[120-123] B-cell PVRL is also characterized by presence of monoclonality of immunoglobulin heavy chain (IgH) gene in minimal 15 malignant cells of a vitreous sample.[124-127] T-cell intraocular lymphomas are extremely rare, but have a high mortality rate.

Intraocular chemotherapy and CNS screening should immediately follow diagnosis of PVRL. Intraocular injection of methotrexate is highly effective in regressing the PVRL lesions, although resistance and toxicity should be monitored. Systemic chemotherapy and whole cranial radiation are indicated if PCNSL is detected. Rituximab, an engineered anti-CD20 monoclonal antibody, is a promising new therapy for B-cell PVRL.[127]

REFERENCES

1. Abu-Yaghi NE, Hartono SP, Hodge DO, et al. White dot syndromes: a 20-year study of incidence, clinical features, and outcomes. Ocul Immunol Inflamm. 2011;19(6):426-30.
2. Jampol LM, Becker KG. White spot syndromes of the retina: a hypothesis based on the common genetic hypothesis of autoimmune/inflammatory disease. Am J Ophthalmology. 2003;135(3):376-9.
3. Vianna RN, Socci D, Nehemy MB, et al. The white dot syndromes. Arq Bras Oftalmol. 2007;70(3):554-62.
4. Crawford CM, Igboeli O. A review of the inflammatory chorioretinopathies: the white dot syndromes. ISRN Inflammation. 2013;2013:ID 783190. [online] Available from http://dx.doi.org/10.1155/2013/783190. [Accessed December, 2017].
5. Vianna R, Van Egmond J, Priem H, et al. Natural history and visual outcome in patients with APMPPE. Bull Soc Belge Ophthalmology. 1993;248(1):73-6.
6. Quillen DA, Davis JB, Gottlieb JL, et al. The white dot syndromes. Am J Ophthalmology. 2004;137(3):538-50. Comment in: Am J Ophthalmology. 2004;138(4):686; author reply 686-7.
7. Deutman AF, Lion F. Choriocapillaris nonperfusion in acute multifocal placoid pigment epitheliopathy. Am J Ophthalmology. 1977;84(5):652-7.
8. Dhaliwal RS, Maguire AM, Flower RW, et al. Acute posterior multifocal placoid pigment epitheliopathy: an indocyanine green angiographic study. Retina. 1993;13(4):317-25.
9. Wilson CA, Choromokos EA, Sheppard R. Acute posterior multifocal placoid pigment epitheliopathy and cerebral vasculitis. Arch Ophthalmology. 1988;106(6):796-800.
10. Gass JD. Stereoscopic Atlas of Macular Diseases: Diagnosis and Treatment, 4th edition. St. Louis: Mosby; 1997.
11. Jampol LM, Sieving PA, Pugh D. Multiple evanescent white dot syndromes. I. Clinical findings. Arch Ophthalmology. 1984;102(5):671-4.
12. Obana A, Kusumi M, Miki T. Indocyanine green angiographic aspects of multiple evanescent white dot syndrome. Retina. 1996;16(2):97-104.
13. Sieving PA, Fishman GA, Jampol LM, et al. Multiple evanescent white dot syndrome. II. Electrophysiology of the photoreceptors during retinal pigment epithelial disease. Arch Ophthalmology. 1984;102(5):675-9.
14. Krill AE, Deutman AF. Acute retinal pigment epitheliitus. Am J Ophthalmology. 1972;74(2):193-205.
15. Baillif S, Wolff B, Paoli V, et al. Retinal fluorescein and indocyanine green angiography and spectral-domain optical coherence tomography findings in acute retinal pigment epitheliitis. Retina. 2011;31:1156-63.
16. Prost M. Long-term observations of patients with acute retinal pigment epitheliitis. Ophthalmologica. 1989;199:84-9.
17. Gass JD. Are acute zonal occult outer retinopathy and the white spot syndromes (AZOOR complex) specific autoimmune diseases? Am J Ophthalmology. 2003;135(3):380-1.
18. Mahajan VB, Stone EM. Patients with an acute zonal occult outer retinopathy-like illness rapidly improve with valacyclovir treatment. Am J Ophthalmology. 2010;150(4):511-8.
19. Cheung MC, Nune GC, Hwang DG, et al. Acute zonal occult outer retinopathy in a patient with graft-versus-host disease. Am J Ophthalmology. 2004;138(6):1058-60.
20. Carrasco L, Ramos M, Galisteo R, et al. Isolation of Candida famata from a patient with acute zonal occult outer retinopathy. J Clin Microbiol. 2005;43(2):635-40.
21. Pisa D, Ramos M, García P, et al. Fungal infection in patients with serpiginous choroiditis or acute zonal occult outer retinopathy. J Clin Microbiol. 2008;46(1):130-5.
22. Gass JD. Acute zonal occult outer retinopathy. Donders Lecture: The Netherlands Ophthalmological Society, Maastricht, Holland, June 19, 1992. J Clin Neuroophthalmol. 1993;13(2):79-97.
23. Francis PJ, Marinescu A, Fitzke FW, et al. Acute zonal occult outer retinopathy: towards a set of diagnostic criteria. Br J Ophthalmology. 2005;89:70-3.
24. Mrejen S, Khan S, Gallego-Pinazo R, et al. Acute zonal occult outer retinopathy: a classification based on multimodal imaging. JAMA Ophthalmology. 2014;132(4):1089-98.
25. Ryan SJ, Maumenee AE. Birdshot retinochoroidopathy. Am J Ophthalmology. 1980;89(1):31-45.
26. Priem HA, Oosterhuis JA. Birdshot chorioretinopathy: clinical characteristics and evolution. Br J Ophthalmology. 1988;72(9):646-9.
27. Priem HA, Kijlstra A, Noens L, et al. HLA typing in birdshot chorioretinopathy. Am J Ophthalmology. 1988;105(2):182-5.
28. Fardeau C, Herbort CP, Kullmann N, et al. Indocyanine green angiography in birdshot chorioretinopathy. Ophthalmology. 1999;106(10):1928-34.
29. Vianna RN, Socci D, Deschênes J, et al. The role of indocyanine green angiography in the diagnosis of birdshot chorioretinopathy. Rev Bras Oftalmol. 2006;65(4):242-5.

30. Priem HA, De Rouck A, De Laey JJ, et al. Electrophysiologic studies in birdshot chorioretinopathy. Am J Ophthalmology. 1988;106(4):430-6.

31. Oh KT, Christmas NJ, Folk JC. Birdshot retinochoroiditis: long-term follow-up of a chronically progressive disease. Am J Ophthalmology. 2002;133(5):622-9.

32. Socci D, Vianna RN, Moura Brasil O. Optic coherence tomography in birdshot chorioretinopathy [poster]. In: World Ophthalmology Congress. São Paulo, 19-24 Feb. 2006.

33. Vitale AT, Rodriguez A, Foster CS. Low-dose cyclosporine therapy in the treatment of birdshot retinochoroidopathy. Ophthalmology. 1994;101(5):822-31.

34. Baltatzis S, Tufail F, Yu EN, et al. Mycophenolate mofetil as an immunomodulatory agent in the treatment of chronic ocular inflammatory disorders. Ophthalmology. 2003;110(5):1061-5.

35. Watzke RC, Packer AJ, Folk JC, et al. Punctate inner choroidopathy. Am J Ophthalmology. 1984;98(5):572-84.

36. Tiffin PA, Maini R, Roxburgh ST, et al. Indocyanine green angiography in a case of punctate inner choroidopathy. Br J Ophthalmology. 1996;80(1):90-1.

37. Campos J, Campos A, Castro Sousa JP. Punctate inner choroidopathy: a systematic review. Med Hypothesis Discov Innov Ophthalmology. 2014;3(3):76-82.

38. Folk JC, Walker JD. Multifocal choroiditis with panuveitis, diffuse subretinal fibrosis, and punctate inner choroidopathy. In: Ryan SJ, Schachat AP, Hinton DR, et al. (Eds). Retina, 4th edition. St. Louis: Mosby; 2006.

39. Patel KH, Birnbaum AD, Tessler HH, et al. Presentation and outcome of patients with punctate inner choroidopathy at a tertiary referral center. Retina. 2011;31(7):1387-91.

40. Nozik RA, Dorsch W. A new chorioretinopathy associated with anterior uveitis. Am J Ophthalmology. 1973;76(5):758-62.

41. Brown J Jr, Folk JC, Reddy CH, et al. Visual prognosis of multifocal choroiditis and panuveitis, punctate inner choroidopathy, and the diffuse subretinal fibrosis syndrome. Ophthalmology. 1996;103(7):1100-5.

42. Vianna RN, Ozdal PC, Souza Filho JP, et al. Long-term follow-up of patients with multifocal choroiditis and panuveitis. Acta Ophthalmology Scand. 2004;82(6):748-53.

43. Spaide RF, Freund KB, Slakter J, et al. Treatment of subfoveal choroidal neovascularization associated with multifocal choroiditis and panuveitis with photodynamic therapy. Retina. 2002;22(5):545-9. Comment in: Retina. 2003;23(3):428.

44. Abu el-Asrar AM. Serpiginous (geographical) choroiditis. Int Ophthalmology Clin. 1995;35:87-91.

45. Gass JD. Stereoscopic Atlas of Macular Diseases: A Funduscopic and Angiographic Presentation. St. Louis, MO: CV Mosby; 1970. p. 66.

46. Weiss H, Annesley WH, Shields JA, et al. The clinical course of serpiginous choroidopathy. Am J Ophthalmology. 1979;87:133-42.

47. Hamilton AM, Bird AC. Geographical choroidopathy. Br J Ophthalmology. 1974;58:784-97.

48. Babel J. Geographic and helicoid choroidopathies: clinical and angiographic study; attempted classification. J Fr Ophthalmology. 1983;6:981-93.

49. Laatikainen L, Erkkilä H. Serpiginous choroiditis. Br J Ophthalmology. 1974;58:777-83.

50. Erkkilä H, Laatikainen L, Jokinen E. Immunological studies on serpiginous choroiditis. Graefes Arch Clin Exp Ophthalmology. 1982;219:131-4.

51. Priya K, Madhavan HN, Reiser BJ, et al. Association of herpesviruses in the aqueous humor of patients with serpiginous choroiditis: a polymerase chain reaction-based study. Ocul Immunol Inflamm. 2002;10:253-61.

52. Gupta V, Agarwal A, Gupta A, et al. Clinical characteristics of serpiginous choroidopathy in North India. Am J Ophthalmology. 2002;134:47-56.

53. Christmas NJ, Oh KT, Oh DM, et al. Long-term follow-up of patients with serpiginous choroiditis. Retina. 2002;22:550-6.

54. Jampol LM, Orth D, Daily MJ, et al. Subretinal neovascularization with geographic (serpiginous) choroiditis. Am J Ophthalmology. 1979;88:683-9.

55. Laatikainen L, Erkkila H. Subretinal and disc neovascularization in serpiginous choroiditis. Br J Ophthalmology. 1982;66:326-31.

56. Lee DK, Suhler EB, Augustin W, et al. Serpiginous choroidopathy presenting as choroidal neovascularization. Br J Ophthalmology. 2003;87:1184-5.

57. Bansal R, Gupta A, Gupta V, et al. Tubercular serpiginous-like choroiditis presenting as multifocal serpiginoid choroiditis. Ophthalmology. 2012;119(11):2334-42.

58. Abu El-Asrar AM, Herbort CP, Tabbara KF. Retinal vasculitis. Ocul Immunol Inflamm. 2005;13:415-33.

59. Jabs DA, Johns CJ. Ocular involvement in chronic sarcoidosis. Am J Ophthalmology. 1986;102:297-301.

60. Obenauf CD, Shaw HE, Sydnor CF, et al. Sarcoidosis and its ophthalmic manifestations. Am J Ophthalmology. 1978;86:648-55.

61. Rothova A. Ocular involvement in sarcoidosis. Br J Ophthalmology. 2000;84:110-6.

62. Nicholas J. Sarcoidosis. Curr Opin Ophthalmology. 2002;13:393-6.

63. Tugal-Tutkun I, Onal S, Altan-Yaycioglu R, et al. Uveitis in Behçet disease: an analysis of 880 patients. Am J Ophthalmology. 2004;138:373-80.

64. Gedik S, Akova YA, Yilmaz G, et al. Indocyanine green and fundus fluorescein angiographic findings in patients with active ocular Behçet's disease. Ocul Immunol Inflamm. 2005;13:51-8.

65. Tugal-Tutkun I. Behcet's uveitis. Middle East Afr J Ophthalmology. 2009;16:219-24.

66. Okada AA. Drug therapy in Behcet's disease. Ocul Immunol Inflamm. 2000;8:85-91.

67. Bullen CL, Liesegang TJ, McDonald TJ, et al. Ocular complications of Wegener's granulomatosis. Ophthalmology. 1983;90:279-90.

68. Spalton DJ, Graham EM, Page NG, et al. Ocular changes in limited forms of Wegener's granulomatosis. Br J Ophthalmology. 1981;65: 553-63.

69. Pulido JS, Goeken JA, Nerad JA, et al. Ocular manifestations of patients with circulating antineutrophil cytoplasmic antibodies. Arch Ophthalmology. 1990;108:845-50.

70. Iida T, Spaide RF, Kantor J. Retinal and choroidal arterial occlusion in Wegener's granulomatosis. Am J Ophthalmology. 2002;133:151-2.

71. Gold DH, Morris DA, Hertrind P. Ocular findings in systemic lupus erythematosus. Br J Ophthalmology. 1972;56:800-4.

72. Jabs DA, Fine SL, Hochberg MC, et al. Severe retinal vaso-occlusive disease in systemic lupus erythematosus. Arch Ophthalmology. 1986;104:558-63.

73. Quillen DA, Stathopoulos NA, Blankenship GW, et al. Lupus associated frosted branch periphlebitis and exudative maculopathy. Retina. 1997;17:449-51.

74. Abu El-Asrar AM, Naddaf HO, Al-Momen A, et al. Systemic lupus erythematosus flare-up manifesting as a cilioretinal artery occlusion. Lupus. 1995;4:158-60.

75. Morgan CM, Foster CS, Gragoudas ES. Retinal vasculitis in polyarteritis nodosa. Retina. 1986;6:205-9.

76. Hsu CT, Kerrison JB, Miller NR, et al. Choroidal infarction, ischemic optic neuropathy, and central retinal artery occlusion from polyarteritis nodosa. Retina. 2001;21:348-51.

77. Takanashi T, Uchida S, Arita M, et al. Ischemic vasculitis in Churg-Strauss syndrome. Report of two cases and review of the literature. Ophthalmology. 2001;108:1129-33.

78. Singh R, Toor P, Parchand S, et al. Quantitative polymerase chain reaction for Mycobacterium tuberculosis in so-called Eales' disease. Ocul Immunol Inflamm. 2012;20(3):153-7.

79. Gieser AS, Murphy RP. Eales' disease. In: Ryan SJ (Ed). Retina, 2nd edition. St. Louis: CV Mosby; 1994. pp. 1503-7.

80. Partal A, Moshfeghi DM, Alcorn D. Churg-Strauss syndrome in a child: retina and optic nerve findings. Br J Ophthalmology. 2004;88:971-2.

81. Rao NA. Pathology of Vogt-Koyanagi-Harada disease. Int Ophthalmology. 2007;27:81-5.

82. Knecht PB, Mantovani A, Herbort CP. Indocyanine green angiography guided management of Vogt-Koyanagi-Harada disease: differentiation between choroidal scars and active lesions. Int Ophthalmology. 2013;33:571-7.

83. Maruko I, Tomohiro I, Sugano Y, et al. Subfoveal choroidal thickness after treatment of Vogt-Koyanagi-Harada disease. Retina. 2011;31:510-7.

84. da Silva FT, Sakata VM, Nakashima A, et al. Enhanced depth imaging optical coherence tomography in long-standing Vogt-Koyanagi-Harada disease. Br J Ophthalmology. 2013;97:70-4.

85. Takahashi H, Takase H, Ishizuka A, et al. Choroidal thickness in convalescent Vogt-Koyanagi-Harada disease. Retina. 2014;34:775-80.

86. Moorthy RS, Inomata H, Rao NA. Vogt-Koyanagi-Harada syndrome. Surv Ophthalmology. 1995;39:265-92.

87. Rajendran R, Evans M, Rao NA. Vogt-Koyanagi-Harada disease. Int Ophthalmology Clin. 2005;45:115-34.

88. Gupta V, Gupta A, Gupta P, et al. Spectral domain cirrus optical coherence tomography of choroidal striations in the acute stage of Vogt-Koyanagi-Harada disease. Am J Ophthalmology. 2009;147:148-53.

89. Arellanes-García L, Hernández-Barrios M, Fromow-Guerra J, et al. Fluorescein fundus angiographic findings in Vogt-Koyanagi-Harada syndrome. Int Ophthalmology. 2007;27:155-61.

90. Fardeau C, Tran TH, Gharbi B, et al. Retinal fluorescein and indocyanine green angiography and optical coherence tomography in successive stages of Vogt-Koyanagi-Harada disease. Int Ophthalmology 2007;27:163-72.

91. Wu W, Wen F, Huang S, et al. Choroidal folds in Vogt-Koyanagi-Harada disease. Am J Ophthalmology. 2007;143:900-1.

92. Bouchenaki N, Herbort CP. The contribution of indocyanine green angiography to the appraisal and management of Vogt-Koyanagi-Harada disease. Ophthalmology. 2001;108:54-64.

93. Miyanaga M, Kawaguchi T, Miyata K, et al. Indocyanine green angiography findings in initial acute pretreatment Vogt-Koyanagi-Harada disease in Japanese patients. Jpn J Ophthalmology. 2010;54:377-82.

94. Rao NA, Gupta A, Dustin L, et al. Frequency of distinguishing clinical features in Vogt-Koyanagi-Harada disease. Ophthalmology. 2010;117:591-9.

95. Maruyama Y, Kishi S. Tomographic features of serous retinal detachment in Vogt-Koyanagi-Harada syndrome. Ophthalmic Surg Lasers Imaging. 2004;35:239-42.

96. Ishihara K, Hangai M, Kita M, et al. Acute Vogt-Koyanagi-Harada disease in enhanced spectral domain optical coherence tomography. Ophthalmology. 2009;116:1799-807.

97. Rao NA. Treatment of Vogt-Koyanagi-Harada disease by corticosteroids and immunosuppressive agents. Ocul Immunol Inflamm. 2006;14:71-2.

98. Paredes I, Ahmed M, Foster CS. Immunomodulatory therapy for Vogt-Koyanagi-Harada patients as first-line therapy. Ocul Immunol Inflamm. 2006;14:87-90.

99. Sakata VM, da Silva FT, Hirata CE, et al. Choroidal bulging in patients with Vogt-Koyanagi-Harada disease in the non-acute uveitic stage. J Ophthalmic Inflamm Infect. 2014;4:6.

100. Rubsamen PE, Gass JD. Vogt-Koyanagi-Harada syndrome. Clinical course, therapy, and long-term visual outcome. Arch Ophthalmology. 1991;109:682-7.

101. Lertsumitkul S, Whitcup SM, Nussenblatt RB, et al. Subretinal fibrosis and choroidal neovascularization in Vogt-Koyanagi-Harada syndrome. Graefes Arch Clin Exp Ophthalmology. 1999;237:1039-45.

102. Ober RR, Smith RE, Ryan SJ. Subretinal neovascularization in the Vogt-Koyanagi-Harada syndrome. Int Ophthalmology. 1983;6:225-34.

103. Albert DM, Diaz-Rohena R. A historical review of sympathetic ophthalmia and its epidemiology. Surv Ophthalmology. 1989;34(1):1-14.

104. Chan CC, Roberge RG, Whitcup SM, et al. 32 cases of sympathetic ophthalmia A retrospective study at the National Eye Institute, Bethesda, Md., from 1982 to 1992. Arch Ophthalmology. 1995;113(5):597-600.

105. Arevalo JF, Garcia RA, Al-Dhibi HA, et al. Update on sympathetic ophthalmia. Middle East Afr J Ophthalmology. 2012;19(1):13-21.

106. Gupta V, Gupta A, Dogra MR. Posterior sympathetic ophthalmia: a single centre long-term study of 40 patients from North India. Eye. 2008;22(12):1459-64.

107. Castiblanco C, Adelman RA. Imaging for sympathetic ophthalmia: impact on the diagnosis and management. Int Ophthalmology Clin. 2012;52(4):173-81.

108. Lubin JR, Albert DM, Weinstein M. Sixty-five years of sympathetic ophthalmia. A clinicopathologic review of 105 cases (1913–1978). Ophthalmology. 1980;87(2):109-21.

109. Chan CC, Benezra D, Rodrigues MM, et al. Immunohistochemistry and electron microscopy of choroidal infiltrates and Dalen-Fuchs nodules in sympathetic ophthalmia. Ophthalmology. 1985;92(4):580-90.

110. Chan CC, Nussenblatt RB, Fujikawa LS, et al. Sympathetic ophthalmia. Immunopathological findings. Ophthalmology. 1986; 93(5) 690-5.

111. Rao NA, Robin J, Hartmann D, et al. The role of the penetrating wound in the development of sympathetic ophthalmia experimental observations. Arch Ophthalmology. 1983;101(1):102-4.

112. Shindo Y, Ohno S, Usui M, et al. Immunogenetic study of sympathetic ophthalmia. Tissue Antigens. 1997;49(2):111-5.

113. Tessler HH, Jennings T. High-dose short-term chlorambucil for intractable sympathetic ophthalmia and Behcet's disease. Br J Ophthalmology. 1990;74(6):353-7.

114. Lau CH, Comer M, Lightman S. Long-term efficacy of mycophenolate mofetil in the control of severe intraocular inflammation. Clin Exp Ophthalmology. 2003;31(6):487-91.

115. Chan CC. Primary intraocular lymphoma: clinical features, diagnosis and treatment. Clin Lymphoma. 2003;4:30-1.

116. Tuailon N, Chan CC. Molecular analysis of primary central nervous system and primary intraocular lymphomas. Curr Mol Med. 2001;1:259-72.

117. Chan CC, Buggage RR, Nussenblatt RB. Intraocular lymphoma. Curr Opin Ophthalmology. 2002;13:411-8.

118. Whitcup SM, de Smet MD, Rubin BI, et al. Intraocular lymphoma. Clinical and histopathologic diagnosis. Ophthalmology. 1993;100:1399-406.

119. Akpek EK, Maca SM, Christen WG, et al. Intraocular-central nervous system lymphoma: clinical features, diagnosis and outcomes. Ophthalmology. 1999;106:1805-10.

120. Velez G, Chan CC, Csaky KG. Fluorescein angiographic findings in primary intraocular lymphoma. Retina. 2002;22:37-43.

121. Chan CC. Molecular pathology of primary intraocular lymphoma. Trans Am Ophthalmology Soc. 2003;101:275-92.

122. Gonzales JA, Chan CC. Biopsy techniques and yields in diagnosing primary intraocular lymphoma. Int Ophthalmology. 2007;27:241-50.

123. Coulpland SE, Bechrakis NE, Anastassiou G, et al. Evaluation of vitrectomy specimens and chorioretinal biopsies in the diagnosis of primary intraocular lymphoma in patients with masquerade syndrome. Graefes Arch Clin Exp Ophthalmology. 2003;241:860-70.

124. Lopez JS, Chan CC, Burnier M, et al. Immunohistochemistry findings in primary intraocular lymphoma. Am J Ophthalmology. 1991;112:472-4.

125. Wolf LA, Reed GF, Buggage RR, et al. Vitreous cytokine levels. Ophthalmology. 2003;110:1671-2.

126. Shen DF, Zhuang Z, LeHoang P, et al. Utility of microdissection and polymerase chain reaction for the detection of immunoglobulin gene rearrangement and translocation in primary intraocular lymphoma. Ophthalmology. 1998;105:1664-9.

127. Rubenstein JL, Fridlyand J, Abrey L, et al. Phase I study of intraventricular administration of rituximab in patients with recurrent CNS and intraocular lymphoma. J Clin Oncol. 2007;25:1350-6.

Chapter 40

Infectious Inflammation

Reema Bansal, Mohit Dogra, Amod Gupta

INTRODUCTION

Cytomegalovirus (CMV) retinitis is the most common ocular manifestation, and the most common cause of visual loss in patients with acquired immunodeficiency syndrome (AIDS).[1-3] The morbidity and mortality associated with AIDS-associated infections have changed with the introduction of highly active antiretroviral therapy (HAART). Differences in the incidence of CMV retinitis, its location, severity of retinitis and patient's immune status have been reported between pre- and post-HAART era.[4] The immunological profile of patients presenting with new CMV retinitis lesions typically includes a low CD4+ count (less than 50 cells/μL) and elevated viral loads, but patients on HAART exhibit a wider range.[3,5] The diagnosis is based on ophthalmoscopic appearance of fundus lesions, characterized by necrotizing retinitis manifesting as white, fluffy lesions, along with retinal hemorrhages and vascular sheathing in three forms: granular, edematous and frosted branch angiitis. The vitreous has minimal or no inflammatory cells. The granular form of CMV retinitis arises in the peripheral retina and extends to the posterior pole (Fig. 40.1). The edematous form has widespread areas of retinal necrosis along with retinal hemorrhages and vascular sheathing (Fig. 40.2). Frosted branch angiitis is associated with retinal vasculitis.

Majority of newly diagnosed cases of CMV retinitis are due to HAART failure. There are fewer chances of retinal detachment, disease progression and fellow eye involvement in HAART-treated patients.[3]

Treatment of CMV retinitis can be local or systemic, and split into two phases: induction and maintenance phase. Local therapy comprises of twice-weekly injections of ganciclovir (2000–4,000 μg/0.1 mL) during the induction phase, followed by weekly injection during the maintenance phase.[6,7] High retinal tissue concentrations of ganciclovir can be achieved without causing systemic bone marrow suppression through intravitreal injections. Induction therapy with foscarnet comprises of six injections (2,400 μg) at 72-hour

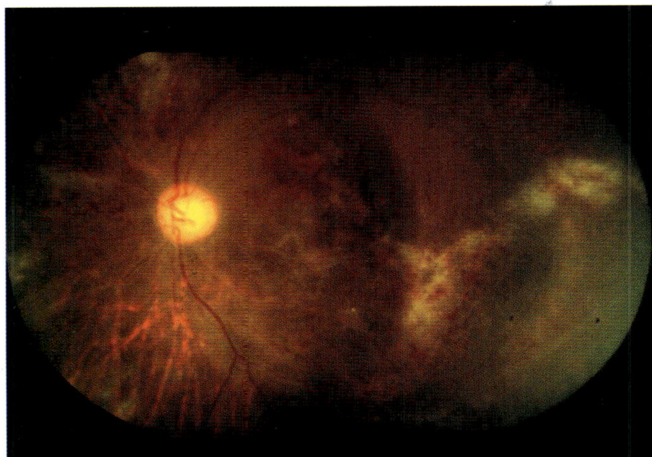

Fig. 40.1: Cytomegalovirus (CMV) retinitis arising in the retinal periphery and spreading to the posterior pole.

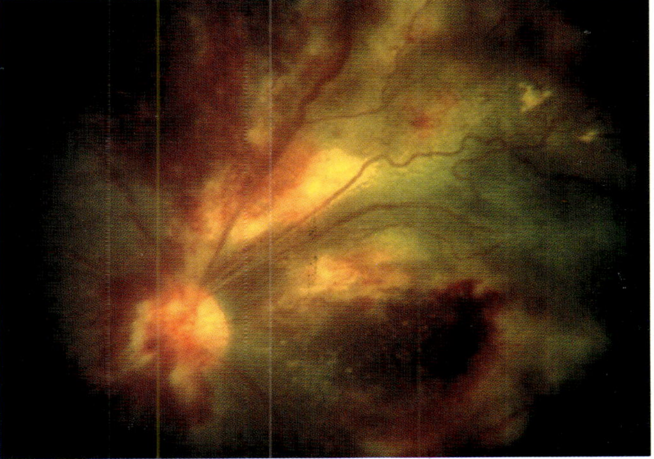

Fig. 40.2: Widespread areas of retinal necrosis along with retinal hemorrhages in a patient with cytomegalovirus (CMV) retinitis (Brushfire appearance).

interval, and maintenance therapy includes weekly injection.[8,9] Intravitreal cidofovir is no longer recommended as it is associated with serious side effects such as iritis, irreversible hypotony, severe visual loss and low efficacy.[10,11] Ganciclovir implant (Vitrasert) consists of a 4.5 mg capsule that releases the drug at the rate of 1 μg/hr for up to 9 months.[12] It is surgically implanted through a pars plana incision and sutured through a transscleral suture.

Systemic treatment is preferred for cases with simultaneous involvement of other organs, or cases with bilateral CMV retinitis, and includes ganciclovir, foscarnet and cidofovir. Systemic therapy in induction phase includes intravenous ganciclovir (5 mg/kg every 12 hours for 14–21 days), or oral valganciclovir (450 mg tablets every 12 hours for 21 days). The latter is equally effective as intravenous ganciclovir.[13,14] The maintenance therapy can be suspended in post-HAART era if the immunological status of the patient improves with a CD4+ count more than 100 cells/mm³ and an undetectable viral load.[15-18] A CD4+ less than 50 cells/mm³ increases the risk of relapse of CMV retinitis. Resistance or intolerance to ganciclovir is an indication for intravenous foscarnet, which is equally effective.[19] Cidofovir is associated with significant side effects (local and systemic).[20]

The treatment strategy of CMV retinitis is individualized for every patient. Introduction of HAART is now being associated with "immune recovery uveitis", a phenomenon representing an exaggerated inflammatory response against the CMV antigens in the retina due to an improvement in the immunological status of the patient. It is manifested as anterior uveitis, vitritis and CME and requires treatment with corticosteroids.[21-23]

ACUTE RETINAL NECROSIS

Acute retinal necrosis (ARN) is classically caused by herpes simplex virus (HSV) or herpes zoster virus (HZV), and may occasionally be caused by CMV or Epstein-Barr virus.[24-30] It was first described in 1971 by Urayama,[31] and later redefined in 1994 by the American Uveitis Society based on clinical features and course of the disease.[32] It manifests as widespread area(s) of confluent or multifocal, full thickness necrotizing retinitis in peripheral retina, circumferential spread of the lesions with rapid progression in the absence of antiviral therapy, occlusive vasculopathy with arterial involvement, and significant vitritis (Figs. 40.3 to 40.5). Anterior uveitis is often present with granulomatous or nongranulomatous inflammation, patches of iris atrophy and secondary glaucoma. There is no racial or sex predilection. It usually occurs unilaterally in immunocompetent individuals, although reports of its occurrence in immunocompromised patients are available. Patients with severe immune dysfunction develop progressive outer retinal necrosis (PORN), the other form of herpetic retinopathy. Vitreous inflammation is minimal in PORN despite severe retinal necrosis, with a tendency to affect the posterior pole. Presence of retinal hemorrhages also distinguishes it from PORN. As compared to ARN, it is often bilateral and less commonly associated with retinal vasculitis and optic neuropathy.[33]

Majority of cases of ARN and PORN are caused by VZV, followed by HSV-1 (in older patients) and HSV-2 (in younger patients).[28,34] Diagnosis is aided by polymerase chain reaction (PCR) of intraocular fluid, which has a high sensitivity and specificity (greater than 95%) for viruses.[35,36] A quick anterior chamber tap offers sufficient volume of aqueous for testing of viral and toxoplasmic DNA. Other diagnostic techniques include antibody detection from serum or ocular fluid.[37-39] Other causes of necrotizing retinitis such as toxoplasmosis, syphilis, PVRL, Behcet's disease, tuberculosis, sarcoidosis, fungal endophthalmitis need to be ruled out by clinical and laboratory clues.

In the absence of timely treatment of ARN, the fellow eye gets involved in about one-third of cases within 6 weeks

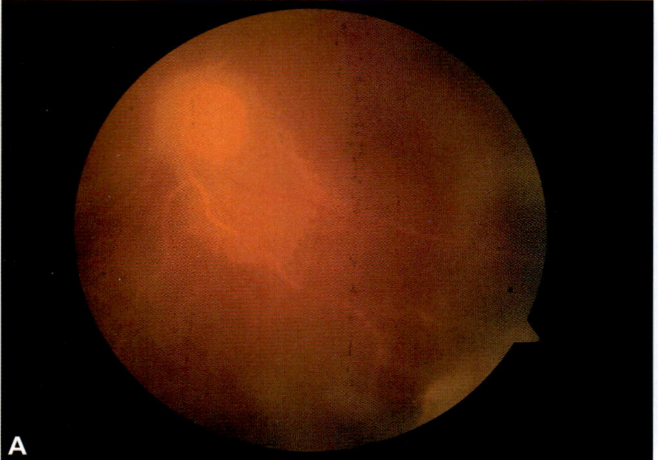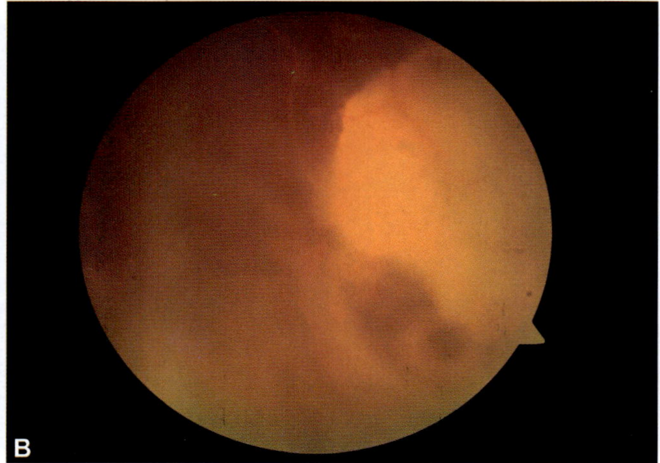

Figs. 40.3A and B: Severe vitritis and tongue-shaped lesions of necrotizing retinitis in peripheral fundus in a patient with acute retinal necrosis (ARN).

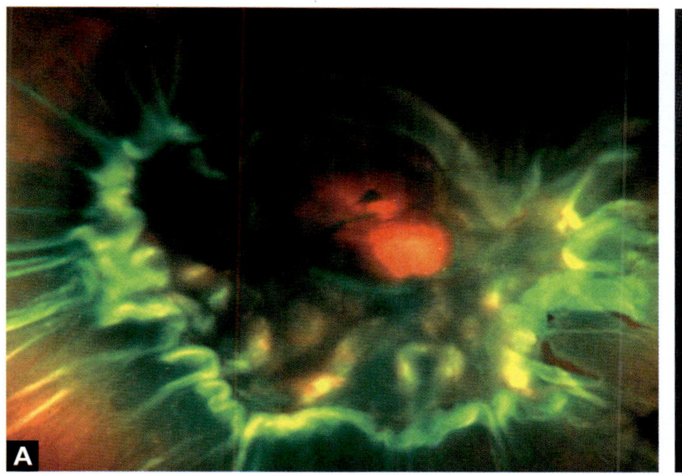

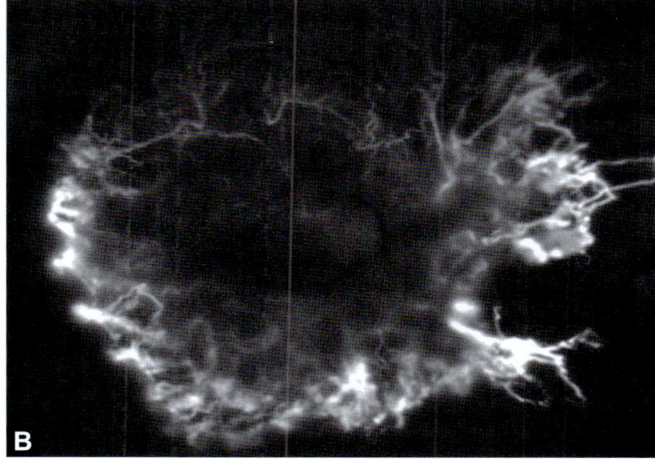

Figs. 40.4A and B: (A) Color fundus picture showing total RRD with necrotic peripheral retna. (B) Occlusive arteritis on FFA in a patient of ARN.

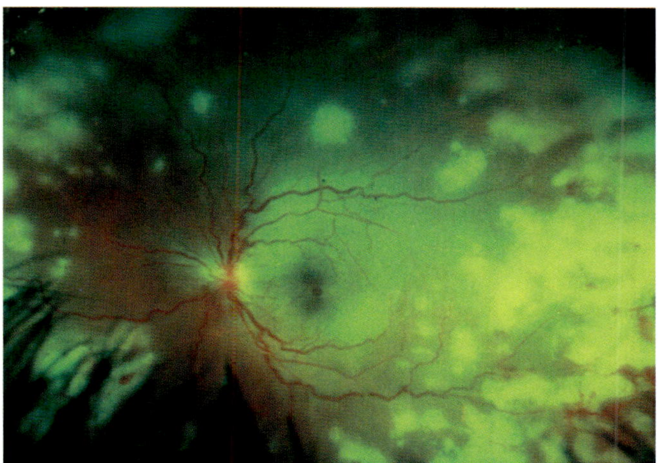

Fig. 40.5: Widefield pseudo-color image of a patient with ARN.

of initial presentation. This has decreased dramatically from 75.3% to 35.1% within 2 years of initial onset,[40] and 13.6% within a mean of 4 years follow up.[41] A further lower rate of fellow eye involvement has been reported as 3.4% within a median of 2 years follow up.[42] The mainstay of medical therapy includes intravenous acyclovir during induction phase (10 mg/kg/day in three divided doses) for 2–3 weeks with inpatient hospitalization and close renal function monitoring, followed by oral acyclovir 800 mg five times/day for 3–4 months.[43,44] As compared to oral acyclovir, newer drugs valaciclovir and famciclovir have greater bioavailability and hence, can achieve systemic levels nearly equal to intravenous acyclovir. Valaciclovir can be given in induction phase at 2 g three times a day. Oral corticosteroids are started about 48 hours after initiating antiviral therapy and tapered according to the clinical response. Some clinicians are using intravitreal injections of foscarnet (1.2–2.4 mg/0.1 mL) and gancicolvir (200–2,000 μg/0.1 mL) as an adjunct to systemic antiviral therapy.[45,46] Due to rare occurrence of ARN, there is lack of randomized clinical trials and no single treatment strategy has been proposed as a standard of care for ARN. With a wide range of antiviral agents currently becoming available, physicians are resorting to single agent therapy or varying combinations of intravenous, oral and intravitreal drugs for initial and long-term treatment of ARN.[42] The outcomes have not been affected by different treatment strategies, but retinal detachment is a common complication of ARN and the visual prognosis generally remains poor.

SYPHILITIC CHORIORETINITIS

Posterior segment involvement in syphilis includes a wide variety of chorioretinal inflammations, manifesting as acute posterior placoid chorioretinitis, multifocal chorioretinitis, retinal vasculitis, intermediate uveitis and panuveitis.[47-49] Acute syphilitic posterior placoid chorioretinopathy (ASPPC), originally described by Gass, is characterized by large, placoid, solitary, subretinal lesions that are pale-yellowish in color.[50-51] They occur during secondary syphilis and result from macular and peripapillary RPE involvement. Differential diagnosis includes APMPPE, serpiginous choroiditis, PVRL, toxoplasmic chorioretinitis and herpetic retinitis. The large size of the lesion and its solitary nature differentiates ASPPC from APMPPE. Patients are often immunocompromised, vitritis is present and the lesions fade centrally.[52] Hyperpigmentation of the RPE in the cicatricial phase produces the characteristic leopard-spot pattern on FA. Multifocal chorioretinitis is associated with significant vitritis, multiple deep, yellowish-gray lesions which may coalesce. Syphilitic retinitis can be difficult to distinguish from necrotizing herpetic retinitis, particularly ARN. It begins as a patchy retinitis, with significant vitritis, vasculitis and panuveitis, very similar to ARN. However, certain characteristics of the syphilitic lesions provide important differentiating clues. Syphilitic lesions arise in the posterior pole, unlike peripheral lesions of ARN. The syphilitic retinitis lesion has an indistinct surface mimicking an exudate, making it difficult to view the underlying retina, while the ARN lesions have a thick surface of the necrotic retina. Serous retinal detachment can sometimes accompany syphilitic retinitis.[53] The mottled appearance of syphilitic lesions becomes more prominent as the lesions heal, while the ARN lesion of retinal necrosis appears homogenous. It may also manifest as neuroretinitis with vasculitis, vitritis, papillitis or optic neuritis.[54,55] The syphilitic lesions respond dramatically to intravenous penicillin. Involvement of the RPE leads to significant scarring as the lesions heal, presenting as pseudo-retinitis pigmentosa. In HIV infected patients with syphilis, ocular involvement is more severe, often bilateral and tends to have a high relapse rate.[52,56] Diagnosis in these patients is challenging due to high false-positive and false-negative rates of serological tests at different levels of immune status.[57,58] A high rate of neurosyphilis is reported in patients with syphilitic uveitis coinfected with HIV.[54,59,60]

Serological testing for syphilis is routinely ordered by most of the clinicians in all kinds of intraocular inflammations, as syphilis is a great masquerade. A combination of nontreponemal [Venereal Disease Research Laboratory (VDRL) and rapid plasma regain, (RPR)] and treponemal [fluorescent treponemal antibody absorption test (FTA-abs) and *Treponema pallidum* hemagglutination (TPHA)] tests is preferred for serologic diagnosis. Following treatment, nontreponemal tests reveal decreasing antibody titers and are used for disease monitoring. Treponemal tests stay positive for lifetime.

Although the CDC recommends lumbar puncture in these patients, neurosyphilis should be suspected in all patients with ocular syphilis.[61] Prompt antibiotic therapy is indicated to stop progression of uveitis in both eyes, prevent visual loss and prevent occurrence of symptomatic neurosyphilis. Acute uveitis is treated (after a negative skin test) with intravenous aqueous crystalline penicillin G 2-4 MU every 4hr or 12–24 MU/day for 10–14 days. For late stage ocular syphilis (tertiary stage), this is supplemented with intramuscular benzathine penicillin G 2.4 MU every week for 3 weeks.

ENDOGENOUS ENDOPHTHALMITIS

Endophthalmitis is an ocular emergency with devastating visual prognosis and multifactorial etiology.[62] "Endogenous endophthalmitis (EE)" or "metastatic endophthalmitis" occurs due to hematogenous spread of the infective organisms that cross the blood retinal barrier to enter the eye from a focus elsewhere in the body.[63,64] It involves infection of the inner coats of the eyeball with progressive vitreous involvement. Much less common than exogenous endophthalmitis, EE constitutes about 2–8% of all endophthalmitis.[65,66] Predisposing factors include certain underlying medical ailments like diabetes mellitus, intravenous drug use, cardiac or liver

disease, indwelling catheters, immune deficiency such as AIDS/organ transplantation/malignancy, post-surgery and recent hospitalization with use of intravenous injections.[67,68] There is no sex or age predilection. While majority of cases have an identifiable organism, few remain unrecognized from ocular/blood/urine cultures. Varying culture positivity rates have been reported from different series.[69-71] The etiology can be bacterial or fungal. Bacterial EE is now on the decline due to a rapid progress in diagnostic and therapeutic modalities including newer antibiotics. However, fungal EE is being increasingly reported due to long survival of terminally ill patients. Nearly 35–65% of all EE are fungal in origin.[69,72-74] While majority of fungal EE occur in immunocompromised individuals, it has also been reported following intravenous infusions of contaminated dextrose solutions in healthy subjects.[68]

The causative fungi include *Candida* and *Aspergillus*, and occasionally *Fusarium, Blastomyces, Histoplasma, Coccidioidomycosis, Cryptococcus* and *Mucormycosis*. About 50–60% of fungal EE are reported to be due to *Candida*, and 24% by *Aspergillus*.[73] The onset is insidious, and commonly presents an initial diagnostic error. While lesions in Candida EE usually begin in retinal periphery and progress slowly to cause an extensive disease, *Aspergillus* EE tends to affect the macula and worsens rapidly.[69,72-74]

Candida EE typically involves the vitreous cavity as the preferred site for its growth. Fluff balls in the vitreous provide a strong clue, which may or may not be associated with focal/multifocal chorioretinitis lesions.[75,76] The spread of the inflammation to the anterior chamber is more severe and rapid in intravenous drug abusers. Aspergillus EE begins as a large abscess, arising from the sub-RPE space, typically in the macular area. It shows a fulminant spread, breaking into the vitreous cavity, and spreading into the anterior segment.[77-79] Hypopyon may be present in few cases (Figs. 40.6A and B). Other causes of fungal EE are rare.[80-83]

The etiology of bacterial EE shows a geographical variation, with gram-positive dominating the developed world and gram-negative affecting the Asian population.[72] Unlike fungal EE, the anterior segment manifestations are more common and severe in bacterial EE with pain, diminished vision, photophobia, lid edema, conjunctival/circumcorneal congestion, hypopyon, corneal edema, loss of red fundus glow, and dense vitreous haze.[84-87] Fundus involvement is severe in the form of subretinal or choroidal abscess. Worse prognosis is associated with certain organisms like *Klebsiella* (requiring enucleation) and Methicillin-resistant *Staphylococcus aureus* (high rates of retinal detachment).[88-90]

A high index of suspicion is required for timely diagnosis of EE. In the setting of poor fundus view, ultrasonography provides important clues in terms of the degree of vitreous exudates, retinal detachment or choroidal abscess. A combined diagnostic/therapeutic vitrectomy is indicated for microbiological analysis of vitreous specimen for fungal/bacterial smears and cultures. Blood and urine cultures are done for

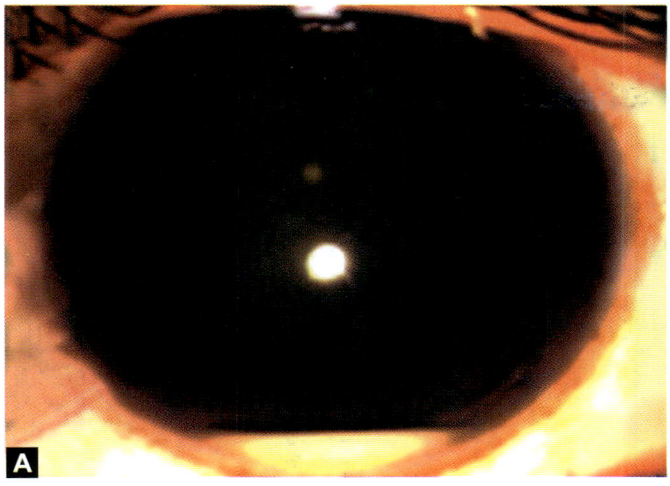
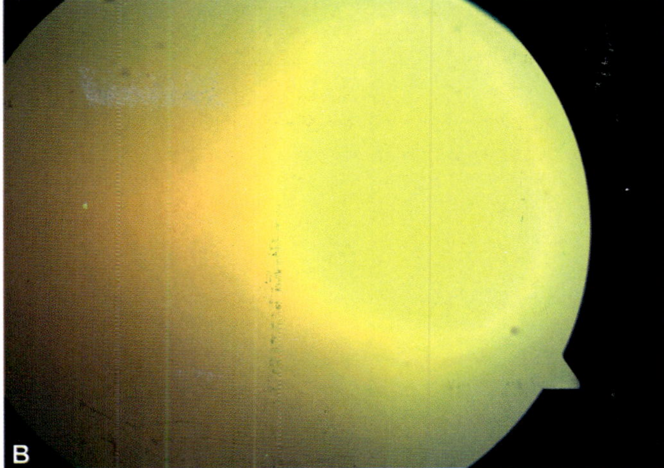

Figs. 40.6A and B: (A) A case of endogenous fungal endophthalmitis presenting with hypopyon dense vitreous exudates precluding retinal evaluation. (B) Following vitrectomy, a large macular scar was revealed.

3 consecutive days although they have a low sensitivity.[91,92] For early results, PCR allows a rapid identification of the organisms.[93] Systemic therapy with oral fluconazole for *Candida* and itraconazole for *Aspergillus* are effective.[91,92] Intravitreal Amphotericin-B (5–10 μg) is used as an adjunct. Newer drug voriconazole is effective as an oral, intravenous or intravitreal treatment. The role of corticosteroids is controversial in EE.[94] Systemic antibiotics for underlying bacteremia are administered soon after drawing the blood cultures. Additionally, intravitreal antibiotic injections and vitrectomy should be promptly performed as an ophthalmic emergency. First-line empirical intravitreal treatment targeting both gram-positive and gram-negative organisms comprises of vancomycin (1 mg/0.1 mL) plus ceftazidime (2.25 mg/0.1 mL).

LYME DISEASE

Ocular involvement in Lyme disease (caused by spirochete *Borrelia Burgdorferi*) is rare, and usually occurs during late phases of the disease. It can range from transient conjunctivitis, episcleritis, keratitis, uveitis, posterior scleritis, orbital myositis, optic neuritis, papilledema, and neuroretinitis.[95-98]

Uveitis can present in a manner similar to syphilis, and includes anterior uveitis, intermediate uveitis, panuveitis with choroiditis, retinal vasculitis, or peripheral multifocal choroiditis.[96,99-102] Vascular occlusion may be associated with retinal vasculitis.[99] Diagnosis is based on medical history of systemic symptoms, living in endemic area, and clinical (ocular and systemic) manifestations. As serological tests lack sensitivity and specificity, other uveitic etiologies should be ruled out. Biopsy from erythema migrans or synovial fluid may help by doing PCR. Treatment involves a combination of beta-lactam plus tetracycline antibiotics and corticosteroids. Doxycycline is the most common antibiotic used for 1–2 months.

TOXOPLASMA RETINOCHOROIDITIS

Uveitis due to toxoplasmosis typically involves the posterior segment. Retinochoroiditis is the most common presentation, causing necrotizing retinitis.[103-106] Children and young adults are mostly affected. Congenital toxoplasmosis is classically bilateral, characterized by a macular scar and absence of vitreous inflammation.[103,104] Primary acquired toxoplasmosis is seen as active retinitis without any previous scar (Figs. 40.7A and B). Recurrent disease is characterized by an active lesion known as satellite lesion, occurring adjacent to an old, pigmented previous scar. The active lesions appear as focal retinitis with blurred margins.[105-108] Vitreous inflammation may be severe enough precluding retinal details, causing "headlight in the fog" appearance (Figs. 40.8A and B). The retinitis lesion can vary in size and may affect the posterior pole or retinal periphery. Healing of the lesion starts at the margins and it resolves from periphery to the center. Pigmentation of the scar occurs with passage of time. While an immunocompetent individual usually develops focal retinitis that is self-limiting, the disease is multifocal, bilateral and progressive in immunocompromised hosts.[109-110]

The other atypical manifestations include neuroretinitis, papillitis, punctate outer retinal toxoplasmosis, multifocal necrotizing retinitis (Figs. 40.9A and B), scleritis or anterior uveitis.[111] An increased vascular response may be seen along the blood vessels in proximity of the lesion or far from it in the form of vascular sheathing. Multiple small deposits of inflammatory debris may be seen on the surface of the arteries known as Kyrieleis plaques, which are highly suggestive of toxoplasmosis. Anterior uveitis may be granulomatous or nongranulomatous. The scar may be complicated by a CNVM, which worsens the visual prognosis further.[112]

Diagnosis is often clinical. Aqueous or vitreous sample may be subjected to PCR or local antibody titers for

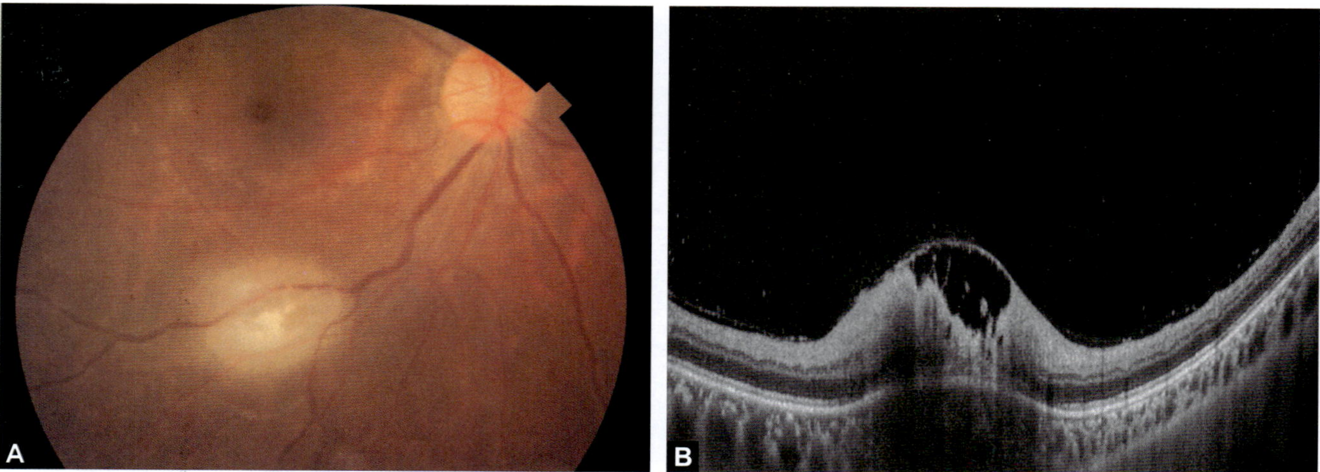

Figs. 40.7A and B: (A) Primary acquired toxoplasmosis with an active retinochoroiditis lesion that is solitary in the absence of any old scar. (B) Swept Source OCT through the lesion.

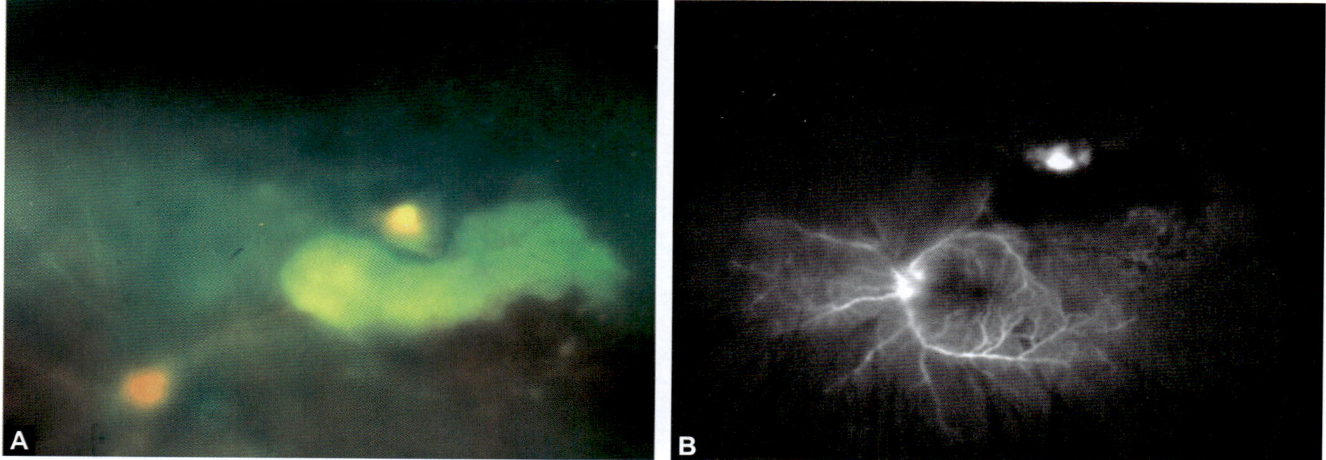

Figs. 40.8A and B: Extramacular toxoplasmosis. (A and B) Clinical picture and FFA picture with typical "Headlight in fog" appearance due to vitritis.

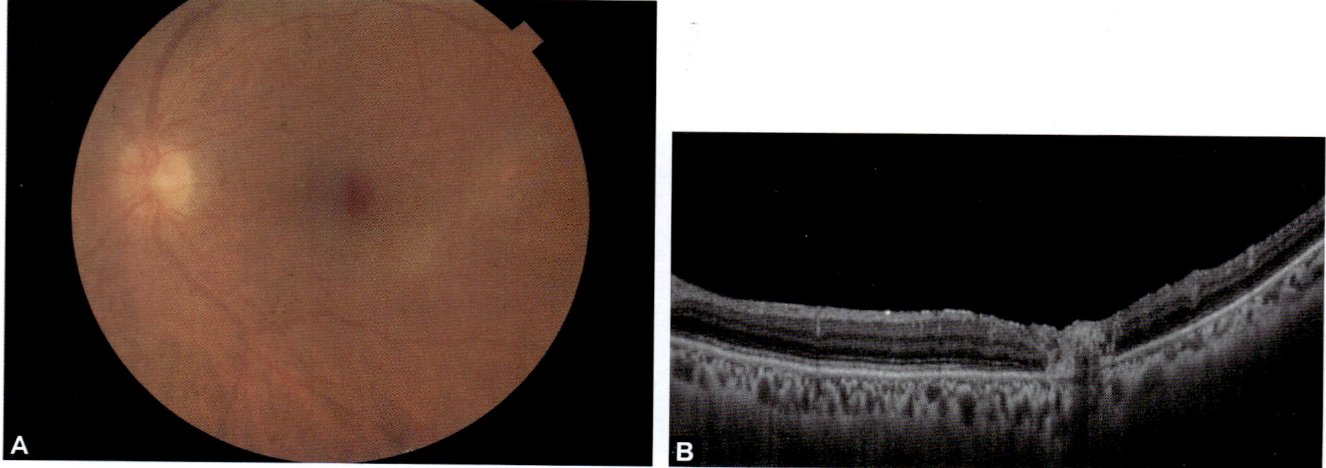

Figs. 40.9A and B: A typical toxoplasmosis lesion with corresponding OCT in a HIV patient.

strengthening the diagnosis.[113-114] Cytological examination of intraocular fluid may reveal tachyzoites or bradyzoites.[115] Serological tests also aid in the diagnosis. The treatment aims at elimination of the parasite and control of intraocular inflammation. A combination of pyrimethamine and sulfadiazine is the most commonly used regimen (classic therapy) along with oral corticosteroids.[116-118] To minimize drug toxicity and allergic reactions, alternative regimens consist of trimethoprim and sulfamethoxazole with corticosteroids, or classic therapy with clindamycin (quadruple therapy). Intravitreal clindamycin with dexamethasone injections offer a good adjunctive therapy, minimizing side effects of systemic medications.[119-120] Spiramycin, azithromycin, clarithromycin and atovaquone are other drugs used as monotherapy or combination therapy.[121-123]

TOXOCARA CHORIORETINITIS

One of the parasitic diseases of the humans, toxocariasis is caused by infection by the eggs of larvae of *Toxocara canis* (dog or fox roundworm) or *Toxocara cati* (cat roundworm).[124] The usual presentation is in children with proximity to pets, or those eating contaminated soil or uncooked food.[125] While majority are asymptomatic infections, toxocariasis has three clinical forms: visceral larva migrans (VLM), ocular larva migrans (OLM) and covert toxocariasis.[126] Young children may develop VLM manifesting as fever, cough, malaise, lymphadenopathy etc. Symptoms of OLM include unilateral visual loss, leukocoria or strabismus. The posterior segment is typically involved with significant vitritis.[127] Three clinical forms of OLM exist: peripheral granuloma, posterior pole granuloma and endophthalmitis. A granuloma involving the periphery or posterior pole is a distinctive feature. Tractional retinal detachment often complicates visual prognosis. The diagnosis is largely clinical. Granuloma represents the retinal site of larval migration. It appears as a dense, yellowish-white mass within the retina along with severe vitritis and a radial fold of retina extending from the granuloma to the optic disc, which is highly characteristic (Fig. 40.10). Retinal vasculitis, optic neuritis and neuroretinitis may rarely occur.[128] Complications like tractional retinal detachment, epiretinal membrane and CNVM worsen the visual prognosis.[129] Vitrectomy is indicated in cases with severe inflammation for anatomical and functional restoration.[130] The role of antihelminthic drugs is controversial.[131,132]

TUBERCULOSIS

Intraocular tuberculosis (IOTB) has protean manifestations and affects any layer of the eye. Posterior segment involvement is the commonest.[133] Multifocal serpiginoid choroiditis is well-documented from endemic as well as nonendemic areas.[134-138] It usually affects young to middle-aged healthy males, with an immunological evidence of latent TB. The

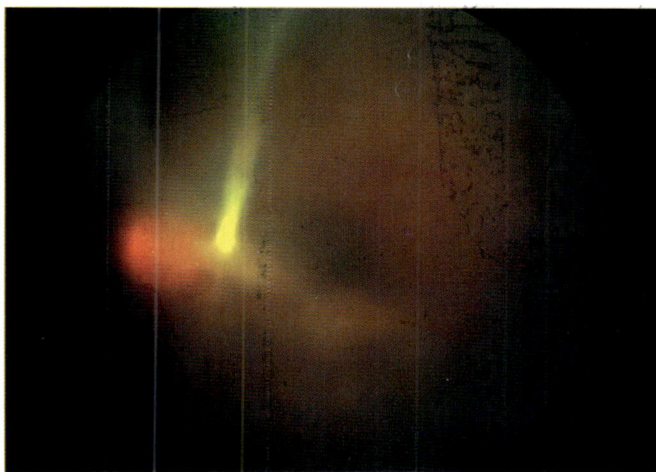

Fig. 40.10: Dense vitritis with a radial retinal fold extending from the optic disc to retinal periphery suggestive of toxocariasis.

disease is often bilateral and associated with vitritis. It typically begins as multifocal, creamish-yellow lesions with indistinct borders in posterior pole and/or periphery and non-contiguous to the optic disc. As the disease progresses, they become confluent. Fluorescein angiography has a typical pattern of an early hypofluorescence and a late hyperfluorescence (Fig. 40.11). On ICGA, the lesions remain hypofluorescent in all phases. Fundus autofluorescence (FAF) is very characteristic, showing four stages as the disease evolves from acute to healed stage.[139] Macula is frequently involved but the fovea escapes the final insult, retaining good final visual acuity although with visual field defect. It responds favorably to antitubercular therapy (ATT) with oral corticosteroids. Its differentiation from the autoimmune classic serpiginous choroiditis is clinical which in contrast, has large solitary lesion, contiguous to the optic disc.[140-145] Vitritis is usually absent and the lesions show relentless progression despite maximum immunosuppressive therapy. Final visual acuity is generally poor because of extensive macular involvement.

Retinal vasculitis is a common presentation of tubercular uveitis and occurs in the absence of concurrent systemic TB. It is usually an occlusive vasculitis which is best demonstrated on FA as ischemic areas of capillary nonperfusion. New vessels may be seen on the optic disc or retina.[146,147] Young and healthy males are more commonly affected. Patients in late stages present with vitreous hemorrhage or tractional retinal detachment. While considering differential diagnosis, a perivascular choroiditis/scar if present, is strongly suggestive of TB vasculitis.[147] Typically, vasculitis is occlusive which is seen on FA as areas of capillary nonperfusion with or without neovascularization in the fundus. Diagnosis is clinical with corroborative evidence of systemic TB in the form of a positive tuberculin skin test (TST), interferon gamma release assays (IGRA), X-ray chest/CT chest. Evidence of *Mycobacterium tuberculosis* DNA by PCR of vitreous/aqueous humor

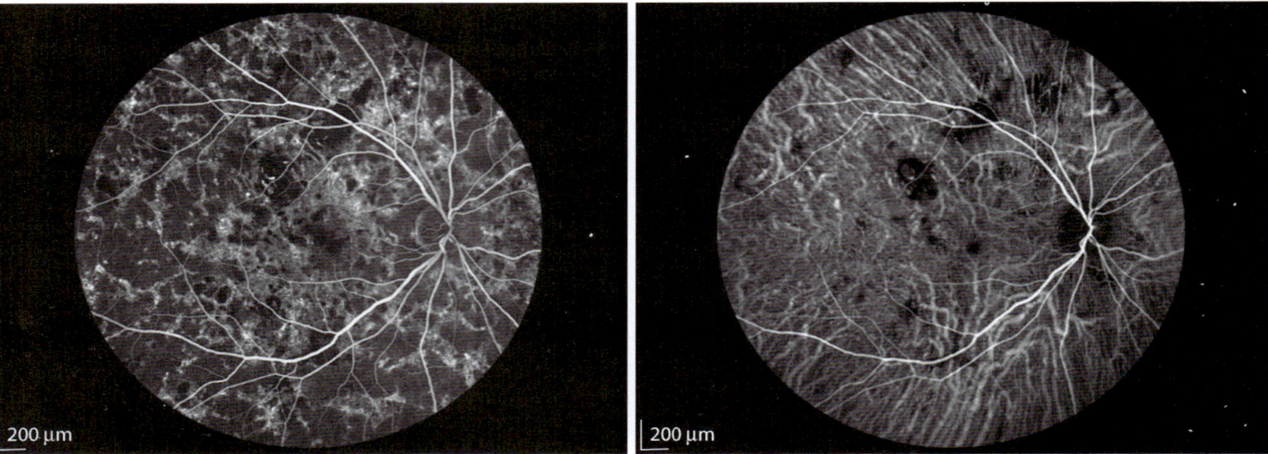

Fig. 40.11: Serpiginous-like choroidopathy. FFA and ICG pictures showing active serpiginoid like lesions with healed ones in the right eye of a tuberculosis patient.

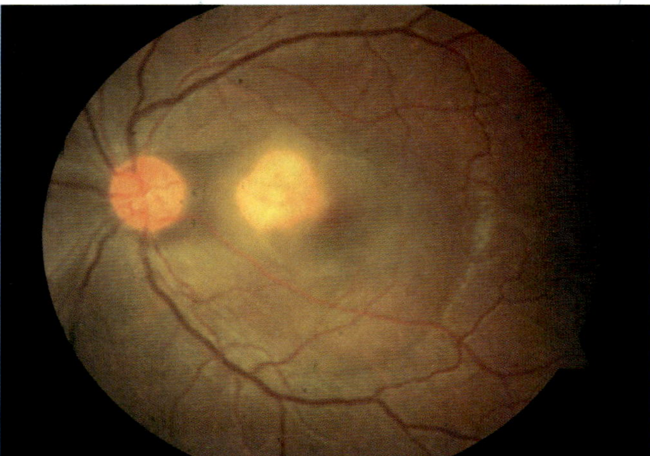

Fig. 40.12: A solitary choroidal granuloma with surrounding exudative retinal detachment in a patient with intraocular tuberculosis.

confirms the diagnosis.[146] Treatment with oral steroids (1 mg/kg/day) and ATT is highly effective.[148] Ischemic retina requires scatter laser photocoagulation. Vitrectomy is indicated for complications such as vitreous hemorrhage, subhyaloid hemorrhage or tractional/combined retinal detachment.

Choroidal tubercles are one of the earliest reported signs in IOTB.[149] About one-third of them may be associated with a negative TST and an immunocompromised state, they may occur as an isolated ocular disease in an otherwise healthy individual.[150] These are located deep in the choroid, may be unilateral/bilateral and manifest as yellowish discrete lesions with ill-defined borders. These are usually solitary but may be few in number. The posterior pole is commonly involved (Fig. 40.12).[150,151] The lesions are typically subretinal usually affecting the posterior pole, 1–5 in number, may be 1–8 disc diameter in size and are raised from the retinal surface.

Subretinal exudation usually surrounds the active lesion. Retinal vasculitis may coexist with tubercles. They demonstrate an early hypofluorescence and late hyperfluorescence on FA. In immunosuppressed individuals, they may not show any signs of inflammation and hence, be asymptomatic. HIV must be ruled out in such patients. They respond favorably to ATT and corticosteroids and heal with a dense scar formation (Figs. 40.13A and B). Occasionally, the granuloma may become vascularized which responds favorably to intravitreal bevacizumab, in addition to ATT and corticosteroids.[152]

If not treated on time, a choroidal tubercle may progress into a large tuberculoma which mimics a subretinal abscess. These are caused due to a rapid multiplication of the bacilli and progressive liquefied caseation necrosis. A subretinal abscess may burst into the vitreous cavity leading to severe intraocular inflammation.[151] Tubercular choroidal granuloma suggest a hematogenous spread and may represent an infective mechanism.[149-151]

REFERENCES

1. Goldberg DE, Smithen LM, Angelilli A, et al. HIV-associated retinopathy in the HAART era. Retina. 2005;25(5):633-49.
2. Kedhar SR, Jabs DA. Cytomegalovirus retinitis in the era of highly active antiretroviral therapy. Herpes. 2007;14(3):66-71.
3. Holland GN, Vaudaux JD, Shiramizu KM, et al. Southern California HIV/Eye Consortium. Characteristics of untreated AIDS-related cytomegalovirus retinitis. II. Findings in the era of highly active antiretroviral therapy (1997 to 2000). Am J Ophthalmology. 2008;145(1):12-22.
4. Lin DY, Warren JF, Lazzeroni LC, et al. Cytomegalovirus retinitis after initiation of highly active antiretroviral therapy in HIV infected patients: natural history and clinical predictors. Retina. 2002;22(3):268-77.
5. Kuppermann BD, Petty JG, Richman DD, et al. Correlation between CD4+ counts and prevalence of cytomegalovirus retinitis and human immunodeficiency virus-related noninfectious retinal vasculopathy in patients with acquired immunodeficiency syndrome. Am J Ophthalmology. 1993;115(5):575-82.

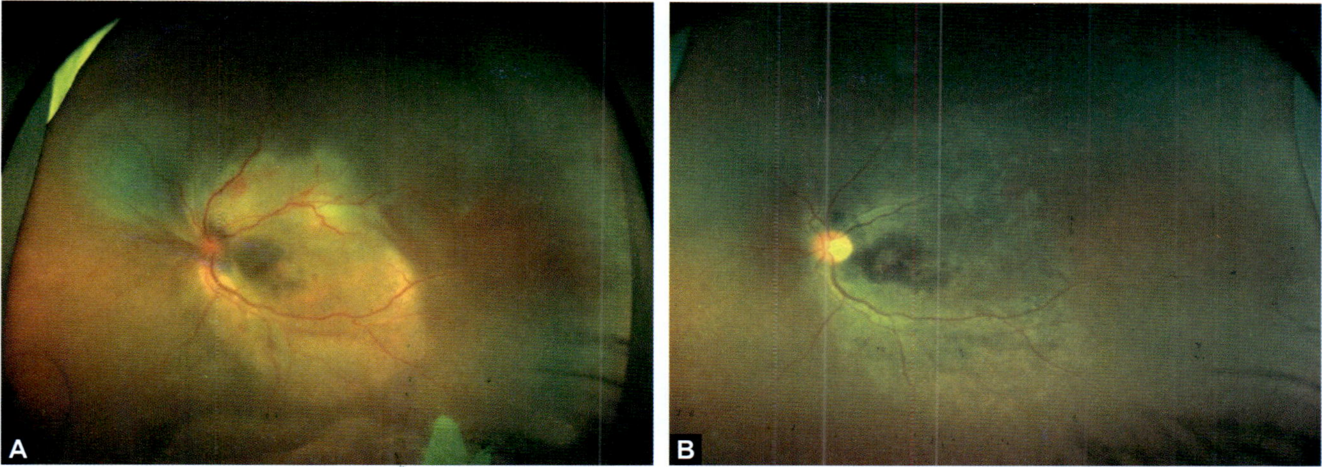

Figs. 40.13A and B: (A) Patient with active tuberculous choroiditis with exudative retinal detachment. (B) Follow-up pseudocolor photograph of the same patient on AKT showing scarring and healing response.

6. Henry K, Cantrill H, Fletcher C, et al. Use of intravitreal ganciclovir (dihydroxypropoxymethyl guanine) for cytomegalovirus retinitis in a patient with AIDS. Am J Ophthalmology. 1987;103(1):17-23.

7. Cochereau-Massin I, Lehoang P, Lautier-Frau M, et al. Efficacy and tolerance of intravitreal ganciclovir in cytomegalovirus retinitis in acquired immune deficiency syndrome. Ophthalmology. 1991;98(9):1348-53.

8. Diaz-Llopis M, Chipont E, Sanchez S, et al. Intravitreal foscarnet for cytomegalovirus retinitis in a patient with acquired immunodeficiency syndrome. Am J Ophthalmology. 1992;114(6):742-7.

9. Lieberman RM, Orellana J, Melton RC. Efficacy of intravitreous foscarnet in a patient with AIDS. N Engl J Med. 1994;330(12):868-9.

10. Rahhal FM, Arevalo JF, Munguia D, et al. Intravitreal cidofovir for the maintenance treatment of cytomegalovirus retinitis. Ophthalmology. 1996;103(7):1078-83.

11. Kupperman B, Wolitz R, Stagg R, et al. A Phase II randomized, double-masked study of intraocular cidofovir for relapsing cytomegalovirus retinitis in patients with AIDS. Presented at the Vitreous Society Annual Meeting; Cancun, Mexico, December 8-12, 1996.

12. Musch DC, Martin DF, Gordon JF, et al. Treatment of cytomegalovirus retinitis with a sustained-release ganciclovir implant. The Ganciclovir Implant Study Group. N Engl J Med. 1997;337(2):83-90.

13. Holland GN, Buhles WC Jr, Mastre B, Kaplan HJ. A controlled retrospective study of ganciclovir treatment for cytomegalovirus retinopathy. Use of a standardized system for the assessment of disease outcome. UCLA CMV Retinopathy. Study Group. Arch Ophthalmology. 1989;107(12):1759-66.

14. Martin DF, Sierra-Madero J, Walmsley S, et al. Valganciclovir Study Group. A controlled trial of valganciclovir as induction therapy for cytomegalovirus retinitis. N Engl J Med. 2002;346(15):1119-26.

15. Whitcup SM, Fortin E, Nussenblatt RB, et al. Therapeutic effect of combination antiretroviral therapy on cytomegalovirus retinitis. JAMA. 1997;277(19):1519-20.

16. Vrabec TR, Baldassano VF, Whitcup SM. Discontinuation of maintenance therapy in patients with quiescent cytomegalovirus retinitis and elevated CD4+ counts. Ophthalmology. 1998;105(7):1259-64.

17. Curi AL, Muralha A, Muralha L, et al. Suspension of anti-CMV maintenance therapy following immune recovery due to highly active antiretroviral therapy. Br J Ophthalmology. 2001;85(4):471-3.

18. MacDonald JC, Torriani FJ, Morse LS, et al. Lack of reactivation of cytomegalovirus (CMV) retinitis after stopping CMV maintenance therapy in AIDS patients with sustained elevations in CD4 T cells in response to highly active antiretroviral therapy. J Infect Dis. 1998;177(5):1182-7.

19. Jacobson MA, O'Donnell JJ, Mills J. Foscarnet treatment of cytomegalovirus retinitis in patients with the acquired immunodeficiency syndrome. Antimicrob Agents Chemother. 1989;33(5):736-41.

20. Lalezari JP, Stagg RJ, Kuppermann BD, et al. Intravenous cidofovir for peripheral cytomegalovirus retinitis in patients with AIDS. A randomized, controlled trial. Ann Intern Med. 1997;126(4):257-63.

21. Murdoch DM, Venter WD, Van Rie A, et al. Immune reconstitution inflammatory syndrome (IRIS): review of common infectious manifestations and treatment options. AIDS Res Ther. 2007;4:9.

22. Kempen JH, Min YI, Freeman WR, et al. Risk of immune recovery uveitis in patients with AIDS and cytomegalovirus retinitis. Ophthalmology. 2006;113(4):684-94.

23. Kenneth H, Hirsch HH, Kaufmann G, et al. Immune reconstitution in HIV infected patients. Clin Infect Dis. 2004;38(8):1159-66.

24. Guex-Crosier Y, Rochat C, Herbort CP. Necrotizing herpetic retinopathies. A spectrum of herpes virus-induced diseases determined by the immune state of the host. Ocul Immunol Inflamm. 1997;5(4):259-65.

25. Lau CH, Missotten T, Salzmann J, et al. Acute retinal necrosis features, management, and outcomes. Ophthalmology. 2007;114(4):756-62.

26. Fisher JP, Lewis ML, Blumenkranz M, et al. The acute retinal necrosis syndrome. Part 1: Clinical manifestations. Ophthalmology. 1982;89(12):1309-16.

27. Muthiah MN, Michaelides M, Child CS, et al. Acute retinal necrosis: a national population-based study to assess the incidence, methods of diagnosis, treatment strategies and outcomes in the UK. Br J Ophthalmology. 2007;91(11):1452-55.

28. Ganatra JB, Chandler D, Santos C, et al. Viral causes of the acute retinal necrosis syndrome. Am J Ophthalmology. 2000;129(2):166-72.

29. Tran TH, Rozenberg F, Cassoux N, et al. Polymerase chain reaction analysis of aqueous humour samples in necrotising retinitis. Br J Ophthalmology. 2003;87(1):79-83.

30. Tran TH, Stanescu D, Caspers-Velu L, et al. Clinical characteristics of acute HSV-2 retinal necrosis. Am J Ophthalmology. 2004;135(5):872-9.

31. Urayama A YN, Sasaki T, Nishiyama Y, et al. Unilateral acute uveitis with periarteritis and detachment. Japan J Ophthalmology. 1971;25:607-19.

32. Holland GN. Standard diagnostic criteria for the acute retinal necrosis syndrome. Executive Committee of the American Uveitis Society. Am J Ophthalmology. 1994;117(5):663-7.

33. Margolis T, Irvine AR, Hoyt WF, et al. Acute retinal necrosis syndrome presenting with papillitis and arcuate neuroretinitis. Ophthalmology. 1988;95(7):935-40.

34. Wong RW, Jumper JM, McDonald HR, et al. Emerging concepts in the management of acute retinal necrosis. Br J Ophthalmology. 2013;97(5):545-52.

35. Cunningham ET Jr, Short GA, Irvine AR, et al. Acquired immunodeficiency syndrome-associated herpes simplex virus retinitis. Clinical description and use of a polymerase chain reaction-based assay as a diagnostic tool. Arch Ophthalmology. 1996;114(7):834-40.

36. Knox CM, Chandler D, Short GA, et al. Polymerase chain reaction-based assays of vitreous samples for the diagnosis of viral retinitis. Use in diagnostic dilemmas. Ophthalmology. 1998;105(1):35-44.

37. Abe T, Tsuchida K, Tamai M. A comparative study of the polymerase chain reaction and local antibody production in acute retinal necrosis syndrome and cytomegalovirus retinitis. Graefes Arch Clin Exp Ophthalmology. 1996;234(7):419-24.

38. de Boer JH, Luyendijk L, Rothova A, et al. Detection of intraocular antibody production to herpes viruses in acute retinal necrosis syndrome. Am J Ophthalmology. 1994;117(2):201-10.

39. de Boer JH, Verhagen C, Bruinenberg M, et al. Serologic and polymerase chain reaction analysis of intraocular fluids in the diagnosis of infectious uveitis. Am J Ophthalmology. 1996;121(6):650-8.

40. Palay DA, Sternberg P Jr, Davis J, et al. Decrease in the risk of bilateral acute retinal necrosis by acyclovir therapy. Am J Ophthalmology. 1991;112(3):250-5.

41. Blumenkranz MS, Culbertson WW, Clarkson JG, et al. Treatment of the acute retinal necrosis syndrome with intravenous acyclovir. Ophthalmology. 1986;93(3):296-300.

42. Kim SJ, Lo WR. Acute retinal necrosis. Ophthalmology. 2008;115(6):1104-6.

43. Tibbetts MD, Shah CP, Young LH, et al. Treatment of acute retinal necrosis. Ophthalmology. 2010;117(4):818-24.

44. Duker JS, Blumenkranz MS. Diagnosis and management of the acute retinal necrosis (ARN) syndrome. Surv Ophthalmology. 1991;35(5):327-43.

45. Morse LS, Mizoguchi M. Diagnosis and management of viral retinitis in the acute retinal necrosis syndrome. Semin Ophthalmology. 1995;10(1):28-41.

46. Luu KK, Scott IU, Chaudhry NA, et al. Intravitreal antiviral injections as adjunctive therapy in the management of immunocompetent patients with necrotizing herpetic retinopathy. Am J Ophthalmology. 2000;129(6):811-3.

47. Meffert SA, Kertes PJ, Lim PL, et al. Successful treatment of progressive outer retinal necrosis using high-dose intravitreal ganciclovir. Retina. 1997;17(6):560-2.

48. Wilhelmus K, Lukehart S. Syphilis. In: Pepose JS, Holland GN, Wilhelmus KN (Eds). Ocular Infection and Immunity. St. Louis, Mosby; 1996. pp. 1435-66.

49. Samson CM, Foster CS. Syphilis. In: Foster CS, Vitale AT (Eds). Diagnosis and Treatment of Uveitis. Philadelphia: WB Saunders; 2002. pp. 235-44.

50. Margo CE, Hamed LM. Ocular syphilis. Surv Ophthalmology. 1992;37(3):203-20.

51. Gass JDM, Braunstein RA, Chenoweth RG. Acute syphilitic posterior placoid chorioretinitis. Ophthalmology. 1990;97(10):1288-97.

52. Baglivo E, Kapetanios A, Safran AB. Fluorescein and indocyanine green angiographic features in acute syphilitic macular placoid chorioretinitis. Can J Ophthalmology. 2003;38(5):401-5.

53. Tran TH, Cassoux N, Bodaghi B, et al. Syphilitic uveitis in patients infected with human immunodeficiency virus. Graefes Arch Clin Exp Ophthalmology. 2005;243(9):863-9.

54. Jumper JM, Machemer R, Gallemore RP, et al. Exudative retinal detachment and retinitis associated with acquired syphilitic uveitis. Retina. 2000;20(2):190-4.

55. McLeish WM, Pulido JS, Holland S, et al. The ocular manifestations of syphilis in the human immunodeficiency virus type 1-infected host. Ophthalmology. 1990;97(2):196-203.

56. Ormerod LD, Puklin JE, Sobel JD. Syphilitic posterior uveitis: correlative findings and significance. Clin Infect Dis. 2001;32(12):1661-73.

57. Oette M, Hemker J, Feldt T, et al. Acute syphilitic blindness in an HIV-positive patient. AIDS Patient Care STDS. 2005;19(4):209-11.

58. Gourevitch MN, Selwyn PA, Davenny K, et al. Effects of HIV infection on the serologic manifestation and response to treatment of syphilis in intravenous drug users. Ann Intern Med. 1993;118(5):350-5.

59. Erbelding EJ, Vlahov D, Nelson KE, et al. Syphilis serology in human immunodeficiency virus infection: evidence for false-negative fluorescent treponemal testing. J Infect Dis. 1997;176(5):1397-400.

60. Levy JH, Liss RA, Maguire AM. Neurosyphilis and ocular syphilis in patients with concurrent human immunodeficiency virus infection. Retina. 1989;9(3):175-80.

61. Becerra LI, Ksiazek SM, Savino PJ, et al. Syphilitic uveitis in human immunodeficiency virus-infected and noninfected patients. Ophthalmology. 1989;96(12):1727-30.

62. Sexually transmitted diseases treatment guidelines 2002. Centers for Disease Control and Prevention. MMWR Recomm Rep. 2002;51(RR-6):1-78.

63. Kresloff MS, Castellarin AA, Zarbin MA. Endophthalmitis. Surv Ophthalmology. 1998;43(3):193-224.

64. Garg SP, Talwar D, Verma LK. Metastatic endophthalmitis: a reappraisal. Ann Ophthalmology. 1991;23(2):74-8.

65. Greenwald MJ, Wohl LG, Sell CH. Metastatic bacterial endophthalmitis: a contemporary reappraisal. Surv Ophthalmology. 1986;31(2):81-101.

66. Chee SP, Jap A. Endogenous endophthalmitis. Curr Opin Ophthalmology. 2001;12(6):464-70.

67. Shrader SK, Band JD, Lauter CB, et al. The clinical spectrum of endophthalmitis: incidence, predisposing factors, and features influencing outcome. J Infect Dis. 1990;162(1):115-20.

68. Okada AA, Johnson RP, Liles WC, et al. Endogenous bacterial endophthalmitis. Report of a ten-year retrospective study. Ophthalmology. 1994;101(5):832-8.

69. Gupta A, Gupta V, Dogra MR, et al. Fungal endophthalmitis after a single intravenous administration of presumably contaminated dextrose infusion fluid. Retina. 2000;20(3):262-8.

70. Binder MI, Chua J, Kaiser PK, et al. Endogenous endophthalmitis: an 18-year review of culture-positive cases at a tertiary care center. Medicine (Baltimore). 2003;82(2):97-105.

71. Chakrabarti A, Shivaprakash MR, Singh R, et al. Fungal endophthalmitis: fourteen years' experience from a center in India. Retina. 2008;28(10):1400-7.

72. Essman TF, Flynn HW Jr, Smiddy WE, et al. Treatment outcomes in a 10-year study of endogenous fungal endophthalmitis. Ophthalmic Surg Lasers. 1997;28(3):185-94.

73. Scheidler V, Scott IU, Flynn HW Jr, et al. Culture-proven endogenous endophthalmitis: clinical features and visual acuity outcomes. Am J Ophthalmology. 2004;137(4):725-31.

74. Puliafito CA, Baker AS, Haaf J, et al. Infectious endophthalmitis: Review of 36 cases. Ophthalmology. 1982;89(8):921-9.

75. Ness T, Pelz K, Hansen LL. Endogenous endophthalmitis: microorganisms, disposition and prognosis. Acta Ophthalmology scand. 2007;85(8):852-6.

76. Baley JE, Annable WL, Kliegman RM. Candida endophthalmitis in the premature infant. J Pediatr. 1981;98(3):458-61.

77. Brod RD, Flynn HW Jr, Clarkson JG, et al. Endogenous Candida endophthalmitis. Management without intravenous amphotericin B Ophthalmology. 1990;97(5):666-74.

78. Weishaar PD, Flynn HW Jr, Murray TG, et al. Endogenous Aspergillus endophthalmitis: Clinical features and treatment outcomes. Ophthalmology. 1998;105(1):57-65.

79. Smith JR, Chee SP. Endogenous Aspergillus endophthalmitis occurring in a child with normal immune function. Eye (Lond). 2000;14(Pt 4):670-1.

80. Myles WM, Brownstein S, Deschenes J. Clinically unsuspected bilateral Aspergillus endophthalmitis. Can J Ophthalmology. 1997; 32(3):182-4.

81. Goldstein BG, Buettner H. Histoplasmic endophthalmitis: a clinicopathologic correlation. Arch Ophthalmology. 1983;101(5): 774-7.

82. Rezai KA, Eliott D, Plous O, et al. Disseminated Fusarium infection presenting as bilateral endogenous endophthalmitis in a patient with acute myeloid leukemia. Arch Ophthalmology. 2005;123(5): 702-3.

83. Lam DS, Koehler AP, Fan DS, et al. Endogenous fungal endophthalmitis caused by Paecilomyces variotii. Eye(Lond). 1999;13(Pt 1):113-6.

84. Gonzales CA, Scott IU, Chaudhry NA, et al. Endogenous endophthalmitis caused by Histoplasma capsulatum var. capsulatum: a case report and literature review. Ophthalmology. 2000;107(4):725-9.

85. Grixti A, Sadri M, Datta AV. Uncommon ophthalmologic disorders in intensive care unit patients. J Crit Care. 2012;27(6):746.e9-22.

86. Jackson TL, Eykyn SJ, Graham EM, et al. Endogenous bacterial endophthalmitis: a 17-year prospective series and review of 267 reported cases. Surv Ophthalmology. 2003;48(4):403-23.

87. Dua S, Chalermskurat W, Miller MB, et al. Bilateral hematogenous Pseudomonas aeruginosa endophthalmitis after lung transplantation. Am J Transplant. 2006;6(1):219-24.

88. Khan A, Okhravi N, Lightman S. The eye in systemic sepsis. Clin Med (Lond). 2002;2(5):444-8.

89. Scott IU, Matharoo N, Flynn HW Jr, et al. Endophthalmitis caused by *Klebsiella* species. Am J Ophthalmology. 2004;138(4):662-3.

90. Sng CC, Jap A, Chan YH, et al. Risk factors for endogenous Klebsiella endophthalmitis in patients with Klebsiella bacteraemia: a case-control study. Br J Ophthalmology. 2008;92(5):673-7.

91. Ho V, Ho LY, Ranchod TM, et al. Endogenous methicillin-resistant *Staphylococcus aureus* endophthalmitis. Retina. 2011;31(3):596-601.

92. Brod RD, Flynn HW Jr. Endophthalmitis: current approaches to diagnosis and therapy. Curr Opin Infect Dis. 1993;6:628-35.

93. Essman TF, Flynn HW Jr, Smiddy WE, et al. Treatment outcomes in a 10-year study of endogenous fungal endophthalmitis. Ophthalmic Surg Lasers. 1997;28(3):185-94.

94. Anand A, Madhavan H, Neelam V, et al. Use of polymerase chain reaction in the diagnosis of fungal endophthalmitis. Ophthalmology. 2001;108(2):326-30.

95. Schulman JA, Peyman GA. Intravitreal corticosteroids as an adjunct in the treatment of bacterial and fungal endophthalmitis. A Review. Retina. 1992;12(4):336-40.

96. Berglöff J, Gasser E, Feigl B. Ophthalmic manifestations in Lyme borreliosis. J Neurcophthalmol. 1994;14:15-20.

97. Copeland RA Jr. Lyme uveitis. Int Ophthalmology Clin. 1990;30(4): 291-3.

98. Lesser RL. Ocular manifestations of Lyme disease. Am J Med. 1995;98(Supp 4A):60-2.

99. Balcer LJ, Winterkorn JM, Galetta SL. Neuro-ophthalmic manifestations of Lyme disease. J Neuroopthalmol. 1997;17(2):108-21.

100. Mikkilä HO, Seppälä IJ, Viljanen MK, et al. The expanding clinical spectrum of ocular Lyme Borreliosis. Ophthalmology. 2000;107(3):581-7.

101. Karma A, Seppälä I, Mikkilä H, et al. Diagnosis and clinical characteristics of ocular Lyme Borreliosis. Am J Ophthalmology. 1995;119(5):127-35.

102. Breeveled J, Rothova A, Kuiper H. Intermediate uveitis and Lyme Borreliosis. Br J Ophthalmology. 1992;76(3):181-2.

103. Lardenoye CW, Van der Lelji A, de Loos WS, et al. Peripheral multifocal chorioretinitis: a distinct clinical entity? Ophthalmology. 1997;104(11):1820-6.

104. Mets MB, Holfels E, Boyer KM, et al. Eye manifestations of congenital toxoplasmosis. Am J Ophthalmology. 1997;123(1):1-16.

105. KodjiKian L, Wallon M, Fleury J, et al. Ocular manifestations in congenital toxoplasmosis. Graefes Arch Clin Exp Ophthalmology. 2006;244(1):14-21.

106. Rothova A. Ocular involvement in toxoplasmosis. Br J Ophthalmology. 1993;77(6):351-7.

107. Bosch-Driessen LE, Berendschot TT, Ongkosuwito JV, et al. Ocular toxoplasmosis: clinical features and prognosis of 154 patients. Ophthalmology. 2002;109:869-78.

108. Hovakimyan A, Cunningham ET Jr. Ocular toxoplasmosis. Ophthalmology Clin North Am. 2002;15(3):327-32.

109. Akstein RB, Wilson LA, Teutsch SM. Acquired toxoplasmosis. Ophthalmology. 1982;89(12):1299-302.

110. Heinemann MH, Gold JM, Maisel J. Bilateral toxoplasma retinochoroiditis in a patient with acquired immune deficiency syndrome. Retina. 1986;6(4):224-7.

111. Moorthy RS, Smith RE, Rao NA. Progressive ocular toxoplasmosis in patients with acquired immunodeficiency syndrome. Am J Ophthalmology. 1993;115(6):742-7.

112. Fardeau C, Romand S, Rao NA, et al. Diagnosis of toxoplasmic retinochoroiditis with atypical clinical features. Am J Ophthalmology. 2002;134(2):196-203.

113. Ben Yahia S, Herbort CP, Jenzeri S, et al. Intravitreal bevacizumab (Avastin) as primary and rescue treatment for choroidal neovascularization secondary to ocular toxoplasmosis. Int Ophthalmology. 2008;28(4):311-6.

114. De Groot-Mijnes JD, Rothova A, Van Loon AM, et al. Polymerase chain reaction and Goldmann-Witmer coefficient analysis are complimentary for the diagnosis of infectious uveitis. Am J Ophthalmology. 2006;141(2):313-8.

115. Garweg JG, Garweg SD, Flueckiger F, et al. Aqueous humor and serum immunoblotting for immunoglobulin types G, A, M, and E in cases of human ocular toxoplasmosis. J Clin Microbiol. 2004;42(10):4593-8.

116. Nijhawan R, Bansal R, Gupta N, et al. Intraocular cysts of Toxoplasma gondii in patients with necrotizing retinitis following periocular/intraocular triamcinolone injection. Ocular Immunol Inflamm. 2013;21(5):396-9.

117. Holland GN, Lewis KG. An update on current practices in the management of ocular toxoplasmosis. Am J Ophthalmology. 2002;134(1):102-14.

118. Bosch-Driessen LH, Verbraak FD, Suttorp-Schulten MS, et al. A prospective, randomized trial of pyrimethamine and azithromycin vs pyrimethamine and sulphadiazine for the treatment of ocular toxoplasmosis. Am J Ophthalmology. 2002;134(1):34-40.

119. Stanford MR, See SE, Jones LV, et al. Antibiotics for toxoplasmic retinochoroiditis: An evidence-based systematic review. Ophthalmology. 2003;110(5):926-31.

120. Soheilian M, Ramezani A, Azimzadeh A, et al. Randomized trial of intravitreal clindamycin and dexamethasone versus pyrimethamine, sulfadiazine, and prednisolone in treatment of ocular toxoplasmosis. Ophthalmology. 2011;118(1):134–41.

121. Kishore K, Conway MD, Peyman GA. Intravitreal clindamycin and dexamethasone for toxoplasmic retinochoroiditis. Ophthalmic Surg Lasers. 2001;32(3):183-92.

122. Vergani P, Ghidini A, Ceruti P, et al. Congenital toxoplasmosis: efficacy of maternal treatment with spiramycin alone. Am J Reprod Immunol. 1998;39(5):335-40.

123. Rothova A, Bosch-Driessen L, van Loon HN, et al. Azithromycin for ocular toxoplasmosis. Br J Ophthalmology. 1998;82(11):1306-8.

124. Pearson PA, Piracha AR, Sen HA, et al. Atovaquone for the treatment of toxoplasma retinochoroiditis in immunocompetent patients. Ophthalmology. 1999;106(1):148-53.

125. Molk R. Ocular toxocariasis: a review of the literature. Ann Ophthalmology. 1983;15(3):216-9.

126. Ellis GS Jr, Pakalnis VA, Worley G, et al. Toxocara canis infestation. Clinical and epidemiological associations with seropositivity in kindergarten children. Ophthalmology. 1986;93(8):1032-7.

127. Shields JA. Ocular toxocariasis: A review. Surv Ophthalmology. 1984;28(5):361-81.

128. Upadhyay MP, Rai NC. Toxocara granuloma of the retina. Jpn J Ophthalmology. 1980;24(3):278-81.

129. Brown DH. Ocular Toxocara Canis Part II. Clinical Review. J Pediatr Ophthalmology. 1970;7(3):182-91.

130. Monshizadeh R, Ashrafzadeh MT, Rumelt S. Choroidal neovascular membrane: a late complication of inactive toxocara chorioretinitis. Retina. 2000;20(2):219-20.

131. Belmont JB, Irvine A, Benson W, et al. Vitrectomy in ocular toxocariasis. Arch Ophthalmology. 1982;100(12):1912-5.

132. Barisani-Asenbauer T, Maca SM, Hauff W, et al. Treatment of ocular toxocariasis with albendazole. J Ocul Pharmacol Ther. 2001;17(3):287-94.

133. Dinning WJ, Gillespie SH, Cooling RJ, et al. Toxocariasis: a practical approach to management of ocular disease. Eye(Lond). 1988;2(Pt 5):580-2.

134. Singh R, Gupta V, Gupta A. Pattern of uveitis in a referral eye clinic in north India. Indian J Ophthalmology. 2004;52(2):121-5.

135. Gupta V, Gupta A, Arora S, et al. Presumed tubercular serpiginouslike choroiditis: clinical presentations and management. Ophthalmology. 2003;110(9):1744-9.

136. Bansal R, Gupta A, Gupta V, et al. Tubercular serpiginous-like choroiditis presenting as multifocal serpiginoid choroiditis. Ophthalmology. 2012;119(11):2334-42.

137. Gan WL, Jones NP. Serpiginous-like choroiditis as a marker for tuberculosis in a non-endemic area. Br J Ophthalmology. 2013;97(5):644-7.

138. Gupta A, Bansal R, Gupta V, et al. Ocular signs predictive of tubercular uveitis. Am J Ophthalmology. 2010;149(4):562-70.

139. Mackensen F, Becker MD, Wiehler U, et al. QuantiFERON TB-Gold—a new test strengthening long-suspected tuberculous involvement in serpiginous-like choroiditis. Am J Ophthalmology. 2008;146(5):761-6.

140. Gupta A, Bansal R, Gupta V, et al. Fundus autofluorescence in serpiginous-like choroiditis. Retina. 2012;32(4):814-25.

141. Laatikainen L, Erkkila H. Serpiginous choroiditis. Br J Ophthalmology. 1974;58(9):777-83.

142. Lim WK, Buggage RR, Nussenblatt RB. Serpiginous choroiditis. Surv Ophthalmology. 2005;50(3):231-44.

143. Weiss H, Annesley WH Jr, Shields JA, et al. The clinical course of serpiginous choroidopathy. Am J Ophthalmology. 1979;87(2):133-42.

144. Gass JDM: Stereoscopic atlas of macular diseases: a funduscopic and angiographic presentation. St Louis: C.V Mosby Co; 1970. pp. 66.

145. Khanamiri HN, Rao NA. Serpiginous choroiditis and infectious multifocal serpiginoid choroiditis. Surv Ophthalmology. 2013;58(3):203-32.

146. Vasconcelos-Santos DV, Rao PK, Davies JB, et al. Clinical features of tuberculous serpiginous-like choroiditis in contrast to classic serpiginous choroiditis. Arch Ophthalmology. 2010;128(7):853-8.

147. Gupta A, Gupta V, Arora S, et al. PCR-positive tubercular retinal vasculitis: clinical characteristics and management. Retina. 2001;21(5):435-44.

148. Gupta A, Bansal R, Gupta V, et al. Ocular signs predictive of tubercular uveitis. Am J Ophthalmology. 2010;149(4):562-70.

149. Bansal R, Gupta A, Gupta V, et al. Role of anti-tubercular therapy in uveitis with latent/manifest tuberculosis. Am J Ophthalmology. 2008; 146(5):772-9.

150. Helm CJ, Holland GN. Ocular tuberculosis. Surv Ophthalmology. 1993;38(3):229 -56.

151. Mansour AM, Haymond R. Choroidal tuberculomas without evidence of extraocular tuberculosis. Graefes Arch Clin Exp Ophthalmology. 1990;228(4):382-3.

152. Gupta V, Gupta A, Sachdeva N, et al. Successful management of tubercular subretinal granulomas. Ocul Immunol Inflamm. 2006;14(1):35-40.

153. Bansal R, Beke N, Sharma A, et al. Intravitreal bevacizumab as an adjunct in the management of a vascular choroidal granuloma. BMJ Case Rep. 2013.

Surgical Retina

Chapter 41

Retinal Detachment

Parveen Sen, Sufiyan Shaikh, Sharan Shetty, Kaustubh Deshmukh

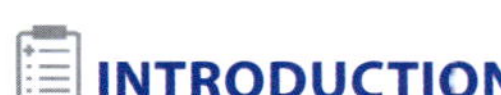 INTRODUCTION

Retina consists of ten layers spanning from the retinal pigment epithelium (RPE) till the internal limiting membrane. All layers of the retina other than the RPE constitute the neurosensory retina. Retinal detachment (RD) implies separation of the neurosensory retina from the underlying RPE. The separation is prone to happen at this level because of the presence of a potential space between these two layers which is due to their separate embryological origin. The RPE is derived from the outer wall of the optic cup while the neurosensory retina is derived from the inner wall of the optic cup.[1]

PATHOGENESIS OF RETINAL DETACHMENT

Accumulation of fluid in the subretinal space (between the neurosensory retina and RPE) occurs when the normal physiological processes responsible to keep the subretinal space dry are overwhelmed. Various anatomical, physiological and metabolic factors are involved in holding the neurosensory retina and RPE together under normal circumstances. These factors include:

- Presence of Na$^+$-K$^+$ ATPase pump on the cell membrane of RPE. This pump actively removes the fluid from the subretinal space into the choroid.[2,3]
- Intraocular pressure (IOP) and osmotic pressure of the extracellular fluid in the choroid cause passive movement of fluid from the vitreous into the choroid.[4]
- Interphotoreceptor matrix (IPM) serves as biological adhesive glue.[5] Once this IPM is breached as in retinal detachment, it takes the reattached retina time to get firmly re-adherent. This is explained by the time IPM needs to develop to actively hold the retina in place again.[6]
- The interdigitation between the RPE microvilli and photoreceptor outer segments also help to hold these two layers together.[7,8]
- Presence of formed, intact, homogenous, healthy vitreous gel acts as a support to the retina. Even in the presence of a full thickness retinal break, retinal detachment may not occur unless the vitreous undergoes liquefaction.[9]

When these factors are overwhelmed by various physiological or pathological processes in the eye, retinal detachment occurs.

TYPES OF RETINAL DETACHMENT

Based on the pathological mechanisms involved, retinal detachment can be of the following types:

- Rhegmatogenous retinal detachment
- Tractional retinal detachment
- Combined retinal detachment
- Exudative retinal detachment

Rhegmatogenous Retinal Detachment

Rhegmatogenous retinal detachment is by far the commonest type. It occurs due to the presence of a *rhegma* (*rhegma* means break/fissure in Greek) (Figs. 41.1A and B).

Usually the following prerequisites are required for the development of a rhegmatogenous retinal detachment:

- Forces that can precipitate a retinal break.
- A rhegma or retinal break.
- Posterior vitreous syneresis or liquefaction.

If vitreous is not liquefied or if adequate traction is not present, retinal detachment may not occur even in the presence of a full thickness break.[10,11] Occurrence of posterior vitreous detachment (PVD) in the eye is an event when all three factors may coexist.

Increased incidence of retinal break formation leading to retinal detachment is associated with myopia (Fig. 41.2),[12] cataract surgery[13] or other intraocular surgeries like penetrating keratoplasty,[14] or even laser-assisted in situ keratomileusis (LASIK).[15]

Hereditary vitreoretinopathies like Marfan syndrome, Ehlers-Danlos syndrome, Wagner's syndrome, Stickler syndrome. Even optic disc abnormalities like Morning glory disc can predispose to retinal detachment (Fig. 41.3). Goldmann-Favre syndrome and X-linked retinoschisis also predispose to RD due to strong and abnormal vitreoretinal adhesions which can lead to retinal break formation.[16-18]

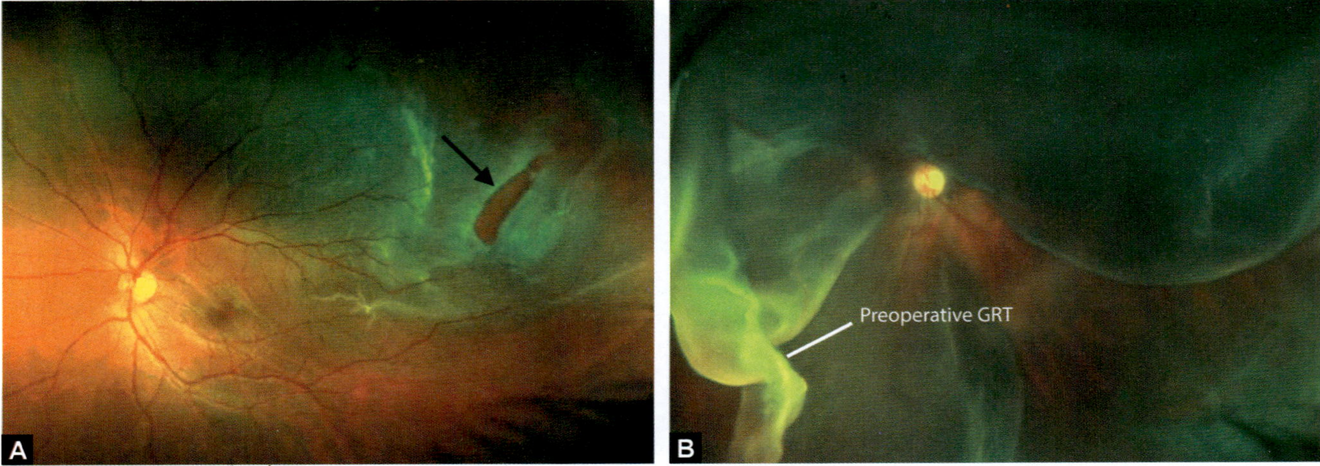

Figs. 41.1A and B: Ultra-widefield image showing rhegmatogenous retinal detachment with retinal corrugations with large superotemporal retinal tear.

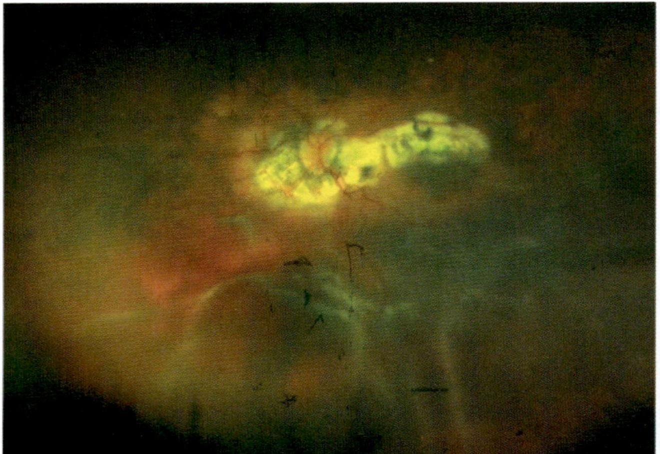

Fig. 41.2: Bullous rhegmatogenous retinal detachment in a pathological myope with focal choroidal atrophy at posterior pole.

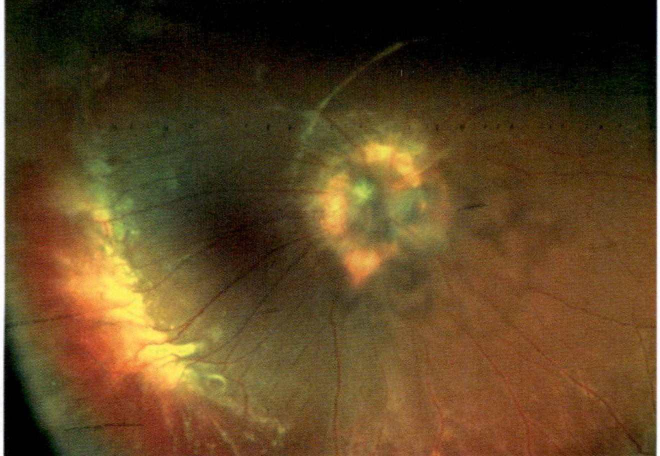

Fig. 41.3: Rhegmatogenous retinal detachment in a child with morning glory disc.

Patients with retinochoroidal coloboma also have an increased incidence (23–42%) of development of retinal break formation.[19] This break formation may be seen at the edge of the coloboma or within the intercalary membrane. These patients must be kept under a regular follow-up.

Rhegmatogenous retinal detachment may also occur after inflammatory or infective retinal disorders (Figs. 41.4A and B) like post regressed tuberculoma, acute retinal necrosis (RD seen in 75% of cases) or cytomegalovirus retinitis.[20,21]

Closed globe trauma also predisposes to rhegmatogenous retinal detachment arising out of breaks from contusion necrosis or retinal dialysis (Figs. 41.5, 41.6 and 41.7).

Tractional Retinal Detachment

This is the second most common form of retinal detachment. This occurs as a result of growth of fibrovascular proliferation on the retinal surface. Mechanical forces exerted by this fibrovascular tissue cause the separation of the retina from the RPE without a retinal break. These tractional retinal detachments (TRDs) are usually concave in configuration (Figs. 41.9A to D). These are not very high or bullous.

In cases like retinopathy of prematurity (ROP) (Fig. 41.8) however, the tractional forces may pull the retina up to the lens. Proliferative diabetic retinopathy, sickle cell disease, venous occlusions, penetrating trauma and advanced retinopathy of prematurity are some of the common causes of tractional retinal detachment.

Combined Retinal Detachment

Strong adhesions and traction may result in the development of a retinal tear or break in a tractional retinal detachment

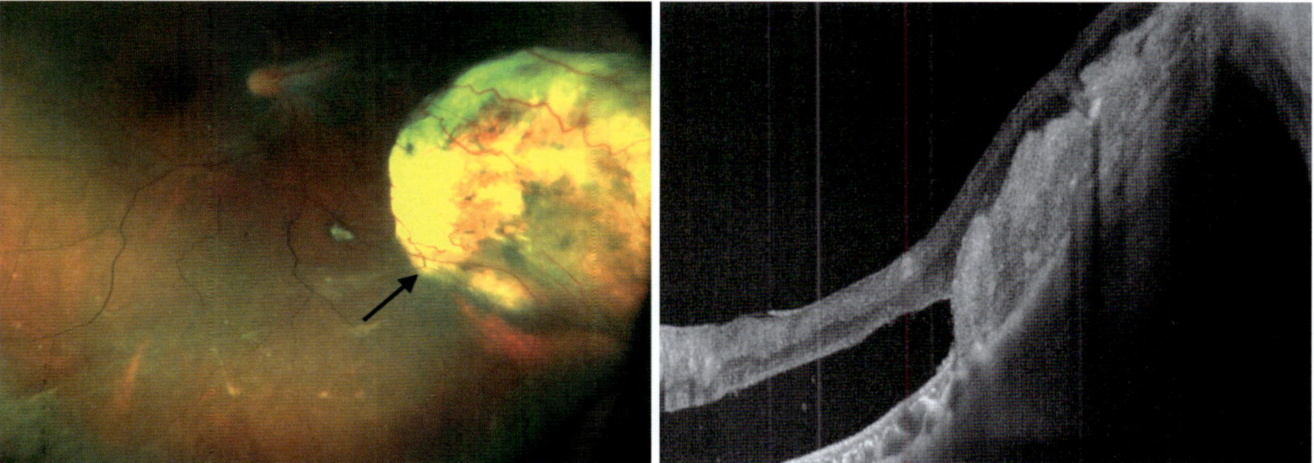

Fig. 41.4A and B: (A) Post regressed tuberculoma (black arrow) with retinal detachment (B) OCT image showing retinal detachment.

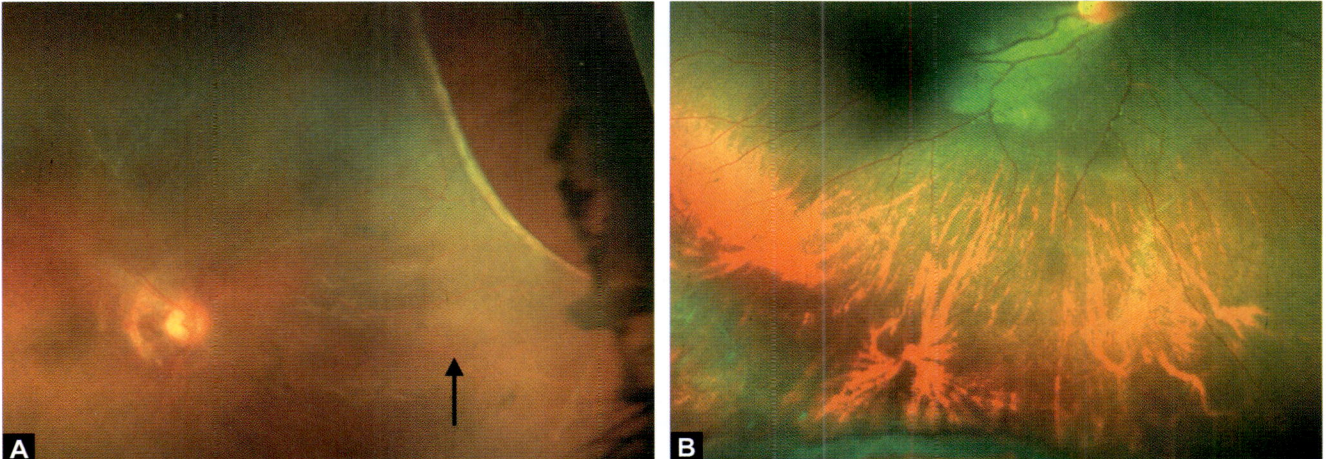

Figs. 41.5A and B: (A) Ultra-widefield image showing post closed globe injury rhegmatogenous retinal detachment with large superonasal dialysis. (B) Inferior vitreous base dialysis (hammock appearance) seen in an eye with closed globe injury. This patient also had a retinal dialysis just anterior to the avulsion site.

leading to a combination of a rhegmatogenous and a tractional retinal detachment (Figs. 41.10A and B).

These breaks are usually seen at the base of the fibrovascular proliferations where the tractional forces are maximal and the retina is thinned out. These are seen commonly in proliferative diabetic retinopathy (PDR), vasoproliferative retinopathies (Eales, post vein occlusions especially BRVO eyes develop a TRD converting overtime to a combined RD, FEVR eyes etc.), proliferative vitreoretinopathy (PVR) and ocular trauma. In these cases though a retinal break is present, the preretinal membranes hold the retina down and bullous RD does not develop. Treatment remains surgical, needing relief of traction and removal of all the preretinal proliferative membranes and laser retinopexy for the retinal breaks.

Exudative Retinal Detachment

Exudative retinal detachment occurs when separation of the neurosensory retina from the underlying RPE develops because of accumulation of subretinal fluid (SRF) due to leakage caused by excessive fluid secretion or compromised health of the RPE so that normal fluid is not absorbed. There is no break in the retina (Figs. 41.11 and 41.12).

Excessive fluid secretion is seen in posterior scleritis, Vogt-Koyanagi-Harada disease, nanophthalmos, malignant hypertension, toxemia of pregnancy and Coats' disease. Malignant melanoma, choroidal hemangioma and metastatic tumors of the choroid are the ocular tumors commonly associated with exudative RD. Idiopathic uveal effusion

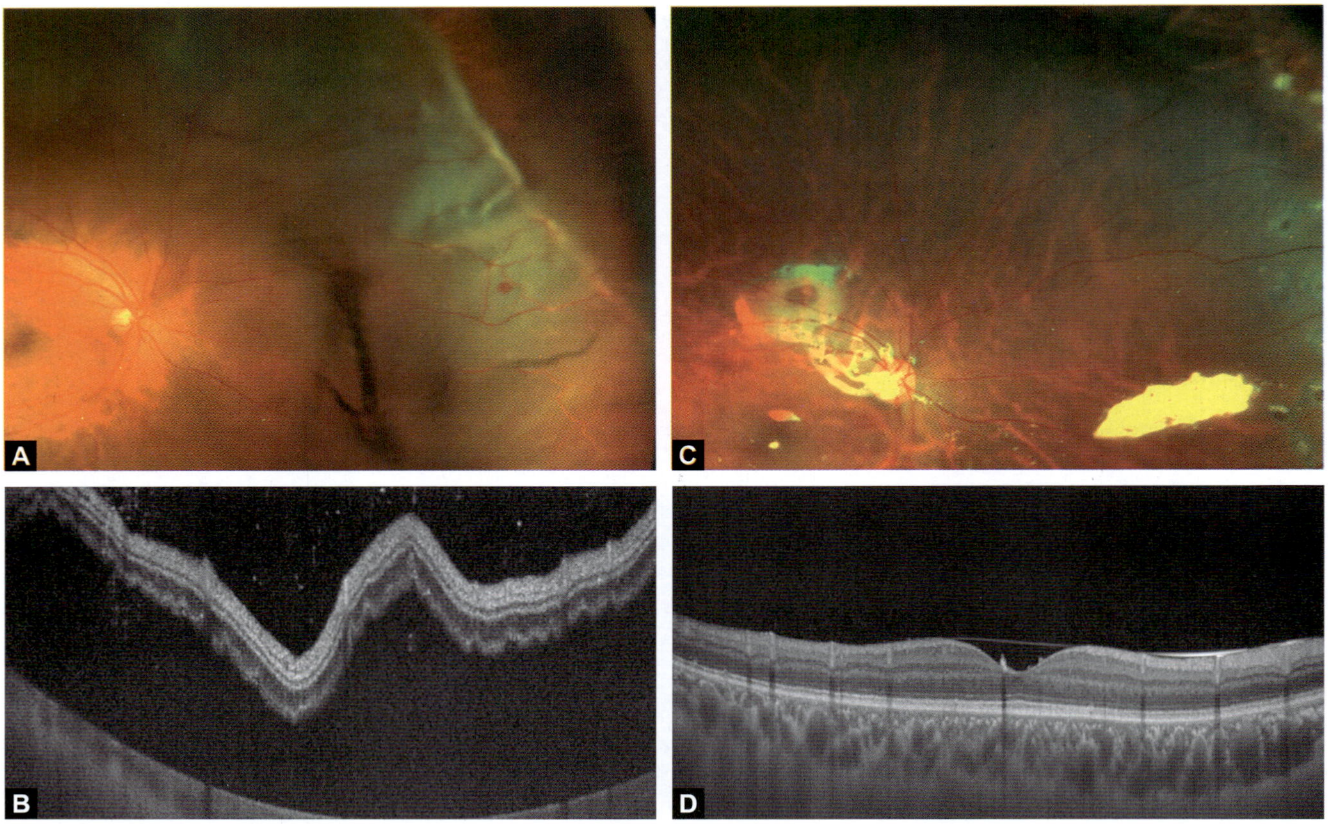

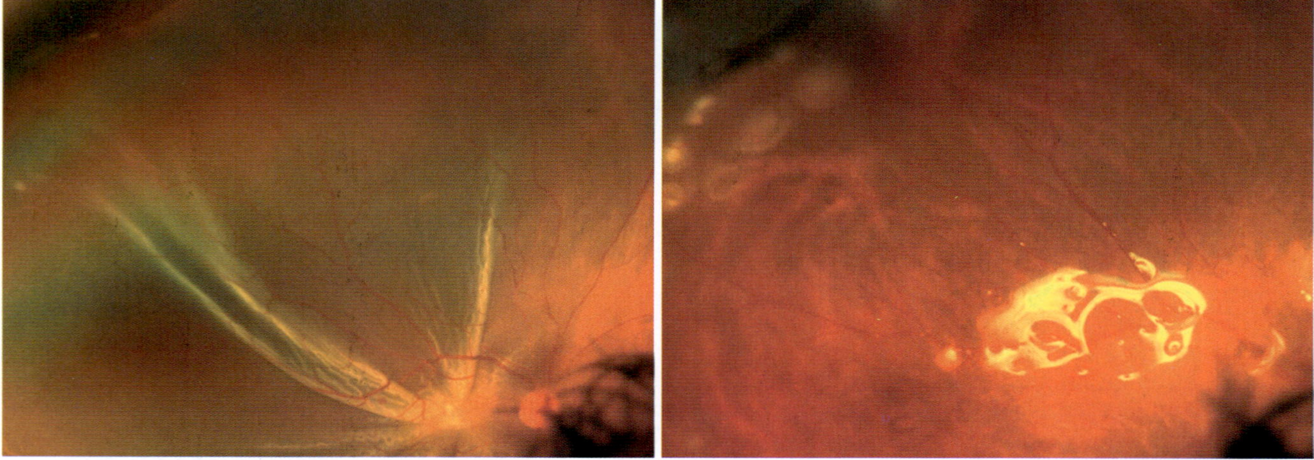

Figs. 41.6A to D: (A) Ultra-widefield image showing superonasal retinal dialysis in right eye with localized retinal detachment, (B) Pre-operative corresponding optical coherence tomography (OCT) image of retinal detachment, (C) Post-op colored image showing settled retina, (D) OCT showing settled retina after surgery.

Fig. 41.7: Fundus photograph showing traumatic retinal dialysis with macular pucker (left), postoperatively settled retina (right).

syndrome causes exudative RD because of obstruction to the choroidal outflow while central serous chorioretinopathy causes exudative RD due to defective metabolic activity of the RPE.[22] Exudative retinal detachment do not usually require surgical intervention. Correction of the underlying pathology typically leads to resolution of these detachments.

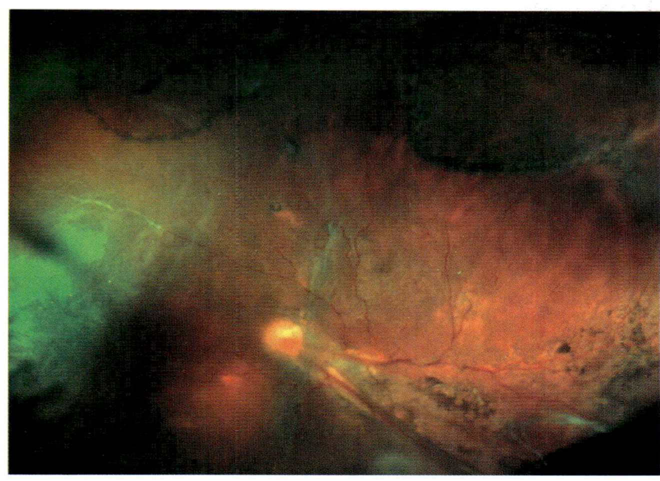

Fig. 41.8: Fundus photograph showing regressed retinopathy of prematurity (ROP) with retinal detachment and dragged retina. Patient was one-eyed having lost his other eye in childhood post ROP surgery.

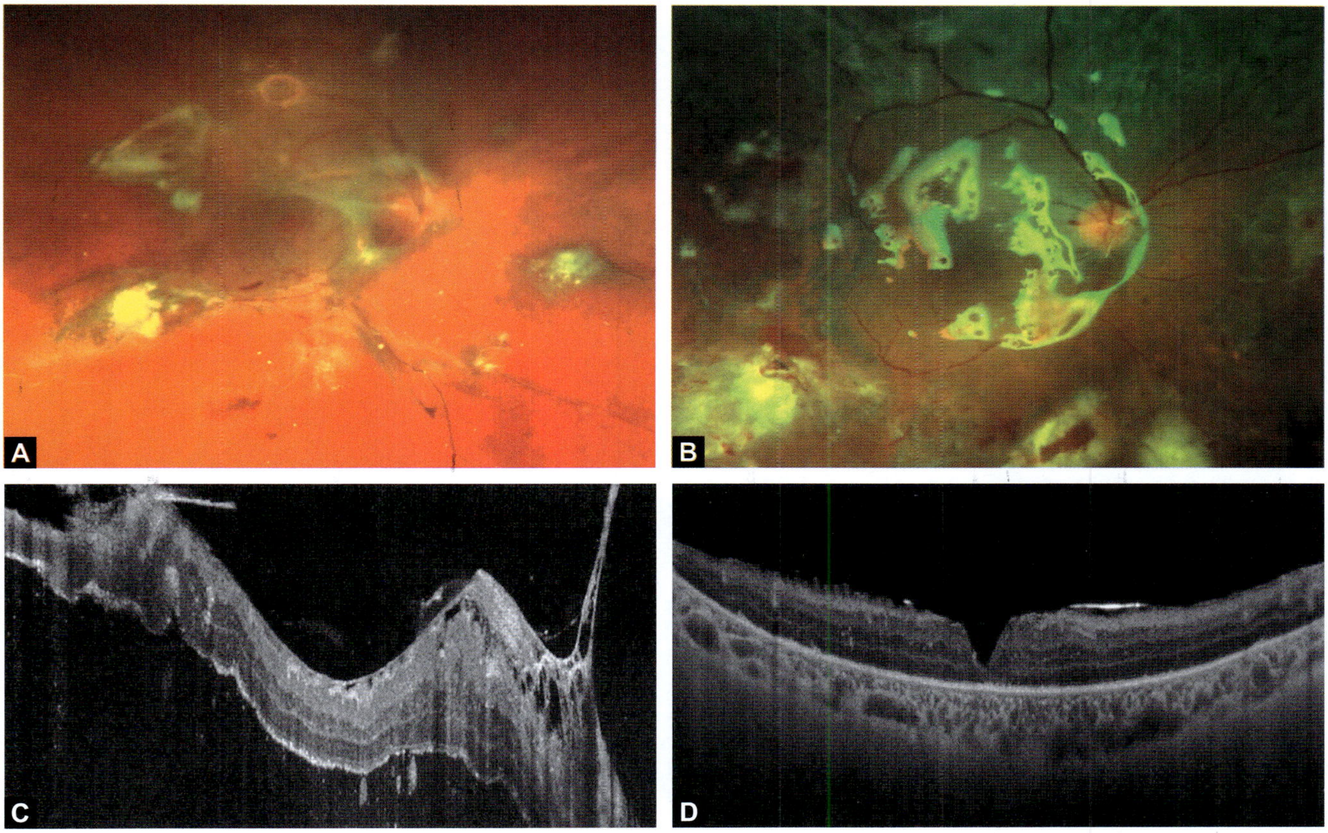

Figs. 41.9A to D: Fundus photograph showing (A) Fibrovascular proliferation at disc and along arcades in case of proliferative diabetic retinopathy (PDR) with tractional retinal detachment. (B) Postoperatively, the retina is attached with laser marks and oil in the vitreous cavity. Bimanual vitrectomy helped to cut and segment areas of complex tractional tissue. (C) Optical coherence tomography (OCT) shows detached macula preoperatively and well-settled retina under oil postoperatively (D).

Subretinal hemorrhage may also cause RD. These hemorrhagic RDs can be seen in cases of ocular trauma or in patients with polypoidal choroidal vasculopathy or choroidal neovascular membranes seen in advanced age related macular degeneration.[23]

Posterior Vitreous Detachment

Posterior vitreous detachment is defined as the separation of the posterior vitreous cortex from the internal limiting membrane of the retina. PVD is a normal physiological process. It is found in 27% of patients aged 60–69 years and in

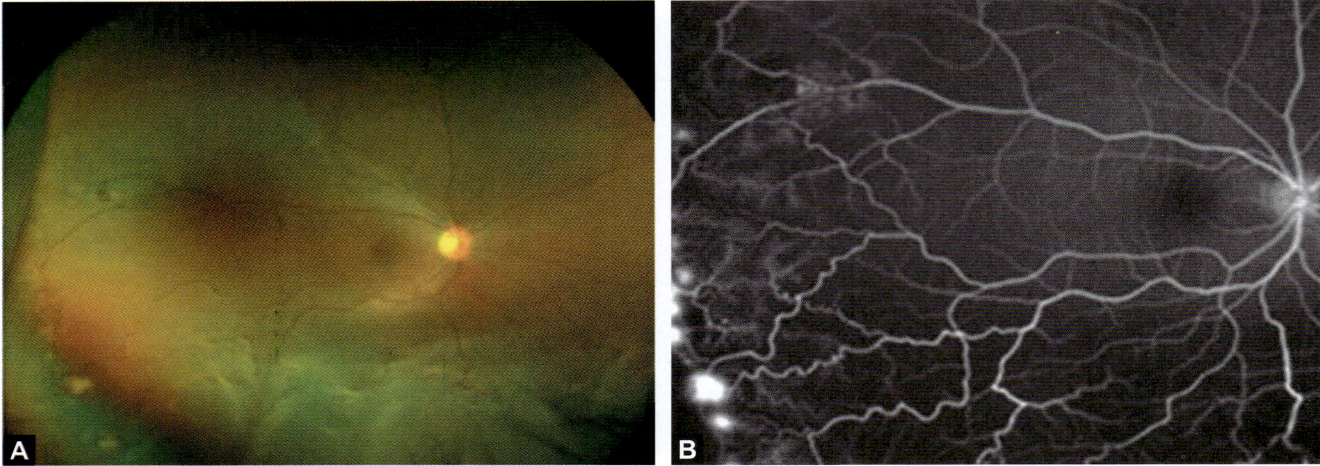

Figs. 41.10A and B: Ultra-widefield image showing (A) Combined retinal detachment with a retinal break temporally in presence of peripheral retinal neovascularization in an eye with familial exudative vitreoretinopathy (FEVR). (B) Fundus fluorescein angiography (FFA) showing leaking peripheral retinal neovascularization in inferotemporal quadrant.

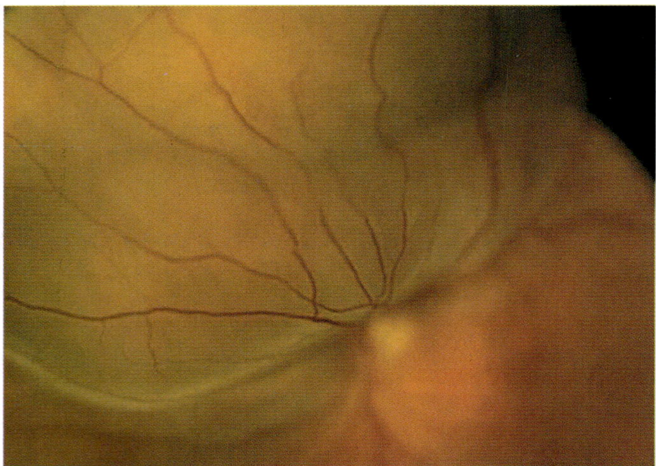

Fig. 41.11: Fundus photograph showing exudative retinal detachment in the absence of retinal break or retinal corrugations.

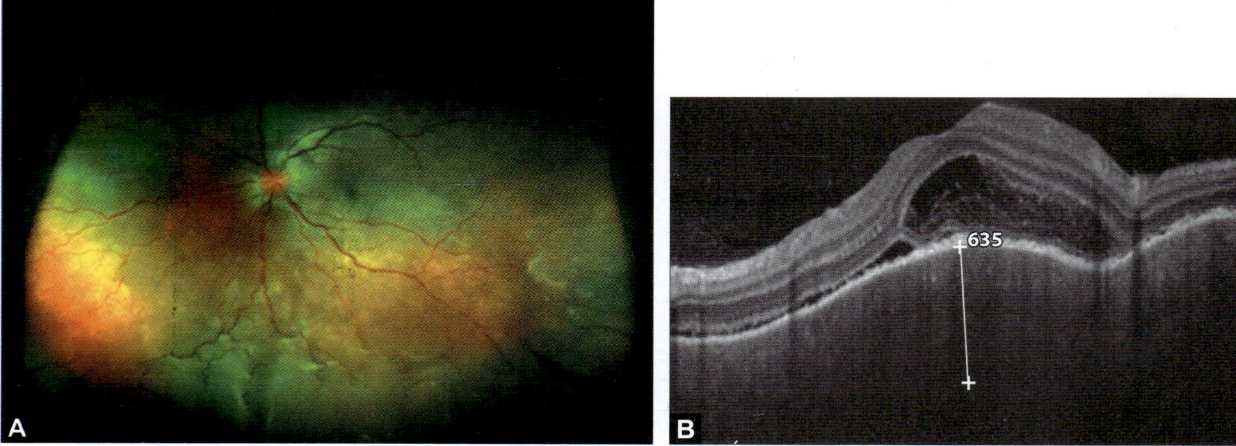

Figs. 41.12A and B: (A) Inferior exudative retinal detachment (RD) on ultra-widefield imaging. (B) Swept-source optical coherence tomography (SS-OCT) showing massive thickening of the choroid with subretinal fibrin.

63% of patients after the age of 70.[24] Myopia, trauma, cataract surgery, yttrium-aluminium-garnet (YAG) capsulotomy, and intraocular inflammation may accelerate its occurrence.[25,26] PVD can be *partial* (incomplete) or *total* (complete). PVD is considered to be partial when some vitreous fibers are still attached to the macula and the optic nerve head and complete once it is totally separated from the optic nerve head as indicated by the presence of *Weiss ring*.

The areas in the eye where the vitreous may be strongly adherent include optic disc margins, major retinal blood vessels and the vitreous base.

Posterior vitreous detachment may be totally asymptomatic or the patient may experience some flashes of light or floaters. Flashes or photopsia are due to the mechanical stimulation of the retina caused by traction exerted on the retina by the vitreous fibers. Floaters are experienced due to shadows cast on the retina by the collapsed vitreous gel, free floating retinal pigment epithelial cells and red blood cells which may enter the vitreous body if a retinal break forms due to the PVD. The most common presenting complaint of patients with PVD is a single large prominent floater in the visual axis generally caused by the *Weiss ring*. Though Weiss ring is considered pathognomonic of PVD, not all patients with a Weiss ring may have a complete vitreous detachment. Vitreous may be separated at the disc leading to the ring but may still be attached elsewhere. Patients may even experience a *shower of floaters* or a drop in vision if PVD is associated with vitreous hemorrhage due to the rupture of any retinal vessel during the vitreous separation.

PATHOPHYSIOLOGY OF POSTERIOR VITREOUS DETACHMENT

Vitreous forms the largest component of the eye. It is colorless and gelatinous. When healthy it is 100% in gel form with a volume of about 4.0 mL. There is no free fluid. It is composed of 98% water and 2% structural proteins and extracellular matrix. The most common structural protein is collagen. Type 2 collagen comprises nearly 75% of the collagen in the vitreous.[27] Other collagen types seen include type 5, 6, 9, 11 and 18.[28] These collagen fibers are aligned parallel to the retinal surface other than at the vitreous base. Hence, peeling of the vitreous from the retinal surface can be done posteriorly but not at the vitreous base where only *shaving* is possible. Structural proteins other than collagen seen in the vitreous include fibrillin (implicated in the pathogenesis of RD in patients with Marfan syndrome) and opticin (an extracellular matrix leucine-rich repeat protein).[27] Other important components of the vitreous include hyaluronan and chondroitin sulfate. They play a crucial role in maintaining the morphology of the vitreous. Hyaluronan serves as both structural and functional role. It has unique biophysical and hydrodynamic properties which influence the vitreous homeostasis and biomechanics.[29] The role of chondroitin sulfate is poorly understood. However, it plays a crucial role in the functioning of vitreous

and its structural stability by binding hyaluronan and other binding proteins.[30]

Collagen fibrils have a natural tendency to aggregate. A network of hyaluronan fills the space between the collagen fibrils and does not allow aggregation of collagen in mammalian vitreous. Also, these thin collagen fibrils have a coating of macromolecules like opticin which, along with the surface features of the collagen fibrils (especially type IX), plays a fundamental role in maintaining gel stability.[31]

The changes which occur with age, in this highly hydrated vitreous matrix, are responsible for retinal disorders including retinal breaks and retinal detachment. With aging the hyaluronic content of the vitreous starts decreasing and the collagen begins to aggregate primarily due to the loss of collagen IX from its surface[32] as well as decrease in the chondroitin sulfate side-chains resulting in an increased exposure of the *sticky* type II collagen.[33] Fragmentation or break down of these collagen fibers causes liquefaction of the vitreous and formation of lacunae leading to *syneresis* and vitreoschisis.[34] Rupture of posterior hyaloid layer allows this liquefied/syneretic vitreous to enter the subhyaloid space separating it from the internal limiting membrane (ILM) of the retina producing a true PVD.

The prevalence of a complete PVD is often overestimated.[35] Despite preoperative biomicroscopic examination suggesting a complete vitreous detachment, a thin layer of cortical vitreous may remain attached to the retina.[36] This is particularly seen in cases of highly myopic eyes due to the presence of *posterior vitreoschisis*.[37] The outer wall of the schisis cavity is difficult to detect clinically as well as on ultrasound, but may be picked on the newer high resolution optical coherence tomography (OCT).

MANAGEMENT OF POSTERIOR VITREOUS DETACHMENT

Posterior vitreous detachment itself does not require any treatment. Some subjects with floaters are however extremely symptomatic. Small incision pars plana vitrectomy has been tried in these patients with nearly 96% subjects feeling relief from symptoms and improvement in visual acuity after surgery.[38,39] However, careful patient selection is very important and the subject should be clearly explained the possible complications of surgery with retinal detachment seen in 10.9% of cases following this procedure.[40,41]

A thorough retinal examination using indirect ophthalmoscope with scleral indentation is necessary to look for any retinal breaks or holes formed during PVD.

Formation of Retinal Break

Retinal break is defined as a full thickness discontinuity of the retinal tissue. Retinal breaks can be retinal tears or retinal holes based on the pathological mechanism involved in the causation of break. Retinal tears are usually associated with dynamic and strong vitreoretinal traction. These typically

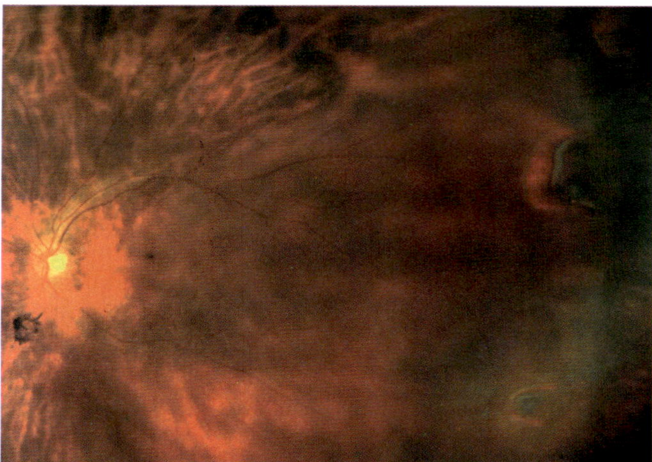

Fig. 41.13: Ultra-widefield image showing superotemporal and inferotemporal superotemporal horse shoe tears with flap with temporal rhegmatogenous retinal detachment.

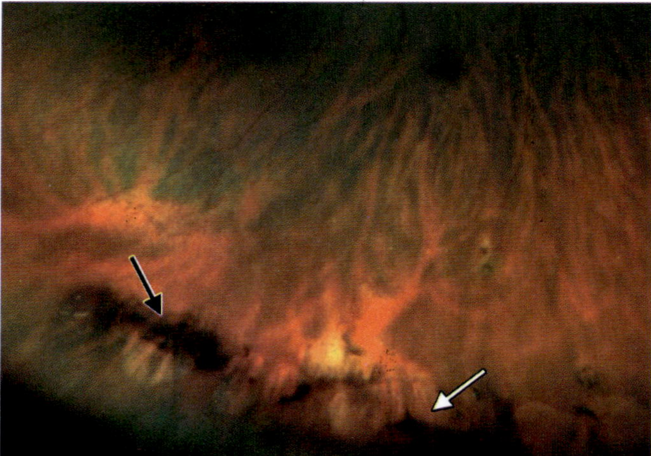

Fig. 41.14: Fundus photograph showing pigmented lattice degeneration (black arrow) with clearly visible paving stone degeneration, identified by pigmented borders and a depigmented center (white arrow).

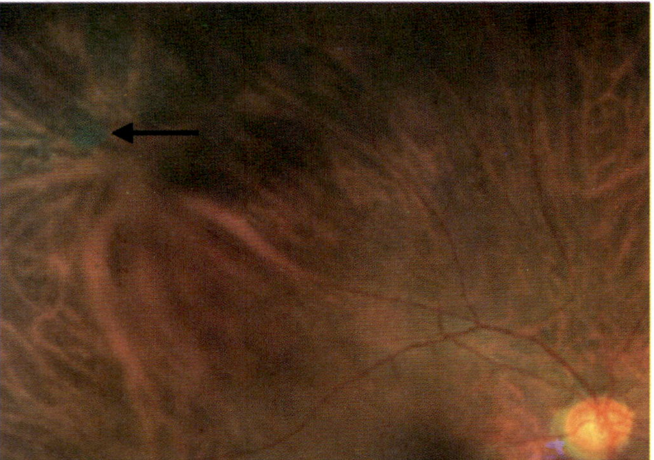

Fig. 41.15: Ultra-widefield image showing superotemporal anteriorly located operculated hole (lasered) with overlying operculum seen in the vitreous cavity (black arrow).

present as a horseshoe shape tear with some vitreous attached on to the anterior flap of the tear (Fig. 41.13).

These horse shoe tears form at the site of strong vitreoretinal adhesions like lattices (Fig. 41.14).

Retinal holes on the other hand are often caused by localized atrophy or degeneration of the retinal layers and are usually not associated with dynamic vitreoretinal traction.[42] A round retinal hole can also form when the vitreous gets detached completely from the edge of the hole as an operculum (operculated break) (Fig. 41.15). An operculum containing some retinal tissue lying in the vitreous is called a *true operculum.*

Retinal breaks that are associated with the symptoms of photopsia or floaters are called *symptomatic* retinal breaks.

These are usually associated with an acute posterior vitreous detachment. Once a break occurs, ocular movements force the fluid vitreous into the subretinal space separating the neurosensory retina from the underlying RPE resulting in a rhegmatogenous retinal detachment.[43,44]

Approximately 10–15% of all patients with an acute symptomatic PVD have at least one retinal break.[45,46] Around 70% of patients who develop a vitreous hemorrhage secondary to PVD would have developed an underlying retinal tear.[47] Vitreous hemorrhage during PVD occurs due to avulsion of a peripapillary vessel or rupture of a retina vessel.[47]

Every retinal tear does not lead to a retinal detachment. Prevalence of only a retinal tear may be as much as 83 times than that of a retinal detachment.[48] Acute symptomatic breaks seen during PVD usually results in retinal detachment. Prompt treatment of these breaks is necessary to prevent retinal detachment.[49]

Also, around 30–50% of patients with a horseshoe tear may result in retinal detachment and prophylactic treatment of these breaks can reduce the incidence of RD by 5–6%.[50] Hence prophylactic treatment of retinal tears should be recommended for symptomatic tears and horseshoe tears.[51-53]

Asymptomatic (not associated with complaints of flashes of light or floaters) operculated holes and atrophic round holes rarely lead to a retinal detachment. These may not be prophylactically treated; however, treatment may be necessary prior to cataract surgery.[49]

Some operculated holes can lead to a subclinical retinal detachment.[54] A subclinical retinal detachment is defined as subretinal fluid extending at least 1 disc diameter (DD) around the break, but no more than 2 DD posterior to the equator. Studies suggest that breaks with a subclinical RD are more likely to have a clinical retinal detachment than without a subclinical retinal detachment.[55] Nearly 31% of the phakic

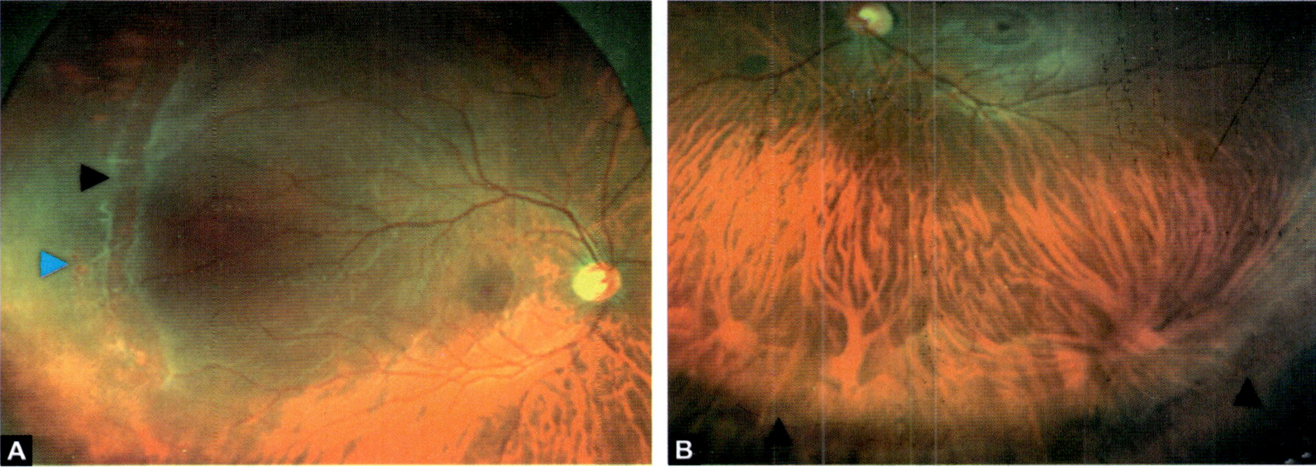

Figs. 41.16A and B: (A) Ultra-widefield pseudocolor photograph showing lattice degeneration (black arrowhead) with hole (blue arrowhead) with temporal retinal detachment. Note the typical cross-hatching of hyalinized vessels over the lesion. (B) Ultra-widefield pseudocolor photograph showing lattice degeneration (black arrowheads) in inferior retinal periphery in the other eye of same patient.

patients with a subclinical retinal detachment (SCRD) progressed to clinical RD, whereas only 5% of the patients with retinal breaks without SCRD progress to clinical RD. Prophylactic treatment for subclinical retinal detachment must be considered.[55]

Retinal detachment in the absence of posterior vitreous detachment may be seen in eyes with retinal dialysis or in eyes with small round retinal holes. RD in these cases is usually shallow and slow to progress. Presence of demarcation lines between the attached and detached retina may be seen in these cases because of the slow progress of RD. PVR may not occur in these eyes because of the tiny *rhegma* and because the formed vitreous does not allow the migration of the RPE cells responsible for PVR, into the preretinal space. Examination of the fellow eye must be done in eyes with round holes because of high chances of bilateral disease with nearly 33% of the eyes having a *mirror image distribution*.[56]

PERIPHERAL RETINAL LESIONS PREDISPOSING TO RETINAL DETACHMENT

Lattice Degeneration

Lattice degeneration is one of the most important visible retinal degeneration predisposing to retinal detachment. It is seen in 6–8% of the general population and up to 30% of cases with phakic RD.[57]

Lattice degeneration typically appears as a sharply demarcated, well-circumscribed patch of excavation or thinning of the inner retinal surface that is circumferentially oriented and is usually associated with liquefaction of the overlying vitreous gel (Figs. 41.16A and B).

Strong vitreoretinal adhesions are usually present along the edges of these lesions. Vitreous traction on these areas during PVD is often responsible for the formation of retinal tears or *edge tears*. Other features that can be seen are white hyalinized vessels in the form of fine crossing white lines, speckled areas of proliferating retinal pigment epithelium, punched out areas of extreme retinal thinning and atrophic retinal holes. The pathophysiology of these retinal lesions is not yet very well understood. Various theories that have been put forward include primary choroidal changes, embryologic vascular anastomosis, vitreous traction due to primary disorder of the vitreous, retinal ischemia, and a primary defect in the internal limiting membrane of the retina. Recent studies have evaluated the structure of lattice degeneration using spectral domain optical coherence tomography (SD-OCT). These studies have shown the presence of U-shaped vitreous traction, retinal thinning, retinal breaks and vitreous membranes.[58]

Full thickness retinal defects were found even in areas without clinically apparent holes, especially at the outer border of the ends of lattice degeneration.[59] Recent studies even implicate that variants in the *COL4A4* gene may contribute to the development of lattice degeneration of the retina.[60]

Snail track degeneration is also believed to be a variant of lattice degeneration. Presence of multiple flecks is seen associated with this form of lattice; origin of these flecks is unknown (Fig. 41.17). Pigmentation along the lattice degeneration is also seen. This pigment comes from the hyperplasia of the RPE. These lesions are treated similarly to lattice degeneration.

Maximum prevalence of lattice degeneration is seen in the second decade of life. Lattice degeneration may be unilateral (54.2%) or bilateral (45.8%) and there is no sex predilection.[61] Though some studies have mentioned that the prevalence of lattice degeneration increases with increasing axial length of the eye,[62,63] others found that the greatest prevalence of lattice degeneration was found in eyes with myopia ranging from

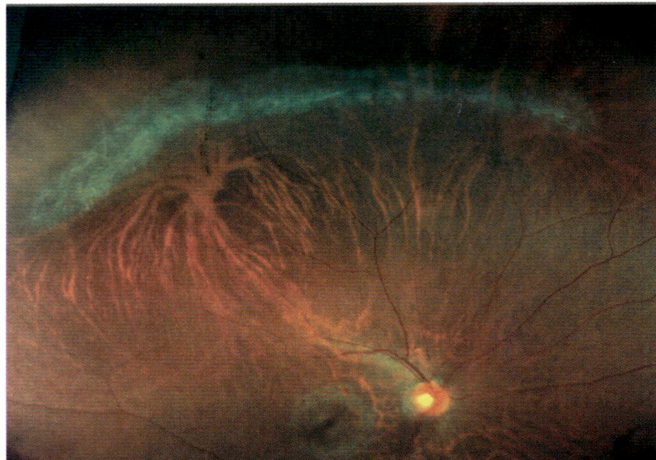

Fig. 41.17: Ultra-widefield image showing snail track degeneration can be noted in superotemporal quadrant with frosted appearance over the oval lesion. Note the absence of cross-hatching.

–6.00 to –8.70 diopters, and the least prevalence of lattice degeneration was found in eyes with a myopia of –24.00 diopters or greater.[61]

Patients with lattice degeneration are mostly asymptomatic and are usually found coincidentally during a routine fundus examination. Symptoms like acute onset of floaters or flashes of light are due to acute posterior vitreous detachment while field defect is due to the presence of retinal detachment. The chances of RD developing in an eye with lattice degeneration has been reported to be less than 1% over an average follow-up of 11 years if retinal detachment had not occurred in the other eye.[64]

Some lattice degenerations may have tiny holes in them. These holes usually occur in the middle of the patch of lattice degeneration. These are usually single and small lying within the body of the lattice. Multiple holes may also be present. These holes may occasionally cause slowly progressive retinal detachment especially in young individuals and more commonly in myopes.[65] The cumulative incidence of retinal detachment from atrophic holes has been found to be 1.5% at the age of 40 years.[66] *Horseshoe* retinal tears or edge tears along the lateral and/or posterior edge of lattice degeneration are almost always due to PVD and are frequently associated with symptoms of flashes and floaters and commonly lead to RD. Lattice degeneration needs to be differentiated from the benign lesions like paving stone degeneration or focal chorioretinal scars. The latter do not cause RD and hence are not treated.

Indications for Prophylactic Treatment of Lattice Degeneration

Presence of lattice degeneration without any symptoms or any associated features like a hole, tear or any subretinal fluid does not constitute a high risk factor for development of retinal detachment in future and hence does not require prophylactic treatment. These patients can be regularly followed up. Lattice degenerations that require treatment are:[67,68]

- Lattice degeneration associated with *edge tear* formed as a result of acute posterior vitreous detachment indicates a high risk factor for development of retinal detachment and hence requires urgent treatment.
- Lattice degeneration associated with atrophic retinal hole with progressively increasing subretinal fluid requires treatment.
- Presence of lattice degeneration in the fellow eye of RD should be given prophylactic treatment.
- Patients with lattice degeneration who have family history of RD.

Avitabile et al.[69] reported that there is a highly statistically significant difference of reduced incidence (P < 0.001) of retinal detachment in the fellow eye (1.2%) when prophylactic treatment is done as compared to the incidence of retinal detachment in the fellow eyes not treated prophylactically (13.4%).

RETINAL TUFTS

Retinal tufts are classified as cystic or noncystic.

Noncystic Retinal Tuft

Noncystic retinal tufts are thin, short and pointed projections of retinal tissue. These are usually present in clusters on the vitreous base. These contain altered retinal cells and proliferated glial tissue. They may be present at birth, and 50% of these tufts are bilateral. Tufts can be seen in all quadrants but most commonly are found in the inferonasal quadrant. Tip of the tuft may break due to degenerative changes forming tiny fragments that may float in the vitreous. They rarely result in full thickness retinal breaks hence do not predispose to rhegmatogenous retinal detachment.[70]

Cystic Retinal Tuft

These are larger than the noncystic tufts and appear as nodular projections extending from the vitreous base. These projections are often surrounded by cystic retinal degeneration. They may appear as single or in clusters. Histologically, these are similar to the noncystic tufts; composed of degenerated retinal cells and proliferated glial tissue along with some degeneration of the adjacent RPE. These are present since birth in 5% of the individuals and can be bilateral in 6% of the patients.[71,72] They do not show any predilection to any of the retinal quadrants. On indirect ophthalmoscopy these cystic tufts are easily distinguishable from the noncystic tufts because of their larger size as well as the surrounding cystic degeneration. It is important to distinguish the two because cystic tufts can lead to formation of retinal tears because of vitreous traction during posterior vitreous detachment. Cystic retinal tufts are the cause for about 7% of the retinal breaks

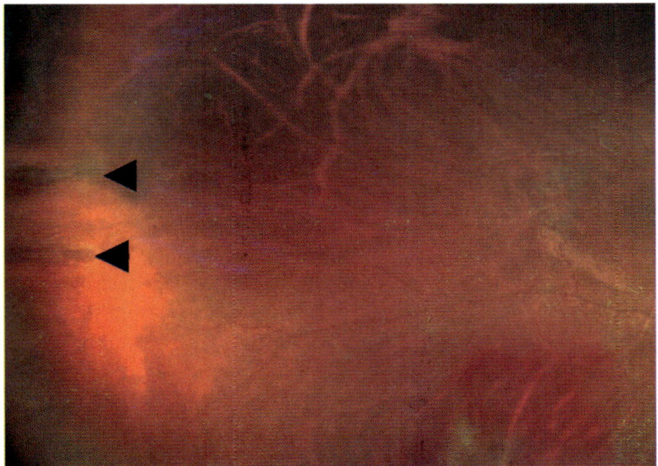

Fig. 41.18: Ultra-widefield pseudocolor photograph showing meridional complex (black arrowheads).

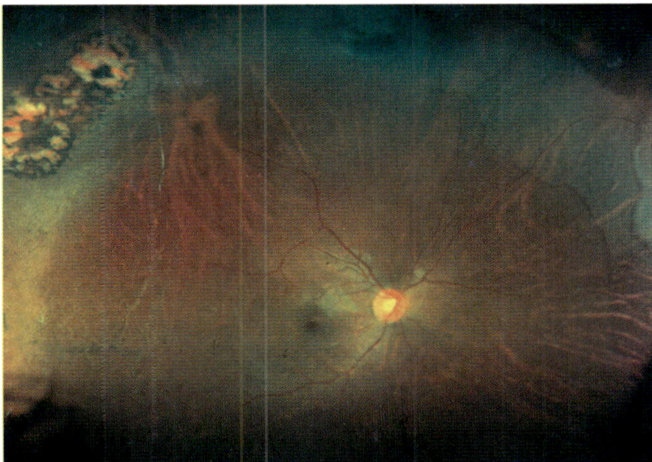

Fig. 41.19: Widefield fundus photograph showing white without pressure area along the superior quadrant between the equator and ora with a sharp posterior border.

leading to retinal detachment, but only 0.18% of the eyes with cystic retinal tufts have been reported to develop retinal detachment.[11] Prophylactic treatment of the cystic tufts without retinal tear is not advised because of the low association with retinal detachment. In another study by Murakami-Nagasako and Ohba,[73] 7.5% of nontraumatic retinal detachments were due to retinal tears associated with cystic retinal tufts.

Other peripheral retinal degeneration that are seen on routine peripheral retinal examination include meridional folds, meridional complex, pars plana cysts, enclosed oral bays, and paving stone retinal degeneration.

Meridional Folds

These are radially oriented ridge like elevations seen on the peripheral retina directed toward the vitreous (Fig. 41.18). These are typically in alignment with the dentate processes of the ora. These thickened retinal folds usually contain cystoid degeneration. These are most commonly seen in the superior nasal quadrant and may be present in 26% of the population and may be bilateral in up to 55% of the patients.[74]

When the dentate processes and ciliary process occur within the same meridian these are called as *meridional complexes*. The retinal fold in these meridional complexes is large and reaches up to the posterior ciliary processes. Usually there is a tiny retinal break at the base of these meridional complexes. These occur in 16% of the population and are bilateral in 58% of the affected patients.[74]

Pars Plana Cysts

These are commonly seen anterior to the ora serrata. These cysts are formed by the cystic fluid accumulation between the pigmented and nonpigmented epithelium.[70] These are not associated with retinal break formation or retinal detachment.

Enclosed Oral Bays

These are uncommon peripheral retinal lesions usually seen along the horizontal meridians both nasally and temporally. They are seen posterior to the ora serrata as islands of nonpigmented pars plana epithelium surrounded by neurosensory retina. Their prevalence is about 6% and 8% of those affected have bilateral lesions.[75]

White without Pressure

These are well-circumscribed areas of whiteness that appear in the peripheral retina without scleral depression. When this white area is seen on scleral depression it is called white with pressure. These are sharply defined and circumferentially oriented between the ora and the equator (Fig. 41.19). Many authors believe white without pressure to be an abnormal light reflex originating from the peripheral retina without any underlying structural changes of the retina.[76] Increased prevalence of these areas have been seen in the fellow eye of giant retinal tear. Many surgeons routinely advocate laser photocoagulation of these areas in the fellow eye of giant retinal tear (GRT).

Paving Stone or Cobble Stone Degeneration

Paving stone retinal degeneration (PSD)[77] is characterized by round shaped single/multiple, well-circumscribed area of depigmentation and retinal thinning, commonly seen between the ora serrata and the equator (Fig. 41.20).

These lesions appear yellow-white, usually with pigmented margins and a size ranging from 0.1 mm to 1.5 mm in diameter. Multiple PSDs may coalesce to form a large lesion with convexly scalloped margins. These frequently reveal prominent underlying choroidal vessels. Histologically these are composed of sharply circumscribed areas of retinal thinning due to loss of the photoreceptor, outer plexiform and

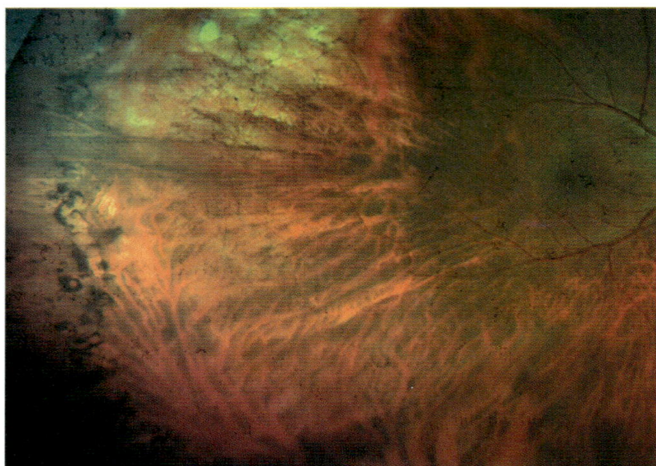

Fig. 41.20: Ultra-widefield pseudocolor image showing paving stone degeneration.

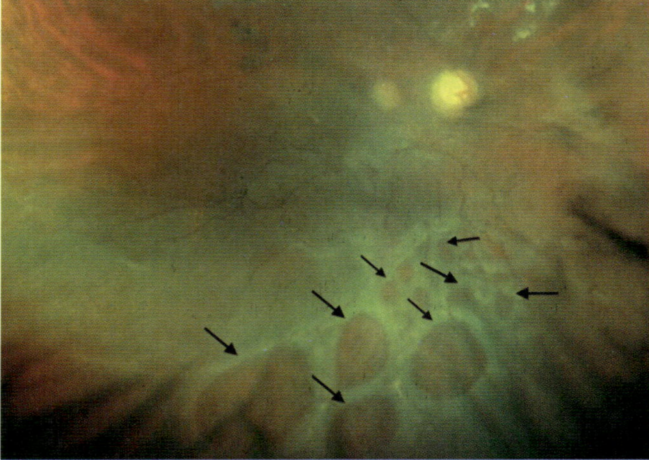

Fig. 41.21: Retinoschisis with large holes in the outer retinal layer with retinal detachment.

outer nuclear layer of the retina. There is absence of external limiting membrane, pigment epithelium and variable loss of choriocapillaris with adherence of retina to Bruch's membrane.[78] PSDs have a predilection for inferior quadrants. Paving stone degeneration is seen in 22% of adult patients, 38% of them have bilateral lesions.[78] These lesion do not lead to retinal breaks hence do not warrant any form of treatment.

RETINOSCHISIS

Retinoschisis is the splitting of neural retina into inner and outer layers. Retinoschisis may be *senile* or congenital X-linked. In senile retinoschisis, the splitting predominantly happens at the level of the outer plexiform layer while in the congenital form the split is seen at the level of the nerve fiber layer.

Senile retinoschisis is not uncommon. It is seen to be an extreme form of cystoid retinal degeneration.[79] It is seen in nearly 7% of eyes in subjects over 40 years of age and up to 16% in subjects over 60 years of age.[80] It is seen to be bilateral in nearly 57% of eyes with maximal involvement of the Inferotemporal quadrant (44.4%).[81]

Rhegmatogenous retinal detachment due to retinoschisis is rare.[82] It can occur in retinoschisis when retinal holes are seen in both the inner as well as outer layers of the schitic retina (Fig. 41.21). Holes only in the outer retinal layer may cause a localized retinal detachment as the fluid in the schisis cavity is viscous and does not spread rapidly. As there is no communication with the vitreous cavity due to an absence of a break in the inner layer, liquefied vitreous does not gain access to the subretinal space. Hence, these detachments may remain localized and rarely require any surgical intervention.[83,84] Cataract surgery is a risk factor for the progression to rhegmatogenous retinal detachment. Most surgeons do serial follow-up of these eyes.[85] Prophylactic laser if required is done to barrage or demarcate the schisis cavity. Some authors in addition also advocate scatter laser to the schisis cavity in an attempt to cause a total collapse of the cavity.[86]

Rhegmatogenous retinal detachment (RRD) with retinoschisis with outer retinal breaks have been treated with cryopexy and scleral buckle. Pars plana vitrectomy with collapse or retinectomy or deroofing of the schitic cavity has been described for progressive retinal detachment following retinoschisis with breaks both in the outer and inner retina.[85]

TREATMENT OF PREDISPOSING LESIONS

Once the decision to do prophylactic treatment has been taken it can be performed using any of the following:

- Laser photocoagulation
- Cryotherapy
- Scleral buckle in case of lattice associated with subclinical retinal detachment.

Laser photocoagulation with indirect laser ophthalmoscope (ILO) is preferred over cryotherapy because it can be done under topical anesthesia and is more comfortable for the patient. It causes minimal destruction of the underlying RPE as well as smaller retinal scars. When doing laser photocoagulation care should be taken to use moderate intensity burns. Very high intensity burns as well as treatment of large areas of lattice degeneration has the potential of inducing posterior vitreous detachment, which can cause large tears and lead to RD. If large areas of lattice need to be treated, the laser can be done in multiple consecutive sittings.

Cryotherapy is preferred in some cases of peripheral dialysis or in some retinal tears with overlying vitreous hemorrhage, which may not allow a complete laser photocoagulation. Also, in cases with associated subretinal fluid, cryotherapy may be more effective. Scleral buckling is rarely necessary. Prophylactic encircling bands for GRT have not been found to be useful.

Diagrammatic presentation of the technique of laser for various peripheral retinal lesions is shown in Figures 41.22 to 41.26.

Complications of Prophylactic Treatment

- Failure to prevent RD.
- Inadvertent laser burns to the healthy retina.
- High intensity large number of burns can induce acute PVD increasing the risk of retinal detachment.

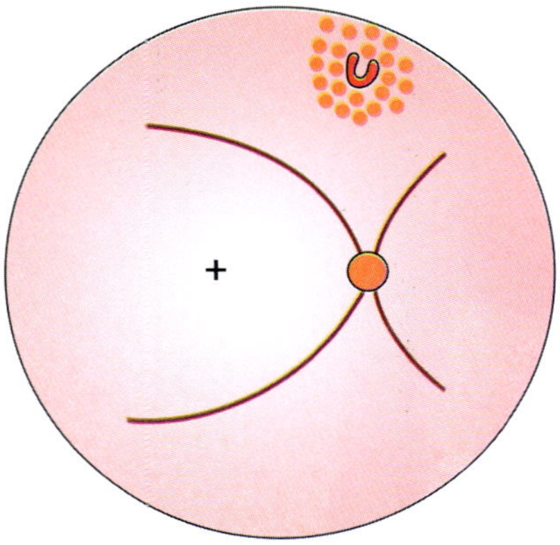

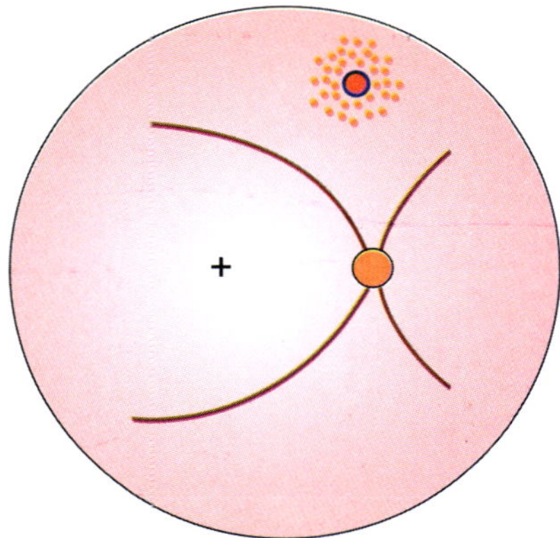

Fig. 41.22: Horseshoe tear should be lasered all around; 2–3 rows of laser should be done especially around the anterior horns.

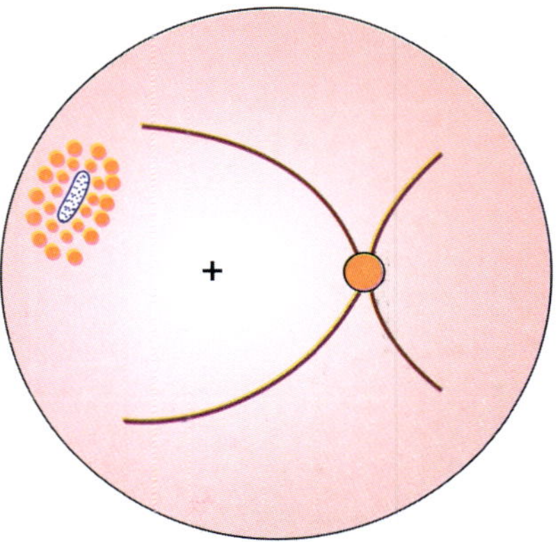

Fig. 41.23: Lattice degeneration should be lasered all around; 2–3 rows of moderate intensity laser photocoagulation should be done.

Fig. 41.24: Atrophic hole or operculated hole if needs treatment, should be lasered all around; 2–3 rows of moderate intensity laser photocoagulation should be done.

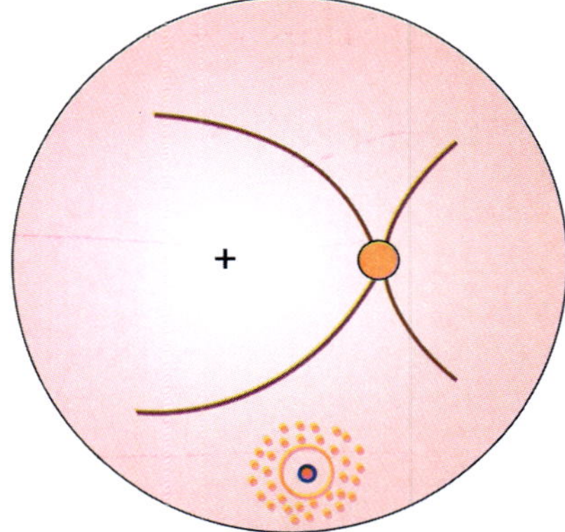

Fig. 41.25: Atrophic hole with subretinal fluid should be lasered all around with 2–3 rows of laser.

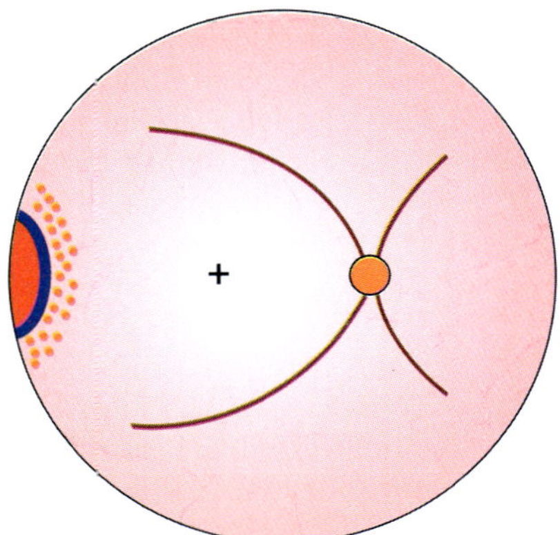

Fig. 41.26: Retinal dialysis should be lasered with 2–3 rows around the posterior edge connecting it to the ora on either side of dialysis.

- Serous choroidal detachment due to excessive laser or cryotherapy.
- Epiretinal membrane formation due to excessive cryotherapy or laser photocoagulation.

Prevention of RRD is important but this decision should be taken in consideration with various aspects like age, presence of myopia, area of retina to be lasered, presence of strong vitreoretinal adhesions in the area to be lasered, aphakia or pseudophakia, and associated vitreoretinopathies. Also, the patient should be properly counseled regarding the signs and symptoms of retinal detachment and explained the need to report early for an ophthalmic examination if any such symptoms are present. Need for a regular periodic follow-up even after prophylactic laser has been done cannot be overemphasized.

Once retinal detachment is seen, the treatment is surgical. Before surgery is done careful examination and planning is necessary. Very few ancillary investigations are necessary and a detailed retinal examination with indirect ophthalmoscope and slit-lamp biomicroscopy is most important.

DIAGNOSIS AND PREOPERATIVE ASSESSMENT OF RETINAL DETACHMENT

Preoperative assessment involves:
- Careful history
- General physical evaluation
- Anterior segment evaluation
- Posterior segment evaluation
- Finding the retinal break
- Ancillary investigations

History

A careful history to elicit the symptoms of flashes of light, floaters, visual field loss, blurring of vision or metamorphopsia should be taken. History of flashes and floaters points toward a symptomatic PVD and a careful examination of the retina to look for retinal breaks with or without retinal detachment should be done. Visual field loss usually described by the patient as a curtain falling in front of the eye is often seen in detachments extending posterior to the equator. Shallow retinal detachments or subclinical retinal detachment may not be associated with this symptom. Blurring of vision or metamorphopsia usually suggests macular involvement. Duration of these symptoms also helps the surgeon to plan the timing of surgery as well as predict a possible visual outcome of the surgery; the same can be used to counsel the patient.

Sometimes patients may not come with the presenting complain of blurring of vision especially in the pediatric age group where monocular blurring of vision goes unnoticed. Children may come with a squint or leukocoria especially if RD has been there for a long period of time.

History of previous ocular surgeries should be recorded. While previous cataract surgery may change the surgical technique (scleral buckle/pars plana vitrectomy), presence of a prior trabeculectomy may necessitate a posterior conjunctival incision. One can expect scarring during muscle manipulation if prior squint surgery has been done. History of prior refractive surgery should be recorded.

Best corrected visual acuity as well as the refractive status of the eye should be determined. It is important to know the degree of myopia to plan the surgery and to prevent the potential complications of high myopia intraoperatively. Also, presence of amblyopia should be ruled out in unilateral myopic patients.

General Physical Evaluation

It is necessary not only to assess fitness to undergo surgical intervention but also to rule out syndromic forms of retinal detachment which may be associated with connective tissue disorders, typical craniofacial anomalies and mental retardation which will have to be addressed during surgery.

Anterior Segment Evaluation

Slit lamp examination should be done to look for conjunctival scarring from previous surgery or trauma, corneal clarity, radial keratectomy marks, scleral thinning, previous surgical wound, iris coloboma or aniridia, anterior uveitis, angle-closure and lens status. Presence of these may need additional medical or surgical treatment or may affect the surgical approach. Eyes with RD usually present with low IOP. High IOP may be seen in Schwartz-Matsuo syndrome.[87] This is characterized by pigment epithelial cells/fragments of photoreceptors blocking the trabecular meshwork and increased/fluctuating IOP. This is more commonly associated with retinal tears around the vitreous base, like retinal dialysis or tears of the nonpigmented epithelium of the pars plana or pars plicata of the ciliary body.[88] Other causes of high IOP include associated glaucoma, trauma, inflammation or presence of associated hemorrhagic choroidal detachment.

Posterior Segment Evaluation

This is done using an indirect ophthalmoscope or slit-lamp biomicroscopy. Attention should be given to reconfirm rhegmatogenous retinal detachment and rule out tractional/exudative retinal detachment or retinoschisis (Table 41.1).

Note should be made of extent, configuration and height of retinal detachment, status of macula, peripheral lesions and their localization, signs of chronic detachment like retinal cysts/subretinal bands/demarcation line, signs of PVR and status of the fellow eye.

Finding the Retinal Break

A successful outcome of any retinal detachment surgery depends upon finding the break. The position of the retinal break can be determined from the configuration of RD especially in cases of a single break. Lincoff et al. showed how distribution of subretinal fluid can point toward the location of a

Table 41.1: Differentiating clinical features of three types of retinal detachment.

Features	Rhegmatogenous retinal detachment	Tractional retinal detachment	Exudative retinal detachment
Schaffer's sign	+	–	–
Posterior vitreous detachment	++	+/–	+/–
Vitreous hemorrhage	+/–	+/–	–
Contour of retinal detachment	Convex	Concave	Convex, Bullous
Surface of retinal detachment	Corrugated	Tethered	Smooth
Presence of shifting fluid	+/– May be seen in long standing retinal detachment within the area of detachment	–	++ Characteristic fluid shift across the retina

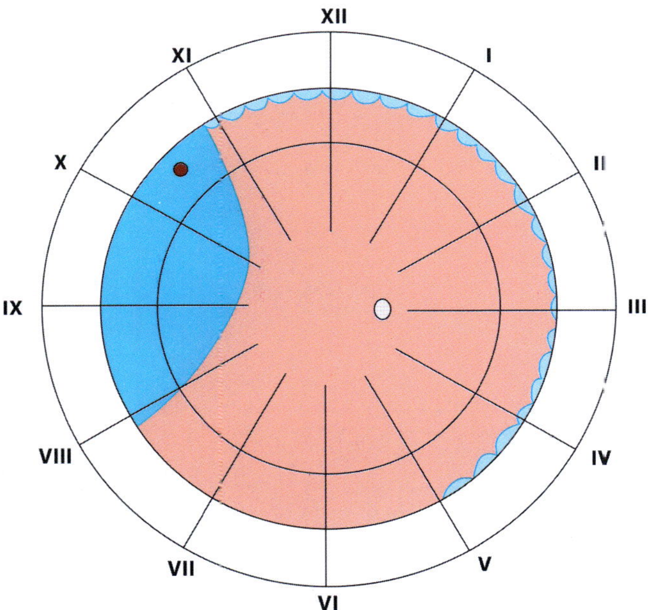

Fig. 41.27: Retinal drawing chart showing detachment involving the upper and lower quadrants but not crossing the vertical meridian. Primary break is likely to be located within 1 and 1/2 clock hours of the highest border of detachment.

Fig. 41.28: Retinal drawing chart showing detachment involving the nasal as well as the temporal inferior quadrants and the level of detachment on both sides is equal. Primary break is likely to be located at 6 o'clock if the detachment is not bullous.

retinal break. It is depicted in the following figures (Figs. 41.27 to 41.31).[89]

In case of multiple breaks, the most superior break in a detachment is designated as the *primary break* because it would produce the same contour if it were a single break.[90] Treatment of all breaks during surgery is however essential for the successful outcome.

Ancillary Investigations

These include ultrasonography (USG) and optical coherence tomography (OCT).

Ultrasound

This may be essential in cases with hazy media to confirm the diagnosis and configuration of retinal detachment (Figs. 41.32 to 41.34), in uncooperative patients, to look for PVD, to look for associated choroidal detachment (Figs. 41.35A and B) axial length measurement, in cases of trauma to look for intraocular foreign body or posterior scleral rupture or retinal incarceration.

Optical Coherence Tomography

It may be done in some cases to look for PVD or to assess the macular status in shallow retinal detachments.

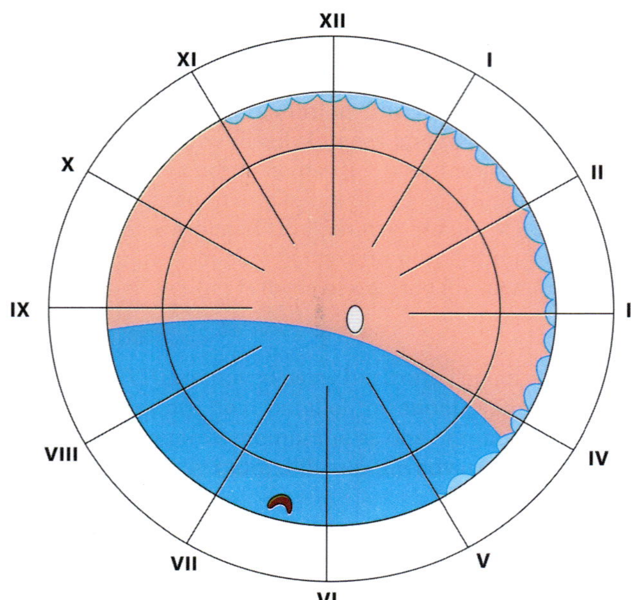

Fig. 41.29: Retinal drawing chart showing detachment involving both the lower quadrants and the level of detachment is higher on one side. Primary break is likely to be located within 1½-clock hour on that side of 6 o'clock hour where detachment is higher.

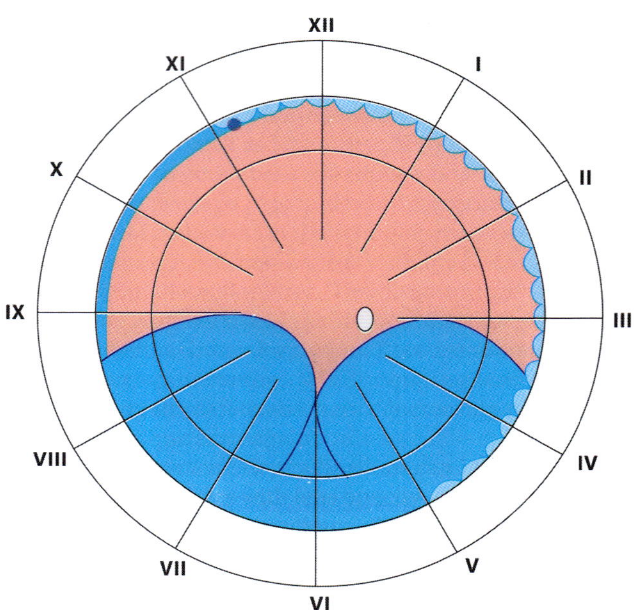

Fig. 41.30: Retinal drawing chart showing bullous detachment involving both the inferior quadrants. Primary break is often above the horizontal meridian with a communicating track of subretinal fluid (SRF) seen leading to the break.

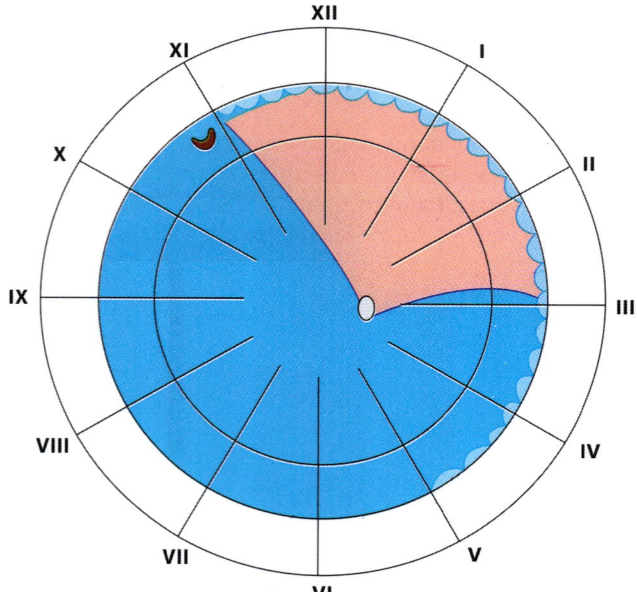

Fig. 41.31: Retinal drawing chart showing subtotal retinal detachment with a superior wedge of attached retina. Primary break is likely to be located within 1½-clock hour of the highest extent of detachment.

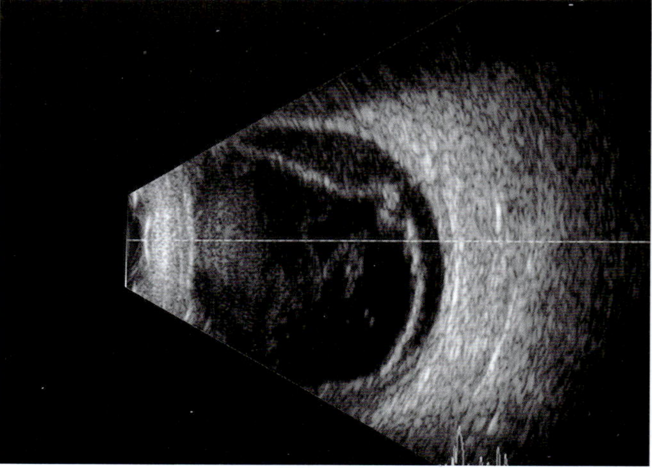

Fig. 41.32: Ultrasound B-scan showing an echogenic membrane attached to disc with smooth configuration, which had poor after movements on kinetic examination, suggestive of retinal detachment (RD) without proliferative vitreoretinopathy (PVR).

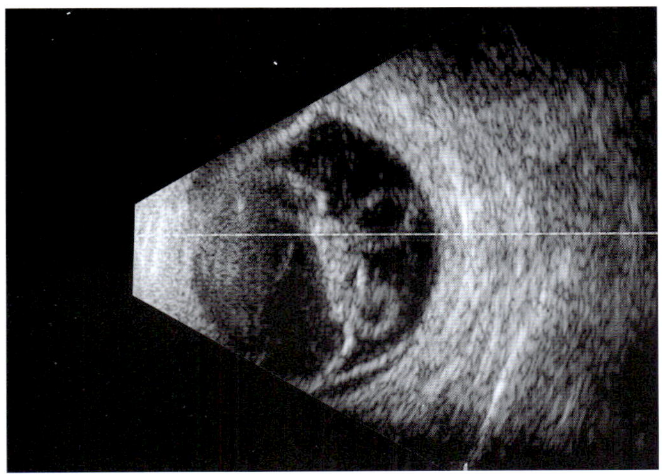

Fig. 41.33: Ultrasound B-scan showing an echogenic membrane attached to disc with intraretinal cysts, which had poor after movements on kinetic examination, suggestive of chronic retinal detachment (RD) with proliferative vitreoretinopathy (PVR).

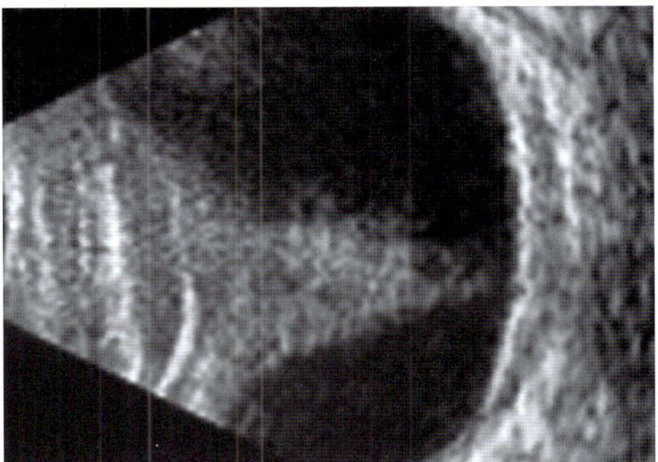

Fig. 41.34: Ultrasound B-scan showing an echogenic membrane attached to disc with closed funnel appearance suggestive of closed funnel retinal detachment (RD) with proliferative vitreoretinopathy (PVR).

PROLIFERATIVE VITREORETINOPATHY

INTRODUCTION

Proliferative vitreoretinopathy is characterized by the growth and subsequent contraction of cellular membranes on both surfaces of the retina in rhegmatogenous retinal detachment.[91] Recognition of this process is extremely important. Presence of PVR can predict the outcome and visual prognosis after retinal detachment surgery. Also, these membranes can exert retinal traction and create new retinal breaks or open up previously successfully closed retinal breaks. They can also compromise the visual outcome by obscuring the macula by forming epimacular membranes. Up to 5–10% of primary rhegmatogenous retinal detachments and up to 75% of post-surgical retinal detachments can be complicated by PVR.[92-98]

 PATHOPHYSIOLOGY OF PROLIFERATIVE VITREOUS RETINOPATHY

Membranes seen in PVR are fibrocellular in composition. These are a result of migration, metaplasia and proliferation of retinal glial cells, retinal pigment epithelium and inflammatory macrophages. Transdifferentiated fibroblast cells lay down collagen which on contraction can lead to elevation of the retina and distortion leading to tractional detachment.[99]

Development of PVR is characterized by
- Cell activation
- Cell metaplasia
- Cell proliferation
- Extracellular matrix elaboration and remodeling
- Contraction of membranes.

Cell Activation

Due to the formation of a retinal break, a large area of the RPE is exposed to the vitreous cavity causing[100,101] RPE cell activation and migration. These cells, move from the subretinal space into the vitreous cavity through the *rhegma*. These cells are usually seen in the vitreous cavity as *tobacco dust*. Proliferation of these cells then occur.[102] Physical-mechanical forces such as cryopexy can exaggerate this response.

Cellular Metaplasia

These RPE and retinal glial cells also undergo metaplasia and transform into myofibroblasts. These myofibroblasts form opaque, contractile membranes.[101-104]

Cellular Proliferation

Under normal circumstances, RPE cells and intraretinal glial cells are in resting phase. These do not proliferate actively. However, in response to ischemic, thermal or mechanical injury, proliferation of these cells start. Proliferation of these myofibroblast like cells on both surfaces of the retina, posterior lens surface, ciliary body and subretinal space result in formation of cellular membranes that are invisible but have contractile properties.

Extracellular Matrix Elaboration and Remodeling

Extracellular matrix of collagen and glycosaminoglycans, along with cellular elements of RPE cells, glial cells, fibroblasts and macrophages form the membranes seen in PVR.[105] Collagen is secreted by the metaplastic RPE cells (fibroblasts) and glial cells as pro-collagen which later on modifies leading to collagen fiber formation. It is the deposition of this collagen which transforms the invisible cellular membranes into whitish preretinal tissue which is seen as star folds on the surface of the retina and as subretinal sheets.

Contraction of Membranes

These mature membranes now exert traction on the retina causing it to pucker up.[105-107]

In addition to the role of RPE cells, inflammation also plays a very important role in the development of PVR. Breakdown of the blood-retinal barrier causes release of serum into the vitreous cavity which causes release of growth factors like platelet derived growth factor-C, transforming growth factor-beta, basic fibroblast growth factor, hepatocyte growth factor, epidermal growth factor, and vascular endothelial growth factor.

A flowchart depicting the important steps in the pathogenesis of PVR is shown below:

CLASSIFICATION OF PROLIFERATIVE VITREORETINOPATHY

Retina Society Classification published in 1983 was the first universally accepted classification for proliferative vitreoretinopathy (Table 41.2).[192]

The Retina Society classification of proliferative vitreoretinopathy as published in 1983 was later updated to accommodate major progress in the understanding of this disease. In the new classification by Machemer et al.[108] only three grades describe severity of the disease (Table 41.3). Posterior and anterior locations of PVR have been emphasized. A more detailed description of type C PVR has been made, by dividing it into focal, diffuse, subretinal, circumferential contraction, and anterior displacement. The extent of the abnormality has been detailed by using clock hours instead of quadrants.

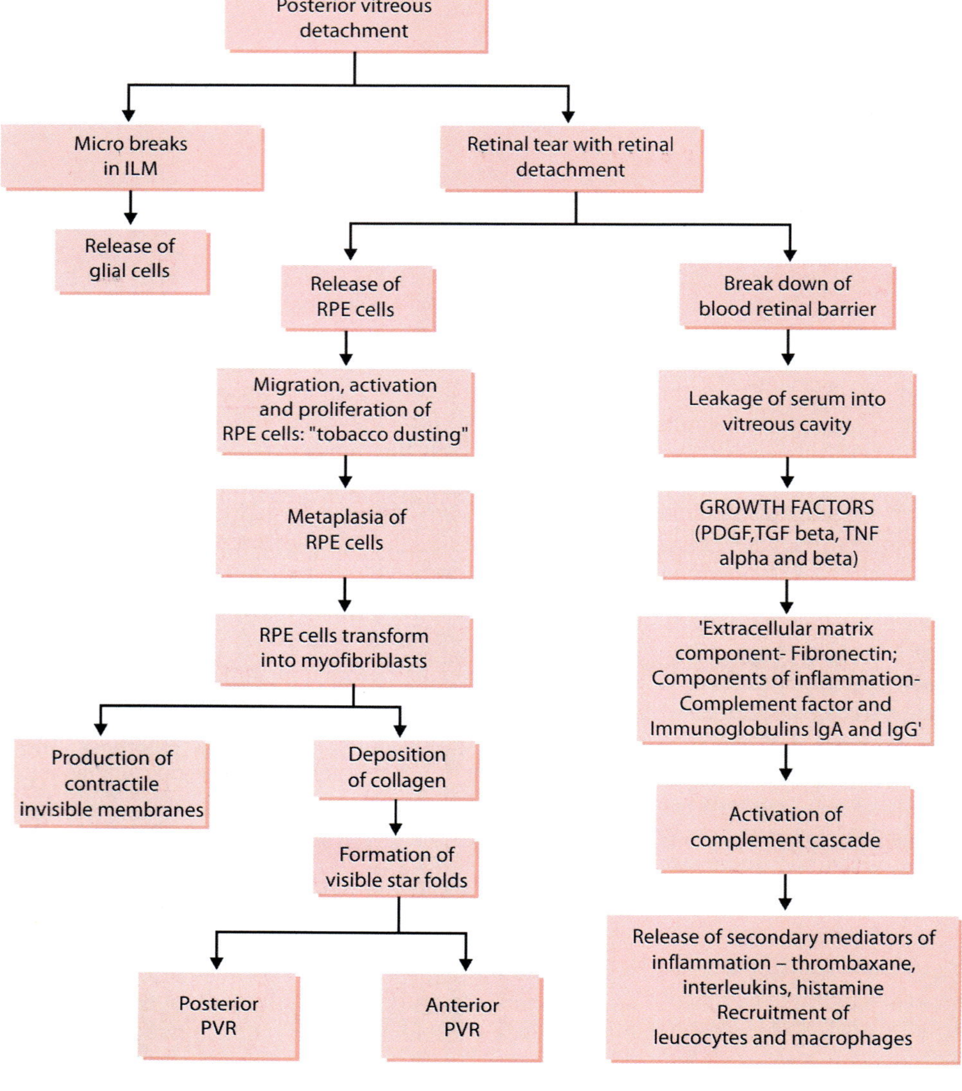

Table 41.2: Stages of proliferative vitreoretinopathy as per Retina Society Classification (1983).

Stage	Description of proliferative vitreoretinopathy
A (minimal)	Vitreous haze, tobacco dusting or vitreous pigments
B (moderate)	Wrinkling of inner retinal surface, rolled edges of retinal breaks, increased vessel tortuosity, increased retinal stiffness
C (marked)	Formation of retinal star folds
C1	Fixed retinal star folds in one quadrant
C2	Fixed retinal star folds in two quadrants
C3	Fixed retinal star folds in three quadrants
D (massive)	Fixed retinal star folds in all quadrants
D1	Wide open funnel configuration
D2	Narrow funnel
D3	Closed funnel (optic nerve head not visible)

Table 41.3: Modification of original Retina Society Classification of proliferative vitreoretinopathy by Machemer (1991).

Grade	Features
A	Vitreous haze, vitreous pigment clumps, or clusters on inferior retina
B (Fig. 41.36)	Wrinkling of retinal surface, decreased mobility of vitreous, retinal stiffness, increased vessel tortuosity, rolled and irregular edge of retinal break
CP1-12	Posterior to equator: focal, diffuse, or circumferential full-thickness retinal folds (Fig. 41.37) or subretinal strands in the form of annular strands or subretinal bands

PREDISPOSING FACTORS

Probability of PVR increases with various factors that increase the vascular permeability. Various risk factors that increase the risk of PVR include:[97,109-112]

- Large retinal tears
- Multiple retinal tears
- Large retinal detachments involving greater than 2 quadrants
- Prolonged retinal detachment
- Uveitis
- Vitreous hemorrhage
- Associated hemorrhagic or serous choroidal detachments

- Aphakia
- Multiple previous surgeries
- Trauma
- Abnormal vitreous as seen in conditions like Wagner syndrome, Stickler syndrome, Marfan syndrome and Familial exudative retinopathy.

Proliferative retinopathy may also develop following various retinal surgical procedures like scleral buckling and pars plana vitrectomy. Surgical procedures involving excessive retinal resection like relaxing retinectomies, macular translocation, ocular tumor resection and implantation of retinal prosthesis may induce rapid and severe PVR.

Surgical causes increasing PVR during scleral buckling and causing secondary or recurrent RD include:

- Excessive cryotherapy during scleral buckling[113]
- Open retinal break
- Choroidal detachment (hemorrhagic or serous)[114]
- Vitreous hemorrhage
- Retinal incarceration or retinal break formation during subretinal fluid drainage.

This is typically seen 4–12 weeks after the surgical procedure. Hence examination must be done at this time to look for any recurrence of RD due to PVR.

Factors predisposing to the development of PVR following PPV include:

- Excessive intraoperative bleeding
- Inability to completely remove the blood
- Choroidal detachment (hemorrhagic or serous)
- Open retinal break
- Inadequate traction relief
- Instrument touch causing retinal or choroidal bleed
- Excessive or high intensity laser photocoagulation which may lead to small multiple Bruch's membrane rupture.
- Large retinectomies, inadequate trimming of the peripheral redundant anterior retinal flaps of large retinal tears or anterior edge of the relaxing retinotomy.
- Excessive use of diathermy
- Impurities in silicone oil causing inflammation
- Postoperative infections or inflammation.

All risk factors for PVR are basically associated with intravitreal dispersion of RPE cells or breakdown of the blood-ocular barrier, which are prerequisite to development of PVR.[115]

Hence uncomplicated and meticulous surgery goes a long way to keep PVR at bay and improve the success rate of RD surgery. It is important to understand these factors and make an effort to reduce PVR because not only does PVR bring down the success rates of RD surgery but also the final visual recovery in these eyes is limited in spite of successful reattachment of the retina.[115]

Surgeons have also used steroid injection intravitreally at the end of the surgery to prevent PVR.[116]

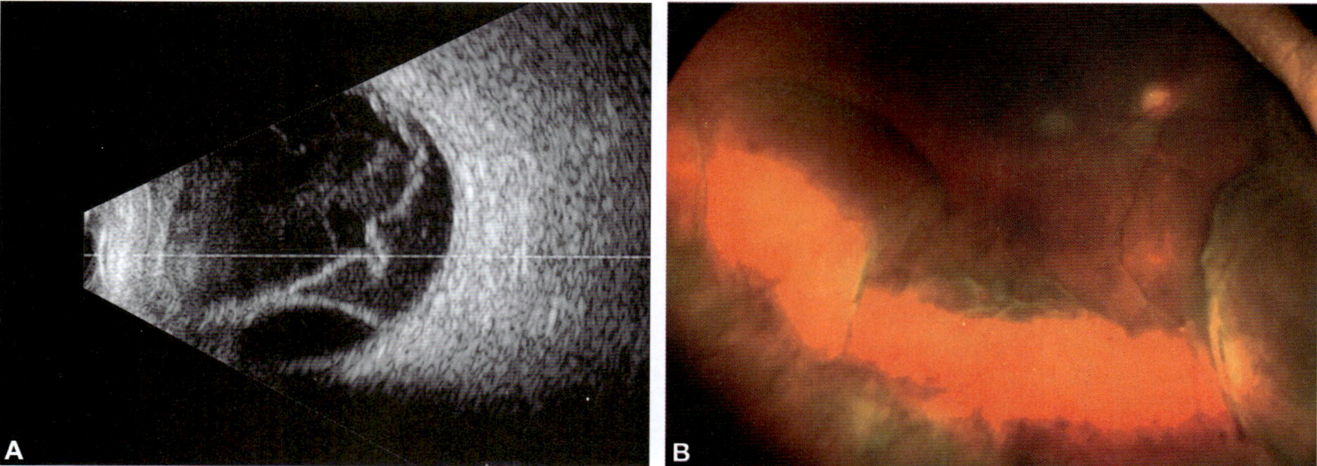

Figs. 41.35A and B: (A) Ultrasound B-scan showing an echogenic membrane attached to disc with poor after movements suggestive of retinal detachment (RD). A smooth membranous mount can be seen inferiorly suggestive of serous choroidal detachment. (B) Ultra-widefield photographs showing retinal detachment with choroidal detachment.

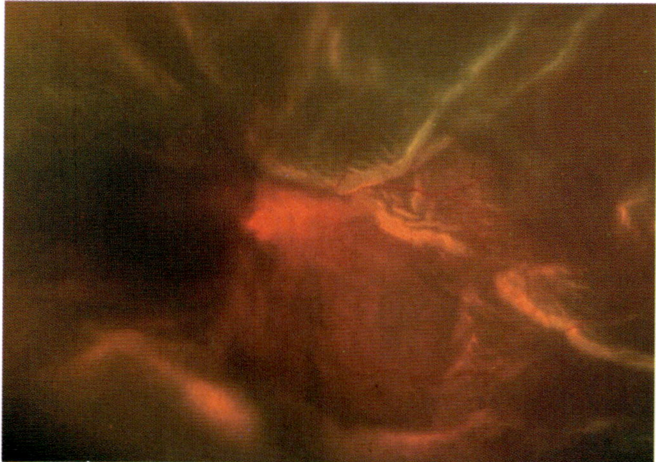

Fig. 41.36: Ultra-widefield pseudocolor photographs of retinal detachment with proliferative vitreoretinopathy showing wrinkling of retina. Note the vitreous haze blurring retinal details.

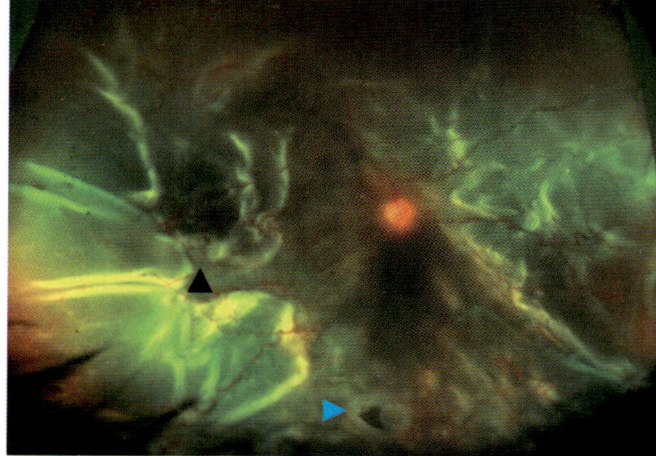

Fig. 41.37: Ultra-widefield pseudocolor image showing total retinal detachment with rolled out edges of break (blue arrowhead) with fixed folds (black arrowhead) proliferative vitreoretinopathy (PVR CP2).

MEDICAL MANAGEMENT OF PROLIFERATIVE VITREORETINOPATHY

Surgery is the only treatment once PVR sets in; it has the potential of affecting the visual and anatomical outcome of RD surgery. Surgical success may be seen in 60–80% of cases with PVR depending on the severity of PVR present.[117] Various pharmacologic therapies have been used by surgeons in an effort to prevent PVR.

Corticosteroids are the most common adjunctive agents used for preventing PVR. Steroids reduce the inflammatory process by reducing the histamine production and inhibiting cellular proliferation. In animal models of PVR, periocular or intravitreal corticosteroid injections have been found to show good results. Intravitreal triamcinolone has been used to prevent postoperative PVR. Jonas et al. found that intravitreal injections of crystalline cortisone could reduce postoperative intraocular inflammation without toxicity to the intraocular structures.[118] Blumenkranz et al.[119] found that steroids have a better inhibitory effect on PVR at higher doses.

However, other studies have shown limited benefit of steroids in preventing PVR.[121] So the potential benefits of use of steroids must be weighed against occurrence of known side effects like glaucoma and cataract.[122]

Given the role of cell proliferation in PVR, antineoplastic drugs that target reproducing cells have also been used to prevent PVR. Agents that have been studied in animal models or cell culture models include 5-fluorouracil (5-FU), daunorubicin, mitomycin, vincristine, and bleomycin sulfate.[123] Among these agents, 5-FU and daunorubicin have been extensively evaluated for prevention of PVR.

5-FU has been used in other ocular surgeries like trabeculectomy and removal of conjunctival lesions. A sustained-release bioerodible device with modifiable release properties for intraocular drug delivery has also been used for delivery of 5-FU in animal eyes.[124] Researchers believe that slow release of the drug by this method reduces the risk of toxicity and increases the efficacy by providing a constant concentration of drug during the active phase of the disease.[124]

A combination of 5-FU with low molecular weight heparin has also been used in the perioperative infusion fluid to prevent the occurrence of PVR following PPV for rhegmatogenous retinal detachment. A randomized controlled trial of combined 5-FU and low-molecular-weight heparin (LMWH) in the management of rhegmatogenous retinal detachment undergoing primary vitrectomy by Wickham et al.[124] concluded that adjuvant therapy with 5-FU and LMWH does not improve the anatomic or visual success rate of PPV for primary retinal detachments. They in fact observed a worse visual outcome in patients presenting with macula-sparing retinal detachments. Hence, they recommended that a combination of 5-FU and LMWH should not be used routinely for primary RRD surgery.[125,126]

Daunorubicin is an anthracycline antibiotic. It acts as a *topoisomerase inhibitor*.[125] An experimental study from our center, using intravitreal daunorubicin concluded that 5 micrograms of intravitreal daunorubicin effectively inhibited PVR in the rabbit eye and the dosage was safe and nontoxic. The half-life of the drug was determined to be about 140 minutes, suggesting a prolonged intravitreal concentration sufficient to prevent fibroblast proliferation.[127] A subsequent prospective, single-center, controlled clinical trial from the same author showed increased settlement of retinal detachment eyes in the daunomycin group versus controls with a statistically significant reduction of vitreous haze in the treatment group.[128] Major drawback of using antineoplastic drugs is because of their potential side effects especially if systemic absorption is seen. Antineoplastic therapies target cells that are biologically active. Creten et al.[129] showed systemic absorption of 5-FU in 2 patients which could be seen for up to 48 hours in the urine after receiving 5-FU through vitrectomy infusion. Hence, caution must be used when using these drugs especially when their efficacy is questionable.

Various other growth factors and cytokines have been implicated in the pathogenesis of PVR leading to targeting specific molecules. Some of the growth factors which have been studied in animal models for inhibiting PVR include protein kinase C, transforming growth factor-beta, epidermal growth factor, microtubules, and platelet-derived growth factor.[130,131] PVR is a multifactorial disease caused by interaction of several cells and various intraocular and extraocular factors. Therefore, therapeutic options based on the inhibition of one factor or phenomenon may be not be successful.[132]

Newer treatment modalities need to be evaluated before PVR can be managed medically. Till then the secret to success lies in meticulous surgery and correct planning.

REFERENCES

1. Chow RL, Lang RA. Review early eye development in vertebrates. Annu Rev Cell Dev Biol. 2001;17:255-96.
2. Cantrill HL, Pederson JE. Experimental retinal detachment. VI. The permeability of the blood-retinal barrier. Arch Ophthalmology. 1984;102(5):747-51.
3. Marmor MF, Negi A. Pharmacologic modification of subretinal fluid absorption in the rabbit eye. Arch Ophthalmology. 1986;104(11):1674-7.
4. Foulds WS. The vitreous in retinal detachment. Trans Ophthalmology Soc UK. 1975;95(3):412-6.
5. Yao XY, Hageman GS, Marmor MF. Retinal adhesiveness is weakened by enzymatic modification of the in vivo. Invest Ophthalmology Vis Sci. 1990;31(10):2051-8.
6. Anderson DH, Guerin CJ, Erickson PA, et al. Morphological recovery in the reattached retina. Invest Ophthalmology Vis Sci. 1986;27(2):168-83.
7. Hageman GS, Marmor MF, Yao XY, et al. The interphotoreceptor matrix mediates primate retinal adhesion. Arch Ophthalmology. 1995; 113(5):655-60.
8. Marmor MF, Yao XY, Hageman GS. Retinal adhesiveness in surgically enucleated human eyes. Retina. 1994;14(2):181-6.
9. Snead MP, Snead DR, James S, et al. Clinicopathological changes at the vitreoretinal junction: posterior vitreous detachment. Eye (Lond). 2008;22(10):1257-62.
10. Bardbury MJ, Landers MB. Pathogenetic mechanisms of retinal detachment. In: Ryan SJ, Wilkinson CP (Eds). Retina. Mosby: St Louis; 2001. pp. 1987-93.
11. Byer NE. Changes in prognosis of lattice degeneration of the retina. Trans Am Acad Ophthalmology Otolaryngol. 1974;78(2):114-25.
12. Curtin BJ. The Myopias. Philadelphia: Harper and Row; 1985. p. 337.
13. Norregaard JC, Thoning H, Anderson TF, et al. Risk of retinal detachment following cataract extraction: results from the international cataract surgery outcomes study. Br J Ophthalmology. 1996;80(8):689-93.
14. Musch DC, Meyer RF, Sugar A, et al. Retinal detachment following penetrating keratoplasty. Arch Ophthalmology. 1986;104(11):1617-20.
15. Arevalo JF, Ramirez E, Suarez E, et al. Rhegmatogenous retinal detachment after laser-assisted in situ keratomileusis (LASIK) for the correction of myopia. Retina. 2000;20(4):338-41.
16. Sharma T, Gopal L, Shanmugam MP, et al. Retinal detachment in Marfan syndrome: clinical characteristics and surgical outcome. Retina. 2002;22(4):423-8.
17. Ang A, poulson AV, Goodburn SF, et al. Retinal detachment and prophylaxis in type 1 Stickler syndrome. Ophthalmology. 2008;115(1):164-8.
18. Weinberg DV, Lyon AT, Greenwald MJ, et al. Rhegmatogenous retinal detachments in children: risk factors and surgical outcomes. Ophthalmology. 2003;110(9):1708-13.
19. Jesberg DO, Schepens CL. Retinal detachment associated with coloboma of the choroid. Arch Ophthalmology. 1961;65:163-73.

20. Ahmadieh H, Soheilian M, Azarmina M, et al. Surgical management of retinal detachment secondary to acute retinal necrosis: clinical features, surgical techniques, and long-term results. Jpn J Ophthalmology. 2003;47(5):484-91.

21. Kerkhoff FT, Lamberts QJ, van den Biesen PR, et al. Rhegmatogenous retinal detachment and uveitis. Ophthalmology. 2003;110(2):427-31.

22. Uyama M, Takahashi K, Kozaki J, et al. Uveal effusion syndrome: clinical features, surgical treatment, histologic examination of the sclera, and pathophysiology. Ophthalmology. 2000;107(3):441-9.

23. el Baba F, Jarrett WH 2nd, Harbin TS Jr, et al. Massive hemorrhage complicating age-related macular degeneration. Clinicopathologic correlation and role of anticoagulants. Ophthalmology. 1986;93(12):1581-92.

24. Steinberg RH. Research update: report from a workshop on cell biology of retinal detachment. Exp Eye Res. 1986;43(5):695-706.

25. Nasir M. The age of onset of posterior vitreous detachment. Surv Ophthalmology. 1995;39(5):426-7.

26. Yonemoto J, Ideta H, Sasaki K, et al. The age of onset of posterior vitreous detachment. Graefes Arch Clin Exp Ophthalmology. 1994; 232(2):67-70.

27. Swann DA, Constable IJ. Vitreous structure. I. Distribution of hyaluronate and protein. Invest Ophthalmology. 1972;11(3):159-63.

28. Bhutto IA, Kim SY, McLeod DS, et al. Localization of collagen XVIII and the endostatin portion of collagen XVIII in aged human control eyes and eyes with age-related macular degeneration. Invest Ophthalmology Vis Sci. 2004;45(5):1544-52.

29. Theocharis DA, Skandalis SS, Noulas AV, et al. Hyaluronan and chondroitin sulfate proteoglycans in the supramolecular organization of the mammalian vitreous body. Connect Tissue Res. 2008;49(3):124-8.

30. Wu YJ, La Pierre DP, Wu J, et al. The interaction of versican with its binding partners. Cell Res. 2005;15(7):483-94.

31. Bishop PN. Structural macromolecules and supramolecular organisation of the vitreous gel. Prog Retin Eye Res. 2000;19(3): 323-44.

32. Le Goff MM, Bishop PN. Adult vitreous structure and postnatal changes. Eye (Lond). 2008;22(10):1214-22.

33. Bishop PN, Holmes DF, Kadler KE, et al. Age-related changes on the surface of vitreous collagen fibrils. Invest Ophthalmology Vis Sci. 2004;45(4):1041-6.

34. Spitzer MS, Januschowski K. Aging and age-related changes of the vitreous body. Ophthalmologe. 2015;112(7):552,554-8.

35. Kuhna F, Aylward B. Rhegmatogenous retinal detachment: a reappraisal of its pathophysiology and treatment. Ophthalmic Res. 2014;51(1):15-31.

36. Morita H, Funata M, Tokoro T. A clinical study of the development of posterior vitreous detachment in high myopia. Retina. 1995;15(2):117-24.

37. Akiba J. Prevalence of posterior vitreous detachment in high myopia. Ophthalmology. 1993;100(9):1384-8.

38. Navarro RM, Machado LM, Maia O Jr, et al. Small-Gauge Pars Plana Vitrectomy for the Management of Symptomatic Posterior Vitreous Detachment after Phacoemulsification and Multifocal Intraocular Lens Implantation: A Pilot Study from the Pan-American Collaborative Retina Study Group. J Ophthalmology. 2015;2015:156910.

39. Mason JO 3rd, Neimkin MG, Mason JO 4th, et al. Safety, efficacy, and quality of life following sutureless vitrectomy for symptomatic vitreous floaters. Retina. 2014;34(6):1055-61.

40. Henry CR, Smiddy WE, Flynn HW Jr. Pars plana vitrectomy for vitreous floaters: is there such a thing as minimally invasive vitreoretinal surgery? Retina. 2014;34(6):1043-5.

41. De Nie KF, Crama N, Tilanus MA, et al. Pars plana vitrectomy for disturbing primary vitreous floaters: clinical outcome and patient satisfaction. Graefes Arch Clin Exp Ophthalmology. 2013;251(5):1373-82.

42. Green WR, Sebag J. Vitreoretinal interface. In: Ryan SJ, Wilkinson CP (Eds). Retina, 3rd edition. Mosby: St Louis; 2001. pp. 1897-906.

43. Machemer R. The importance of fluid absorption, traction, intraocular currents, and chorioretinal scars in the theory of rhematogenous retinal detachments. Am J Ophthalmology. 1984;98:681-93.

44. Machemer R, Williams JM Sr. Pathogenesis and therapy of traction detachment in various retinal vascular diseases. Am J Ophthalmology. 1988;105(2):170-81.

45. Linder B. Acute posterior vitreous detachment and its retinal complications. Acta Ophthalmology. 1966;87:1-108.

46. Tasman WS. Posterior vitreous detachment and peripheral retinal breaks. Trans Am Acad Ophthalmology Otolaryngol. 1968;72(2): 217-24.

47. Lindgren G, Lindblom B. Causes of vitreous hemorrhage. Curr Opin Ophthalmology. 1996;7(3):13-9.

48. Jaffe N. Complications of acute posterior vitreous detachment. Arch Ophthalmology 1968;79(5):568-71.

49. Davis MD. Natural history of retinal breaks without detachment. Arch Ophthalmology. 1974;92(3):183-94.

50. Colyear BH Jr, Pischel DK. Clinical tears in the retina without detachment. Am J Ophthalmology. 1956;41(5):773-92.

51. Byer NE. Clinical study of retinal breaks. Trans Am Acad Ophthalmology Otolaryngol. 1967;71(3):461-73.

52. Neumann E, Hyams S, Barakai S. Conservative management of retina breaks: a follow-up study of subsequent retinal detachment. Br J Ophthalmology. 1972;56(6):482-6.

53. Combs JL, Welch RB. Retinal breaks without detachment: natural history, management and long-term follow-up. Trans Am Ophthalmology Soc. 1982;80:64-97.

54. Byer NE. Subclinical retinal detachment resulting from asymptomatic retinal breaks: prognosis for progression and regression. Ophthalmology. 2001;108(8):1499-503.

55. Kazahaya M. Prophylaxis of retinal detachment. Semin Ophthalmology. 1995;10(1):79-86.

56. Ung T, Comer MB, Ang AJ, et al. Clinical features and surgical management of retinal detachment secondary to round retinal holes. Eye (Lond). 2005;19(6):665-9.

57. Wilkinson CP. Interventions for asymptomatic retinal breaks and lattice degeneration for preventing retinal detachment. Cochrane Database Syst Rev. 2014;9:CD003170.

58. Manjunath V, Taha M, Fujimoto JG, et al. Posterior lattice degeneration characterized by spectral domain optical coherence tomography. Retina. 2011;31(3):492-6.

59. Kothari A, Narendran V, Saravanan VR. In vivo sectional imaging of the retinal periphery using conventional optical coherence tomography systems. Indian J Ophthalmology. 2012;60(3):235-9.

60. Meguro A, Ideta H, Ota M, et al. Common variants in the COL4A4 gene confer susceptibility to lattice degeneration of the retina. PLoS One. 2012;7(6):e39300.

61. Celorio JM, Pruett RC. Prevalence of lattice degeneration and its relation to axial length in severe myopia. Am J Ophthalmology. 1991;111(1):20-3.

62. Cheng SC, Lam CS, Yap MK. Prevalence of myopia-related retinal changes among 12–18 year old Hong Kong Chinese high myopes. Ophthalmic Physiol Opt. 2013;33(6):652-60.

63. Lam DS, Fan DS, Chan WM, et al. Prevalence and characteristics of peripheral retinal degeneration in Chinese adults with high myopia: a cross-sectional prevalence survey. Optom Vis Sci. 2005;82(4):235-8.

64. Byer NE. Long-term natural history of lattice degeneration of the retina. Ophthalmology. 1989;96(9):1396-401.

65. Wilkinson CP, Rice TA. Retinal Holes within Lattice Degenration: Michels Retinal Detachment. St Louis: Mosby; 1997. pp. 29-100.

66. Sasaki K, Ideta H, Yonemoto J, et al. Risk of retinal detachment in patients with lattice degeneration. Jpn J Ophthalmology. 1998; 42(4):308-13.

67. Wilkinson CP. Evidence-based analysis of prophylactic treatment of asymptomatic retinal breaks and lattice degeneration. Ophthalmology. 2000;107(1):12-5.

68. Wilkinson C. Interventions for asymptomatic retinal breaks and lattice degeneration for preventing retinal detachment. Cochrane Database Syst Rev. 2012;3:CD003170.

69. Avitabile T, Bonfiglio V, Reibaldi M, et al. Prophylactic treatment of the fellow eye of patients with retinal detachment: a retrospective study. Graefes Arch Clin Exp Ophthalmology. 2004;242(3):191-6.

70. Spencer LM, Foos RY, Straatsma BR. Meridional folds, meridional complexes, and associated abnormalities of the peripheral retina. Am J Ophthalmology. 1970;70(5):679-714.

71. Byer NE. Relationship of cystic retinal tufts to retinal detachment. Dev Ophthalmology. 1981;2:36-42.

72. Byer NE. Cystic retinal tufts and their relationship to retinal detachment. Arch Ophthalmology. 1981;99(10):1788-90.

73. Murakami-Nagasako F, Ohba N. Phakic retinal detachment associated with cystic retinal tuft. Graefes Arch Clin Exp Ophthalmology. 1982;219(4):188-92.

74. Spencer LM, Foos RY, Straatsma BR. Meridonal folds and meridional complexes of the peripheral retina. Trans Am Acad Ophthalmology Otolaryngol. 1969;73(2):204-21.

75. Spencer LM, Foos RY, Straatsma BR. Enclosed bays of the ora serrate. Relationship to retina tears. Arch Ophthalmology. 1970;83(4):421-5.

76. Byer NE: The Peripheral Retina in Profile—A Stereoscopic Atlas. Torrance, CA: Criterion Press; 1982. p. 112.

77. Shukla M, Anuja OP. White with pressure (WWP) and white without pressure (WWOP) lesions. Indian J Ophthalmology. 1982;30(3):129-32.

78. O'Malley PF, Allen RA, Straatsma BR, et al. Paving-stone degeneration of the retina. Arch Ophthalmology. 1965;73:169-82.

79. Zimmerman LE, Spencer WH. The pathologic anatomy of retinoschisis,with a report of two cases diagnosed as malignant melanoma. Arch Ophthalmology. 1960;63:10-9.

80. Byer NE. Clinical study of senile retinoschisis. Arch Ophthalmology. 1968;79(1):36-44.

81. Buch H, Vinding T, Nielsen NV. Prevalence and long-term natural course of retinoschisis among elderly individuals: the Copenhagen City Eye Study. Ophthalmology. 2007;114(4):751-5.

82. Byer NE. Long-term natural history study of senile retinoschisis with implications for management. Ophthalmology. 1986;93(9): 1127-37.

83. Byer NE. The natural history of senile retinoschisis. Trans Am Acad Ophthalmology Otolaryngol. 1976;81:458.

84. Shanmugam MP, Nagpal A. Foveal schisis as a cause of retinal detachment secondary to macular hole in juvenile X-linked retinoschisis. Retina. 2005;25(3):373-5.

85. Muqit MM, Xue K, Patel CK. National survey of progressive symptomatic retinal detachment complicating retinoschisis in the United Kingdom. Eye (Lond). 2013; 27(12):1425-6.

86. Yassur Y, Feldberg R, Axer-Siegel R, et al. Argon laser treatment of senile retinoschisis. Br J Ophthalmology. 1983;67(6):381-4.

87. Matsuo T. Photoreceptor outer segments in aqueous humor: key to understanding a new syndrome. Surv Ophthalmology. 1994;39(3): 211-33.

88. Matsuo T, Muraoka N, Shiraga F, et al. Schwartz-Matsuo syndrome in retinal detachment with tears of the nonpigmented epithelium of the ciliary body. Acta Ophthalmology Scand. 1998;76(4):481-5.

89. Lincoff H, Gieser R. Finding the retinal hole. Arch Ophthalmology. 1971;85(5):565-9.

90. Saxena S, Lincoff H. Finding the retinal break in rhegmatogenous retinal detachment. Indian J Ophthalmology. 2001;49(3):199-202.

91. The Retina Society Terminology Committee. The classification of retinal detachment with proliferative vitreoretinopathy. Ophthalmology. 1983;90:121.

92. Speicher MA, Fu AD, Martin JP, et al. Primary vitrectomy alone for repair of retinal detachments following cataract surgery. Retina. 2000 20(5):459-64.

93. Duquesne N, Bonnet M, Adeleine P. Preoperative vitreous hemorrhage associated with rhegmatogenous retinal detachment: a risk factor for postoperative proliferative vitreoretinopathy? Graefes Arch Clin Exp Ophthalmology. 1996;234(11):677-82.

94. Greven CM, Sanders RJ, Brown GC, et al. Pseudophakic retinal detachments. Anatomic and visual results. Ophthalmology. 1992;99(2):257-62.

95. Girard P, Mimoun G, Karpouzas I, et al. Clinical risk factors for proliferative vitreoretinopathy after retinal detachment surgery. Retina. 1994;14(5):417-24.

96. Gartry DS, Chignell AH, Franks WA, et al. Pars plana vitrectomy for the treatment of rhegmatogenous retinal detachment uncomplicated by advanced proliferative vitreoretinopathy. Br J Ophthalmology. 1993;77(4):199-203.

97. Bonnet M, Fleury J, Guenoun S, et al. Cryopexy in primary rhegmatogenous retinal detachment: a risk factor for postoperative proliferative vitreoretinopathy? Graefes Arch Clin Exp Ophthalmology. 1996;234(12):739-43.

98. Heimann H, Bornfeld N, Friedrichs W, et al. Primary vitrectomy without scleral buckling for rhegmatogenous retinal detachment. Graefes Arch Clin Exp Ophthalmology. 1996;234:561-8.

99. Ryan SJ. The pathophysiology of proliferative vitreoretinopathy and its management. Am J Ophthalmology. 1985;100(1):188-93.

100. Vidaurri-Leal JS, Glaser BM. Effect of fibrin on morphologic characteristics of retinal pigment epithelial cells. Arch Ophthalmology. 1984;102(9):1376-9.

101. Campochiaro PA, Bryan JA III, Cpnway BP, et al. Intravitreal chemotactic and mitogenic activity implications of blood retinal barrier break down. Arch Ophthalmology. 1986;104:1685-7.

102. Campochiaro PA, Glaser BM. Mechanism involved in retinal pigment epithelial cell chemotaxis. Arch Ophthalmology. 1986; 104(2);277-80.

103. Glaser BM, Cardin A, Biscoe B. Proliferative vitreoretinopathy. The mechanism of development of vitreoretinal traction. Ophthalmology. 1987;94(4):327-32.

104. Miller B, Miller H, Patterson R, et al. Retinal wound healing, cellular activity at the vitreoretinal interface. Arch Ophthalmology. 1986;104(2):281-5.

105. Machemer R. Massive periretinal proliferation, a logical approach to therapy. Trans Am Ophthalmology Soc. 1977;75:556-86.

106. Kirmani M, Ryan SJ. Invitro measurement of contractile force of transvitreal membranes formed after penetrating ocular injury. Arch Ophthalmology. 1985;103(1):107-10.

107. Blumenkranz MS, Hartzer M. Contractile mechanism in proliferative vitreoretinopathy (PVR). Invest Ophthalmology Vis Sci. 1986; 27:188.

108. Machemer R, Aaberg TM, Freeman HM, et al. An updated classification of retinal detachment with proliferative vitreoretinopathy. Am J Ophthalmology. 1991;112(2):159-65.

109. Bonnet M. Clinical findings associated with the development of postoperative PVR in primary rhegmatogenous retinal

detachment. In: Heimann K, Wiedemann P (Eds). Proliferative Vitreoretinopathy. Heidelberg, Germany: Kaden-Verlag; 1989. pp. 8-20.

110. Bonnet M. Clinical factors predisposing to massive proliferative vitreoretinopathy in rhegmatogenous retinal detachment. Ophthalmologica. 1984;188(3):148-52.

111. Cowley M, Conway BP, Campochiaro PA, et al. Clinical risk factors for proliferative vitreoretinopathy. Arch Ophthalmology. 1989;107(8):1147-51.

112. Duquesne N, Bonnet M, Adeleine P. Preoperative vitreous hemorrhage associated with rhegmatogenous retinal detachment: a risk factor for postoperative proliferative vitreoretinopathy? Graefes Arch Clin Exp Ophthalmology. 1996;234(11):677-82.

113. Dai Y, Wu Z, Sheng H, et al. Identification of inflammatory mediators in patients with rhegmatogenous retinal detachment associated with choroidal detachment. Mol Vis. 2015;21:417-27.

114. Nagasaki H, Shinagawa K, Mochizuki M. Risk factors for proliferative vitreoretinopathy. Prog Retin Eye Res. 1998;17(1): 77-98.

115. Tseng W, Cortez RT, Ramirez G, et al. Prevalence and risk factors for proliferative vitreoretinopathy in eyes with rhegmatogenous retinal detachment but no previous vitreoretinal surgery. Am J Ophthalmology. 2004;137(6):1105-15.

116. Gagliano C, Toro MD, Avitabile T, et al. Intravitreal Steroids for the Prevention of PVR After Surgery for Retinal Detachment. Curr Pharm Des. 2015;21(32):4698-702.

117. Heimann H, Bartz-Schmidt KU, Bornfeld N, et al. Scleral buckling versus primary vitrectomy in rhegmatogenous retinal detachment: a prospective randomized multicenter clinical study. Ophthalmology. 2007;114(12):2142-54.

118. Jonas JB, Hayler JK, Panda-Jonas S. Intravitreal injection of crystalline cortisone as adjunctive treatment of proliferative vitreoretinopathy. Br J Ophthalmology. 2000;84(9):1064-7.

119. Blumenkranz MS, Claflin A, Hajek AS. Selection of therapeutic agents for intraocular proliferative disease. Cell culture evaluation. Arch Ophthalmology. 1984;102(4):598-604.

120. Shi H, Guo T, Liu PC, et al. Steroids as an adjunct for reducing the incidence of proliferative vitreoretinopathy after rhegmatogenous retinal detachment surgery: a systematic review and meta-analysis. Drug Des Devel Ther. 2015;9:1393-400.

121. Tano Y, Chandler D, Machemer R. Treatment of intraocular proliferation with intravitreal injection of triamcinolone acetonide. Am J Ophthalmology. 1980;90(6):810-6.

122. Salah-Eldin M1, Peyman GA, el-Aswad M, et al. Evaluation of toxicity and efficacy of a combination of antineoplastic agents in the prevention of PVR. Int Ophthalmology. 1994;18(2):53-60.

123. Borhani H, Peyman GA, Rahimy MH, et al. Suppression of experimental proliferative vitreoretinopathy by sustained intraocular delivery of 5-FU. Int Ophthalmology. 1995;19(1):43-9.

124. Wickham L, Bunce C, Wong D, et al. Randomized controlled trial of combined 5-fluorouracil and low-molecular- weight heparin in the management of unselected rhegmatogenous retinal detachments undergoing primary vitrectomy. Ophthalmology. 2007;114(4):698-704.

125. Kumar A, Nainiwal S, Sreenivas B. Intravitreal low molecular weight heparin in PVR surgery. Indian J Ophthalmology. 2003;51(1):67-70.

126. Kumar A, Tewari HK, Bathwal DP, et al. Experimental inhibition of proliferative vitreoretinopathy in retinal detachment using daunorubicin. Indian J Ophthalmology. 1994;42(1):31-5.

127. Kumar A, Nainiwal S, Choudhary I, et al. Role of daunorubicin in inhibiting proliferative vitreoretinopathy after retinal detachment surgery. Clin Experiment Ophthalmology. 2002;30(5):348-51.

128. Wiedemann P, Hilgers RD, Bauer P, et al. Adjunctive daunorubicin in the treatment of proliferative vitreoretinopathy: results of a multicenter clinical trial. Daunomycin Study Group. Am J Ophthalmology. 1998;126(4):550-9.

129. Creten O, Spileers W, Stalmans P. Systemic resorption of 5-fluorouracil used in infusion fluid during vitrectomy. Bull Soc Belge Ophtalmol. 2007;(303):37-41.

130. Er H, Turkoz Y, Mizrak B, et al. Inhibition of experimental proliferative vitreoretinopathy with protein kinase C inhibitor (chelerythrine chloride) and melatonin. Ophthalmologica. 2006;220(1):17-22.

131. Lei H, Hovland P, Velez G, et al. A potential role for PDGF-C in experimental and clinical proliferative vitreoretinopathy. Invest Ophthalmology Vis Sci. 2007;48(5):2335-42.

132. Pastor JC, de la Rua ER, Martin F. Proliferative vitreoretinopathy: risk factors and pathobiology. Prog Retin Eye Res. 2002;21(1): 127-44.

Chapter 42

Basic Principles and Laser Delivery Systems

Atul Kumar, Kavitha Duraipandi, Raghav Ravani, Sagnik Sen

INTRODUCTION

The concept of creating a retinal burn was first conceived by Dr Gerhard Meyer-Schwickerath in 1949, when he took patients to the roof of his laboratory on a sunny day and through a series of condensing lenses focused sunlight on their retina to treat melanomas (Meyer-Schwickerath, 1960). As the technique was cumbersome, nonsolar sources were sought. By the early 60s, Xenon arc photocoagulator became available and was effective for sealing retinal breaks and treating tumors, but with large-spot sizes and deeper heavy burns destroying most layers of the retina and choroid.

Laser (an abbreviation for "Light Amplification by Stimulated Emission of Radiation") is a light source capable of emitting a powerful monochromatic and highly coherent beam of electromagnetic radiation. The principle of stimulated emission of a photon of electromagnetic radiation was first theoretically proposed by Albert Einstein in 1917. Electromagnetic radiation of a single frequency or single wavelength thus eliminating chromatic aberration is called as monochromatic. Coherent beam implies that all the photons in the beam are in phase with each other.

Zaret reported the use of a pulsed ruby laser in the field of ophthalmology in 1961 for the first time to treat retinal breaks and proliferative diabetic retinopathy (PDR). He used a monocular direct ophthalmoscope to deliver the laser.[1] Later in 1968, L'Esperance introduced argon laser.[2] Since then, the field of ophthalmology has witnessed a rapid explosion in terms of the tremendous advances in laser technology. The introduction of lasers to treat ocular disorders has revolutionized the field of ophthalmology.

LASER PHYSICS

It is necessary to understand the nature of photons, atoms, and the interactions of atoms and photons to understand the working of a LASER. Light is comprised of individual "wave packets" called photons. Each photon has a characteristic frequency. The energy of the photon is proportional to its frequency.[3] Higher the frequency, more is the energy possessed by the photon. As the term denotes, a laser is derived by the excitation of electrons by a photon of light. The excited electrons, on reverting to a lower energy level, emit energy in the form of radiation. The matter, composed of the atoms and molecules, at low temperatures is in the lowest and thereby the most stable level or "ground state". As the temperature increases, more and more atoms jump to the higher energy levels. This is described as the Boltzmann energy distribution, according to which the higher energy level always has fewer molecules populating it than a lower level. Now, if a light beam of a suitable wavelength is introduced into the medium, the beam will become attenuated and the photons will get absorbed by the atoms, which get excited to a higher energy level. Subsequently, the atoms spontaneously decay to a lower level and emit photons in random directions. There is an energy difference between the orbits of the electrons. This energy is required to excite an electron to a higher level and the same amount of energy will be lost when the electron fall back to the original orbit. Interaction of photons and atoms can lead to:

- Absorption
- Spontaneous emission
- Stimulated emission.

Stimulated emission results when a photon passes close to an electron with high energy. The photon stimulates the electron to emit another photon. This causes the electron to lose energy and fall to a lower energy level. Thus, it is essential that the stimulating photon must possess energy equal to the energy difference between the higher and lower orbits of the electron. Following such a successful interaction we get two photons and an electron in a lower energy level.

Since this requires the electrons which interact with the photons to be in a higher energy state, this is not a random process like spontaneous emission. A feature of stimulated emission is that the emitted photon has the same frequency and phase as the stimulating photon. This makes the emitted radiation coherent.[4]

Most of the electrons of atoms are in a low-energy orbit. However, to generate a laser we require more electrons in higher energy orbits. This is called *"population inversion"*. It is essential to understand this phenomenon, which is in fact, reverse of the Boltzmann distribution—"population inversion", i.e. more atoms are in the higher energy levels than in a lower level. It can be achieved by introduction of the following:

- Electrical discharge
- Optical pump using a xenon arc lamp or another laser.

In a medium with population inversion, the introduction of a beam of light leads to subsequent emission of photons, which are in phase and coherent with each other and also the exciting light beam. So, the two prerequisites for the emission of a laser beam are:

1. Population inversion of the medium
2. A light beam of correct wavelength introduced to stimulate the excited atom into emitting light that is coherent with the exciting light beam.

Population inversion can be achieved when the proportion of atoms of a substance in a higher energy state are more than those decaying into lower energy states. This increases the rate of stimulated emission. This chain reaction is amplified by surrounding the medium with two mirrors, one of which is totally reflective and the other one typically partially reflective, an arrangement called a resonator.[5] To constrain the direction of radiation release, the excited atoms are contained in a laser cavity.

Thus, laser is monochromatic, in phase, coherent, collinear and with limited divergence.

Lasers can be classified into various types depending on the laser materials and laser–tissue interactions (Table 42.1). They include solid state and gas lasers. The action of lasers includes photocoagulation, photodisruption, photoablation, photovaporization and photochemical interactions.

CONTINUOUS AND PULSED LASERS

Lasers can be made to emit light in a continuous or pulsed manner. Pulsed lasers have a higher power, as the energy is concentrated in a very short time period. For example, Neodymium-doped:yttrium aluminum garnet (Nd:YAG) and excited dimer (excimer). A continuous laser, on the other hand, is of lower power as it delivers more overall energy over a relatively long time, e.g. argon lasers, krypton lasers, diode lasers and dye lasers.

SEMICONDUCTOR LASERS

These are made by joining a p-type (atom with a relative deficiency of electrons) material with n-type (atom with excess electrons) material to produce a p-n junction. Heat built-up is very detrimental to semiconductors and this limits the output. Only a limited number of wavelengths are available for such lasers.

PHOTODISRUPTIVE LASERS

Energy is used to raise electrons to a higher energy metastable state in photodisruptive lasers, just as in continuous wave lasers. There are two main ways the laser cavity can be switched—(1) Q switching or (2) lock mode methods. The functional difference between these two modes is not important for clinical use. These lasers concentrate energy that is used to pump electrons into a light pulse, which lasts to the order of 10^{-8} seconds or less. Even though the total energy delivered may be only 1 mJ, the concentrating effect of the short duration creates an irradiance of millions of watts. This produces an optical breakdown and formation of plasma from molecules of the tissue in a region confined to the focus point of the laser. This can be used to cut or perforate without coagulating tissue. The most common photodisruptive laser used in ophthalmic practice is the Nd:YAG laser. Because of the extremely high-energy densities produced, photodisruptive lasers do not depend on the absorbing pigments to produce optical breakdown. This allows us to cut clear tissue such as vitreous fibers, lens capsule and posterior hyaloid phase.

CHOICE OF WAVELENGTH

A number of wavelengths are available to the ophthalmic surgeon. The reasons to pick one wavelength over another are

Table 42.1: Laser–tissue interaction.

	Thermal effect		Photochemical effect	Ionizing effect
Photocoagulation	Photoablation	Photovaporization	Photoradiation	Photodisruption
E.g. Argon, Kr	E.g. Excimer	E.g. Carbon dioxide	E.g. Dye	Nd:YAG (1064)
Frequency-doubled Nd:YAG (532)	Holmium: YAG	—	Gold vapor	—
Dye	Frequency-doubled dye	—	Diode (689)	—
Diode (810)	—	—	—	—

(Kr: Krypton; Nd:YAG: Neodymium-doped:yttrium aluminum garnet).

mostly theoretical, but the over-riding concern is an attempt to increase the therapeutic index. One wavelength, argon blue, should not be used, as blue light is more likely to be scattered and has the potential to be absorbed by the xanthophylls in the macula causing unintended macular damage (Table 42.2).

Xanthophyll pigment of the retina absorbs blue light but passes green, yellow and red. Hemoglobin absorbs blue, green and yellow light, but does not absorb red as well. Melanin in retinal pigment epithelium (RPE) and the choroid absorb all visible wavelengths.

Longer (toward red) wavelengths are scattered less and therefore penetrate the cloudy media better. Longer wavelengths (like diode), owing to their increased penetrance, are frequently more painful.

Yellow laser has among its advantages, minimal scatter through nuclear sclerotic lens, low-xanthophyll absorption and little potential for photochemical damage. It has more utility in destroying vascular structures while causing minimal damage to adjacent pigmented tissue.

The key pigments found in ocular tissues are:
- Melanin, which has excellent absorption by green, yellow, red and infrared wavelengths.
- Macular xanthophyll absorbs blue but minimally absorbs yellow or red wavelengths.
- Hemoglobin easily absorbs blue, green and yellow with minimal absorption of red wavelength.

LASER LENSES

The most common lenses used to enable slit-lamp delivery of photocoagulation are either planoconcave lenses or high-plus power lenses.
- *Planoconcave lenses*: Image obtained is erect, has a high resolution, but the retinal area seen is small. The angulations of mirrors of a Goldmann three-mirror planoconcave lens are 59°, 67° and 73° (prototype: Goldmann three-mirror lens).
- *High-power plus lenses*: Image obtained is inverted, with some loss of resolution as compared to the above lenses, but provide a wider field of view. The planoconcave lenses

do not magnify the laser spot size selected, but high-plus power lenses magnify the spot size (depending on the lens used).

Selection of laser setting parameters (spot size, power, and duration of laser delivery) depends on the area of retina to be treated, clarity of ocular media and fundus pigmentation. Smaller spot size and longer duration exposures require less power setting. Macular laser treatment usually requires spot size of 100 µm, low-power setting (just visible "laser take") to prevent overheating of retinal tissue and consequent nerve fiber layer damage.

Commonly Used Laser Lenses for Retinal Photocoagulation

Panretinal Laser Lenses (Table 42.3)

Table 42.3: Panretinal laser lenses.

	Panretinal laser lenses (Fig. 42.1)	Use	Laser spot magnification factor (LSMF)	Field of view
a.	Volk TransEquator	PRP	1.43	122°
b.	Mainster Standard	PRP	1.05	90°
c.	Rodenstock Panfundoscope	PRP	1.40	120°
d.	Mainster Wide Field Lens	PRP	1.47	125°
e.	Mainster Ultra field PRF	PRP	1.89	140°
f.	Volk QuadrAspheric	PRP	1.97	130°
g.	Volk Super Quad 160	PRP	2.0	160°

(PRP: Panretinal photocoagulation).

Table 42.2: Wavelengths of different element.

Diode	810 nm
Krypton red	647 nm
Krypton yellow	568 nm
Frequency doubled Nd:YAG	532 nm
Argon green	514 nm
Argon blue	485 nm

(Nd:YAG: Neodymium–doped:yttrium aluminum garnet).

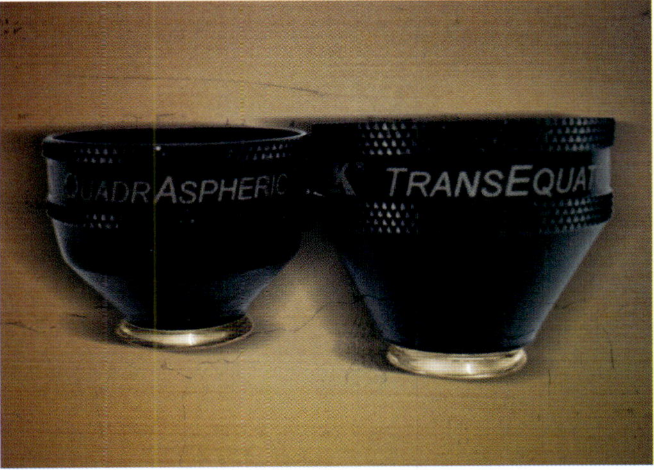

Fig. 42.1: Volk QuadrAspheric and TransEquatorial lenses.

Focal Laser Lenses (Table 42.4)

Table 42.4: Focal laser lenses.

	Focal laser lenses	Use	LSMF	Field of view
a.	Goldmann three-mirror lens: • Central region—for posterior pole • Three-angled mirrors: → 59° − 67° − 73°	posterior pole corresponds to central region Ora Serrata Equator	1.80	35°
b.	Volk area centralis	Posterior pole	0.95	82°
c.	Ocular PDT lens	Posterior pole	1.6	80°
d.	Volk PDT lens	Posterior pole	1.5	80°

(LSMF: Laser spot magnification factor; PDT: Photodynamic therapy).

Cleaning, Disinfection and Sterilization of Laser Lenses

Cleaning

- Use a mild cleaning solution—diluted liquid soap and water, or alcohol and wipe with soft cotton cloth.
- Use isopropyl alcohol tissue wipes to clean laser lenses.

Disinfection

- Glutaraldehyde 2% aqueous solution can be used, soak time 15–20 minutes and then wash in distilled water.
- Sodium hypochlorite (10 parts water and 1 part bleach)—soak for 10 minutes. Then wash with distilled water.
- Merthiolate (1:1000)—soak for 5 minutes, wash with distilled water.

Sterilization

- Ethylene oxide sterilization is recommended. (Never autoclave or boil lenses).

ANESTHESIA FOR LASER THERAPY

Topical anesthesia is sufficient in most of the patients for performing majority of the laser procedures. In some patients, peribulbar or retrobulbar anesthesia may be needed to facilitate delivery of laser photocoagulation.

The amount of pain experienced by the patient depends on the laser wavelength used. Infrared diode laser treatment (810-nm wavelength) often causes more pain to the patient than frequency-doubled Nd:YAG laser and may require a peribulbar or retrobulbar block to obviate the pain.

LASER DELIVERY SYSTEM

Meyer-Schwickerath was the first person to treat diabetic retinopathy (DR) with retinal photocoagulation in the 1950s. The present-day laser machines have evolved immensely since then. Initial photocoagulators utilized incandescent light, which was polychromatic and had a low efficiency. The invention of laser changed all this and became a major tool for treatment of many retinal vascular disorders.

After selecting the wavelength of the laser to be used, the treating physician needs to decide the mode of laser power delivery. Various laser delivery systems are available.

Laser can be delivered through three types of approaches:

1. *Slit lamp biomicroscope (Fig. 42.2)*: The most common and popular delivery system. Laser parameters viz.—power, exposure time and spot size can be changed.
2. *Laser indirect ophthalmoscope (LIO) (Figs. 42.3A and B)*: Green and diode lasers are delivered through a fiber optic cable. This method of laser delivery is ideal for photocoagulation of peripheral retinal breaks, degenerations, and in children under general anesthesia. However, they are unsuitable for focal or grid laser of macula. Laser spot size is varied by changing the dioptric strength of the hand-held condensing lens and by the refractive status of the eye. The spot size in a hypermetropic eye is smaller than in an emmetropic eye; whereas, the spot size in a myopic eye is larger than in an emmetropic eye.

In LIO,

Retinal spot size = (Power of condensing aspheric lens × Image plane spot size)/60

3. *Intraoperative laser endoscope*: Green and diode lasers can be delivered through fiber optic endoscope during vitrectomy. It works best for photocoagulation of neovascularization (NVE), retinal breaks and degenerations.

The most common route of delivery of laser is transpupillary, either performed on a slit lamp using specialized contact

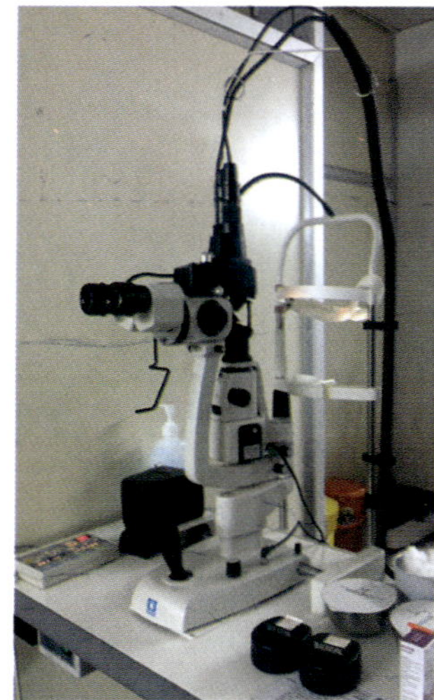

Fig. 42.2: Slit lamp laser with delivery facility.

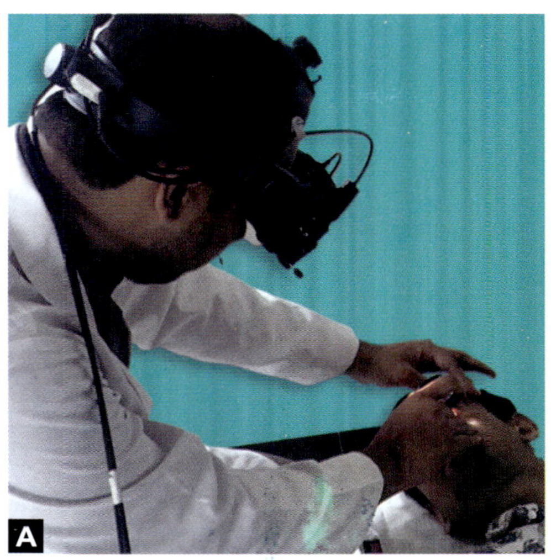 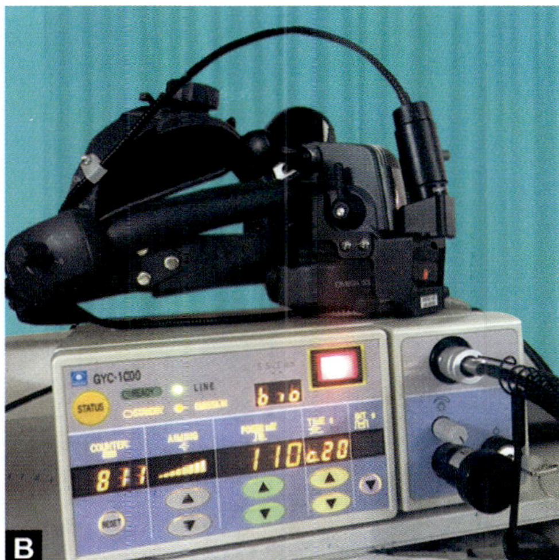

Figs. 42.3A and B: Use of a laser indirect ophthalmoscope (LIO).

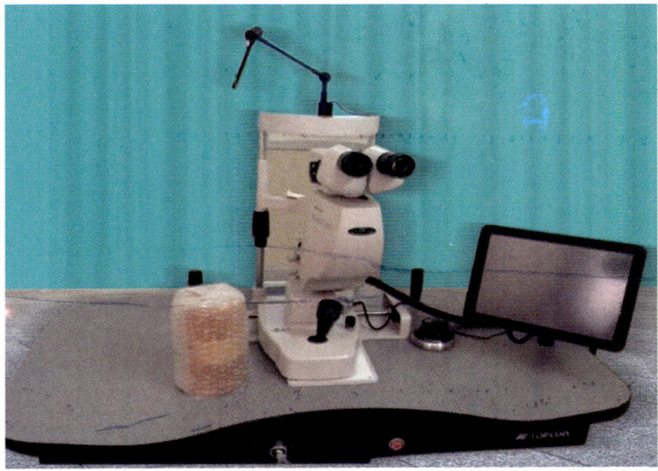

Fig. 42.4: The PASCAL® (Pattern Scan Laser) system.

laser lenses, or with binocular indirect ophthalmoscopy without contact lenses. The latter offers a wider field of view and is helpful for peripheral retinal lesions, e.g. lattices and atrophic holes. Transscleral application of laser using contact probes is also described, e.g. cyclodestructive procedures in glaucoma.

Temporal modes for laser delivery have been described in the recent years. Currently, the majority of retinal photocoagulation is achieved using continuous mode where laser is emitted at a sustained energy level for a given period of time. The downside to this mode of laser delivery is the passive thermal damage to adjacent retinal tissue due to diffusion. The delayed enlargement of laser scars up to 300% the size of the original laser spot can have detrimental effects if the fovea gets involved. This led to the development of subthreshold micropulse mode, which limits the amount of damage to adjacent tissue by delivering laser energy in ultrashort pulses (microseconds) with adjustable on and off times. The length of these pulses needs to be shorter than the thermal relaxation time of the target tissue, thereby minimizing damage to the normal surrounding retinal tissue.

Laser delivery can vary as per single spot treatment or a patterned PASCAL® treatment.

PASCAL® (Pattern Scan Laser) Photocoagulator

Introduction

The PASCAL® (Pattern Scan Laser) coagulation system by OptiMedica Corporation, USA, is a fully integrated pattern scan laser system. This machine can provide multispot therapy with up to 56 simultaneous spot applications on the retina in prefixed configurations such as squares and arcs. Depending on the pathology to be treated, a suitable pattern and spot number can be selected to deliver a faster and more efficient therapy.[6] In 2005, the company received Food and Drug Administration (FDA) clearance for its PASCAL® laser for use in standard photocoagulation procedures.

Benefits of using such a multispot laser compared to single spot photocoagulation are—reduced treatment time, improved precision, safety and patient comfort.[7] The pattern array options include single spot, square arrays, octants, quadrants, macular grid and arcs. The laser used is frequency-doubled Nd:YAG diode-pumped solid state with a wavelength of 532 nm. The aiming beam used is 630–650 nm diode laser.

Instrument

PASCAL® system includes (Fig. 42.4):
- Touchscreen user interface
- Pattern scanner technology
- Advanced optics slit lamp
- Slit lamp-mounted micromanipulator
- Dual slit lamp-mounted rotary power controls

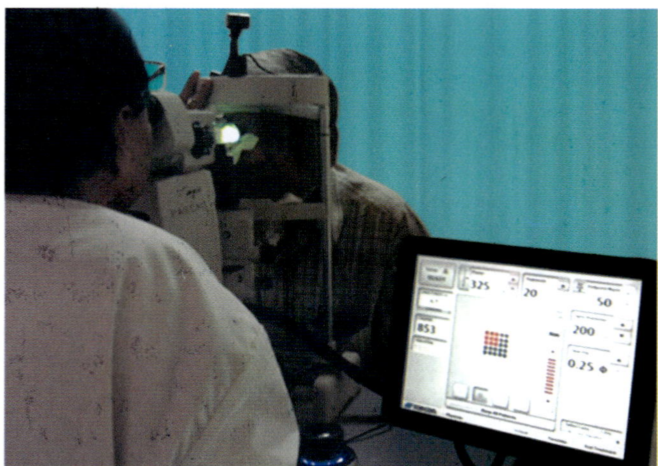

Fig. 42.5: The PASCAL® (Pattern Scan Laser) laser in use with a 9 spot pattern, power 325 mW, pulse duration 20 ms, and spot size 200 μ. The shorter pulse duration in this laser decreases risk of pain during the procedure.

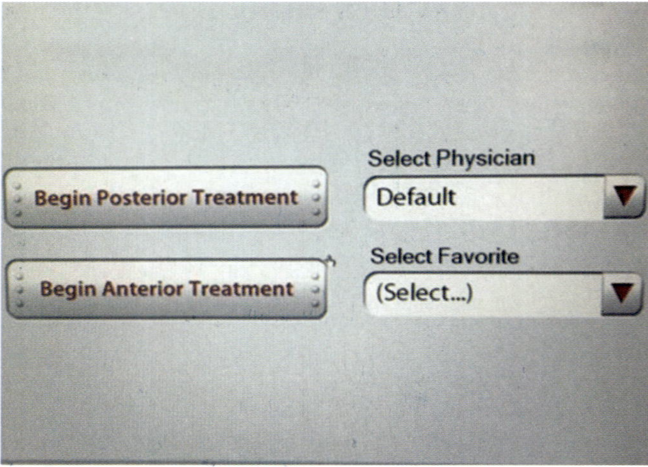

Fig. 42.6: Touchscreen user interface of PASCAL® (Pattern Scan Laser) displaying the available treatment modalities.

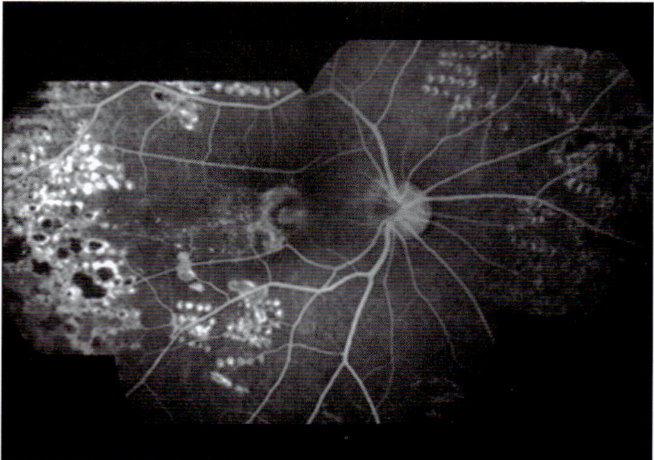

Fig. 42.7: 16 spot array of equidistant patterned laser are visible on fluorescein angiography (FA).

- Precision Spot™ laser
- Compatible LIO.

The laser emission is controlled by a foot switch. The control panel is a liquid crystal display (LCD) provided with a touchscreen control for the selection of laser parameters, such as aiming beam intensity, laser spot size, power, duration and system status (Figs. 42.5 and 42.6).

Different predetermined pattern types can be selected as described below (Figs. 42.7 to 42.9).

- *Arrays*: Panretinal photocoagulation (PRP)—2 × 2 to 5 × 5 spot pattern delivery per foot pedal depression. Best suited for PDR.
- *Triple arcs*: The radius of the arcs can be varied, thus aiding in treating retinal tears and peripheral retinal degeneration.

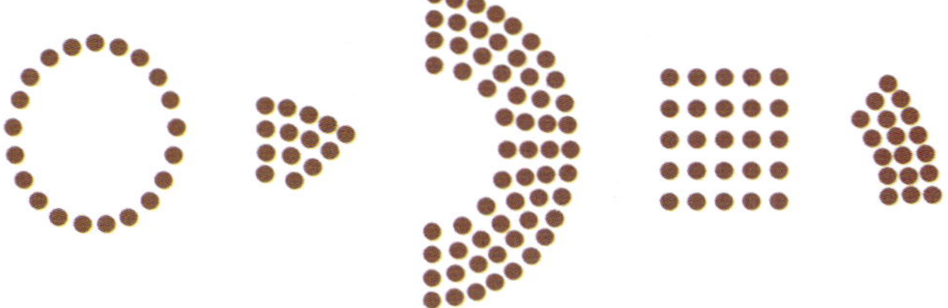

Fig. 42.8: Various patterns available for laser with PASCAL® (Pattern Scan Laser).

- *Focal/modified macular grids*: Macular treatments—pattern subset of the macular grid with four concentric arcs.
- *Full macular grids*: Macular treatments—pattern of four concentric rings totaling 56 spots encircles the fovea. Smallest spot pattern diameter is greater than 2,000 μm ("safety zone").
- *Single spot*: Conventional treatment.

Endpoint Management Using PASCAL® Laser (Fig. 42.10)

Endpoint management (EpM) allows for the control of the laser energy relative to titration level providing considerable advantage especially when treating close to the fovea. The titration algorithm for EpM begins by defining the laser power required to produce a barely visible burn at a pulse duration of 20 ms. This energy is taken as 100% and all other pulse energies are expressed as a percentage of this titration threshold.

At 30% energy level, only a single RPE cell in the center of the 200 μm spot is damaged. With EpM, some spots in a grid treatment pattern can be set at 100% (or above) to mark the location of the subvisible treatment with an immediately visible reference. EpM allows the physician to consistently

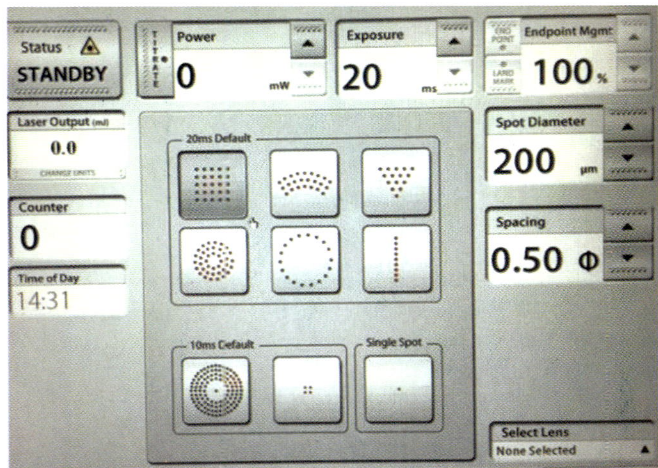

Fig. 42.9: Touchscreen user interface displaying pattern, power, spot size and other parameters of laser delivery.

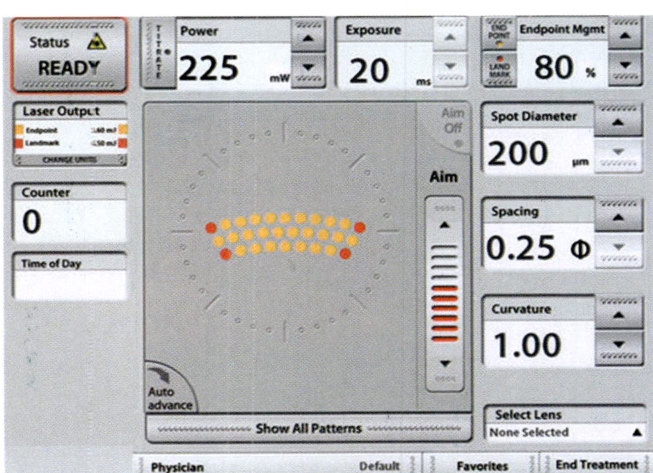

Fig. 42.10: PASCAL® (Pattern Scan Laser) control panel depiction of the four corners of threshold burns and subthreshold burns within it (endpoint management—EpM).

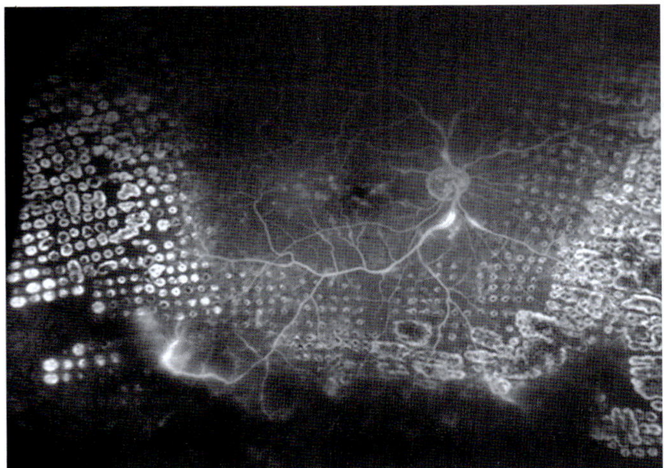

Fig. 42.11: Equidistant PASCAL® (Pattern Scan Laser) patterned laser spots on ultrawide-field fluorescein angiography (UWFA).

operate within therapeutic range when performing subvisible treatments. It is especially helpful in terms of reducing the side effects when doing single sitting PRP.

To easily recognize the treated area, the edge of the array of burns is done with 100% laser power to get a barely visible burn. By providing a landmark, it helps in avoiding previously treated areas. Immediately following the application of barely visible or subthreshold laser, the complete array of spots can be mapped using fundus autofluorescence (FAF) imaging. FAF helps in knowing the spatial distribution of the burns and guides retreatment. EpM makes it easier to obtain highly localized burns with minimal axial and lateral spread. Therefore, it reduces side effects like pain, visual field impairment and minimizes outer retinal damage and RPE atrophy.

Advantages of PASCAL® Photocoagulation over Conventional Single Spot Lasers

PASCAL® photocoagulation provides rapid, efficient and precise laser treatment over vast areas of the retina using multiple spots in a rapid successive order. The pattern and number of spots can be adjusted depending on the desired location. The burns created by a PASCAL® laser are more precisely spaced and uniform as compared to conventional laser systems (Fig. 42.11). The gradation of retinal burns is the same but can be titrated more easily.

This rapid therapy is believed to cause less patient discomfort by shortening the duration of the laser treatment, thereby increasing patient compliance.

Semicircular pattern is better suited for photocoagulation of retinal periphery and standard square pattern is ideal for retinal midperiphery. Circular pattern is suitable for treating retinal holes/breaks. It has a short-learning curve and is easy to use. Visual field defects are less pronounced with this technique probably due to reduced heat diffusion toward the choroid and inner retina.

Disadvantages

Patient's cooperation is critical as multiple spots are delivered in successive order after activation. Sudden movements by patients can result in coagulation of unintended locations.

More power may also be required, as the spot size is usually kept small, so is the duration of laser delivery.

Conclusion

Thus, PASCAL® photocoagulation enables improved efficiency, less treatment time, safe treatment with increased patients and physician comfort.

NAVILAS LASER SYSTEM

Navigated Laser Treatment

Navigated retinal laser therapy is a relatively new concept in retinovascular disease therapy introduced to ensure greater accuracy in laser spot application compared to traditional laser treatment. The Navilas Laser System (OD-OS GmbH-FDA approved) (Fig. 42.12) is the first navigated retinal laser to reach the clinic and integrates real-time fundus imaging with computer-based image-guided 577-µm retinal laser therapy. Navilas enables the delivery of a preplanned, target-assisted and digitally documented focal navigated treatment, including microsecond pulsing and high-speed navigated panretinal laser photocoagulation. Studies have reported a 92% hit rate with the navigated laser versus 72% with conventional laser when targeting microaneurysm, reduced retreatment rate using navigated laser in patients with diabetic macular edema (DME) and PDR, and that procedure time and accuracy of treatment was independent of operator experience. Unlike any other retina laser, Navilas offers focal treatment without a contact lens and infrared illumination for unsurpassed patient comfort. A large field of view and assisted pattern positioning greatly improve speed in panretinal and focal treatments.

With the Navilas, it is also important that the user is good with information technology and computer systems. It is also important to note that when performing focal treatment with the Navilas, the time commitment for the surgeon is a little longer, perhaps an extra 2 or 3 minutes due to the planning and imaging phase, although for the patient the actual treatment time is shorter.

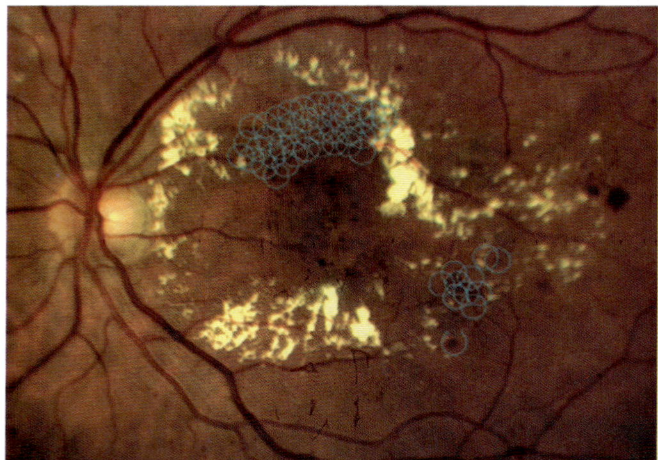

Fig. 42.12: Real-time fundus imaging and computer-based image-guided laser spots, sketch of which is seen on the fundus photo.

ENDOLASER PHOTOCOAGULATION

The endolaser is a critical component of vitreoretinal surgery. Endolaser coagulation is a method by which the laser light is brought directly inside the eye through a fiber optic cable connected to the laser delivery console for treatment to the retina. When the surgeon is performing an intraocular surgery and a need for coagulation exists, the laser light is directed toward the desired area through a probe and photocoagulation is performed (Figs. 42.13A to D).

For retinal breaks, laser is applied all around encircling the tear. Subretinal fluid under the break must be completely removed for the RPE to effectively absorb the laser energy. Endolaser can be performed through air, silicone oil and perfluorocarbon liquids. With the wide-angle intraoperative viewing systems, it is easier and safer to reach the far

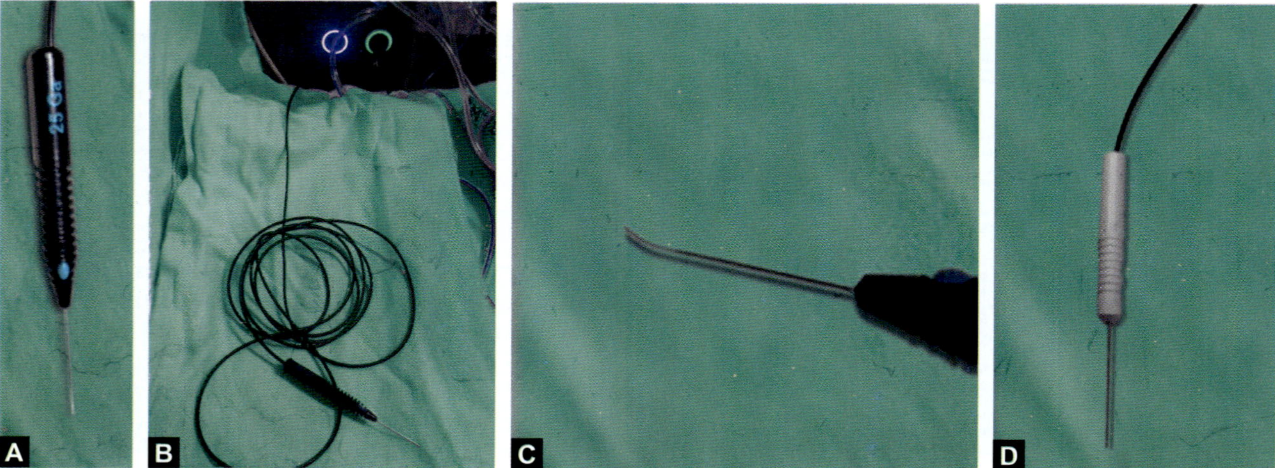

Figs. 42.13A to D: (A to C) show a 25G Alcon endolaser probe. The flexible curved tip makes it easy to access the peripheral retina. The other end of the probe is attached to a groove on the Alcon Constellation vitrectomy system (B). Figure (D) shows a 25G/0.5-mm laser probe (straight tip) from DORC®.

periphery of the retina. Curved small-gauge endolaser probes further enhance the surgeon's ability to laser up to the ora serrata and beyond when needed.

Endolaser probes are available in several forms such as—straight/curved, blunt/tapered, simple/aspirating, and even illuminating.[8-10] The most commonly used is the straight probe with a blunt or tapered tip. The curved tip helps in accessing the anterior-superior retina or peripheral retina near the surgeon's dominant hand with ease.

Illuminating probes help the surgeon to free the opposite hand for use of another instrument like forceps/scissors; particularly useful in diabetic cases. Although the downside of this is the limited range of illumination compared to the standard endoilluminator.[4]

Aspirating tips can be used to drain subretinal fluid or blood from the edge of retinal holes during laser application, helping in keeping the media clear.[5]

23G and 25G endolaser probes are now available for MIVS (microincision vitrectomy surgery) that enhance postoperative comfort for the patient. 25G probes are overly flexible, lack rigidity, and thus are unable to easily maneuver the globe position during surgery. 25+G instruments are more rigid and easy to maneuver.

LASER PHOTOCOAGULATION FOR POSTERIOR SEGMENT DISORDERS

The basic light–tissue interactions include:
- Thermal
- Photochemical effect
- Photovaporization
- Ionizing effects.

Thermal Effects

These occur when visible or infrared light is absorbed by pigments present in the tissue. This leads to denaturation of proteins and tissue destruction (photocoagulation). The temperature rise is proportional to light absorption in that tissue, which is directly proportional to the amount of pigment present in the tissue. The light absorption by hemoglobin leads to thrombus formation and shrinkage of collagen in the wall of a blood vessel, thus closing the blood vessels.

Absorption of laser energy results in a 10–20°C temperature rise.[11] This temperature rise is highly localized and limited to within 1 mm of the burn's center. Most of the thermal damage created during posterior segment laser is due to absorption of energy by melanin in the RPE and choroid. Various lasers can induce photocoagulation, such as—argon green laser (514 nm), argon blue-green laser (488 nm), krypton red laser (647 nm), ruby red laser (694 nm), diode laser (810 nm near infrared), rhodamine 6G organic tunable dye laser (570–630 nm yellow to red) and the frequency-doubled Nd:YAG laser (532-nm green).[12]

Photochemical Effects

Photosynthesis and bleaching of rhodopsin are a few examples of normal physiologic photochemical reactions.[13] Laser is said to have a photochemical effect, if the laser light leads to formation or destruction of chemical bonds.

Photovaporization

Application of laser irradiation higher than those required for photocoagulation to target tissue causes rapidly expansion of water vapor, which can cause tissue disruption (photovaporization). This results from a microexplosion when the temperature of water rises above the boiling point. Photovaporization is usually also accompanied by photocoagulation and provides hemostasis. The CO_2 laser (10,600-nm wavelength irradiation) effectively vaporizes tissues.[14] Vaporization can also occur following an overly intense argon burn.

Ionizing Effects

High irradiance by short-pulsed laser energy can ionize material and disintegrate it into a collection of ions and electrons called plasma.[15] The electrons are stripped away from atoms and molecules. This rapidly expanding plasma produces shock waves, which can mechanically disrupt tissues. The plasma formed can be considered a fourth state of matter, which has the mechanical properties of gas and electrical properties of a metal. Femtosecond laser works on this principle.

ABLATIVE PHOTODECOMPOSITION

Ultraviolet (UV) radiation shorter than 300 nm causes chemical reactions in biological tissues. If tissues are exposed to high-energy UV light in a short-time interval, their surface can be removed layer-by-layer with precision and is a controllable process. This can be achieved by an excimer laser, which has sufficient energy to break chemical bonds at the target site. The excimer laser wavelength for corneal ablation is 193 nm (argon fluoride). This entire procedure of corneal reshaping and modeling is called photorefractive keratectomy.[16]

PHOTODYNAMIC THERAPY

This therapy is most commonly being used in ophthalmology for treatment of choroidal neovascularization and some tumors.

Principle

Photodynamic therapy (PDT) involves intravenous injection of a hematoporphyrin derivative dye. The dye is selectively taken up and retained in the new vessels/tumor. This is then treated with 689-nm red light from a laser source. The interaction of the dye with the laser releases singlet oxygen, which causes destruction of tissues.[17] The gold vapor laser is a useful alternative laser for such a therapy.

Indications

- Choroidal neovascular membrane (CNVM) secondary to wet age-related macular degeneration (AMD) or CNVM from any other cause (up to 5,400 μm in size)
- CNVM due to polypoidal choroidal vasculopathy (PCV)
- Retinal angiomatous proliferation (RAP)
- Retinal pathologies like choroidal hemangioma, retinal hamartoma, choroidal melanoma, chronic central serous chorioretinopathy (CSCR), vasoproliferative tumor and angiomatous lesions secondary to systemic diseases (VHL).

Technique of Verteporfin Dye Injection and Application of Laser

- Written informed consent.
- Fundus fluorescein angiography is done (not less than 72-hour old), late venous phase frames are selected where the entire neovascular membrane fills up and greatest linear diameter (GLD) of lesion is calculated.
- PDT laser spot size = GLD + 1,000 μ. Dose of verteporfin = 6 mg/m².
- Nomogram is available for dose calculation based on body mass index (BMI).
- Reconstitute each vial of Visudyne with 7 mL of sterile water for injection to provide 7.5 mL containing 2 mg/mL. Reconstituted Visudyne must be protected from light and used within 4 hours. It is an opaque dark green solution.
- The volume of reconstituted Visudyne required to achieve the desired dose of 6 mg/m² body surface area is withdrawn from the vial and diluted with 5% dextrose for injection to make a total infusion volume of 30 mL (e.g. if dose is 4.5 mL then the drug is diluted with 25.5 mL of 5% dextrose). After dilution, protect from light and use within a maximum of 4 hours.
- This 30 mL is then infused slowly over 10 minutes with the help of an infusion pump with anesthesiologist standby, in a dark room.
- Wait for 5 minutes after the infusion is over; subsequently, laser of 689 nm is applied for 83 seconds (both eyes can be treated in same session).
- Patient is advised to stay indoors at home avoiding sunlight and halogen light sources for 4–5 days as verteporfin is a photosensitive dye and cause skin burns in sunlight. Patient is informed about discoloration of urine, tears and sweat.

Safety of Photodynamic Therapy

- Photosensitivity reactions
- Adverse events at the injection site (such as pain, edema, hemorrhage or inflammation)
- Backache during dye infusion

- If extravasation occurs, protect the site from light
- Transient visual disturbances.

The most serious and sight-threatening of the ocular side effects is an acute severe acuity decrease, described as a loss of more than or equal to 20 letters occurring within 7 days of PDT administration, owing to choroidal ischemia and infarction, damage to retinal tissues and subretinal hemorrhage.[18]

Modifications of Standard Photodynamic Therapy Protocols to Improve Efficacy and Safety

Studies evaluating several new approaches to better utilize PDT in the treatment of subfoveal AMD were identified in the literature review. These included both modifications in the dose of the laser energy used for photoactivation of verteporfin and assessment of patient progress by optical coherence tomography (OCT).

ALTERATION IN THE LIGHT DOSE OF THE ACTIVATING LASER

Collateral damage to adjacent retinal structures is much reduced compared to that seen with thermal laser photocoagulation; however, PDT is not an innocuous procedure and leads to severe choroidal ischemia, which may turn permanent with loss of central vision. Reducing laser fluence by decreasing either exposure time or intensity on the safety and efficacy of PDT has been evaluated. Encouraging outcomes from this approach have already been observed in the Verteporfin in Minimally classic CNVM (VIM) trial, in which lower fluence produced significant treatment benefits. More recently, Michels et al. compared the administration of PDT at standard fluence (with a reduced fluence of 25 J/cm² or decreasing the intensity to 300 mW), or the exposure time to 42 seconds.[19] In the patients receiving standard fluence, choriocapillaris nonperfusion observed on late indocyanine green chorioangiography (ICG) at week 1 lasted for up to 3 months. In contrast, patients receiving a reduced fluence of 25 J/cm² (in both groups) were found to have complete CNVM closure; however, without the accompanying reduction in choroidal perfusion.

CLINICAL USE OF LASER PHOTOCOAGULATION

Photocoagulation is perhaps the most commonly performed laser procedure in ophthalmology. In the posterior segment, photocoagulation is used for treating numerous conditions such as PDR, DME, choroidal neovascularization, retinal breaks and retinal detachments, and CSCR.

Laser Management of Diabetic Retinopathy

Photocoagulation for DR was first employed by Meyer-Schwickerath.[20] To date, treatment with laser photocoagulation remains the cornerstone for management of diabetic maculopathy and proliferative retinopathy. The argon blue-green and now the green lasers are the most widely used in the treatment of DR, though more recently solid state frequency-doubled 532-nm YAG (green) lasers, dye yellow and diode lasers are also being used to a large extent. The treating physician must ensure a systemically stable patient before starting the laser sessions.

Laser Management of Proliferative Retinopathy

Fibrovascular proliferation on or within 1 disc diameter of the disc is referred to as neovascularization of the disc (NVD). Such a proliferation at any other site on the retina or in the vitreous is referred to as neovascularization elsewhere (NVE). Most of the neovascularizations in DR are observed around the arcades or between the arcades and the equator. Contraction of vitreous attachment to these areas of fibrovascular proliferation can lead to hemorrhage in the posterior hyaloid space or into the vitreous cavity. A further traction on the retina can lead to a tractional retinal detachment. If this progresses further, a secondary retinal break formation leading to a secondary rhegmatogenous retinal detachment occurs. Development of new vessels in the anterior chamber angle or on the iris can be extremely detrimental, as this leads to an increased intraocular pressure. This condition is called neovascular glaucoma (NVG) and is very resistant to treatment.

Diabetic retinopathy has been classified into *five levels* according to the international clinical DR disease severity scale:[21]

1. No apparent retinopathy
2. Mild nonproliferative diabetic retinopathy (NPDR, only microaneurysms)
3. Moderate NPDR
4. Severe NPDR [including any of—intraretinal hemorrhage in all 4 quadrants with atleast 20 in each, venous beading in ≥ two quadrants, intraretinal microvascular abnormalities (IRMA) ≥ one quadrant, but no new vessel proliferation]
5. Proliferative retinopathy (defined by neovascularization and/or vitreous/preretinal hemorrhage).

The Diabetic Retinopathy Study (DRS) established that treatment with photocoagulation reduced the risk of severe vision loss (SVL) by over 50% in cases of PDR with high-risk characteristics.[22] SVL was defined as visual acuity less than 5/200 in two consecutive follow-up visits at least 4 months apart.[22]

The DRS and the early treatment diabetic retinopathy study (ETDRS)[23] were both prospective, randomized controlled, multicentric studies, which provide proof of the efficacy of laser photocoagulation for DR.

High-risk PDR was defined as any one of the following (by the DRS):[22]

- Mild NVD with vitreous hemorrhage.
- Moderate-to-severe NVD with or without vitreous hemorrhage (showing ¼ to ⅓ disc area)
- Moderate (½ disc area) NVE with vitreous hemorrhage.

High-risk PDR was also defined by any combination of three of the four retinopathy risk factors:

- Presence of vitreous/preretinal hemorrhage
- Presence of new vessels
- Location of new vessels on/near optic disc
- Moderate-to-severe extent of new vessels.

Panretinal photocoagulation is indicated for any eye with DRS high-risk characteristics, rubeosis iridis or NVG. When regular follow-up of the patient is doubtful or when one eye has had a bad outcome due to DR or in a one-eyed patient or in pregnant women, we do perform laser of eyes with PDR without high-risk characteristic or even with severe NPDR according to suggestions given by the ETDRS. If both PDR and CSME coexist then there is always a risk of the macular edema worsening after PRP. In such a scenario, if the PDR is not severe, we can perform laser for macular edema first and do PRP after 4 weeks. If the case demands urgent PRP then we can club the macular laser with the first sitting of PRP. With the advent of antivascular endothelial growth factor (VEGF) agents, we can also treat them first with an anti-VEGF agent and subsequently start the laser in 2–3 weeks.

The intensity of the laser burn can be titrated depending upon the clinical appearance of the burn. Table 42.5 gives the correlation of the color of burn and its intensity.

Panretinal photocoagulation usually comprises a total of approximately 1,800 applications of 500 µ retinal spot size of 0.1–0.2-second duration moderate-intensity burns. The power is initially kept low (around 100–150 mW) and gradually increased to achieve the desired endpoint of moderate-intensity burns (40.6). Treatment extends nasally from 500 µ nasal to optic disc, superior and inferiorly from just within the temporal arcades and temporally from 2DD temporal to the fovea and anteriorly slight anterior to the equator all around. Close (one burn width apart), but nonconfluent burns are applied for PRP. Peripheral nonelevated NVE are treated focally with confluent burns.

The PRP is usually completed in three sessions over a 2–3-week interval (Fig. 42.14). Inferior half of the retina is photocoagulated first, as this area may not be visible, if vitreous hemorrhage occurs before completion of PRP. The number of PRP sessions and the time taken to perform each session can be reduced using a multispot laser.

We use the Volk QuadrAspheric lens for the mid-periphery and Volk TransEquatorial lens for posterior pole treatment (*see* Fig. 42.1). With these lenses, the view is inverted and reversed, and these allow for a magnification of the size of the burn delivered. The spot size setting on the slit lamp delivery system must take into account the magnification factor.

Table 42.5: Chorioretinal burn intensity.	
Light	Barely visible retinal blanching
Mild	Faint white retinal burn
Moderate	Opaque, dirty-white retinal burn
Heavy	Dense-white retinal burn

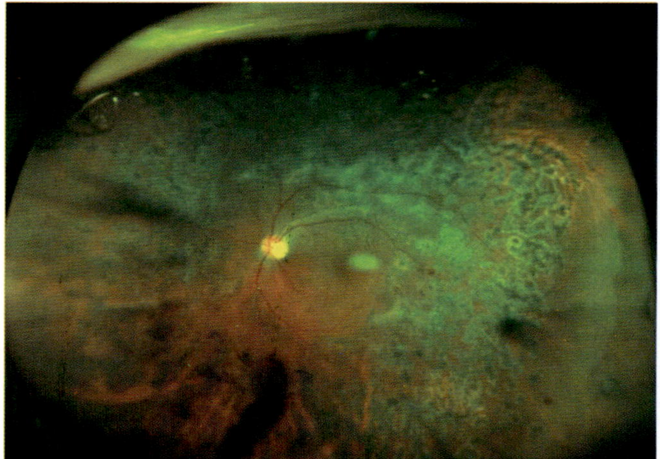

Fig. 42.14: Optos color picture showing lasered proliferative diabetic retinopathy.

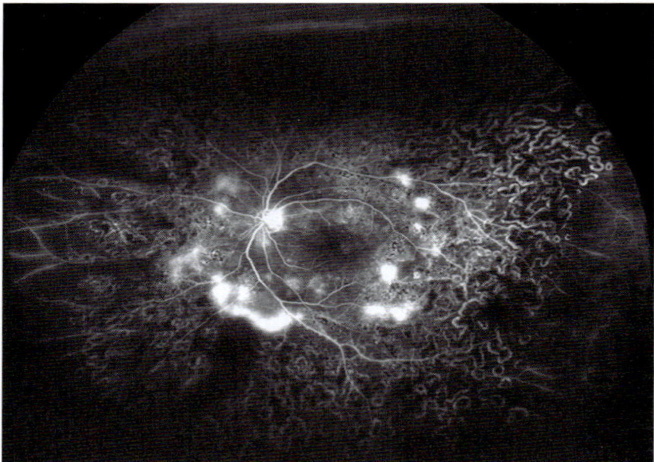

Fig. 42.15: Ultra-wide field angiography (UWFA) image reveals peripheral capillary dropout areas with persisting neovascularization of the disc/neovascularization elsewhere (NVD/NVE).

Panretinal photocoagulation results in regression of NVD and NVE (complete regression of neovascularization was seen in only 21% of eyes at 1-year follow-up in the DRS) and minimizes the risk of vitreous bleed and other complications like tractional retinal detachment. Persistent NVD requires fill-in treatment and this is extended more peripherally usually with the Goldmann three-mirror lens or LIO. In severe cases, peripheral cryoablation can be added and lightly pigmented scars can be treated over with laser again. Persistent or fresh NVE (Fig. 42.15) can also be treated with confluent laser burns. If new vessels persist despite maximal treatment, it is best to observe the patient. If vitreous hemorrhage occurs, it is usually mild and tends to clear spontaneously. Nonlasered eyes with vitreous hemorrhage should be operated early (approximately 2–3 months) to avoid continuing vasoproliferation under the overlying vitreous/subhyaloid hemorrhage.

All wavelengths are equally effective in inducing regression of PDR. The green wavelengths are generally better tolerated, since the longer diode wavelengths are absorbed deeper in the retina and choroid and can potentially cause more pain. The longer red wavelengths are better able to penetrate through hazy media, which can be due to a dense cataract or vitreous hemorrhage.

The role of PRP for pre-PDR is not very clearly established. Treatment is recommended, if the other eye shows changes of PDR, or has had a vitreous hemorrhage or in one-eyed patients.

Q. How does Laser Photocoagulation help in Regression of Proliferative Diabetic Retinopathy?

Ans. Some hypotheses which have been proposed for this are:[24]
- Laser converts hypoxic retina into anoxic retina. This reduces VEGF production.
- As RPE is the highest consumer of oxygen, laser reduces the oxygen requirement of the retina itself by ablating the RPE cells.
- Laser may improve the transport of oxygen through RPE itself.
- It may liberate vasoinhibitive factors.
- It could also induce a posterior vitreous detachment (PVD) and relieve traction on the fibrovascular proliferation.

Panretinal photocoagulation is not without side effects. It can lead to delayed dark adaptation and restriction of peripheral visual fields. Worsening of traction on retina due to an increase in the fibrous component of the proliferation or induction of a partial PVD following PRP can cause a secondary retinal detachment or vitreous hemorrhage. To avoid such complications, it is best to divide the entire treatment into sessions and give around 1,000 burns per session. This also reduces the risk of development of cystoid macular edema (CME), choroidal effusion, exudative retinal detachment and angle closure.

Patients may experience pain after the treatment session. This may be due to the laser energy itself or sometimes it could be due to angle closure caused by choroidal effusion and anterior ciliary body rotation. Patients are followed up after 4–6 weeks following the completion of the PRP.

For eyes, which do not show any regression of proliferative retinopathy or if retinopathy progresses despite treatment, supplemental treatment is advocated.

Additional laser is performed using similar parameters to the original treatment sessions. Tighter PRP with application of laser burns between previous burns and treatment of any previously skipped areas is performed during retreatment. Peripheral cryopexy (ARC) or preferably indirect laser ophthalmoscopy is used to fill in the peripheral retina.

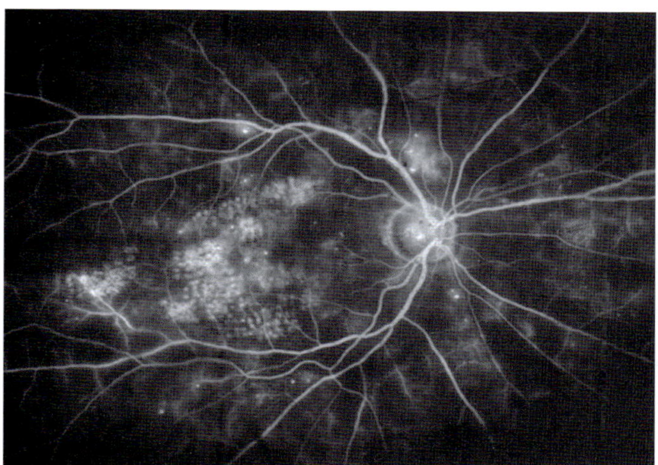

Fig. 42.16: FFA image showing macular grid laser done for diffuse diabetic macular edema.

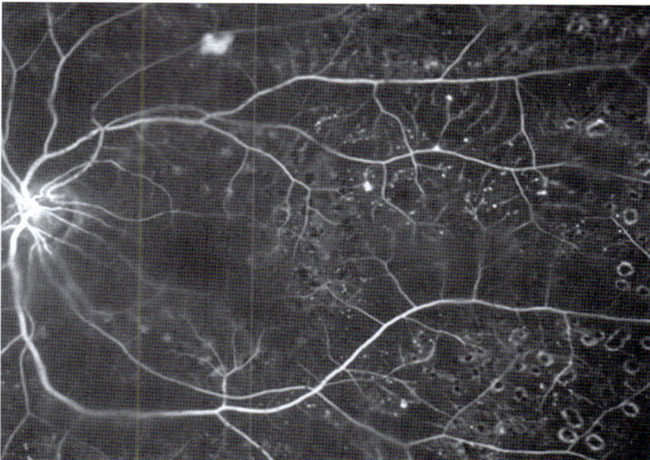

Fig. 42.17: Fundus image showing focal laser of the leaking microaneurysms at the macula in diabetic macular edema. Focal NVE is visible in the superior quadrant.

Anti-VEGF agents and/or vitrectomy should be promptly considered in patients who have already received adequate laser and still appear to have florid and advancing proliferative disease.

Laser Management of Macular Edema

Macular edema is the most important cause of visual loss due to DR. It can be diagnosed clinically by performing a careful slit lamp biomicroscopic examination (using +90D or +78D). Objective quantification and detailed assessment of type and cause of macular edema is possible using OCT and fluorescein angiography.

Diffuse macular edema is conventionally treated with grid laser photocoagulation (Fig. 42.16). 100-µ burns of light intensity are placed one burn width apart staying 500 µ away from the foveal center and the disc margin and extending up to 3,000 µ from the macular center. Modified macular grid (usually performed) excludes the area of the papillomacular bundle. If macular edema persists on follow-up examination and if vision is worse than 6/12 with a good perifoveal capillary network, focal treatment up to 300 µ from fovea can be considered.

Focal treatment of leaking microaneurysms can be combined with grid laser or can be performed as a standalone procedure (Fig. 42.17), if indicated on fluorescein angiogram. Treatment within the papillomacular bundle can be done as long as the leaking points are more than 500 µ from the disc and also fovea. Retreatment, when required, is usually considered at least 3–4 months after initial laser photocoagulation.

Argon green, double frequency Nd:YAG (514 nm or 532 nm) and yellow wavelengths are the commonly used lasers for treatment of diabetic maculopathy, while blue is generally avoided for macular lasers due to the presence of xanthophyll pigment, which absorbs blue wavelength. Adequate treatment of the maculopathy results in obliteration of the microvascular lesions, resolution of edema, absorption of hard exudates, and stabilization or improvement of visual acuity.

Possible complications, which can further reduce vision following grid laser, are inadvertent foveal burn and secondary choroidal neovascularization. Secondary CNVM usually results from using inappropriately high-laser power and small spot sizes close to the fovea (leading to rupture of Bruch's membrane). Apart from laser, other therapeutic modalities like intravitreal injection of anti-VEGF agents and steroids have been recently employed for managing DME.

The DRCR.net studied the effects of anti-VEGF (ranibizumab) with prompt or deferred laser and triamcinolone with prompt laser alone in a multicentric and randomized clinical trial of 854 eyes with DME involving the center of the macula with vision impairment,[25] and found that ranibizumab along with prompt or deferred laser was better than prompt laser alone (with 95% confidence intervals favoring ranibizumab with deferred laser) and suggested that addition of ranibizumab may result in a favorable anatomical and functional outcomes in eyes with center involving DME with vision impairment.[25]

They also noted that eyes receiving ranibizumab or triamcinolone in addition to laser were less likely to progress to PDR. Thus these cases were also less likely to develop vitreous hemorrhage and required PRP less often. This was suggestive of an additional benefit of anti-VEGF agents and triamcinolone (other than a decrease in macular edema). The main drawback of the treatment with intravitreal injections is the need for repeated treatments. This reduces compliance and many patients may not be willing for such an invasive therapy. For such cases, laser still remains the mainstay for management and stabilization of DME.

Coexistent Macular Edema and Proliferative Disease

Major studies like DRS and ETDRS showed that full-scatter photocoagulation may exacerbate macular edema leading to moderate-visual loss.[22,23] When maculopathy coexists with PDR, it is better to treat macular edema and wait for

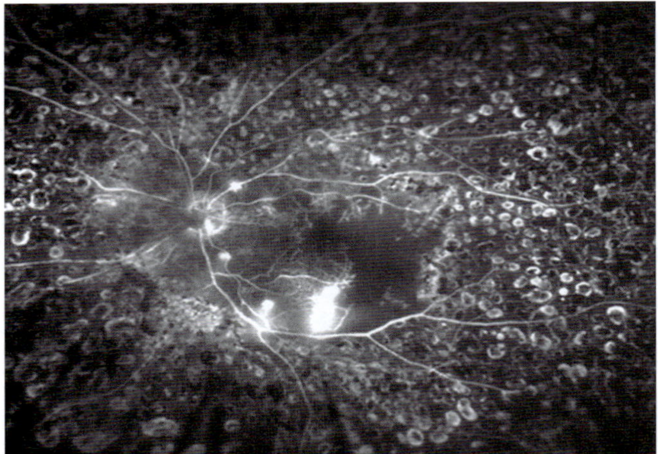

Fig. 42.18: A case of lasered proliferative diabetic retinopathy with neovascularization elsewhere (NVE) and macular ischemia on fundus fluorescein angiography imaging.

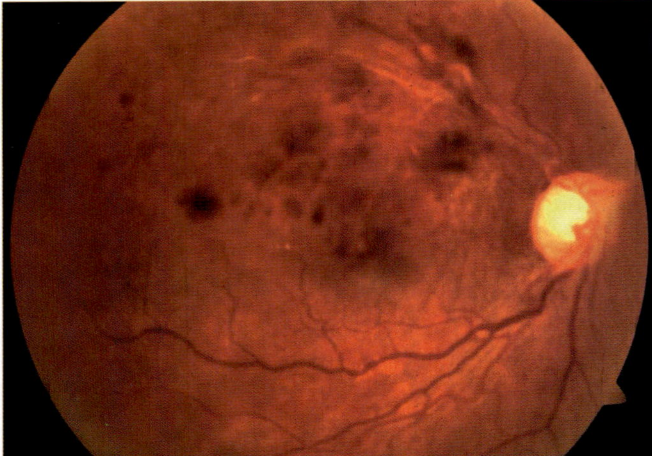

Fig. 42.19: Clinical fundus picture of a case of recent branch retinal vein occlusion (BRVO) showing marked retinal hemorrhages and macular exudates.

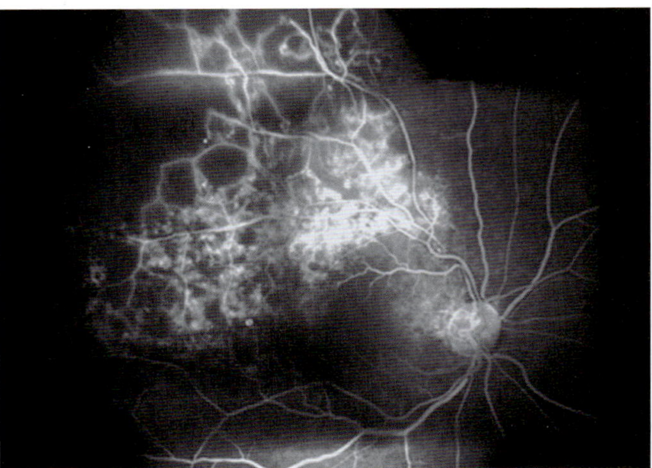

Fig. 42.20: Fundus fluorescein angiography (FFA) of a case of branch retinal vein occlusion (BRVO) showing capillary nonperfusion areas.

4–6 weeks before PRP (Fig. 42.18). This reduces the risk of exacerbation of edema after PRP.

All patients undergoing laser photocoagulation should have periodic comprehensive ocular examination to detect and treat any other retinal or ocular problem. When there is significant cataract with coexisting retinopathy, one should attempt to treat retinopathy first. In case, media clarity does not permit proper assessment and laser of the retinopathy, laser therapy can be undertaken as early as possible following cataract extraction. This can be as early as within 1 week following an uncomplicated phacoemulsification procedure.

Laser Treatment in Venous Occlusion

Laser plays an important role in the management of branch and central vein occlusion, which represent the second most frequent retinal vascular disorders, after DR. The amount of visual and retinal damage is related to the geographical area drained by the occluded vein, the extent of occlusion, and the ability of the surrounding vessels to develop collaterals.

In the acute phase, fluorescein angiography may not be helpful as many intraretinal hemorrhages are present, which obscure the surrounding retinal vessels and underlying retina and make interpretation difficult. Vascular occlusions are seriously blinding diseases, since most of the patients develop complications of ischemia leading to NVG.

Proper and timely referral for management of any underlying systemic condition should be done by the treating retinal physician. Standardized treatment protocols for managing vascular occlusions and its sequelae are still evolving.

Branch Retinal Vein Occlusion

Two most significant vision-threatening complications of branch vein occlusion are macular edema and retinal/optic disc neovascularization (Figs. 42.19 to 42.22). The Branch Vein Occlusion Study[26,27] (BVOS) does not recommend extensive systemic laboratory investigations in patients with a typical branch retinal vein occlusion (BRVO). In atypical cases, i.e. young patients, bilateral cases, or patients with a personal or family history of thromboembolism, certain laboratory studies may be of use—prothrombin time, activated partial thromboplastin time, protein S, factor V Leiden, antithrombin III, protein C, serum homocysteine, antinuclear antibody, lupus anticoagulant, anticardiolipin and serum protein electrophoresis.[28]

Macular Edema

The BVOS showed the efficacy of grid laser photocoagulation in the treatment of BRVO-related macular edema. They

Angio (Superficial)   Angio (Deep)

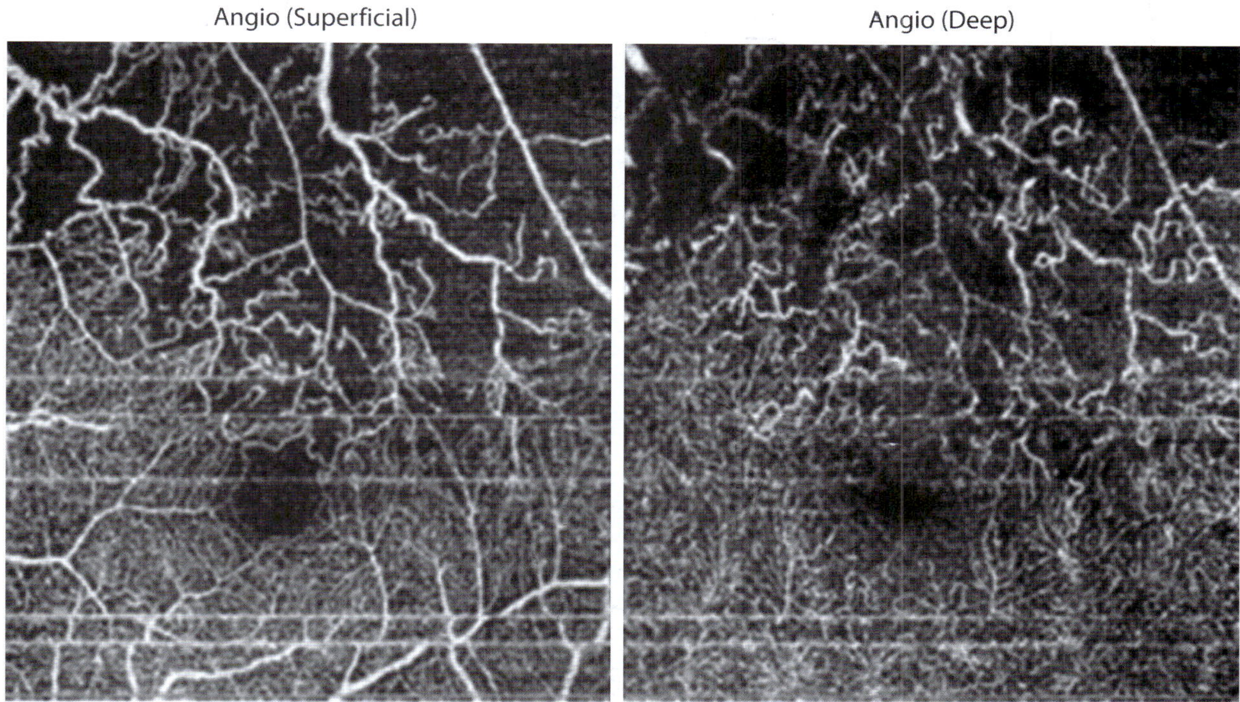

Fig. 42.21: Macular ischemia is clearly visible on optical coherence tomography ang ography (OCTA) imaging.

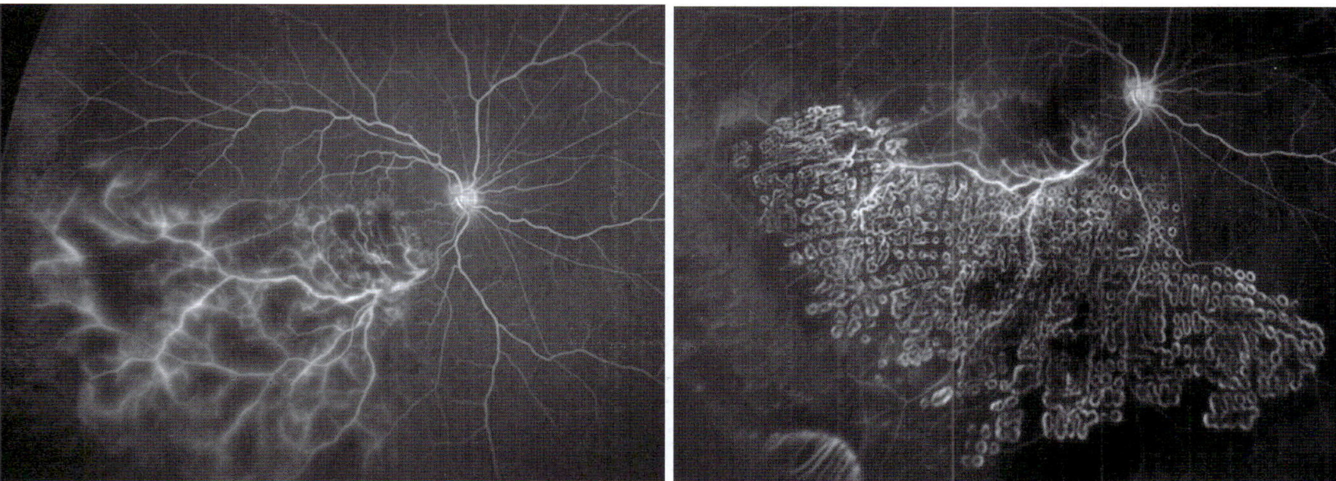

Fig. 42.22: Young essent al hypertensive, pre- and postlaser inferotemporal branch retinal vein occlusion (BRVO) on fundus fluorescein imaging. Retinal ischemia is evident in left picture.

performed grid photocoagulation in the first 12 months of onset of the occlusion, which helped in maintaining or improving vision in a larger number of patients (65% vs 35%) as compared to the natural course.[27]

According to the study, laser photocoagulation in a grid pattern should be performed in cases of BRVO of at least 3 months duration but no longer than 18 months duration, if there is late leakage at the fovea on fluorescein angiography and visual acuity is 6/12 or worse. The laser should be performed after resolution of most of the intraretinal hemorrhages at the macula. Intravitreal triamcinolone acetonide (IVTA) may help in supplementing the laser treatment.

Though a recent SCORE study did not find any benefit of IVTA over grid laser in cases of BRVO.[29]

If the fluorescein angiogram reveals macular nonperfusion suggesting an ischemic macula then laser may not be of much use and only observation is to be done.

Laser burns are placed one burn width apart, beginning 500 μ from the foveal avascular zone (FAZ) and extending to the edge of the macular edema but not further peripheral than the large-arcade vessels. Uninvolved macula is also spared. Spot size of 100 μ (increase to 200 μ near the arcades) and duration of 0.1 second is selected. Mild-intensity retinal burns are applied. Photocoagulation should be avoided over retinal hemorrhages due to the risk of iatrogenic inner retinal damage. Patient is followed up after 3 months. At that time, treat any residual areas of leakage, if macular edema is still present, especially if no improvement in vision has occurred.

Retinal or Disc Neovascularization

Usually in eyes with large branch vein occlusions, 50% develop significant capillary nonperfusion (CNP greater than 5-disc diameters) and of these patients, only 50% develop retinal or disc neovascularization. Many authors have shown that scatter photocoagulation in the affected eyes can lessen the likelihood of vision loss from vitreous hemorrhage. BVOS study also studied the utility of sector scatter retinal laser photocoagulation in reducing the risk of development of neovascularization and vitreous hemorrhage.[26]

It showed that scatter laser would be advisable to perform only after retinal neovascularization has developed, as it would probably be unwise to treat many patients for the prevention of neovascularization since more than 50% will never develop this problem. As and when scatter laser is performed in a case with BRVO, it is carried out only in the ischemic areas.

Once neovascularization has occurred and treatment is contemplated, the patient should still be informed that he or she still has a 30% chance of developing a vitreous hemorrhage even after treatment. The laser parameters used are similar to that used in a case of PDR undergoing PRP. The laser spots size of 200 μ is selected at the posterior pole. Laser spots are applied only throughout the region involved by the branch retinal vein occlusion in a sector fashion, extending no closer than 2 disc diameters from the center of the fovea. Macular grid (as previously described) is combined in the same sitting, if indicated. Blue-green and green wavelengths are effective in treating fresh BRVO and may prove to be a better wavelength option than krypton red laser wavelength.

Laser-induced chorioretinal anastomosis has also been described to treat BRVO.[30] The anastomosis aims to create an alternate drainage channel through the choroid bypassing the normal retinal drainage in the area of the obstructed vein. However, this procedure lacks repeatability and reliability in creating an anastomosis (most series report a 30–50% success rate). It can also have complications such as vitreous hemorrhage, development of an iatrogenic CNVM or even a choroidovitreal neovascularization and even tractional retinal detachment.

Central Retinal Vein Occlusion (Fig. 42.23)

Scattered panretinal hemorrhages with venous dilation and tortuosity establishes the diagnosis of central retinal vein occlusion (CRVO). It is important to determine the degree of nonperfusion in CRVO, as there is a significant risk of development of iris neovascularization and subsequent NVG. The other common complication is macular edema, the diagnosis of which depends on clinical appearance (macular edema is almost always present in an eye with an acute episode of CRVO). Fundus fluorescein angiography (FFA) in the acute phase of CRVO shows delayed transit time for fluorescein entry into the venous system. FFA is also helpful in determining the extent of capillary nonperfusion.

Central retinal vein occlusion can be ischemic or nonischemic. Cases of ischemic CRVO are at a higher risk of developing iris or angle neovascularization (NVI/NVA) or retinal neovascularization. If on FFA, an area of over 10-disc diameters of nonperfusion is present, a higher risk of the neovascular complications exists. According to the CRVO study, the risk of developing anterior segment neovascularization increases with the extent of capillary nonperfusion.[31] It is said to be around 16% in cases of more than 20-disc areas of nonperfusion and 52% in cases with more than 74-disc areas of nonperfusion.

Electroretinogram (ERG) "a" and "b" wave amplitude values and ratios of b/a-wave amplitude less than one or markedly depressed b-wave amplitude also suggests an ischemic CRVO. Marked relative afferent pupillary defect (RAPD) on testing with neutral density filters and poor-visual acuity on presentation (<6/60) are also indicators of ischemic CRVO.

In addition to the total area of retinal nonperfusion (Fig. 42.24), the three other risk factors for developing NVI/NVA/

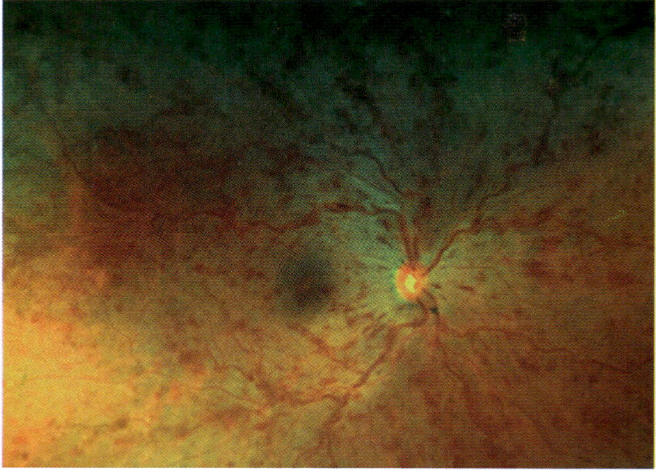

Fig. 42.23: Ultra-widefield (UWF) color picture of fresh central retinal vein occlusion (CRVO) right eye.

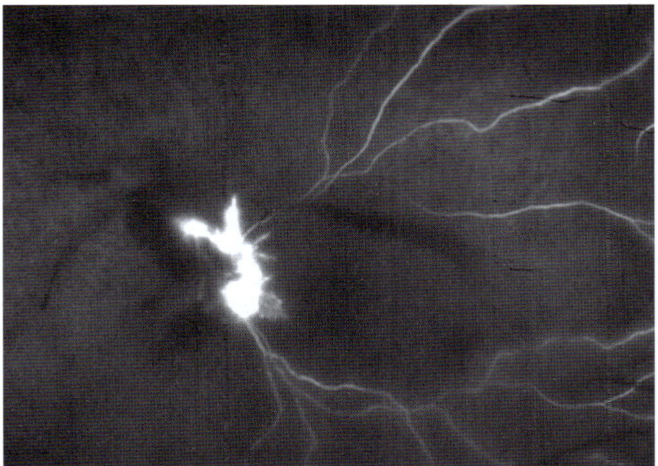

Fig. 42.24: Central retinal vein occlusion (CRVO)–fundus fluorescein angiography showing severe retinal ischemia with neovascularization of the disc (NVD).

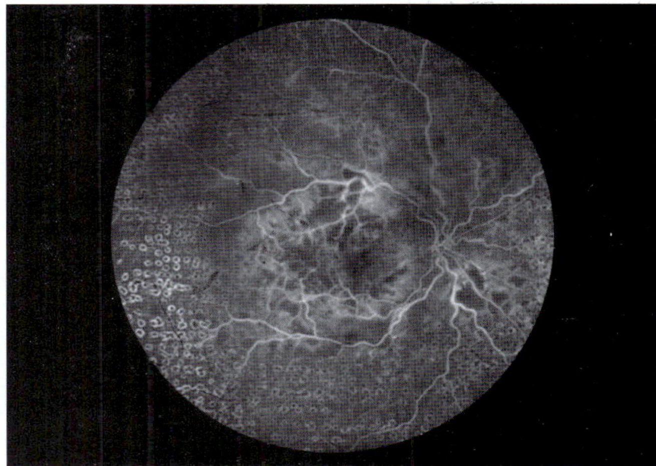

Fig. 42.25: Extensive panretinal photocoagulation of the capillary nonperfusion (CNP) areas in a case of central retinal vein occlusion (CRVO).

NVD/NVE include marked amount of retinal hemorrhages, duration of CRVO less than 1 month, and male gender. If there are no risk factors present, the chance of developing any neovascularization is less than 5%; whereas with three risk factors, the incidence increases to 80%.

Panretinal photocoagulation has been demonstrated by numerous studies to prevent iris and retinal neovascularization. The collaborative CRVO study group (1991–1994) carried out a prospective randomized clinical trial to test the efficacy of PRP in the:[31]

- Prevention of iris and retinal neovascularization
- Study the natural course of the disease—importance of undilated slit lamp examination of iris was found helpful in early detection of NVI.
- Study the role of macular grid treatment for post-CRVO macular edema—they concluded that laser has no role in reducing macular edema.
- Evaluate the role of ERG in CRVO—b:a amplitude ratio less than 1 was suggestive of ischemic CVO.

Twenty percent of eyes treated with prophylactic PRP developed anterior segment neovascularization, whereas this occurred in 35% of untreated eyes. Untreated eyes have a greater chance of regression in response to subsequent treatment. Therefore, it is recommended that patients be followed carefully for the development of iris or angle neovascularization (NVI/ANV). If either develops, extensive PRP (similar parameters as in a case of PDR) should be performed.

Extensive PRP (Fig. 42.25) is performed in these eyes, because a marked amount of retinal ablation helps to decrease the amount of vasoproliferative agent produced by the ischemic retina. In patients who cannot be followed carefully and have at least one risk factor, prophylactic PRP can be considered. Full treatment is completed in one or two sessions over 2–3 weeks. Patients should be examined monthly until regression of the rubeosis iridis occurs. If needed,

retreatment can be performed at 3–4 months. If marked retinal hemorrhages do not improve, use of red or infrared laser can be considered.

Most cases of ischemia develop within first 6 months, therefore the iris and angle should be examined monthly prior to dilation for that period, then every 2 months for the 1st year. After 1 year, the chances of developing an ischemic form of CRVO decrease markedly.

The CRVO study did not find any role of grid pattern photocoagulation for managing macular edema in CRVO. However, there was some improvement of vision of patients with a CRVO who were younger than 60 years. Worsening of vision with treatment occurs for those older than 60 years. Based on these findings, macular grid treatment for macular edema after CRVO should be offered only to those with age 60 years or younger after discussing that there might be slight-to-none improvement in the visual acuity. A useful alternative is IVTA to manage post CRVO macular edema. Low-dose IVTA has been found to be effective in reducing macular edema in cases of CRVO with minimal risks of complications.[32]

Macular treatment by laser shows anatomical improvement in the macular thickening/edema, but usually does not show improvement in visual acuity. Grid treatment should cover only all of the areas of leaking capillaries within 2-disc diameters of the foveola and should never extend within the FAZ. The macular grid treatment is given for edema with duration longer than 3 months and parameters are used as in BRVO macular edema patients as described previously in this chapter.

Photocoagulation in Retinal Vasculitis

Once the venous inflammation subsides or is brought under control by oral steroids, the proliferative retinopathy produced as a sequel can be managed satisfactorily by photocoagulation. The principle is very similar to the management of

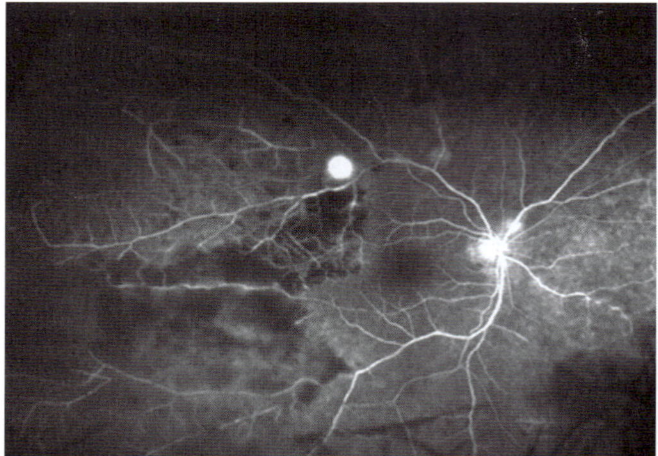

Fig. 42.26: Fundus fluorescein angiography (FFA) image showing postinflammatory vein occlusion with ischemic retina.

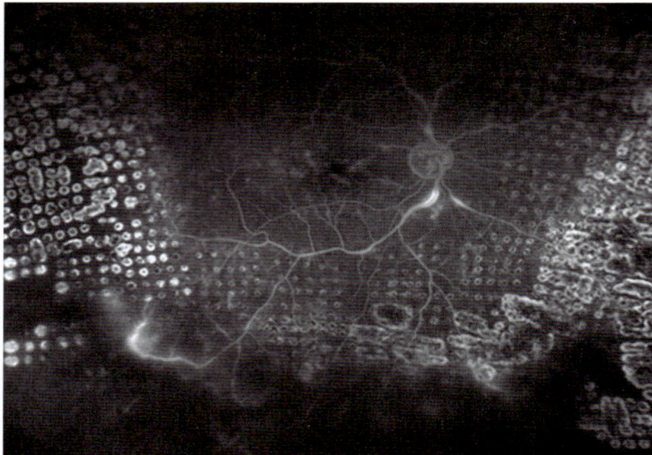

Fig. 42.27: Fundus fluorescein angiography (FFA) image of left eye with idiopathic vasculitis (Eales disease) with sheathing of vessels and laser marks along the retinal periphery.

BRVO (Fig. 42.26). The special situations in retinal vasculitis (more often than not, Eales disease in the Indian context) are:

- Presence of multiple postinflammatory BRVO's in one eye itself.
- Development of disc neovascularization (NVD) as a consequence.
- The development of new vessels elsewhere is also common.

Etiologically, causes of retinal vasculitis include toxoplasmosis, pars planitis, Behcet's disease, viral retinitis [including acute retinal necrosis (ARN), cytomegalovirus (CMV) retinitis, etc.], sarcoidosis, collagen vascular disorders [e.g. systemic lupus erythematosus (SLE), grant cell arteritis, etc.], syphilis and Lyme disease among others.[11,14]

As a rule, it is better to prevent a significant neovascular growth than to regress it. Preventing neovascularization is occasionally possible. If the amount of inflammation can be well controlled, then the progression to neovascularization may be checked as well. The concept is prevention of the inflammation and vascular occlusion before peripheral retina becomes ischemic. Once the conditions for ischemia prevail then the angiogenic stimulus for neovascularization is set into motion. PRP is also effective for eyes with iris neovascularization, particularly if applied before angle neovascularization develops.

The macular edema of vasculitic origin is inflammatory and usually responds to corticosteroid use. Laser is very rarely, if ever, needed for this type of edema (Fig. 42.27). Photocoagulation of paracentral telangiectasia can be effective in controlling the macular edemas or circinate maculopathy causing decreased vision.

Principle of Photocoagulation in Eales Disease

Neovascularization, once identified, is usually treated. Argon laser photocoagulation of the peripheral retina may be performed with a contact lens, indirect ophthalmoscope delivery or by endolaser. The argon green laser creates burns centered on the RPE. Red wavelengths are better absorbed by choroidal pigment, so for an effective retinal burn with red wavelengths to be produced, more choroidal damage occurs. The red wavelength is not absorbed as much by hemoglobin or yellow lens pigment. Consequently, the advantage of using red wavelength is that it can penetrate through vitreous hemorrhage or nuclear cataracts more effectively than the green wavelength.

Once the venous inflammation subsides, it leaves an ischemic retina, which poses the danger of vascular proliferation—proliferative retinopathy. On fluorescein angiography, areas of capillary closures, increased permeability of the capillary system and growth of new vessels are suggestive of persistent ischemia. Selective retinal ablation of the ischemic retina, by scatter photocoagulation, gives good results and, if needed, peripheral cryotherapy can be used. Peripheral cryotherapy has some special indications.

- When pupil is small and it is difficult to laser the peripheral retina.
- When vitreous hemorrhage settles over the lower periphery and impedes the completion of laser treatment.
- When in spite of repeated laser new vessels do not regress.

Eales disease is often associated with massive neovascular proliferation both in the periphery of the retina and at the posterior pole, which includes optic disc neovascularization.[23] A peripheral scatter photocoagulation can produce a regression of these new vessels. However, unless one follows certain principles of anchoring photocoagulation, the massive gliosis, which replaces the regressing new vessels, on contraction can cause several unfortunate complications like:

- Tractional detachment of the macula
- Occurrence of retinal breaks near the base of the fibrovascular tissue. These could then lead to a secondary rhegmatogenous retinal detachment

- Contracting glial tissue around the posterior pole may wrinkle the retina leading to epiretinal membrane formation and cystoid macular degeneration.

Applying anchoring laser all around extensive fibrovascular proliferation first followed by completion of scatter laser may help to minimize or eliminate some of these complications.[33]

Scatter laser effectively treats many forms of neovascularization. Laser burns are placed about one lesion width apart in areas of retina thought to be ischemic (sector scatter) or throughout the peripheral retina (panretinal). Exactly how scatter laser causes neovascularization to regress is not known. Perhaps the balance of angiogenic and inhibitory factors is changed, or perhaps loss of the outer retina allows oxygen to reach previously ischemic inner retina. In any case, photocoagulation suppresses the neovascular signal and treatment is often effective.

Laser Principles for Treating Fibrovascular Proliferation around Posterior Pole

In the first sitting, moderate-to-severe intensity burns of 200–300 μ are placed around the neovascular tissue along the temporal blood vessels. All extensions are similarly surrounded. After about 2–3 weeks when the photocoagulation scars are well formed, anchoring the retina to the underlying choroid; peripheral retinal ablation is carried out by scatter photocoagulation of mild-to-moderate intensity, in more than one sitting, till new vessels regress. Sometimes, in cases with florid new vessels or when vitreous hemorrhage does not permit adequate photocoagulation, peripheral cryotherapy could conclude the regressive process. Once the retina around the neovascular lesions is properly "anchored", regression by peripheral retinal ablation with photocoagulation or cryotherapy or both is safer.

Laser Principles for Treating Fibrovascular Proliferation in Periphery (Fig. 42.28)

The first step is again surrounding the neovascular lesion with moderate-to-severe grade photocoagulation spots of 200–300 μ. Besides anchoring, photocoagulation is also carried out along the draining venules. This step prevents retinal breaks around the point where the draining veins are pulled up when the shrinking vascular mass is pulled up into the vitreous. If the new vessels are found to be bleeding or are suspected to be on the verge of bleeding (too vascular), the crimping of the feeding arterioles is also carried out. Some peripheral photocoagulation can be done at this stage anterior to the neovascular tissue, as this is usually the ischemic zone, which stimulates NVE formation.

Treatment should extend 1.5 mm anterior and posterior and 1 clock hour to either side of the neovascularization in case of sector scatter laser. Any fresh areas of neovascularization found on follow-up should be treated with supplemental photocoagulation.

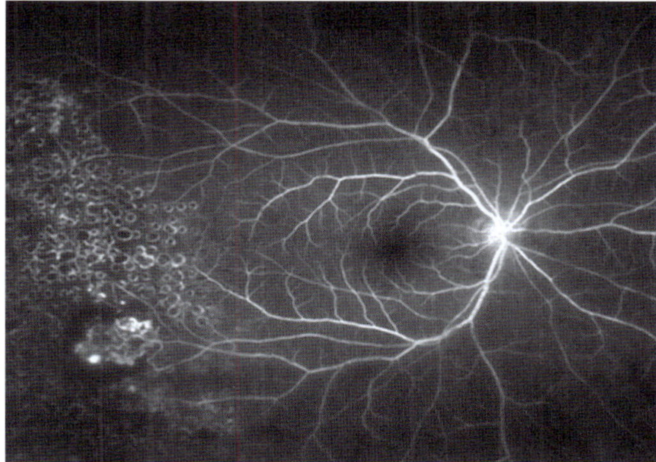

Fig. 42.28: Laser 4–5 rows are closely placed surrounding the fibrovascular growth and anterior as this area has ischemia and must be treated with laser.

The patients need to be reviewed after 3–4 weeks to see for regression or progression of neovascularization. The patient should be instructed to review SOS in case of any fall in vision during the follow-up. The patient can develop complications due to neovascularization immediately after laser and before the full regression of these abnormal vessels. These complications as in case of DR could be vitreous hemorrhage and retinal detachment. Anterior segment neovascularization can also develop. If left untreated, this leads to NVG with resultant severe visual loss and, occasionally, even loss of the eye. There is no treatment modality as of now to prevent capillary nonperfusion. We recommend mandatory triple mirror examination in both the eyes of Eales disease patients to detect and manage early changes of the disease process and limit its complications.

Scatter laser photocoagulation causes significant inflammatory leukocyte–endothelial interactions in the untreated half of the retina also.[34] Leukocyte accumulation in the untreated half of the retina is said to increase after photocoagulation and peaks at 24 hours after photocoagulation.[24] Retinal vascular permeability also increases in the untreated half. These changes may increase retinal edema in untreated retina. Thus, it may be best to give a short course of systemic steroids (2–3 days) after scatter photocoagulation to reduce this inflammatory reaction. To summarize, acute inflammation should be controlled prior to retinal laser photocoagulation. Always examine the apparently normal fellow eye of the patient with great concern as peripheral disease may not be symptomatic and timely laser photocoagulation can prevent many of the sight-threatening complications of this ischemic process. Direct laser treatment of flat retinal new vessels can be done. Sectoral photocoagulation helps in regression of neovascularization following vasculitis. Anchoring photocoagulation can help to prevent complications of laser in such cases. It is not essential to do a pan retinal scatter in all cases of peripheral neovascularization secondary to retinal vasculitis.

Central Serous Chorioretinopathy

Central serous chorioretinopathy manifests commonly as a neurosensory detachment at the macula. This was first described in middle-aged men. The visual acuity is usually modestly reduced and is often correctable to 6/6 with addition of a weak "plus" lens. There is an acquired hyperopic shift because neurosensory detachment causes the retina to be closer to the focal point of the eye. This gives rise to disparity between the subjective and objective refraction of the eye. The patient notices metamorphopsia and decreased vision. The former results from Stiles–Crawford effect, which states that if retinal photoreceptors are not properly oriented, they do not transduce light signals accurately.

Positive relative scotoma and impaired dark adaptation are also commonly associated. Scotoma is usually paracentral. Threshold Amsler grid test and macular threshold perimetry will detect subclinical scotoma in almost all cases of CSCR.

Fundus examination shows a loss of the foveal reflex and small well-defined zone of elevated neurosensory retina. There may be associated small spots of retinal pigment epithelial atrophy. In some cases, subretinal whitish fibrin deposition is also visible. Occasionally, patients have massive neurosensory detachments. These may be seen in patients who are using corticosteroids, usually after an organ transplant or for treatment of an autoimmune disorder. Discontinuing the steroids stops the leakage and leads to slow resolution of the detachment.

Chronic form of CSCR is more aggressive. There is a greater tendency for recurrence with nonresolution of the neurosensory detachment. The fluid has a tendency to track down to the inferior periphery, but almost never reaching up to the ora serrata (most important differentiating feature for rhegmatogenous retinal detachment).

Fluorescein angiography helps to detect either active foci of detachment or evidence of previous injury to the RPE. In active CSCR, FFA shows a spot or area of hyperfluorescence surrounded by increasing fluorescence in the later stages of the angiogram (inkblot leak). The classic smokestack appearance (Figs. 42.29 to 42.31) is seen only rarely. This type of leak probably occurs as the warmer fluorescein associated serum rises into the cooler overlying neurosensory detachment, and then diffuses throughout the neurosensory detachment. Fluorescein rises as it is lighter than subretinal fluid and also because of an osmotic pressure gradient caused by different protein concentrations. This produces a smokestack pattern. The leak seen more commonly is a circular expanding diffusion (inkblot) of fluorescein from the leaking area. Most common site of leakage is superonasal to the foveal center.

Optical coherence tomography provides immense information about CSCR detachments and their resolution over time. OCT scanning (Fig. 42.30) reveals a classical neurosensory detachment. Follow-up OCT helps to monitor the disease process and resolution. In fact, repeat FFAs, which are an invasive modality, can be avoided and only OCT performed on serial visits.

Often leakage stops spontaneously and the neurosensory detachment is slowly resorbed. For the first episode, it is probably best not to treat the patient immediately but to have the patient return in 1 month. At the return visit, if active leakage is still seen, treatment can be considered. It must be remembered that there is a possibility, up to 15% chance that a CNVM could develop after treatment. The CNVM may also develop spontaneously (with a much lesser incidence), but it is better to wait for up to 3–4 months.

Corticosteroids have to be strictly avoided in CSCR, as these may increase the risk of recurrence. About 80% of eyes with CSCR can resolve on their own with the visual acuity improving to 6/6 within 1–6 months. Remaining 20% last longer but resolve within 12 months, if no continuous insult is present in the form of steroid use. It must be remembered that treating the lesion with laser hastens recovery but does not affect chances of recurrence and the final visual acuity achieved. Laser treatment has been reported to result in suboptimal recovery of contrast sensitivity in comparison to cases that resolve spontaneously (Fig. 42.32). The prerequisites for laser photocoagulation are vision of less than 6/12 with a well-defined leakage point on FFA that is at least 500 µ from the fovea. The indications for the laser treatment in CSCR could be:

- Angiographic leak persisting beyond 4 months
- In recurrent CSCR to hasten visual recovery and decrease the risk of chronic RPE decompensation
- Bilateral CSCR—treat only one eye
- Patients' occupational needs
- Other eye vision impaired due to an episode of CSCR.

Early treatment is performed only after comparing the fluorescein angiograms and OCT images from the first and second visits to ensure that there is still active leakage and that there is no evidence of growth of the area of active leakage, which would be suspicious for a growing CNVM. In addition, patients should be questioned carefully about the use of any medication that could predispose them to the development or perpetuation of CSCR. If the leakage is within 500 µ of the foveal center, laser photocoagulation is not considered, because the laser spot can cause a central scotoma after resolution of the neurosensory detachment.

The protocol for laser in CSCR is similar to that for focal macular laser in CSME. Longer wavelength lasers are preferred. Carefully visualize the fovea before activating the laser. Locate the leakage spot and activate the laser. Use a 100-µ spot for most cases. Smaller sized spot has higher chance for later CNVM development. Place a couple of test burns close to the arcade to determine the power required. Use 0.1 second or less interval and burn with power adjusted to obtain a barely perceptible gray burn. Then place three or four burns on the

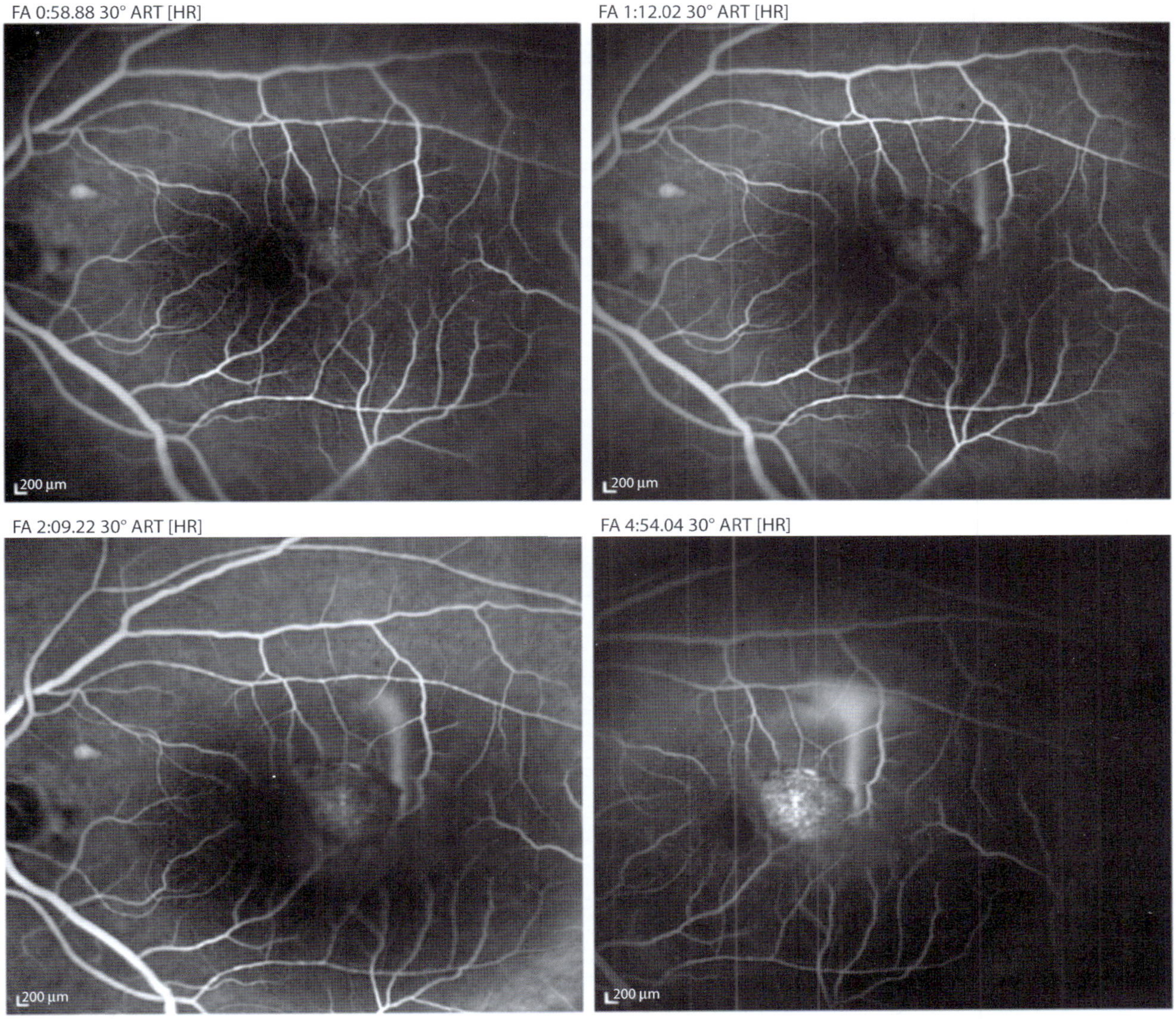

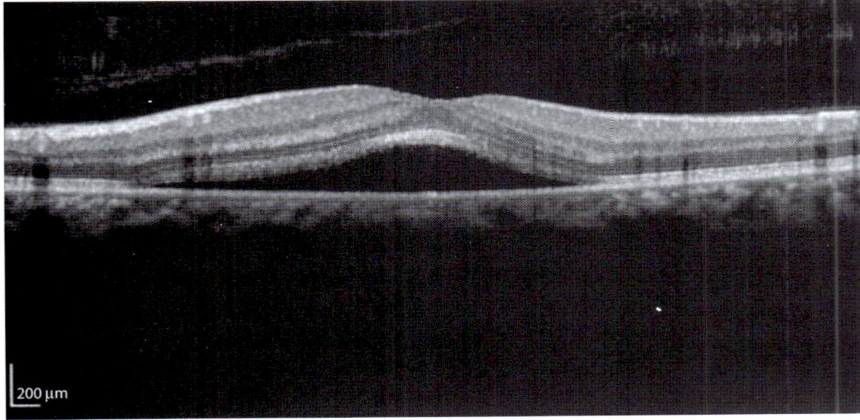

Fig. 42.29: Central serous detachment—early smokestack leak visible on fundus fluorescein angiography (FFA).

Fig. 42.30: Line scan (optical coherence tomography) is showing central neurosensory detachment.

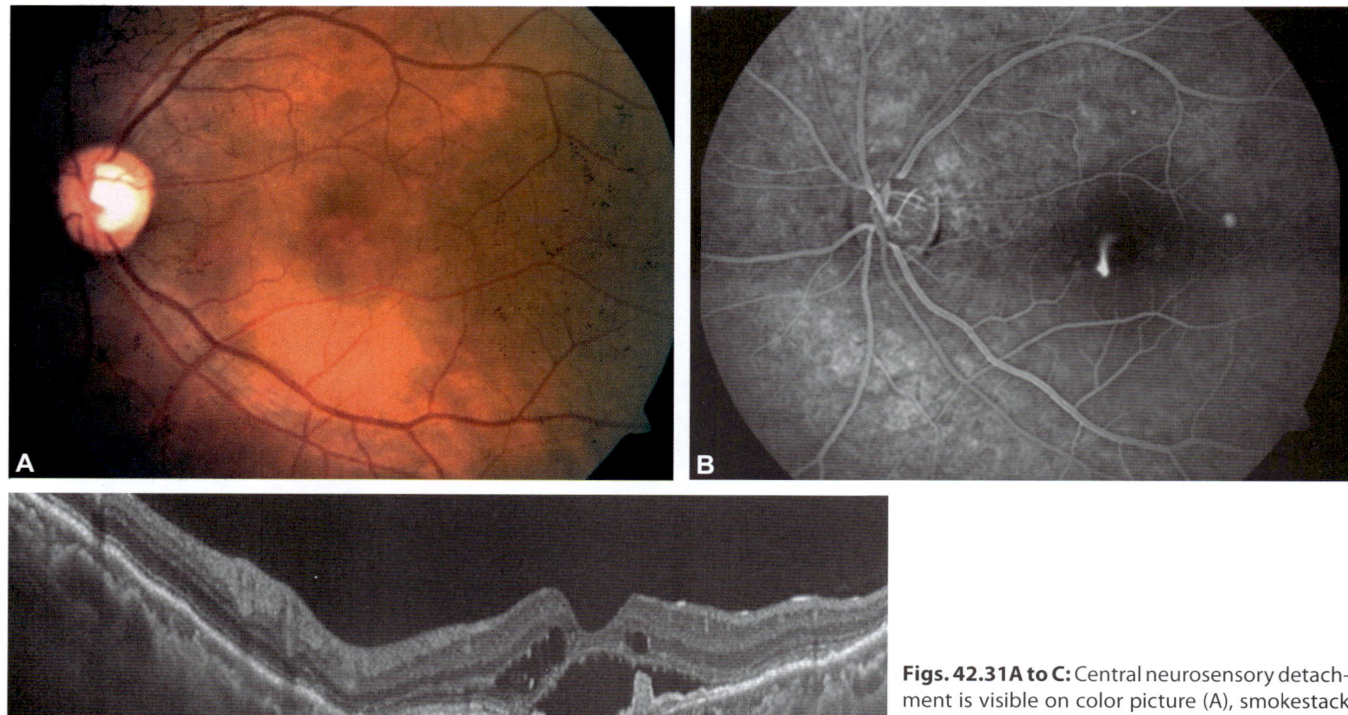

Figs. 42.31A to C: Central neurosensory detachment is visible on color picture (A), smokestack leak on fluorescein angiography (FA) (B) and optical coherence tomography (OCT) (C) shows subretinal leak with early thumb-like PED and obvious choroidal thickening

Role of Photodynamic Therapy in Chronic Central Serous Chorioretinopathy

Acute cases of CSCR usually undergo spontaneous remission with favorable visual outcome as opposed to chronic cases of CSCR where symptoms persist for months or years together. This persistent detachment of fovea leads to atrophic degeneration of the retina and RPE, with poor visual recovery even after the detachment resolves. Laser photocoagulation can lead to neovascularization; hence, PDT may be an ideal choice in chronic CSCR.

In CSCR, there is ischemic congestion and hyperpermeability of the choriocapillaris, and therefore, a modality of treatment like PDT aimed at this level is helpful. Studies have shown improvement or stable visual acuity after PDT in patients with CSCR. Subretinal fluid has been shown to reduce with reduction of leakage on FFA and an improvement in vision has been documented after PDT (Figs. 42.33 to 42.35). Thus, PDT allows for faster resolution of the neurosensory retinal detachment than laser. ICG-guided treatment with PDT was first demonstrated to be efficacious by Yannuzzi et al.[35] PDT using Visudyne has also now being reported to manage chronic CSCR leaks. ICG angiography is preferred prior to PDT treatment, as the leaky and diseased choriocapillaris are outlined by ICG imaging and the PDT

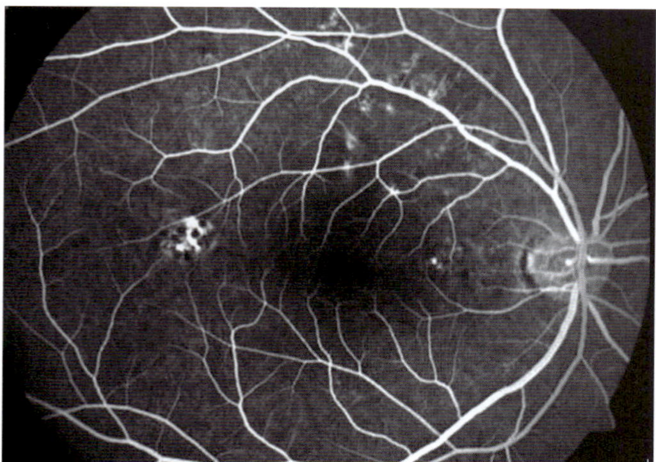

Fig. 42.32: Fundus fluorescein angiography image showing focal laser of the leak in a case of chronic chronic central serous chorioretinopathy (CSCR).

leakage spot. Re-evaluate the patient after 6 weeks. There is approximately 20% chance of recurrence after an episode of CSCR.

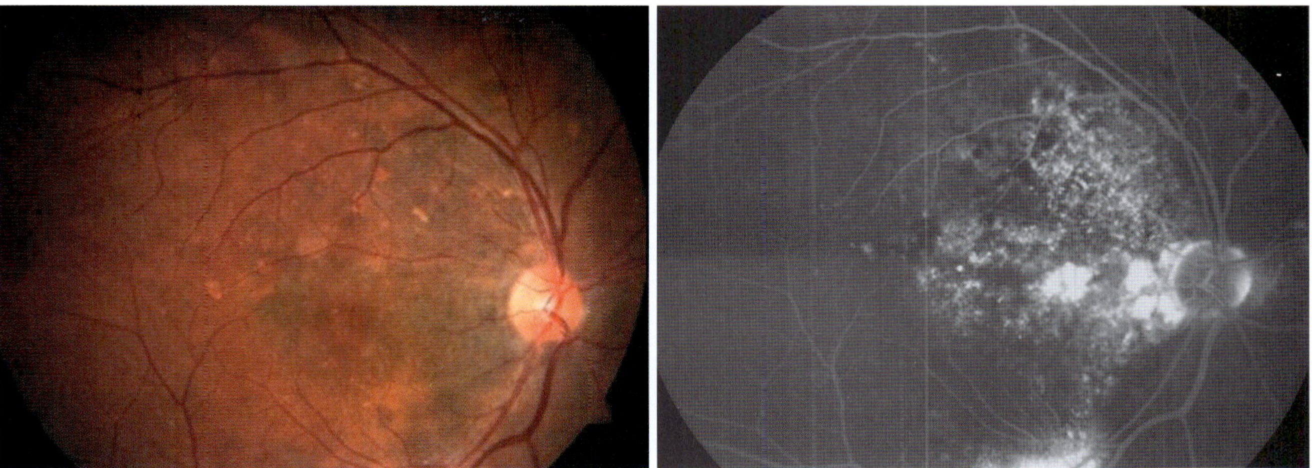

Fig. 42.33: Clinical picture and fundus fluorescein angiography (FFA) showing leak in a case of chronic central serous chorioretinopathy (CSCR) (prephotodynamic therapy).

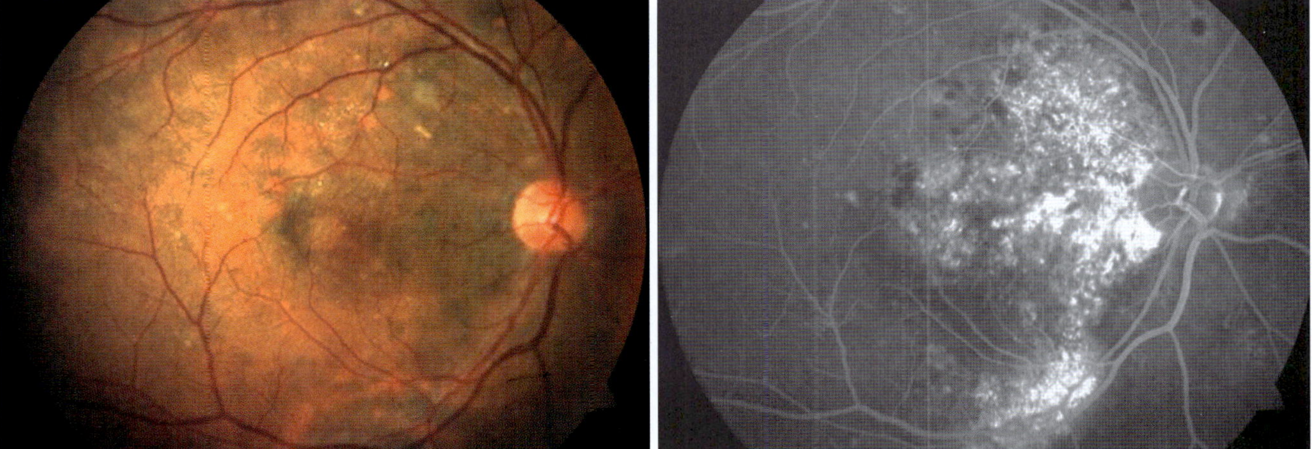

Fig. 42.34: Clinical picture and fundus fluorescein angiography (FFA) of the same patient postphotodynamic therapy (PDT) 4 weeks.

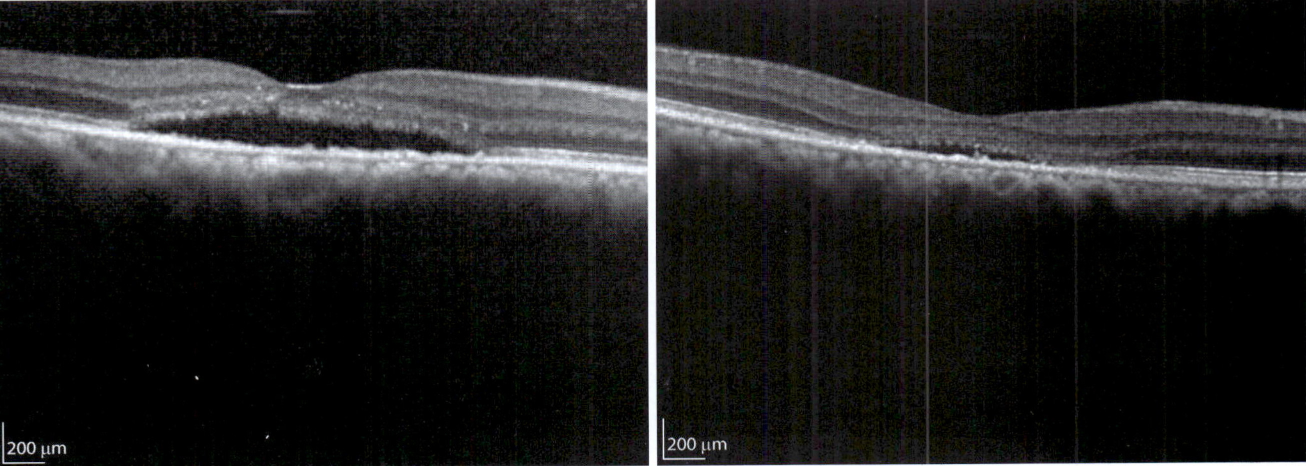

Fig. 42.35: Pre- and postphotodynamic therapy (PDT) optical coherence tomography (OCT) images showing resolution of chronic central serous chorioretinopathy (CSCR) post-PDT treatment.

laser beam is aimed to target this area. A study done by Piccolino et al. in 2003 showed resolution of CSCR leak in 81% eyes post-PDT treatment. Visual acuity improved by one to four lines in 11 eyes and was unchanged in five eyes.[36]

Half-fluence Photodynamic Therapy

There are various ways of administrating PDT. PDT is usually performed in the "standard" fluence and dose (10-minute infusion of verteporfin dose 6 mg/m², exposure duration—83 seconds of 689-nm light wavelength spot; exposure of 600 mW/cm², 5 minutes half after infusion, and yielding 50 J/cm² fluence). To perform fluence PDT, the dose of the drug is kept the same but the energy or fluence is halved (25 J/cm² over a duration of 83 seconds). On the other hand, in half-dose PDT, the amount of drug infused is halved (3 mg/m²), and the duration and power of the laser application are not changed (50 J/cm² for 83 seconds). A multicenter and retrospective study has shown that the half-fluence PDT is as effective as conventional PDT and it also reduces the adverse effects of PDT on choriocapillaris perfusion and retinal thickness.[37] Some studies have shown similar results with both low-fluence PDT and PDT with half-dose verteporfin in cases of chronic CSCR with good long-term outcomes.[28,38] In our experience half-fluence PDT is a promising modality for treating cases of chronic CSCR with leaks around the fovea.

Disadvantages

Photodynamic therapy can cause damage to the choroid, especially the choriocapillaris and the RPE. It may not be that effective in eyes not showing intense hyperfluorescence on ICG angiography. Patients with significant leakage in the late frames of ICG angiography show a good response.

The most important differential diagnosis is CNVM and retinal pigment epithelial detachments. CNVM usually occurs in association with AMD, so it is important to examine the rest of the fundus and the fellow eye to see if other signs may lead to a different diagnosis. If there are drusen present and the patient is elderly, the diagnosis may be CNVM. One should look carefully for the subretinal blood and re-evaluate the early phases of angiogram for evidence of a classic CNVM resembling a lacy fluorescein pattern that increases in fluorescence. If PED is present then performing laser is almost contraindicated because of much increased incidence of development of CNVM in the treated area. OCT angiography is a new modality, which may help to distinguish a case of CSCR from that of CNVM.

TRANSPUPILLARY THERMOTHERAPY

It was considered an alternative to PDT for treatment of subfoveal CNVM (Table 42.6). However, it was seen to cause much more scarring and is now seldom used for this purpose. In cases of tumors, transpupillary thermotherapy (TTT) may be effective alone only for small tumors (up to 4 mm in basal diameter and 2 mm in thickness).

Indications

- Occult CNVM in wet AMD
- Retinoblastoma
- Choroidal hemangioma
- Choroidal melanoma.

Contraindication

- Dry AMD
- Choroidal neovascular membrane within 200 μm of the optic disc
- Subfoveal CNVM with good visual acuity.

Table 42.6: Distinguishing features between photodynamic therapy (PDT) and transpupillary thermotherapy (TTT).[7]

Features	PDT	TTT
Laser and wavelength (nm)	Diode, 689	Diode, 810
Laser–tissue interaction	Photoradiation	Photothermal
Indications	Classic subfoveal CNVM	Occult subfoveal and juxtafoveal CNVM Retinoblastoma Choroidal hemangioma Choroidal melanoma
Temperature rise (Intralesional)	2°C	10°C
Exposure duration	83 seconds	60 seconds
Postlaser special restrictions	Avoid phototoxicity	Nil restrictions
Side effects	Pain at injection site due to extravasation Backache	Nil
Treatment cost	Expensive	Inexpensive

(CNVM: Choroidal neovascular membrane).

Mode of Action

Transpupillary thermotherapy employs a large spot size, low-irradiance diode laser (810 nm—infrared). The temperature rises to a maximum of 10°C within the lesion following exposure. This causes endothelial thrombosis and occlusion of the neovascular membrane, through release of free radicals, and without collateral damage to the overlying photoreceptors.

Parameters Used

- *Spot size*: 0.8 mm/1.2 mm/2 mm/3 mm.
- *Exposure time*: 60 seconds (fixed)
- *Power*: 200–600 mW (aim is to get a subthreshold burn).

CONVENTIONAL LASERS IN AGE-RELATED MACULAR DEGENERATION

Age-related macular degeneration is the most important cause of blindness in the West and is of increasing importance in most other countries and races. It accounts for 26–30% of all blind registrations in the UK. It is a bilateral and asymmetrical disease. The average age of loss on vision in one eye in this disease is around 65. The chances of involvement of the second eye increase by about 12% every year.[39,40] Studies have identified few factors, which determine the risk of progression to neovascular AMD.[41]

Low-risk non-neovascular AMD:
- Small hard drusen and minimal pigment epithelial abnormalities in macula
- 10% will progress to high-risk non-neovascular group over 5 years.

Intermediate-risk non-neovascular AMD:
- Excessive medium-sized drusen or more than or equal to 1 large drusen
- 18% progress to advanced AMD over 5 years.

High-risk non-neovascular AMD:
- Soft drusen, confluent drusen, both distinct and indistinct large drusen, and pigment epithelial abnormalities
- 15.6% risk of developing CNVM over 3 years.

Advanced AMD:
- Geographical atrophy involving center of macula
- Features of CNVM (neovascular AMD).

Patients who present with reduced acuity or blurred vision, distortion (metamorphopsia), discrete scotomas and reading difficulties, especially those over 65 years of age, should be suspected of having CNVM and or AMD or both. Once identified as being at risk on a screening retinal examination, all patients should receive an Amsler grid for home screening, although Amsler grid testing is not particularly reliable.

Studies have also identified risk factors for development of CNVM in the fellow eye:[42]
- More than 5 drusen
- Focal hyperpigmentation

- Large drusen (>64 µ)
- Systemic hypertension.

If all the above factors are present, the chance of developing a CNVM in the fellow eye in the next 5 years is around 87%. The 5-year incidence is a mere 7%, if none of the above mentioned risk factor is present. It is important to remember that these values are for the incidence in the fellow eye.

Classification of Choroidal Neovascular Membrane

Topographic classification:
- Extrafoveal (≥200 µ from foveal center)
- Juxtafoveal (1–199 µ from foveal center)
- Subfoveal (involving foveal center).

Angiographic classification:
- Classic
- Occult.

Idiopathic polypoidal choroidal vasculopathy (IPCV) and retinal angiomatous proliferans (RAP) are newly described variants of wet AMD.

Management of Age-related Macular Degeneration

Drusen

Many eyes with drusen maintain normal vision throughout life. Some may suffer mild-to-moderate visual loss. Development of focal hyperpigmentation and confluent drusen increase the risk of subsequent vision loss. In such patients, FA and OCT must be performed urgently and the lesion treated according to the findings. New technology in the form of OCT angiography is also proving helpful in investigating such cases noninvasively. Various studies have shown direct laser of drusen present at least 400 µ away from the fovea or indirect treatment of drusen by giving two vertical rows of laser 400 µ away may help in disappearance of drusen without improvement in vision. However, due to possible risks of laser-induced CNVM or scotomas developing after this treatment, it is not recommended. Use of subthreshold laser burns in such cases has been proposed by few authors.[43] Prophylactic treatment of AMD trial (PTAMD) was a multicenter, prospective and randomized controlled trial to determine the effects of subthreshold 810-nm-diode laser treatment on the rate of development of choroidal neovascularization and visual acuity in cases with multiple large drusen in one eye and a preexisting neovascular AMD lesion in the other.[44] They found that laser rather increased the risk of developing CNVM in fellow eyes. Thus, they advised against using prophylactic subthreshold diode laser treatment for large drusen.

Dry Age-related Macular Degeneration

Apart from provision of low-vision aids, there is no effective treatment. Refraction, cataract surgery (if required), dietary supplements, and home Amsler grid monitoring and regular retina evaluation might help.

Exudative Age-related Macular Degeneration

Retinal pigment epithelial detachment may resolve spontaneously, but it must be remembered that 66% can harbor a CNVM. Presence of CNVM warrants laser photocoagulation. The aim of treatment is to destroy the CNVM, but minimize laser damage to the fovea.

In the FAZ, heat dispersion, as related to circulation rate, is very low. Hence, the photothermal effect of lasers increases considerably. RPE cells have tight junctions, thus occluding the flow of elements from the choriocapillaris to the sensory neuroepithelium. Laser applied in high energy or in very small spots can break or destroy these junctions and aggravate the pathology. RPE cells damaged by the thermal effect of photocoagulation can, in turn, lead to destruction of rods and cones, which are metabolically dependent on the RPE. The action of laser on the retinal and choroidal vascular networks does not depend exclusively on wavelength, but also on the oxygen content of hemoglobin.

Selections of Lasers

- Blue light—not preferred, as it is absorbed much more by xanthophylls in the macula, by hemoglobin in the blood vessels and by a nuclear cataract, besides being scattered more than longer wavelengths.
- Green argon light (514 nm or pea-green 532 nm)—preferred, as it is absorbed primarily by the pigment epithelium. Hence, a burn of mild-to-moderate intensity is limited to the outer retinal layers. It can completely destroy CNVM. However, because it is absorbed by hemoglobin, it can cause some damage to the inner retinal layers and normal retinal vessels. These are therefore especially hazardous to use in the event of subretinal blood because of absorption and spread of thermal damage. These are more useful in hypopigmented eye, recurrent CNVM from an atrophic laser burn scar, and a CNVM originating from idiopathic juxtafoveal retinal telangiectasis (JXT).
- Diode laser—preferred, as it causes maximum damage to the RPE and choroid. Clinical results for juxtafoveal lesions may be slightly superior to argon green. It is also much less scattered by lens opacities and vitreous opacities. This does spare the inner retina and theoretically may cause less overall tissue damage.

In the present era of anti-VEGF agents, laser is mostly used only for extrafoveal CNVM.

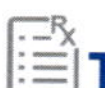

Treatment Protocol

Preoperative tracing of the CNVM and its retinal vascular landmarks from the pretreatment angiogram is useful. This allows accurate localization of a CNVM in relation to foveal center. This is critical because inadequately treated CNVM is a major cause of treatment failure, especially when treating juxtafoveal lesions. The drawing can be made manually or by digitized angiographic analysis.

A good general rule is—further the CNVM from the fovea, larger the spot size used for its treatment. The same is true for patient cooperation; the more cooperative the patient, the longer and larger the spot size. This enables us to have a "slow and homogenous burn" rather than a short, intense, explosive or hazardous one.

Angiogram must not be older than 72 hours for planning laser treatment. This is because the vascular component has a high-growth rate reaching up to 10 μ per day and therefore may rapidly increase in extent. Delayed presentation (from first symptom to retinologist consultation) deteriorates the outcome. Patients presenting within 2 weeks of first symptom have up to 80% chance of having treatable lesion, while the same reduces to 10% in case the patient presents after 4 months of first symptom.

Laser using 100–200 μ spots, time 0.1 second and power 200–300 mW. High-intensity burns should be used, the endpoint being a slightly white or whitish reaction. Spots of 50 μ as well as high short intensity should not be employed because of the risk of hemorrhage or rupture of the Bruch's membrane.

The perimeter of the CNVM is treated initially with overlapping burns and then the entire area is covered. The treatment must extend at least 100 μ beyond the margin of the CNVM. Repeat FFA is carried out 14 days after treatment to ensure that the obliteration of the CNVM is complete. If leakage is persisting, it suggests presence of residual CNVM. Any new CNVM after 2 weeks at the edge of the treated area is considered a recurrence. Retreatment is often necessary. The patient is warned to present urgently, if the vision drops suddenly, as this usually signifies a recurrence.

When treating peripapillary CNVM, at least one and one-half clock hours of the temporal side of the disc should be spared to prevent nerve fiber bundle defects. In addition, treatment for CNVM should not be extended closer than 100 μ to the optic nerve to avoid thermal necrosis of the disc tissue.

Fresh intraretinal hemorrhage possibly related to thermal retinal capillary damage (usually seen during the 1st week) should not be confused with subretinal hemorrhage associated with residual CNVM. RPE hyperplasia induced by photocoagulation can be differentiated from granular early sub-RPE CNVM by fluorescein angiogram; the former is hypofluorescent, while the latter is hyperfluorescent. Visual acuity may or may not improve, but metamorphopsia decreases.

Macular photocoagulation study was a landmark study on the effects of laser photocoagulation in cases of CNVM.[45]

The main results of the study are as follows:

Argon laser photocoagulation for extrafoveal CNVM:

- Laser treatment is beneficial in preventing or delaying loss of visual acuity for at least 5 years.
- The relative risk of severe visual loss (losing six or more lines from baseline visual acuity) among untreated eyes compared with laser treated eyes was 1.5 from 6 months to 5 years after entry (P = 0.001).

- After 5 years, untreated eyes had lost a mean of 7.1 lines of visual acuity; while laser treated eyes had lost 1.2 lines.
- Recurrent neovascularization was observed in 54% laser treated eyes by the end of 5 years.
- Almost 80% of all recurrences occur within 1 year of initial treatment.
- Frequent follow-up in the initial 2 years after treatment needed.

Krypton laser photocoagulation for CNVM:
- After 3 years, 49% of treated eyes, in contrast to 58% of untreated eyes, had severe visual loss.
- Average visual acuity of treated and untreated eyes was 20/200 and 20/250, respectively.
- The benefit of laser treatment was largest among patients who had no evidence of hypertension.
- There was no apparent benefit in hypertensive patients.
- Thirty-two percent treated eyes showed persistent neovascularization detected within 6 weeks of initial treatment.
- Additional 47% were expected to develop neovascularization over 5-year period.
- Both persistence and recurrence were accompanied by an increased frequency of severe visual loss.
- Persistence rate, among eyes having more than 10% of the foveal side of CNVM not covered by treatment, was twice as high as in eyes having more extensive coverage.
- Patients having a fellow eye with a CNVM or scar, 20 or more drusen in the central macula, or a dry AMD at initial visit had more recurrences than those without these characteristics.
- Persistent neovascularization and associated severe visual loss may be reduced by covering the entire lesion with treatment.
- Krypton laser treatment, while beneficial in many eyes, is not the perfect treatment.

 Postprocedural Management

The patient should be re-examined, including an appropriate angiogram, at 2 weeks and again 4–6 weeks later. After 2 weeks, the patient should be encouraged to check the Amsler grid at home to monitor any changes in central vision. Since the recurrence rate is high, the patient should be seen again at 3 months, 6 months, 12 months and 18 months after initial laser treatment.

At the initial 2-week examination, exudative manifestations should be resolving. Subretinal fluid usually reabsorbs faster than subretinal lipid or blood. The laser scar should be flat, though the central aspect of the scar may remain slightly thickened. Leakage at the edge of the scar, especially when accompanied by thickening of the RPE, is suggestive of residual CNVM.

At the 6-week examination and thereafter, the treatment site should be flat and the subretinal fibrosis contracted. A successful laser ablation of CNVM corresponds histopathologically to a scar in which proliferation of fibrocytes (with collagen production) and RPE cells (hyperplasia) are found and in which capillaries are present only external to the Bruch's membrane. Functional visual success depends significantly on the patient's ability to adapt to scotomas.

Recurrent Choroidal Neovascular Membrane (Fig. 42.36)

New or nonresolving metamorphopsia reported by the patient, often associated with decreased visual acuity, warrants immediate re-examination. Natural scarring within the CNVM prior to laser treatment and CNVM composed of more than 25% fibrous tissue carries a decreased risk of recurrence. Any recurrence associated with the edge of the photocoagulation burn is referred to as a "marginal recurrence".

Angiographic findings in cases of recurrence are variable and rarely show lacy hyperfluorescence with late pooling, as

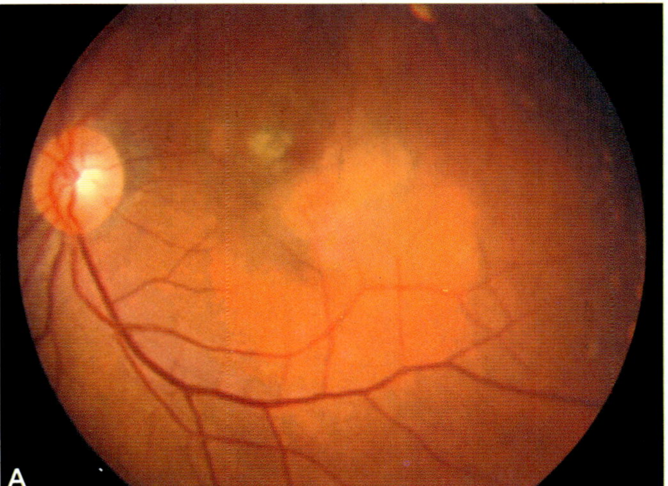
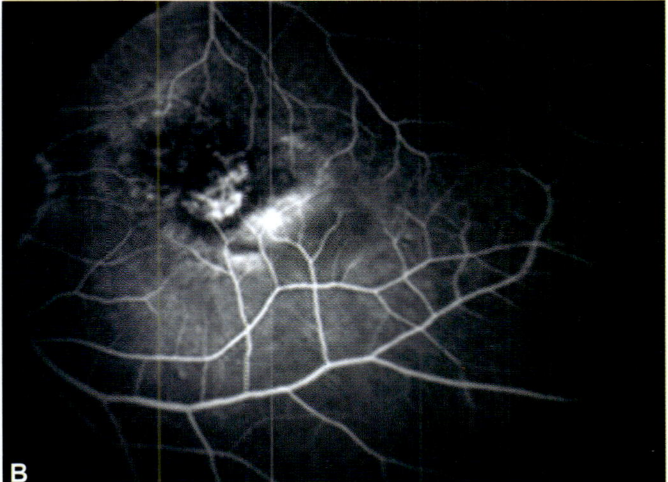

Figs. 42.36A and B: Color fundus image (A) and fundus fluorescein angiography (B) of a patient with recurrent CNV within the scar after PDT.

is seen in classic CNVM. Normal fluorescence due to intact choriocapillaris perfusion beneath the atrophic RPE at the margin of the burn must be differentiated from a recurrence. Late staining of the sclera in this region also occurs but does not intensify or spread as much as in recurrent CNVM.

Photodynamic Therapy

The treatment of wet AMD changed dramatically with introduction of PDT with verteporfin. Though PDT has been used in various medical specialties, its use originated from cancer research. Its use did not gain much popularity due to toxicity and skin photosensitivity. In ophthalmology, verteporfin has been approved for use of PDT in patients with macular degeneration, ocular histoplasmosis, myopic and idiopathic choroidal neovascularization.

It probably acts by causing direct endothelial cell damage, with platelet adhesion and degranulation. This initiates local vascular thrombosis and occlusion of the new vessels. PDT releases singlet oxygen and other free radicals. The photosensitizing dye on stimulation by laser is excited from the electronic ground state to a higher level. On returning back to its ground state, it releases energy. This energy breaks down the surrounding oxygen and other elementary compounds into singlet oxygen and other charged particles that can lead to vascular thrombosis and occlusion.

The first dye used for this type of treatment was hematoporphyrin dye. Recent studies have used benzoporphyrin or texaphyrin dye. These dyes are lipophilic and accumulate in proliferating vascular endothelial cells, perhaps because replicating endothelial cells have a higher concentration of lipophilic molecules. The endothelial cells of growing neovascular membranes can be destroyed by activating the accumulated dye with a laser whose wavelength is absorbed by the dye. Liposome-encapsulated benzoporphyrin derivative (verteporfin) is a modified porphyrin with an absorption maximum near 689 nm.[46,47] The effectiveness of treatment depends on a number of factors. These are wavelength, the metabolic profile of the dye and vehicle used in the dye.

The procedure of performing PDT is a "two-step process". It first involves infusion of the photosensitizing dye followed by application of appropriate wavelength of light to the site of the target tissue. The dose of the dye depends on the patient's weight and total body surface area (Fig. 42.37). After injecting the dye over 10 minutes and further waiting for 5 minutes, the laser is applied for around 83 seconds. These time intervals have been calculated to ensure maximum amount of dye in the CNVM. A later application of laser, while the dye is still in the retinal vessels, can cause complications like unwanted neovascular occlusion and neurosensory infarction.

The size of the lesion is calculated from the fluorescein angiogram. Lesions less than 5,400 μ in greatest linear dimension can be treated by a single spot. The beam size is kept least 500 μ beyond the margins of the neovascular complex

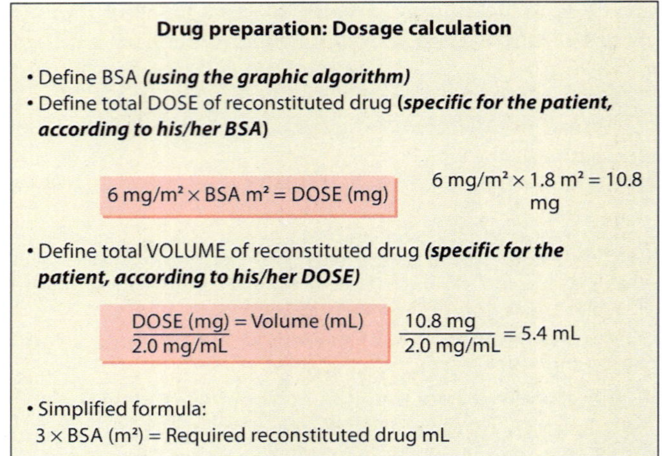

Fig. 42.37: Drug preparation for photodynamic therapy. (BSA: Body surface area).

on either side. Dose of the light energy is 50 J/cm², while the dose rate is 600 mW/cm². The drug is infused over 10 minutes and laser delivery is started 5 minutes later (15 minutes from initiation of injection). Unlike a thermal laser, post-PDT no visible change is seen on the fundus.

Multiple sessions of PDT may be required for treating CNVM (Figs. 42.38 to 42.42). After 1 year of treatment with benzoporphyrin (verteporfin) dye, approximately 60% of patients retain stable vision, compared with 45% of patients using a placebo. This therapy is also used for juxtafoveal photocoagulation for juxtafoveal CNVM.

Postprocedural precautions are to be followed diligently. Photosensitivity normally persists for 24–48 hours. Protective sunglasses should be worn immediately post-treatment. The patient should not expose his/her skin to sunlight or yellow bulb light post-therapy for 2–3 days. Treatment card/wristband should be carried to alert emergency crews of photosensitivity of patient in case of emergency.

Side effects of PDT are few but can be serious. Extravasations of the dye can cause localized tissue inflammation and injection. Infusion-related problems are reported in about 15% of patients. Photosensitivity reactions can occur in around 3% of patients undergoing PDT. There is mild-to-moderate sunburn in patients who had sun exposure within 24 hours of dye infusion. Back pain is a peculiar side effect of this treatment modality. This back pain may be related to possible changes or fluctuations in blood pressure and resolves with the patient standing up.

Optical coherence tomography proves an excellent guidelines for determining the efficacy of PDT treatment and serial follow-up, besides also contributes in decision making for retreatment.

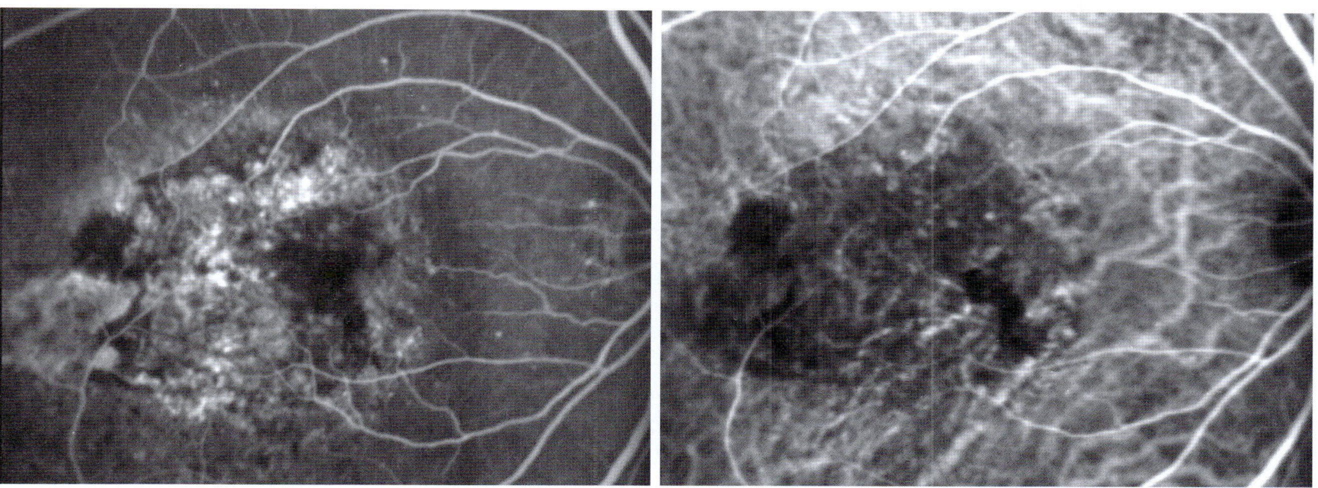

Fig. 42.38: Fundus fluorescein angiography (FFA) and indocyanine green chorioangiography (ICG) in a case of polypoidal choroidal vasculopathy. Note the numerous hyperfluorescent polyps on ICG angiography image (prephotocynamic therapy treatment).

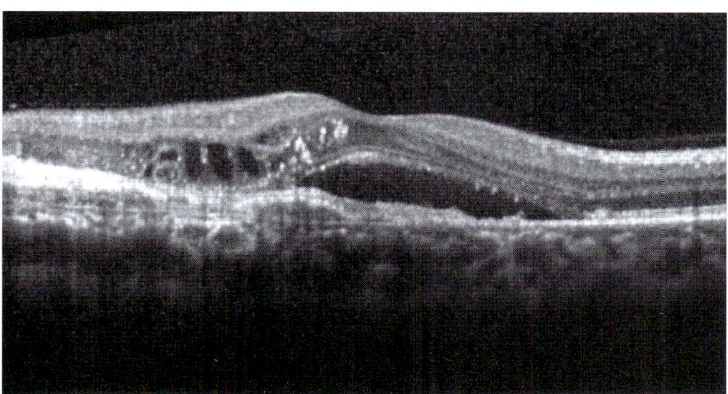

Fig. 42.39: Spectral domain optical coherence tomography (SD-OCT) showing choroidal neovascular membrane (CNVM) complex lesion (prephotodynamic therapy treatment).

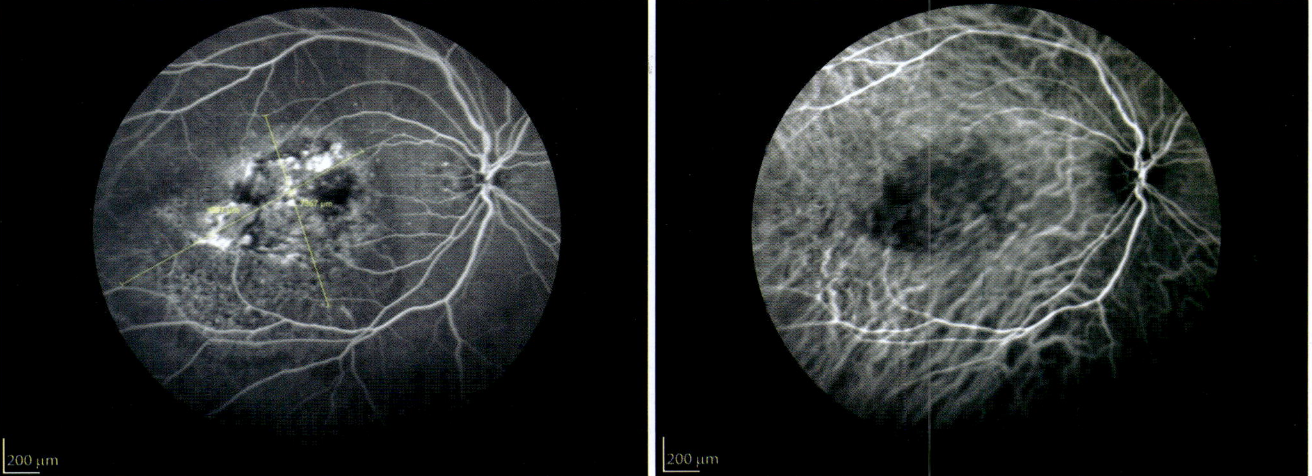

Fig. 42.40: Fundus fluorescein angiography (FFA) and indocyanine green chorioangiography (ICG) postphotodynamic therapy 4 weeks showing reduction in lesion size diameter and regression of polyps.

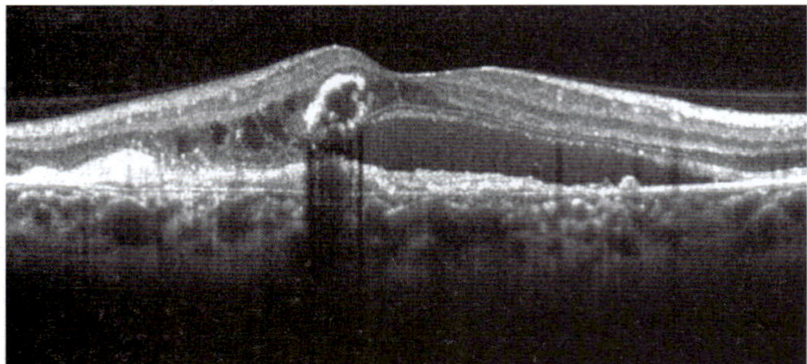

Fig. 42.41: Spectral domain optical coherence tomography (SD-OCT) postphotodynamic therapy 4 weeks showing little resolution of subretinal fluid.

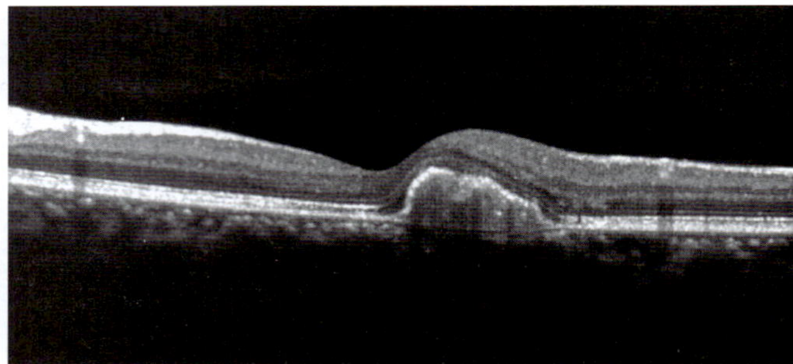

Fig. 42.42: Line scan (optical coherence tomography) showing markedly hyper-reflective lesion (suggestive of scar) with resolution of subretinal fluid.

LASER MANAGEMENT IN MISCELLANEOUS RETINAL DISORDERS

Retinal Artery Macroaneurysm

These are acquired often multiple, round or fusiform dilations of retinal arterioles. Hypertension, female sex and past history of vein occlusions are considered significant risk factors. Hemorrhages (pre-, intra- and subretinal) and retinal exudation is usually associated.

In acute presentations, the angiogram may not demonstrate the typical, nodular dilation of the involved artery in the early frames because of the presence of overlying vitreous and surrounding intraretinal hemorrhage. In later phases, there is often an area of hyperfluorescence appearing along involved artery. With clearing of the associated hemorrhage, the macroaneurysm becomes increasingly visible. ICG angiography may be helpful in examining patients with overlying vitreous hemorrhage.

Retinal arterial macroaneurysm (RAM) is treated to reduce the possibility of hemorrhage or to reduce macular exudation. Once it bleeds, it is likely to spontaneously resolve. Subretinal bleed, if it occurs, may cause permanent loss of vision. Also, macular edema and lipid exudation contribute to permanent vision loss. It is difficult to decide, which aneurysms are likely to bleed. Pulsatile aneurysms and large ones without much fibrosis are more likely to bleed.

A RAM may be directly treated with large laser spot of at least 200–500 µ burns and exposure time of 0.2–0.5 seconds. Power should be adjusted to produce a gentle whitening of the lesion. Laser can also be applied around the RAM in 2–3 overlapping rows.

Subhyaloid Hemorrhage

Hemorrhage under the posterior hyaloid or internal limiting membrane (ILM) at the macula is a cause of potential visual loss. It can be seen with PDR, RAM, Eales disease, trauma or Valsalva retinopathy. A membranotomy can be created in such cases using the double frequency Nd:YAG laser burn at the inferior margin of the entrapped blood to drain it into the vitreous cavity (Fig. 42.43). The YAG-hyaloidotomy (as is commonly referred) is done using single pulses of gradually increasing energy until drainage of the hemorrhage occurs. Drainage may not occur, if the blood is clotted or if adequate energy is not used.

Treatment of such eyes is usually performed, if the premacular hemorrhage persists for long or the occupation of the patient demands early recovery of binocular vision and stereopsis; or again, if early visual rehabilitation is required in patients with poor vision in the fellow eye. Most of such cases may resolve with observation alone. If YAG-hyaloidotomy does not help, surgical intervention might be needed.

Coats' Disease

Coats' disease (retinal telangiectasia) is characterized by vascular anomalies including telangiectatic vessels, microaneurysms, capillary dilatations, peripheral areas of capillary nonperfusion; and in some cases, significant exudation leading to bullous exudative detachments. Usually seen toward the end of first decade, a male preponderance and unilaterality of the disease are classic. It may mimic retinoblastoma, which has to be excluded by investigations like ultrasound and CT scan.

Treatment of Coats' disease is restricted to extensive laser photocoagulation (Fig. 42.44) or cryotherapy to reduce the lipid leakage and also to prevent NVI and subsequent NVG. Prognosis, however, stays guarded in such eyes.

Retinopathy of Prematurity

Laser photocoagulation is the primary therapeutic modality for nonregressing retinopathy of prematurity (ROP). Laser is initiated according to early treatment of ROP (ETROP) guidelines.[48]

Good pupillary dilation helps to achieve adequate laser. Pupillary dilation is done by application of a combination of 0.5% tropicamide and 2.5% phenylephrine drops. The entire avascular retina anterior to the ridge is ablated with moderate intensity nearly confluent burns. The laser should be done

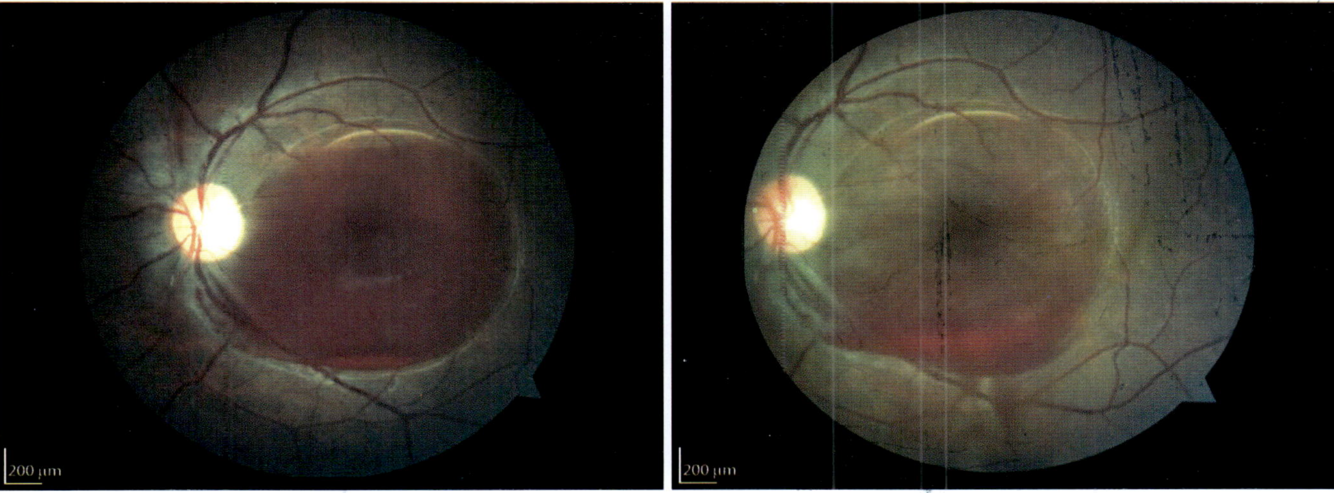

Fig. 42.43: Clinical fundus picture showing subhyaloid blood being drained with hyaloidotomy.

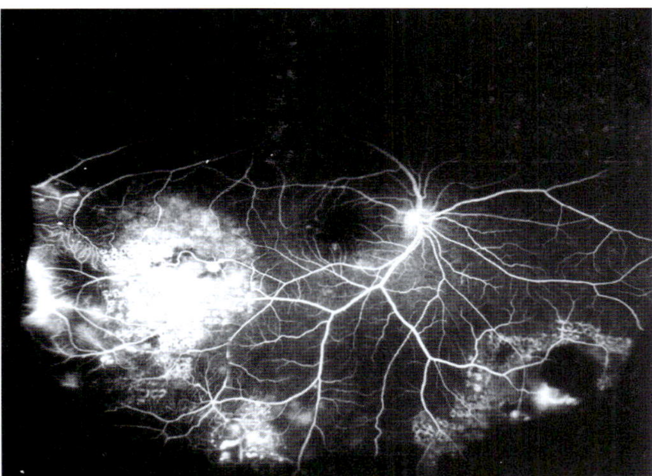

Fig. 42.44: Wide-field angiography of a lasered Coats' disease with persisting exudation.

till the ora anteriorly and all the capillary nonperfusion areas should be covered. Infrared diode laser or frequency double Nd:YAG laser delivered by an indirect ophthalmoscope is used (Fig. 42.45). Treat as much area as possible without indentation first and with minimal rotation of the globe. Try to complete the full treatment in one sitting. If follow-up at 1 week shows skip areas or disease progression, retreatment should be performed. A +28D lens is preferable for evaluation and lasering ROP cases for a wider view of the periphery.

A neonatologist/anesthetist specially trained to handle such small babies in case of an emergency should be physically present when the procedure is being performed.

Laser Vitreolysis

This can be used for cutting discrete, avascular and taut vitreoretinal bands causing traction toward the macula. Nd:YAG laser has been used for this. Large vessels in the vitreous membrane should be avoided, so as to prevent hemorrhage, although vascular closure with photocoagulation may be attempted prior to Nd:YAG laser vitreolysis. The aiming beam is focused on the vitreous lesion to be cut, using energy of 10 mJ or above and multiple (up to 6) pulses per burst. Energy is delivered to a stretched portion of the vitreous band. Multiple treatment sessions are usually needed to sever the desired vitreous structure.

Retinal Breaks

Not all breaks need to be treated. Breaks with evidence of significant vitreous traction are much more likely to lead to retinal detachment than those without traction. In this regards, flap tears are of greatest concern. Operculated holes and atrophic holes need treatment, if symptomatic. Generally, any such lesion in the fellow eye of a patient who has suffered a retinal detachment in one eye needs to be treated.

Objective of applying laser around a retinal break is to create a chorioretinal adhesion around the break. Laser creates a more rapid adhesion and liberates fewer retinal pigment epithelial cells during treatment than cryotherapy. Pigmentary reaction around the break should be checked approximately 1–2 weeks after treatment. Patients are at risk for additional breaks, particularly within first 3 months of symptoms and thus a follow-up should be planned accordingly.

Laser spot size of around 300–500 µ with 0.2 second burn duration should be used. Aim at moderate retinal whitening. Two or three nearly confluent rows of photocoagulation burns should be placed into attached retina up to margin of the break (Fig. 42.46). Treatment should adequately cover even the anterior aspect of the break. This can be achieved using a panfundoscopic-type lens or LIO. Laser can also be useful for preventing the spread of small retinal detachments or for delimiting a persistent retinal detachment following failed

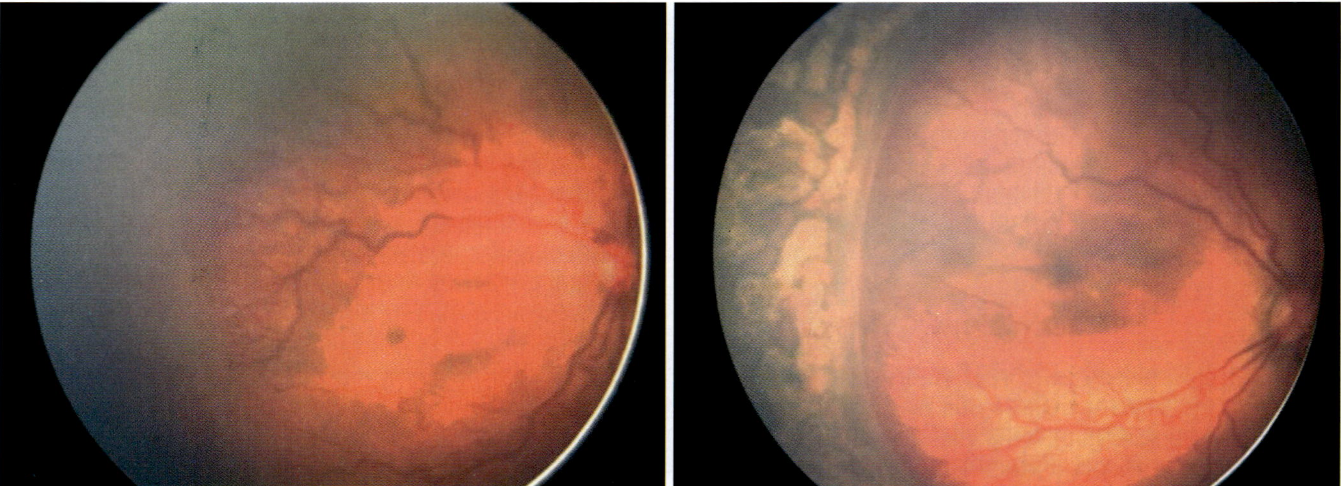

Fig. 42.45: Clinical fundus image showing flat neovascularization in a case of retinopathy of prematurity (ROP); lasers spots delivered by indirect laser ophthalmoscope are visible anterior to neovascular ridge.

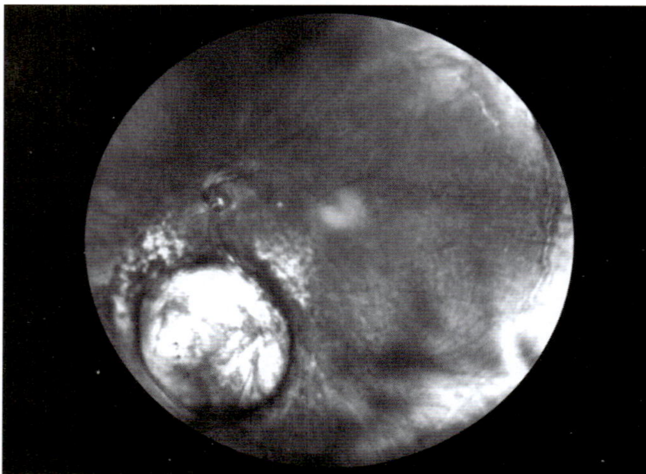

Fig. 42.46: Fundus red free image showing laser delimitation in a type-III choroidal coloboma eye.

scleral buckling surgery. Similarly, the retinochoroidal colobomas should be laser delimited; especially if detected before 15 years of age or if the fellow eye has retinal detachment due to coloboma. The laser spot settings are similar to those used for laser around retinal breaks. The extreme anterior retinal periphery of the coloboma at the ora can sometimes not be delimited even with laser indirect delivery system. In such cases, cryopexy of the coloboma edge at the normal retina–ora junction can be considered. Care is taken to avoid the actual or presumed fovea at the edge of the coloboma.

Idiopathic Juxtafoveal Retinal Telangiectasis (Fig. 42.47)

Idiopathic parafoveal telangiectasia (IPT) is characterized by the presence of focal microaneurysms or saccular dilatation of some portion of the juxtafoveal capillary network. Three types have been described Group 1—unilateral congenital (A) JXT with exudation or idiopathic (B) JXT where exudation is not common. Group 2 is bilateral acquired parafoveal telangiectasia and is often seen in diabetics, and is the most common form. Group 3 is bilateral IPT, where progressive obliteration of the perifoveal network occurs. Glucose tolerance test is abnormal in nearly 35% of patients with unilateral disease and 60% of patients with bilateral disease.

Laser is indicated for group 1 telangiectasis with visual loss due to macular edema or lipid exudation. Group 1 unilateral JXT represents a mild form of Coats' disease and shows unilateral, easily visible telangiectasis and intraretinal exudation. This type is nonfamilial in origin. Macular grid should be performed in such cases, especially those with foveal lipid. Groups 2 and 3 JXT are usually bilateral and do not respond to laser photocoagulation.

Retinal Cavernous Hemangioma

This is a hamartomatous retinal or optic nerve head (ONH) tumor composed of thin-walled dilated vessels. Treatment is usually unnecessary unless subretinal or vitreous hemorrhage causes visual loss. Confluent laser can successfully obliterate the tumor.

Choroidal Hemangioma (Figs. 42.48 to 42.51)

This is also a hamartomatous tumor occurring in two forms. Cases may have only circumscribed hemangiomas not associated with any systemic disease or diffuse choroidal hemangiomas associated with systemic disease as in Sturge-Weber syndrome. Laser is performed, if serous/exudative detachment involves or threatens to involve the macula. Obliteration should not be attempted. The entire tumor surface should be covered with light-to-moderately intense burns placed 1-burn-width apart and spot size of 300–500 μ. Duration of laser exposure per spot is usually kept at 0.3–0.7 seconds.

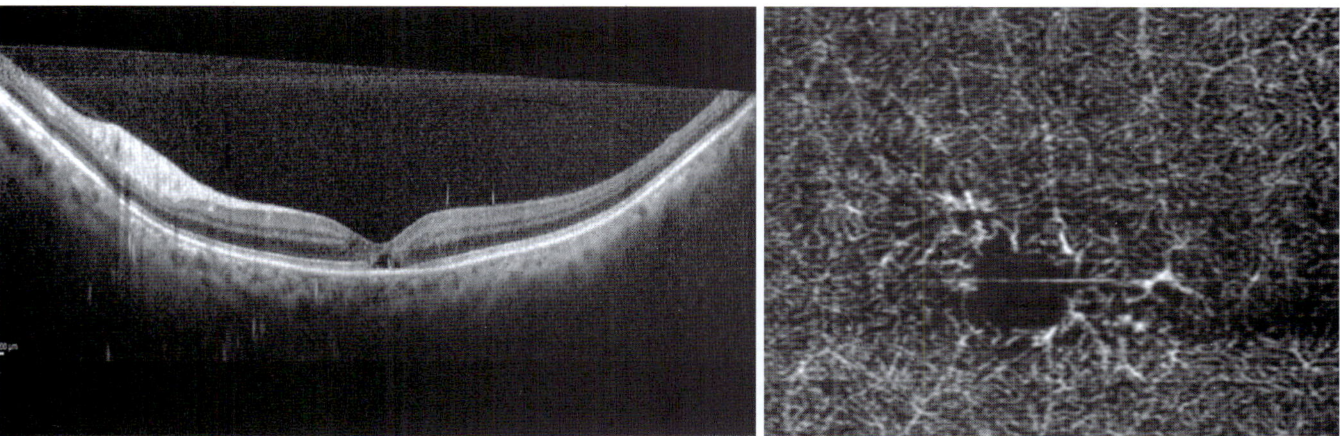

Fig. 42.47: Spectral domain-optical coherence tomography (SD-OCT) shows tissue defect at the fovea secondary to loss of outer nuclear layer and ellipsoid zone in type 2 macular telangiectasia. OCT angiography also reveals the structurally abnormal capillaries.

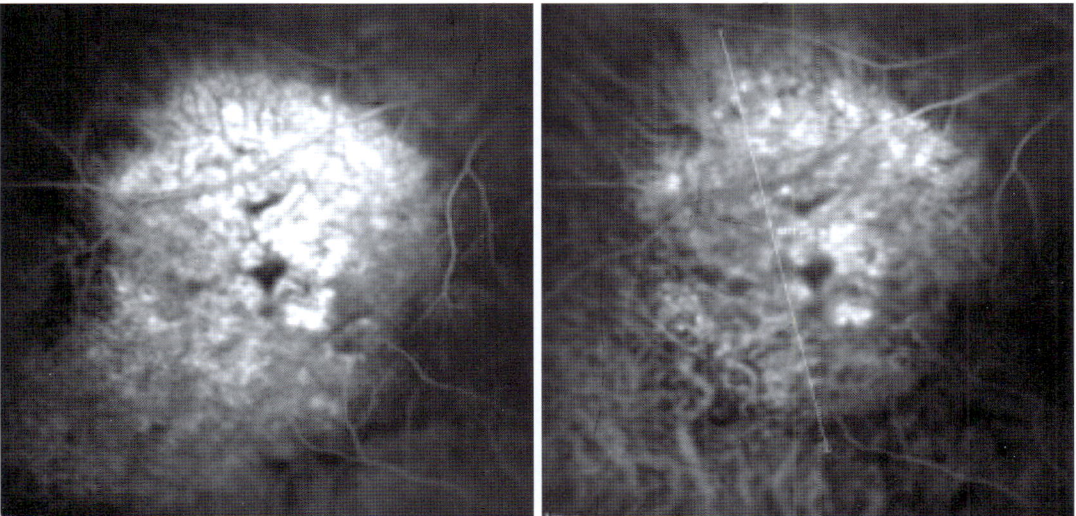

Fig. 42.48: Fundus fluorescein angiography (FFA) and indocyanine green chorioangiography (ICG) showing a circumscribed choroidal hemangioma (lesion diameter 677 μ).

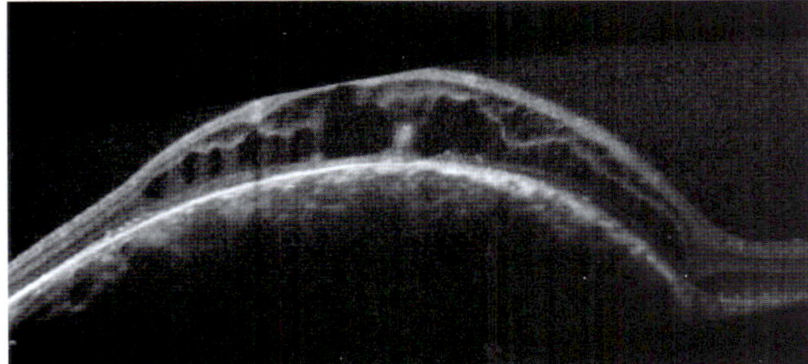

Fig. 42.49: Spectral domain-optical coherence tomography (SD-OCT) of circumscribed choroidal hemangioma depicting a smooth and gently sloping choroidal mass.

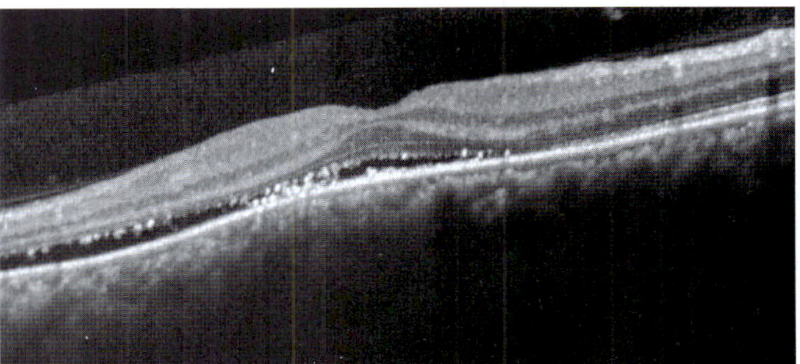

Fig. 42.50: Spectral domain-optical coherence tomography (SD-OCT) scan showing subretinal fluid in a case of choroidal hemangioma (pre-photodynamic therapy).

Alternatively, PDT with Visudyne has been successfully used to treat the lesion. Alternatively, non-responding hemangiomas can be treated with double dose (12 mg/m), or even double duration (166 secs) full-fluence PDT with satisfactory outcomes as we have observed in some of our treated eyes.

Retinoblastoma (Fig. 42.52)

It is most common primary intraocular tumor of childhood. Laser photocoagulation is indicated for small extrapapillary retinoblastoma located at least 3 mm from foveola, confined to neurosensory retina without vitreous seeding. Laser can be used to treat primary tumor or as supplemental treatment when initial radiotherapy or cryotherapy has been performed. Intense laser burns should surround the tumor with a 1-mm rim of confluent treatment.

Optic Disc Pit Maculopathy (Fig. 42.53)

Fluid from a temporally present ONH pit can track under the neurosensory retina and cause a macular detachment.

Lasering the edge of the ONH may help to reabsorb the fluid and flatten the detachment. Though presently, the most accepted management option is vitrectomy with ILM peeling sparing the fovea, and inversion of the ILM flap into the pit.

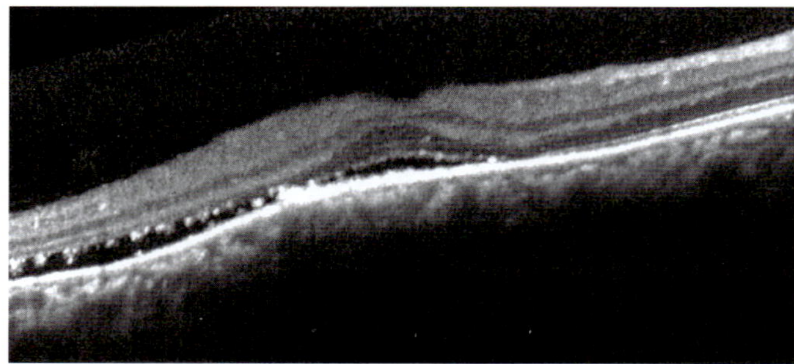

Fig. 42.51: Spectral domain-optical coherence tomography (SD-OCT) scans showing little resolution of subretinal fluid in a case of choroidal hemangioma (postphotodynamic therapy—2 months).

SUBTHRESHOLD LASERS

SUBTHRESHOLD LASERS

INTRODUCTION

Laser has been the gold standard for various retinal disorders especially DME since the first publication from the ETDRS in 1985. Laser may be needed multiple times to effectively treat these disorders. Laser photocoagulation is applied to the retinal lesion centered on the RPE. The heat from the laser burn radiates into the surrounding RPE, the retina and the choroid, thus coagulating and denaturing the proteins within the cell. Photoradiation reaction produced surrounding this burn leads to temperature rise and changes the surrounding tissue that may be temporary, permanent or slowly progressive in nature. The photocoagulation scar will enlarge, so that the area between two adjacent photocoagulation scars may

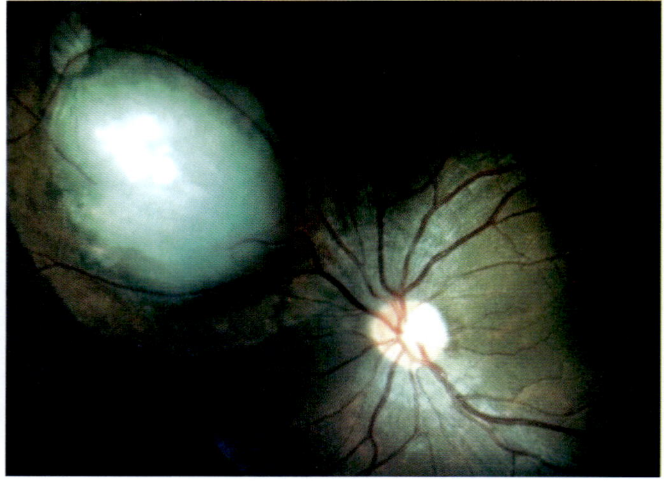

Fig. 42.52: Clinical picture of retinoblastoma with surrounding laser burns.

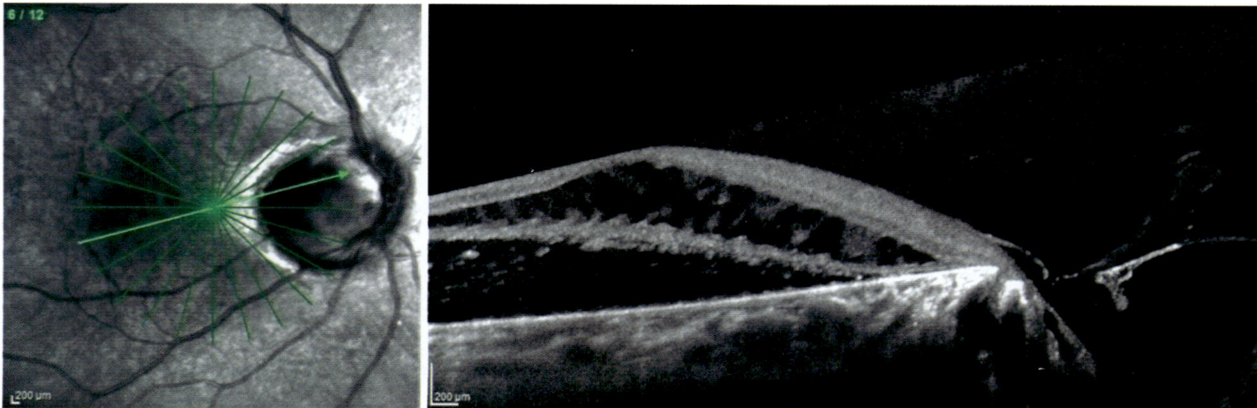

Fig. 42.53: Spectral domain-optical coherence tomography (SD-OCT) showing inferotemporal optic disc pit and serous macular detachment of the right eye.

become confluent with loss of function of the intervening retina.

There are several shortcomings of conventional laser, the most important being scarring. For instance, a standard laser burn enlarges by 16% per year for up to 4 years. The annual scar expansion rate (16.5%) continues for up to 4 years following PRP.[49] The application of laser to the visible endpoint photocoagulation causes thermal damage to areas adjacent to the target RPE. In 1990, Pankratov reported a design to deliver laser energy in short pulses ("micropulses") rather than as a continuous wave. Subthreshold diode micropulse laser photocoagulation (SDM) serves as invisible retinal phototherapy for retinal disorders.

RATIONALE

The main determinant of the retinal thermal lesion size is the duty cycle when other parameters like retinal spot size, energy and pulse duration are the same. Lower duty cycle means lower repetition rate implying less heat and less thermal damage to the retina. Conversely, higher the duty cycle, more the lesions produced and more is the heat production.

The energy absorption and thermal diffusion to the surrounding retinal tissue can be minimized by using a longer wavelength near infrared 810-nm diode laser. By micropulsing the 810-nm diode laser and reducing the frequency of laser micropulses by lowering the duty cycle, heat energy can be directly applied to the RPE, thus lowering the thermal damage. Cellular events occur at one-half to one-fourth of the laser exposure levels needed to produce a clinically obvious lesion and these are adequate to cause VEGF downregulation.[50,51] Mainster postulated that as RPE cells were 10–14 μm in height, laser exposures of 0.7 ms or lesser result in thermal effects localized within these cells. On the other hand, manual or automated pattern conventional photocoagulators have comparatively longer exposures times (at least 50 times longer). The risk of hemorrhages and post-treatment choroidal neovascularization is increased, as most of the laser energy is delivered in a single 0.7-ms pulse.

Instead of a single pulse, in micropulse photocoagulation, laser energy is delivered in a burst or "envelope" of micropulses, thus limiting the time for heat conduction to raise the temperature in the adjacent retinal tissue thereby significantly reducing collateral damage.

It delivers a subthreshold laser that is above the threshold of biochemical effect but below the threshold of a visible destructive lesion, thus preventing progressive enlargement of laser scars leading to scotoma and loss of color vision.[52] In this micropulse mode, the laser is delivered in micropulses (microseconds), which are shorter than the thermal relaxation time of the target tissue (RPE). Hence, the temperature rise is insufficient to cause ancillary damage to the surrounding normal retinal tissue. The usage of lower energy levels targeting the RPE causes sublethal injury rather than destruction. The cytokines released from the recovering RPE cells causes the effects of photocoagulation.[53]

UNDERLYING WORKING PRINCIPLE

Laser by inducing thermal retinal destruction of the diseased retina reduces metabolic demand, decreases the production of vasoactive substances like VEGF, and increases the oxygen tension.

Subthreshold diode micropulse laser photocoagulation works in absence of retinal damage as opposed to the previously held notion that thermal retinal damage is necessary to offer a therapeutic benefit. The near-infrared laser affects many cells, altering the biological behavior at cellular levels through a variety of intracellular receptors, which further improve cell function and reduce inflammation.

Subthreshold diode micropulse laser photocoagulation selectively targets and avoids lethal thermal damage to the RPE and surrounding retina. The targets RPE cells rather than being eliminated, aid in the therapeutic response by releasing cytokines.

DOSING OF SUBTHRESHOLD DIODE MICROPULSE LASER PHOTOCOAGULATION

As per the American National Standards Institute (ANSI) recommendations, for the SDM laser to be both clinically effective and safe, the key parameters are as follows:

- A low-duty cycle (5% or less)
- A small-spot size to minimize heat accumulation
- Sufficient power to produce retinal laser exposures
- High-density treatment of the pathological retina with contiguous laser spots to maximize the therapeutic benefit or "high-density" SDM as invisible retinal phototherapy for DME.[54,55]

SUBTHRESHOLD DIODE MICROPULSE LASER FOR DIABETIC RETINOPATHY

Despite, major advances in the surgical and pharmacological management of DR since the publication of the landmark studies like Diabetic Retinopathy Study (DRS, 1976); Early Treatment of Diabetic Retinopathy Study (ETDRS, 1985), and laser photocoagulation of the retina remains the cornerstone of treatment in the management of DR.

In 1997, Friberg and Karatza initiated the use of micropulse laser in DME.[8] In 2005, Luttrell et al. published their experience of using subthreshold micropulse 810-nm diode laser for DME with complete and contiguous treatment of the entire edematous area without tissue damage.[56,57] Since then, various studies have demonstrated micropulse laser to be as efficacious as the conventional laser.[58-60]

There is an alteration in RPE cytokine expression induced by the laser, which is responsible for the slower but long-lasting benefits seen in DME with subthreshold micropulse diode laser.[61,62]

The 810-nm diode laser is minimally absorbed and negligibly scattered by cataract, vitreous hemorrhage, intraretinal blood, fundus pigmentation, and even severely edematous neurosensory retina, thus providing a wide therapeutic window.

WAVELENGTH VARIATION IN RETINAL LASER THERAPY

Retinal laser therapy has undergone tremendous changes in laser mediums, laser delivery systems and mostly in the wavelengths used. This has helped in achieving better patient compliance along with increasing the safety and efficacy of the laser therapy.

In 1960, Maiman at Hughes Aircraft in California produced a functioning laser for the first time with "ruby" red light output of approximately 694-nm wavelength. Meyer-Schwickerath reported his first xenon-arc photocoagulator in 1956.[63] It did not gain popularity as it was polychromatic, required long exposures and was difficult to focus the beam to a small spot. This paved the way for the targeted treatments using ruby laser (694-nm wavelength), which did not go a long way due to the following disadvantages—it required a high-power pumping source, had low efficiency, and resulted in hemorrhage caused by intense chorioretinal damage. The laser output occurred in the form of pulses of microsecond duration. The advent of argon laser revolutionized retinal photocoagulation. Studies like DRS proved argon laser to be equally efficacious to xenon arc laser and produced less adverse effects.[64]

There are various pigments present in human retina—namely xanthophylls (420–500 nm) within the neurosensory retina, melanin (400–1,000 nm) within the retinal pigment epithelial cells and choroidal melanocytes, and hemoglobin (450–550 nm) within red blood cells. Thus, the peak absorbance of these pigments varies. The macular xanthophylls minimally absorb green (495–570 nm) and yellow (570–590 nm) wavelengths, thus proving to be safe in treating macular pathologies.

The argon laser can be tuned providing a wide range of wavelengths from 457 nm to 528 nm. Argon laser uses both the blue (488-nm wavelength) and green (514-nm wavelength) light emissions, which are absorbed by both hemoglobin and melanin pigments, present in the retina. The chief disadvantages are the requirement of large amounts of power along with lower efficacy. Soon, the air-cooled Nd:YAG frequency-doubled lasers (532-nm wavelength) replaced the argon lasers. The solid state lasers have offered an advantage of being portable and less expensive. Presently, this is the laser of choice for treating DR and vascular occlusions.

The dye lasers represent a futuristic development. In a dye laser, the laser crystal is replaced by a dye cell. Dye lasers are tunable and by changing the dye and some optics, one can usually get the entire visible and near infrared spectrum. The downsides of the dye lasers are that they cannot be operated in a light-stabilized mode, are expensive, and these are cumbersome and hazardous to change the dye from time to time.

There are very few studies reporting clinical differences between green and yellow laser wavelength in retinal practice.

ADVANTAGES OF YELLOW LASER OVER GREEN LASER

The yellow laser has a better uptake by hemoglobin when compared with green. This property makes it suitable to treat microaneurysms with less damage to the underlying RPE. Also, the yellow-wavelength laser requires less power to produce the same clinical response relative to the green laser therapy.

The retinal pathologies can be visualized through the dense hemorrhage more easily than with green wavelengths, as it can penetrate vitreous hemorrhage more than the green. This is especially helpful in treating DR with vitreous hemorrhage and to treat a break with bleed obstructing the view. The use of red-free filter during treatment makes the identification of the fovea and microaneurysms easier. This helps in the inadvertent laser of the fovea and helps to apply precise focal laser energy.

The new Iridex yellow laser can also perform a micropulse treatment. The micropulse ability to administer a sharp 50-μm spot allows very meticulous focal treatment in cases of DME. This treatment has an additional advantage of causing minimal scarring with minimal scar expansion with time.

LASER VITREOLYSIS FOR SYMPTOMATIC VITREOUS FLOATERS

Laser vitreolysis is a noninvasive painless outpatient department (OPD) procedure, which involves the application of nanosecond pulses of high-energy laser light (nano-pulsed YAG laser, energy used is often 4.0-5.0 mJ) to evaporate the vitreous opacities and to sever the vitreous strands. During this process, the laser energy evaporates the collagen and hyaluronic molecules to form a gas. The end result is that the floater is removed and/or reduced to a size that no longer impedes vision. The goal is basically functional improvement and prospective trial to evaluate the safety and efficacy of YAG laser vitreolysis for symptomatic floaters arising from posterior vitreous detachment would be needed.

A recent study (JAMA Ophthalmology 2017, in press) compared sham vitreolysis with YAG laser vitreolysis and some of the results of this short-term study are given below.

Study Design

The single-center trial randomized 52 eyes to receive one session of YAG laser (n = 36) or sham (16). The primary outcomes were subjective changes using various scales to quantify visual disturbance.

Outcomes

At 6 months, all outcome measures including symptoms, visual disturbances and vision-related quality of life supported the efficacy of YAG vitreolysis (all P < 0.001). Best corrected visual acuity (BCVA), however, was no different between groups (P = 0.94).

The authors documented one case of intraocular lens (IOL) pitting in the YAG laser group and one retinal tear in the control group. No serious complications or adverse events were noted.

Limitations

The biggest limitations are the small sample size and the short follow-up. As one of the reported risks of YAG vitreolysis is retinal detachment, longitudinal follow-up with a larger group would be needed to exclude this and other potential adverse events. In addition, this study only allowed one treatment session; whereas in real clinical practice, it may require more than a single laser session to adequately address the patient's symptoms and pathology.

Clinical Significance

While the results from this study are encouraging, I would not alter my clinical practice yet. Larger randomized trials with longer follow-up will be necessary to assess the efficacy and safety of YAG laser vitreolysis for symptomatic floaters.

LASER HAZARDS

Every health professional using lasers should bear in mind its hazards and make sure that adequate safety measures are taken. Laser hazards can be divided into two types:

1. *Beam hazards*: Inflicted ocular and cutaneous injury.
2. *Nonbeam hazards*: They arise due to laser devices itself or its interaction with the surgical environment. This includes fire hazards, plume hazards and electrical hazards.

There are four classes of lasers based on intensity of laser (Table 42.7).

Safety Standards

Laser safety standards for medical applications exist in many countries. In addition to the safety guidelines that exist in

Table 42.7: Classification of lasers—classification system as specified by the International Electrotechnical Commission (IEC) 60825-1 standard.

Class	US: FDA/CDRH	ICE 60825 (Amendment 2)
Class 1	• No known hazards to eye or skin *during normal operation* • Note: Service operation may require access to hazardous embedded lasers	
Class 1M	N/A	• No known hazards to eye or skin, unless collecting optics are used
Class 2a	• Visible lasers not intended for viewing • No known hazards up to maximum exposure time of 1000 seconds	N/A
Class 2	• Visible lasers • No known hazard with 0.25 seconds (aversion response)	
Class 2M	N/A	• No known hazard with 0.25 seconds (aversion response) unless collecting optics are used
Class 3a	• Similar to Class 2 with the exception that collecting optics cannot be used to directly view the beam • Visible only	N/A
Class 3R	N/A	• Replaces Class 3a (with different limits) • 5 × Class 2 limit for visible • 5 × Class 1 limit for some invisible
Class 3B	• Medium-powered (visible or invisible) • Intrabeam and specular eye hazard • Generally not a diffuse or scatter hazard • Generally not a skin hazard	
Class 4	• High powered lasers (visible or invisible) • Acute eye and skin hazard intrabeam, specular and scatter conditions • Non-beam hazard (fire, toxic fumes, etc.)	

(FDA: Food and Drug Administration; CDRH: Center for Devices and Radiological Health).

different countries, the IEC has a technical note (IEC 60825-8-1999-11) on the safe use of medical lasers. In the USA, there are two safety standards, which apply to medical lasers—(1) the American National Standard for the Safe Use of Lasers in the Health Care Environment, ANSI Z136.3-1996,[65] which is a voluntary consensus standard for users; and (2) a Federal Regulation that applies to laser manufacturers (21 CFR1040), issued by the Food and Drug Administration (FDA).[66]

Class 1 may be thought of as "eye-safe" lasers; Class 2 is a 1-mW (or less) visible laser (e.g. an aiming beam); Class 3 is a significant eye hazard (e.g. an Nd:YAG photodisruptor). Protective eye wear is required for direct viewing; and Class 4 is a skin hazard as well (e.g. all photocoagulators capable of exceeding 500 mW total average power). Hazard control measures are assigned to each class by the ANSI standard.[67]

An ocular hazard depends on the wavelength of the laser used. The anterior segment absorbs ultraviolet light (200–400 nm), mid-infrared (1,400–3,000 nm), and far-infrared (3,000–10,600 nm) range of wavelengths. Posterior segment absorbs light emitted in the range of visible spectrum (400–760 nm) and near-infrared (760–1400 nm). Retinal injury largely results due to absorption by melanin and to a lesser extent by xanthophylls and hemoglobin.

Commonly used terminology in laser hazard management includes:
- *Maximum permissible exposure limit (MPE)*: It is the maximum energy to which an individual can be exposed safely.
- *Nominal hazard zone (NHZ)*: It is the area surrounding the laser, which has exposure greater than normal MHE.

Lasers used in posterior segment include:
- Argon green lasers
- Diode lasers
- Double frequency Nd:YAG laser.

Complications can be divided as those specific to laser, and those due to its ocular effects.

Argon lasers have poor electrical efficiency and require a water-cooling system. Diode lasers (e.g. TTT) have the disadvantage of poor focusing due to light being more divergent (divergent cone angle). Around 20% of laser emission is absorbed by RPE compared to 90% in argon laser use. Hence, five times higher energy is required. Since energy absorption is poor by RPE, much of it is transmitted to choroid stimulating nerve endings causing pain. It must be remembered that laser scars increase in size with time.

OCULAR HAZARDS (FIG. 42.54)

Normally, the upper lids and the brow ridge help to protect the eye against radiations (UV, visible and infrared-radiant energy) from the natural environment. As compared to the skin, it is well known that the eye is more susceptible to optical hazards than the skin. The potential hazards depend upon

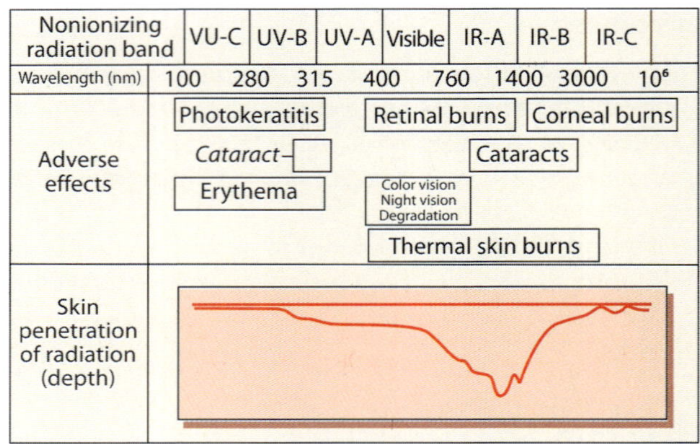

Fig. 42.54: Tissue interaction of lasers.[68] (UV: Ultraviolet; IR: Infrared).

the laser wavelength and the temporal and geometrical characteristics of the exposure.
- Ultraviolet cataract (~295–325 nm to 400 nm). Mostly due to chronic exposure.
- Ultraviolet photokeratoconjunctivitis (wavelengths of ~180–400 nm) also known as "welder's flash" or simply "photokeratitis", one aspect of "snow-blindness".
- Skin cancers arising from chronic exposure to UV radiation, mostly UV-B (280–315 nm), but also demonstrated due to UV-A.
- Thermal injury to the retina (400–1,400 nm) caused by lasers, like a focused, very intense xenon–arc source resulting in a blind spot (scotoma).
- Blue-light photochemical injury to the retina (principally 400–550 nm blue light) also called as "blue light" photoretinitis, e.g. solar retinitis and welder's maculopathy, leading to a permanent scotoma.
- Near-infrared thermal hazards to the lens (approximately 800–3,000 nm) in patients working in industries (glass and steel workers exposed to infrared irradiances).
- Others include thermal injury of the cornea and conjunctiva (approximately 1,400 nm to 1 mm), thermal injury of the skin (approximately 400 nm to 1 mm). Laser-induced thermal injury is seen from most Class 4 lasers.

OCULAR EFFECTS

- Decrease in visual acuity
- Visual fields defects
- Diminished color vision and contrast sensitivity
- Reduced dark adaptation and nyctalopia
- A very brief exposure to high-density energy producing heat in tissue causing chorioretinal distortion and bleeding.

Cornea

- Corneal epithelial defect/erosions due to contact lens-induced trauma
- Photokeratoconjunctivitis.

Iris and Lens

- Iritis or iris burns
- Lenticular opacification
- Transient uveitis.

Retina

- Accidental foveal and disc injury
- Retinal nerve fiber layer thinning
- Retinal hole
- Bruch membrane rupture (when small spot size of less than 50 µ)
- Choroidal hemorrhage
- Choroidal neovascularization
- Vitreous, preretinal and subhyaloid hemorrhage
- Subretinal fibrosis.

Due to Breakdown of Blood Retinal Barrier

- Macular edema
- Choroidal effusion mostly seen in 1st week, usually asymptomatic but may cause angle closure especially in predisposed eyes like hyperopic eyes with shallow chamber
- Exudative retinal detachment.

Contraction of Fibrovascular Tissue

- This may lead to tractional retinal detachment.

Injury to Long Posterior Ciliary Nerves

- Inadvertent laser injury of long posterior ciliary nerves can cause paresis of accommodation and mydriasis.

Skin and Teeth Hazards

- Skin injury can range from erythema to overt burns.
- Dental enamel melting and resolidification at high fluence, and cracking, charring, flaking and discoloration at low fluence.

Ocular injury may not only result from direct viewing of the beam but also from exposure to light reflected or scattered.

Ocular protective devices are hence to be used by the professionals who may be exposed to the laser. They are chosen based on the wavelength of the radiation used. They can be made of coated glass material or from polymeric materials.

PHOTODYNAMIC THERAPY

Most common systemic side effects are infusion-related pain and minor allergic reactions. Life-threatening allergic reactions are rare. Exposure to sunlight has to be avoided for 3 days following the procedure. The ocular side effects are secondary CNVM, persistent hypoperfusion of the choriocapillaris and pigmentary changes over the treated area due to RPE damage.

OCCUPATIONAL LASER HAZARDS

The source of accidental ocular exposure is most frequently a reflected beam. Laser beam reflections can occur from the flat or curved surfaces, which are characteristic of contact lenses and from the metallic intraocular instruments. To avoid these, most of the surgical instruments are now black anodized or sandblasted to roughen the surfaces, so as to reduce the harmful reflections. The potential hazards to both the patient and the surgical staff can be minimizing by undertaking few preventive steps depending upon the type of laser.

Since laser wavelengths in the UV and infrared spectral regions are invisible, the presence of hazardous reflections could go unnoticed as opposed to the argon and the Nd:YAG (sometimes referred to as the "potassium titanyl phosphate—KTP") lasers, which emit highly visible, blue-green, thus in some respects, pose a lesser potential hazard.

Safety of the Treating Physician

Usually, the target issue is viewed through the optics of a slit lamp biomicroscope, endoscope, operating microscope, etc the optics of which attenuate the reflections. Thus, the surgeon is not normally susceptible to injury. But if the laser beam is viewed accidentally, the surgeon will be just as much at risk as any other person in the room.

Patient Safety

Accidental exposure to the patient due to the misdirection of the laser beam should be avoided. The use of the standby mode or proper placement of the laser foot-switch can help to reduce the number of laser hazards. The LIO delivery system poses more problems than the slit lamp delivery systems, since the beam is not as well controlled as the latter and can be directed anywhere. A momentary misfiring can prove to be hazardous. Hence, laser eye protectors are mandatory for bystanders or visitors in the treatment room. A warning light or sign should be displayed during laser use.

Thus, fortunately, most of the hazards by the ophthalmic lasers are well understood and can be prevented by taking certain precautions.

REFERENCES

1. Zaret MM, Mreinin GM, Schmidt H, et al. Ocular lesions produced by an optical maser (laser). Science. 1961;134:1525.
2. L'Esperence FA. Ophthalmic Lasers. St Louis: CV Mosby; 1989.
3. Reed BC. Quantum Mechanics: A First Course. Winnipeg: Wuerz; 1990. pp. 1-35.
4. Lipson SG, Lipson H, Tannhauser DS. Optical Physics, 3rd edition. Cambridge: Cambridge University Press; 1995. pp. 423-5.
5. Siegman AE. Lasers. 2nd edition. Mill Valley, CA: University Science Books; 1986. pp. 558-891.
6. Blumenkranz MS, Yellachich D, Andersen DE, et al. Semiautomated patterned scanning laser for retinal photocoagulation. Retina. 2006;26:370-6.

7. Gupta A, Gonzales CR; PASCAL Study Group. Novel Delivery of Laser Therapy with the PASCAL (Pattern Scanning Laser) Photocoagulator. IOVS ARVO J. 2007;48(13). [online] Available from http://iovs.arvojournals.org/article.aspx?articleid=2386710. [Accessed December, 2017].

8. Chang S. Multifunction endolaser probe. Am J Ophthalmology. 1992;114:648-9.

9. Awh CC, Schallen EH, de Juan E. An illuminating laser probe for vitreoretinal surgery. Arch Ophthalmology. 1994;112:553-4.

10. Peyman GA, D'Amico DJ, Alturki WA. An endolaser probe with aspiration capability. Arch Ophthalmology. 1992;110:718.

11. Coonan P, AiE. The early treatment of diabetic retinopathy. In: AiE, Freeman WR (Eds). Ophthalmology Clinics of North America: New Developments in Retinal Disease. Philadelphia: WB Saunders; 1990. pp. 359-72.

12. Diabetic Retinopathy Study Research Group. Photocoagulation treatment of proliferative diabetic retinopathy: the second report of Diabetic Retinopathy Study findings. Ophthalmology. 1978;85:82-106.

13. ETDRS Research Group. Treatment Techniques and clinical guidelines for photocoagulation of diabetic macular edema. ETDRS Report No. 2. Ophthalmology. 1987;94:761-74.

14. Khosla PK, Tewari HK, Atul K, et al. Contrast sensitivity in diabetic retinopathy after pan retinal photocoagulation. Ophthalmic Surg. 1994;25(8):284-6.

15. Tewari HK, Gupta V, Kumar A, et al. Efficacy of diode laser for managing diabetic macular edema. Acta Ophthalmology. 1998;76:363-6.

16. Tewari HK, Ravindranath, Atul K. Diode laser scatter photo-coagulation in diabetic retinopathy. Ann Ophthalmology. 2000; 32(2):110-2.

17. Tewari HK, Wagh VB, Sony P, et al. Macular thickness evaluation using the OCT in normal Indian eyes. Ind J Ophthalmology. 2004;52:199-204.

18. Verteporfin in Photodynamic Therapy (VIP) Study Group. Verteporfin therapy of subfoveal choroidal neovascularization in age-related macular degeneration: 2-year results of a randomized clinical trial including lesions with occult with no classic choroidal neovascularization. VIP Report 2. Am J Ophthalmology. 2001;131:541-60.

19. Michels S, Hansmann F, Geitzenauer W, et al. Influence of treatment parameters on selectivity of verteporfin therapy. Invest Ophthalmology Vis Sci. 2006;47:371-6.

20. Meyer-Schwickerath GRE. The history of photocoagulation. Aust N Z J Ophthalmology. 1989;17:427-34.

21. Wilkinson CP, Ferris FL, Klein RE, et al. Proposed international clinical diabetic retinopathy and diabetic macular edema disease severity scales. Ophthalmology. 2003;110(9):1677-82.

22. Diabetic Retinopathy Research Group. Photocoagulation treatment of proliferative diabetic retinopathy. Clinical application of Diabetic Retinopathy Study (DRS) findings, DRS report number 8. Ophthalmology. 1981;88:583-600.

23. Early Treatment Diabetic Retinopathy Study Research Group. Early photocoagulation for diabetic retinopathy. ETDRS report number 9. Ophthalmology. 1991;98:766-85.

24. Stefánsson E, Machemer R, de Juan E Jr, et al. Retinal oxygenation and laser treatment in patients with diabetic retinopathy. Am J Ophthalmology. 1992;113(1):36-8.

25. Elman MJ, Bressler NM, Qin H, et al. Expanded 2-year follow-up of ranibizumab plus prompt or deferred laser or triamcinolone plus prompt laser for diabetic macular edema. Ophthalmology. 2011;118(4):609-14.

26. Branch Vein Occlusion Study Group. Argon laser scatter photocoagulation for prevention of neovascularization and vitreous hemorrhage in branch vein occlusion. Arch Ophthalmology. 1986;104:34-41.

27. BVOS Group. Argon Laser photocoagulation for macular edema in branch vein occlusion. Am J Ophthalmology. 1984;98(3):271-82.

28. Kanski JJ, Milewski SA. Diseases of the Macula. A Practical Approach. London: Mosby; 2002.

29. SCORE Study Research Group. A randomized trial comparing the efficacy and safety of intravitreal triamcinolone with standard care to treat vision loss associated with macular edema secondary to branch retinal vein occlusion: the Standard Care vs Corticosteroid for Retinal Vein Occlusion (SCORE) study report 6. Arch Ophthalmology. 2009;127(9):1115-28.

30. Fekrat S, Goldberg MF, Finkelstein D. Laser-induced chorioretinal venous anastomosis for nonischemic central or branch retinal vein occlusion. Arch Ophthalmology. 1998;116(1):43-52.

31. The CVOS Group. Natural history and clinical management of central vein occlusion. Arch Ophthalmology. 1997;115:486-91.

32. SCORE Study Research Group. A randomized trial comparing the efficacy and safety of intravitreal triamcinolone with observation to treat vision loss associated with macular edema secondary to central retinal vein occlusion: the Standard Care vs Corticosteroid for Retinal Vein Occlusion (SCORE) study report 5. Arch Ophthalmology. 2009;127(9):1101-14.

33. Das TP, Biswas J, Atul K, et al. Eales Disease. Ind J Ophthalmology. 1993;42(1)1-18.

34. Nonaka A, Kiryu J, Tsujikawa A, et al. Inflammatory response after scatter laser photocoagulation in nonphotocoagulated retina. Invest Ophthalmology Vis Sci. 2002;43(4):1204-9.

35. Yannuzzi LA, Slakter JS, Gross NE, et al. Indocyanine green angiography-guided photodynamic therapy for treatment of chronic central serous chorioretinopathy: a pilot study. Retina. 2003;32(Suppl 1):288-98.

36. Cardillo Piccolino F, Eandi CM, Ventre L, et al. Photodynamic therapy for chronic central serous chorioretinopathy. Retina. 2003;23(6):752-63.

37. Shin JY, Woo SJ, Yu HG, et al. Comparison of efficacy and safety between half-fluence and full-fluence photodynamic therapy for chronic central serous chorioretinopathy. Retina. 2011;31(1):119-26.

38. Alkin Z, Perente I, Ozkaya A, et al. Comparison of efficacy between low-fluence and half-dose verteporfin photodynamic therapy for chronic central serous chorioretinopathy. Clin Ophthalmology. 2014;8:685-90.

39. Bressler SB, Bressler NM, Gragoudas ES. Age-related macular degeneration: drusen and geographic atrophy. In: Albert DM, Jakobiec FA (Eds). Principles & Practice of Ophthalmology, 2nd edition. Philadelphia: Saunders; 2000. p. 198201991.

40. Abugreen S, Muldrew KA, Stevenson MR, et al. CNV subtype in first eyes predicts severity of ARM in fellow eyes. Br J Ophthalmology. 2003;87(3):307-11.

41. Choroidal neovascularization Prevention Trial Research Group. Laser treatment in eyes with large drusen: short-term effects seen in a pilot randomized clinical trial. Ophthalmology. 1998;105:11-23.

42. Macular Photocoagulation Study Group. Risk factors for choroidal neovascularization in the second eye of patients with juxtafoveal or subfoveal choroidal neovascularization secondary to age-related macular degeneration. Arch Ophthalmology. 1997;115(6):741-7.

43. Bessho K, Rodanant N, Bartsch DU, et al. Effect of subthreshold infrared laser treatment for drusen regression on macular autofluorescence in patients with age-related macular degeneration. Retina. 2005;25(8):981-8.

44. Friberg TR, Musch DC, Lim JI, et al.; PTAMD Study Group. Prophylactic treatment of age-related macular degeneration report number 1: 810-nanometer laser to eyes with drusen. Unilaterally eligible patients. Ophthalmology. 2006;113(4):622.

45. Macular Photocoagulation Study (MPS) Group. Evaluation of argon green vs krypton red laser for photocoagulation of subfoveal choroidal neovascularization in the macular photocoagulation study. Arch Ophthalmology. 1994;112(9):1176-84.

46. Kramer M, Miller JW, Michaud N, et al. Liposomal benzoporphyrin derivative verteporfin photodynamic therapy. Selective treatment of choroidal neovascularization in monkeys. Ophthalmology. 1996;103(3):427-38.

47. Schnurrbusch UE, Jochmann C, Einbock W, et al. Complications after photodynamic therapy. Arch Ophthalmology. 2005;123(10):1347-50.

48. Good WV; Early Treatment for Retinopathy of Prematurity Cooperative Group. Final Results of the Early Treatment for Retinopathy of Prematurity (ETROP) Randomized Trial. Trans Am Ophthalmology Soc. 2004;102:233-48.

49. Maeshima K, Utsugi-Sutoh N, Otani T, et al. Progressive enlargement of scattered photocoagulation scars in diabetic retinopathy. Retina. 2004;24(4):507-11.

50. Mainster MA. Laser tissue interactions: future laser therapies. Diabetic Retinopathy: Approaches to a Global Epidemic. Association for Research in Vision and Ophthalmology Summer Research Conference 2010; 31 July. Bethesda MD: Natcher Center, National Institutes of Health; 2010.

51. Mainster MA. Decreasing retinal photocoagulation damage: Principles and techniques. Semin Ophthalmology.1999;14:200-9.

52. Sivaprasad S, Elagouz M, McHugh D, et al. Micropulsed diode laser therapy: Evolution and clinical applications. Surv Ophthalmology. 2010;55:516-30.

53. Dorin G. Subthreshold and micropulse diode laser photocoagulation. Semin Ophthalmology. 2003;18:147-53.

54. Sramek C, Mackanos M, Spitler R, et al. Non-damaging retinal phototherapy: dynamic range of heat shock protein expression. Invest Ophthalmology Vis Sci. 2011;52(3):1780-7.

55. American National Standards Institute. American national standard for the safe use of lasers, ANSI Z136.12000. Washington, DC: American National Standards Institute. 2000.

56. Friberg TR, Karatza EC. The treatment of macular disease using a micropulsed and continuous wave 810-nm diode laser. Ophthalmology. 1997;104:2030-8.

57. Luttrull JK, Musch DC, Mainster MA. Subthreshold diode micropulse photocoagulation for the treatment of clinically significant diabetic macular oedema. Br J Ophthalmology. 2005;89:74-80.

58. Akduman L, Olk RJ. Subthreshold (invisible) modified grid diode laser photocoagulation in diffuse diabetic macular edema (DDME). Ophthalmic Surg Lasers. 1999;30:706-14.

59. Figueira J, Khan J, Nunes S, et al. Prospective randomized controlled trial comparing subthreshold micropulse diode laser photocoagulation and conventional green laser for clinically significant diabetic macular oedema. Br J Ophthalmology. 2009;93:1341-4.

60. Ulbig MW, McHugh DA, Hamilton AM. Diode laser photocoagulation for diabetic macular oedema. Br J Ophthalmology. 1995;79:318-21.

61. Gao X, Xing D. Molecular mechanisms of cell proliferation induced by low power laser irradiation. J Biomed Sci. 2009;16:4.

62. Mascud S, Heidari GK, Alireza R, et al. Two year results of a randomized trial of intravitreal bevacizumab alone or combined with triamcinolone versus laser in diabetic macular edema. Retina. 2012;32:314-21.

63. Meyer-Schwickerath G. Light Coagulation: a method for treatment and prevention of the retinal detachment. Albert Von Graefes Arch Ophthalmology. 1954;156(1):2-34.

64. The Diabetic Retinopathy Study Research Group. Photocoagulation treatment of proliferative diabetic retinopathy: clinical application of Diabetic Retinopathy Study (DRS) findings, DRS Report Number 8. Ophthalmology. 1981;88(7):583-600.

65. American National Standards Institute (ANSI). Safe Use of Lasers in Health Care Facilities ANSI Standard Z136.3-1996. New York, NY: ANSI; 1996.

66. US Food and Drug Administration (FDA). Laser Performance Standard, Title 21, Code Federal Regulations, Part 1040 (21CFR1040). Washington, DC: Government Printing Office; 1986.

67. Sliney DH, Trokel SL. Medical Lasers and Their Safe Use. New York, NY: Springer Verlag; 1993.

68. Fankhauser F, Kwasniewska S. Textbook of Lasers in ophthalmology. Basic, Diagnostic and Surgical Aspects—A Review. Netherland: Kugler Publication; 2003.

Chapter 43

Scleral Buckling

Parveen Sen, Sufiyan Shaikh, Sharan Shetty, Kaustubh Deshmukh

HISTORY OF RETINAL DETACHMENT SURGERY

Scleral indentation or buckling was first introduced by Ernst Custodis in 1953. He used surface diathermy for treatment of breaks followed by closure with a polyviol explant sutured onto the overlying sclera.[1,2] Scleral necrosis was a major complication of surface diathermy. To overcome this, Meyer-Schwickerath proposed the use of xenon arc photocoagulation immediately or 1–2 days after explant placement.[3] Lincoff did revolutionary work by introducing cryotherapy for retinal surgery.[4] This did not require retrobulbar anesthesia as in xenon arc photocoagulation and was better acceptable by the patients. Lincoff also introduced silicone sponges and spatula needle for scleral suturing.[5,6]

Charles Schepens introduced implants to reduce vitreous traction, which were buried in the bed of lamellar scleral dissection.[7] He pioneered the use of encircling element to permanently decrease vitreous traction.[8] He invented the binocular indirect ophthalmoscope making it possible to directly visualize and treat the retinal breaks. Lincoff later developed the technique of temporary balloon buckling where an inflatable balloon catheter was placed in sub-Tenon's space under the retinal break and removed after a week following resolution of subretinal fluid.[9] This avoided many complications of permanent buckling procedure.

The basic principle of scleral buckle (SB) is to close the communication between the vitreous cavity and subretinal space. This is achieved by:

- Identification of all the retinal breaks
- Closure of these breaks by creating a chorioretinal adhesion between the neurosensory retina and the retinal pigment epithelium (RPE)
- To support these retinal breaks externally by a scleral explant
- Use of an encircling element to reduce the circumferential traction.

PRINCIPLES OF SCLERAL BUCKLING

Overview of Forces Acting on Retina

Scleral buckle alters the forces that produce a retinal tear and detachment and enhances the forces that promote retinal attachment.

Forces that Lead to Retinal Tears and Detachment and Effect of Scleral Buckle

Retinal tears and detachment occurs due to combination of forces namely, vitreous traction, fluid movement with saccades and epiretinal proliferation.

Vitreous Traction and Effect of Scleral Buckle

Vitreous tractional forces include gravitational force of vitreous body onto retina, inertial force from vitreous to retina during ocular saccades and vitreoretinal traction at sites of cellular proliferation. Vitreous traction may be exerted in radial, tangential or oblique direction. Radial traction on retina is more likely to cause breaks than tangential traction. Vitreous traction causes elevation of retinal breaks and allows fluid from vitreous cavity to enter the subretinal space and cause detachment.

Indentation of sclera by buckle decreases vitreous traction and possibly changes the direction of vitreous traction on the retinal tear. Circumferential buckles decrease transretinal vitreous traction by decreasing the diameter and circumference of the vitreous base according to Hook's law. This law states that the force of stretch in a spring is proportional to the distance of stretch.

Fluid Movement and Effect of Scleral Buckle

Fluid currents occurring with rotational eye movements cause fluid to funnel into the subretinal space through the retinal break elevated by vitreous traction.[10] Once detachment occurs, continued fluid influx maintains the detachment.

Scleral indentation displaces the preexisting subretinal fluid away from the break and decreases the distance between RPE and retinal break. Retinal reattachment force is inversely proportional to the cube of distance from the neurosensory retina (retinal break) and RPE on the buckle.[11] So, closer the break is from RPE, greater is the force promoting retinal reattachment. Also indentation displaces vitreous fluid away from break and allows solid vitreous gel to plug the break.

Epiretinal Membranes, Breaks and Effect of Scleral Buckle

Cellular epiretinal membranes (ERMs) create tangential as well as radial vectoral forces on the retina. Tractional retinal detachment (RD) occurs if radial tension is more than the adhesive force of RPE to retina.

Scleral buckle reverses the direction of radial inward force of ERM on retina to an outward force with greater magnitude which promotes reattachment. This occurs due to a smaller radius of curvature of sclera over the buckle element than the radius of curvature of a normal concave eyeball.

Forces that Promote Retinal Attachment

Physiological Adhesion between Retina and Retinal Pigment Epithelium

The most important factor maintaining retinal attachment is RPE pump, which actively pumps out fluid from subretinal space.[12] Other factors are viscous mucopolysaccharide substance between RPE and photoreceptors, oncotic pressure difference between choroid and subretinal space and hydraulic forces on the retina.[13,14]

Thermal CR Adhesions

Diathermy, cryopexy and laser photocoagulation are different modalities for creation of chorioretinal adhesions. Final adhesion of these modalities has similar strength but the rapidity of onset of adhesion formation is maximum with laser.[15,16]

Preoperative Assessment

Preoperative evaluation should include a carefully elicited history, systemic examination, anterior and posterior segment examination. Important things that should be noted include macular status (attached or detached or threatened), presence of vitreous detachment, number and position of the retinal breaks and significant ocular co-pathologies.

Note should be made about the stability of the intraocular lens in pseudophakic eyes as well as the presence of peripheral capsular opacification. If significant peripheral opacification is seen peripheral view may become hazy leading to "missed" retinal breaks.

Missed retinal breaks are an important cause of surgical failure and thus the preoperative examination should be very thorough. Even when a break has been found, it is essential to do a complete examination of the retina as most RDs have more than one break.

A fundus drawing detailing the retinal breaks and other easily recognizable lesions on the retina is drawn with attention to their exact location and relation to optic disc, macula and other visible landmarks like pigmentation and vortex veins. This is of utmost importance. It helps in formulation of a tentative plan of surgery. These drawings can be referred to in the operation theater as well to facilitate surgery.

Assess Surgical Feasibility

Few situations where SB will probably be the first choice amongst many vitreoretinal surgeons include:

- Fresh rhegmatogenous retinal detachment (RRD) due to a retinal break anterior to the equator that is easily accessible to scleral buckling technique.
- No signs of proliferative vitreoretinopathy (PVR). Buckle surgery alone may work in cases with PVR C1 or less.
- RRD in young phakic patients without any posterior vitreous detachment (PVD).
- RRD secondary to retinal dialysis usually secondary to blunt trauma. Usually these eyes have no PVD and a broad and shallow "buckle" best supports retinal dialysis.[17]
- RRD due to retinal breaks in the inferior quadrant because the tamponading effect of silicone oil or intraocular gas may be inadequate for these inferior breaks.

Scleral buckle should not be the procedure of choice in case of RD with extensive PVR (more than one quadrant), posterior PVR, extensive conjunctival scarring, posterior breaks (posterior to equator) and coexisting macular hole.

Anesthesia

Peribulbar anesthesia is the preferred choice for scleral buckling procedures. A 1:1 mixture of lignocaine and bupivacaine used with adjunctive Hyalase provides excellent and long-lasting anesthesia and akinesia. General anesthesia is considered for pediatric patients and uncooperative patients. Sub-Tenon's anesthesia can be used as adjunct to general anesthesia to prevent vagal stimulation and for analgesia in immediate postoperative period.[18] It can also be used as top-up anesthesia with peribulbar anesthesia when its effect starts wearing off.[19]

TECHNIQUE OF SCLERAL BUCKLING

Surgical Steps

Peritomy

Circumferential limbal peritomy with radial relieving incisions is the preferred incision.[20] The conjunctiva is adherent to the sclera at the limbus, so the radial incisions to enter the subconjunctival plane have to be made just behind the limbus. The conjunctiva becomes friable with age and care must be taken to avoid tearing and buttonholing. Non-toothed forceps are used to grasp the conjunctiva. A blunt-tipped spring scissor is used to make the incision through the conjunctiva and Tenon's capsule down to the sclera. A modification of this technique with the circumferential incision 3–4 mm behind the limbus leaves a frill that may be useful during closure (Figs. 43.1 and 43.2). The extent of the peritomy depends on the size of the buckle planned. A 360° peritomy is usually required if an encircling element is also placed.

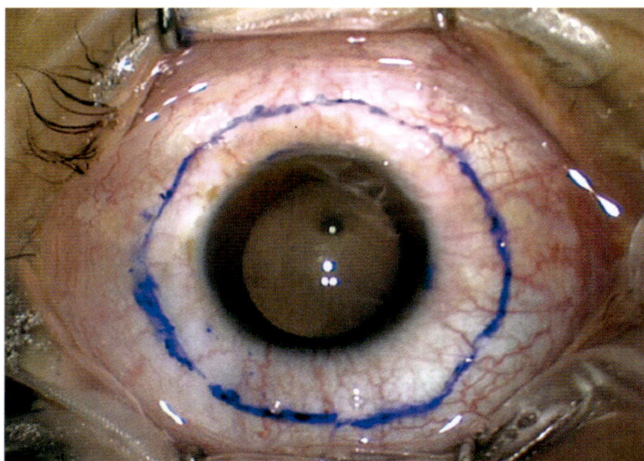

Fig. 43.1: Desired area of conjunctival peritomy is marked with dye at 3–4 mm from limbus.

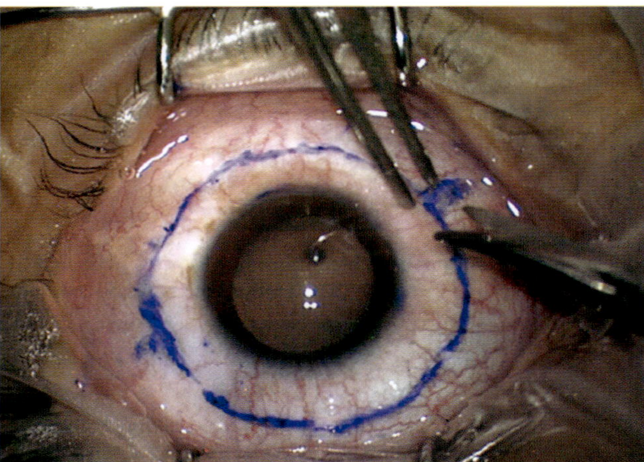

Fig. 43.2: Peritomy with blunt forceps to hold the conjunctiva and sharp conjunctival scissor.

Slinging Recti

Between two and four rectus muscles are slung depending on the planned size of the buckle and whether encircling element is to be placed. The muscle is engaged with a sweeping posterior and circumferential movement around the globe using a muscle hook (Fig. 43.3). Very posterior movement can damage the vortex veins.

The muscle hook is inserted just behind the insertion of the muscle taking care to avoid the oblique muscles. The superior oblique muscle runs laterally from the trochlea to its insertion under the superior rectus. Passage of a superior rectus muscle hook from the temporal side of the muscle reduces the risk of inadvertently "hooking" the superior oblique. The inferior oblique muscle passes under the lateral rectus muscle. The chance of inadvertently hooking it while passing a muscle hook under the lateral rectus is reduced by passing the hook from the superior side. Cotton suture or braided silk suture is passed under the muscle (Fig. 43.4).

Break Localization

Careful scleral indentation is done under indirect ophthalmoscope using a fine blunt tipped instrument such as Gass scleral indenter.[21] Once the indent is seen to correspond to the position of a retinal break, this point is marked with a surgical marker pen.

Errors in break localization may lead to buckle malposition. Localization errors tend to be radial rather than circumferential. If a retinal break is highly elevated, parallax errors may make the break seem more posterior than it truly is. Parallax errors may be avoided by draining subretinal fluid and then reforming the globe with air, i.e. the DACE procedure (explained under drainage of subretinal fluid).[22]

Retinopexy

The indent from the explant closes retinal breaks but retinopexy is required to produce an enduring bond between the

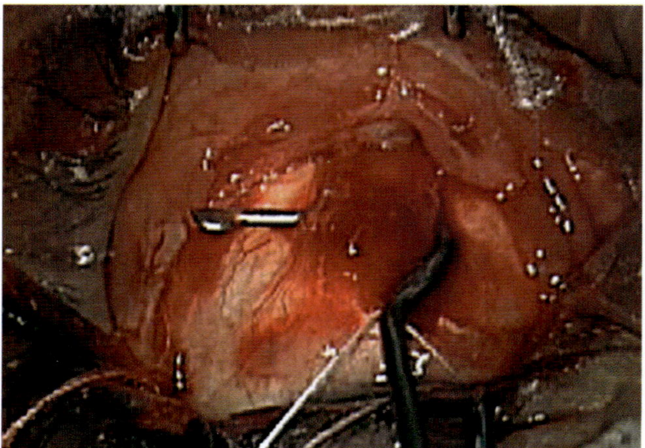

Fig. 43.3: Inferior rectus muscle is being hooked with muscle hook from medial to lateral side close to the insertion of muscle to avoid damage to vortex vein.

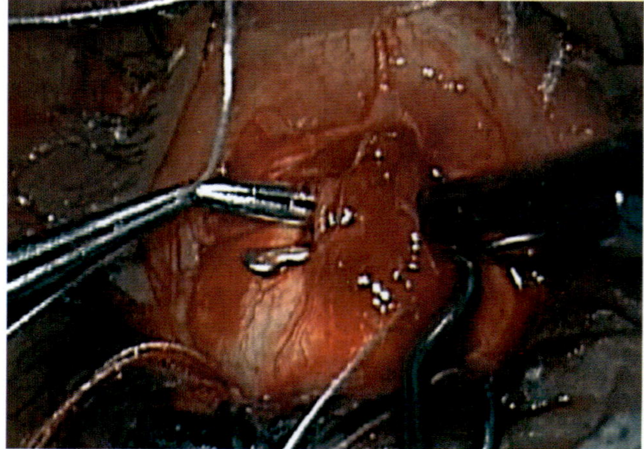

Fig. 43.4: Cotton suture is being used to bridle the inferior rectus muscle.

retina and the RPE. Cryotherapy, diathermy and photocoagulation create chorioretinal scars to seal the retinal breaks.

Retinopexy was initially achieved using diathermy in association with lamellar scleral dissection and scleral implants. Cryotherapy has supplanted diathermy because it can be performed without scleral dissection. Cryotherapy is the recommended method currently.

All breaks and areas of retinal degeneration are treated with transscleral cryotherapy applied under direct visualization. Scleral depression is done to approximate RPE and retina. Treatment is done in form of a single row of near confluent burns around the breaks. Freezing is terminated as soon as the retina blanches and starts to whiten. Cryotherapy probe is allowed to thaw before moving away from scleral surface.

Cryotherapy burns should not extend onto large areas of the bare choroid otherwise it causes pigment dispersion into the vitreous cavity. Treated retina is difficult to visualize immediately after thawing and can lead to overtreatment by treating the same area multiple times. Inadvertent posterior cryotherapy can occur when indentation is seen with the shaft instead of the tip of the cryotherapy probe. This can be prevented by starting the indentation with the tip of the probe anteriorly near the ora and then gradually moving posteriorly under visualization.

It is even possible to perform laser photocoagulation of retinal breaks through a gas bubble in the postoperative period in eyes with an attached retina.

Choice of Explant

Various materials like fascia lata, autografts or homografts like temporalis fascia, cartilage and Dura mater have been used for scleral buckling in the past. These are more of historical interest now.

The most commonly used material today is the silicone rubber. It is biologically inert and can be left in the eye indefinitely. Silicone explants used in buckling surgery includes band, sponge and tires.[23] Scleral buckles or tires may be placed circumferential or radial in orientation. Circumferential buckles provide support in the region of vitreous base where vitreous traction is usually most severe (Fig. 43.5). They support multiple areas of pathology. However, with shortening of eye-wall, radial retinal folds commonly occur and may cause fish-mouthing phenomenon.

Radial buckles provide localized support for a retinal tear and prevent fish mouthing. They are preferred for more posterior retinal breaks.

If circumferential segmental buckle is planned, suture limbs are placed parallel to limbus (Fig. 43.6). The posterior bite is usually placed at least 3 mm behind the posterior most extent of retinal break on sclera. Anterior bite is placed 10 mm anterior to posterior bite usually just anterior to the posterior margin of vitreous base. A silicone tire of adequate width to cover the break is used. The further apart the suture bites are placed and tighter they are tied, more will be the indentation.

Sponges have been typically used for posterior radial breaks/horse shoe tears especially those associated with "fish mouthing". Sponges can give a much higher and posterior buckle effect as compared to a solid buckle tire. But silicone sponges are associated with higher incidence of astigmatism.[24] Also silicone sponges have communicating air cells in them which may serve as a nidus for infection. Hence, postoperative infection and extrusion are more common with the use of silicone sponges as compared with solid tires.[25,26]

Polyhydroxyethyl acrylate (hydrogel), a synthetic sponge has also been used for scleral buckling.[27] It has micropores that absorb antibiotics and slowly release them over a period

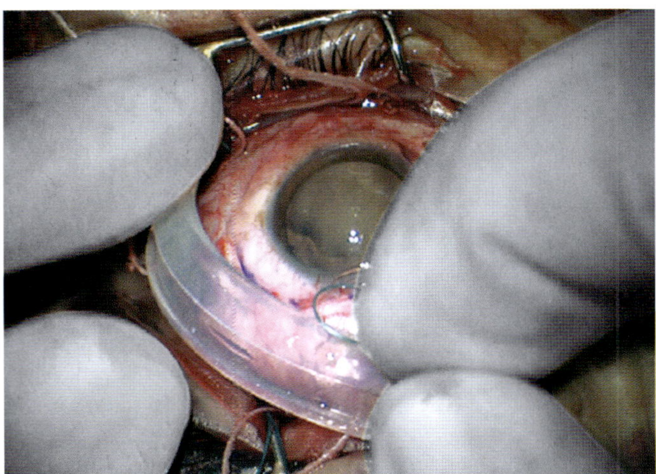

Fig. 43.5: An asymmetric 276 number silicone tire of 90° circumferential extent.

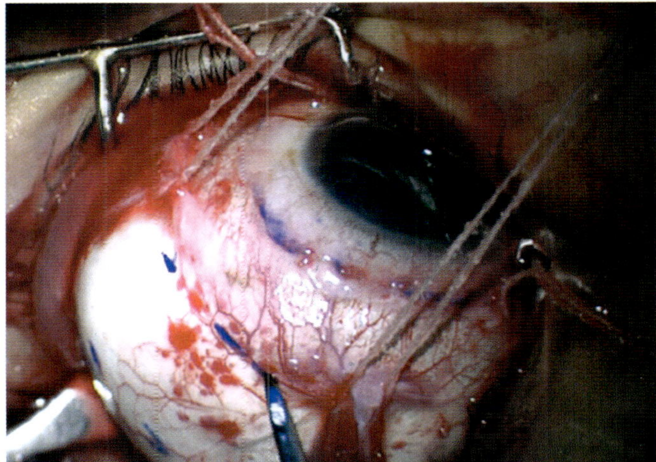

Fig. 43.6: For circumferential buckles, mark for posterior bite of mattress suture is taken at least 3 mm behind the localized break and anterior bite is 10 mm anterior to posterior bite.

of time; thus reducing the risk of buckle infection. However, foreign body granulomatous reactions are still known.

Encircling Element or Belt Buckle

An encircling number 240, 41 or 42 silicone band is passed beneath the recti muscles circumferentially to provide 360 degree indent of modest width and height. Single mattress suture usually suffice in each quadrant. Suture bites should be placed just far apart to allow free movement of the band. Narrower bites limit the movement while wider bites may allow band to move anteriorly than desired. Band is usually intended to support breaks but can be placed in the area of vitreous base. If a high indent is required then two broad mattress sutures may be put in each quadrant.

The ends of the encircling band are either sutured with each other or joined with silicone Watzke sleeve (Fig. 43.7). Later adjustment of length of band can be done in case of sleeve.

Scleral Sutures

Explants are sutured to sclera with 5-0 nonabsorbable synthetic mattress suture attached to spatulated needle. Buckle suture commonly used is 5-0 Prolene because it is nonbiodegradable and durable. Mattress sutures are preferred over crossover sutures because the former give a better scleral indentation. Scleral passes are planned at a depth of one-half to two-thirds with at least 6 mm length in case of tires and sponges. Shorter pass may suffice for encircling band. The needle tip must be visualized at all times during its passage through the sclera (Fig. 43.8).

Inadvertent scleral perforation during passage of buckle sutures is seen in 5% of cases undergoing SB.[28] If scleral perforation does happen it can cause escape of subretinal fluid (SRF), which causes hypotony. Straightening of the eyeball and injecting saline into the vitreous cavity immediately make up the loss of fluid followed by inspection of the site of perforation using indirect ophthalmoscopy. If retinal break is seen it will also need to be treated with cryotherapy and will need to be supported by a SB if RRD is seen around it. If retinal break happens in attached retina additional cryopexy is enough. On examination with indirect ophthalmoscope, if a lot of subretinal hemorrhage/choroidal hemorrhage is seen one may need to switch to PPV.

Sutures are tied at this stage using Slipknot's (Fig. 43.9). If intraocular pressure (IOP) is seen to increase following suture tying paracentesis through the anterior chamber is done (Fig. 43.10). Indirect ophthalmoscope examination is repeated at this stage to look for:

- Adequate coverage of the retinal breaks with the buckle
- Adequate indentation of the SB
- Reassess the amount and distribution of the SRF to decide the need for SRF drainage
- Decide on the location for SRF drainage.

MANAGEMENT OF SUBRETINAL FLUID

Subretinal fluid may or may not be drained depending upon whether responsible breaks can be easily and nearly completely closed with buckling effect alone.

Non-drainage: This procedure is effective if summit of buckle lies within 3 mm of retinal break at that location. It is commonly undertaken in RD with single break that can be easily approximated close to RPE during scleral indentation. Scleral buckle may always be repositioned and readjusted if break buckle summit relation is skewed.

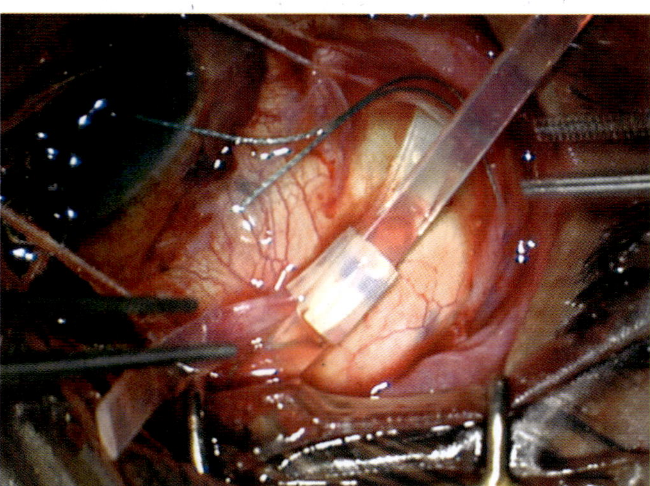

Fig. 43.7: Silicone sleeve can be used for the final tie of encircling band.

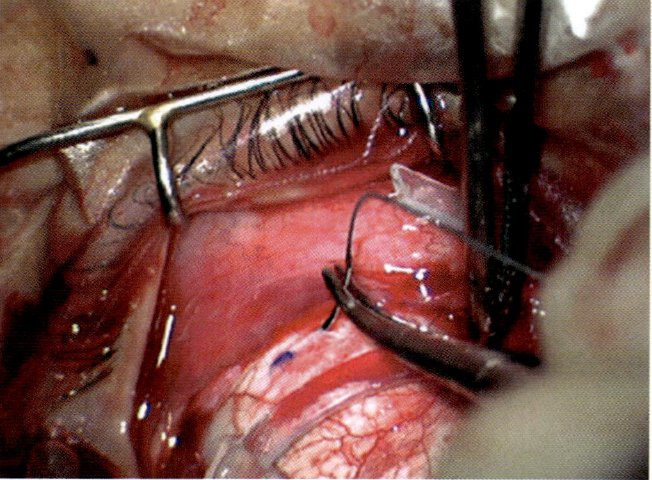

Fig. 43.8: Needle tip should be visible throughout its course in the sclera to prevent scleral perforation (Jameson's rule).

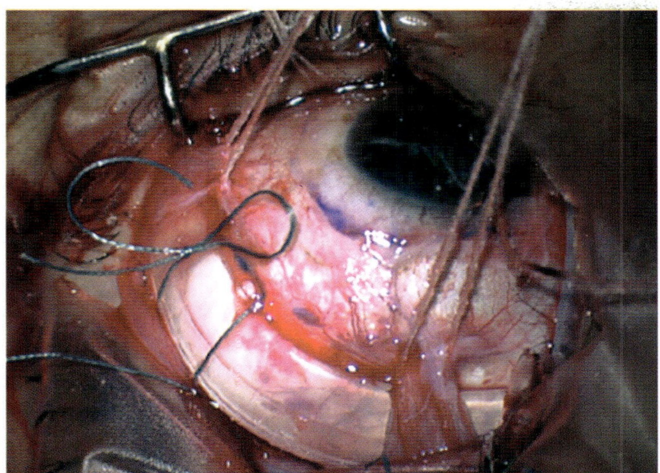

Fig. 43.9: Slip-knots are put temporarily for circumferential scleral buckle with 5-0 Ethibonc suture.

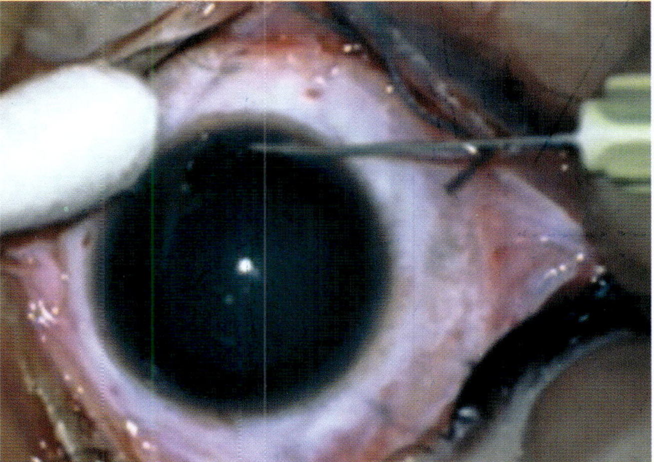

Fig. 43.10: Anterior chamber (AC) paracentesis is done with 30-G needle over a 2 cc syringe with plunger out. Needle is inserted away from center tangentially to prevent inadvertent lens injury.

Perfusion of optic nerve head should be checked at the time of tightening of scleral sutures. Frequently with high IOP, pulsations of central retinal artery (CRA) are observed. If pulsations are not seen and perfusion is questioned, additional digital pressure applied to globe can elicit pulsations if IOP is lower to start with. Otherwise scleral sutures may have to be relaxed.

Drainage: Indications of drainage include old RD with thick SRF, bullous RD, eyes with poor RPE function (myopic eyes, retinitis pigmentosa), early PVR, inferior RD, glaucomatous optic neuropathy and aphakic RD. In very high RRD, apposition of RPE to neurosensory retina is difficult with buckle effect alone. The DACE technique (Drain-Air-Cryo-Explant) has been used in these cases successfully.[22] However cryo application and visualization through the gas can be challenging. Hence, this technique has not gained popularity.

Drainage is performed at a site depending upon the configuration of RD. Additional factors that govern this include location of breaks, location and configuration of buckle, location of vitreoretinal traction and ease of exposure of proposed site. Usual locations include just above or below medial or lateral rectus as major choroidal vessels can be avoided. Drainage is performed away from the site of retinal breaks to avoid vitreous incarceration. Drainage is done at or slightly anterior to equator and site should preferably be supported by explant. Drainage is also avoided at the site of excessive cryotherapy. Cryotherapy may increase choroidal congestion leading to choroidal hemorrhage.[29]

Scleral cut-down or needle drainage may be adopted. The original method of SRF drainage by scleral cut-down was described by Schepens and is widely used. In cut-down procedure, a 3–4 mm radial scleral incision is made until choroid is observed. Avoiding any large vessel, choroid is then perforated with a 10-0 suture/flat diathermy probe keeping it perpendicular to the ocular coats. This choroidotomy can also be made with the help of high intensity laser beam.[30] Modest pressure is applied while doing so until a sudden give-away occurs and subretinal fluid starts to drain. Diathermy needle is withdrawn soon and pressure is applied on the globe to maintain IOP and facilitate complete drainage. Sudden and significant increase in IOP is avoided to prevent retinal incarceration. Presence of pigment granules in draining SRF indicates the last of SRF is exiting. Sclerotomy site is closed with suture once drainage ceases.

In needle technique originally introduced by Charles, a 25 g hypodermic needle attached to a tuberculin syringe is used to perforate sclera and choroid tangentially simultaneously. Even ophthalmoscopic visualization may also be done during this step using 20 diopter lens and indirect ophthalmoscope. Burton et al. reported increased incidence of subretinal hemorrhage with the needle drainage technique.[31]

Azad et al. described a modified needle drainage technique involving use of a 26-G disposable long needle attached to a 2 mL syringe without the plunger.[32] This needle is inserted perpendicularly into the sclera for not more than 2 mm and spontaneous drainage of SRF allowed. They noticed reduced incidence of subretinal hemorrhage as compared to the conventional drainage technique.

The site of drainage is quickly inspected for evidence of subretinal or choroidal bleed, retinal or vitreous incarceration and iatrogenic retinal break formation. Now, if RPE is not in contact with break and SRF remains, additional drainage may be attempted.

A major complication of subretinal fluid drainage is choroidal hemorrhage. Subretinal blood tends to gravitate to the most dependent area of subretinal fluid—the macula if this is detached. It can have serious consequences for visual recovery. First the IOP is elevated, either by tightening sutures or intravitreal injection. The patient's head may also be tilted toward the drain site. Later, subfoveal hemorrhage may be displaced pneumatically or removed subsequently by vitrectomy.[33]

Dry tap or failure of SRF drainage may occur due to drainage at the site where SRF is absent/minimal or failure to perforate the choroid completely.

Retinal incarceration at the site of drainage may happen because of sudden egress of SRF. As a result the retina quickly comes to reattach with the RPE even before complete fluid drains. To avoid retinal incarceration one must ensure that the IOP is maintained adequately at all times. If retinal incarceration happens, a retinal star fold may be visible at the site of drainage. It is better to avoid repositing the retina and support the area of incarceration with an explant and do a cryopexy in case of a retinal break.

Adjustment of Buckle Height

Following drainage, optimal buckle effect is created by adjusting scleral sutures and length of the band. If IOP remains low and break—buckle indent relation is good then sutures are permanently tied (Fig. 43.11).

Fish mouthing can happen because of high indentation effect of circumferential buckle especially in repair of RRD due to Hubble Space Telescopes (HSTs).[34] Radial retinal folds communicating the vitreous cavity with the subretinal space are seen. This can be managed by decreasing the height of the circumferential buckle or by placing a radial buckle or silicone sponge over the break and underneath the SB. Another technique is intravitreal injection of expansile 0.3 mL of C3F8 followed by appropriate patient positioning.[34]

Intravitreal Gas Injection

Gas injection may be performed together with scleral buckling to tamponade retinal break internally. This is performed after drainage but usually before localization and cryotherapy of break. However, this impairs the visualization of fundus through the gas bubble. Therefore gas is injected only after breaks are well treated and positioned on the buckle. Eye must be soft before injection of large amount of gas bubble. Either sulfur hexafluoride (SF6) or perfluoropropane (C3F8) gas can be injected. Gas is injected briskly with help of a 30-G needle attached to a tuberculin syringe at appropriate distance from the limbus. Disc perfusion has to be checked as mentioned before.

Intravitreal Balanced Salt Solution Injection

Balanced salt solution (BSS) can also be injected to restore globe tension after drainage during buckle suture adjustment.

Closure

Before closure, assess for:
- Optic nerve head perfusion
- Any complication at the drainage site
- Adequacy of buckle height
- All retinal breaks are flat on the buckle
- Rule out any other missed break.

7-0 vicryl sutures can be used to close the peritomy wound by running or interrupted technique. Episclera should be included into the bites to prevent posterior retraction of conjunctiva.

Outcomes

Single operation anatomical success rate of scleral buckling are up to 90%.[35] Primary failure can occur due to inadequate buckling effect, missed or new breaks and PVR. Reoperation (scleral buckling) is also usually successful unless PVR is the cause of failure where vitrectomy is preferred.

Good preoperative visual acuity is the most important predictor of both anatomical and visual outcome. Macula on RD has a better anatomical and visual prognosis than macula off case.[36]

ADVERSE EFFECTS AND COMPLICATIONS

Intraoperative Complications

Corneal Edema

This may occur because of prolonged elevated IOP especially during scleral indentation and while passing the silicone tire. This can be tackled by mechanically rolling a dry cotton tip applicator firmly across the cornea. If the edema persists, the central corneal epithelium is gently scraped with a blunt iris repositor.

Inadvertent Scleral Perforation

Scleral perforation can occur during the passage of buckle suture. This is avoided by avoiding the areas of scleral thinning, careful passage of sutures and use of spatulated needles (discussed earliar).

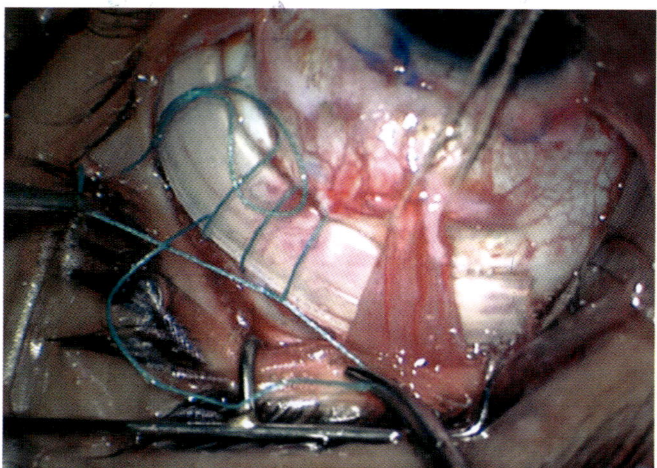

Fig. 43.11: After ensuring good break buckle relation and normal intraocular pressure (IOP), scleral buckle sutures are permanently tied.

Central Retinal Artery Occlusion

This is a rare but a potentially devastating complication that can occur because of increased IOP that is seen during tightening of buckle sutures or due to injection of large volume of expansile intravitreal gas.

It is important to visualize the optic nerve head during the procedure as well as at the conclusion. If the optic nerve is seen to be pale and the optic nerve pulsations are absent immediate paracentesis should be done; if no pulsations are seen, the IOP is increased by applying digital pressure on the globe. If pulsation now appear (induced pulsations), it suggests normal IOP. However, if pulsations are still not visible then it suggests an increased IOP and paracentesis should be done and buckle sutures should be loosened.

Postoperative Complications

Choroidal Detachment

It is a common postoperative complication of scleral buckling surgery seen in about 5%.[37] Predisposing factors are older age, high blood pressure, hypotony due to SRF drainage, elevated vortex vein pressure due to vortex vein compression and damage to the choroidal vessels due to excessive cryotherapy or laser photocoagulation.[38] It is usually seen 24–48 hours postoperatively which increases over a few days and then resolves spontaneously in around 2 weeks. Treatment is by frequent topical and systemic steroids and cycloplegics.

Change in Refractive Error

Use of encircling band in scleral buckling causes a myopic change in refractive error.[39,40] Each 1 mm increase in axial length causes a myopic shift of –2.75 diopter. Radial buckles affect refraction variably but less than circumferential buckles. Significant astigmatism occurs if buckle is quite anterior.[39] Patient with good postoperative vision can have significant anisometropia and aniseikonia.

Recurrent Retinal Detachment/Failure of Surgery

Primary failure of surgery is known to occur if retina does not settle within 2 weeks. Recurrence of disease occurs if retina has once settled but later redetachment occurs. Recurrent RD following SB occurs in 9–25% cases with the cause of recurrence commonly being an associated open break.[41] If extensive PVR is present, then vitrectomy should be undertaken. If recurrence occurs due to new breaks or inadequate buckling effect, revision of surgery can be done.

Glaucoma

Open angle glaucoma occurs after SB due to steroid response. Angle closure after SB occurs due to forward displacement of lens-iris diaphragm without pupillary block.[42] This does not respond to iridotomy or miotic therapy (which tends to exacerbate it). Most cases resolve after 1 week with conservative measures including steroids, cycloplegia, and ocular hypotensive agents.

Epiretinal Membrane

Macular ERM causing distortion of architecture occurs in 2–17% of cases.[43] These are a common cause of poor visual acuity in postoperative period. Grade 2 ERM (thick ERM causing macular pucker) should be removed with vitrectomy and ERM peeling.

Extrusion/Infection

These typically present several weeks or months postoperatively with redness, pain and purulent discharge. Buckle exposure may be occult but purulent discharge can be expressed in usually most cases through area of conjunctival dehiscence. Infection and extrusion are often associated. Radial sponges have a greater risk than circumferential ones.[44] In most cases microorganisms gain access to the explants through conjunctival dehiscence over protruding segment of buckle or suture. Most commonly isolated organisms are coagulase-positive staphylococci and occasionally Gram-negative bacteria but mycobacterial and polymicrobial infections have also been documented.[45]

Closure of Tenon's capsule and conjunctiva in separate layers may be the best way to prevent these complications. Definitive treatment is removal of the explant. Provided adequate retinopexy has been performed recurrent RD is unusual. Buckle exposure tends to follow a relatively chronic course but occasionally patients develop acute sight-threatening complications such as endophthalmitis or scleritis requiring urgent removal.

Migration

Encircling bands may intrude into the vitreous cavity and occur with the use of supramid thread as encircling material or a tightly placed belt-buckle (Fig. 43.12). The buckle could also migrate over the surface, usually anteriorly. Migration

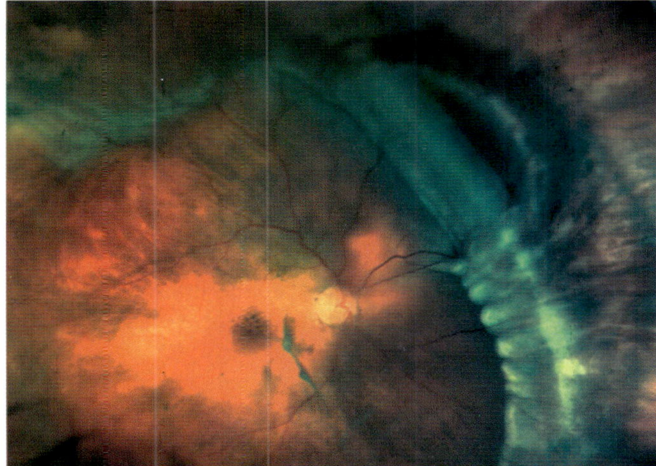

Fig. 43.12: Ultra-widefield color image shows intrusion of scleral buckle into the vitreous cavity.

anteriorly may affect rectus muscle function and even cause the band to migrate anteriorly and extrude through the limbal conjunctiva.

Strabismus/Diplopia

Extraocular muscle imbalance occurs in up to 25% of patients undergoing SB.[46] Responsible causes may include surgical trauma to muscle, mechanical disturbances by location and shape of explant and abnormal adhesion between muscle and sclera or Tenon's capsule.

Anterior Segment Ischemia

Very high indentation and rectus disinsertion can compromise uveal circulation leading to anterior segment ischemia rarely. Patients with sickle cell disease are at particularly high risk.[47] Presenting features are corneal edema, pain, anterior chamber flare, and a deep anterior chamber. Intraocular pressure may be high. Mild cases may be managed with topical steroids but severe cases need loosening or division of the band.

MODIFICATIONS IN SCLERAL BUCKLING

Intrascleral Buckling

Intrascleral buckles involve lamellar dissection to create a partial thickness scleral bed.[27,48,49] The implant is placed in the bed and the flaps are then closed over the top with sutures. An encircling band is usually used, attached directly to the surface of the sclera in the areas not undermined. Drainage is performed usually within the bed. Advantage of this procedure include less chance of infection and extrusion of implant and drainage can be done easily in the bed of implant. Disadvantages include need for scleral dissection and risk of intrusion of implant. This technique is not commonly performed.

Chandelier-assisted Scleral Buckling

Scleral buckling may fail in some patients with pseudophakia or aphakia due to impaired visualization of peripheral retina with indirect ophthalmoscope compared to those who are phakic. Endoilluminator-assisted scleral buckling (EASB) is a boon for such situations.[50,51] Chandelier-assistance obviates the need for indirect ophthalmoscopy. The operating microscope and wide-angle viewing systems provide an improved view of the peripheral retina with oblique lighting to perhaps improve identification of peripheral breaks. Wide-field viewing may also make subretinal fluid needle drainage safer as it may decrease the risk of losing the view of the needle, which may occur with indirect ophthalmoscopy. Moreover, chandelier-buckling permits all team members to share the same surgical view, which improves both surgeon-team communication and teaching.

REFERENCES

1. Custodis E. Bedeutet die Plombenaufnahung auf die Sklera einen Fortschritt in der operativen Behandlung der Netzhautablösung? Ber Deutsch Ophthal Ges. 1953;58:102-5.
2. Custodis E. Scleral buckling without excision and with polyviol implant. In: Schepens CL (Ed). Importance of Vitreous Body with Special Emphasis on Reoperations. St. Louis: CV Mosby; 1960. pp. 175-82.
3. Meyer-Schwickerath G. Light Coagulation. St. Louis: CV Mosby; 1960. pp. 1-113.
4. Lincoff HA, Mclean JM, Nano H. Cryosurgical treatment of retinal detachment. Trans Am Acad Ophthalmology Otolaryngol. 1964;68:412-32.
5. Lincoff HA, Baras I, Mclean J. Modifications to the custodis procedure for retinal detachment. Arch Ophthalmology. 1965;73:160-3.
6. Lincoff HA, Nano H. A new needle for scleral surgery. Am J Ophthalmology. 1965;60:146-8.
7. Schepens CL, Okamura ID, Brockhurst RJ. The scleral buckling procedures. I. Surgical techniques and management. AMA Arch Ophthalmology. 1957;58(6):797-811.
8. Schepens CL, Okamura ID, Brockhurst RJ, et al. Scleral buckling procedures. V. Synthetic sutures and silicone implants. Arch Ophthalmology. 1960;64:868-81.
9. Lincoff HA, Kreissig I, Hahn YS. A temporary balloon buckle for the treatment of small retinal detachments. Ophthalmology. 1979;86:586-96.
10. Rosengren B, Osterlin S. Hydrodynamic events in the vitreous space accompanying eye movements. Significance for the pathogenesis of retinal detachment. Ophthalmologica. 1976;173:513-24.
11. Hammer ME. Retinal re-attachment forces created by absorption of subretinal fluid. Doc Ophthalmology Proc Ser. 1981;25:61-75.
12. Lincoff H. The rationale for radial buckling. Mod Probl Ophthalmology. 1974;12:484-91.
13. Berman ER, Bach G. The acid mucopolysaccharides of cattle retina. Biochem J. 1968;108:75-88.
14. Negi A, Marmor MF. The resorption of subretinal fluid after diffuse damage to the retinal pigment epithelium. Invest Ophthalmology Vis Sci. 1983;24:1475-9.
15. Bloch D, O'Connor P, Lincoff H. The mechanism of the cryosurgical adhesion. 3. Statistical analysis. Am J Ophthalmology. 1971;71:666-73.
16. Yoon YH, Marmor MF. Rapid enhancement of retinal adhesion by laser photocoagulation. Ophthalmology. 1988;95:1385-8.
17. Jan S, Hussain Z, Khan U, et al. Retinal detachment due to retinal dialysis: surgical outcome after scleral buckling. Asia Pac J Ophthalmology (Phila). 2015;4:259-62.
18. Bergman L, Bäckmark I, Ones H, et al. Preoperative sub-Tenon's capsule injection of ropivacaine in conjunction with general anesthesia in retinal detachment surgery. Ophthalmology. 2007;114:2055-60.
19. Mein CE, Flynn HW Jr. Augmentation of local anesthesia during retinal detachment surgery. Arch Ophthalmology. 1989;107:1084.
20. King LM Jr, Schepens CL. Limbal peritomy in retinal detachment surgery. Arch Ophthalmology. 1974;91:295-8.
21. Gass JD. Scleral marker for retinal detachment surgery. Arch Ophthalmology. 1966;76:700-1.
22. Gilbert C, McLeod D. D-ACE surgical sequence for selected bullous retinal detachments. Br J Ophthalmology. 1985;69:733-6.
23. Chhablani J, Nayak S, Jindal A, et al. Scleral buckle infections: microbiological spectrum and antimicrobial susceptibility. J Ophthalmic Inflamm Infect. 2013;3:67.

24. Harris MJ, Blumenkranz MS, Wittpenn J, et al. Geometric alterations produced by encircling scleral buckles. Biometric and clinical considerations. Retina. 1987;7:14-9.

25. McMeel JW, Naegele DF, Pollalis S, et al. Acute and subacute infections following scleral buckling operations. Ophthalmology. 1978;85:341-9.

26. Hahn YS, Lincoff A, Lincoff H, et al. Infection after sponge implantation for scleral buckling. Am J Ophthalmology. 1979;87: 180-5.

27. Das T, Namperumalsamy P. Scleral buckling with hydrogel implant. Indian J Ophthalmology. 1991;39:41-3.

28. Brown P, Chignell AH. Accidental drainage of subretinal fluid. Br J Ophthalmology. 1982;66:625-6.

29. Pearce IA, Wong D, McGalliard J, et al. Does cryotherapy before drainage increase the risk of intraocular haemorrhage and affect outcome? A prospective, randomised, controlled study using a needle drainage technique and sustained ocular compression. Br J Ophthalmology. 1997;81:563-7.

30. Ryan EH Jr, Arribas NP, Olk RJ, et al. External argon laser drainage of subretinal fluid using the endolaser probe. Retina. 1991;11: 214-8.

31. Burton RL, Cairns JD, Campbell WG, et al. Needle drainage of subretinal fluid. A randomized clinical trial. Retina. 1993;13:13-6.

32. Azad R, Kumar A, Sharma YR, et al. Modified needle drainage. A safe and efficient technique of subretinal fluid drainage in scleral buckling procedure. Indian J Ophthalmology. 2004;52:211-4.

33. Rubsamen PE, Flynn HW Jr, Civantos JM, et al. Treatment of massive subretinal hemorrhage from complications of scleral buckling procedures. Am J Ophthalmology. 1994;118:299-303.

34. Norton EW. Intraocular gas in the management of selected retinal detachments. Trans Am Acad Ophthalmology Otolaryngol. 1973;77:OP85-98.

35. Schwartz SG, Kuhl DP, McPherson AR, et al. Twenty-year follow-up for scleral buckling. Arch Ophthalmology. 2002;120:325-9.

36. Khanzada MA, Wahab S, Hargun LD. Impact of duration of macula off rhegmatogenous retinal detachment on visual outcome. Pak J Med Sci. 2014;30:525-9.

37. Verma L, Venkatesh P, Chawla R, et al. Choroidal detachment following retinal detachment surgery: an analysis and a new hypothesis to minimize its occurrence in high-risk cases. Eur J Ophthalmology. 2004;14:325-9.

38. Auriol S, Mahieu L, Arné JL, et al. Risk factors for development of choroidal detachment after scleral buckling procedure. Am J Ophthalmology. 2011;152:428-32.e1.

39. Cetin E, Ozbek Z, Saatci AO, et al. The effect of scleral buckling surgery on corneal astigmatism, corneal thickness, and anterior chamber depth. J Refract Surg. 2006;22:494-9.

40. Okada Y, Nakamura S, Kubo E, et al. Analysis of changes in corneal shape and refraction following scleral buckling surgery. Jpn J Ophthalmology. 2000;44:132-8.

41. Chignell AH, Talbot J. Absorption of subretinal fluid after nondrainage retinal detachment surgery. Arch Ophthalmology. 1978;96:635-7.

42. Perez RN, Phelps CD, Burton TC. Angel-closure glaucoma following scleral buckling operations. Trans Sect Ophthalmology Am Acad Ophthalmology Otolaryngol. 1976;81:247-52.

43. Tanenbaum HL, Schepens CL, Elzeneiny I, et al. Macular pucker following retinal detachment surgery. Arch Ophthalmology. 1970;83:286-93.

44. Deckule S, Reginald A, Callear A. Scleral explant removal: the last decade. Eye (Lond). 2003;17:697-700.

45. Pathengay A, Karosekar S, Raju B, et al. Microbiologic spectrum and susceptibility of isolates in scleral buckle infection in India. Am J Ophthalmology. 2004;138:663-4.

46. Farr AK, Guyton DL. Strabismus after retinal detachment surgery. Curr Opin Ophthalmology. 2000;11:207-10.

47. Ryan SJ, Goldberg MF. Anterior segment ischemia following scleral buckling in sickle cell hemoglobinopathy. Am J Ophthalmology. 1971;72:35-50.

48. Tolentino FI, Roldan M, Nassif J, et al. Hydrogel implant for scleral buckling. Long-term observations. Retina. 1985;5:38-41.

49. Borrás A, Meerhoff A. Ten years' experience with intrascleral gelatin implants in retinal detachment. Am J Ophthalmology. 1972;73:390-3.

50. Seider MI, Nomides REK, Hahn P, et al. Scleral buckling with chandelier illumination. J Ophthalmic Vis Res. 2016;11:304-9.

51. Gogia V, Venkatesh P, Gupta S, et al. Endoilluminator-assisted scleral buckling: our results. Indian J Ophthalmology. 2014;62:893-4.

Chapter 44

Pneumatic Retinopexy

Atul Kumar, Devesh Kumawat, Raghav Ravani, Sagnik Sen

INTRODUCTION

In current clinical scenario the procedures most commonly performed by retinal surgeons for management of rhegmatogenous retinal detachment (RRD) include scleral buckling (SB), pars plana vitrectomy (PPV), and pneumatic retinopexy (PR) with success rate of up to 95%, 71–92%, and 64%, reported respectively in the literature.[1-3] PR has gained popularity because it can be performed as an outdoor procedure without any need for incisions and is much less expensive than SB and PPV. However, it requires good patient selection and cannot be used universally for all cases of RRD. PR is done as the primary procedure in nearly 14–17% of cases.[4]

PRINCIPLE OF PNEUMATIC RETINOPEXY

Pneumatic retinopexy involves injection of expansile gas into the vitreous cavity followed by cryopexy or laser photocoagulation. This tamponades the retinal breaks, preventing further egress of vitreous fluid into the subretinal space. The existing fluid is absorbed by the retinal pigment epithelium. PR is a minimally invasive surgical procedure for treatment of selected cases of RRD. Hilton and Grizzard first introduced it in 1986 following which it has been used worldwide for the treatment of simple retinal detachment.[5] When compared to SB and PPV, PR has the advantage of minimal tissue trauma, less invasive, rapid recovery, and reduced financial burden on the patient because of reduced hospital stay.[6,7]

Patient selection is of utmost importance in the success of this procedure. Classical indications for PR include:

- RRD due to a single break not more than 1 clock hour in size
- Multiple breaks not more than 1 clock hour apart
- Superior breaks (located in superior 8 clock hours of the retina)
- Clear media to allow cryopexy/indirect laser photocoagulation
- Proliferative vitreoretinopathy (PVR) not more than grade B (retina society terminology)
- Cooperative patient to maintain postoperative positioning.

Recently expanded indications for PR include RRDs with inferior retinal breaks (post-procedure positioning may become very difficult), breaks larger than 1 clock hour, multiple breaks more than 1 clock hour apart up to 3 clock hours, and PVR changes not exceeding grade C2.[8] Though surgeons have used PR for these indications, the success rates come down rapidly.[9] Though higher success rates have been seen in phakic eyes[10] PR can also be done in aphakic and pseudophakic eyes if above selection criteria are met.

A relatively new indication of PR, which is becoming increasingly popular, is as a rescue procedure in case of retinal detachment post SB or vitrectomy, due to a superior break.[11-13]

Preprocedure Examination

Before the start of the procedure, slit lamp anterior segment examination should be done to look for conjunctival integrity at the area to be used for gas injection, corneal clarity, anterior chamber depth, angle closure, lens status, and intraocular pressure (IOP). Also, in aphakic and pseudophakic eyes care must be taken to look for presence of any vitreous strands in the anterior chamber which may make paracentesis difficult during the procedure. Posterior segment should be examined for media clarity, retinal break—location, size, and number, extent of subretinal fluid, presence of lattice degenerations in area of attached retina especially inferior, and any PVR changes. Also the patient should be counseled regarding the importance of post procedural positioning for the success of surgery.

TECHNIQUE OF PNEUMATIC RETINOPEXY

Anesthesia and Asepsis

Patient is seated comfortably in front of a slit lamp or can even be done in the lying down position. PR is routinely performed under topical anesthesia or local anesthesia if patient is not cooperative for topical anesthesia. Anesthetic eye drops (proparacaine) are instilled into the conjunctival cul-de-sac. The eyelids are kept closed for about 5–10 minutes. An eyelid speculum is then inserted and a drop of 5% povidone iodine is then instilled especially over the area of the intended injection site.

Control of Intraocular Pressure before Gas Injection

Anterior chamber paracentesis can be done prior to the injection of intraocular gas. 0.2–0.3 mL of aqueous tap is done using a 27 G or 30 G needle. This avoids the postoperative rise of IOP and also facilitates the smooth injection of the gas into the vitreous cavity; thus preventing "fish egg formation" (multiple small intravitreal gas bubbles).

Intraocular Gas Injection

The gas injection can be done in any quadrant though most surgeons prefer inferotemporal quadrant. Also it is better to avoid the area of bullous retinal detachment to avoid accidental retinal break formation and injection of the gas into the subretinal space. The gas should be injected using 30 G needle 3–3.5 mm posterior to the limbus (3 mm in aphakic, 3.5 mm in pseudophakic, and 4 mm in phakic eyes). Care must be taken to avoid lens touch during the gas injection. This is best done with the needle pointing toward the midvitreous cavity. The gas injection should be made in a moderately brisk and continuous fashion so that the tip of the needle remains within the gas bubble at all times. This helps in the formation of a single large bubble.

The needle is then quickly removed and cotton tipped applicator is used to seal the puncture site to prevent escape of gas out of the vitreous cavity.

The IOP is checked again digitally; if noted to be high then anterior chamber paracentesis can be repeated.

Choice and Volume of Injected Gas

Most commonly used gases are SF6 (sulfur hexafluoride) or C3F8 (perfluoropropane) (Fig. 44.1). 100% SF6 doubles its volume in 24–36 hours and remains in the vitreous cavity for 10–14 days; around 0.5–0.6 mL of SF6 is injected as an expansile gas bubble. 100% C3F8 quadruples its volume in 48–72 hours and remains in vitreous cavity for 4–6 weeks; 0.3 mL of C3F8 is injected as an expansile gas bubble.[14] The gas bubble expands slowly which allows time for equilibration of IOP during the first few days after injection.

Control of Intraocular Pressure after Gas Injection

After the gas injection, optic nerve head perfusion should be checked with indirect ophthalmoscope. If pulsation at the optic nerve is not seen initially but appears after slight increase in digital pressure it indicates normal IOP. If pulsations do not appear even on increase in digital pressure it indicates high IOP and paracentesis should be repeated till normal perfusion is observed (Fig. 44.2).

Assessing the Size and Adequacy of the Gas Bubble

Indirect ophthalmoscopy should be done at the end of the injection to assess the size of gas bubble and to look for any complications at the site of gas injection. If fish eggs are formed then a gentle tap at the eye wall by cotton tipped applicator may coalesce the tiny gas bubbles giving rise to a single bubble (Fig. 44.3).

Post Injection Positioning

Post-procedure positioning is extremely important to achieve adequate tamponade of the retinal break and prevent further egress of vitreous fluid into the subretinal space till adequate retinopexy happens. Patient should be sufficiently educated regarding the utmost importance of positioning for the success of this procedure.

In case of a bullous retinal detachment where the subretinal fluid extends almost up to the macula, placing

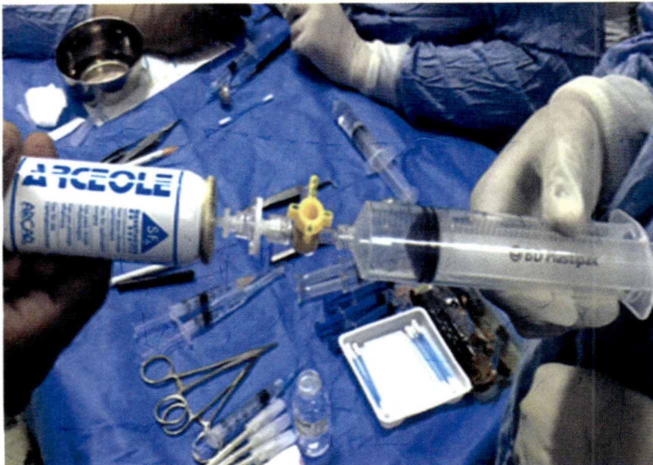

Fig. 44.1: Procedure to load 100% gas (SF6 in this case) using three way stopcock before intravitreal injection.

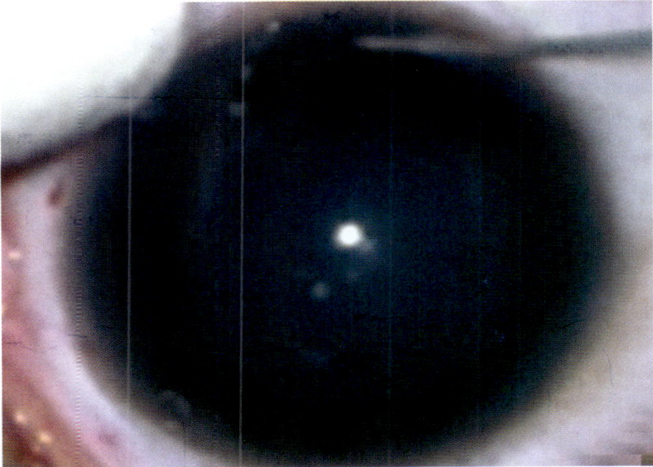

Fig. 44.2: Assessing the intraocular pressure (IOP) and performing paracentesis.

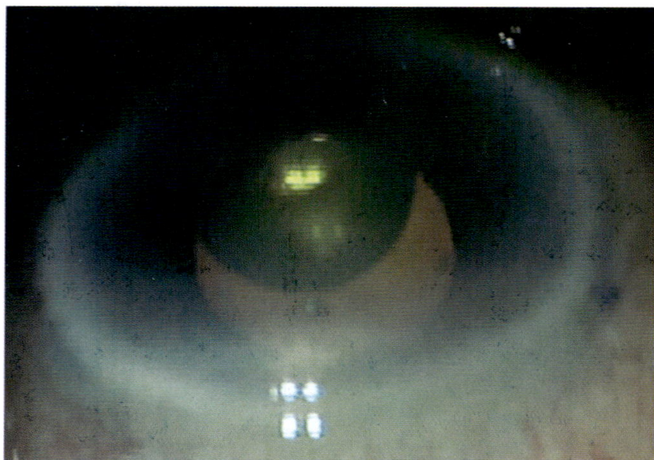

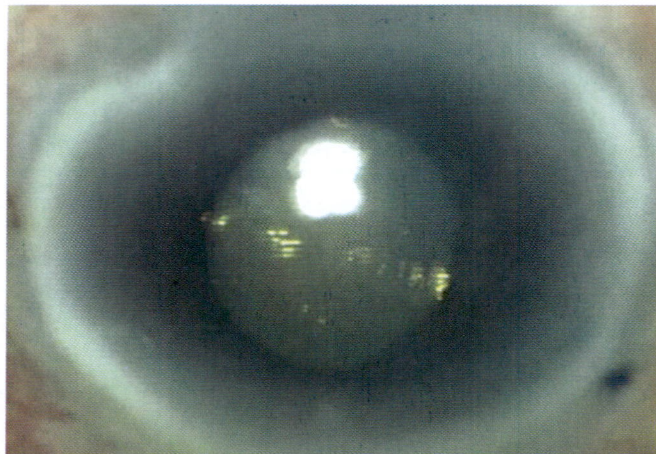

Fig. 44.3: Coalescence of multiple bubbles into a single gas bubble in vitreous cavity following gentle tap with cotton tipped applicator following injection of intravitreal gas for pneumatic retinopexy.

a bubble against the detachment may push fluid into the macula with subsequent detachment of the macula.

"Steamroller" maneuver can be performed to prevent the subretinal fluid from tracking under the macula. After the gas bubble is injected, the patient's head is turned face-down in a direction planned so as to ensure that the bubble traverses only the attached retina while reaching the macula. Over 1–10 minutes, the patient's head position is gradually changed such that the retinal break is at the highest position so that the bubble moves toward the retinal break, pushing the subretinal fluid out into the vitreous cavity thus causing retinal flattening.

Also patient should be instructed not to sleep on the back for prolonged periods of time to prevent cataract formation due to contact between the lens and the gas bubble. Air travel and deep sea diving also should be avoided for as long as the gas remains in the vitreous cavity.

Laser Retinopexy

Once the retina around the break is attached, laser retinopexy can be done. Laser indirect ophthalmoscope is the best possible method to achieve laser retinopexy. Cryopexy can also be done. It causes excessive inflammation but the advantage is that it can be done in most cases even before the injection of the gas. Following this, patient is advised to maintain strict positioning for next few days to allow firm chorioretinal adhesion. IOP should be monitored. Maximum spike of IOP is expected at 6 hours post injection of the gas.

OUTCOMES OF PNEUMATIC RETINOPEXY

A single-operation success rate of PR is up to 80%, with 98% final attachment rates with one or more operations. Success

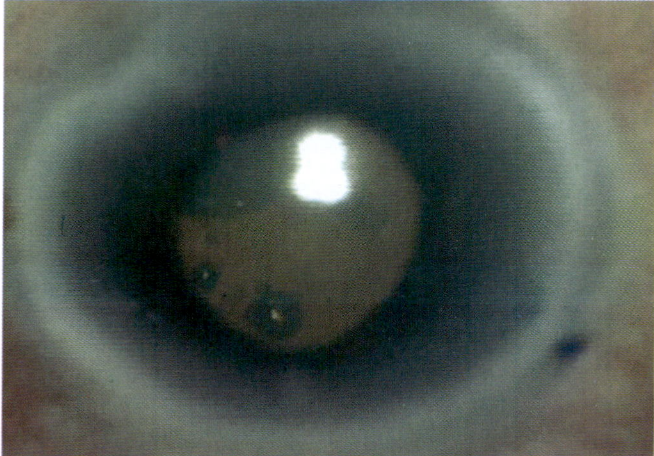

Fig. 44.4: Intravitreal gas injection for pneumatic retinopexy showing formation of fish eggs, due to multiple bubbles.

of a single operation is adversely affected by the presence of multiple retinal breaks, more than 50% retinal detachment and pseudophakia/aphakia. Second surgery requiring SB after a failed PR does not adversely affect the final visual outcome compared with SB alone.

COMPLICATIONS OF PNEUMATIC RETINOPEXY

Fish Eggs

Multiple small gas bubbles or "fish eggs" (Fig. 44.4) can occur with faulty injection technique and especially when large retinal break is present, the gas can migrate under the retina. This can be prevented by placing the needle tip vertical and shallow in vitreous cavity, keeping the injection site uppermost and injecting at moderately brisk speed. The bubbles usually coalesce spontaneously within 24 hours. Alternatively,

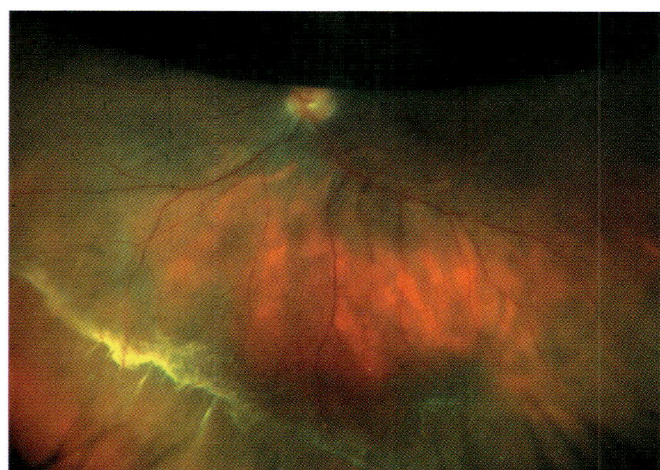

Fig. 44.5: An eye with failed pneumoretinopexy with redetachment inferiorly, and the starting of a linear proliferative vitreoretinopathy (PVR) fixed folds are visible on color fundus image.

flicking the eye gently with a cotton tipped applicator will cause the bubble to coalesce.

Gas Entrapment

Gas bubble can remain trapped at the injection site in the canal of Petit (between the anterior hyaloid, the lens and zonules, and the pars plana epithelium). When this happens the gas will be visible behind the lens in the form of a partial ring, described as the "bagel," "donut," or "sausage" sign. No treatment is required when the amount of gas trapped is small. If a large amount of gas is trapped, face down positioning is advised for a day, subsequently as the gas expands it will float up the macula. A 27-gauge needle can also be used to remove the trapped bubble by passing it into the gas bubble through the injection site.

Subretinal Gas

The gas bubble can be maneuvered back through the retinal break if the retinal break is larger than the bubble. Under indirect ophthalmoscopic visualization, the bubble can be teased out of the retinal break by using scleral depression and forcing it out. If this maneuver fails and the amount of subretinal gas is very less, it may be left as such. The detachment may still resolve if proper positioning is maintained as the intravitreal gas will outlast the subretinal gas. Large amounts of gas can be removed by passing a needle into the subretinal space transclerally.

Other complications include increased IOP, new retinal break formation, progression of cataract (38%),[15] PVR, and epiretinal membrane formation. Suprachoroidal gas has also been rarely seen.[16] However, in a multicenter clinical trial, PVR developed in 3% of eyes managed with PR compared with 5% in the SB control group. So there is inadequate evidence to support the concern of PVR being stimulated by intravitreal gas.

Causes of Failure (Fig. 44.5)

Previously undetected, untreated break, new break formation and PVR are the most common causes of failure of PR. Unrelieved vitreous traction along with expansile gas in the vitreous cavity can lead on to formation of new breaks especially in the areas of strong vitreous traction like lattice degeneration. This is particularly common in the inferior quadrant. The majority of new breaks appear within the first postoperative month.

CONCLUSION

Pneumatic retinopexy can be the procedure of choice for the repair of RRD, but in carefully selected cases. The failure rate is reasonably high and this procedure is largely given up.

REFERENCES

1. Fraser S, Steel D. Retinal detachment. BMJ Clin Evid. 2010;2010:710.
2. Han DP, Mohsin NC, Guse CE, et al. Comparison of pneumatic retinopexy and scleral buckling in the management of primary rhegmatogenous retinal detachment. Southern Wisconsin Pneumatic Retinopexy Study Group. Am J Ophthalmology. 1998;126(5):658-68.
3. Sodhi A, Leung LS, Do DV, et al. Recent trends in the management of rhegmatogenous retinal detachment. Surv Ophthalmology. 2008;53(1):50-67.
4. Hwang JC. Regional practice patterns for retinal detachment repair in the United States. Am J Ophthalmology. 2012;153(6):1125-8.
5. Hilton GF, Grizzard WS. Pneumatic retinopexy. A two-step outpatient operation without conjunctival incision. Ophthalmology. 1986;93(5):626-41.
6. Mandelcorn ED, Mandelcorn MS, Manusow JS. Update on pneumatic retinopexy. Curr Opin Ophthalmology. 2015;26(3):194-9.
7. Ellakwa AF. Long term results of pneumatic retinopexy. Clin Ophthalmology. 2012;6:55-9.
8. Goldman DR, Shah CP, Heier JS. Expanded criteria for pneumatic retinopexy and potential cost savings. Ophthalmology. 2014;121(1):318-26.
9. Rootman DB, Luu S, Conti SM, et al. Predictors of treatment failure for pneumatic retinopexy. Can J Ophthalmology. 2013;48:549-52.
10. Chan CK, Lin SG, Nuthi AS, et al. Pneumatic retinopexy for the repair of retinal detachments: a comprehensive review (1986–2007). Surv Ophthalmology. 2008;53(5):443-78.
11. Friberg TR, Eller AW. Laser pneumatic retinopexy for repair of recurrent retinal detachment after failed scleral buckle: ten years experience. Ophthalmic Surg Lasers. 2001;32(1):13-8.
12. Modi YS, Townsend J, Epstein AE, et al. Pneumatic retinopexy for retinal detachment occurring after prior scleral buckle or pars plana vitrectomy. Ophthalmic Surg Lasers Imaging Retina. 2014;45(5):409-13.
13. Petrushkin HJ, Elgohary MA, Sullivan PM. Rescue Pneumatic Retinopexy in Patients with Failed Primary Retinal Detachment Surgery. Retina. 2015;35(9):1851-9.
14. Lincoff H, Kreissig I, Brodie S, et al. Expanding gas bubbles for the repair of tears in the posterior pole. Graefes Arch Clin Exp Ophthalmology. 1982;219:193-7.
15. Feng H, Adelman RA. Cataract formation following vitreoretinal procedures. Clin Ophthalmology. 2014;8:1957-65.
16. Uji A. Suprachoroidal gas injection as a complication of pars plana vitrectomy confirmed by computed tomography. Clin Ophthalmology. 2012;6:533-6.

Chapter 45

Vitreous Substitutes

Raghav Ravani, Anin Sethi, Atul Kumar

INTRODUCTION

The vitreous is a transparent, hydrophilic gelatinous structure that makes up approximately 80% of the volume of the eye and fills the space between the lens and the retina.[1] The molecular and biochemical structure along with age-related physiological and pathological changes have been discussed in the chapter "Clinical anatomy and physiology of retina" of the book. Apart from maintenance of normal turgor of the globe, the vitreous plays an important role in nourishment of the eye and providing hydrostatic pressure for maintaining normal retinal attachment. Anomalous posterior vitreous detachment plays an important role in various vision-threatening conditions like macular hole, retinal tears, retinal detachment, vitreomacular traction, etc. With tremendous advancement in instrument design and techniques of vitreoretinal surgery since Machemer first described vitrectomy surgery, removal of vitreous or vitrectomy has become the mainstay of surgeries performed for various vitreoretinal pathologies.[2] Since vitreous humor cannot regenerate, the vitreous cavity must be filled with a substitute that closely resembles vitreous in both structure and function during and after surgery.

THE IDEAL VITREOUS SUBSTITUTE

The ideal vitreous substitute should mimic the native vitreous in both form and function (Box 45.1).[3,4] Like vitreous, it should be optically clear. It should be biocompatible and immunologically inert without being biodegradable inside the eye. It should permanently stay in the vitreous cavity after one-time injection maintaining the physiologic range of intraocular pressure (IOP) and providing support to the intraocular tissues by allowing exchange of ions, electrolytes, and nutrition thereby maintaining the physiological concentration gradient of various substances without inducing any toxic reactions. From a surgical point of view, it should be readily available at an affordable cost, stable for long-term storage, easily injectable through small gauge syringe/port, and easily manageable during surgery. The substitutes in clinical use have been

Ideal vitreous substitute
- Inert and biocompatible
- Should resemble vitreous in its physical and chemical properties
- Should be easily injectable and removable through a small port
- Cheap and easily accessible
- Should maintain its optical properties and transparency in the postoperative period.

created with the intention of acting as a retinal tamponade rather than matching the characteristics of the vitreous body.

HISTORY

One of the earliest mention of the use of vitreous substitutes dates back to 1911 when air was injected into the vitreous cavity for retinal reattachment.[5,6] Pneumatic retinopexy was first introduced by Lincoff, and later popularized by Hilton and Grizzard.[7] As air had the disadvantage of being absorbed quickly, other longer acting gases were tried and sulfur hexafluoride and perfluorocarbons [like perfluoroethane (C2F6), perfluoropropane (C3F8), etc.] became the most commonly used intraocular gases. The use of intraocular substitutes has become indispensible with advent of three port microincision vitrectomy surgery. Perfluorocarbon liquid (PFCL), initially a blood substitute was examined as a possible vitreous substitute in 1980s.[8] Chang pioneered its use in humans as an intraoperative tool to manipulate the retina in complicated retinal detachments. The use of silicone oil (SO) in treating retinal detachment was introduced even before the introduction of pars plana vitrectomy by Paul Cibis, and was injected in nonvitrectomized eyes to overcome tractional forces.[9]

CLASSIFICATION OF VITREOUS SUBSTITUTES

A functional classification which has surgical applications has been described as: (1) vitreous substitutes as temporary fillers of vitreous cavity during the surgical procedure to maintain the ocular tone; (2) vitreous substitutes used as surgical tools themselves during different steps of vitreoretinal surgery, removed at the end of surgery; (3) vitreous substitutes left inside the eye after vitreoretinal surgery with different permanence time.[10,11] Classification based on molecular state includes: (1) gases (air, SF6, and C3F8); (2) liquids (balanced salt solution, SO, PFCL, semifluorinated alkanes, and SO/semifluorinated alkanes combination); (3) experimental vitreous substitutes (hydrogels, implants, and cell culture).

GASES

No single gaseous substitute is ideal or fulfills all the desired properties of an ideal vitreous substitute. Many products have been investigated for intraocular use.[10-14] Commonly used are air, sulfur hexafluoride (SF6), and perfluoropropane (C3F8). The clinically important properties of gas include expansion ratio, nonexpansile concentration, and intraocular longevity. The comparison of important physical properties of the most commonly used gases is shown in Table 45.1.

Properties, Effects, and Functions of Gases

The main mechanism behind the use of gases in retinal detachment is that the bubble makes an arc of contact with the retina and prevents water from gaining access to the subretinal space via the retinal breaks. The surface tension of the gas bubbles ensures that the gas covers the break till chorioretinal adhesions develop due to laser or cryotherapy and seal the break permanently. The high-interfacial tension between gas and fluid makes sure that the gas stays as one bubble and prevents it from passing subretinal through small retinal breaks. The higher buoyancy of gas as compared to SO makes it take the shape of vitreous cavity and assume a flat bottom as opposed to the rounded shape of SO. This means that most of the volume of gas having higher buoyancy makes contact with the retina instead of forming a meniscus which has a lesser area of contact with the retina.

Functions of intraocular gas includes: (1) providing internal tamponade; (2) flattening of retina; (3) replacing globe volume; and (4) reducing intraocular currents.

Intraocular Gas Bubble Dynamics of an Expansile Gas

An expansile gas after injection undergoes three phases before complete absorption. These are the phase of expansion (Fig. 45.1A), phase of equilibrium (Fig. 45.1B), and phase of dissolution (Fig. 45.1C).

Phase of Expansion

Due to a difference in partial pressure of nitrogen within the bubble and outside the bubble, pure gases absorb nitrogen and expand following injection into the vitreous. The rate of

Table 45.1: Comparison of physical properties of different types of gaseous vitreous substitutes.

Gas	Chemical formula	Expansion volume of 100% gas	Time for expansion of 100% gas	Duration of tamponade	Isoexpansile concentration
Air	—	—	—	5–7 days	—
Sulfur hexafluoride	SF6	Twice the injected amount	1–2 days	2 weeks	20%
Perfluoropropane	C3F8	Three to four times the injected amount	3–4 days	6–8 weeks	14%

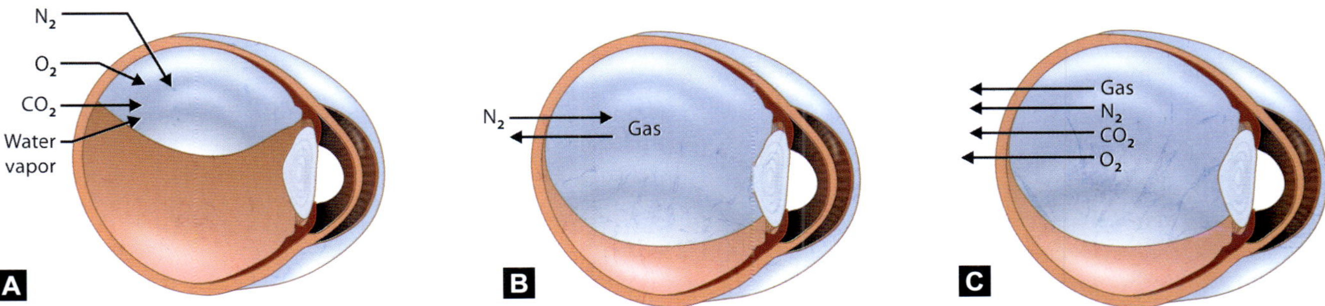

Figs. 45.1A to C: Different phases of gas resorption in vitreous cavity.

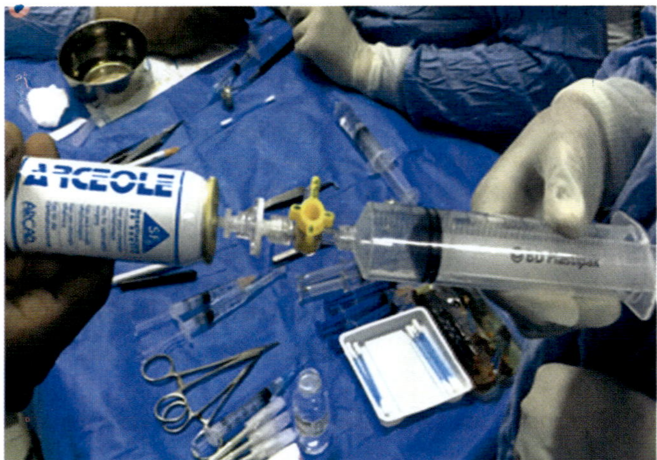

Fig. 45.2: Picture shows 10cc of SF6 gas being withdrawn in a 50cc syringe, filled with 40cc air to give a final concentration of nonexpansile 20% SF6.

expansion is maximum in the initial 6–8 hours after injection. The maximum size of the bubble is reached when equilibrium is reached between gases diffusing into and out of the bubble, i.e. 1–2 days for SF6 and 3–4 days for C3F8, which is thus a critical period of monitoring and maintaining IOP.

Phase of Equilibration

The beginning of this phase is marked by equalization of partial pressure of nitrogen within the bubble and outside it (i.e. vitreous cavity).

Phase of Dissolution

The longest phase of the dynamics is characterized by dissolution of gases into the vitreous and thereby a decrease in volume of the gas bubble.

Clinical Applications and Indications of Gaseous Vitreous Substitutes

Various indications for intraocular gas injection are:
- Pneumatic retinopexy (using pure gas)
- Internal tamponade with vitrectomy for cases of retinal detachment [nonexpansile concentration (Fig. 45.2)]
- Internal tamponade with vitrectomy in macular hole surgery (nonexpansile concentration)
- Displacement of fresh subretinal hemorrhage (using pure gas) with or without recombinant tissue plasminogen activator (rt-PA)
- Retinal detachment surgery with scleral buckling as additional internal tamponade or for flattening fish-mouthing of breaks.

Postoperative Care and Precautions in Case of Gaseous Substitutes

- Head positioning to ensure that the break is located at the uppermost position of the eye. This is one of the most important postoperative measures to ensure proper apposition of the break with the expansile gas (e.g. pneumatic retinopexy). Similarly prone or face down posturing with expansile gas is advocated for displacement of submacular hemorrhage. In certain cases prone positioning may also be required to avoid complications like pupillary block glaucoma or optic capture of an intraocular lens (IOL).
- Worsening of vision immediately after surgery should be emphasized in the preoperative counseling of patients with good vision as the vision drops due to diffraction and glare, which reverses after resorption of the gas.
- In the postoperative period sudden changes in altitude may lead to changes in gas bubble size. This might compromise the aqueous outflow facility and lead to an increase in IOP. This may be sudden and significant enough leading to a central retinal artery occlusion. Thus, sudden changes in altitude like air travel, scuba diving, or fast ascent to a high altitude should not be permitted till complete dissolution of the gas bubble.

Side Effects and Complications of Gaseous Substitutes

Cataract

The most common type of cataract seen is a feathery posterior subcapsular cataract. The incidence is especially more with pure gases and longer acting gases.[13] Cataract is usually mild and resolves spontaneously.

Corneal Decompensation

Prolonged contact of the gas bubble to endothelium leads to decompensation, especially in aphakic and pseudophakic eyes with a ruptured posterior capsule.

Increased Intraocular Pressure

This is specially seen with expansile concentration of gases with reported incidence varying from 26% to 59%.[15] This is mainly due to inability of aqueous outflow to compensate for the bubble expansion. Infrequently, secondary glaucoma occurs due to angle closure from prolonged anterior displacement of iris-lens diaphragm.

Hypotony

Intraoperative and postoperative hypotony can result due to leak from the sclerotomy site, which in turn may lead to choroidal effusion or hemorrhage.

LIQUID SUBSTITUTES

Balanced Salt Solution

It is most commonly used as irrigating fluid to replace the lost vitreous volume intraoperatively during vitrectomy. It has also been commonly used as a medium for drugs used for pupillary dilatation, anti-inflammatory effects or hemostasis. To prevent postoperative proliferative vitreoretinopathy, drugs like low-molecular weight heparin and 5-fluorouracil (5-FU) have also been used recently in infusion fluids.

Silicone Oil

Paul Cibis in 1960s described use of SO for retinal detachment by injecting it intraocularly in nonvitrectomized eyes.[16] It is now one of the most important components of vitreoretinal surgery, especially for complex retinal detachments (Fig. 45.3).

Chemical Properties of Silicone Oil

Silicone oil can be classified into lighter-than-water SO and heavier-than-water SO.

Chemically, amongst the lighter-than-water SO, the most common form is a polymer made of repeating units of siloxane [-Si-O-] (i.e. silicon and oxygen) bonded with two methyl chains forming polydimethylsiloxane (PDMS). This has a specific gravity of 0.97 and is thus lighter than water. Heavier-than-water SO is in fact a mixture of PDMS and semi-fluorinated alkanes or alkenes instead of two methyl side chains. For example, a polysiloxane unit could bind with a methyl and a trifluoropropyl group to form poly trifluoropropyl methylsiloxane, also called as fluorosilicone oil.[17] These have a specific gravity of about 1.23–1.3. When impurities like unpolymerized residual monomers, cyclic forms of siloxane, oligomeric or polymeric chains, and residual catalysts are removed, the resultant SO is called as highly purified SO. Commercially available SOs are grouped according to and differ in their average viscosities (which in turn depends on average molecular weight or amount of high molecular weight polymers).

Physical Properties of Silicone Oil

The physical properties of different types of SO are different based on its chemical composition.

Specific gravity: All PDMS irrespective of chain length or molecular weight (and viscosity), have a specific gravity of 0.97, which is lighter than aqueous or water (with specific gravity of 1.01 and 1.00, respectively). Thus, they float on water/aqueous.

Buoyancy: The tamponade effect of SO depends on buoyancy and thus on area in contact with retina and size and shape of bubble as discussed in section on tamponade with gases.

Surface tension and interfacial tension: Surface tension is the force acting on the surface that tries to and reduces the surface for a given volume. Surface tension between two immiscible liquids is termed as interfacial tension. With regard to SO (or any tamponade), interfacial tension refers to the force that keeps a bubble as a whole.[18] The effectiveness of SO is enhanced by presence of a single bubble. The interfacial tension decreases when oil is in contact with physiological fluid, blood, or presence of impurities.[19] The oil bubble remains intact as a single bubble till interfacial tension is above 6 mN/m (milli-Newton/meter).

Viscosity: It is defined as the resistance offered by a fluid against getting deformed under shear stress. SO viscosity as mentioned earlier is directly proportional to chain length.

Indications of Silicone Oil Use

1. *Retinal detachment with proliferative vitreoretinopathy*: The Silicone Study—a multicenter prospective randomized control clinical trial comparing the effect of SO with intraocular gases in management of retinal detachment associated with proliferative vitreoretinopathy (PVR) grade C3 or above found SO better than SF6 and similar to C3F8 in anatomic success (reattachment) after retinal detachment.[20,21] Incidence of complications like hypotony and keratopathy were less with SO as compared to SF6. In subgroup analysis, SO showed initial good results but later showed a deteriorating trend. However, with advent of newer SOs with various viscosities and use of PFCL for complicated surgeries, the success with SO has improved since the SO study.
2. *Retinal detachment with giant retinal tear (GRT) (Figs. 45.4A and B):* The use of SO in retinal detachment with GTR without PVR is controversial. Studies have shown good anatomical success with either SO or gas as a tamponade in GTRs,[22,23] with some showing 100% success with SO as a tamponade.[24] The posterior flap of GRT being free from vitreous adhesion is highly mobile.

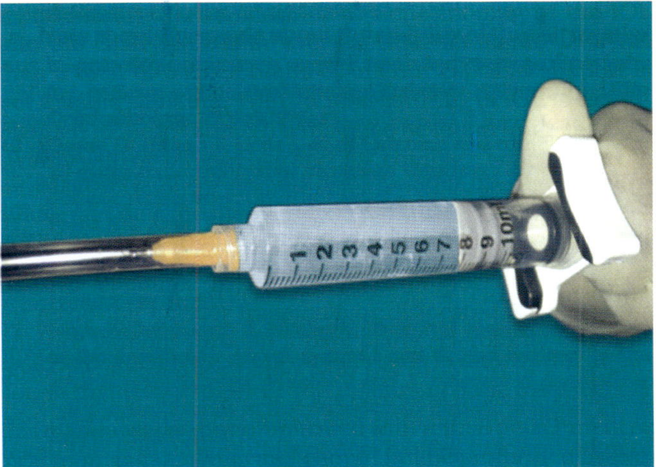

Fig. 45.3: Viscous fluid injector (VFI) containing silicone oil for automated injection of silicone oil into the vitreous cavity.

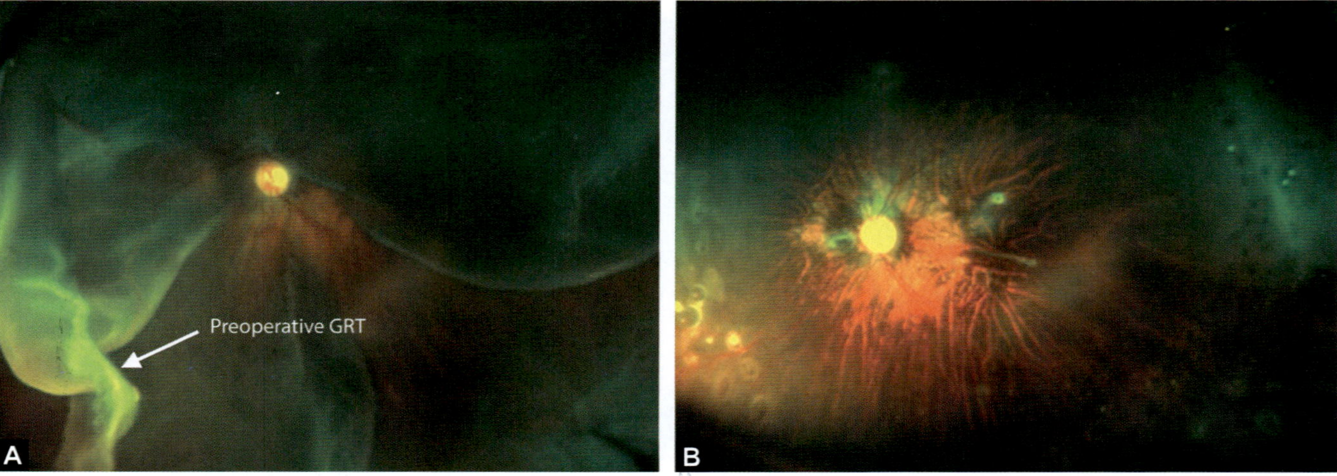

Figs. 45.4A and B: Shows a preoperative giant retinal tear (GRT) eye, and after surgery the retina is settled with oil in the vitreous cavity.

With advent of PFCL and its use in unfolding the posterior retinal flap of GRT followed by endophotocoagulation, PFCL-SO exchange reduces the risk of slippage during the surgery.[22]

3. *Pediatric retinal detachments*: Silicon oil tamponade is commonly used in complicated pediatric retinal detachments associated with trauma, retinopathy of prematurity (ROP), or choroidal coloboma.

4. *Endophthalmitis*: A prospective randomized control trial by Azad et al., comparing vitrectomy with and without SO, for cases of post-traumatic endophthalmitis suggested that a significant number of patients achieved vision of 20/200 or better vision in the group, where SO was used as a tamponade (58% vs 8%).[25] Thus, apart from being used as an internal tamponade, SO also may have antimicrobial activity.

5. *Tractional retinal detachment with severe proliferative diabetic retinopathy*: Advantages of SO in such complicated surgeries for proliferative diabetic retinopathy are:
   - Rapid visual recovery for the patient
   - Immediate media clarity for fundus evaluation
   - Reduces postoperative vitreous hemorrhage
   - Prevents vascular endothelial growth factor (VEGF) movement from posterior to anterior segment
   - Internal tamponade in case of iatrogenic breaks.

6. *Inability to maintain position postoperative positioning*: Adequate fill of SO may make it a better substitute than air or gas for patients that are incapable of strict postoperative positioning, e.g. in children or in adults with physical impairment.

7. *Postoperative air travel or travel to high altitude*: The time for SO removal is mostly around 3–6 months, when the retina is attached and retinal traction is absent.[26] Anatomic outcomes and visual acuity remain stable from 6–24 months of oil injection. This may suggest its potential for longer term use.[27]

Complications of Silicone Oil

Corneal decompensation and keratopathy: Prolonged duration of intraocular SO may result in keratopathy which may be seen either in the form of band shaped keratopathy (BSK) in earlier stages or bullous keratopathy and corneal decompensation in late stages. The incidence of keratopathy with SO as found in the SO study was 27% at 2 years.[28] The risk factors identified were aphakia or pseudophakia, need for resurgery and presence of neovascularization of iris (NVI).

Glaucoma: The main causes of postoperative rise in IOP with SO are:
- *Pupillary block glaucoma*: It is seen in aphakic patients in the early postoperative period, especially in cases where an inferior peripheral iridotomy (Ando's PI) is not patent. SO being lighter than water, can block the pupil when the patient is in the supine position. If the PI is not functioning, aqueous accumulates behind the iris and cannot enter the anterior chamber (AC) if it is blocked by the SO bubble. This in turn leads to further aqueous accumulation behind the iris and progression of the block. This may be treated by neodymium-doped yttrium aluminum garnet (Nd:YAG) PI or surgical PI to relieve the pupillary block.[29,30]

Silicone oil overfill: It is one of the causes of immediate rise in IOP postsurgery. On examination, AC is often shallow with secondary angle closure seen in some aphakic patients. On clinical examination, an overfill in phakic or pseudophakic patient may be seen as oil in front of crystalline or IOL protruding through the pupil.[31] Overfill is especially seen if an encirclage is applied or tightened after SO insertion leading to severe glaucoma.

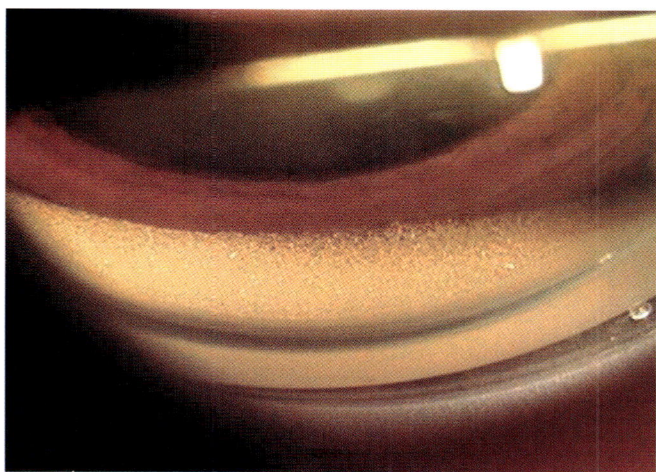

Fig. 45.5: Gonioscopic photograph of superior angle showing emulsified silicone oil globules.

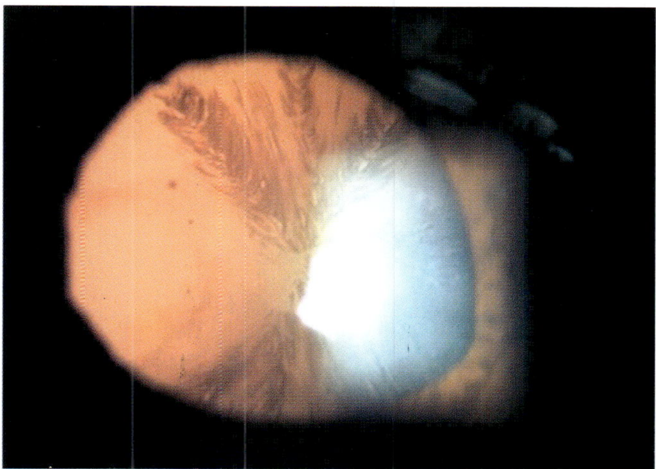

Fig. 45.6: Retroillumination photograph showing early feathery cataract following vitrectomy with silicon oil tamponade.

- *Migration of silicone oil in anterior chamber*: It can be avoided by ensuring patent PI in aphakic eyes, use of IOL along with SO insertion in aphakia, maintenance of intact posterior capsule, early removal of SO before emulsification, avoiding overfill and intraoperative use of viscoelastic in AC to prevent or to displace back small bubble back into vitreous cavity.
- *Secondary open angle glaucoma*: It may be due to mechanical blockage of trabecular meshwork by emulsified SO (Fig. 45.5) or due to trabeculitis induced by it.
- *Treatment of raised intraocular pressure with silicon oil*: Medical management remains the initial treatment of choice, followed by surgery if uncontrolled. Glaucoma drainage devices seem preferable over trabeculectomy, as subconjunctival SO may induce fibrosis due to foreign body reaction. SO removal for control of IOP could be beneficial and has been tried, but with variable results. Some researchers have found the rise in IOP to be reversible after removal of in situ SO, while some on the other have reported persistence of raised IOP even after SO removal.[32-35] Trans-scleral cyclodiode photocoagulation (TSCP) can be used to lower IOP in refractory cases, but the sustainability of its IOP-lowering effect is debatable.[36-39]

Cataract: Cataract formation in patients undergoing vitrectomy with SO is almost inevitable. The mechanism of cataract formation is multifactorial. This may be due to vitrectomy itself or surgical trauma or due to SO. Though initially it was thought that cataract occurs in patients with long-term SO, studies have shown cataract formation in relatively young patients within 2 years even following early removal of SO.[40] Mechanisms by which SO induces cataract may include impaired metabolic exchange across posterior capsule or direct toxicity of SO. Type of cataract may include posterior feathery cataract in the early postoperative period (Fig. 45.6), posterior subcapsular cataract, and progression of nuclear sclerosis.

Emulsification: It occurs when the surface energy of dispersed SO bubbles is reduced in presence of surfactants which may be phospholipids, lipoproteins and cellular debris. As the shear viscosity and hence the extensional viscosity of higher viscosity SOs (e.g. 5,000 cSt) is more than that of 1,000 cSt, the tendency to disperse and thus emulsify is less.[41] Emulsified SO in turn may lead to glaucoma, inflammation, and other side effects. The time frame for development of emulsification varies and may depend on various factors like intactness of blood-ocular barrier, amount of inflammation, completeness of oil fill, properties of SO used, etc.; but can occur as early as 1 week postoperative to typically about few months after surgery. SO with higher viscosity or low viscosity SO on addition of very-high-molecular-weight polymers have lower rate of emulsification.[42]

Perfluorocarbon Liquid

The advent and use of PFCL has greatly improved anatomic success rates in patients with complicated retinal detachments. As discussed earlier in the history of vitreous substitutes, the use of PFCL was pioneered by Chang in 1987.[43]

Biochemical Structure of Perfluorocarbon Liquid

Perfluorocarbon liquid is composed of carbon-fluoride bonds forming a synthetic fluorinated hydrocarbon, which may be arranged either in straight chains (C_5-C_9) or cyclically (C_5-C_{17}). Some of the PFCLs investigated for potential ophthalmic use are perfluoro-n-octane (C_8F_{18}), perfluorodecalin ($C_{10}F_{18}$) and perfluorophenantherene ($C_{14}F_{24}$).[44-49] Perfluoro-n-octane (C_8F_{18}) has been US Food and Drug Administration (FDA) approved for intraocular use.

Table 45.2: Physical properties of commonly used perfluorocarbon liquids.

Properties	Perfluorooctane	Perfluorophenanthrene	Perfluorodecalin
Chemical formula	C_8F_{18}	$C_{14}F_{24}$	$C_{10}F_{18}$
Molecular weight (g/mol)	438.06	624	462
Specific gravity (g/cm³)	1.76	2.03	1.94
Viscosity (cSt at 25°C)	0.8	8.03	2.7
Surface tension (dyne/cm at 25°C)	14	16	16
Refractive index	1.27	1.33	1.31
Vapor pressure (mm Hg at 37°C)	50	<1	13.5

Physical Properties of Perfluorocarbon Liquid

Certain physical properties of PFCL make it a useful tool for vitreoretinal surgery. These include:
1. It is colorless.
2. It is odorless.
3. It is optically clear.
4. *It has a low viscosity*: This allows for easy injection and aspiration intraoperatively even with smaller gauge instruments.
5. *Higher density and specific gravity than water*: This allows it the settle down on the retina, which enables the surgeon to use it as a third hand. PFCL has revolutionized surgery for GTRs as PFCL can be used to unroll the flap of a GRT and flatten the retina.[50]
6. *Low surface tension and high interfacial tension*: It reduces risk of subretinal migration by keeping the PFCL in a single bubble.
7. *Different refractive index from fluid/saline*: It creates a visible PFCL-fluid interface that helps in intraocular PFCL visibility, maneuvering, and helps in complete and easy removal.
8. *Higher boiling point than water, stable at high temperature and does not absorb wavelengths of commonly used lasers*: It allows for endophotocoagulation under PFCL, especially useful in GRT.
9. *Immiscible with silicon oil*: It allows PFCL-SO exchange thereby reducing the risk of posterior flap slippage in GRT.

The physical properties of the commonly used PFCL are shown in Table 45.2.

Indications for Perfluorocarbon Liquid

Complicated retinal detachment with proliferative vitreoretinopathy: With introduction of use of PFCL in vitreoretinal surgery, dissection of membranes and removal of PVR from posterior pole has improved which increases anatomic success rate especially when used along with encircling buckle to relieve anterior traction.[51-53] PFCL aids in visualization of membranes and delineating area requiring further peeling apart from flattening the posterior pole and opening up the funnel in severe PVR. Moreover, PFCL helps to displace the vitreous anteriorly, and also provides a clear interface between PFCL and vitreous fluid; thereby helping to shave the vitreous base. PFCL can also be used along with triamcinolone acetonide for better vitreous base shaving.[54] After relieving traction till the anterior retina, endophotocoagulation under PFCL can be done which is later followed by PFCL-air exchange followed by internal tamponade.

Giant retinal tears: Treatment of GTRs has changed drastically following the introduction of PFCL. In pre-PFCL area, maneuvers like use of Stryker table as described by Peyman were used to roll the patient into prone position intraoperatively to unfold the retinal flap with help of intraocular gas bubble with obvious difficulties and a low success rates.[55,56] Intraoperative use of PFCL helps in gentle manipulation and unfolding of the posterior flap of the tear and permits endophotocoagulation under PFCL bubble itself, thereby significantly improving the success rate of the surgery (Figs. 45.7A and B).[57] After thorough vitrectomy and endophotocoagulation under PFCL, PFCL-SO exchange can be done to prevent slippage of posterior flap (Figs. 45.8A and B). A low rate of slippage has been reported using the technique described by Li and Wong.[58] Previous studies have described use of PFCL for prolonged internal tamponade, but in view of potential intraocular toxicity and other intraocular complications, this is rarely done.[59,60]

Ocular trauma with or without retained intraocular foreign body: Use of PFCL in post-traumatic cases has multiple advantages.[61] Apart from stabilizing the retina and maintaining a clear media during vitrectomy; it displaces the pre-retinal, subretinal, or suprachoroidal bleed. It assists in the removal of incarcerated retina. Also it facilitates the removal of posteriorly dislocated crystalline or cataractous lens or IOL or intraocular foreign body (IOFB).

Posteriorly dislocated lens/intraocular lens: Perfluorocarbon liquid is often used in the management of posteriorly dislocated crystalline/cataractous lens and lens fragments. PFCL

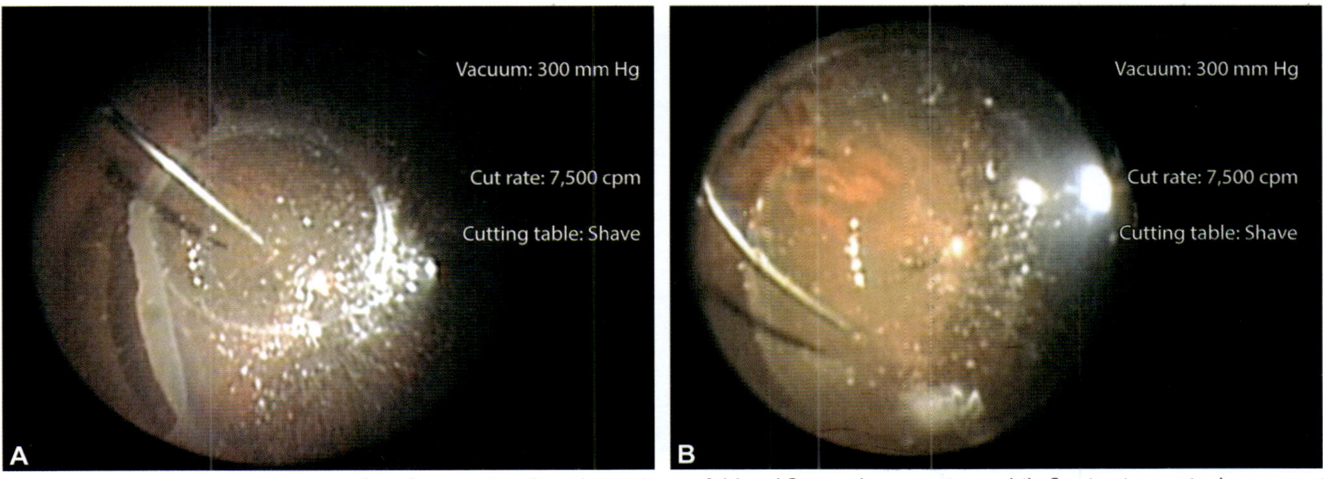

Figs. 45.7A and B: Intraoperative use of perfluorocarbon liquid (PFCL) to unfold and flatten the posterior mobile flap in giant retinal tear associated retinal detachment.

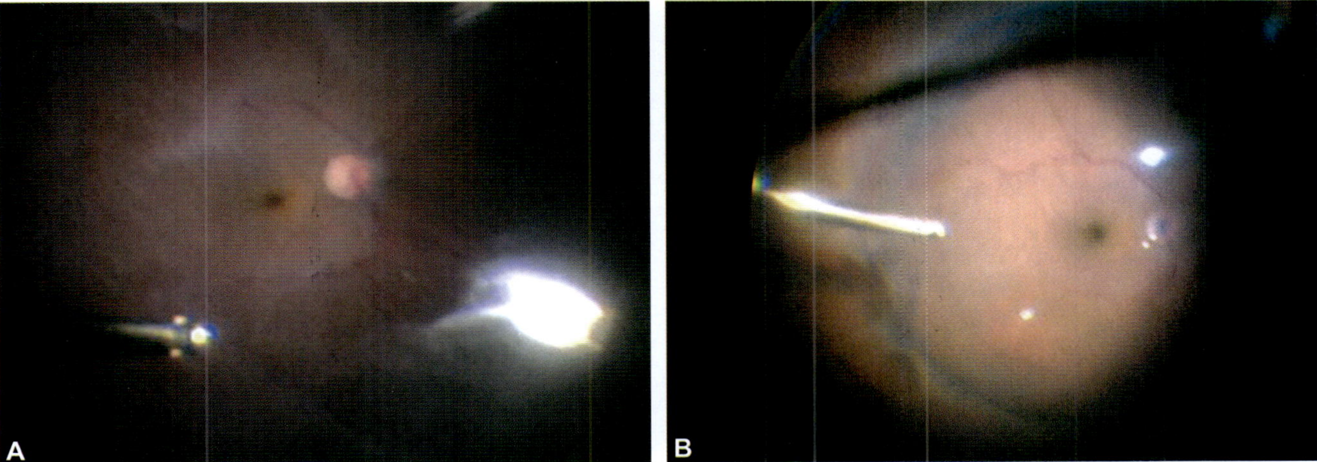

Figs. 45.8A and B: (A) Chandelier illumination being used in a case of pars plana vitrectomy for giant retinal tears associated retinal detachment. (B) Direct perfluorocarbon liquid (PFCL)-silicone oil exchange being done with extrusion of PFCL bubble from the posterior pole and simultaneous injection of silicone oil.

acts as a "cushion" against transmitted ultrasound energy of phacofragmatome to prevent damage to macula and help to levitate lens matter away from the retina into the midvitreous where it can safely be fragmented by a cutter or fragmentome (Fig. 45.9). In some cases with hard cataract or cases associated with retinal detachment, PFCL may be used to float the whole lens into the AC and express it out of the corneal/scleral wound.[62,63] PFCL may be used to float up a dropped IOL and then it can be grasped from an anterior incision and further be removed or repositioned into the sulcus.

Other indications: Other indications for use of PFCL may include retinal detachment associated with diabetic retinopathy/choroidal coloboma/ROP and displacement of submacular hemorrhage etc.[64-67]

Complications

Subretinal perfluorocarbon liquid: This can occur intraoperatively in case PFCL breaks into numerous small globules while injecting or due to a jet of fluid from the infusion post. It can also occur in cases of giant/large retinal tears if PFCL injection is done before complete relief of traction over the break/retina.

Subretinal PFCL may eventually reach under the fovea with time if left untreated (Figs. 45.10A and B). This can cause a central scotoma and permanently damage the retinal function in long standing cases.[68,69] Long-standing subretinal PFCL has also been reported to cause retinal hole formation.[70] Various methods have been described for removal of subretinal/subfoveal PFCL bubble. We use a 41G translocation

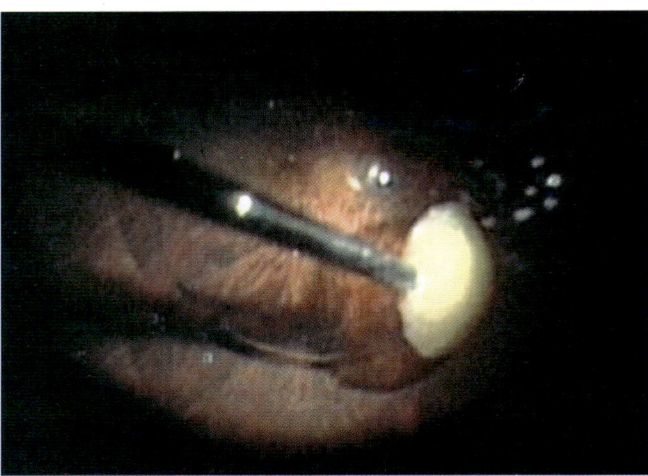

Fig. 45.9: Use of perfluorocarbon liquid to levitate or displace posteriorly dislocated nucleus for phacofragmentation to prevent ultrasound related macular damage.

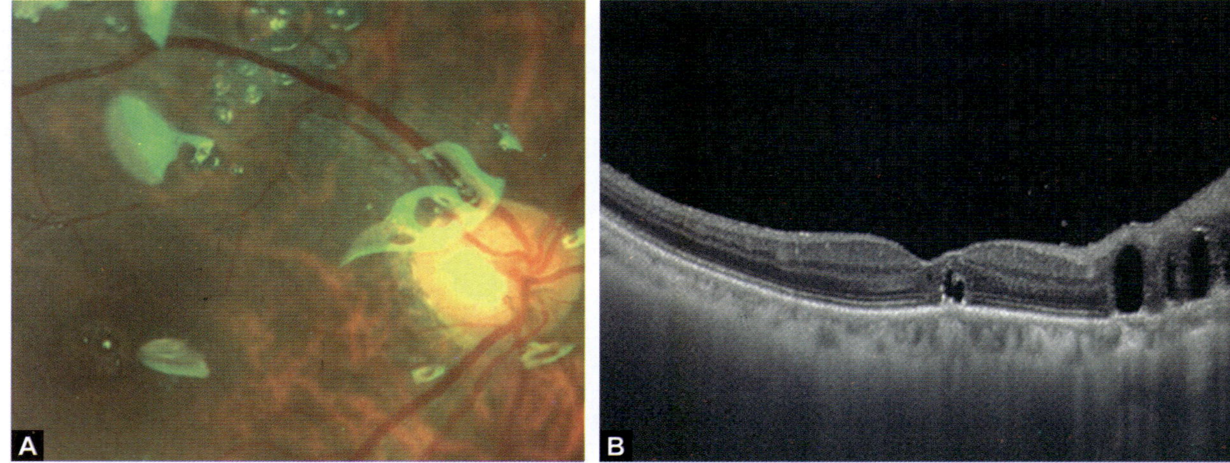

Figs. 45.10A and B: (A) Pseudocolor image and (B) optical coherence tomography (OCT) showing multiple subretinal perfluorocarbon liquid (PFCL) bubbles at fovea and at superotemporal arcade in oil filled eye with attached retina.

needle with self- sealing retinotomy to aspirate the PFCL bubble under intraoperative optical coherence tomography (OCT) guidance.

Intraocular toxicity: The incidence of incomplete removal of PFCL ranges from 0.9% to 11.1%, resulting in toxicity. Retained intraocular PFCL may be seen over the retina or as a fluid level inferiorly on the retina with the patient in a sitting position or as small bubbles in the inferior angle. Toxicity of PFCL may be either mechanical or chemical.

Mechanical toxicity is seen due to prolonged compression from the retained PFCL due to its high specific gravity. This may lead to histological changes like loss of outer plexiform layer, displacement of photoreceptor nuclei into the outer segments and atrophy of the retinal pigment epithelium.[48] These atrophic changes are postulated to occur due to the exclusion of water from the retinal surface leading to disruption of potassium siphoning mechanism of the Müller cells.

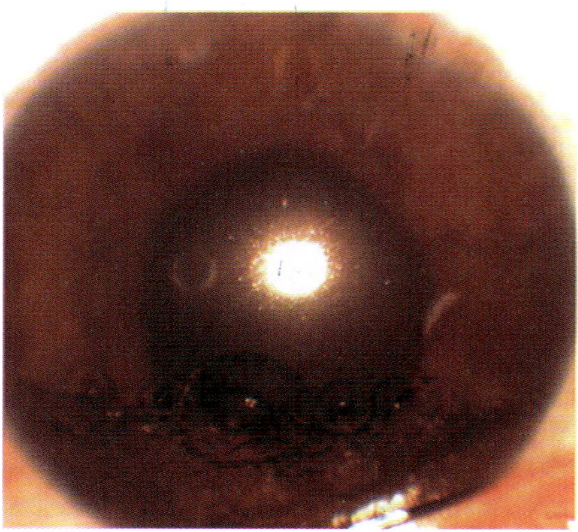

Fig. 45.11: Retained perfluorocarbon liquid (PFCL) bubbles in an eye operated for retinal detachment (RD). Patient presented to us with history of operated RD surgery and oil fill. On examination, projection of light rays was inaccurate on all sides with no glow and PFCL bubbles in the anterior chamber (AC).

Chemical toxicity may be attributed to the high oxygen carrying capacity of PFCL and due to the presence of polar impurities.[71] The high oxygen carrying capacity may either lead to vasoconstriction of retinal blood vessels or may cause direct toxicity leading to damage of the retinal vessels.[71-73]

Other complications like retained PFCL in AC may lead to visual disturbances, endothelial cell loss and rise in IOP (*see* Fig. 45.11).[74]

REFERENCES

1. Sebag J, Balazs EA. Morphology and ultrastructure of human vitreous fibers. Invest Ophthalmology Vis Sci. 1989;30:1867-71.
2. Machemer R, Buettner H, Norton EW, et al. Vitrectomy: a pars plana approach. Trans Am Acad Ophthalmology Otolaryngol. 1971;75(4):813-20.
3. Maruoka S, Matsuura T, Kawasaki K, et al. Biocompatibility of polyvinylalcohol gel as a vitreous substitute. Curr Eye Res. 2006;31(7-8):599-606.
4. Pruett RC, Schepens CL, Swann DA. Hyaluronic acid vitreous substitute. A six-year clinical evaluation. Arch Ophthalmology. 1979;97(12):2325-30.
5. Ohm J. Uber die Behandlung der Netzhautablosung durch operative Entleerung der subretinalen Flussigkeit und Einspritzung von Luft in den Glaskorper. Graefes Arch Clin Ophthalmology. 1911;79:442-50.
6. Rosengren B. Results of treatment of detachment of the retina with diathermy and injection of air into the vitreous. Acta Ophthalmology. 1938;16:573-9.
7. Hilton GF, Grizzard WS. Pneumatic retinopexy: a two-step outpatient operation without conjunctival incision. Ophthalmology. 1986;93:626-41.
8. Haidt SJ, Clark LC Jr, Ginsberg J. Liquid perfluorocarbon replacement of the eye. Invest Ophthalmology Vis Sci. 1982;22:233.
9. Dufour R. Experience with Intraocular Silicone Injection: New and Controversial Aspects of Retinal Detachment Surgery. New York: Harper & Row; 1968. p. 377.
10. Lincoff A, Lincoff H, Iwamoto T, et al. Perfluoro-butane—a gas for a maximum duration retinal tamponade. Arch Ophthalmology. 1983;101:460-2.
11. Lincoff A, Lincoff H, Solorzano C, et al. Selection of xenon gas for rapidly disappearing retinal tamponade. Arch Ophthalmology. 1982;100:996-7.
12. Vygantas CM, Peyman GA, Daily MJ, et al. Octafluorocyclobutane and other gases for vitreous replacement. Arch Ophthalmology. 1973;90:235-6.
13. Fineberg E, Machemer R, Sullivan P, et al. Sulphur hexafluoride in owl monkey vitreous cavity. Am J Ophthalmology. 1975;79:67-76.
14. Killey MP, Edelhauser HF, Aaberg TM. Intraocular sulfur hexafluoride and octofluorocyclobutane. Arch Ophthalmology. 1978;96:511-5.
15. Sabates WI, Abrams GW, Swanson DE, et al. The use of intraocular gases: the results of sulfur hexafluoride gas in retinal detachment surgery. Ophthalmology. 1981;88:447-54.
16. Cibis PA, Becker B, Okun E, et al. The use of liquid silicone in retinal detachment surgery. Arch Ophthalmology. 1962;68:590-9.
17. Wolf S, Schon V, Meier P, et al. Silicone oil–RMN3 mixture ("heavy silicone oil") as internal tamponade for complicated retinal detachment. Retina. 2003;23:335-42.
18. Feynman RP, Leighton RB, Sands M. The Feynman Lectures on Physics, 7th edition. Reading, MA: Addison-Wesley; 1972.
19. Yamanaka A, Matsuda T, Nakamae K, et al. Interfacial Aspects of Liquid Silicone as an Artificial Vitreous Body. Vail, CO: Fifth Vail Vitreoretinal Seminar; 1986.
20. McCuen BW 2nd, Azen SP, Stern W, et al. Vitrectomy with silicone oil or perfluoropropane gas in eyes with severe proliferative vitreoretinopathy. Silicone Study Report 3. Retina. 1993;13:279-84.
21. Vitrectomy with silicone oil or sulfur hexafluoride gas in eyes with severe proliferative vitreoretinopathy: results of a randomized clinical trial. Silicone Study Report 1. Arch Ophthalmology. 1992;110:770-9.
22. Mathis A, Pagot V, Gazagne C, et al. Giant retinal tears: surgical techniques and results using perfluorodecalin and silicone oil tamponade. Retina. 1992;12:x7-10.
23. Unlu N, Kocaoglan H, Acar MA, et al. The management of giant retinal tears with silicone oil. Eur J Ophthalmology. 2003;13:192-5.
24. Leaver PK, Lean JS. Management of giant retinal tears using vitrectomy and silicone oil/fluid. Trans Ophthalmology Soc UK. 1981;101(1):189-91.
25. Azad R, Ravi K, Talwar D, et al. Pars plana vitrectomy with or without silicone oil endotamponade in posttraumatic endophthalmitis. Graefes Arch Clin Exp Ophthalmology. 2003;241:478-83.
26. Pastor JC. Proliferative vitreoretinopathy: an overview. Surv Ophthalmology. 1998;43:3-18.
27. Azen SP, Scott IU, Flynn HW Jr, et al. Silicone oil in the repair of complex retinal detachments. A prospective observational multicenter study. Ophthalmology. 1998;105:1587-97.
28. The incidence of corneal abnormalities in the silicone study. Silicone Study Report 7. Arch Ophthalmology. 1995;113:764-9.
29. Ando F. Intraocular hypertension resulting from pupillary block by silicone oil. Am J Ophthalmology. 1985;99:87-8.
30. Bartov E, Huna R, Ashkenazi I, et al. Identification, prevention and treatment of silicone oil pupillary block after an inferior iridectomy. Am J Ophthalmology. 1991;111:501-4.
31. Jackson TL, Thiagarajan M, Murthy R, et al. Pupil block glaucoma in phakic and pseudophakic patients after vitrectomy with silicone oil injection. Am J Ophthalmology. 2001;132:414-6.
32. Han L, Cairns JD, Campbell WG, et al. Use of silicone oil in the treatment of complicated retinal detachment: results from 1981–1994: Aust NZ J Ophthalmology. 1998;26:299-304.
33. Budenz DL, Taba KE, Feuer WJ, et al. Surgical management of secondary glaucoma after pars plana vitrectomy and silicone oil injection for complex retinal detachment. Ophthalmology. 2001;108:1628-32.
34. Jonas JB, Knorr HL, Rank RM, et al. Intraocular pressure and silicone oil endotamponade. J Glaucoma. 2001;10:102-8.
35. Flaxel CJ, Mitchell SM, Aylward GW. Visual outcome after silicone oil removal and recurrent retinal detachment repair. Eye. 2000;14:834-8.
36. Ghazi-Nouri SM, Vakalis AN, Bloom PA, et al. Long-term results of the management of silicone oil-induced raised intraocular pressure by diode laser cycloablation. Eye (Lond). 2005;19:765-9.
37. Han SK, Park KH, Kim DM, et al. Effect of diode laser trans-scleral cyclophotocoagulation in the management of glaucoma after intravitreal silicone oil injection for complicated retinal detachments. Br J Ophthalmology. 1999;83:713-7.
38. Kumar A, Dada T, Singh RP, et al. Diode laser trans-scleral cyclophotocoagulation for glaucoma following silicone oil removal. Clin Experiment Ophthalmology. 2001;29:220-4.
39. Gangwani R, Liu DT, Congdon N, et al. Effectiveness of diode laser transscleral cyclophotocoagulation in patients following silicone oil-induced ocular hypertension in Chinese eyes. Indian J Ophthalmology. 2011;59:64-6.
40. Leaver PK, Grey RHB, Garner A. Complications following silicone-oil injection. Mod Probl Ophthalmology. 1979;20:290-4.
41. Williams RL, Day M, Garvey MJ, et al. Increasing the extensional viscosity of silicone reduces the tendency for emulsification. Retina. 2010;30:300-4.
42. Crisp A, de Juan E Jr, Tiedeman J. Effect of silicone oil viscosity on emulsification. Arch Ophthalmology. 1987;105:546-50.

43. Chang S. Low viscosity liquid fluorochemicals in vitreous surgery. Am J Ophthalmology. 1987;103:38-43.

44. Bourke RD, Simpson RN, Cooling RJ, et al. The stability of perfluoro-n-octane during vitreoretinal procedures. Arch Ophthalmology. 1996;114:537.

45. Sparrow JR, Matthews GP, Iwamoto T, et al. Retinal tolerance to intravitreal perfluoroethylcyclohexane liquid in the rabbit. Retina. 1993;13:56-62.

46. Azzolini C, Brancato R, Trabucchi G, et al. Endophotocoagulation through perfluorodecalin in rabbit eyes. Int Ophthalmology. 1994;18:33.

47. Batman C, Cekic O. Effects of the long-term use of perfluoro-phenanthrene on the retina. Ophthalmic Surg Lasers. 1998;29:144-6.

48. Chang S, Zimmerman NJ, Iwamoto T, et al. Experimental vitreous replacement with perfluorotributylamine. Am J Ophthalmology. 1987;103:29-37.

49. Bryan JS, Friedman SM, Mames RN, et al. Experimental vitreous replacement with perfluorotri-n-propylamine. Arch Ophthalmology. 1994;112:1098.

50. Schulman JA, Peyman GA, Blinder KJ, et al. Management of giant retinal tears with perfluoroperhydrophenanthrene (Vitreon). Jpn J Ophthalmology. 1993;7:70-7.

51. Banker AS, Freeman WR, Vander JF, et al. Use of Perflubron as a new temporary vitreous substitute and manipulation agent for vitreoretinal surgery. Retina. 1996;16:285.

52. Carroll BF, Peyman GA, Mehta NJ, et al. Repair of retinal detachment associated with proliferative vitreoretinopathy using perfluoroperhydrophenanthrene (Vitreon). Can J Ophthalmology. 1994;29:66-9.

53. Coll GE, Chang S, Sun J, et al. Perfluorocarbon liquid in the management of retinal detachment with proliferative vitreo-retinopathy. Ophthalmology. 1995;102:630-8.

54. Veckeneer M, Wong D. Visualising vitreous through modified trans-scleral illumination by maximising the Tyndall effect. Br J Ophthalmology. 2009;93:268-70.

55. Peyman GA. A new operating table for the management of giant retinal breaks. Arch Ophthalmology. 1981;99:498-9.

56. Cairns JD, Campbell WG. Vitrectomy techniques in the treatment of giant retinal tears: A fexible approach. Aust NZ J Ophthalmology. 1988;16:209-14.

57. Kreiger AE, Lewis H. Management of giant retinal tears without scleral buckling: use of radical dissection of the vitreous base and perfluoro-n-octane and intraocular tamponade. Ophthalmology. 1992;99:491-7.

58. Li KK, Wong D. Avoiding retinal slippage during macular translocation surgery with 360 retinotomy. Graefes Arch Clin Exp Ophthalmology. 2008;246:649-51.

59. Foster RE, Smiddy WS, Alfonso ED, et al. Secondary glaucoma associated with retained perfluorophenanthrene. Am J Ophthalmology. 1994;118:253-5.

60. Millsap CM, Peyman GA, Mehta NJ, et al. Perfluoroperhydro-phenanthrene (Vitreon®) in the management of giant retinal tears: Results of a collaborative study. Ophthalmic Surg. 1993;24:759-63.

61. Alfaro DV, Liggett PF. Perfluorocarbon liquid in the management of traumatic retinal detachment: advantages of PFCs in traumatic retinal detachment. Vitreoretinal Surg Technol. 1993;15:1-2.

62. Lewis H, Blumenkranz MS, Chang S. Treatment of dislocated crystalline lens and retinal detachment with perfluorocarbon liquid. Retina. 1992;12:299-304.

63. Brod RD, Flynn HW Jr, Clarkson JG, et al. Management options for retinal detachment in the presence of a posteriorly dislocated intraocular lens. Retina. 1990;10:50-6.

64. Mathis A. The use of perfluorodecalin in diabetic vitrectomy. Retina. 1992;1:28-9.

65. Lee KJ, Peyman GA, Paris CL, et al. Management of retinal detachment associated with choroidal coloboma using pertluoroperhydrophenanthrene (Vitreon) Ophthalmic Surg. 1992;23:563-4.

66. Millsap CM, Peyman GA, Ma PE, et al. The surgical management of retinopathy of prematurity using a perfluorocarbon liquid. Int Ophthalmology. 1994;18:97-100.

67. Lambert HM, Capone A Jr, Aaberg TM, et al. Surgical excision of subfoveal neovascular membranes in agerelated macular degeneration. Am J Ophthalmology. 1992;13:257-62.

68. Le Tien V, Pierre-Kahn V, Azan F, et al. Displacement of retained subfoveal perfluorocarbon liquid after vitreoretinal surgery. Arch Ophthalmology. 2008;126:98-101.

69. Tewari A, Eliott D, Singh CN, et al. Changes in retinal sensitivity from retained subretinal perfluorocarbon liquid. Retina. 2009;29:248-50.

70. Cohen SY, Dubois L, Elmaleh C, et al. Retinal hole as a complication of long standing subretinal perfluorocarbon liquid. Retina. 2006;26:843-4.

71. Kobuch K, Menz DH, Dresp JH, et al. New substances for intraocular tamponades:perfluorocarbon liquid, hydrofluorocarbon liquid and hydrofluorocarbon-oligomers in vitreoretinal surgery. Graefe's Arch Clin Exp Ophthalmology. 2001;239:635-42.

72. Kobuch K, Fuchs B, Tomi A, et al. The influence of O_2 and CO_2 concentrations in perfluorocarbon liquid as vitreous substitutes on the retinal perfusion. Invest Ophthalmology Vis Sci. 1999;40:4052.

73. Kobuch K, El Batarny A, Ueda N, et al. Perfluorophenanthrene causes vascular and neural damage in the rabbit eye. Invest Ophthalmology Vis Sci. 1997;38:3111.

74. Elsing SH, Fekrat S, Green WR, et al. Clinicopathologic findings in eyes with retained perfluoro-n-octane liquid. Ophthalmology. 2001;108:45-8.

Chapter 46

Pars Plana Vitrectomy

Atul Kumar, Devesh Kumawat, Raghav Ravani

HISTORY AND EVOLUTION OF VITRECTOMY

Pars plana vitrectomy involves surgical removal of vitreous gel by introducing instruments through pars plana region using three ports, placed 3–4 mm posterior to the limbus. One port is used for infusion of balanced saline solution, which maintains the intraocular pressure (IOP) intraoperatively. The remaining ports are used to introduce instruments to illuminate the posterior segment and manipulate the intraocular tissues.

Vitrectomy is performed using an operating microscope with a contact lens or noncontact lens viewing system. Direct and indirect lenses are available to aid fundus viewing. The advantages of indirect visualization include a wider viewing angle as well as better visualization through media opacities, miotic pupils, and gas-filled eyes. The direct viewing systems allow greater magnification and enhanced stereopsis but at the expense of a smaller field of view.

A recent advance in vitreous surgery has been the development of minimally invasive transconjunctival vitrectomy systems [23- or 25- or 27-gauge (G) systems]. Unlike sclerotomies made using standard 19G or 20G instruments, those made using the 23G or 25G or 27G technique are self-sealing and generally do not require suture closure, thereby eliminating the risk of suture-related complications.

Advantages of small-gauge vitrectomy over large-gauge vitrectomy include reduced patient discomfort and inflammation, faster wound healing and postoperative recovery, conjunctival preservation, easier instrument exchange shortened operative time, and better operating room efficiency.[1-3] Potential disadvantages include an increased risk of postoperative hypotony, endophthalmitis, increased iatrogenic retinal tears, and epithelial down growth.[1,4]

SURGICAL STEPS IN VITREORETINAL SURGERY

Surgical Preparation

Standard surgical draping of eye is done after cleaning with povidone-iodine solution (10% solution for skin and 5% solution for cul-de-sac). Conventional 20G surgery requires conjunctival dissection prior to sclerotomy incision with microvitreoretinal (MVR) blade. Infusion cannula is typically placed through a sclerotomy inferotemporally made 3.5–4 mm posterior to limbus in phakic eyes and 3–3.5 mm in aphakic or pseudophakic eyes (Fig. 46.1). Sclerotomy incision should enter in the pars plana region.

Trocars are used to make pars plana sclerotomy entries (Fig. 46.2). Trocar needle can be 20G/23G/25G/27G. Microcannulas made up of polyamide, are preloaded on the needle trocars. Microcannula can be valved or nonvalved. Valved cannulas eliminate the need for repeated placement and removal of plugs during instrument withdrawal or exchange, besides maintaining IOP and reducing turbulence within vitreous cavity.

Combined components of the trocar needle, microcannula, and trocar handle are referred to as the trocar or cannula assembly. This system maintains alignment between the entry holes in conjunctiva and sclera as well as provides unobstructed instrument access.

Self-retaining infusion cannulae of different sizes according to microcannula (20G or 23G or 25G or 27G) is used to introduce irrigating solution into the vitreous cavity (Fig. 46.3). Cannulae can be 4 mm or 6 mm in length. Standard surgery requires a 4 mm cannula. Longer cannulae can be used for aphakic or pseudophakic eyes or high myopes or eyes with peripheral choroidal detachment or endophthalmitis to minimize the risk of the cannula being in subretinal space.

Additional sclerotomy sites are made in superonasal and superotemporal quadrants. These sites should be ideally 160°–180° apart to facilitate manipulation (Fig. 46.4).

Vitrectomy

The goal of the vitrectomy is to remove the centrally formed vitreous first and then move gradually towards the periphery. Vitreous is strongly adherent at the vitreous base straddling the ora serrata. This vitreous is usually not removed during vitrectomy. Incision of the central vitreous gel is performed initially. Illumination probe and cutter are inserted through the remaining port sclerotomies. The illumination probe is to

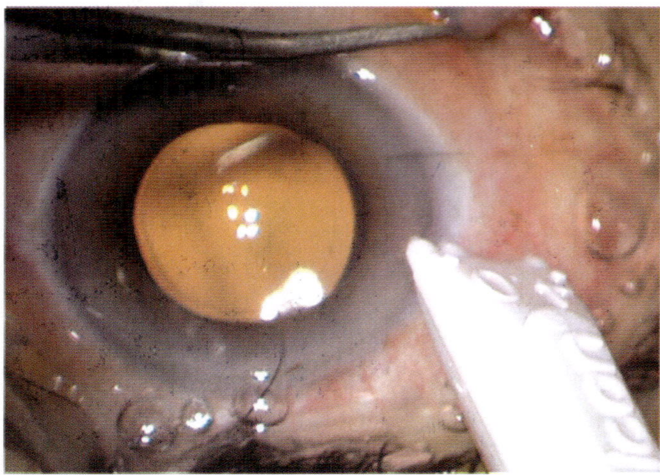

Fig. 46.1: Trocar is inserted at 3.5 mm from limbus in a pseudophakic patient.

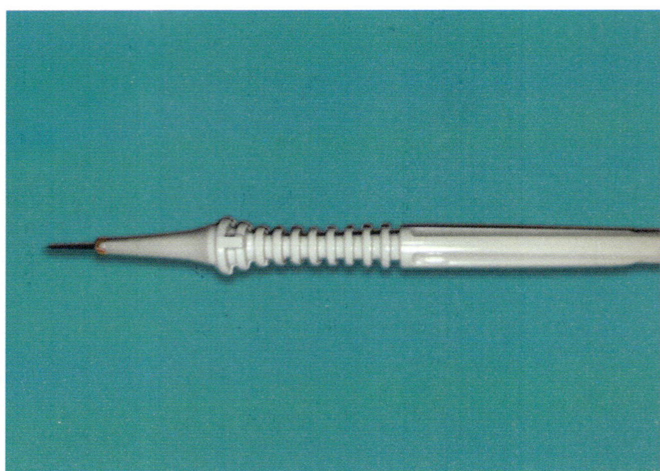

Fig. 46.2: 23G trocar with valved microcannula.

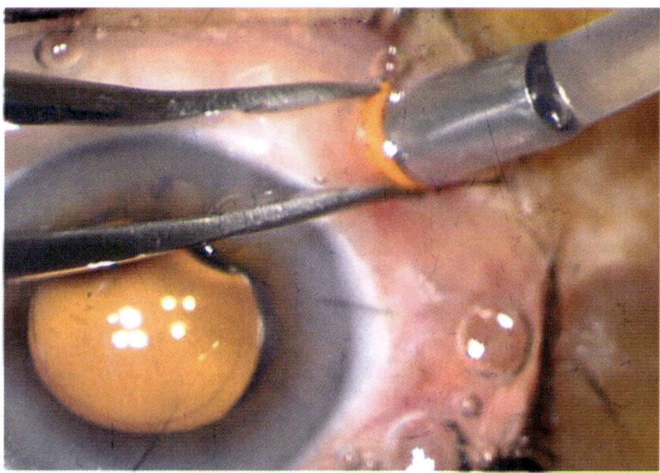

Fig. 46.3: Self-retaining infusion cannula.

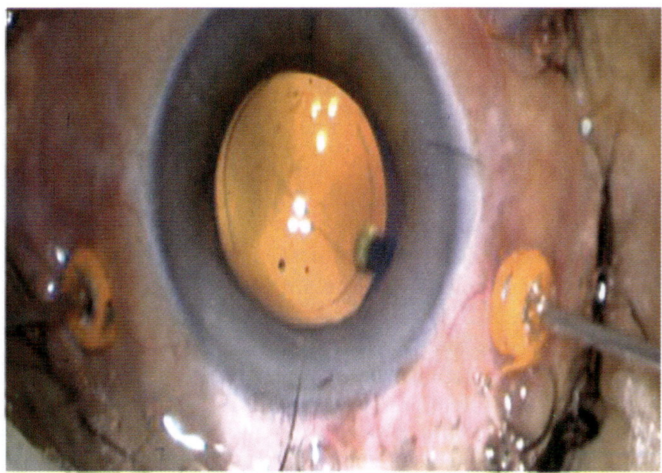

Fig. 46.4: Sclerotomy ports at 160° to each other.

be kept at a distance from the cutter, so that the tip of the cutter is well illuminated and a greater field of view is obtained (Fig. 46.5).

Once within the vitreous cavity, foot pedal of the vitrectomy console is depressed to begin aspiration and cutting. The cutting port on the vitreous cutter should face the vitreous to be cut at all times. Vitreous cutters utilize suction and inclusive shearing force to cut vitreous.[5] These can be of two broad types—electrodynamic cutter or pneumatic cutter. Electrodynamic cutters are heavy, can cause fatigue and exacerbate tremors. Pneumatic cutters are lighter with the added advantage of being cheap. Based on the mechanism of cutting, there are three types of cutters:[5] (1) rotating mechanism, (2) oscillating mechanism or Peyman type—it has less shearing effect, so considered to be better than the first one, and (3) Guillotine type—it has two tubes, an outer fixed tube and an inner tube that can slide. The inner tube cuts the vitreous by sliding across the port and the vitreous is aspirated through an opening present on the outer tube.

Vitrectomy Modes

The earlier pneumatic driven cutter was based on spring return mechanism in which the diaphragm inside the probe was pushed by an air pulse (port closed position). This pulse also compressed a spring which then forced the diaphragm back to the open port position. The spring return mechanism limited the control over the duty cycle (DC). DC is the percentage of time the port is open during each cut cycle (DC = open port time/time of a cut cycle). As cut speed increases, the DC decreases.

The newer dual pneumatic probes use two separate air lines to open and close the vitrectomy port. With these, DC

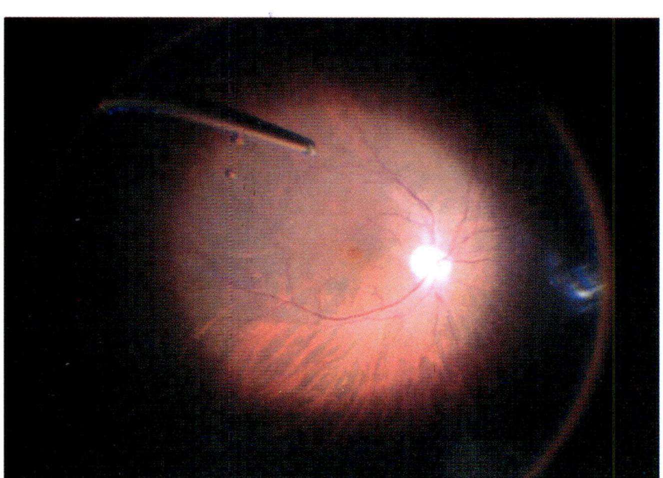

Fig. 46.5: Illumination probe is held close to the port for a wider field of view.

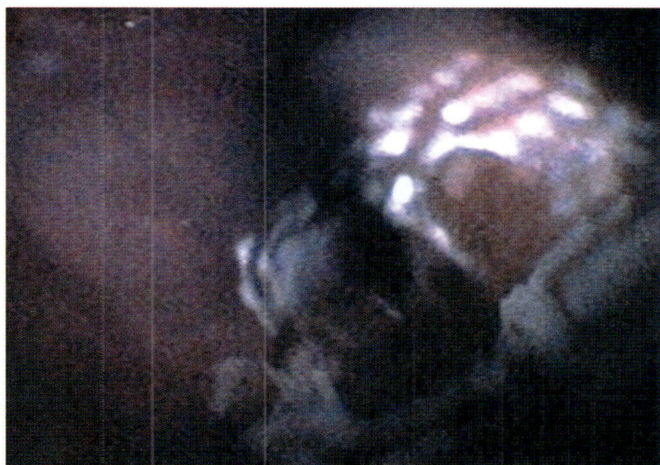

Fig. 46.6: Scleral depression.

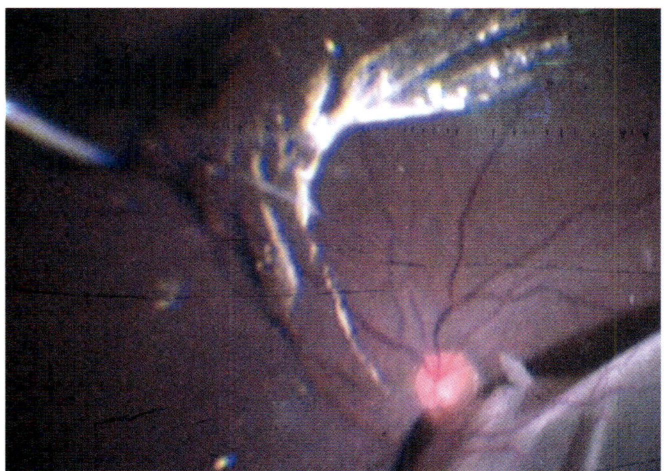

Fig. 46.7: Triamcinolone acetonide assissted PVD induction. (PVD: Posterior vitreous detachment).

can be controlled independent of the cut rate with three customized modes:[5] "core mode" (the port remains open most of the time), 50/50 mode (the port is open 50% of the time), and "shave mode" (the port remains closed for the most of the time). Besides cut rate and aspiration, one can use these vitrectomy modes to control the flow rate.

The instruments are held steady in the vitreous cavity so that the vitreous is allowed to come to the vitreous cutter. Excessive movement of the instruments should be avoided as it will lead to traction and peripheral retinal tears. When the vitreous appears to stop migrating towards the cutter, the cutter is advanced posteriorly to engage any remaining vitreous. Scleral depression by the assistant with cotton tip applicator or metallic scleral depressor permits trimming of the vitreous towards the peripheral vitreous base (Fig. 46.6). Vitreous shaving is done at the area of vitreous base without causing any retinal traction.

The goal of vitrectomy surgery for retinal detachment is not only core vitrectomy, but to remove cortical vitreous adherent to retinal breaks, directly drain the subretinal fluid, tamponade the breaks (with air, gas, or silicone oil), and create chorioretinal adhesions around each retinal break with endolaser photocoagulation or cryopexy also. Subretinal fluid drainage is usually done using active suction using vitrector or passive aspiration using a flute needle or backflush attached to Zivojnovic style backflush handle (Fig. 46.7).

Removal of Posterior Hyaloid

Posterior vitreous face has strong attachment at the vitreous base, optic nerve head, along the vessels, and areas of abnormal chorioretinal adhesions. Any undue traction on the hyaloid will be transmitted to the vitreous base and can result in retinal tears at the posterior margin of vitreous base. Posterior hyaloids is typically engaged in the peripapillary region where the potential for damage to the retina is less.[6] It can be done with either the vitreous cutter or soft tip silicone cannula attached to active suction. Intravitreal triamcinolone can be used for better visualization of cortical vitreous and aids in complete hyaloid removal. Once engaged hyaloid is lifted toward the center of vitreous cavity, it gets detached from the optic nerve head in the form of Weiss ring (Fig. 46.8).

Membrane Removal

The intraoperative use of dyes [indocyanine green (ICG), brilliant blue G (BBG), and trypan blue] or visualization techniques (triamcinolone acetonide crystals) helps in easy identification and removal of internal limiting membrane (ILM) and epiretinal membranes (ERMs). ICG and BBG dyes selectively stain the ILM (Figs. 46.9A and B), while trypan blue stains the epiretinal membranes as well.

Various types of vitreoretinal forceps are available for intraocular manipulation. End grasping forceps have jaws at the tip to hold tissues at the edge only and are used for ERM peeling. ILM forceps are a type of end grasping forcep but with fine tips with smaller jaws, which help in picking up of delicate tissues like ILM (Figs. 46.10A and B). On the other hand, serrated forceps have large flat grasping blades without jaws, which help in strong grip over tissues while managing proliferative vitreoretinopathy (PVR). These are used in tough ERM peeling and retinal pucker release.

Tano's diamond dusted membrane scraper (DDMS Tano, Synergetics TM, USA) helps to find the edge of the ERMs. It is a highly flexible silicone tube whose tip is coated with inert diamond dust (Fig. 46.11). Perfectly suited for both ILM and ERM removal, the diamond dusted, soft silicone tip finds and grasps the edge of the membrane quickly and easily presents it for forceps-assisted removal.

Horizontal scissors are used for delamination during ERM removal. Their cutting edge moves conformal to the retinal surface. Their blades can have a gentle curve or can be straight, with angle of 30° or 45° to the shaft. *Vertical scissors* have vertical blades with pointed tips that move along the axis of shaft. Proximal blade moves down toward the fixed distal blade to cut the tissue vertically. These are used for ERM segmentation.

If PVR is present as in rhegmatogenous retinal detachment (RRD), it may be necessary to peel all the ERMs and remove subretinal membranes or bands to complete the retinal reattachment. In cases of extensive PVR, a relaxing retinotomy or retinectomy may be required.

Internal Drainage of Subretinal Fluid

Subretinal fluid in RRD cases is removed through the original breaks or retinotomy made with diathermy using a flute or back flush needle in the presence of air irrigation. *Charles flute needle* consists of a blunt needle attached to a detachable handle (Fig. 46.12). It is used for controlled passive extrusion of fluid during internal drainage of subretinal fluid. Internal channel leads to an exit port on the side of handle. Egress of

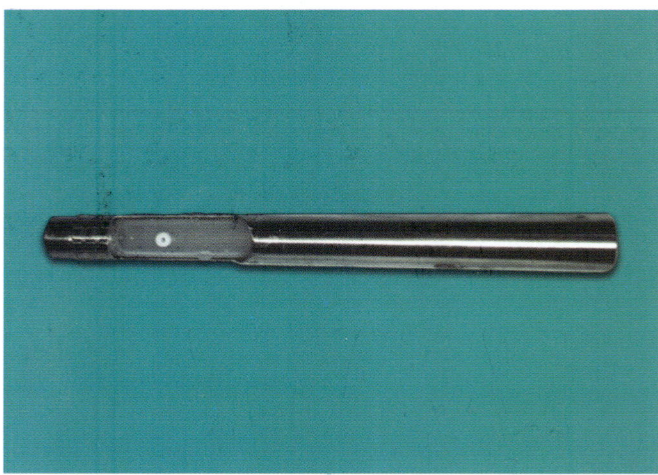

Fig. 46.8: Zivojnovic style backflush handle.

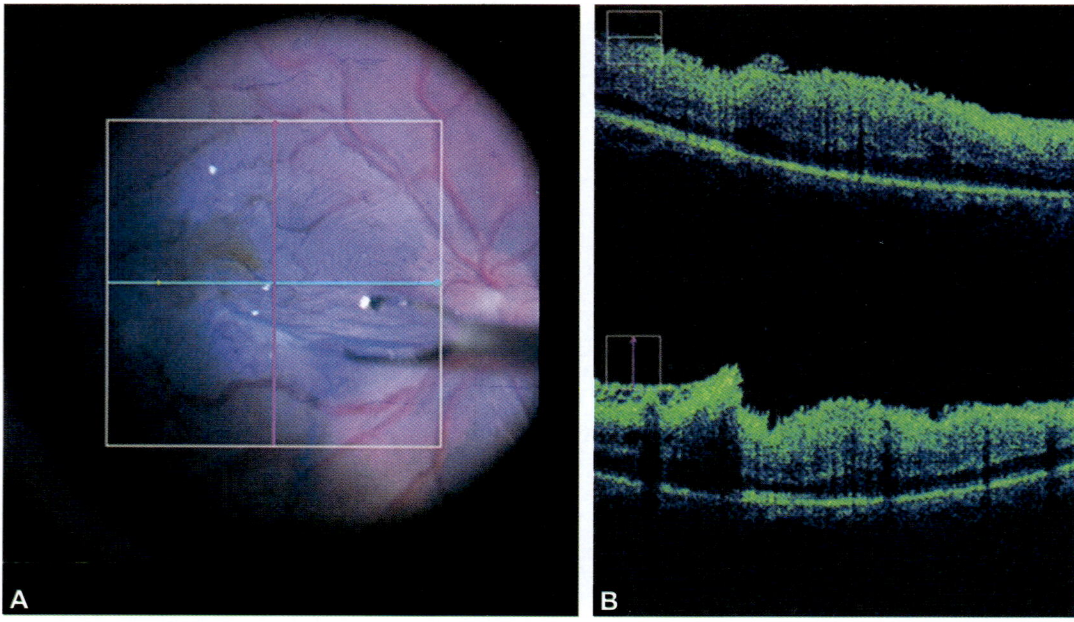

Figs. 46.9A and B: ILM stained with brilliant blue G dye. iOCT-guided ILM peeling.
(ILM: Internal limiting membrane; iOCT: Intraoperative optical coherence tomography)

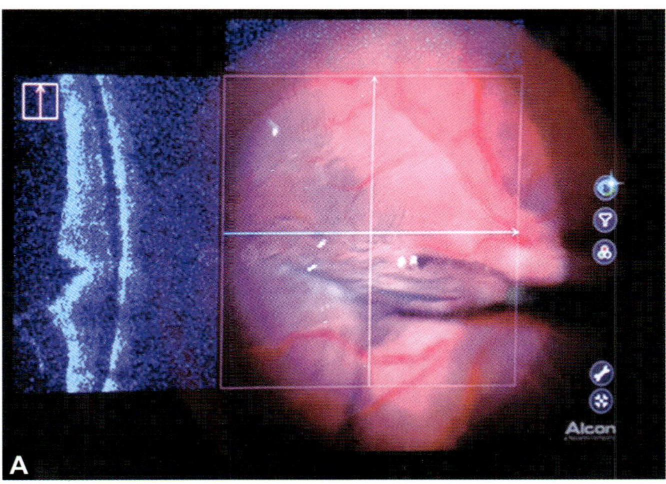 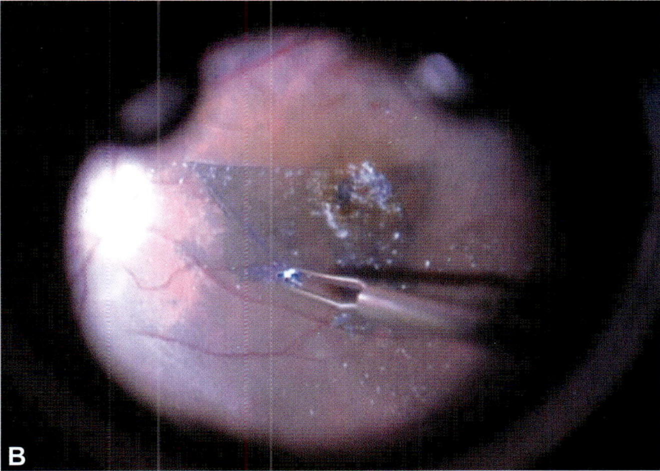

Figs. 46.10A and B: (A) Three-dimensional visualization-guided peeling of ILM Blue dye-stained ILM; (B) ILM peeling using ILM forceps. (ILM: Internal limiting membrane).

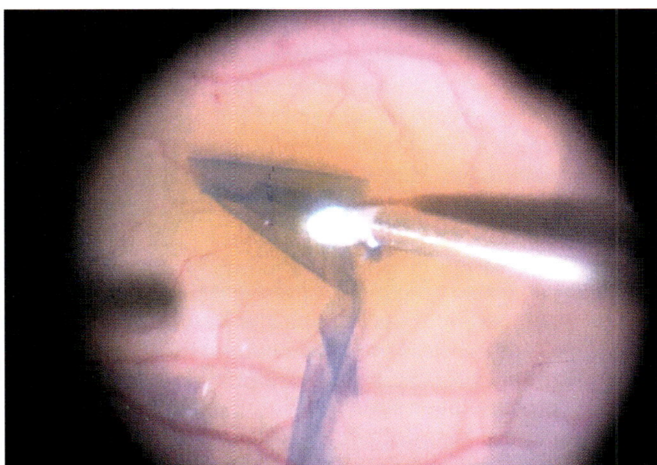

Fig. 46.11: Tano's diamond dusted membrane scraper.

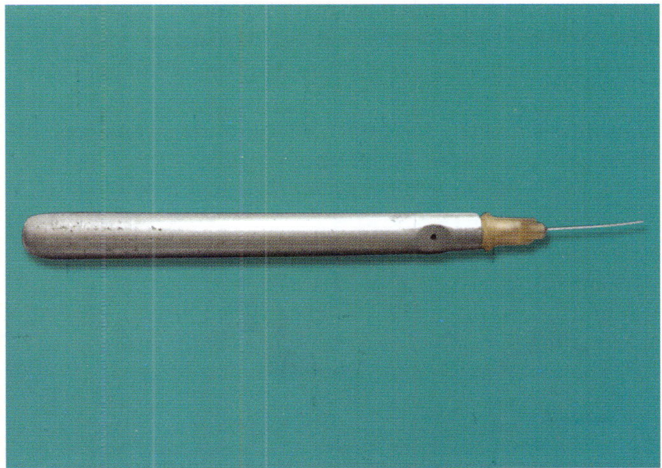

Fig. 46.12: Charles flute needle—blunt needle attached to a detachable handle.

fluid occurs when cannula tip is in fluid and exit port is open, driven by infusion pressure which is above the atmospheric pressure. The blunt tip can be replaced with a soft silicone tip needle as well with decreased risk of iatrogenic retinal damage. *Back flush* is a modified flute handle with large silicone reservoir (Fig. 46.13). Pressure on this reservoir leads to retrograde flushing of the fluid or accidently aspirated or incarcerated tissues. It can be used with either blunt or soft tip needle.

Peripheral Retinal Inspection

360° careful retinal periphery inspection should be done to rule out any advertent retinal breaks or retained cortical vitreous. Scleral depression by the assistant helps in easy peripheral retinal visualization.

Interface Vitrectomy

It is a technique described for vitrectomy at the interface between vitreoretinal tissue and substances immiscible in aqueous media like air, gas, or silicone oil.[7,8] It is performed after near complete vitrectomy and fluid-air exchange to enhance the visualization of the vitreous base. The cutter is placed within the vitreous base with the port directed away from the retina and vitrectomy performed using shave mode (Fig. 46.14).

The filtered air injected in vitreous cavity provides tamponade, dampens retinal motion, keeps the edges of retinal break together due to surface tension, air–vitreous interface provides visualization of any residual vitreous and provides a wider field

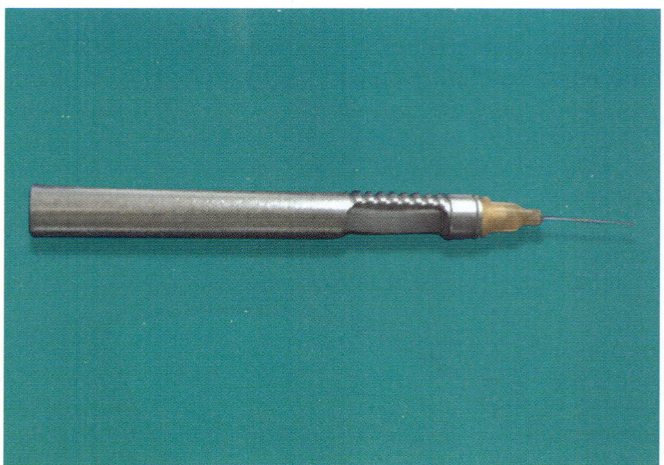

Fig. 46.13: Back flush—modified flute handle with large silicone reservoir.

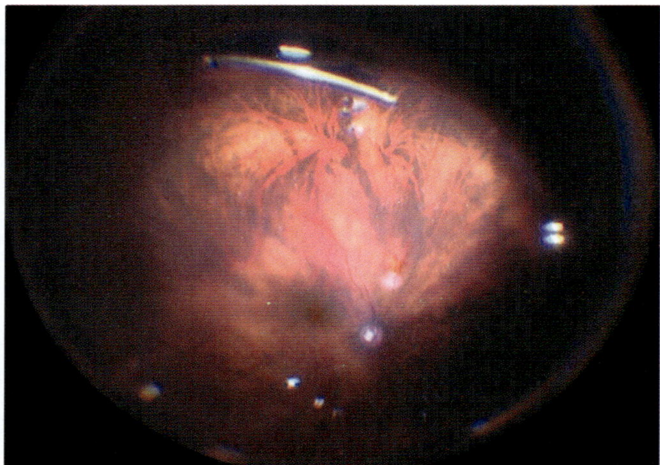

Fig. 46.14: Shave vitrectomy at retinal periphery using vitrectomy cutter.

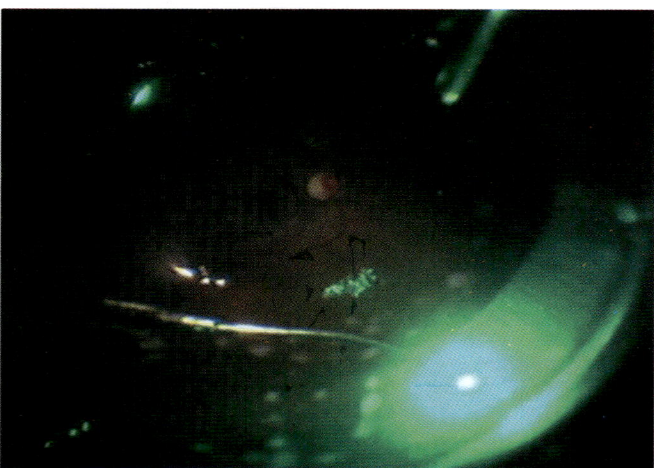

Fig. 46.15: Laser photocoagulation using double frequency Nd:YAG endolaser.
(Nd:YAG: Neodymium-doped Yttrium Aluminium Garnet).

of view.[7] It also confines any intraoperative bleeding to the interface region only. Silicone oil has also been used for interface vitrectomy as it causes dampening of retinal motion and better visualization of the residual vitreous.[7]

Retinopexy

The breaks and retinotomy site are marked by endodiathermy. Endophotocoagulation can be performed under air or a perfluorocarbon liquid (PFCL) bubble, once retina is flat (Fig. 46.15). Two–three rows of laser burns are applied around each break and peripheral retinal degenerations.

Endotamponade

Various vitreous substitutes are available to replace the vitreous after vitrectomy like air, sulfur hexafluoride (SF_6), perfluoropropane (C_3F_8) (Figs. 46.16A to D), silicone oil, and balanced salt solution. These provide retinal tamponade and replace the vitreous with optically clear media. Complex vitreoretinal cases like extensive PVR or giant retinal tears may require long-term tamponade in the form of C_3F_8 or silicone oil.

Closure

Sclerotomy ports are closed with the overlying conjunctiva with absorbable 7-0 Polyglactin suture (e.g. Vicryl™, Ethicon Inc. manufacturer).[9] Initially, superonasal and superotemporal port entries are closed and the infusion line is removed at last. Subconjunctival injection of antibiotic steroid combination is given at the end.

Transconjunctival Sutureless Vitrectomy or Minimally Invasive Vitrectomy Surgery

The advantages of transconjunctival sutureless vitrectomy over conventional 20G surgery include less corneal astigmatism, shorter surgical time, and less inflammation induced by surgery, eventually leading to more patient comfort and postoperative recovery.

Due to excessive flexibility of the instruments, the original minimally invasive vitrectomy surgery (MIVS) procedure (25G), introduced in year 2002, had certain drawbacks. There was difficulty in dissecting the peripheral vitreous, shaving the vitreous base, and in rotating the eye. Potential disadvantages included an increased risk of postoperative hypotony, endophthalmitis, increased iatrogenic retinal tears and epithelial down growth.

Some of these problems were solved by the introduction of 23G instruments. These instruments had greater rigidity, better illumination and fluidics making manipulation of the peripheral retina easier. The newer 25G+ system has more

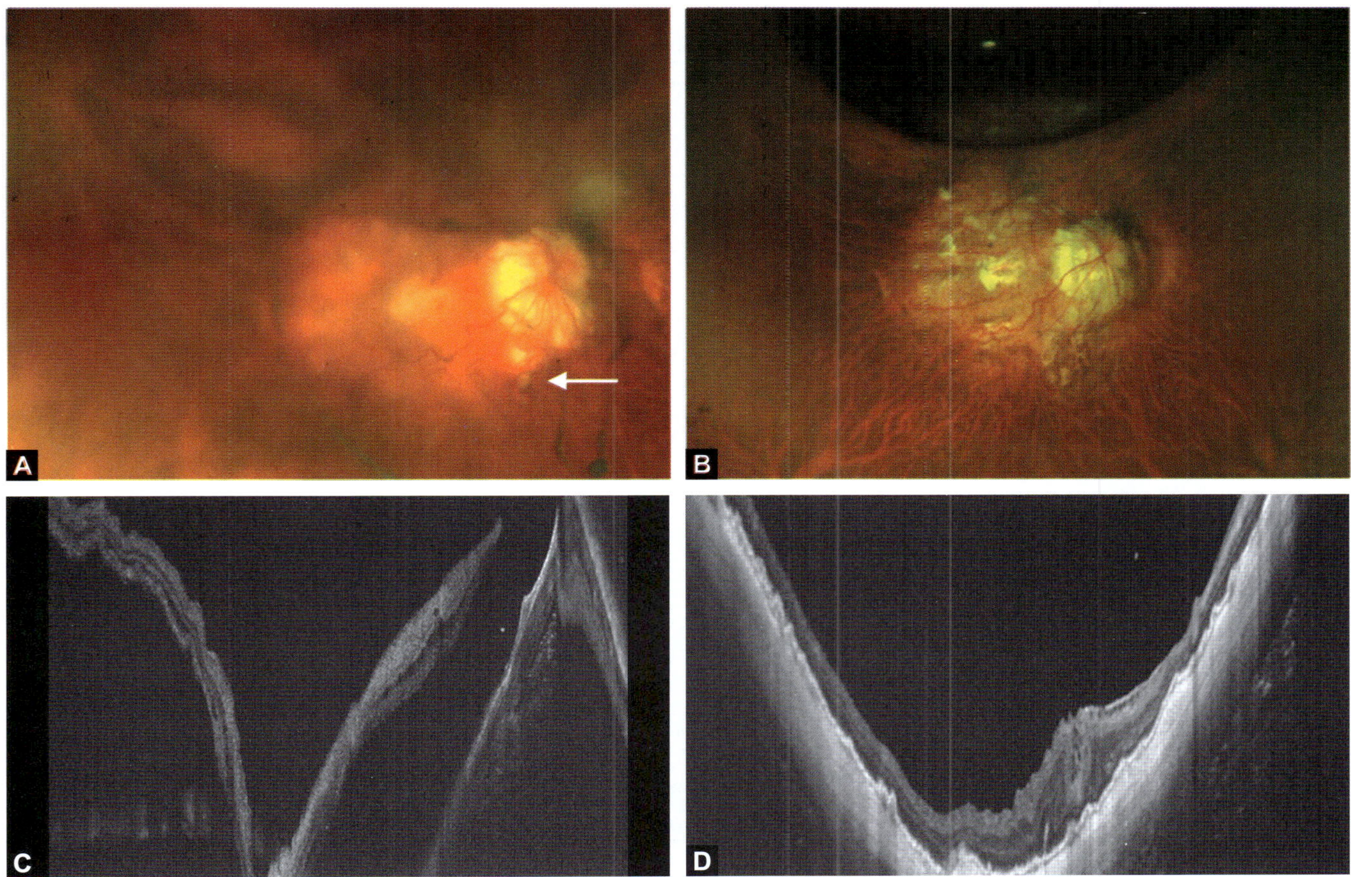

Figs. 46.16A to D: Fundus and OCT imaging shows (A and C) inferior 6 o'clock peripapillary retinal break (white arrow) in a high myopic RD and (B and D) settled retina postvitrectomy, laser and C_3F_8 gas injection.
(RD: Retinal detachment; C_3F_8: Perfluoropropane; OCT: Optical coherence tomography)

rigid instruments with an increase in inner diameter improving the infusion flow rates as well as illumination.

Complications of Pars Plana Vitrectomy

The most common complication of vitrectomy surgery is development of cataract, most commonly nuclear sclerosis.[10,11] More than 90% of eyes in patients over age 50 will develop visually significant nuclear sclerotic cataract within 2 years of vitrectomy surgery.[11] Vitrectomy also increases the long-term risk of open-angle glaucoma by 10–20%.[12] Other complications of pars plana vitrectomy include iatrogenic retinal tears which may lead to retinal detachment, lens touch with instruments leading to intraoperative cataract, subretinal perfluorocarbon, retinal and/or vitreous incarcerations, recurrent vitreous hemorrhage and endophthalmitis.[10] Endophthalmitis after vitrectomy is rare, but it is more common in patients with diabetes and in eyes with retained intraocular foreign bodies.

REFERENCES

1. Fujii GY, De Juan E, Humayun MS, et al. Initial experience using the transconjunctival sutureless vitrectomy system for vitreoretinal surgery. Ophthalmology. 2002;109(10):1814-20.
2. Fujii GY, De Juan E, Humayun MS, et al. A new 25-gauge instrument system for transconjunctival sutureless vitrectomy surgery. Ophthalmology. 2002;109(10):1807-12.
3. Oshima Y, Wakabayashi T, Sato T, et al. A 27-gauge instrument system for transconjunctival sutureless microincision vitrectomy surgery. Ophthalmology. 2010;117(1):93-102.e2.
4. Ibarra MS, Hermel M, Prenner JL, et al. Longer-term outcomes of transconjunctival sutureless 25-gauge vitrectomy. Am J Ophthalmology. 2005;139(5):831-6.
5. de Oliveira PRC, Berger AR, Chow DR. Vitreoretinal instruments: vitrectomy cutters, endoillumination and wide-angle viewing systems. Int J Retina Vitreous. 2016;2:28.
6. Kelly NE, Wendel RT. Vitreous surgery for idiopathic macular holes. Results of a pilot study. Arch Ophthalmology. 1991;109(5):654-9.

7. Sigler EJ, Charles S, Calzada JI. Interface vitrectomy. Retina. 2014;34(3):616-7.

8. Charles S. Vitrectomy techniques for complex retinal detachments. Taiwan J Ophthalmology. 2012;2(3):81-4.

9. Oyagi T, Emi K. Vitrectomy without scleral buckling for proliferative vitreoretinopathy. Retina. 2004;24(2):215-8.

10. Banker AS, Freeman WR, Kim JW, et al. Vision-threatening complications of surgery for full-thickness macular holes. Vitrectomy for Macular Hole Study Group. Ophthalmology. 1997;104(9):1442-52.

11. Cherfan GM, Michels RG, de Bustros S, et al. Nuclear sclerotic cataract after vitrectomy for idiopathic epiretinal membranes causing macular pucker. Am J Ophthalmology. 1991;111(4):434-8.

12. Chang S. LXII Edward Jackson lecture: open angle glaucoma after vitrectomy. Am J Ophthalmology. 2006;141(6):1033-43.

Chapter 47

Giant Retinal Tears

Atul Kumar, Devesh Kumawat, Raghav Ravani, Hemant K Joshi

DEFINITION

A giant retinal tear (GRT) is a full-thickness retinal break, which extends circumferentially for more than or equal to 3 clock hours (≥90°) in the presence of a posteriorly detached vitreous.[1,2]

Why Giant Retinal Tears Need Special Consideration?

Giant retinal tears need special mention because of some special characteristics—(1) they rapidly lead to extensive retinal detachment, (2) posterior flap has a tendency to roll over, fold or invert, (3) they have increased risk of proliferative vitreoretinopathy, (4) they require meticulous surgery to prevent complications, (5) they have several ocular and systemic associations, (6) fellow eye involvement occurs frequently, and (7) redetachments occur frequently in these cases.

CLASSIFICATION

Scott classified GRTs into three types based on their location with emphasis on pathophysiology and required management: equatorial, equatorial with posterior extensions, and oral.[3] Equatorial GRTs are most common and have posterior extensions give posterior flaps extra mobility and tendency to invert or fold. Oral type is least common.

Schepens classified GRTs on the basis of etiology into idiopathic, traumatic, lattice-related, and iatrogenic types. Iatrogenic GRTs are known to occur after heavy diathermy or photocoagulation,[4] pars plana vitrectomy (PPV),[5] and refractive surgeries.[6,7]

Based on the configuration, GRTs may be classified as—(1) GRT without detachment; (2) GRT with detachment with (a) flat posterior flap, (b) rolled posterior flap (Figs. 47.1A and B), and (c) inverted posterior flap; and (3) GRT with detachment with associated posterior extensions (radial rips) at or within the tear margin.[8]

GIANT RETINAL TEARS VERSUS DIALYSIS

Distinction of GRT from giant retinal dialysis (GRD) is important. In GRD, retina disinserts from the ora serrata and vitreous remains attached to the posterior margin of the break,

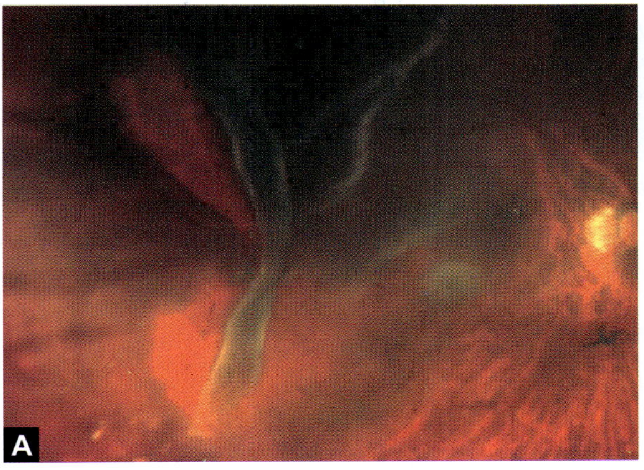

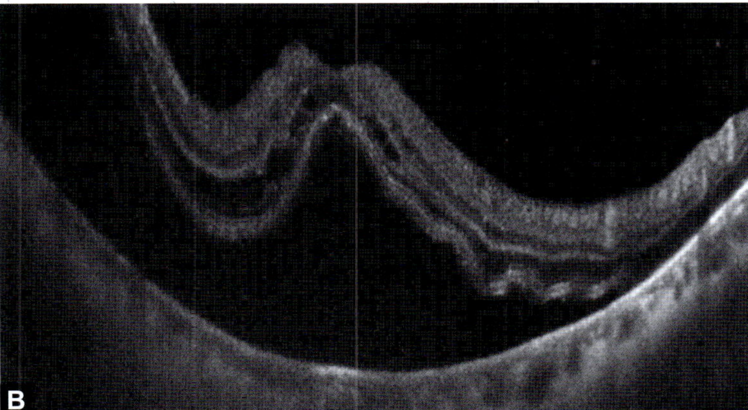

Figs. 47.1A and B: (A) shows optos ultra-widefield pseudocolor image of a patient with GRT and rolled posterior flap; (B) Swept source OCT image of the same patient shows neurosensory detachment at macula. (GRT: Giant retinal tear; OCT: Optical coherence tomography).

thereby a posterior vitreous detachment (PVD) is usually absent. This prevents inversion of the the posterior margin in GRD from inverting. GRDs usually have a good prognosis as they are amenable to scleral buckling or even peripheral cryotherapy.

On the other side, GRTs have strong vitreous adhesion to the anterior margin of break with posterior margin being free from vitreous attachment. Due to gravity and intrinsic retinal elasticity, posterior flap inverts over itself. GRTs pose numerous surgical challenges and outcomes are not as good as GRD.

EPIDEMIOLOGY

The annual incidence of GRT has been estimated to be between 0.094 and 0.114 per 100,000 individuals as per British Giant Retinal Tear Epidemiology Eye Study (BGEES).[9] The Scottish retinal detachment study reported an annual GRT incidence of 0.15 per 100,000 individuals.[10]

Males constitute majority of the patients (65–91%).[1,9,11] In BGEES, the mean age was 42 years.[9] Most GRTs are idiopathic. Common predisposing conditions include trauma, hereditary vitreoretinopathies and high myopia.[4,12] Bilateral nontraumatic cases have been reported to present in up to 13% of cases.[1,11,13] Freeman reported a rate of 6.6% GRT in the fellow eye at presentation and an additional 6.2% developing GRT over follow-up (average follow-up 3.7 years; maximum follow-up 16 years).[1]

PATHOGENESIS AND NATURAL HISTORY OF IDIOPATHIC GIANT RETINAL TEAR

Giant retinal tear occurs due to dynamic vitreous traction at areas of retinal abnormality which usually is an area of white without pressure (WWOP).[1] These areas have dense vitreous condensation and these increase in extent and density over time. The posterior border of WWOP is well defined with thick inelastic vitreous attachment. In addition, in such eyes, central vitreous liquefies early leaving a shrunken gel anteriorly and thin layer of vitreous cortex posteriorly.[14] This gel contains dense bands attached anteriorly. PVD usually stops at this border leading to focal vitreoretinal adhesion and traction. This subsequently causes a neurosensory retinal tear. The anteriorly directed vitreous traction then "rips" the abnormal retina circumferentially.[1,14] Thus, the pathogenesis of GRT is similar to that of a smaller tear with difference only in the area of retinal abnormality.

Giant retinal tears are characterized by intense ocular inflammation due to blood retinal barrier breakdown. Hypotony develops quickly due to increased uveoscleral outflow. Large bare retinal pigment epithelium (RPE) surface predispose to greater release of RPE cells which undergo transdifferentiation into myofibroblasts.[15] Initially, the posterior flap is freely mobile but as proliferative vitreoretinopathy (PVR) sets in, it becomes stiff and begins to roll. If left untreated, the size of GRTs increases with subsequent extension of the RD.

RISK FACTORS

The risk factors for GRTs along with their pathogenesis are mentioned in Table 47.1.

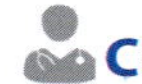 CLINICAL FEATURES

Giant retinal tears have associated rhegmatogenous retinal detachments (RRD) in about 44–92% cases.[9,11,13,15] Presenting visual acuity depends on the status of macula and configuration of GRT flap in relation to macula. Macula-off

Table 47.1: Etiopathogenesis in giant retinal tears.

S. No.	Risk factor	Pathogenesis
1.	Trauma (closed globe)	Shearing force at vitreous base and PVD induction
2.	Trauma (open globe)	Vitreous incarceration and traction
3.	Cataract surgery	PVD induction, aggressive maneuvering, and vitreous traction
4.	Vitrectomy	Vitreous base traction (conventional 20G instruments)
5.	Refractive surgery	High myopia population, shearing force at vitreous base with suction, and shock waves from excimer laser
6.	Myopia	Early PVD, excessive lattice degeneration, and WWOP
7.	Hereditary vitreoretinopathies (Wagner, Stickler, and Marfan syndrome)	Congenital vitreoretinal abnormalities and early PVD
8.	*Rare causes:* Buphthalmos, microspherophakia, retinoschisis, acute retinal necrosis, and endophthalmitis.	

(PVD: Posterior vitreous detachment; WWOP: White without pressure).

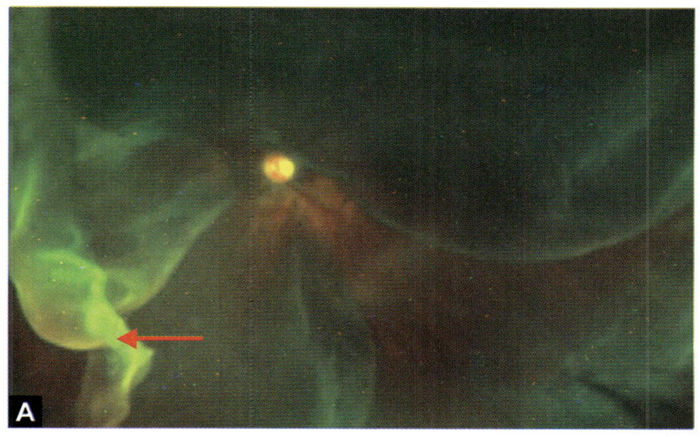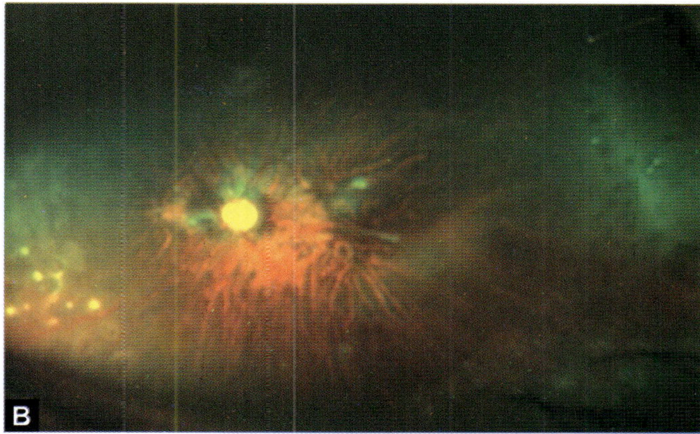

Figs. 47.2A and B: Ultra- widefield pseudocolor image -(A) preoperative giant retinal tear with retinal detachment with rolled edges (red arrow) and (B) postoperative pseudocolor image showing attached retina.

RDs usually have a visual acuity between counting fingers (CF) and light perception (LP).[11,13,16] GRT flap covering the macula also leads to poor presenting visual acuity.[11,13,16]

Tobacco dusting in vitreous cavity is present in all cases.[13] Vitreous hemorrhage may also result if tear involves the retinal vessels. Most GRTs have less than 180° circumferential extent.[9,17,18] Location of GRT varies with inferotemporal and superonasal quadrants being commonly involved in traumatic cases (Figs. 47.2A and B).[19,20]

The posterior flap may invert over the optic disc or the macula, thereby the full extent of the associated RD may not be ascertained. Posterior tears or radial rips may exacerbate the inversion of flap. PVR occurs quickly and frequently because of large area of RPE being exposed and increased liberation of RPE cells into vitreous.[21]

Fundus of the fellow eye should be examined thoroughly to look for any predisposing lesion including WWOP areas which are significant in fellow eye of GRT cases.

INVESTIGATIONS

B-scan ultrasonography of the posterior segment helps in determining the location and extent in cases with media obscuring vitreous hemorrhage. Also it can help to differentiate between GRT and GRD. A classical "double linear echo" sign is seen in GRT with two high-amplitude linear echoes, one extending from the optic disc and other usually lying almost parallel to it (inverted posterior flap).[22] In addition, PVD and inverted posterior flap can be seen, which helps in differentiating it from GRD.[22]

Axial length of the other eye should be measured to determine if high myopia is the cause. Systemic examination should be done for relevant associated syndromes.

MANAGEMENT

Surgery

Prior to the advent of PPV, numerous strategies were adopted for management of GRT associated RRD like binocular occlusion,[4] retinal incarceration,[4] retinal tacks,[23] transscleral suturing,[24] and scleral buckling.[25] However, with introduction of PPV, flap manipulation and complete vitrectomy became possible under direct wide-field visualization.

The surgical principles involved in the management include complete vitrectomy, unfolding of the retinal flap, sealing the tear with chorioretinal adhesion, and providing long term intraocular tamponade.

Vitrectomy

Pars plana vitrectomy has a higher success rate than previously attempted surgeries and is the treatment of choice for GRT.[11,26,27] Despite advances in the surgical techniques and endotamponade agents, GRTs pose challenges due to their complex anatomy, risk of retinal slippage, formation of a new tear, and extension of the existing tear due to PVR. Recurrent detachments have been reported to occur in up to as high as 45% of the cases.[18,28]

Conventional 20G vitrectomy with perfluorocarbon liquid (PFCL) use has been reported to have up to 94% final attachment rates in GRT associated RD.[27] Smaller-gauge vitrectomy has evolved over time and exhibit several advantages compared to conventional 20G surgery including lesser retinal mobility, lesser vitreous traction, easy manipulation of tissues and PVR management, over and above improved wound anatomy and reduced postoperative pain and inflammation.[29,30] 25G PPV can achieve excellent attachment rates in eyes with GRT associated retinal detachment.[31]

The entire circumference of the vitreous base is thoroughly vitrectomized, as the anterior edge of the giant tear has condensed vitreous gel which needs to be removed. Meticulous peripheral vitrectomy reduces occurence of new breaks and incidence of anterior PVR. To dissect the vitreous base, optimal visualization is essential which is possible only with a fully dilated pupil, good scleral indentation by the assistant, or using wide-angle viewing systems. Proliferative tissue and epiretinal membrane should be removed with the help of vitreous base shaving using a vitrectomy cutter.

Lensectomy or Lens Aspiration

Crystalline lens is removed when cataract, lens subluxation or anterior PVR is present. Clear lens extraction in these cases remains controversial, with claims of ease of visualizing the anterior edge of tear and improved access to vitreous base. Ability to see the peripheral retina is greatly enhanced by wide-angle viewing systems in phakic as well as pseudophakic eyes, making lensectomy unnecessary for this particular indication.

ROLE OF PERFLUOROCARBON LIQUID

The introduction of PFCL supplanted all previous techniques for unrolling and repositioning inverted GRT.[8] PCFLs having a high specific gravity with relatively low viscosity allow for precise, controlled, and accurate repositioning of the retina with minimal manipulation (Figs. 47.3A and B).

The retina is mobilized by membrane peeling. Subsequently liquid perfluorooctane is injected over the disc after unfolding the inverted retinal flap to visualize the disc. Care should be taken to prevent the injection of multiple bubbles by ensuring that the tip of injection needle is always within the PFCL bubble and the size of the bubble is gradually increased as subretinal and vitreous cavity fluid is aspirated out of the vitreous cavity.

Endophotocoagulation or Cryotherapy

With the retina fully attached under PFCL, eight to ten rows of endophotocoagulation of 200–500 micron spot size are applied to the posterior edge and anterior retinal flap and at least five rows are placed in the fundus periphery not involved in giant tear.

Cryotherapy can also be used to treat the GRT edges up to the ora, especially if it is very anterior.

Gas-fluid Exchange

The PFCLs can then be directly exchanged with gas or silicone oil. If the surgeon is sure of total vitreous base removal, and drying of free retinal edges, air-PFCL exchange followed by gas or silicon oil exchange may also be done. A flute needle with a soft silicone tip is positioned at the edge of the giant break as air enters the vitreous cavity. The anterior retina is flattened as the bubble descends toward the perfluorocarbon meniscus. Fluid should be aspirated at the edge of the break, at the air or perfluorocarbon interface, to prevent posterior slippage of retina. Slippage may occur when persistent subretinal fluid is trapped posteriorly by descending air bubble causing the retina to slide. It is important to maintain adequate intraocular pressure during PFCL-air exchange to prevent posterior slippage of retina.

Perfluorocarbon Liquid-oil Exchange

Alternatively, a direct silicone oil - PFCL exchange can be done to decrease the chances of slippage of retina (Figs. 47.4A and B). Both PFCL and silicone oil being hydrophobic extrudes fluid at the PFCL-oil interface.[32] Presence of fluid at the PFCL-oil interface at the area of tear allows entry of fluid into subretinal space and cause retinal slippage.[32] With panoramic viewing, aspiration of PFCL should be started at the edge of the giant tear using a silicone tipped blunt needle.

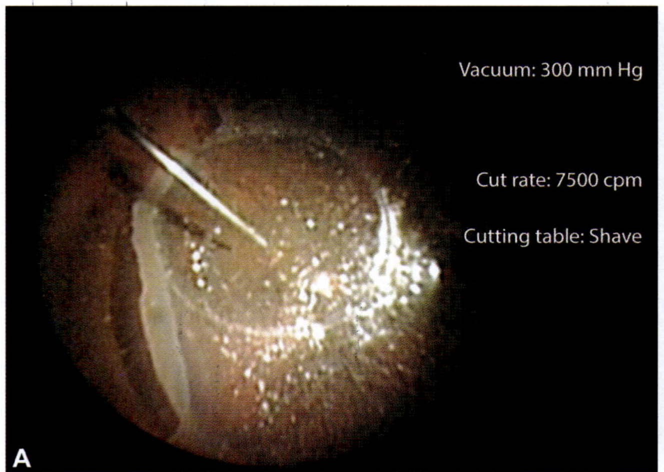

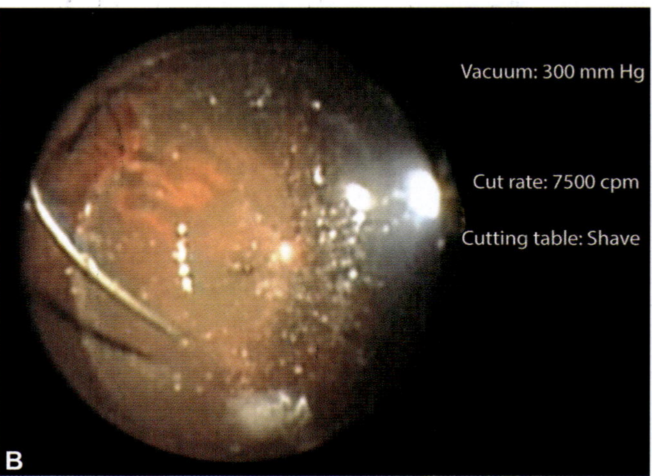

Figs. 47.3A and B: Intraoperative use of PFCL to unfold the flap in giant retinal tear with retinal detachment. (PFCL: Perfluorocarbon liquid).

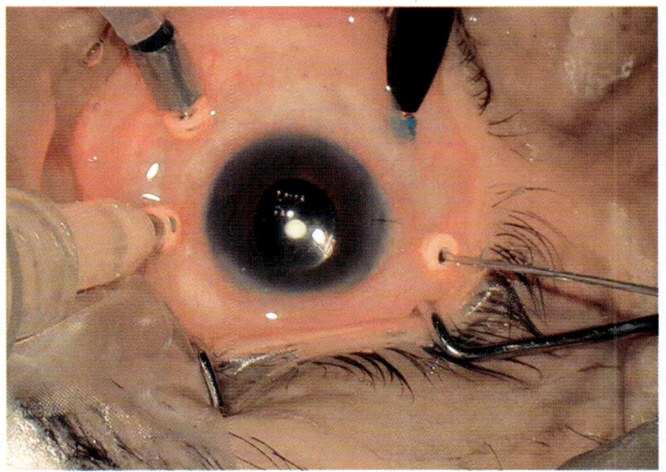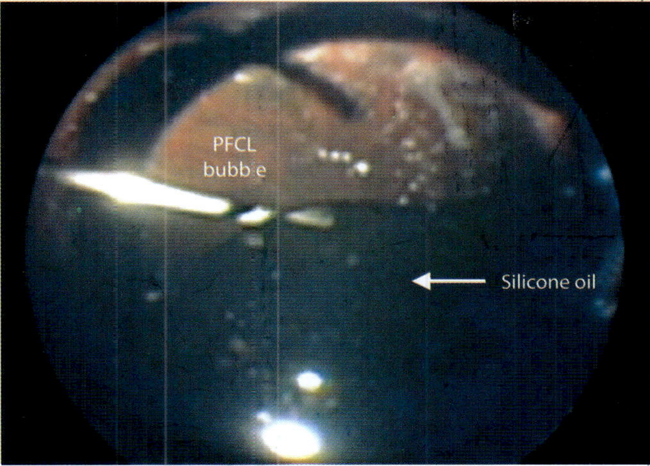

Fig. 47.4: Bimanual technique of chandelier assisted PFCL-oil exchange in a case of giant retinal tear with detachment. (PFCL: Perfluorocarbon liquid).

As the silicon oil-PFCL interface descends and covers the edge of the tear, the liquid overcomes any residual intrinsic elastic forces that may result in posterior slippage. The aspirating tip is then placed just below the anterior surface of the PFCL as the oil continues to fill the vitreous cavity.

ROLE OF ENCIRCLING ELEMENT

The use of encircling scleral band in GRT is controversial. Some studies have reported higher redetachment rates with encirclage due to redundant retinal folds, fish-mouthing and increased posterior retinal slippage.[29,33] While others report a lack of encircling element to be associated with a higher rate of redetachment.[34,35]

COMPLICATIONS

Posterior slippage of a giant tear after successful reapproximation indicates residual fluid at the margin of the tear and requires a repeat PFCL exchange with careful anterior drainage. Incidence of intraoperative slippage has been noted to vary from 10.7% to 49%.[14,28] Postoperative slippage may also occur. This can be managed by careful post-operative head positioning and by additional posterior retinopexy with laser.

Retention of PFCL bubble can lead to retinal toxicity occurring within 1–3 days of retention, hence its total removal is prudent, to prevent its toxic damage to the retina. Removal of PFCL from vitreous cavity is simplified by allowing the eye to remain air-filled for approximately 5 minutes after removal of visible droplets. The high vapor pressure of this substance allows for evaporation from retinal surface and any PFCL entrapped elsewhere in the periphery gravitates to the posterior pole from where it can be easily aspirated.

The most important postoperative complication in giant tear surgery is recurrent detachment principally due to development of proliferative vitreoretinopathy, reported to occur in 49.4% and 31.5% of patients in two separate studies.[14,28] Visually significant postoperative epimacular membranes developed in 7.4% and 15% of patients in these series and reoperation was often required, despite successful repair of a giant tear.

OUTCOMES

Single surgery anatomical success rate of 88% and 92% have been reported in GRT with 23G PPV by Pitcher et al.[36] and Kunikata et al.[37] respectively (mean follow-up of 17 and 12 months, respectively). Randolph et al.[38] reported anatomical success rate of 91.3% with 25G PPV with medium term PFCL endotamponade in GRT (mean follow-up 33 months). Randolph et al. reported a final mean corrected distance visual acuity (CDVA) of 1.08 ± 0.81 logMAR units with visual improvement only in 48% eyes.[38]

PROPHYLAXIS

Fellow eyes of nontraumatic GRT cases often show vitreoretinal pathology on presentation with risks as high as of GRT occuring in these fellow eyes.[9] However, there exists no evidence to support or refute use of 360 prophylactic treatment in the fellow eyes.[12]

Freeman noted several high-risk characteristics in fellow eyes of GRTs—high myopia (≥10 diopters), increasing WWOP areas, and increasing condensation of the vitreous base.[1] The objective in management of such high-risk fellow eyes is to relieve the vitreous traction. A prophylactic scleral buckle in phakic eye with an attached retina may be required in high risk individuals.[1] 360° retinopexy, either in the form of cryopexy or laser photocoagulation may also be considered.[13,39]

REFERENCES

1. Freeman HM. Fellow eyes of giant retinal breaks. Trans Am Ophthalmology Soc. 1978;76:343-82.
2. Kanski JJ. Giant Retinal Tears. Am J Ophthalmology. 1975;79(5):846-52.
3. Scott JD. Giant tear of the retina. Trans Ophthalmology Soc UK. 1975;95(1):142-4.
4. Schepens C, Dobble J, Mc M. Retinal detachments with giant breaks: preliminary report. Trans Am Acad Ophthalmology Otolaryngol. 1962;66:471-9.
5. Shinoda H, Nakajima T, Shinoda K, et al. Jamming of 25-gauge instruments in the cannula during vitrectomy for vitreous haemorrhage. Acta Ophthalmology. 2008 1;86(2):160-4.
6. Navarro R, Gris O, Broc L, et al. Bilateral giant retinal tear following posterior chamber phakic intraocular lens implantation. J Refract Surg. 2005;21(3):298-300.
7. Ozdamar A, Aras C, Sener B, et al. Bilateral retinal detachment associated with giant retinal tear after laser-assisted in situ keratomileusis. Retina. 1998;18(2):176-7.
8. Albert DM, Miller JW, Azar DT. Giant retinal tears. In: Albert DM, Miller JW, Azar DT (Eds). Albert & Jakobiec's Principles and Practice of Ophthalmology. Philadelphia: Saunders Elsevier; 2008. p. 2351.
9. Ang GS, Townend J, Lois N. Epidemiology of giant retinal tears in the United Kingdom: the British Giant Retinal Tear Epidemiology Eye Study (BGEES). Invest Ophthalmology Vis Sci. 2010;51(9):4781-7.
10. Mitry D, Singh J, Yorston D, et al. The predisposing pathology and clinical characteristics in the Scottish retinal detachment study. Ophthalmology. 2011;118(7):1429-34.
11. Ambresin A, Wolfensberger TJ, Bovey EH. Management of giant retinal tears with vitrectomy, internal tamponade, and peripheral 360 degrees retinal photocoagulation. Retina. 2003;23(5):622-8.
12. Ang GS, Townend J, Lois N. Interventions for prevention of giant retinal tear in the fellow eye. Cochrane Database Syst Rev. 2012; 2:CD006909.
13. Ghosh YK, Banerjee S, Savant V, et al. Surgical treatment and outcome of patients with giant retinal tears. Eye (Lond). 2004;18(10):996-1000.
14. Schepens CL, Freeman HM. Current management of giant retinal breaks. Trans Am Acad Ophthalmology Otolaryngol. 1967;71(3): 474-87.
15. Leaver PK, Cooling RJ, Feretis EB, et al. Vitrectomy and fluid/silicone-oil exchange for giant retinal tears: results at six months. Br J Ophthalmology. 1984;68(6):432-8.
16. Kreissig I, Lincoff H, Stanowsky A. The treatment of giant tear detachments using retrohyaloidal perfluorocarbon gases without drainage or vitrectomy. Graefes Arch Clin Exp Ophthalmology. 1987;225(2):94-8.
17. Verstraeten T, Williams GA, Chang S, et al. Lens-sparing vitrectomy with perfluorocarbon liquid for the primary treatment of giant retinal tears. Ophthalmology. 1995;102(1):17-20.
18. Scott IU, Murray TG, Flynn HW, et al. Outcomes and complications associated with giant retinal tear management using perfluoro-n-octane. Ophthalmology. 2002;109(10):1828-33.
19. Cox MS. Retinal breaks caused by blunt nonperforating trauma at the point of impact. Trans Am Ophthalmology Soc. 1980;78:414-66.
20. Aylward GW, Cooling RJ, Leaver PK. Trauma-induced retinal detachment associated with giant retinal tears. Retina. 1993; 13(2):136-41.
21. Machemer R. Proliferative vitreoretinopathy (PVR): a personal account of its pathogenesis and treatment. Proctor lecture. Invest Ophthalmology Vis Sci. 1988;29(12):1771-83.
22. Jalkh AE, Jabbour N, Avila MP, et al. Ultrasonographic findings in eyes with giant retinal tears and opaque media. Retina.. 1983;3(3):154-8.
23. Ando F, Kondo J. A plastic tack for the treatment of retinal detachment with giant tear. Am J Ophthalmology. 1983;95(2): 260-1.
24. Federman JL, Shakin JL, Lanning RC. The microsurgical management of giant retinal tears with trans-scleral retinal sutures. Ophthalmology. 1982;89(7):832-9.
25. Machemer R, Aaberg TM, Norton EW. Giant retinal tears. II. Experimental production and management with intravitreal air. Trans Am Ophthalmology Soc. 1969;67:394-414.
26. Batman C, Cekiç O. Vitrectomy with silicone oil or long-acting gas in eyes with giant retinal tears: long-term follow-up of a randomized clinical trial. Retina. 1999;19(3):188-92.
27. Chang S, Lincoff H, Zimmerman NJ, et al. Giant retinal tears. Surgical techniques and results using perfluorocarbon liquids. Arch Ophthalmology Chic Ill 1960. 1989;107(5):761-6.
28. Kertes PJ, Wafapoor H, Peyman GA, et al. The management of giant retinal tears using perfluoroperhydrophenanthrene. A multicenter case series. Vitreon Collaborative Study Group. Ophthalmology. 1997;104(7):1159-65.
29. Oshima Y, Wakabayashi T, Sato T, et al. A 27-gauge instrument system for transconjunctival sutureless microincision vitrectomy surgery. Ophthalmology. 2010;117(1):93-102.e2.
30. Rizzo S, Barca F, Caporossi T, et al. Twenty-seven-gauge vitrectomy for various vitreoretinal diseases. Retina . 2015;35(6):1273-8.
31. Kumar V, Kumawat D, Bhari A, et al. Twenty-five-gauge pars plana vitrectomy in complex retinal detachments associated with giant retinal tear. Retina. 2017.
32. Wong D, Williams RL, German MJ. Exchange of perfluorodecalin for gas or oil: a model for avoiding slippage. Graefes Arch Clin Exp Ophthalmology. 1998;236(3):234-7.
33. Khan MA, Shahlaee A, Toussaint B, et al. Outcomes of 27 Gauge Microincision Vitrectomy Surgery for Posterior Segment Disease. Am J Ophthalmology. 2016;161:36-43.e1-2.
34. Lee SY, Ong SG, Wong DWK, et al. Giant retinal tear management: an Asian experience. Eye (Lond). 2009;23(3):601-5.
35. Tsang CW, Cheung BTO, Lam RF, et al. Primary 23-gauge transconjunctival sutureless vitrectomy for rhegmatogenous retinal detachment. Retina. 2008;28(8):1075-81.
36. Pitcher JD, Khan MA, Storey PP, et al. Contemporary Management of rhegmatogenous retinal detachment due to giant retinal tears: a consecutive case series. Ophthalmic Surg Lasers Imaging Retina. 2015;46(5):566-70.
37. Kunikata H, Abe T, Nishida K. Successful outcomes of 25- and 23-gauge vitrectomies for giant retinal tear detachments. Ophthalmic Surg Lasers Imaging. 2011;42(6):487-92.
38. Randolph JC, Diaz RI, Sigler EJ, et al. 25-gauge pars plana vitrectomy with medium-term postoperative perfluoro-n-octane for the repair of giant retinal tears. Graefes Arch Clin Exp Ophthalmology. 2016;254(2):253-7.
39. Meyer-Schwickerath G. Prevention and giant tears. Bibl Ophthalmology. 1967;72:345-6.

Chapter 48

Surgery for Proliferative Diabetic Retinopathy

Pramod S Bhende, Atul Kumar, Vineet Mutha

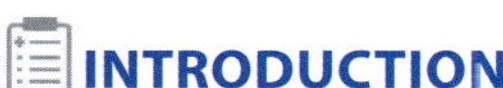 INTRODUCTION

Diabetic retinopathy is primarily a disease of retinal microvasculature, and is characterized by progressive retinal ischemia resulting in development of new blood vessels in the late phase [proliferative diabetic retinopathy (PDR)].[1,2] If left unattended, this stage progresses to develop contractile epiretinal fibrocellular membranes, often resulting in vitreoschisis and/or partial detachment of posterior cortical vitreous and progressive retinal detachment secondary to the areas of fibrovascular proliferation (FVP).

This progressive traction on the friable neovascular tissues can lead to pre-retinal or vitreous hemorrhage (VH). Further fibrosis of vitreous membranes and worsening of traction leads to tractional retinal detachment (TRD) of variable extent.[3,4] In case macula is involved in the TRD, there is a marked deterioration of vision. The continued vitreoretinal traction may also cause retinal breaks in areas of previous tractional detachments resulting in combined tractional and rhegmatogenous retinal detachment (CRD) with rapidly progressive severe vision loss.[5] Clinically, patient may present with advanced stage of disease not amenable for medical management. Few patients, despite medical management, may progress to an advanced disease where surgical intervention is required.

Robert Machemer performed his first vitrectomy in a patient with nonresolving VH secondary to PDR in 1970.[6] Since then, surgical interventions for PDR have continued to evolve.[7] With accumulated experience, recent advances in technology and improved instrumentation, improved instrumentation, emergence of antivascular endothelial growth factors (anti-VEGFs) and better understanding of the pathoanatomy, the spectrum of indications for surgical management in PDR have expanded many folds. Newer vitrectomy machines with better fluidics and intraocular pressure (IOP) control, smaller gauge instruments (23G, 25G, and 27G),[8-10] high-speed vitreous cutters with cut rate up to 7,500 cuts per minute, with port optimization, multifunctional instruments, and wide angle visualization systems with better and brighter illumination sources, have made vitreoretinal surgeries safer and quicker. Intraoperatively, there is now a reduced need for multiple instrument exchanges and safer reach to more peripheral retina. With availability of anti-VEGFs agents, eyes with more severe and florid FVP can be taken up for surgery, with reduced risk of intra and postoperative complications and acceptable functional outcomes.

PATHOANATOMY

The understanding of biochemical mechanisms and pathoanatomy of PDR is very crucial.[11-15] Careful assessment and understanding of vitreoretinal relationship is of paramount importance in these eyes for planning of surgery. Anomalous vitreous adhesions can have several possible configurations. Posterior vitreous detachment (PVD) can be absent, minimal, incomplete, and rarely complete.

Vitreoschisis is defined as lamellar separation or splitting of the posterior cortical vitreous. It is a spontaneous event during evolution of PDR. It can be easily misinterpreted as complete PVD on echography in eyes with media opacity. Evidence of persistent traction on the retina, in presence of PVD, is a clue to suspect vitreoschisis. This is due to adherence of outer cortical vitreous to the retina (*second layer*). The thin outer layer of vitreoschisis lines the surrounding retina to certain distance before joining with inner layer of vitreoschisis (Figs. 48.1A and B). Recognition of vitreoschisis and removal of this "second layer" is important for the complete relief of vitreoretinal traction and success of surgery in diabetic eyes.[16-18]

Progressive vitreoretinal traction may cause retinal breaks in areas of previous attachments resulting in CRD (Fig. 48.2).

TYPES OF VITREORETINAL ADHESIONS

The vitreoretinal attachments can be focal or broad. Focal attachment indicates point foci of attachment usually along arcades and can be single (Fig. 48.3A) or multiple (Fig. 48.3B) and is associated with *tent like or hammock like* localized TRD. A broad vitreoretinal adhesion can be a flat large FVP on the posterior pole or may involve peripheral retina

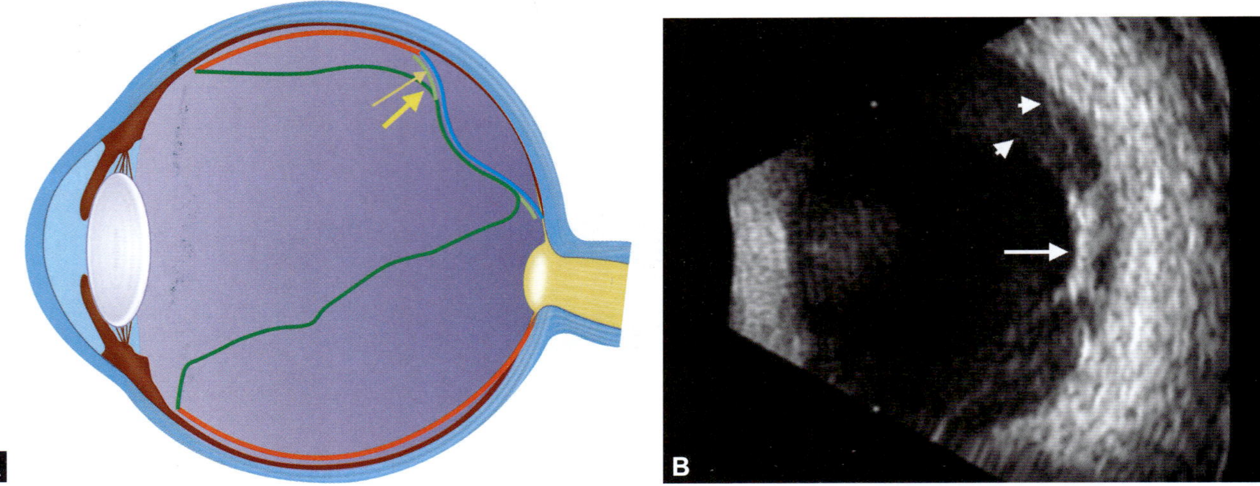

Figs. 48.1A and B: (A) Pictorial representation of vitreoschisis with table top tractional retinal detachment, showing the layers of inner cortical vitreous (thick yellow arrow) and outer cortical vitreous (thin yellow arrow) adherent to retina and causing tractional detachment. (B) B-scan ultrasonography of such a case with arrowheads pointing to vitreoschisis cavity layers and arrow pointing to table top tractional RD.

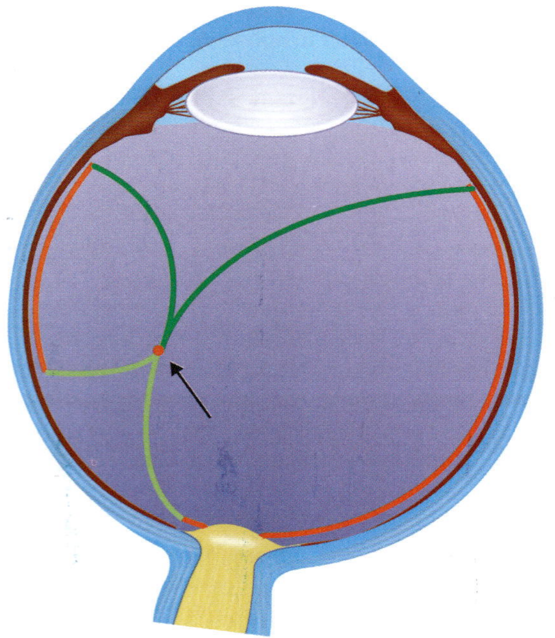

Fig. 48.2: Schematic diagram showing combined tractional and rhegmatogenous retinal detachment due to retinal break (red dot) formation at the base of focal vitreoretinal traction (black arrow) in a eye with proliferative diabetic retinopathy.

(Fig. 48.3C). Depending on status of PVD, underlying retina can be either attached or detached giving typical *"table-top"* configuration to TRD. Persistent and prolonged vitreous traction can also lead to *tractional retinoschisis*. Generally schitic retina is thin and atrophic and resists flattening even after tractional elements have been relieved. Visual gain in these eyes is very guarded even after successful surgery.

INDICATIONS FOR SURGICAL INTERVENTION IN PROLIFERATIVE DIABETIC RETINOPATHY

Based on the surgical goal, the indications for the vitrectomy can be grossly divided into three groups:

1. *To clear the media opacity*:
   - Nonresolving intraocular hemorrhage (vitreous, sub-hyaloid, and premacular)
   - Dense asteroid hyalosis, preventing laser photocoagulation (PHC) for PDR
2. *For tractional effects*:
   - TRD involving or threatening macula
   - CRD
   - Dense premacular fibrosis
   - Macular edema associated with taut posterior hyaloid
   - Progressive FVP even with adequate laser PHC
3. *Other or additional indications (often after vitrectomy)*:
   - Recurrent VH with/without anterior hyaloidal fibrovascular proliferation (AHFVP)
   - Ghost cell/hemolytic glaucoma
   - Submacular hard exudates
   - Recurrent retinal detachment (TRD or CRD)
   - Fibrinoid syndrome (FS)
   - Epiretinal membrane (ERM).

Nonclearing Vitreous Hemorrhage

Vitreous hemorrhage (Fig. 48.4) is no longer the commonest indication for vitrectomy in diabetic eyes. Widespread use of scatter retinal laser photocoagulation (PRP) has reduced the incidence of severe nonclearing VH. The aim of surgery in these eyes is to clear the optical media. Generally, there will be an associated incomplete PVD with underlying FVP of variable severity. Preoperative ultrasonography helps to assess the status of underlying retina and V-R relationship. Laser to

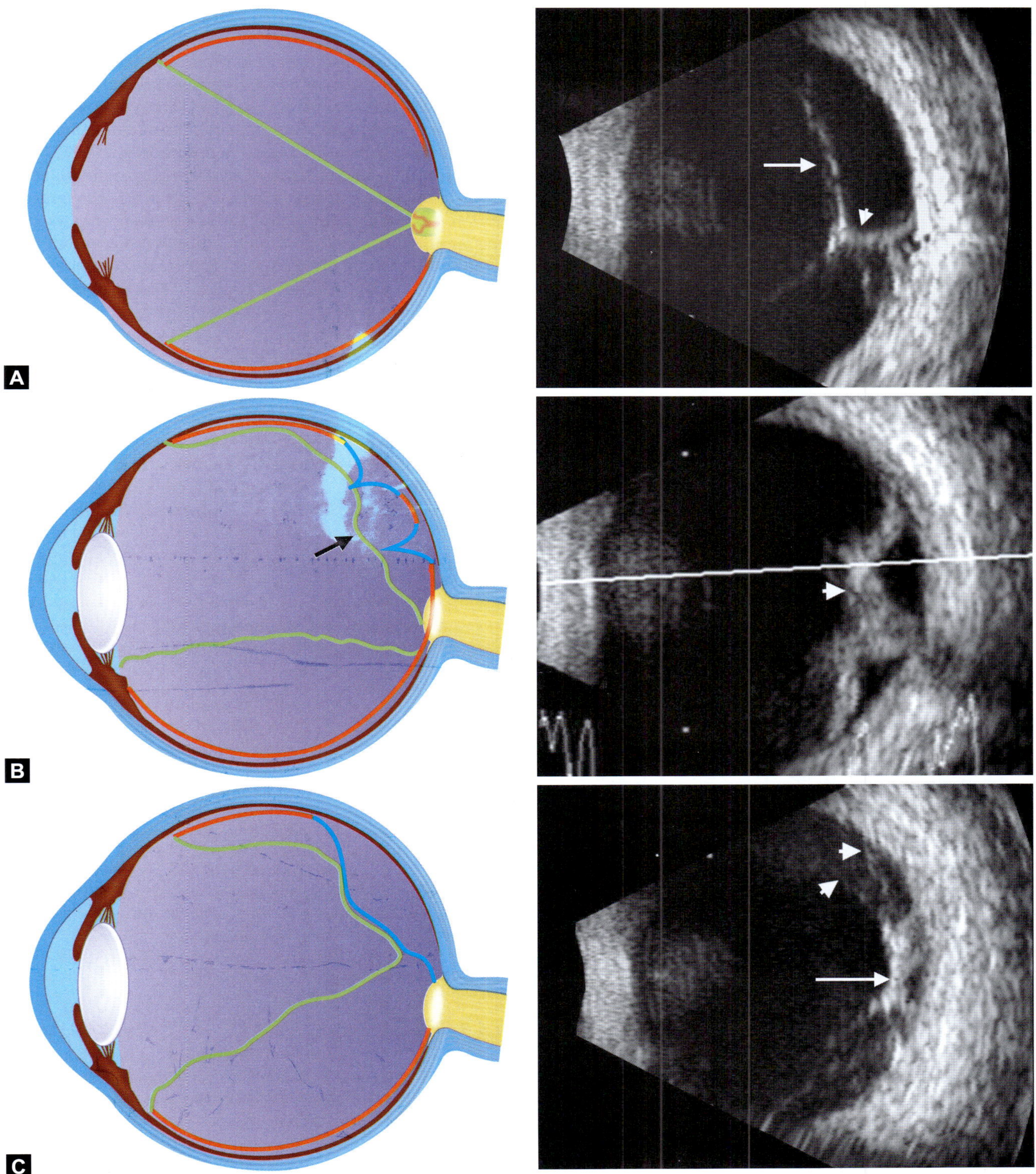

Figs. 48.3A to C: Schematic diagrams of various types of vitreoretinal adhesions in PDR along with corresponding ultrasonographic findings (A) Focal (arrowhead in the image on right) or single point attachment causing tent like TRD seen along with posterior cortical vitreous (arrow) (B) Multiple point attachments causing hammock like TRD (black arrow in image on left and white arrowhead in image on right) (C) Broad vitreo-retinal attachment (white arrow) causing table top TRD along with layers of vitreoschisis (arrowheads).

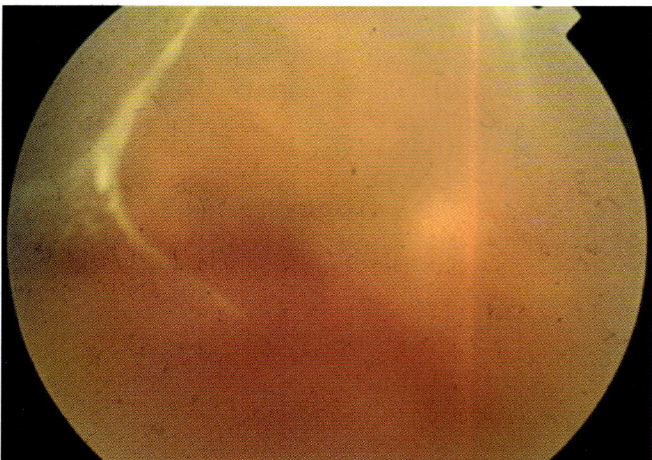

Fig. 48.4: Nonclearing vitreous hemorrhage in proliferative diabetic retinopathy.

the ischemic retina towards the end of surgery, minimizes the incidence of recurrent VH. Early surgery is indicated in eyes with recurrent hemorrhage,[19,20] bilateral involvement, one eyed patients, eyes with no prior PRP, and in eyes with underlying RD. The Diabetic Retinopathy Vitrectomy Study (DRVS) demonstrated the benefit of early vitrectomy in terms of better final visual acuity in eyes of subjects having type I diabetes.[21] Surgery for VH can be delayed in eyes with complete PVD and an attached retina, history of good prior PRP and in patient with unstable general condition. With the advent of improved surgical instrumentation, given the reduced systemic risk of surgery, improved visual, and anatomic outcomes with newer techniques, surgeons are now performing vitrectomies for VH at times well before 3 months duration, which was previously the well-accepted standard time-limit for observing cases of VH.[22,23]

Tractional Retinal Detachment

At present, TRD involving macula is the commonest indication and probably accounts for more than 40% of vitrectomies performed for diabetic retinopathy. Based on the area involved, TRD can be extramacular, extramacular but threatening the macula, and macular. TRDs tend to remain stable over prolonged periods of time and patients with extramacular TRD can safely be observed at regular intervals. Reported rate of progression of TRD to involve macula is 13% in 1 year, 21% in 2 years, and 23% by 3rd year.[3,20,24,25] Indication for vitrectomy in these eyes are: TRD involving macula, extramacular TRD with documented progression towards the macula (threatening the macula) (Figs. 48.5A to D), and TRD behind VH precluding the evaluation of the macula.

Combined Tractional and Rhegmatogenous Retinal Detachment

Combined tractional and rhegmatogenous retinal detachment is seen in around 7–35% of eyes undergoing vitrectomy for complications of diabetic retinopathy. Progressive fibrosis and contraction of active proliferation and vitreous membranes can lead to retinal break formation, converting TRD into CRD. Contraction of the retina due to heavy laser treatment in presence and adjacent to TRD can also lead to iatrogenic break formation corresponding to the laser burn. In eyes with CRD, typically there is incomplete PVD with single oval break adjacent to FVP or area of VR traction (Figs. 48.6A to D). Occasionally, there may be a flap tear (suggestive of anteroposterior traction) or slit or round break without flap or operculum (suggestive of tangential traction). In few eyes, configuration of detachment is suggestive of CRD, but thick preretinal FVP, retinal fold(s) or vitreous hemorrhage/opacity may preclude detection of a break preoperatively.

These patients may present with sudden onset, painless and rapidly progressive loss of vision. There may be a past history of laser PHC. These eyes need early surgery, regardless of the macular status.

Progressive Fibrovascular Proliferation

It is commonly seen in young type I diabetics. In these eyes, extensive FVP progresses despite adequate PRP. PVD is usually absent and there is higher incidence of recurrent VH.[26,27] Visual loss depends on the area involved but overall prognosis is not good. Intravitreal injection of anti-VEGF followed by early vitrectomy may be helpful in these eyes.[28]

Recurrent Vitreous Hemorrhage

About 10–30% of the eyes undergoing vitrectomy for PDR can have recurrent bleeding and 30–40% of these may need revision surgery to clear the hemorrhage. The rebleed could be early or persistent (up to 3 weeks postsurgery) or late onset (2–6 months postsurgery with a brief period of clear vitreous cavity).

Early hemorrhage could be due to oozing from surface bleeders or cut ends of new vessels and stumps of residual fibrovascular tissues or from sclerotomy site ooze. Leaching of red blood cells (RBCs) from uncut vitreous gel in the periphery, residual anterior vitreous and clot lysis also contributes to persistent hemorrhage. This blood usually clears spontaneously.

Sclerotomy site neovascularization (NV), AHFVP, and recurrent retinal NV are commonly responsible for late or recurrent hemorrhage. Ultrasound biomicroscopy (UBM) is helpful in identification of AHFVP and FVP at sclerotomies in these eyes.[29]

Possible treatment options could be anterior retinal cryopexy (ARC) with or without anti-VEGF injection,[28,30-32] outpatient fluid air exchange, vitreous lavage with cutting of proliferative membranes during surgery, and dissection of FVP at the sclerotomy sites and AHFVP followed by good retinal ablation.

Adequate removal of vitreous gel during primary surgery, with special attention to the vitreous base and anterior vitreous, including Wiegert's ligament, removal of all vitreoretinal traction and meticulous dissection of all fibrovascular

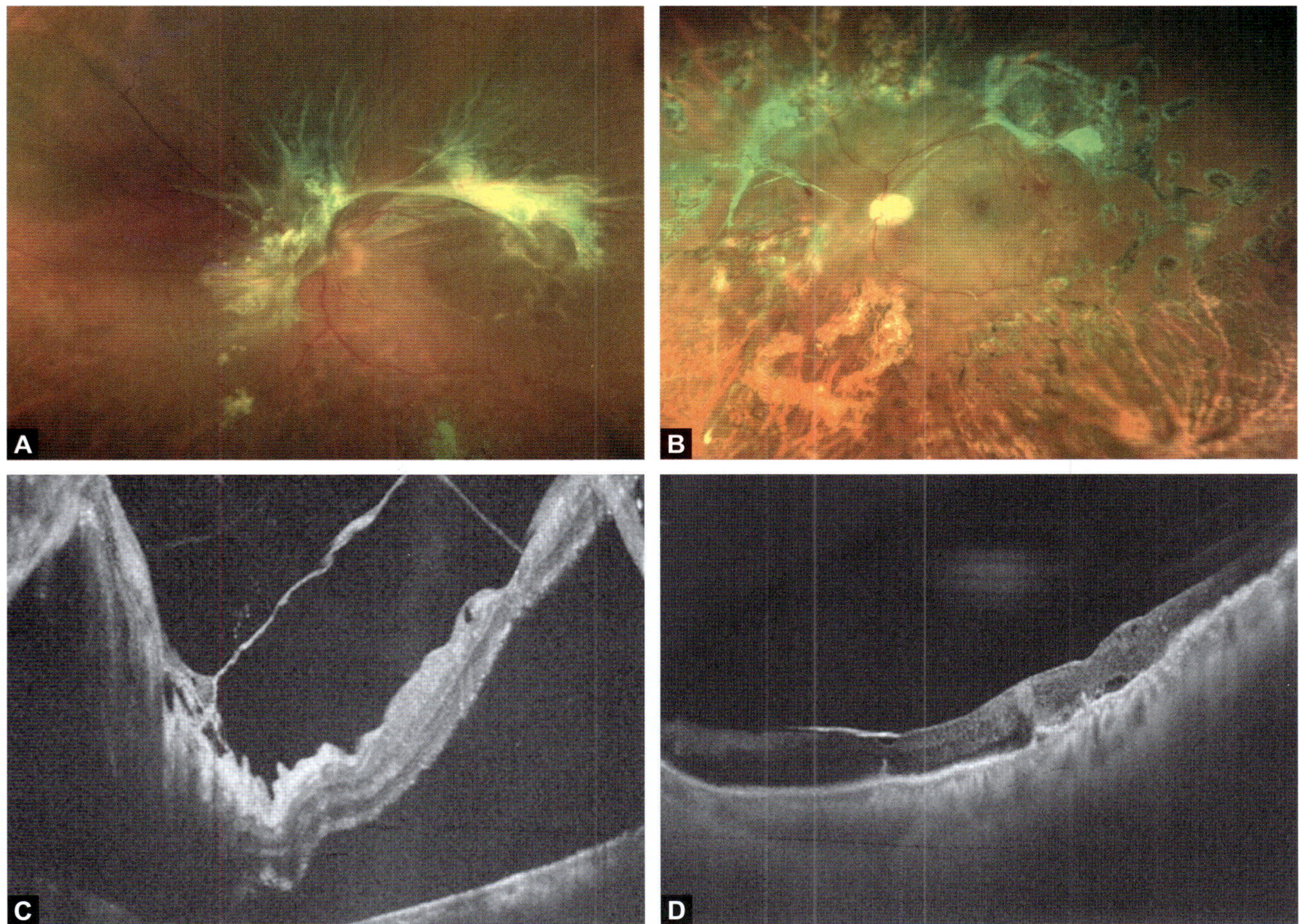

Figs. 48.5A to D: Macular tractional retinal detachment along the superotemporal arcade with striae extending to and threatening the macula. Postoperatively retina as settled on color picture and swept-source optical coherence tomography (SS-OCT).

tissues, good hemostasis during surgery, and adequate PRP to ischemic retina is helpful to minimize the risk of recurrent bleeding.

PREOPERATIVE EVALUATION

It should include both ocular and systemic parameters.

Systemic Status

Stable general condition and good metabolic control before surgery is very important. High and uncontrolled blood sugar increases the risk of postsurgery infection and also delays wound healing. Good control of systemic hypertension minimizes the risk of intra- and postoperative bleeding. In patients with chronic renal failure and on dialysis for the same, the surgery can be scheduled between two dialysis sessions. For patients on antiplatelet or anticoagulation therapy, internist should be consulted before stopping the treatment.

Ocular Status

Comprehensive eye examination should be performed before surgery. It is important to look for media clarity, pupillary dilatation, anterior segment NV and lens status. Knowledge of severity and extent of FVP, extent of TRD/CRD and PVD helps surgeon in planning the steps of surgery. Preoperative vision, status of the optic disc and macula is indicative of functional prognosis. Macular detachment is associated with an increased risk of unfavorable functional outcome and is an indication for early surgery.[33]

In eyes with media opacity, *ultrasonography* provides information regarding status of PVD and VR relationship, vitreoschisis, and presence/absence of retinal detachment including its extent and configuration. *UBM* is helpful in identifying presence of AHFVP and proliferation at sclerotomies in eyes with recurrent vitreous hemorrhage following vitrectomy (Fig. 48.7).[29]

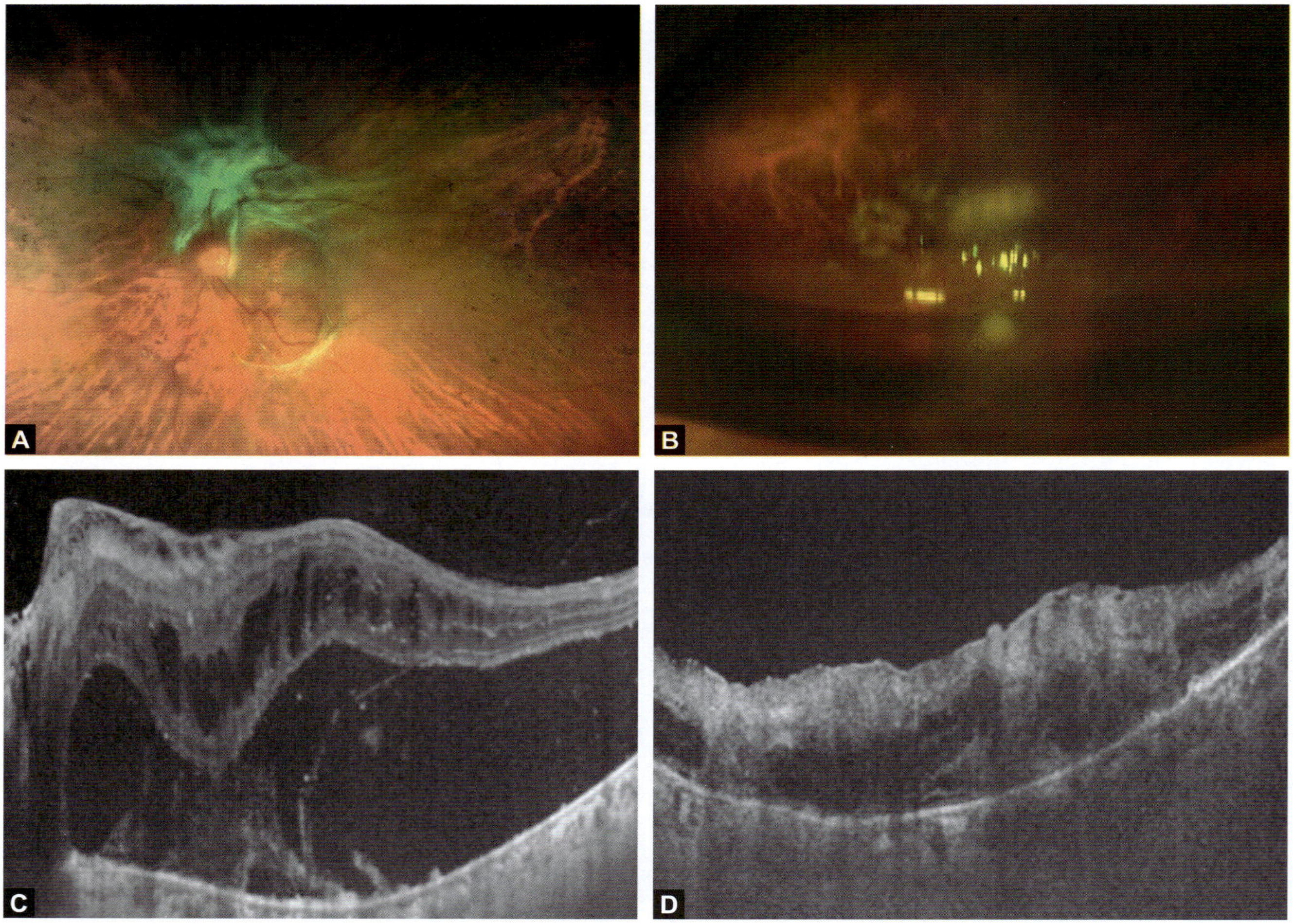

Figs. 48.6A to D: Combined tractional and rhegmatogenous retinal detachment. Retinal detachment is convex anteriorly on color picture (A) and optical coherence tomography (OCT) (B). Postoperatively (C and D) the gas filled eye shows a nearly settled retina on 1st postoperative day.

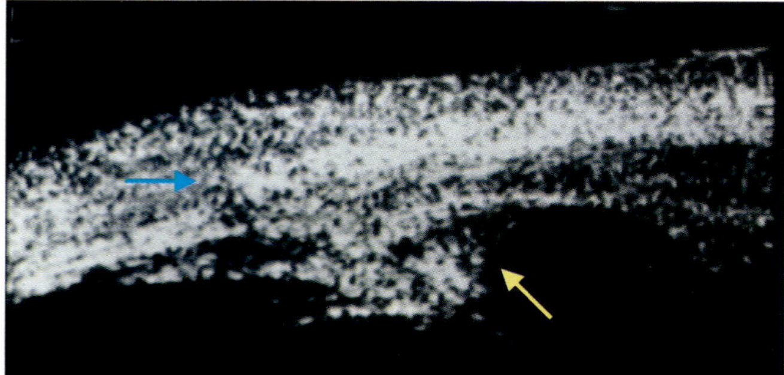

Fig. 48.7: Ultrasound biomicroscopy image of sclerotomy site (blue arrow) in a diabetic patient with recurrent hemorrhage after pars plana vitrectomy. Note the fibrovascular proliferation (yellow arrow) at the inner side of sclerotomy site.

SURGICAL TECHNIQUES

There is angiographic evidence that complete removal of the vitreous increases retinal circulation with better oxygen diffusion to the inner retina leading to reduced ischemic drive and reduced stimulus for NV.

Variable surgical anatomy, compromised visibility and higher risk of intra- and postoperative complications make diabetic vitrectomy as one of the most challenging condition. Over past few years, microincision vitrectomy surgery (MIVS) with wide angle visualization system has been a preferred technique for vitrectomy.[34,35] Generally, standard 3 port pars plana approach is preferred but an additional sclerotomy can be made for a chandelier light, in special situations, to perform bimanual surgery.

Goals of the Surgery

- To remove all the media opacities
- To relieve the vitreoretinal traction (both anterior-posterior and tangential)
- To stabilize the diabetic neovascular process by removing vitreous scaffold, by removing surface NV and applying laser to ischemic retina.

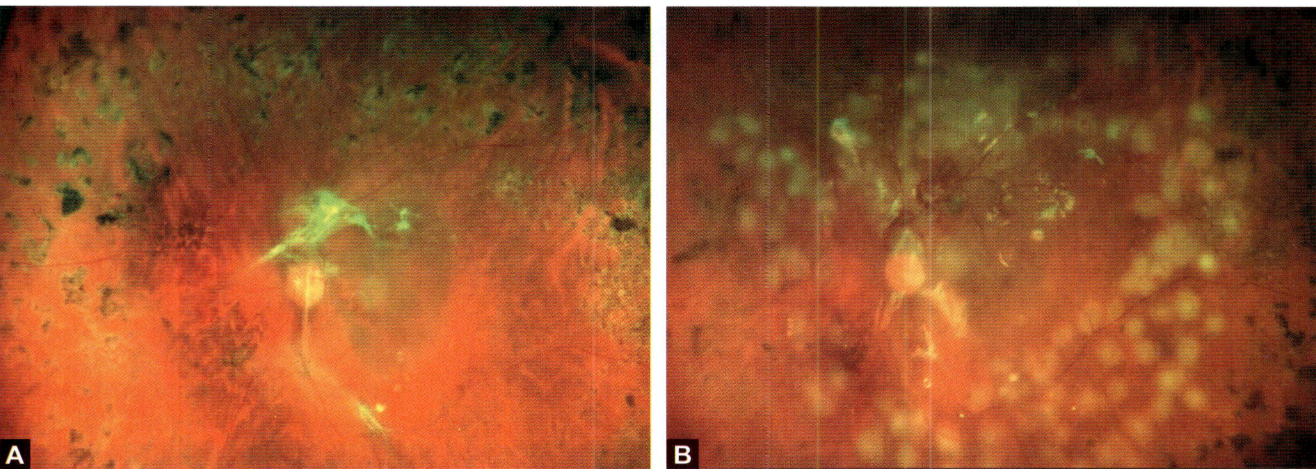

Figs. 48.8A and B: (A) Diabetic tractional retinal detachment (TRD) with macular detachment. (B) Status post vitrectomy retina is flat and well-attached with silicone oil in vitreous cavity.

Local anesthesia is preferred for most of the cases. Good pupillary dilation is essential for better visualization and better peripheral approach during surgery. If necessary, intracameral adrenaline or iris hooks can be used to dilate pupil adequately by pharmacological/mechanical means.

Key Surgical Steps

- Core vitrectomy/clear sclerotomy sites
- Opening of post hyaloid/truncation of cone
- Removal of subhyaloid hemorrhage
- Membrane dissection
- Control of bleeding
- Laser PHC/cryotherapy
- Intraocular tamponade if needed.

Typically vitreous removal is initiated at and around the sclerotomies followed by anterior, mid and posterior vitrectomy. Initial vitrectomy can be performed under direct visualization with microscope using coaxial illumination.

Special care is needed to avoid accidental lens trauma in phakic eyes. Cataract surgery, if needed, can also be combined with vitreous surgery. Phacoemulsification with intraocular lens (IOL) implantation is the preferred choice. Cataract removal can be done at the beginning or after vitrectomy depending on surgeons' and patient's comfort and discretion.

In eyes with incomplete PVD, preoperative ultrasonography may help in choosing safe meridian for posterior hyaloidotomy during vitrectomy. Trimming of vitreous membranes, bridging FVP and vitreous base helps in releasing anteroposterior traction along with clearing of media opacities (Figs. 48.8 and 48.9).

Membrane Removal

Preretinal membrane removal is the most important step for success of surgery in diabetic eye. It helps in the release of tangential and membrane induced surface traction. The

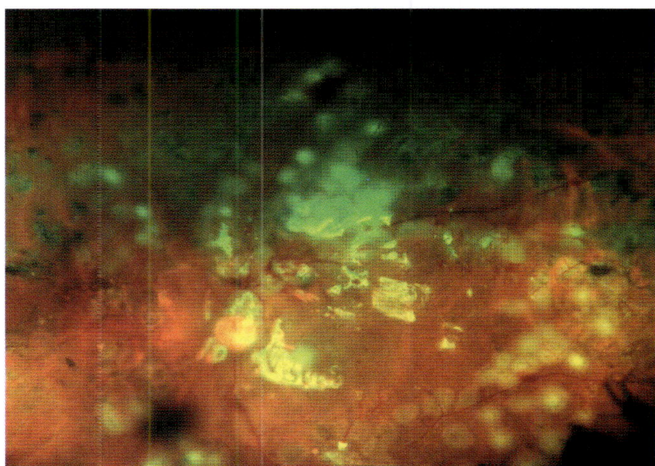

Fig. 48.9: Postvitrectomy in diabetic tractional retinal detachment (TRD) with vitreous hemorrhage. Picture shows attached retina with laser marks under oil.

challenges for the surgeon are, thin ischemic retina, massive florid NV, bleeding of variable severity, and risk of iatrogenic retinal break(s) (20–45%).[36-38]

For membrane peeling, various techniques have been described. Though superficially, each technique represents different approach, eventually all achieve the same objective in a different order. In fact, in most of the cases, selected technique is a combination of all basic techniques.[36-38]

The two main basic techniques are *segmentation* and *delamination.*

Segmentation

After relief of anteroposterior traction, bridging sheet of large ERM can be divided (segmented) into smaller islands before its removal. A vertical scissors is an instrument of choice.

Scissor blades are kept at right angle to the retina. The lower blade of scissor is inserted between retina and the membrane. It acts as blunt dissector to separate the membrane from underlying retina before cutting. The technique is relatively easy to practice. The disadvantages are, more intraoperative bleeding due to cutting across the blood vessels and higher risk of reproliferation and rebleeding in postoperative period due to left over isolated proliferative tissues. With advent of newer machines, smaller gauge and port optimization, now-a-days vitreous cutter is more often used for segmentation.

Delamination

Preretinal FVP is removed using horizontal or curved scissors. Scissor blades are held parallel to retinal plane to transect epicenters to remove membrane as one or more large sheets. Though technically more difficult, the advantages of delamination are less intraoperative bleeding and more complete removal of the membranes, minimizing risk of reproliferation. In eyes with very extensive and florid membranes, bimanual dissection of ERM can be performed using multifunction instruments or using chandelier light source through a fourth sclerotomy. Bimanual technique is very useful when retina is mobile as in CRD.

To reach correct plane for dissection, it is important to identify *second membrane* (outer layer of vitreoschisis). The dissection can be initiated either from periphery and towards the center or vice versa depending on configuration of RD, extent of the membrane, configuration of PVD, availability of the instruments, and surgeons' experience.

An MIVS with better fluidics and port optimization, allows surgeons to work closer to the retina for closer vitreous shave. The smaller probes can fit under the membranes to be used as pic/forceps (with suction) for dissection and then can be switched to cutting mode for membrane removal (*lift, suck,* and *cut*). For bimanual dissection, forceps can be held in one hand and cutter can be used as scissors in the other to dissect the membranes and cut the epicentres, minimizing or almost eliminating the need of scissors.

Other Techniques

1. *Sub-ERM approach*: The cutter is placed between retina and ERM with port facing the membrane to protect retina during membrane removal.
2. *Conformal delamination*: It is performed by feeding ERM into the port at the leading edge of the membrane. The angle of the cutter port is adjusted to feed the ERM into the port keeping it away from the retina. This technique is useful for removal of thick membranes.
3. *Foldback technique*: It is also known as "*top of ERM approach*". Fibrovascular tissues are approached from a reverse angle. The cutter is placed over the ERM near the edge. Active suction and simultaneous cutting forces the membrane to "foldback" into the port for its removal without exerting traction on the retina. As the cutter is

over the membrane, risk of iatrogenic retinal break is minimized. The technique is useful for removal of thin, flexible membranes with weaker attachments. However, this technique cannot be used in eyes with mobile retina.

4. *Visco dissection*: It is not a new technique. Viscoelastic material is injected between retina and FV membrane to get better cleavage plane, identify epicenters and to create space for dissection. Injection of viscoelastic helps in hemostasis and also enhances visibility by keeping blood away from dissection area. The disadvantage is injection at wrong plane or use of excess force during injection may lead to retinal break formation. Because of smaller gauge and port optimization, MIVS requiring less separation, increasing the safety and hence increasing popularity of this technique once again.
5. *Lens management*: Crystalline lens can be retained as far as possible. In eyes with lens opacity, cataract surgery can be combined with vitrectomy. Phacoemulsification with larger capsulorrhexis and in the bag implantation of IOL, with larger optic size, is preferred.

ADDITIONAL PROCEDURES

- *Scleral buckling*: In eyes with peripheral FVP with unrelieved traction, segmental buckle or encirclage to support the FVP, can help to counter the traction and avoid sacrifice of the crystalline lens.[36,38] Another indication for buckling would be presence of peripheral retinal break, preexisting, or iatrogenic, with unrelieved traction.
- *Retinectomy*: It is indicated in eyes with unrelieved traction with/without break with firm FVP—retinal adhesion. The entire FVP—retina complex can be excised to relieve the traction.
- *Internal tamponade*: Tamponade is not needed in eyes when there is no retinal break. Both, long-acting gas or silicone oil can be used as internal tamponade. As in conventional rhegmatogenous retinal detachment, choice of tamponading agent is influenced by type, location, size, number of retinal break/s, and how effectively the traction is relieved. In one-eyed patients or when there is need for air travel, silicone oil is preferred as an internal tamponade.

ANTIVASCULAR ENDOTHELIAL GROWTH FACTOR AS AN ADJUNCT TO VITRECTOMY

In eyes with florid FVP, intravitreal injection of anti-VEGF agent causes rapid regression of NV.[28] The most used anti-VEGF is Bevacizumab. Fibrous regression following intravitreal injection makes surgery technically easier (Figs. 48.10A and B) as:

- FVP would readily separate from the retina,
- *There is less intraoperative bleeding so*: (1) Reduced endodiathermy usage and reduced postoperative inflammation, (2) Better intraoperative visualization decreases

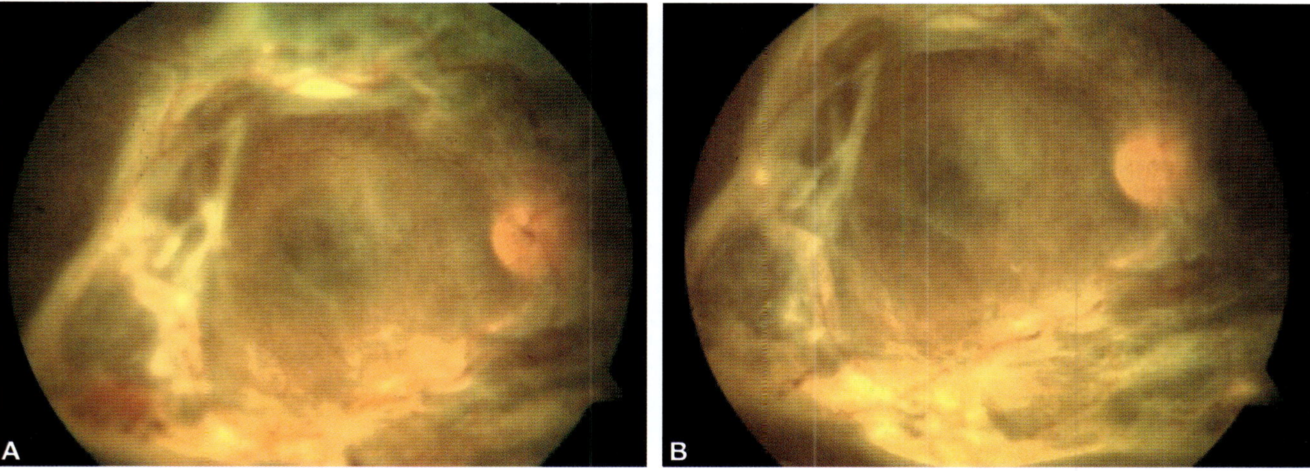

Figs. 48.10A and B: Course of proliferative diabetic retinopathy with active fibrovascular proliferation (FVP) following intravitreal bevacizumab injection. (A) Condition at baseline. (B) Regression of vascular component of FVP at day 4 post intravitreal bevacizumab injection.

overall surgical time, (3) Fewer tool exchanges again reduce surgery time and risk of sclerotomy related iatrogenic complications, and (4) More complete removal of fibrovascular tissues reduce risk of recurrent postoperative hemorrhage leading to overall improved anatomical and functional outcomes.[39-42]

With anti-VEGFs, the balance among different growth factors may tip toward fibrosis inducing factors [e.g. fibroblast growth factor (FGF)] causing contraction and thickening of the fibrous components and worsening of the traction and TRD (Figs. 48.10A and B).[43] Reactivation of the vascular proliferation can occur anytime after 2 weeks. Hence, the ideal window for surgery is between 3 days to 2 weeks, preferably between 5th and 10th day after injecting anti-VEGF agent.

SURGICAL COMPLICATIONS

Corneal Edema

Diabetic eyes have corneal epithelial abnormalities leading to poor adhesion between epithelial layers.[44] These eyes are prone for intraoperative corneal edema and postoperative nonhealing epithelial defects. Corneal epithelial scrapping should be avoided in these eyes as far as possible. Frequent lubrication of the corneal epithelium using viscoelastics to prevent corneal drying, minimizing the duration of surgery, and avoiding elevated IOP during surgery can minimize the risk of this complication. Avoiding contact visualization systems also helps to minimize the risk of corneal complications.[45]

Bleeding

The commonest source of intraoperative bleeding is cut ends of NV fronds. Excessive intraoperative bleeding can hamper progress of the surgery and also pose the risk of recurrent bleeding and exaggerated fibrinous response in postoperative period. In majority of the cases, there is mild ooze which stops spontaneously or by increasing intraocular infusion pressure. Few cases may need diathermy of elevated bleeding points. Presurgery and intraoperative good control of systemic hypertension reduces the risk of intraoperative bleeding.

Retinal Break(s)

The incidence of iatrogenic break(s) during vitrectomy ranges from 27% to 50%.[46-48] Break(s) occur more frequently during membrane surgery or during removal of adherent blood clots. Steps to minimize the risk of iatrogenic breaks include:

- Good debulking of peripheral vitreous before initiating membrane surgery
- Controlled movements with moderately high magnification for membrane surgery
- To identify vitreoschisis and define epicenters before cutting
- Avoid direct peeling of membranes.

If present, the break(s) should be marked with diathermy. Continuing dissection away from the break and working towards the break minimizes the risk of tearing retina and further enlargement of the break. If retina becomes very mobile, bimanual dissection is helpful. Once a break is created, it is necessary to relieve the traction completely before attempting fluid air exchange to reattach the retina. Supplemental scleral buckle or retinectomy can be performed to relieve the traction, if needed.

Iris and Angle Neovascularization

With advanced instrumentation and techniques, the incidence of iris and angle NV has significantly reduced with proportionately reduced incidence of neovascular glaucoma (NVG).[49,50] Possible risk factors include preexisting neovascularization of the iris (NVI), absence of preoperative PRP, and postoperative retinal detachment. Intravitreal injection of anti-VEGF supplemented with additional laser PHC or ARC may help in regression of both NVI and neovascularization of the angle (NVA). However, it does not help in controlling IOP in angle closure stage of NVG.

Complete vitrectomy with good debulking of peripheral vitreous followed by adequate laser PHC can reduce the risk of NVI and NVG. Eyes with preexisting rubeosis usually need very extensive laser PHC.[51] Functional and anatomical prognosis is generally poor in advanced stage of NVG (angle closure) even with glaucoma shunt surgery.

Fibrinoid Syndrome

Diabetic eyes have compromised blood-retinal barrier (BRB). Vitrectomy causes further breakdown of BRB and can lead to severe fibrinous in anterior chamber and vitreous cavity. Young diabetics with poor systemic control are more prone to have FS and generally have poor prognosis. Good control of diabetes prior to surgery and frequent use of topical steroid to minimize inflammation following surgery may help to reduce the risk of FS.

Anterior Hyaloidal Fibrovascular Proliferation

It is one of the serious and vision threatening complication following diabetic vitrectomy. The reported incidence is 15%.[52] Patients typically present with late onset (usually 3–8 weeks after surgery) recurrent intraocular hemorrhage. Other presenting features could be extensive NVI, hyphema, FVP over lens capsule, and/or anterior hyaloid face. Excessive contraction of FVP may cause detachment of peripheral retina and choroid leading to hypotony.

Ultrasound biomicroscopy is a useful diagnostic tool to detect AHFVP.[29,53] If left untreated, these eyes eventually lead to gross hypotony and phthisis. Though intravitreal injection of anti-VEGF and supplemental laser or ARC can be tried, most of these eyes need revitrectomy with meticulous dissection of vascular membranes over pars plana and ciliary body area. Lens or IOL may need to be sacrificed to approach these peripheral membranes. Extensive laser to skip areas and peripheral retina including part of pars plana needs to be performed. Silicone oil can be used as internal tamponade, if needed.

RESULTS

The DRVS was a landmark study which clearly showed the benefit of early vitrectomy; however, the study was concluded before advent of endolaser PHC and other advances in instrumentations and techniques. In eyes with VH, DRVS had shown that early vitrectomy resulted into 20/40 or better vision in 25% eyes when compared to deferred group (15% eyes).[54] The beneficial effect was seen only in type I diabetics. In eyes with severe FVP, 44% patients achieved 20/40 or better vision following early vitrectomy, in DRVS.[25]

Table 48.1: Outcomes of PPV for complications of PDR as studied in DRVS.

Complication	Outcome (% of eyes)		
	Increase in VA	Final VA > 20/200	NLP
VH	69–84	40–62	5–17
FVP	70	70	11
TRD	59–80	21–58	11–19
CRD	32–55	25–36	9–23

(PPV: Pars plana vitrectomy; PDR: Proliferative diabetic retinopathy; DRVS: Diabetic retinopathy vitrectomy study; VH: Vitreous hemorrhage; FVP: Fibrovascular proliferation; TRD: Tractional retinal detachment; CRD: Combined tractional and rhegmatogenous retinal detachment; NLP: No light perception; VA: Visual acuity).

Advances in techniques and instrumentation, now allow handling of more complicated cases with overall improved anatomical and functional outcomes. Results vary with underlying pathology and the time period studied (Table 48.1).

In eyes with VH, reported single surgery anatomical success rate is 85–90%.[47] Eyes with macula sparing TRD have relatively better anatomical success when compared to TRD involving macula.[3,55] However, eyes with prolonged macular detachment have poor anatomical and functional outcomes. If operated early, eyes with CRD have better anatomical success rate compared to TRD, but have higher incidence of recurrent retinal detachment.[56]

Visual outcome following surgery does not correlate with anatomical success and depends on status of the macula and optic nerve. VH without TRD has better visual prognosis than TRD and CRD. Visual acuity of 20/200 or better could be achieved in 47–57% of eyes with TRD.[57] Following vitrectomy for CRD, vision improves in 53–70% of eyes, but 20/200 or better vision could be achieved only in 20–36% of eyes.[5,33,56,58] Eyes with CRD with rapid progressive loss of vision generally report early for treatment; hence, retina is relatively healthy with final better functional outcome. CRD group also had the highest number of no *light perception* eyes in DRVS.

Predictors of favorable vision following vitrectomy are younger age, better preoperative vision (5/200 or more), absence of NVI, previtrectomy PRP, well-perfused attached macula or short duration of macular detachment, and absence of florid FVP.[26] Long-term visual and anatomic results are stable in 83–92% of diabetic eyes with successful result achieved for the first 6 months after vitrectomy.[59-61]

In 25–40% of the patients who had vitrectomy in one eye, will eventually develop complications of PDR in the fellow eye, needing vitrectomy within next 4 years, indicating need for long-term follow-up.

SUMMARY

Pan retinal photocoagulation is still the established first-line treatment for PDR. TRD and CRD are the commonest indication for vitrectomy in PDR. Extramacular TRD can safely be observed. Although, various surgical techniques have been described, often a combination of most given techniques is required. MIVS, with improved fluidics and port optimization along with better illumination sources and wide angle visualization systems, allows vitrector to be used *not only as cutter*, but also as forceps, scissors and a pic, reducing the need for ancillary instrumentation and making surgery safer and less time-consuming. In eyes with severe and extensive FVP with anticipated intraoperative risk of excessive bleeding, preoperative intravitreal injection of anti-VEGFs help to minimize intraoperative complications and to achieve more complete membrane removal, leading to improved long-term functional and anatomical outcomes. However, final visual outcome ultimately depends on macular involvement.

REFERENCES

1. Arnos AF, McCarty DJ, Zimmet P. The rising global burden of diabetes and its complications: Estimates and projections to the year 2010. Diabet Med. 1997;14:S1-85.
2. Klein R, Klein BE, Moss SE, et al. The Wisconsin epidemiologic study of diabetic retinopathy. IV. Diabetic macular edema. Ophthalmology. 1984;91:1464-74.
3. Rice TA, Michels RG, Rice EF. Vitrectomy for diabetic traction retinal detachment involving the macula. Am J Ophthalmology. 1983;95:22-33.
4. Eliott D. Proliferative diabetic retinopathy: principles and techniques of surgical treatment. Amsterdam: The Netherlands Elsevier Inc; 2006.
5. Rice TA, Michels RG, Rice EF. Vitrectomy for diabetic rhegmatogenous retinal detachment. Am J Ophthalmology. 1983;95:34-44.
6. Machemer R, Buettner H, Norton EW, et al. Vitrectomy: a pars plana approach. Trans Am Acad Ophthalmology Otolaryngol. 1971;75:813-20.
7. Machemer R. Reminiscences after 25 years of pars plana vitrectomy. Am J Ophthalmology. 1995;119:505-10.
8. Altan T, Acar N, Kapran Z, et al. Transconjunctival 25-gauge sutureless vitrectomy and silicone oil injection in diabetic retinal detachment. Retina. 2008;28:1201-6.
9. Sato T, Emi K, Bando H, et al. Faster recovery after 25-gauge microincision vitrectomy surgery than after 20-gauge vitrectomy in patients with proliferative diabetic retinopathy. Clin Ophthalmology. 2012;6:1925-30.
10. Ozone D, Hirano Y, Ueda J, et al. Outcome and complications of 25-gauge transconjunctival sutureless vitrectomy for proliferative diabetic retinopathy. Ophthalmologica. 2011;226:76-80.
11. Frank RN, Amin RH, Eliott D, et al. Basic fibroblast growth factor and vascular endothelial growth factor are present in epiretinal and choroidal neovascular membranes. Am J Ophthalmology. 1996;122:393-403.
12. Meyer-Schwickerath R, Pfeiffer A, Blum WF, et al. Vitreous levels of the insulin-like growth factors I and II, and the insulin-like growth factor binding proteins 2 and 3, increase in neovascular eye disease. Studies in nondiabetic and diabetic subjects. J Clin Invest. 1993;92:2620-5.
13. Frank RN, Amin R, Kennedy A, et al. An aldose reductase inhibitor and aminoguanidine prevent vascular endothelial growth factor expression in rats with long-term galactosemia. Arch Ophthalmology. 1997;115:1036-47.
14. Adamis AP, Miller JW, Bernal MT, et al. Increased vascular endothelial growth factor levels in the vitreous of eyes with proliferative diabetic retinopathy. Am J Ophthalmology. 1994;118:445-50.
15. Davis MD. Vitreous contraction in proliferative diabetic retinopathy. Arch Ophthalmology. 1965;74:741-51.
16. Meredith TA, Kaplan HJ, Aaberg TM. Pars plana vitrectomy techniques for relief of epiretinal traction by membrane segmentation. Am J Ophthalmology. 1980;89:408-13.
17. Schwartz SD, Alexander R, Hiscott P, et al. Recognition of vitreoschisis in proliferative diabetic retinopathy: a useful landmark in vitrectomy for diabetic traction retinal detachment. Ophthalmology. 1996;103:323-8.
18. Chu TG, Lopez PF, Cano MR, et al. Posterior vitreoschisis: an echographic finding in proliferative diabetic retinopathy. Ophthalmology. 1996;103:315-22.
19. Joussen AM, Joeres S. Benefits and limitations in vitreoretinal surgery for proliferative diabetic retinopathy and macular edema. Dev Ophthalmology. 2007;39:69-87.
20. Helbig H. Surgery for diabetic retinopathy. Ophthalmologica. 2007;221:103-11.
21. Early vitrectomy for severe vitreous hemorrhage in diabetic retinopathy. Four-year results of a randomized trial: Diabetic Retinopathy Vitrectomy Study Report 5. Arch Ophthalmology. 1990;108:958-64.
22. Yanyali A, Celik E, Horozoglu F, et al. 25-Gauge transconjunctival sutureless pars plana vitrectomy. Eur J Ophthalmology. 2006;16:141-7.
23. Misra A, Ho-Yen G, Burton RL. 23-gauge sutureless vitrectomy and 20-gauge vitrectomy: a case series comparison. Eye. 2009;23:1187-91.
24. Charles S, Flinn CE. The natural history of diabetic extramacular traction retinal detachment. Arch Ophthalmology. 1981;99:66-8.
25. Two-year course of visual acuity in severe proliferative diabetic retinopathy with conventional management. Diabetic Retinopathy Vitrectomy Study (DRVS) report #1. Ophthalmology. 1985;92:492-502.
26. de Bustros S, Thompson JT, Michels RG, et al. Vitrectomy for progressive proliferative diabetic retinopathy. Arch Ophthalmology. 1987;105:196-9.
27. Early vitrectomy for severe proliferative diabetic retinopathy in eyes with useful vision. Clinical application of results of randomized trial— Diabetic Retinopathy Vitrectomy Study Report 4. The Diabetic Retinopathy Vitrectomy Study Research Group. Ophthalmology. 1988;95:1321-34.
28. Avery RL, Pearlman J, Pieramici DJ, et al. Intravitreal bevacizumab (Avastin) in the treatment of proliferative diabetic retinopathy. Ophthalmology. 2006;113:1695.e1-15.
29. Bhende M, Agraharam SG, Gopal L, et al. Ultrasound biomicroscopy of the sclerotomy sites after pars plana vitrectomy for diabetic vitreous haemorrhage. Ophthalmology. 2000;107:1729-36.
30. Spaide RF, Fisher YL. Intravitreal bevacizumab (Avastin) treatment of proliferative diabetic retinopathy complicated by vitreous hemorrhage. Retina. 2006;26:275-8.
31. Huang YH, Yeh PT, Chen MS, et al. Intravitreal bevacizumab and panretinal photocoagulation for proliferative diabetic retinopathy associated with vitreous hemorrhage. Retina. 2009;29:1134-40.
32. Diabetic Retinopathy Clinical Research Network. Randomized clinical trial evaluating intravitreal ranibizumab or saline for vitreous hemorrhage from proliferative diabetic retinopathy. JAMA Ophthalmology. 2013;131:283-93.
33. Bhagat N, Zarbin M. Recent Innovations in Medical and Surgical Retina. Asia Pac J Ophthalmology (Phila). 2015;3:171-9.
34. Goldenberg DT, Hassan TS. Small gauge, sutureless surgery techniques for diabetic vitrectomy. Int Ophthalmology Clin. 2009;49:141-51.

35. Hubschman JP, Gupta A, Bourla DH, et al. 20-, 23-, and 25-gauge vitreous cutters: performance and characteristics evaluation. Retina. 2008;28:249-57.

36. Charles S. Vitreous Microsurgery, 3rd edition. Philadelphia, US: Lippincott Williams & Wilkins; 2002. pp. 107-25.

37. Michels RG. Proliferative diabetic retinopathy. Pathophysiology of extraretinal complications and principles of vitreous surgery. Retina. 1981;1:1-17.

38. Han DP, Pulido JS, Meiler WF, et al. Vitrectomy for proliferative diabetic retinopathy with severe equatorial fibrovascular proliferation. Am J Ophthalmology. 1995;119:563-70.

39. Ishikawa K, Honda S, Tsukahara Y, et al. Preferable use of intravitreal bevacizumab as a pretreatment of vitrectomy for severe PDR. Eye. 2009;23:108-11.

40. Yeoh J, Williams C, Allen P, et al. Avastin as an adjunct to vitrectomy in the management of severe PDR: a prospective case series. Clin Experiment Ophthalmology. 2008;36:449-54.

41. Chen E, Park CH. Use of intravitreal bevacizumab as a preoperative adjunct for TRD repair in severe PDR. Retina. 2006;26:699-700.

42. Rizzo S, Genovesi EF, Di Bartolo E, et al. Injection of intravitreal bevacizumab (Avastin) as a preoperative adjunct before vitrectomy surgery in the treatment of severe PDR. Graefes Arch Clin Exp Ophthalmology. 2008;246:837-42.

43. Arevalo JF, Maia M, Flynn HW, et al. TRD following intravitreal bevacizumab (Avastin) in patients with severe PDR. Br J Ophthalmology. 2008;92:213-6.

44. Chen WL, Lin CT, Ko PS, et al. In vivo confocal microscopic findings of corneal wound healing after corneal epithelial debridement in diabetic vitrectomy. Ophthalmology. 2009;116:1038-47.

45. Virata SR, Kylstra JA, Singh HT. Corneal epithelial defects following vitrectomy surgery using hand-held, sew-on, and noncontact viewing lenses. Retina. 1999;19:287-90.

46. Yorston D, Wickham L, Benson S, et al. Predictive clinical features and outcomes of vitrectomy for proliferative diabetic retinopathy. Br J Ophthalmology. 2008;92:365-8.

47. Gupta B, Wong R, Sivaprasad S, et al. Surgical and visual outcome following 20-gauge vitrectomy in proliferative diabetic retinopathy over a 10-year period, evidence for change in practice. Eye. 2012;26:576-82.

48. Farouk MM, Naito T, Sayed KM, et al. Outcomes of 25-gauge vitrectomy for proliferative diabetic retinopathy. Graefes Arch Clin Exp Ophthalmology. 2011;249:369-76.

49. Kadonosono K, Matsumoto S, Uchino E, et al. Iris neovascularization after vitrectomy combined with phacoemulsification and intraocular lens implantation for proliferative diabetic retinopathy. Ophthalmic Surg Lasers. 2001;32:19-24.

50. Helbig H, Kellner U, Bornfeld N, et al. Rubeosisiridis after vitrectomy for diabetic retinopathy. Graefes Arch Clin Ophthalmology. 1998; 236:730-3.

51. Stringa M, Ivanisevic M. Comparison between efficacy of full and mid scatter (panretinal) photocoagulation on the course of diabetic rubeosis iridis. Ophthalmologica. 1993;207:144-7.

52. Lewis H, Abrams GW, Williams GA. Anterior hyaloidal fibrovascular proliferation after diabetic vitrectomy. Am J Ophthalmology. 1987;104:607-13.

53. Berinstein DM, Garretson BR, Williams GA. Ultrasound biomicroscopy in a case of anterior hyaloidal fibro-vascular proliferation. Ophthalmic Surg Lasers. 2000;31:69-70.

54. Early vitrectomy for severe vitreous hemorrhage in diabetic retinopathy. Two-year results of a randomized trial. Diabetic Retinopathy Vitrectomy Study reports 2. The Diabetic Retinopathy Vitrectomy Study Research Group. Arch Ophthalmology. 1985;103:1644-52.

55. Tao Y, Jiang YR, Li XX, et al. Long-term results of vitrectomy without endotamponade in proliferative diabetic retinopathy with tractional retinal detachment. Retina. 2010;30:447-51.

56. Hsu YJ, Hsieh YT, YehPT, et al. Combined Tractional and Rhegmatogenous Retinal Detachment in Proliferative Diabetic Retinopathy in the Anti-VEGF Era. J Ophthalmology. 2014;2014:917375.

57. Meier P, Wiedemann P. Vitrectomy for traction macular detachment in diabetic retinopathy. Graefes Arch Clin Exp Ophthalmology. 1997;235:569-74.

58. Yang CM, Su PY, Yeh PT, et al. Combined rhegmatogenous and traction retinal detachment in proliferative diabetic retinopathy: Clinical manifestations and surgical outcome. Can J Ophthalmology. 2008;43:192-8.

59. Rice TA, Michels RG. Long term anatomical and functional results of vitrectomy for diabetic retinopathy. Am J Ophthalmology. 1960;90:297.

60. Blankenship GW. Stability of parsplana vitrectomy results for diabetic retinopathy complcations. A comparison of five year and six month post vitrectomy findings. Arch Ophthalmology. 1981; 99:1009-12.

61. Blankenship GW, Machemer R. Long-term diabetic vitrectomy results. Report of 10 year follow-up. Ophthalmology. 1985;92:503-6.

Complications of Vitreoretinal Surgery

Parveen Sen, Sufiyan Shaikh, Sharan Shetty, Kaustubh Deshmukh

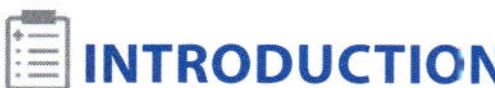 **INTRODUCTION**

The field of vitreoretinal surgery (VR surgery) has seen several advances in the past few decades. With improvement in instrumentation and technology, the indications for surgery have also expanded. Patients who were previously deemed inoperable can now hope to have some functional vision secondary to these advances. There has been an increase in the number of indications with even patients with good preoperative vision opting for surgery. Hence, it is important to avoid or manage complications as both the patients and surgeons have very-high expectations.

Complications of VR surgery, both straightforward and complex, can be broadly classified into those involving the anterior segment and posterior segment. Other ways to classify include intraoperative, postoperative or delayed complications, and whether instrument, technique, or iatrogenic related. With the appropriate preparation and management, VR surgery complications can be minimized and resolved. This chapter provides a brief overview of etiopathogenesis and treatment of complications of VR surgery.

INTRAOPERATIVE COMPLICATIONS

Anesthesia Complications

Many patients who undergo VR surgery have myopic eyes or are on anticoagulants. To avoid anesthesia related complications, it is important to examine the operative eye prior to surgery and carefully review the patient's medications. Those on anticoagulants or antiplatelet drugs need not discontinue their routine medication. However, the risk-benefit ratio should be considered by the treating surgeon. Local anesthetic techniques are now far more commonly used than general anesthesia for VR surgery.[1] It is safer to adopt the peribulbar and sub-Tenon's anesthesia in such patients when feasible. The darkened theater environment, the age and associated medical conditions of many of these patients, and the risk of precipitating abnormal cardiac rhythms from drugs and the oculocardiac reflex mandate continuous

monitoring.[2] The use of nitrous oxide (NO) during general anesthesia in gas-filled eyes may have disastrous visual results caused by gas expansion and elevated intraocular pressure (IOP). Patients must be advised of the potentially catastrophic results of undergoing general anesthesia before their intraocular gas bubble has resorbed.[3]

A rare complication of peribulbar and other needle blocks is retrobulbar and peribulbar hemorrhage. When severe, this can lead to visual loss secondary to orbital compression and impairment of ophthalmic artery circulation. While arterial hemorrhage can cause rapid proptosis and raised IOP, concealed hemorrhage in which blood remains within the muscular cone, produces elevations in IOP without visible evidence of orbital hemorrhage.[4] It is imperative that immediate external ocular external pressure is applied when there is a suspicion of such a complication. Additional interventional treatment like intravenous mannitol, lateral canthotomy, and anterior chamber paracentesis may be used when deemed necessary.[1] The incidence of direct globe injury and the risk of perforation is higher in myopia and resurgeries, because the sclera is thinner and is often associated with a staphyloma. Globe perforation can present with vitreous hemorrhage, pain, hypotony, retinal detachment (RD), or sudden increases in IOP (Fig. 49.1). Needle perforations tend to be associated with poorer visual outcomes and the surgeon needs to be aware of the possibility of this complication to take immediate remedial measures. A more controlled method is the parabulbar block, where the conjunctiva is cut open (small radial peritomy (1–2 mm) near the near fornix and a mixture of lignocaine and bupivacaine is then injected by passing a 1-inch blunt, curved irrigating cannula along the inferior sub-Tenon's space and the anesthetic slowly injected when the cannula is posterior enough. This technique has high efficacy and safety.

Injury to the Recti

A rare complication of 360° peritomy is rectus muscle injury, which is more likely to occur, if the peritomy is more than 2 mm posterior to the limbus. It can be prevented by

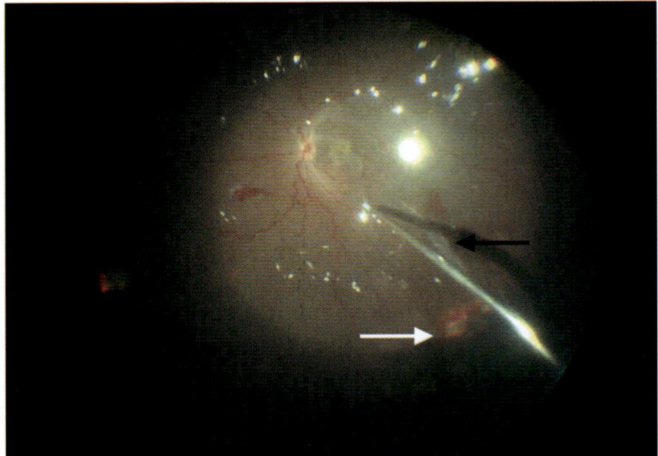

Fig. 49.1: Intraoperative photograph showing retinal fold (black arrow) with superotemporal perforation site (white arrow) with macular ischemia in a case of needle perforation with retinal detachment.

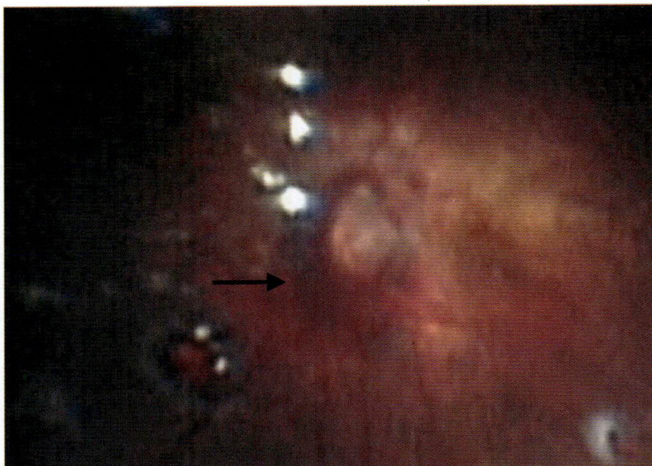

Fig. 49.2: Subretinal bleed around optic disc (arrow) due to superonasal drainage retinotomy.

performing a peritomy 1–2 mm from the limbus, which preserves the limbal stem cells and facilitates a cosmetic closure.

Subretinal Bleed

Subretinal bleed is a rare but known complication of VR surgery. It may happen at one of many steps like inadvertent full thickness entry into the sclera while passing encirclage or explant sutures, external drainage procedure in buckling surgery, inadvertent injury to major vessels or choroid during vitrectomy, retinotomy, or retinectomy procedures (Fig. 49.2). Subretinal bleed in the periphery may not require active intervention. However, those involving posterior pole or macula needs warrant its removal or displacement.

Suprachoroidal Detachment or Hemorrhage

Suprachoroidal hemorrhage (SCH) is an abrupt accumulation of blood in the potential space between the choroid and the sclera (suprachoroidal space), usually associated with ocular surgery. Its presentation can be variable, ranging from small localized suprachoroidal hematomas to massive SCH. It is also referred as expulsive hemorrhage, a term first coined by Terson in 1894.

The incidence of SCH is relatively low as it is an uncommon complication of intraocular surgery. The reported incidence of SCH during various surgical procedures varies from 0.05% to 6.2%.[5] In 1991 Speaker et al. reported an incidence of SCH of 0.41% in VR procedures.[6] Risk factors include a history of glaucoma, axial length greater than 25 mm, aphakia, pseudophakia, external drainage of subretinal fluid, cryotherapy, coughing or "bucking" on the endotracheal tube during general anesthesia, and intraoperative systemic hypertension.[6-11] Previous pars plana vitrectomy (PPV) has been described as a significant risk factor for SCH. Systemic risk factors include hypertension, atherosclerosis, diabetes, and advanced age.[12]

Massive SCH occurs secondary to intraoperative ocular hypotony. Acute hypotony causes rupture of short or long posterior ciliary arteries causing severe SCH. This forced separation of choroid from the sclera will cause more bleeding by damaging more vessels and exacerbating the process.[10] Large IOP fluctuations can often occur during aspiration of subretinal fluid, phacofragmentation, and inadvertent needle penetration of the globe during scleral buckle placement.[13] Localized choroidal hematomas may occur by direct damage to the choroid by instruments during subretinal proliferative membrane removal or drainage of subretinal fluid.

The diagnosis of intraoperative massive SCH is self-evident.[5] Early signs include—a sudden increase in the IOP with firming of the globe, loss of the red reflex and shallowing of the anterior chamber with forward displacement of the iris and lens or lens implant, with or without prolapse of the intraocular contents through the surgical wound.

Management

It is recommended to perform a detailed and complete examination of previously described risk factors to decrease the chances of SCH. In spite of all preventive measures, massive SCH can be an inevitable event. If either choroidal hemorrhage or effusion occurs intraoperatively the procedure is to be terminated and wound to be closed as quickly as possible.[14] Surgical wound closure should be attempted by any means. If closure cannot be achieved immediately, thumb should be placed on the eye to tamponade, it immediately. Acute drainage of the SCH is difficult because blood in suprachoroidal space clots rapidly. Lakhanpal et al. proved that the creation of draining sclerotomies immediately is detrimental to eyes.[5]

Nitrous oxide (NO): The use of NO during general anesthesia in patients with a preexisting intraocular gas bubble can

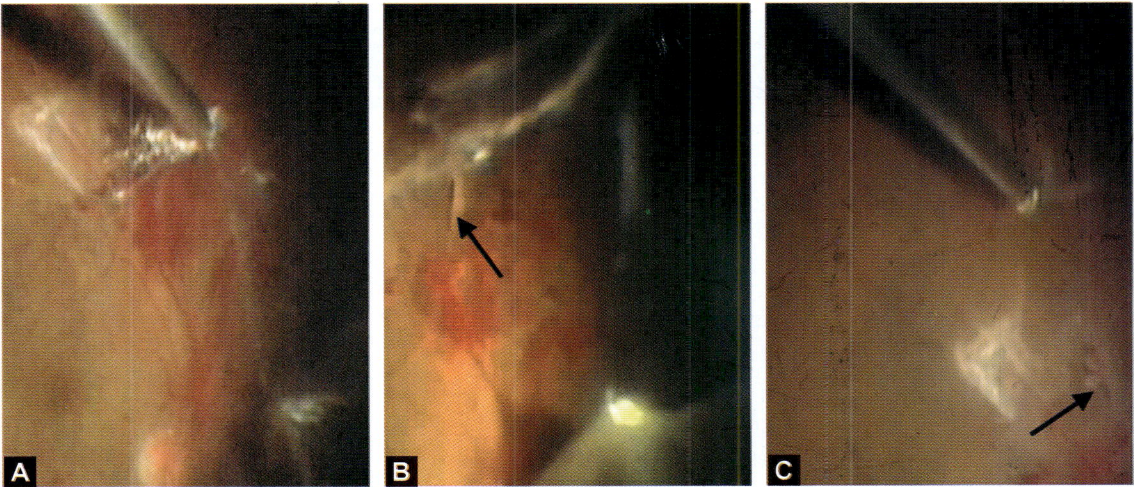

Figs. 49.3A to C: Intraoperative image shows iatrogenic break (black arrows) during PVD induction. (PVD: Posterior vitreous detachment).

lead to elevated IOP, which is intractable and can lead to a central artery occlusion. NO being highly soluble will diffuse quickly into intraocular gas bubbles causing a rapid expansion of the intraocular gas bubble and subsequent rise in IOP. In cats, ventilation with NO has been found to cause a threefold increase in the volume of an intraocular SF6 bubble and a twofold increase in the volume of an intraocular air bubble.[6,7]

This complication can be prevented by discontinuing NO ventilation 15 minutes before the gas-fluid exchange. It is very important, therefore, to notify the anesthesiologist ahead of time before performing an air-fluid exchange under general anesthesia, to insure that NO is not used as an anesthetic.

Air-fluid Exchange Complications

During VR surgery, fluid in the vitreous cavity is replaced by air. Although being a simple procedure, complications can still occur. One of them being damage to the retina during air infusion.[15,16] Preceding the air infusion, if the IOP is high it may lead to damage to the retina contralateral to the infusion cannula, usually seen as a whitening in the superonasal quadrant when the cannula is in the inferotemporal quadrant. During aspiration, mechanical trauma to the optic nerve head may occur. In a case report, three patient developed permanent peripheral temporal visual field defects after vitrectomy with air fluid exchange.[17] Possible mechanism in these cases being mechanical trauma to the optic nerve head by the extrusion instrument. This trauma can be minimized by using a soft tip cannula under clear visualization.

Iatrogenic Retinal Breaks

Iatrogenic retinal breaks generally occur as a consequence of VR procedures. Two types of retinal breaks are being described—(1) those occurring at the entry sites and (2) those occurring elsewhere in the retina.[18] Underlying mechanism

for entry site break is thought to be traction on the vitreous base either during insertion or removal of the instruments or a result of vitreous incarceration at the sclerotomy site. While retinal breaks elsewhere results from traction to the retina by the vitreous cutter or a result of surgically induced posterior vitreous detachment (PVD) (Figs. 49.3 and 49.4).

The frequency of iatrogenic retinal breaks during PPV has been reported to range from 0% to 24% with post-PPV RD occurring in 0–15.8%.[18-21]

Surgically induced PVD can result in small peripapillary retinal hemorrhages as that area has strong VR attachments. These hemorrhages normally resolve spontaneously. If a small break is suspected endodiathermy should be utilized to facilitate visualization and argon laser is used to treat it at the end of surgery. The risk of retinal breaks can be reduced by doing peripheral vitrectomy under air as it provides better visualization.[22] Also air stabilizes the retina against the aspiration force of the cutter due to the spring like property thereby reducing chances of break.

Phototoxicity

First described in six patients who developed a characteristic macular lesion involving outer retina within a few weeks following cataract extraction, subsequently replaced by mottling.[23] More oval-shaped lesions are associated with Tungsten filament sources, whereas fiber optic microscope illuminators usually produce a more homogenous, round lesion.

Iatrogenic phototoxicity during vitrectomy has been reported both from the endoilluminator and the operating microscope.[24,25] Lesions caused by the endoilluminator are usually larger and have well-defined borders as compared to the lesions caused by the operating microscope.[25] The amount

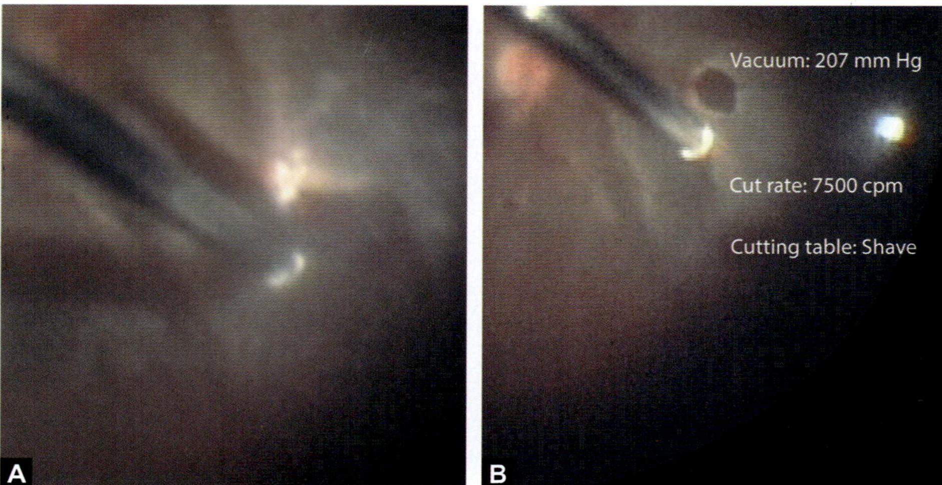

Figs. 49.4A and B: Intraoperative image showing iatrogenic break created while performing peripheral vitrectomy.

of ocular damage following iatrogenic phototoxicity depends on various factors like the wavelength of light used, the power of the light source, and the duration of use. One study with long-term follow-up of patients with phototoxicity found the average duration of surgery to be 109 minutes.[26] Increased chances of phototoxicity with wavelengths less than 515 nm have been in animal stuides.[27-29] Exposure to the operating microscope light should be minimized as much as possible. However, in regards to recent advances with light-emitting diode (LED) being the source of light risk of iatrogenic phototoxicity has considerably decreased.

Subretinal or Suprachoroidal Cannula

Subretinal or suprachoroidal cannula insertion commonly occurs in cases of choroidal detachment and/or bullous RD. It can occur during cannula insertion in any of the three ports. Prompt visualization and correction can prevent dreadful complications like iatrogenic choroidal and total RD (Figs. 49.5A to D).

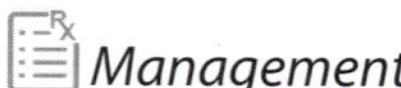

Management

In cases of choroidal detachment or bullous RD, it is advisable to avoid routine position of cannula insertion and choosing an area with minimal detachment. Entry of infusion cannula should be checked before starting infusion. A longer infusion cannula (6 mm) has also been recommended in cases of ciliochoroidal detachment.

POSTOPERATIVE COMPLICATIONS

Wound-related Complications

Sclera, outer coat of eyeball gets damaged whenever an eye surgery is performed on the exterior and interior eye. Pars plana route used during the procedure induces stress and

strain on the sclera and makes the sclera edge weak and makes it difficult to perform a correct and strong suture. Use of 25-gauge vitrectomy within trocars during vitrectomy procedure has decreased the direct damage to sclera edges. Thick sclera stitches may damage overlying conjunctiva and develop ulceration and erosion of overlying layer. Sclerotomy sites should be free of silicone oil, vitreous and small particles to avoid damage to sclera and overlying conjunctiva and to prevent development of complications like traction, chronic inflammation, conjunctival cyst formation, etc. There are concerns of potential wound leakage and hypotony with 25-gauge sutureless vitrectomy. A report on 140 consecutive cases using a 25-gauge vitrectomy system found a requirement of suturing the sclerotomy in 7.1% of all cases.[30] Another group reported on 70 consecutive patients undergoing 25-gauge vitrectomy and found comparable rates of postoperative hypotony.[31] The wound should be inspected well before closure, so as to prevent postoperative hypotony and further complications like endophthalmitis.

Corneal Complications

Silicone oil is the most common internal tamponade used during VR procedures and should be removed once the purpose of tamponade is achieved in order to minimize its long-term complications. Two most common complications are calcific band shaped keratopathy and corneal edema (Fig. 49.6). Band-shaped keratopathy is common in young age and it may occur when silicone oil comes in contact with cornea endothelium. The keratopathy is thought to be result of pH changes caused by reduced flow across the cornea.[32]

However, introduction of Ando iridectomy has reduced its incidences[33] and this complication is largely confined to eyes with severe trauma, hypotony, aniridia, or aphakia. Ando iridectomy is an iridectomy at 6 o'clock position that prevents

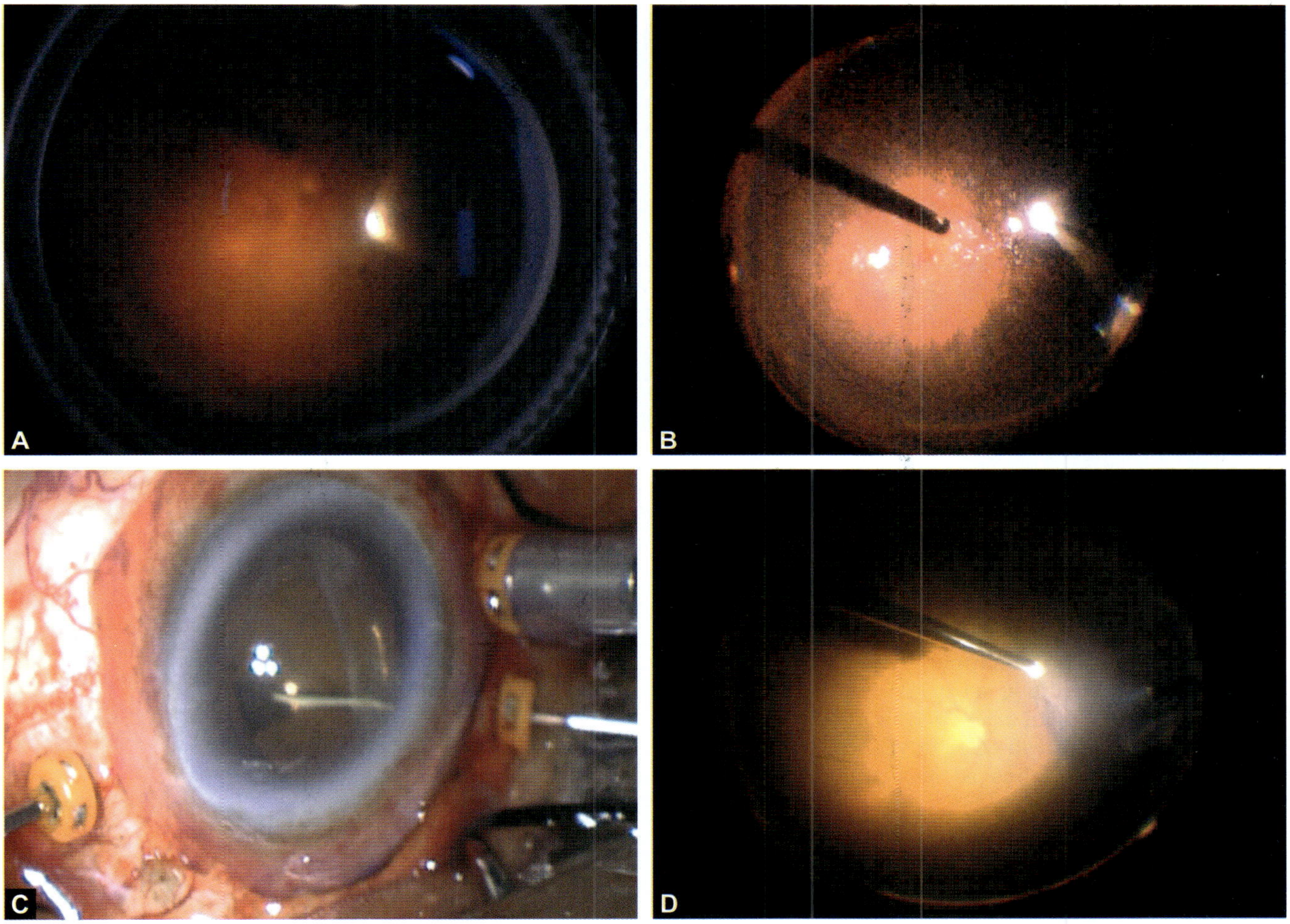

Figs. 49.5A to D: Intraoperative images showing (A) Subretinal cannula; (B) suprachoroidal cannula; (C) Intraoperative management of subretinal cannula using 26 G needle; and (D) Cannula in the vitreous cavity.

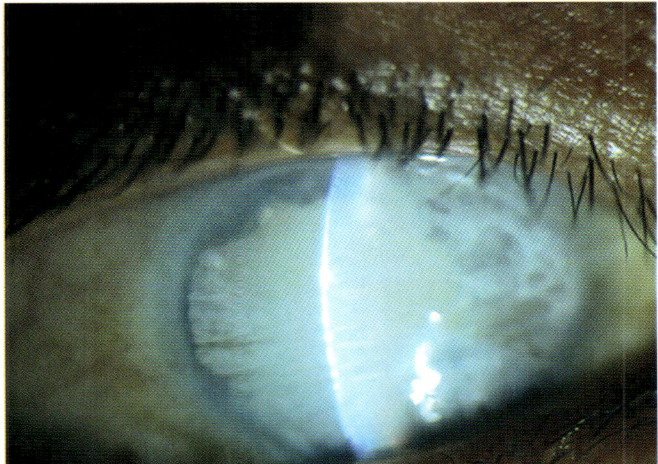

Fig. 49.6: Anterior segment photograph showing band-shaped keratopathy in an eye with operated VR surgery. (VR: Vitreoretinal).

silicone oil from entering anterior chamber.[34] Silicone oil will not enter anterior chamber as long as it does not create a pupillary block. With an existing pupillary block silicone oil will accumulate behind iris diaphragm at the lowest part of posterior segment. During waking hours, this is at 6 o'clock position, which is followed by building up of pressure by aqueous production and that forces silicone oil through the pupil and results in an oil-filled anterior chamber. In such situation, iridectomy at 6 o'clock prevents a pupillary block and thereby prevents entry of silicone oil in anterior chamber.

Treatment options for band-shaped keratopathy include chemical chelation with 1–2% ethylenediaminetetraacetic acid (EDTA)[35] following mechanical removal of the epithelium, excimer laser phototherapeutic keratectomy,[36] amniotic membrane grafting after surgical removal of keratopathy, and in severe cases keratoplasty may be needed to restore the vision.

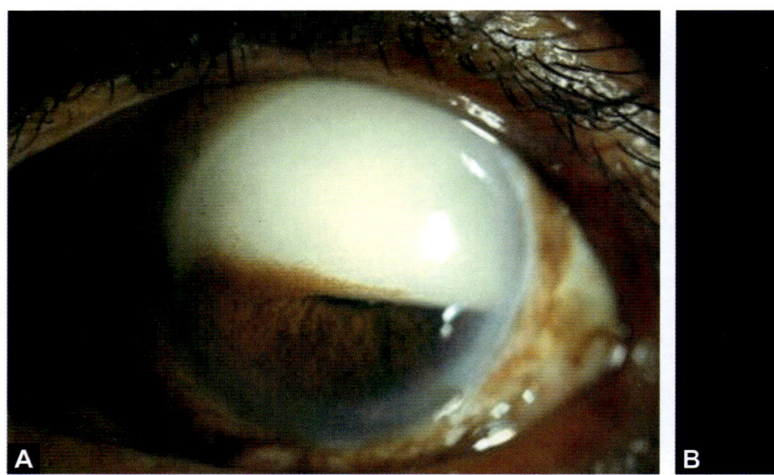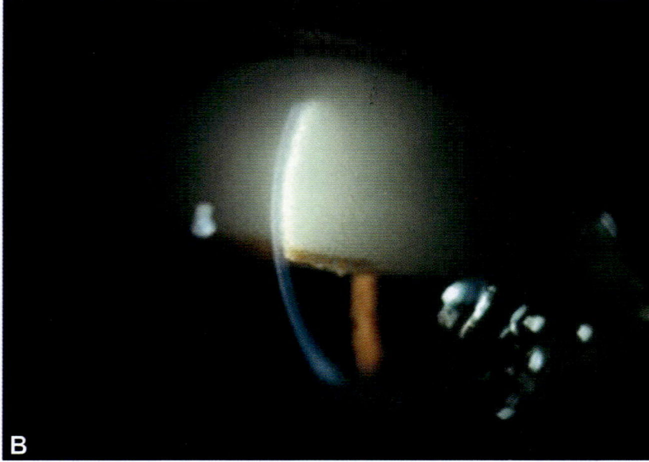

Figs. 49.7A and B: Anterior segment photograph of a patient showing hyperoleon (inverse hypopyon).

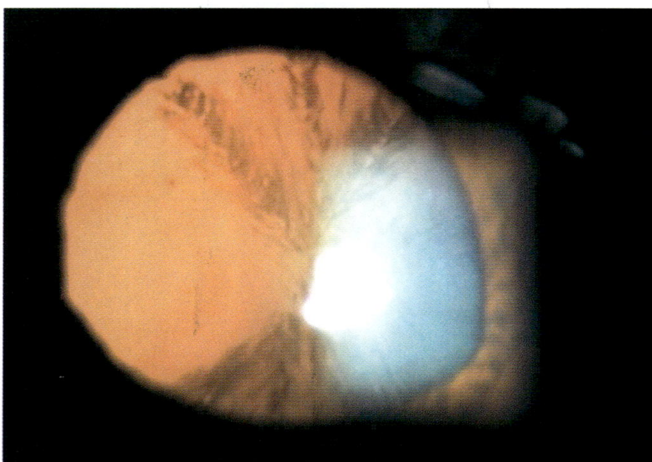

Fig. 49.8: Retroillumination showing feathery cataract following vitrectomy surgery.

Hyperoleon

Silicone oil acts as an internal tamponade to keep the retinal layers approximate. Due to its high surface tension, silicone oil does not enter the subretinal space, also it prevents the entry of fluid into the subretinal space.[37] As the surface tension decreases, the silicone oil globule begins to emulsify. Decrease in surface tension can be due to inflammatory agents and blood that sweeps in after surgery. Emulsified silicone oil does not serve its purpose as an effective tamponade and can present in the form of hyperoleon, i.e. the appearance of oil in the anterior chamber (Figs. 49.7A and B). Long-standing silicone oil in anterior chamber damages cornea in long run and especially endothelial layer.

Silicone oil removal should be planned to prevent further damage. In aphakic and pseudophakic patients, the hyperoleon is removed with the suction of the vitreous cutter. In phakic patients, the hyperoleon is removed with a 26-gauge needle mounted on an open plunger syringe via the limbus. Multiple fluid air exchanges are required to remove silicone oil globules trapped in the retroiridial plane to prevent further damage.

Cataract

Cataract is the most frequent complication following vitrectomy procedure. Cataract can either develop secondary to the internal tamponades used or directly related to the surgical procedure. The accidental contact of the surgical instruments with the lens during the procedure is responsible for rapid onset of cortical opacities that could be seen already at the end of surgery.[37] Long-standing internal tamponades induce progressive changes in lens and gradually develops cataract (Fig. 49.8).[38] If accidental injuries develop cataract then the surgeon should decide as to whether cataract surgery can be performed. If the surgeon decides to operate cataract at the same sitting thorough knowledge about phacodynamics is required as vitrectomized eyes behave very differently from normal eye. Progressive cataracts can be performed electively and at a later date as and when cataract becomes visually disturbing.

Glaucoma

Increased IOP secondary to various mechanisms is a frequent complication of vitrectomy surgery.

- *Hemolytic glaucoma*: Not very common with advances in vitrectomy instruments. It is transient and self-limited due to simple trabecular occlusion by cell debris. Majority of cases can be managed by ocular hypotensive agents.
- *Air-gas and silicone oil pupillary block*: Gas and silicone oil have high surface tension and cause pupillary block. The continuous production of aqueous in retroiridial space thereby pushes iris forward and blocks the angle thereby raising IOP. If not addressed early, it may result in permanent angle closure. Generally, Ando iridectomy is performed intraoperatively to prevent this complication.

Proper postoperative positioning can also prevent development of this complication. Ocular hypotensives can be use, but severe cases need surgical intervention to deepen the anterior chamber.

- *Silicone oil emulsification*: Emulsified oil globules can block and damage the trabecular meshwork because of long-term toxicity.
- *Neovascular glaucoma*: It develops secondary to ischemia of retina or posterior segment structures following VR procedure. The basic process underlying iris neovascularization should be addressed and treated to reduce vascular endothelial growth factor (VEGF) cascade. Patients should be treated aggressively managed with ocular hypotensives. If medical management is unable to achieve pressure less than 35 mm Hg, the cyclophotocoagulation with panretinal photocoagulation (PRP) should be planned.[39] Filtering procedure usually fails unless there is complete involution of neovascularization and inflammation. Patient with no perception of light (PL) vision can be managed by steroids and cycloplegics. Retrobulbar alcohol injection might be required for painful blind eye.[40]
- *Open angle glaucoma*: Generally open angle glaucoma gets aggravated following vitrectomy procedure. It appears that this type of glaucoma is secondary to the trauma suffered by the trabecular meshwork from the infusion fluid, cells, cytokines, protein, and debris. Open angle glaucoma can be managed by topical medications but it may require surgery.

Retained Perfluorocarbon Liquid

Perfluorocarbon liquids (PFCLs) are a commonly used intraocular tamponade in the management of RD repair, particularly when dealing with proliferative vitreoretinopathy or giant retinal tears. Surgical complications secondary to intraoperative use of PFCL are rare. Toxicity occurs due to postoperative retention of the PFCL (Fig. 49.9). Retained intraocular PFCL can cause secondary glaucoma, central scotomas can occur from retained subfoveal PFCL.[41,42] Retinal pigment epithelial (RPE) and photoreceptor toxicity have been demonstrated in an animal model with retained subretinal PFCL.[43]

Corneal toxicity in the form of loss of endothelial cells, stromal inflammation, and corneal vascularization has been demonstrated in aphakic rabbit eyes that were injected with PFCLs.[44] Risk of retention of PFCL increases in cases with large peripheral retinotomies greater than 120°, lack of a saline rinse after PFCL removal.[45] Saline rinse after removal of PFCL likely forms a microscopic residual layer of perfluorocarbon liquid posteriorly that can then be aspirated later.

Buckle Infection

Improper conjunctival wound closure can lead to wound gape and subsequent pathogenic organisms can infect the wide buckle and even the belt buckle. The incidence varies from 0.5% to 5% approximately as reported in literature.[46] Coagulase-positive and coagulase-negative *Staphylococci* are implicated as the most common organisms causing buckle infection.

A constant red eye with discharge and pain is the feature seen in such patients, and the only curative treatment is removal of the buckle (70–90% of cases). At times the buckle or silicon band migrates anteriorly due to improper suturing and gets exposed leading to infection. Chronic buckle infection can erode and cause necrosis of the sclera, which may lead onto uveal tissue prolapse or buckle intrusion into the vitreous cavity rarely (Fig. 49.10).

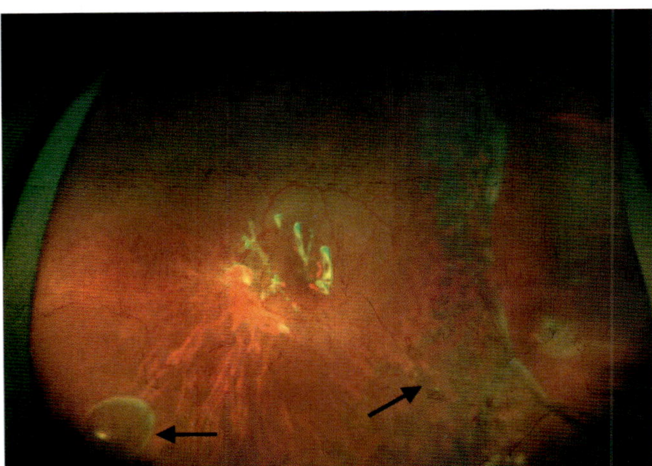

Fig. 49.9: Ultra-widefield image showing multiple subretinal PFCL (arrows) following VR surgery for giant retinal tear. (PFCL: Perfluorocarbon liquid; VR: Vitreoretinal).

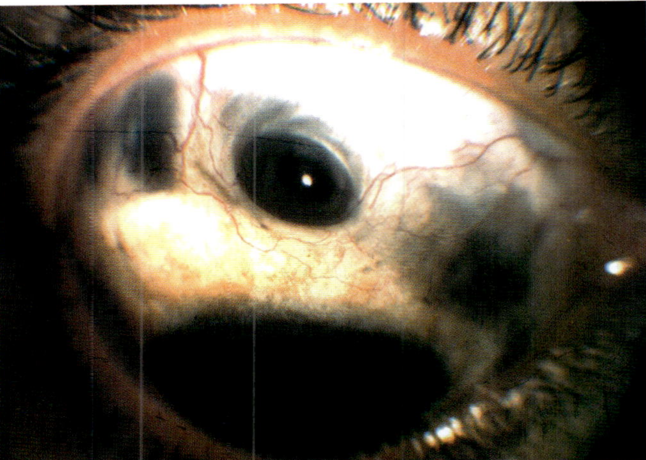

Fig. 49.10: Uveal prolapse in an eye, which had an infected silicon buckle and band removal a few months back and referred to our center.

Endophthalmitis

With the advent of sutureless vitrectomy, although the operating duration has decreased complications, such as endophthalmitis, appear to be increased marginally compared to the more "standard" 20-gauge vitrectomy system.[46] A retrospective comparison of the incidence of endophthalmitis in more than 8,000 patients undergoing either 25- or 20-gauge procedures found a 12-fold increased risk in the 25-gauge vitrectomy group.[46] The increased incidence and risk may be related to inferior wound closure and postoperative hypotony when compared to sutured 20-gauge sclerotomy incisions.[47]

Overall incidence of endophthalmitis following vitrectomy procedure is very less (0.03%).[48] Onset of endophthalmitis symptom is reported within 4 days in half of the cases, demonstrating that it is actually an acute disease, whereas only 13% presented with delayed onset endophthalmitis.[49] First step in management is identification of the causative agent. Vitreous tap should be taken and sent for culture and sensitivity analysis. Meanwhile patient should be treated on empirical therapy against gram-negative and gram-positive organisms, which includes vancomycin (1 mg/0.01 mL), ceftazidime (2.25 mg/0.01 mL), and dexamethasone (400 µg/0.01 mL). Steroids should be avoided, if fungal etiology is suspected. Once diagnosed then the patient needs to be treated aggressively as per usual endophthalmitis management guidelines. Some authors have recommended the use of antibiotics routinely in the infusion fluid. The literature also recommends subconjunctival injection of antibiotics against gram-negative and gram-positive organisms at the end of the procedure. However, vitrectomy is advised only in severe cases with aforementioned intravitreal antibiotics.

Aminoglycoside Toxicity

Aminoglycosides are used intravitreally for the treatment of endophthalmitis as well as subconjunctivally for antibiotic prophylaxis. In high concentrations, aminoglycosides have been reported to cause an acute, toxic ischemic retinopathy.[50] Severe retinal vascular occlusion and optic neuropathy can occur often leading to permanent severe visual loss. Even subconjunctival injection is associated with complication.[51,52] Other antibiotics like cefazolin, ceftazidime, or vancomycin can be used to avoid aminoglycoside related toxicity.[53,54]

Like all ocular surgery, VR surgery is not devoid of complications. However, the majority of them can be presented with careful planning and decision making. Discussing the specific needs of VR surgery with the anesthesiologist well in advance will prevent unwanted patient movement during critical maneuvers as well the use of NO when performing an air-fluid exchange. Other preventable measures include minimizing exposure to the operating microscope light or endoilluminator, appropriate monitoring of intraocular infusion pressure, especially when performing an air-fluid exchange. Lastly, the surgical team should always label all intraocular fluids used prior to the start of surgery and these should be double-checked by the surgeon before use.

REFERENCES

1. Palte HD. Ophthalmic regional blocks: management, challenges, and solutions. Local Reg Anesth. 2015;8:57-70.
2. Kong K, Kirkby G. Anaesthesia for vitreo-retinal surgery. Curr Anaesth Cri Care. 2010;21(4):174-9.
3. Fu A, Mcdonald H, Eliott D, et al. Complications of general anesthesia using nitrous oxide in eyes with preexisting gas bubbles. Retina. 2002;22(5):569-74.
4. Edge KR, Nicoll JM. Retrobulbar hemorrhage after 12,500 retrobulbar blocks. Anesth Analg. 1993;76(5):1019-22.
5. Lakhanpal V. Experimental and clinical observations on massive suprachoroidal haemorrhage. Trans Am Ophthalmology Soc. 1993;91:545-652.
6. Wolf GL, Capuano C, Hartung J. Nitrous oxide increases intraocular pressure after intravitreal sulfur hexafluoride injection. Anesthesiology. 1983;59(6):547-8.
7. Wolf GL, Capuano C, Hartung J. Effect of nitrous oxide on gas bubble volume in the anterior chamber. Arch Ophthalmology. 1985;103(3):418-9.
8. Speaker M, Guerriero P, Met J, et al. A case-control study of risk factors for intraoperative suprachoroidal expulsive hemorrhage. Ophthalmology. 1991;98(2):202-10.
9. Sharma T, Virdi DS, Parikh S, et al. A case-control study of suprachoroidal hemorrhage during pars plana vitrectomy. Ophthalmic Surg Lasers. 1997;28(8):640-4.
10. Hawkins WR, Schepens CL. Choroidal detachment and retinal surgery. Am J Ophthalmology. 1966;62(5):813-9.
11. Piper JG, Han DP, Abrams GW, et al. Perioperative choroidal hemorrhage at pars plana vitrectomy. A case-control study. Ophthalmology. 1993;100(5):699-704.
12. Tabandeh H, Sullivan PM, Smahliuk P, et al. Suprachoroidal hemorrhage during pars plana vitrectomy. Risk factors and outcomes. Ophthalmology. 1999;106(2):236-42.
13. Pollack A, McDonald H, Ai E, et al. Massive suprachoroidal hemorrhage during pars plana vitrectomy associated with Valsalva maneuver. Am J Ophthalmology. 2001;132(3):383-7.
14. Moshfeghi D, Kim B, Kaiser P, et al. Appositional suprachoroidal hemorrhage: A case-control study. Am J Ophthalmology. 2004;138(6):959-63.
15. Brown P, Chignell AH. Accidental drainage of subretinal fluid. Br J Ophthalmology. 1982;66(10):625-6.
16. Campbell J. Expulsive choroidal hemorrhage and effusion: a reappraisal. Ann Ophthalmology. 1980;12:332-42.
17. Yang SS, McDonald HR, Everett AI, et al. Retinal damage caused by air-fluid exchange during pars plana vitrectomy. Retina. 2006;26(3):334-8.
18. Welch J. Dehydration injury as a possible cause of visual field defect after pars plana vitrectomy for macular hole. Am J Ophthalmology. 1997;124(5):698-9.
19. Melberg N, Thomas M. Visual field loss after pars plana vitrectomy with air/fluid exchange. Am J Ophthalmology. 1995;120(3):386-8.
20. Jackson TL, Donachie PHJ, Sparrow JM, et al. United Kingdom National Ophthalmology Database Study of Vitreoretinal Surgery: Report 1; Case mix, complications, and cataract. Eye (Lond). 2013;27(5):644-51.
21. de Bustros S, Thompson J, Michels R, et al. Vitrectomy for idiopathic epiretinal membranes causing macular pucker. Br J Ophthalmology. 1988;72(9):692-5.

22. Moore J, Kitchens J, Smiddy W, et al. Retinal breaks observed during pars plana vitrectomy. Am J Ophthalmology. 2007;144(1):32-6.

23. Dogramaci M, Lee E, Williamson T. The incidence and the risk factors for iatrogenic retinal breaks during pars plana vitrectomy. Eye (Lond). 2012;26(5):718-22.

24. Reibaldi M, Rizzo S, Avitabile T, et al. Iatrogenic retinal breaks in 25-gauge vitrectomy under air compared with the standard 25-gauge system for macular diseases. Retina. 2014;34(8):1617-22.

25. McDonald H, Irvine A. Light-induced maculopathy from the operating microscope in extracapsular cataract extraction and intraocular lens implantation. Ophthalmology. 1983;90(8):945-51.

26. McDonald H, Harris M. Operating microscope-induced retinal phototoxicity during pars plana vitrectomy. Arc Ophthalmology. 1988;106(4):521-3.

27. Michels M, Lewis H, Abrams G, et al. Macular phototoxicity caused by fiberoptic endoillumination during pars plana vitrectomy. Am J Ophthalmology. 1992;114(3):287-96.

28. Postel E. Long-term follow-up of iatrogenic phototoxicity. Arc Ophthalmology. 1998;116(6):753-7.

29. Ham W, Mueller H, Ruffolo J, et al. Sensitivity of the retina to radiation damage as a function of wavelength. Photochem Photobiol. 1979;29(4):735-43.

30. Lawwill T. Three major pathologic processes caused by light in the primate retina: a search for mechanisms. Trans Am Ophthalmology Soc. 1982;80:517-79.

31. Buykkmihci N. Photic retinopathy in the dog. Exp Eye Res. 1981;33(1):95-109.

32. Lakhanpal RR, Humayun MS, de juan E jr, et al. Outcomes of 140 consecutive cases of 25-gauge transconjunctival surgery for posterior segment disease. Ophthalmology. 2005;112(5):817-24.

33. Kreiger A. Sclerotomy complications following pars plana vitrectomy. Br J Ophthalmology. 2001;85(1):121-2.

34. Beekhuis W, Ando F, Zivojnovic R, et al. Basal iridectomy at 6 o'clock in the aphakic eye treated with silicone oil: prevention of keratopathy and secondary glaucoma. Br J Ophthalmology. 1987;71(3):197-200.

35. Al-Jazzaf A, Netland P, Charles S. Incidence and management of elevated intraocular pressure after silicone oil injection. J Glaucoma. 2005;14(1):40-6.

36. Laganowski H, Leaver P. Silicone oil in the aphakic eye: the influence of a six o'clock peripheral iridectomy. Eye (Lond). 1989;3(Pt 3):338-48.

37. Kobayashi W, Yokokura S, Hariya T, et al. Two percent ethylenediaminetetraacetic acid chelation treatment for band-shaped keratopathy, without blunt scratching after removal of the corneal epithelium. Clin Ophthalmology. 2015;9:217-23.

38. Sharma N, Mannan R, Sinha R, et al. Excimer laser phototherapeutic keratectomy for the treatment of silicone oil–induced band-shaped keratopathy. Eye Contact Lens. 2011;37(5):282-5.

39. Yanoff M, Duker J, Augsburger J. Ophthalmology. St. Louis, MO: Mosby; 2008. p. 533.

40. Saxena S, Gopal L. Fluid vitreous substitutes in vitreoretinal surgery. Ind J Ophthalmology. 1996;44(4):191-206.

41. Dangda S, Kumar H, Singh K, et al. Neovascular glaucoma. Delhi J Ophthalmology. 2015;26(2):138-49.

42. Lim K, Kim S, Yang S. Retrobulbar alcohol injection for orbital pain relief in blind: a case report. Europ J Anaesthesiol. 2014;31:232.

43. Lesnoni G, Rossi T, Gelso A. Subfoveal liquid perfluorocarbon. Retina. 2004;24(1):172-6.

44. Foster R, Smiddy W, Alfonso E, et al. Secondary glaucoma associated with retained perfluorophenanthrene. Am J Ophthalmology. 1994;118(2):253-5.

45. Marmor M. Control of subretinal fluid: experimental and clinical studies. Eye (Lond). 1990;4(2):340-4.

46. Moreira H, de Queiroz J, Liggett P, et al. Corneal toxicity study of two perfluorocarbon liquids in rabbit eyes. Cornea. 1992;11(5):376-9.

47. Garcia-Valenzuela E, Ito Y, Abrams G. Risk factors for retention of subretinal perfluorocarbon liquid in vitreoretinal surgery. Retina. 2004;24(5):746-52.

48. Chhablani J, Nayak S, Jindal A, et al. Scleral buckle infections: microbiological spectrum and antimicrobial susceptibility. J Ophthalmic Inflamm Infect. 2013;3:67.

49. Kunmoto D, Kaiser R. Wills eye retina service. Incidence of endophthalmitis after 20- and 25-gauge vitrectomy. Ophthalmology. 2007;114(12):2133-7.

50. Gupta OP, Weichel ED, Regillo CD, et al. Postoperative complications associated with 25-gauge. pars plana vitrectomy. Ophthalmic Surg Lasers Imaging. 2007;38(4):270-5.

51. Dave VP, Pathengay A, Schwartz S, et al. Endophthalmitis following pars plana vitrectomy: a literature review of incidence, causative organisms, and treatment outcomes. Clin Ophthalmology. 2014;8:2183-8.

52. Kernt M, Kampik A. Endophthalmitis: pathogenesis, clinical presentation, management, and perspectives. Clin Ophthalmology. 2010;4:121-35.

53. McDonald H, Schatz H, Allen A, et al. Retinal toxicity secondary to intraocular gentamicin injection. Ophthalmology. 1986;93(7):871-7.

54. Loewenstein A, Zemel E, Vered Y, et al. Retinal toxicity of gentamicin after subconjunctival injection performed adjacent to thinned sclera. Ophthalmology. 2001;108(4):759-64.

Chapter 50

Posterior Dislocation of Lens

Devesh Kumawat, Vineet Mutha, Nasiq Hasan, Atul Kumar

POSTERIORLY DISLOCATED LENS (FIG. 50.1)

The incidence of posterior migration of nuclear or cortical matter during cataract surgery is around 0.1–0.3%, the odds being almost similar with phacoemulsification, small incision cataract surgery and extracapsular cataract extraction.[1] Likelihood of nucleus drop increases in eyes with posterior polar cataract and postintravitreal injections or pars plana vitrectomy due to damaged posterior capsule. A good preoperative evaluation and intraoperative care can prevent lens matter drop.

Traumatic dislocation usually follows a closed globe injury, though post open globe injury has also been described. Tell-tale signs are its association with other signs of blunt injury such as traumatic mydriasis with sphincter tears, vitreous hemorrhage, commotio retinae, retinal dialysis, angle recession and choroidal ruptures. Usually complete dislocation occurs with 360° of zonular rupture. In eyes with vitreous hemorrhage, ultrasonography becomes a key modality for diagnosis (Fig. 50.2).

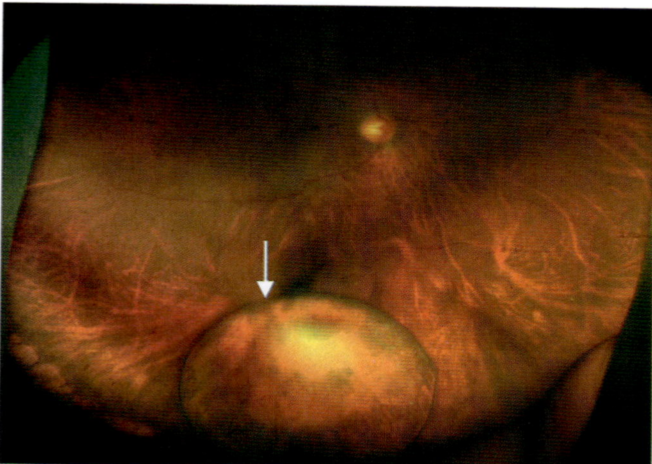

Fig. 50.1: Ultra-widefield fundus photograph showing dropped lens in a case of spontaneous lens dislocation (white arrow).

Spontaneous dislocation of lens without any intraocular intervention has also been described, although their contribution is only 0.8–2% of total cases.[2] Clearing the dilemma of confusing terms, dislocation means lens is outside the patellar fossa while subluxation means lens is displaced within the patellar fossa and ectopia lentis is a type of subluxation with intact but stretched zonules. Common risk factors are listed in Box 50.1.

Risk Factors (Box 50.1)

Box 50.1: Risk factors of dropped lens nucleus or lens matter.

A. Complicated cataract surgery (most common): Post posterior capsular rent or Bag dialysis
B. Trauma
C. Spontaneous dislocation (Fig. 50.1)
1. *Anterior*: Weill-Marchesani syndrome with microspherophakia
   - Spherophakia
   - Malignant glaucoma
   - Phacomorphic glaucoma
   - Ectopia lentis due to Marfan syndrome/homocysteinuria/other rare causes
2. *Posterior*: Ectopia lentis due to Marfan syndrome/homocysteinuria/other rare causes
   - Pseudoexfoliation syndrome
   - Hypermature cataract
   - Chronic uveitis
D. *Rare causes*: Idiopathic, electric injury, use of ocriplasmin, vitrectomized eye

Role of an Anterior Segment Surgeon

Lens matter drop occurs most frequently during nucleus chopping, when an accidental rupture of posterior capsule may occur. It may also occur while hydrodissection in a posterior polar cataract and white or mature cataract. Another important cause is accidental posterior capsular tear when a spontaneous tear in the capsule during capsulorrhexis extends to periphery in intumescent cataracts (Argentinian flag sign). Thus, these high risk situations should be taken into account during preoperative evaluation. A written informed

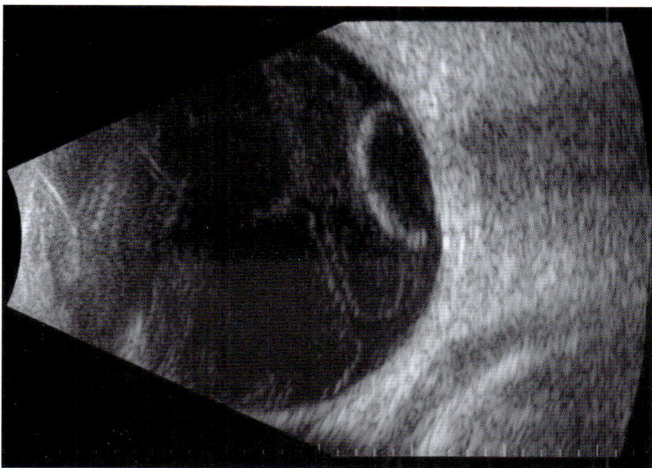

Fig. 50.2: Ultrasonography (USG) B-scan showing posteriorly dislocated lens in the vitreous cavity.

consent should be taken from the patient explaining the risk of lens drop, which may require the surgeon to leave patient aphakic and may require a n additional surgery, e.g. pars plana vitrectomy, secondary IOL implantation, etc.

Complications are a part and parcel of any surgery but the outcomes depend on how well surgeon manages them. Despite adequate precautions, if the operating surgeon notices any lens matter sinking to the posterior segment, *no attempts should be made to fish out posteriorly migrating fragments*, as it increases the chances of future retinal detachment via a retinal break through vitreous pull. The first and foremost steps are stabilization of anterior chamber with dispersive viscoelastics such as Viscoat, decreasing bottle height thereby decreasing the irrigation pressure and *call for help/ vitreoretinal opinion*.

Anterior vitrectomy should be done so that there are no vitreous strands in the wound or touching endothelium. Vitreous visibility can be increased with diluted triamcinolone. If sulcus is available, a single piece polymethymethacrylate (PMMA) lens with large optic or a three-piece posterior chamber intraocular lens (PCIOL) should be placed in sulcus and wound closed with 10-0 nylon. In case of deficient anterior capsular rim, patient can be left aphakic. If vitreoretinal backup is available, then pars plana vitrectomy with phacofragmentation can be completed in the same sitting and if the latter is not available then patient should be explained and referred to a vitreoretinal surgeon.

In case the lens is only subluxated, then use of capsular tension rings (CTRs) and Cionni rings have been described which are used in 3–6 and more than 6 clock hours of subluxation, respectively. For more than 9 clock hours of subluxation, an intracapsular cataract extraction (ICCE) is recommended.

Clinical Manifestations

Inflammation caused due to dropped lens matter is directly proportional to its size and manipulation done during the cataract surgery. Delayed referral may also worsen the situation. Usually patient complains of "no visual improvement" or "visual loss" after cataract surgery and a constant large floater in the superior field which may change its position with posture. On slit-lamp examination, one can find corneal edema, anterior chamber reaction and vitreous strands. Extensive inflammation may lead to an increase in intraocular pressure. Fundus examination with retinal periphery screening should be done as peripheral retinal breaks may occur due to vitreous pull.

Indications for Surgical Intervention

- *Extensive inflammation*: Should be initially controlled with corticosteroids both oral and topical, even intravenous pulse therapy can be given in rare cases of intense inflammation. If there is no improvement within 2–3 days then an intervention is indicated.
- *Size of nuclear fragment:* Dropped fragment of size more than 2 mm or volume more than 20% of total nucleus should be removed even in the absence of inflammation.[3] Smaller fragments can be sequentially observed with careful follow-up as there is always a minimal risk of retinal detachment.
- *Secondary glaucoma:* Uncontrolled glaucoma with multiple anti-glaucoma medications is another important indication. Prostaglandin analogs should not be used as they increase the inflammation as well as the risk of macular edema.
- Retinal detachment and endophthalmitis along with dropped lens matter are indications for early intervention.

Medical treatment comprises of topical antibiotics, steroids, cycloplegics, antiglaucoma medications and hyperosmotic agents (5% sodium chloride).

Surgical Technique (Figs. 50.3 and 50.4)

A 23G or 25G pars plana vitrectomy with posterior vitreous detachment (PVD) induction is primarily required before entering with a 20G fragmatome (Fig. 50.4)—the posterior segment ultrasonic fragmenter designed for removing harder pieces of the lens nucleus. An alternative to this fragmatome, used by some surgeons, is a phacoemulsification probe with an amputated sleeve. Fragmatome cannot cut vitreous and thus a thorough vitrectomy is required prior to its introduction in the eye (Figs. 50.3A to C). After a complete vitrectomy and release of lens fragments all around, the lens fragments tend to settle at the posterior pole. In this scenario, perfluorocarbon liquid (PFCL) can be used to float the nucleus away from the retina prior to engaging the fragment (Fig. 50.3D). It helps the surgeon in two ways: firstly, it decreases the force with which lens matter hits the macula and more importantly it dampens the phacoemulsification energy reaching the macula. If PFCL is not available, then phaco power should not go beyond 50% and vacuum must not exceed beyond

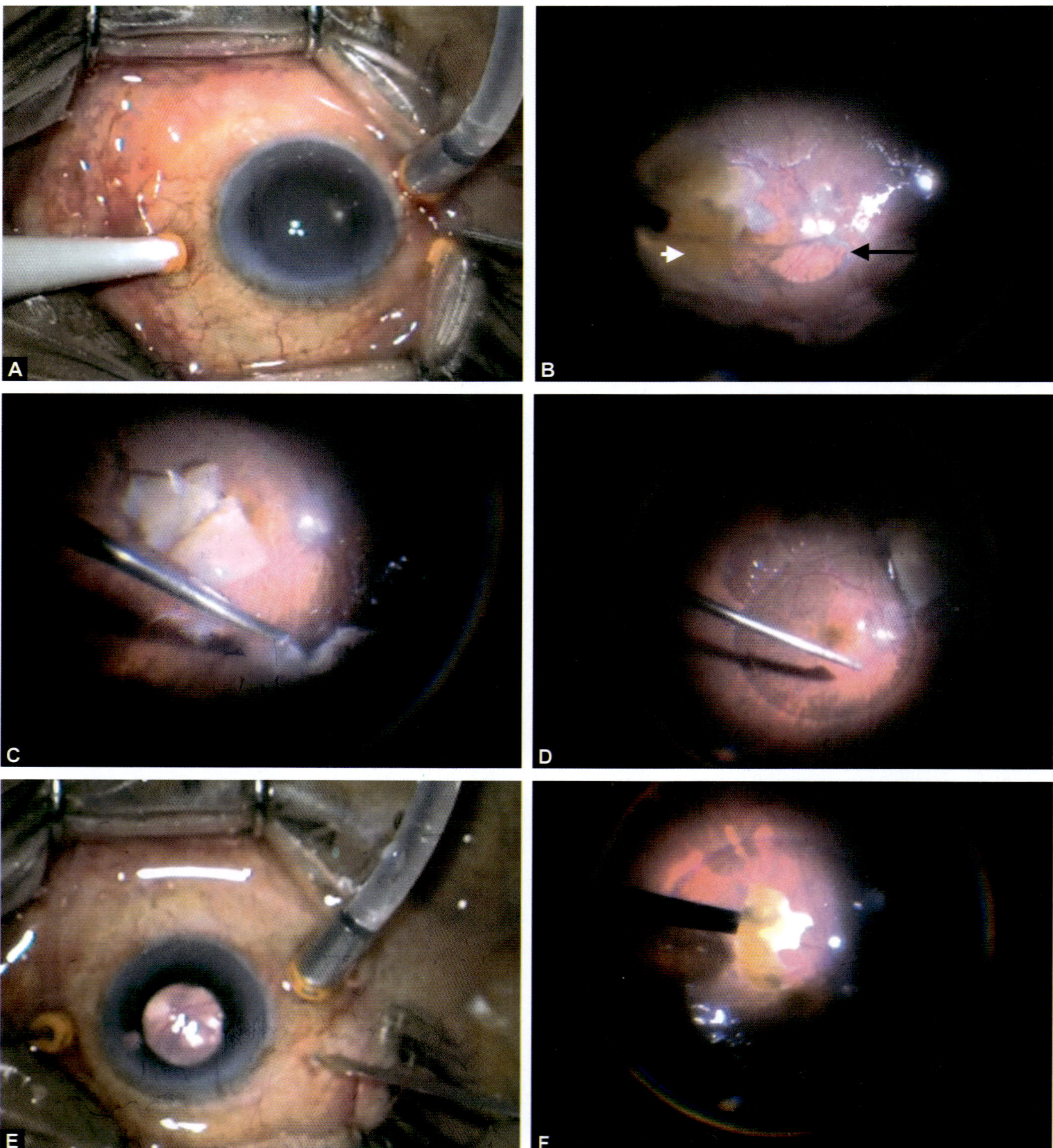

Figs. 50.3A to F: Technique of phacofragmentation surgery: (A) Standard 23G pars plana ports (B) Triamcinolone assisted posterior vitreous detachment (PVD) (Weiss ring : Black arrow) with dropped nucleus matter in vitreous (white arrowhead) (C) Complete peripheral vitrectomy (D) Injection of perfluorocarbon liquid (PFCL). (E) Sclerotomy being enlarged to accomodate the 20G phacofragmatome. (F) Impaled phaco tip into lens matter during phacofragmentation.

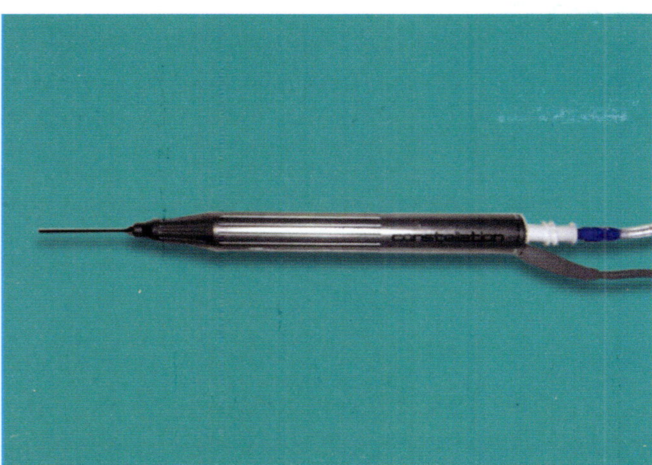

Fig. 50.4: 20G probe used for phacofragmentation with constellation vitrectomy system (Constellation Vision System, Alcon Laboratories, Inc., Forth Worth, TX, USA).

80 mm Hg. Many authors have described similar prognosis even without the use of PFCL.[4]

After vitrectomy, superotemporal port can be removed and extended with a microvitreoretinal (MVR) blade or a new MVR entry can be made just above the superotemporal port (Fig. 50.3E). Then intravitreal 20G fragmatome is used, and nucleus matter is fragmented and aspirated with power settings of 50–70% and vacuum settings of 80–150 mm Hg (Fig. 50.3F), while if only cortical matter is present, it can be cut and easily aspirated with vitrectomy cutter itself. After removal of lens fragments, it is mandatory to check the entry site as there can be associated retinal tear which should be lasered.

Other techniques described are:

- Perfluorocarbon liquid-assisted levitation of dropped nucleus and delivery via corneal wound which is generally used for advanced cataracts which require very high phaco power.
- Endoilluminator-assisted chopping described at our center in which endoillumination probe is used to divide the lens bimanually along with fragmatome which reduces the required phaco power.[5]

Visual rehabilitation can be done with multipiece or 6.5 mm PMMA PCIOL in sulcus, if anterior capsular rim is intact and anterior chamber intraocular lens (ACIOL) or scleral fixated intraocular lens (SFIOL), if the sulcus is deficient depending on the size of constricted pupil. If the specular microscopy reveals endothelial cell count less than 1,000/mm^3, it is best to leave eye aphakic and rehabilitate patient with the use of aphakic glasses or contact lenses.

Prognosis and Postoperative Complications

Prognosis is very good with visual acuity better than 20/40 in 60–80% cases but a lot depends on the initial management by the anterior segment surgeon.[6] According to a study at our center, there was no difference between cases of nucleus drop operated early (<2 weeks) and late (>2 weeks) after the complicated cataract surgery when visual acuities were compared. Also, pseudophakic status at the time of fragmentation was found to cause relatively less endothelial cell loss (Unpublished data).

Complications of Phacofragmentation Surgery

- Glaucoma
- Corneal edema
- Persistent inflammation
- Retinal detachment

POSTERIORLY DISLOCATED INTRAOCULAR LENS

Displacement of intraocular lens (IOL) from its normal location (in the capsular bag) may occur, varying from decentration to dislocation into the vitreous cavity. This may occur at the time of cataract surgery, or it may develop in the postoperative period.

Intraoperative dislocation occurs if IOL is inserted in the presence of large posterior capsular defect or IOL haptic gets misplaced. Early postoperative dislocation occurs few days or weeks after surgery and results from spontaneous IOL haptic rotation away from area of posterior capsule support or dehiscence of zonules. Late dislocation, months or years after surgery, generally occurs following trauma or spontaneous loss of zonular support.[7]

Intraocular lens dislocation has been reported to occur in 0.2–2.8% of cataract surgeries. A retrospective cohort study identified a cumulative risk of IOL dislocation following cataract extraction of 0.1% after 10 years, 0.2% after 15 years, 0.7% after 20 years, and 1.7% after 25 years.[8]

Pathophysiology

Intraocular lens dislocation can be subdivided into early and late dislocation (Table 50.1). Early dislocation occurs within 3 months of cataract surgery, whereas late dislocation occurs more than 3 months after cataract extraction.[9]

Clinical Features

Patients with dislocated IOLs present with variable symptoms.

- Patients may complain of decreased vision, glare, diplopia, streaks of light, haloes, photosensitivity and ghost images.
- Pain and red eye due to inflammation are more common complaints in patients with ACIOL decentration than PCIOL dislocation.
- Decentration causes unwanted optical images caused by either a centering hole or the edge of the optic within the pupil.
- Freely mobile IOL in the vitreous cavity may lead to an unusual complaints of floaters or optical effects or sometimes can develop into pupillary block glaucoma.

Table 50.1: Pathogenesis and causes of early and late intraocular lens (IOL) dislocation.

	Early cases	*Late cases*
Time following cataract surgery	<3 months	≥3 months (even years after uncomplicated cataract surgery)
Pathogenesis	Inadequate IOL fixation within the secure capsular bag	Progressive zonular insufficiency and capsular bag contraction
Predisposing factors	Tearing of the posterior capsule and rupture of the equatorial zonules	Aging, pseudoexfoliation syndrome, high myopia, uveitis, trauma, retinitis pigmentosa, diabetes mellitus, atopic dermatitis, connective tissue disorders, and previous vitreoretinal surgery or acute angle-closure glaucoma attack

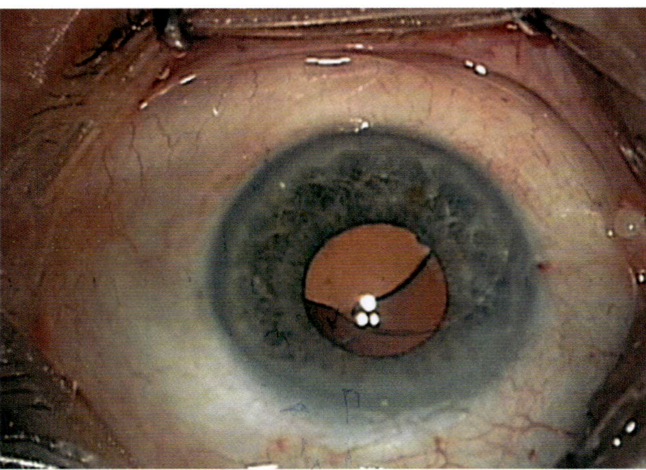

Fig. 50.5: Clinical photograph showing posteriorly dislocated intraocular lens (IOL) with one haptic adherent to iris.

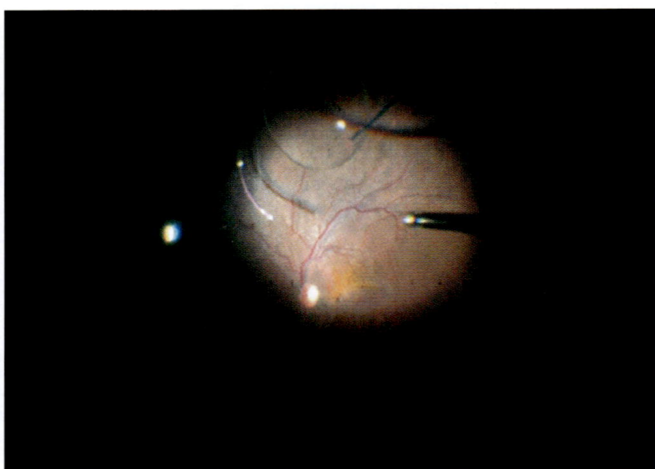

Fig. 50.6: Posteriorly dislocated intraocular lens (IOL) with retinal detachment.

- A sudden loss of vision can occur with dislocated IOL secondary to uncorrected aphakia, retinal detachment, cystoid macular edema, or vitreous hemorrhage.

Posteriorly dislocated IOL usually lies meshed into the anterior vitreous with one haptic still adherent to the capsule or iris (Fig. 50.5).

Therefore, it may cause a vitreous hemorrhage by mechanical damage to ciliary blood vessels. Posterior dislocation of IOL may cause retinal detachment (Fig. 50.6) or cystoid macular edema secondary to vitreous changes and traction.

Preoperative Evaluation

The key points that should be looked into are:
- Best corrected visual acuity in aphakic state
- Corneal status including corneal clarity and specular microscopy
- Intraocular pressure
- Iris and pupil status with white-to-white diameter (if ACIOL is planned after PCIOL explants)
- Residual capsular rim support and its extent (if IOL repositioning in sulcus is planned)
- Dilated posterior segment evaluation including peripheral examination for retinal breaks/dialysis/detachment
- Mobility and fixation points of IOL
- Axial biometry-axial length and keratometry (if IOL exchange is planned).

Management

Observation

Observation may be recommended for dislocated IOLs if following conditions are met:
- Patient is asymptomatic
- There is no evidence of inflammation
- The IOL is not mobile
- There are no retinal complications, and
- Patient is satisfied with aphakic spectacle correction or contact lenses.

Also observation can be considered when patient has other comorbid medical and ocular conditions which prohibit further surgical intervention or if the patient elects not to pursue further surgery.

In case of decentered PCIOL where symptoms of visual discomfort are limited to evening due to dilated pupil, these patients can be treated conservatively by using a topical miotic such as pilocarpine 0.5–1%. Such patients should be given a trial of miotic before considering IOL repositioning or removal.

Indications for Surgical Intervention

Decentered IOL: Treatment should include repositioning, explanting, or exchanging the decentered IOL.[10] Patient's symptoms, visual demands, and expectations are the factors which play a pivotal role in deciding the approach.

Intraocular lens reposition: This should be attempted if sufficient capsule and intact zonules are present to support the IOL. A helpful maneuver is the *bounce test* where the optic is pushed gently towards each haptic to ensure spontaneous recentration. Alternatively IOL can be repositioned with help of McCannel sutures (trans-iris fixation).

Intraocular lens explantation: IOL explantation without secondary IOL implantation may be required in certain cases.

Intraocular lens exchange: Wrong IOL power calculation is the most common indication for exchange of an IOL. Also deformed IOL due to uneven capsular fibrosis may make simple rotation inefficient to properly recenter the IOL. The IOL may be exchanged for an ACIOL, a sulcus-fixated IOL with or without McCannel sutures, a trans-scleral sutured PCIOL, or a posterior iris-claw IOL.[11]

Dislocated intraocular lens: Surgical removal of dislocated IOL should be considered when there is visual loss, inflammation, retinal detachment and vitreous incarceration in the cataract wound associated with cystoid macular edema.

Several surgical options like IOL removal, exchange or repositioning can be considered. Repositioning of the IOL into the ciliary sulcus or over capsular remnants with less than a total of 6 clock hours of inferior capsular support is not a stable situation. Trans-scleral suturing of IOL is recommended in these cases. CTR may also be found migrated posteriorly with or without bag and IOL complex, which has to be removed via anterior chamber or sclera (Fig. 50.7).

Various Techniques for Retrieval of IOL

Assisted levitation: In 1996, Kelman proposed a technique for retrieving nuclear fragments or dislocated IOLs into the anterior vitreous through a pars plana sclerotomy called as posterior-assisted levitation with the insertion of a cyclodialysis spatula, a needle, or a viscosurgical device.[12] However, this maneuver can be complicated with retinal detachment or cystoid macular edema and should not be performed in current scenario.

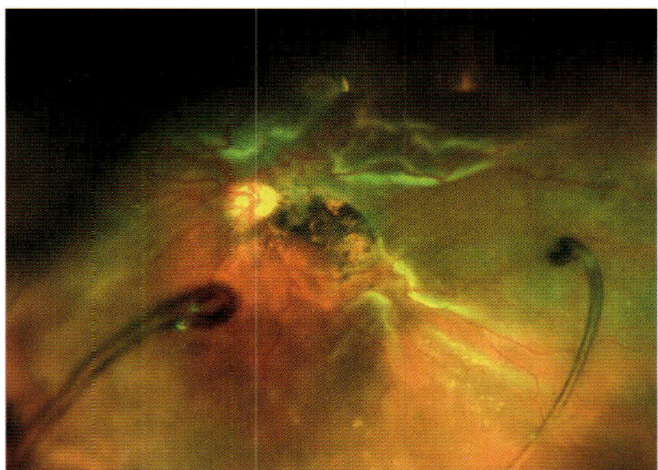

Fig. 50.7: Dropped capsular tension ring with total rhegmatogenous retinal detachment (RRD) seen on color fundus image.

Vitrectomy followed by forceps-assisted removal: If trans-scleral suturing of the IOL is planned, modifications are made into the usual placement of the sclerotomies. Two triangular-shaped scleral flaps are made which are 180° apart across the horizontal meridian. Then, two sclerotomies are made under the flaps 1–1.5 mm posterior to the limbus. The infusion cannula is sutured to the usual position. Thorough vitrectomy is performed and especially removing all vitreous and capsular attachments to the IOL, making it freely mobile. The posterior hyaloid is separated from retina, if still attached. This allows the IOL to gently fall over the posterior pole of the eye.

If positioning holes are present, the IOL may be engaged through them by the pick or hook. After elevating the IOL in the mid-vitreous cavity, it is held by its optic using end grasping forceps or diamond-coated forceps. The IOL can then be repositioned in the sulcus or the IOL can then be delivered into the anterior chamber followed by its removal through a limbal incision.

Perfluorocarbon liquid-assisted retrieval: Liquid perfluorocarbons can also be used to float the IOL at the pupillary plane and then remove it through limbal incision.[13] It is generally advised to perform a thorough vitrectomy which includes separation of the posterior hyaloid from retina, before PFCL is injected. PFCL floats up the IOL. It is then grasped from a limbal approach and delivered. It can also be repositioned in the sulcus, if there is sufficient capsular remnant. Whenever PFCL is used, the IOLs tend to shift laterally, because the upper surface of the PFCL bubble in the eye is convex thereby not allowing IOLs to be in the middle where convexity is the highest. Thus, the IOL slides off to periphery and gets engaged with residual vitreous and damages peripheral retina. Therefore, a moderately thorough shaving of the vitreous base should be carried out prior to any attempts to float the lens. If a retinal detachment is present, PFCLs become very useful. The PFCL bubble helps in attaching the retina by displacing the subretinal fluid out through the retinal break, displaces the subretinal fluid through the retinal breaks reattaching the retina. It also cushions the retina by preventing direct contact between the retina and the IOL.

Other Techniques

Silicone soft-tipped cannula can be used for manipulating the IOL but it may cause inadvertent vitreoretinal traction, hence is not used.

Intraocular lens repositioning: Once the IOL is engaged, it is elevated to bring it to the posterior chamber and one of the haptics can be placed in front of the iris, the other in the sulcus. Subsequently, the IOL can be rotated into place through a limbal stab incision using a sinskey hook. The IOL can be positioned in the sulcus without any suturing if more than 6 clock hours of inferior capsular support is present; otherwise intrascleral haptic fixation, trans-scleral or iris sutures have to be put.

Intraocular lens exchange: An IOL with a broken haptic or optic must be removed through a limbal incision or pars plana route. Removal through the pars plana comes with the increased risk of choroidal bleeding and retinal detachment. In such cases the surgeon has the choice of suturing a posterior IOL or inserting an ACIOL.

In certain cases, in addition to the posteriorly dislocated IOL, an ACIOL may be present making the surgical management more difficult, especially, if associated with a retinal detachment. The ACIOL can be removed and the dislocated IOL can then be repositioned in the sulcus or sutured or the ACIOL can be reinserted. Another option is to remove the dislocated IOL through the pars plana route and leave the ACIOL in situ.

REFERENCES

1. Mathai A, Thomas R. Incidence and management of posteriorly dislocated nuclear fragments following phacoemulsification. Indian J Ophthalmology. 1999;47(3):173-6.
2. Freissler K, Küchle M, Naumann GO. Spontaneous dislocation of the lens in pseudoexfoliation syndrome. Arch Ophthalmology. 1995;113(9):1095-6.
3. Fastenberg DM, Schwartz PL, Shakin JL, et al. Management of dislocated nuclear fragments after phacoemulsification. Am J Ophthalmology. 1991;112(5):535-9.
4. Verma L, Gogoi M, Tewari HK, et al. Comparative study of vitrectomy for dropped nucleus with and without the use of perfluorocarbon liquid. Clinical, electrophysiological and visual field outcomes. Acta Ophthalmology Scand. 2001;79(4):354-8.
5. Kumar V, Takkar B. Intravitreal phacoemulsification using torsional handpiece for retained lens fragments. J Ophthalmic Vis Res. 2016;11(3):268-70.
6. Borne MJ, Tasman W, Regillo C, et al. Outcomes of vitrectomy for retained lens fragments. Ophthalmology. 1996;103(6):971-6.
7. Schneiderman TE, Johnson MW, Smiddy WE, et al. Surgical management of posteriorly dislocated silicone plate haptic intraocular lenses. Am J Ophthalmology. 1997;123(5):629-35.
8. Pueringer SL, Hodge DO, Erie JC. Risk of late intraocular lens dislocation after cataract surgery, 1980–2009: A Population-Based Study. Am J Ophthalmology. 2011;152(4):618-23.
9. Davis D, Brubaker J, Espandar L, et al. Late in-the-bag spontaneous intraocular lens dislocation: evaluation of 86 consecutive cases. Ophthalmology. 2009;116(4):664-70.
10. Jakobsson G, Zetterberg M, Sundelin K, et al. Surgical repositioning of intraocular lenses after late dislocation: complications, effect on intraocular pressure, and visual outcomes. J Cataract Refract Surg. 2013;39(12):1879-85.
11. Gonnermann J, Klamann MK, Maier AK, et al. Visual outcome and complications after posterior iris-claw aphakic intraocular lens implantation. J Cataract Refract Surg. 2012;38(12):2139-43.
12. Schutz JS, Mavrakanas NA. Posterior-assisted levitation in cataract surgery. Curr Opin Ophthalmology. 2010;21(1):50-4.
13. Yu Q, Liu K, Su L, et al. Perfluorocarbon liquid: its application in vitreoretinal surgery and related ocular inflammation. BioMed Res Int. 2014;2014:250323.

Chapter 51

Postoperative Endophthalmitis

Chaitra Jayadev, Raghav Ravani, Atul Kumar

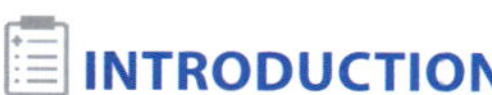 INTRODUCTION

An intraocular inflammation which predominantly affects the inner spaces of the eye and their contents, i.e. the vitreous and/or the anterior chamber which is either infectious or noninfectious in origin. Most cases are exogenous where the organisms are introduced into the eye via trauma, surgery, or an infected cornea. Endogenous endophthalmitis occurs when the eye is seeded via the bloodstream. Patients will usually have systemic manifestations of the underlying disease but sometimes present only with eye symptoms. In endophthalmitis, the infection remains confined to the eye and does not serve as a source of bacteremia or fungemia. However in panophthalmitis, infection spreads from the globe of the eye to the adjacent soft tissues of the orbit. Most cases of endophthalmitis present acutely, within hours to a few days of symptoms. Endophthalmitis is a medical emergency, as delay in treatment may result in permanent vision loss.

CLASSIFICATION

The classification of endophthalmitis is described in Flowcharts 51.1 and 51.2.

ENDOPHTHALMITIS BURDEN

A study of 278 patients with culture proven endophthalmitis presenting in a 6 years period from 1996 to 2001 at the Bascom Palmer Eye Institute, Miami, Florida, USA reported acute postoperative endophthalmitis in 103 of 278 (37%), chronic postoperative endophththalmitis in 97 of 278 (35%), total postoperative endophthalmitis in 200 of 278 (72%), posttraumatic in 37 of 278 (13%), and endogenous in 22 of 278 (8%). Remaining causes being miscellaneous (e.g. keratitis) and unknown.[1]

A tertiary eye care hospital in eastern India found 107 patients of endophthalmitis between December 2006 and January 2009, out of which 46 (43.0%) patients had postoperative (PO), 43 (40.2%) had post-traumatic (PT) and 18 (16.8%) had endogenous (EG) endophthalmitis.[2]

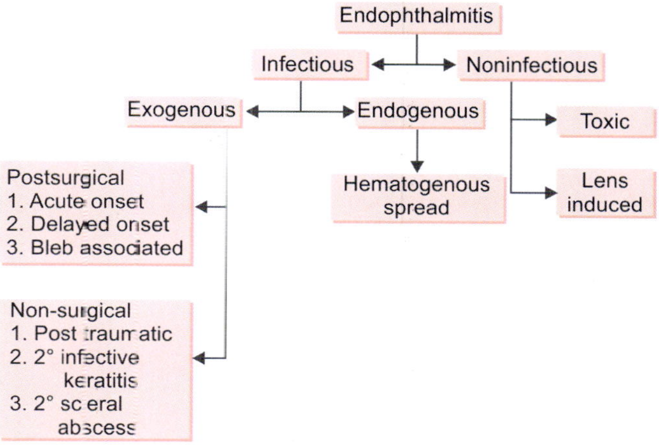

Flowchart 51.1: Classification of endophthalmitis (based on etiology).

Flowchart 51.2: Classification of endophthalmitis based on presentation and causative organism

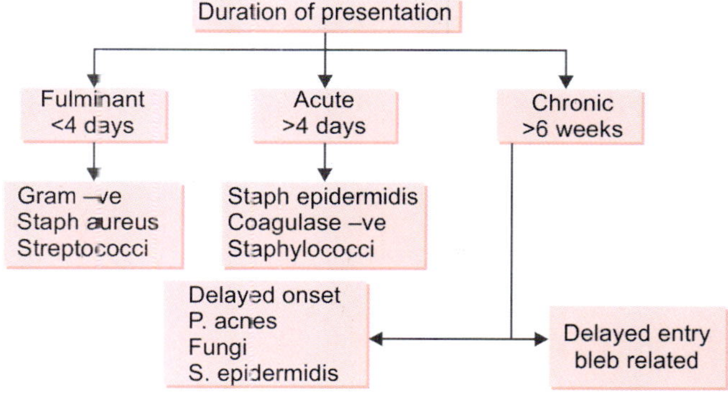

A study reported 955 patients with endophthalmitis in a period between January 1997 and December 2006. Out of the 955 patients, 625 (65.45%) were cases of postoperative endophthalmitis, 217 (22.72%) were post-penetrating ocular injuries and 71 (7.43%) were cases of endogenous

endophthalmitis. Other causes were endophthalmitis post-microbial keratitis and post-scleral abscess. 424 (44.4%) of the 955 cases were culture proven cases of endophthalmitis.[3]

Jambulingam et al.[4] in their study of postoperative cases of endophthalmitis from 2000 to 2007, reported 98 such cases, the distribution of which according to the onset was as follows: acute onset endophthalmitis cases—90 in number, out of which 67 were post-cataract, 8 were post-PKP and 15 were post other intraocular surgeries. Late onset (after 6 weeks) cases were 8 in number, out of which 3 were post-cataract, 2 were post-PKP and 3 were post other intraocular surgeries.

Global rates of endogenous endophthalmitis have been reported to be approximately 2–8% of all cases of endophthalmitis.[5]

Chakrabarti et al. reported 113 cases of fungal endophthalmitis from their center from January 1992 to December 2005. They categorized them into: post-cataract surgery (53 patients), post-trauma (48 patients), and endogenous (12 patients) groups. *Aspergillus* species was the most common (54.4%) agent isolated.[6]

Kim et al.[7] reported a total of 40 eyes from 30 patients with fungal endophthalmitis who presented at their center over a period from January 2007 to October 2013. *Candida* species were the most common causative organism in 35 of the 40 eyes. Endogenous and exogenous endophthalmitis were observed in 33 and 7 eyes, respectively.

POST-CATARACT ENDOPHTHALMITIS

Various factors have played significant role in lowering the rate of endophthalmitis in post-cataract patients.

Intracameral injection of antibiotics (e.g. cefuroxime, moxifloxacin etc.) as prophylaxis against endophthalmitis is commonly employed world-over now.

European Society of Cataract and Refractive Surgeons (ESCRS) have reported a decrease in endophthalmitis rates in nine European countries from 0.35% before prophylactic intracameral cefuroxime injection to 0.05% after its use. Similar findings have been noted in various other reports (Table 51.1).[19]

POST-INTRAVITREAL INJECTION ENDOPHTHALMITIS

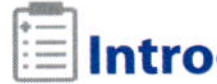 ### Introduction

Intravitreal injections have a very important place in management of exudative age-related macular degeneration (ARMD), diabetic macular edema, edema due to venous occlusions and many other conditions. The drugs that are most commonly administered by the intravitreal route are anti-vascular endothelial growth factors (VEGFs) and steroids. The anti-VEGF drugs most commonly used are bevacizumab and ranibizumab. The steroids most commonly used are triamcinolone acetonide and dexamethasone implant for its longer duration of action. Ranibizumab is supplied directly by the manufacturer in individual vials for intraocular use. Bevacizumab is widely used off-label to treat these same diseases, it is not available as single dose vials and therefore for economic purposes it is routinely aliquoted into ready-to-use syringes by compounding pharmacies or at the institution of administration.

The most dreaded complication following intravitreal injection or following any intraocular surgery for that matter is endophthalmitis. VanderBeek et al. reviewed 406,380 injections in 75,249 patients in a large national US medical claims database performed between 2003 and 2012. There were

Table 51.1: Postcataract endophthalmitis.

Study	Date of collection	Number of cases	%	Location
Leopold[8]	1920–1940	Meta-analysis	2	
Allen and Mangiaracine[9]	1958–1962	22/20,000	0.09	
Aaberg[10]	1984–1994	34/41,654	0.07	
West[11]	1994–2001	1,026/477,627	0.21	
Jensen[12]	1997–2007	40/29,276	0.14	
Moshirfar[13]	2003–2005	14/20,013	0.07	
Freeman[14]	1996–2005	754/510,690	0.15	
Jambulingam[4]	2000–2007	70/131,904 45 in PKE, 20 in ECCE, 5 in SICS	0.053	Southern India
Ravindran[15]	2007–2008	38/42,426	0.09	Southern India
Sheng[16]	1995–2009	140/233,115	0.06	China
Wykoff[17]	1995–2009	8/28,568	0.03	
Levison[18]	2011	Meta-analysis	0.001–0.3	Global

(PKE: Phacoemulsification cataract extraction; ECCE: Extracapsular cataract extraction; SICS: Small incision cataract surgery).

Table 51.2: Percentage of Endophthalmitis as reported in various trials.

Study (Year)	Percentage of endophthalmitis
MARINA (2006)[23]	0.05%
ANCHOR (2009)[24]	0.05%
RISE (2012)[25]	0.038%
RIDE (2012)[25]	0.038%
DRCR.net (2007)[26]	0.05%
SCORE (2007)[26]	0.05%
CATT: Ranibizumab (2012)[27]	0.04%
CATT: Bevacizumab (2012)[27]	0.07%

Table 51.3: Culture status in global cases of endophthalmitis.

	Bevacizumab	Ranibizumab
Endophthalmitis cases	103	79
Cases cultured	94	57
Culture positive	30	24
Culture negative	64	33

Table 51.4: Endophthalmitis in US and Europe.

	US	Europe
Injections	172,991	119,477
Endophthalmitis cases	80 (0.046%)	33 (0.028%)
Cases cultured	77 (96.25%)	21 (63.64%)
Culture positive cases	22	8
Culture negative cases	55	13

73 (rate = 0.019% or 1/5,283 anti-VEGF injections) and 24 (rate = 0.13% or 1/778 steroid injections) cases of endophthalmitis among anti-VEGF and steroid injections, respectively. They reported that the odds ratio (OR) for endophthalmitis occurring after steroid injection was 6.92 (95% confidence interval, 3.54–13.52, p <0.001) times higher than with anti-VEGF injections.[20]

A review of 534 English language articles of varying design, published from 2006 to November 2013, reported global endophthalmitis risk following intravitreal anti-VEGF injections. Out of a total of 445,503 anti-VEGF injections, endophthalmitis was seen in 0.058% (103 in 176,124) of bevacizumab injections versus 0.029% (79 in 269,379) of ranibizumab injections.[21]

A tertiary care center in southern India reported the rate of endophthalmitis following anti-VEGF (bevacizumab and ranibizumab) and intravitreal triamcinolone acetonide (IVTA) injections between January 1, 2010, and December 31, 2014. A total of 17,359 intravitreal injections were administered between January 2010 and December 2014, which included 9,932 bevacizumab injections, 4,108 ranibizumab injections, and 3,319 IVTA injections. Of the 17,359 intravitreal injections administered, 13 (0.07%) eyes presented with clinical features of endophthalmitis. Endophthalmitis was noted in 8 (0.08%) cases after bevacizumab, 1 (0.02%) case after ranibizumab, and 4 (0.12%) cases after IVTA.[22] There have been reports of sporadic cases of endophthalmitis following intravitreal Ozurdex injections. Endophthalmitis rates as reported across various landmark trials are given in Table 51.2.

Etiology

Sigford et al.[21] in their study have discussed the various organisms isolated from the endophthalmitis cases and also the rate of culture negative cases.

Organisms isolated from culture positive cases were *Staphylococcus epidermidis*, coagulase-negative *Staphylococcus*, *Staphylococcus aureus*, Streptococcus species, *Enterococcus faecalis*, *Haemophilus influenzae*, Haemophilus (unspecified), *Propionibacterium acnes*, unknown organisms etc. with Staphylococcus species being the most common causative organism (Tables 51.3 and 51.4).

A study of 13 cases of endophthalmitis postintravitreal injection found 3 patients showing Gram positive cocci and 3 showing Gram-negative bacilli; with KOH stain being negative for all the patients. In 5 of the patients, PCR was positive. Four of these patients were positive for eubacterial genome, and 1 patient was positive for both Eubacterium genome and Propionibacterium acnes. Out of the 4 patients who showed culture positivity, three cases showed Staphylococcus organism and one showed *Acinetobacter calcoaceticus*. They were sensitive to vancomycin, gentamicin, clindamycin, and cefotaxime. However, ceftazidime was resistant in 3 of the 4 cases and penicillin in 1 of the 2 cases. They had a cluster endophthalmitis of 5 patients all of whom were culture and Gram staining negative. On bacteriological evaluation of the vial for these cases, Burkholderia was isolated.[22]

In a study, 17 out of the 199 cases of endophthalmitis were following intravitreal injections of anti-VEGF agents. It represented 8.5% of endophthalmitis (17/199 cases). Intraocular cultures yielded positive results in 75% of postinjection cases, with the majority associated with coagulase-negative Staphylococcus. Consistent with prior literature, a case of *Streptococcus viridans* displayed more rapid onset and progression. Details were available for 16 patients only. Ten cases were post-bevacizumab injection and 6 post-ranibizumab injection.[28]

There is an increase in streptococcal endophthalmitis following intravitreal injections compared with that following cataract surgery.[29,30]

Recently, a majority of patients from a cluster of 21 patients referred to our tertiary care center suffering from postinjection endophthalmitis following injection of bevacizumab from a single vial showed *Stenotrophomonas maltophilia* as the causative agent. The organism was also isolated from the vial, and is an emerging nosocomial infection causing endophthalmitis.[31]

A recent publication from our center described safe and effective guidelines for intravitreal use of bevacizumab in Indian scenario and reinforced the best practice guidelines formulated and issued by VRSI (Vitreo Retina Society of India), AIOS (All India Ophthalmological Society), and Dr Rajendra Prasad Centre for Ophthalmic Sciences, AIIMS New Delhi, India to avoid such dreaded complications like cluster endophthalmitis especially with use of bevacizumab.[31]

Risk Factors

Type of injection plays a role in the incidence of endophthalmitis as mentioned earlier. Intravitreal steroids have increased incidence of postprocedure infection as opposed to intravitreal administration of anti-VEGF. Intravitreal bevacizumab (available as 100 mgs/ml multidose vial) has higher incidence of infection compared to intravitreal ranibizumab due to compounding of bevacizumab as multiple injections can be administered from a single vial of the same.

As shown in epidemiology section the incidence of endophthalmitis is more with intravitreal steroid injections as compared to intravitreal anti-VEGF injections.

Site of injection also plays an important role in predisposing an eye to endophthalmitis. Roth et al.[32] used 10,834 injections in 1302 eyes of 1017 patients. 33 eyes were injected directly superiorly, 8038 superotemporally, 700 superonasally, 1970 inferotemporally, 87 inferonasally, and 6 eyes directly inferiorly. Five eyes developed presumed infectious endophthalmitis; two of which grew positive bacterial cultures from the vitreous samples. Four of the five (80%) eyes with endophthalmitis were injected inferiorly, even though 80.9% of the total study cohorts were injected superiorly. The risk ratio associated with inferior location is 17.0 (95% confidence interval: 1.9 to >100) with a p-value = 0.011.

A study reported that none of the lid speculum use, conjunctival displacement or hemisphere of injection affected risk of endophthalmitis.[33] McCannel[34] suggested that the surgical field may be contaminated by oropharyngeal flora. Wen et al. subsequently showed that speaking from above while injecting produces more bacterial colonies on a blood agar culture plate than speaking while wearing a surgical mask.[35]

Presentation

The mean duration between the injection and time of presentation was 4 days (range, 1–14 days). The common presenting symptoms are decreased visual acuity, pain, and redness in all the patients (Fig. 51.1). The most common signs are hypopyon, corneal edema, vitritis and increased intraocular pressure. A study reported presence of diabetes as a common potential predisposing risk factor. They had five cases of

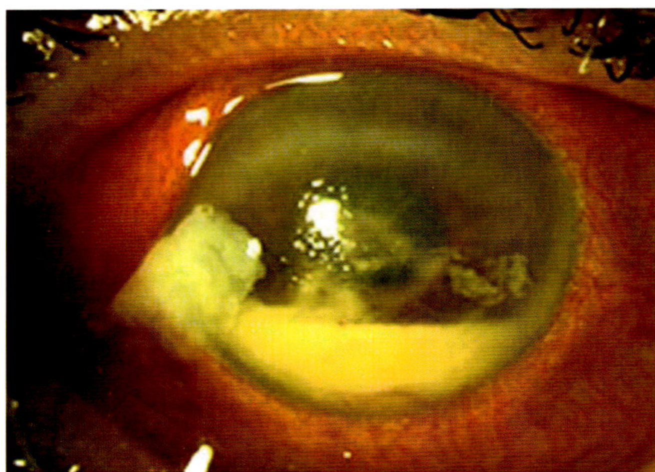

Fig. 51.1: Acute onset endophthalmitis postintravitreal injection.

cluster endophthalmitis where intravitreal bevacizumab was given from the same vial to five patients.[22]

Diagnosis and Prevention

There have been some reports of culture-negative sterile endophthalmitis after intravitreal bevacizumab injection for different retinal pathologies, resembling toxic anterior segment syndrome (TASS-like) seen after intraocular surgery.[36-38] A case series of such patients presenting with sterile endophthalmitis following intravitreal injection and successful treatment with intravitreal antibiotics along with topical antibiotics and steroids has been reported from our center, highlighting the possibility of sterile endophthalmitis following intravitreal injection of bevacizumab and its management.[39] However, *Streptococcus viridans*, a component of human oral flora has been reported to be present three times more often in postinjection endophthalmitis (PIE) as compared to postsurgical endophthalmitis.[40] Thus, PIE has early presentation and worse prognosis, especially with *Streptococcus viridans*. The incidence is especially more in office-based setting as compared to the operating-room setting. An ultrasound B-scan will confirm the inflammatory component of the condition along with choroidal thickness, vitreous membranes or retinal detachment. AC tap, vitreous tap or a vitreous biopsy can be taken to ascertain the microorganism causing endophthalmitis and treatment is given accordingly. Proper preoperative screening, intraoperative precautions (Figs. 51.2A to D) and sterilization (Figs. 51.3A and B) helps to reduce the incidence of endophthalmitis.

The compounding of the bevacizumab drug increases the risk of postprocedural endophthalmitis. Various ways have been described for using the drug.[41]

Preoperative Precautions

- A written informed consent explaining the procedure and the risks involved is to be taken. The use of off label

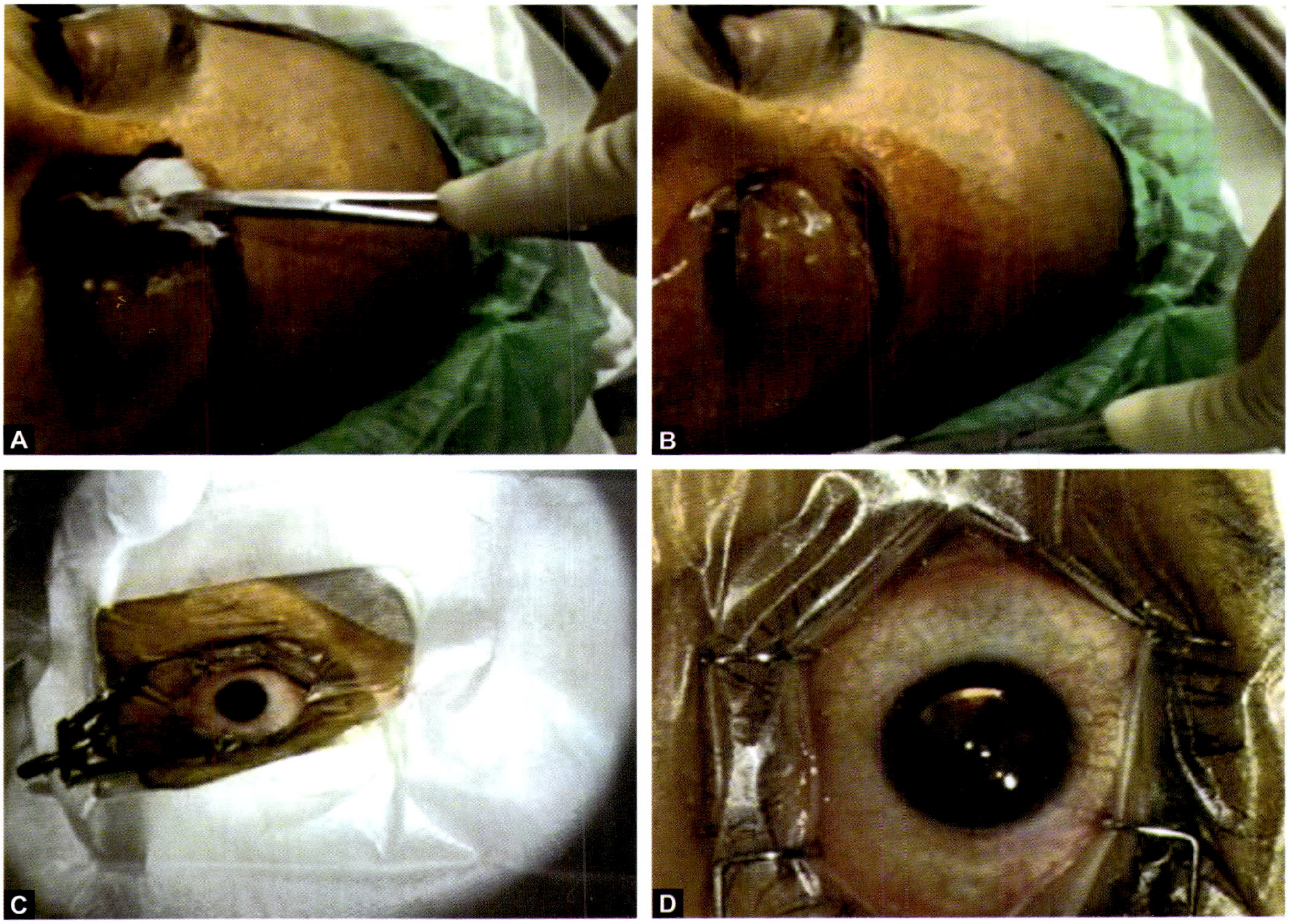

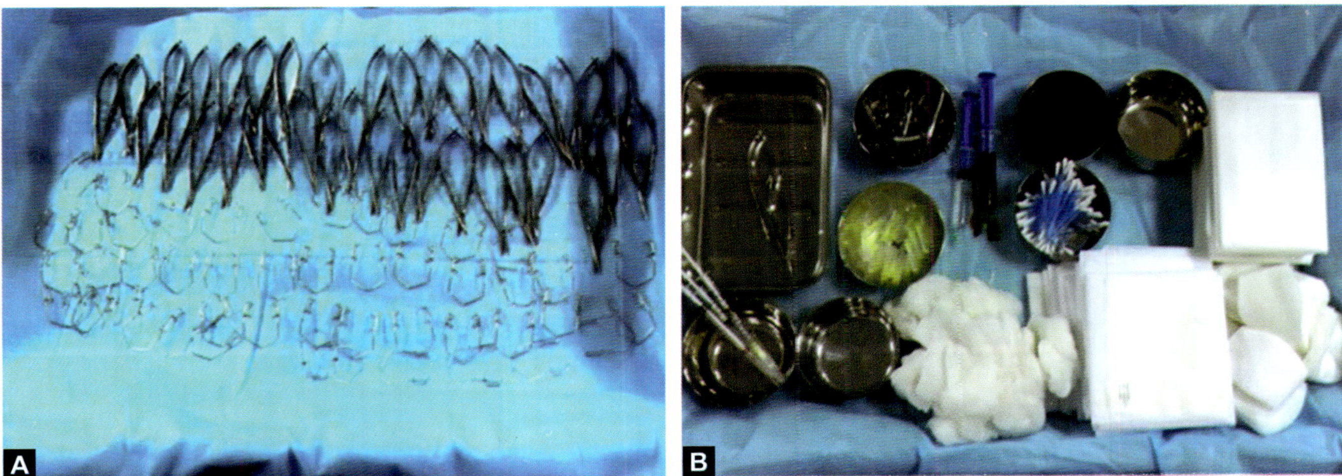

Figs. 51.2A to D: Image showing proper proper cleaning and draping before intravitreal injection.

Figs. 51.3A and B: Image showing sterile instruments (one for each patient) (A) and arrangement of instrument trolley in operating room for intravitreal injection at a tertiary center (B).

drugs has to be included and explained to the patient. Thorough preoperative screening and control of risk factors like localized adnexal infection or systemic condition are mandatory

- Each patient should be given clean OT gown, protective cap, and shoecover before entering the preoperative holding area/OT
- In the preoperative holding area/or on table, the periocular skin should be cleaned with povidone-iodine 10% solution
- Surgical/procedural time-out to verify patient's name, intravitreal agent, and laterality should be practiced before injection in each patient
- Bilateral injections are not recommended. Injection in the other eye should be spaced at least one to 2 weeks apart
- *Prophylactic topical antibiotics*: There is a lack of evidence to support pre-, peri-, or postinjection topical antibiotics. In fact, one of the studies showed a trend toward higher incidence.[42] However, a short course of postprocedure prophylactic antibiotic may be used on surgeon's personal experience and discretion.

Intraoperative Precautions

- *Location:* The procedure should be performed in an OT setting, and not in an office setting[30]
- *Cleaning and draping:* Use 10% povidone-iodine to clean skin and ocular adnexa, 5% povidone-iodine for instillation into cul-de-sac with contact time of at least 3 minute. Drape the surgical area using sterile linen and a single use plastic eye drape
- A speculum should be used to prevent contact of the eyelashes and eyelid margins with the injection site and the needle
- Topical anesthetic drops should be preferred over anesthetic gel as the latter may interfere with povidone-iodine contact with the conjunctiva/injection site
- Reapply povidone-iodine after anesthetic drop use. The last agent to be applied before injection should be povidone-iodine (5%)
- The surgeon/staff/patient should minimize speaking on table during preparation or during the injection procedure to minimize the spread of aerosolized droplets containing oral contaminants (e.g. *Streptococcus viridans*)[30,43]
- Conjunctival displacement and quadrant chosen for injection have no effect on the risk of infection[33]
- Routine anterior chamber paracentesis is not recommended.

Drug Procurement

- Drugs should be purchased from authorized dealers with proper receipt
- Batch number of each vial should be noted in a register before opening the vial and the records should be maintained which might help to track before opening it

- Cold chain should be maintained at each stage (2–8°C, never freeze the vial), especially at dealer's storage facility, transport to the hospital and in the hospital with proper temperature log maintenance.

Multiple Injections from One Vial (Bevacizumab)

Numerous trials performed worldwide that enrolled thousands of patients have shown similar efficacy and safety of intravitreal bevacizumab compared to other anti-VEGF. Bevacizumab being cheaper and available as 4 mL vial has an added advantage of decreasing the economic burden of treatment by significantly reducing the cost of therapy, especially in our country with limited access to resources by the population. Options for multiple injections from a vial are:[31,41]

- *Ideally:* Compounding pharmacy to prepare single-dose ampoules/aliquots. This should be practiced in sterile dispensing Good Manufacturing Practice (GMP) facility (class 10 and class 10,000 environment) under laminar flow hood. Figure 51.4 shows air curtains and laminar flow-hood facility (Class 10) at our center for sterile dispensing of bevacizumab vial into single dose ampoules (Fig. 51.5).
- Prepare multiple syringes by single puncture of vial under the laminar hood. The syringes should be stored at proper temperature in sterile container. Such syringes may be stored with minimal degradation of anti-VEGF activity.[44] Two such syringes are to be sent for culture. The syringes for injection may be used if culture is negative. Discard the stored syringes after 2 weeks.
- In case facility for the above two is not available then upto seven patients may be pooled on the day of injection. After proper scrubbing and using aseptic technique, seven aliquots of around 0.2 mL per syringe (one syringe for one patient) are to be prepared inside the OT by single puncture of the vial. The syringes are to be recapped with fresh sterile needles. Syringes are to be kept on a sterile surface. These are to be used only for the patients in the same session. Discard the vial—it is *not* to be reused or repunctured.

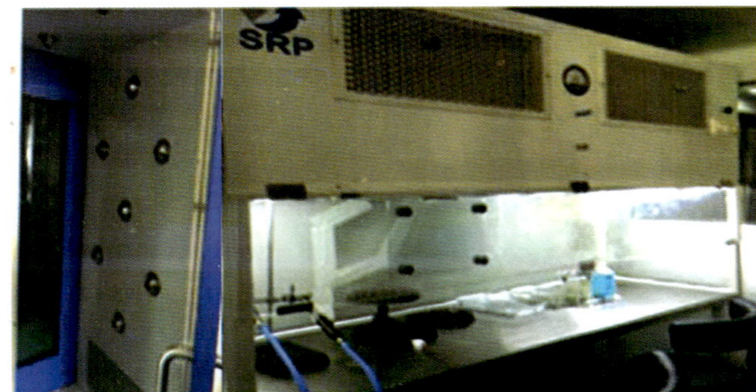

Fig. 51.4: Image showing air curtains and laminar flow hood facility at the ocular pharmacology laboratory at our center, for preparation of single dose Avastin® anti-VEGF ampoules.

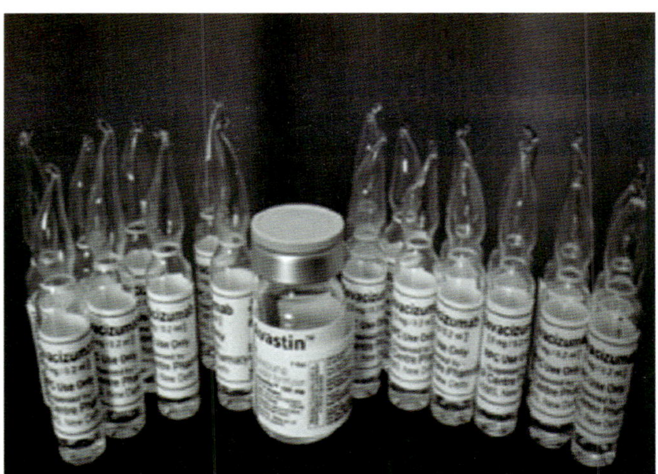

Fig. 51.5: Image shows compounding of Bevacizumab vial into single dose ampoules for individual patient use prepared at our center.

Cold chain has to be maintained. Bevacizumab can be stored at 2–8°C for 45 days. The study by Bakri et al.[44] showed that the drug can be kept in capped disposable 1 ml syringes when stored at 2–8°C with minimal loss of efficacy over 1 month.

Preparation of similar aliquots/or single injection ampoules in a sterile environment under a laminar hood is also described (Fig. 51.4). They have stressed the importance of oblique scleral entry over perpendicular injection to prevent reflux of vitreous and wick related endophthalmitis.[45-48]

Patients should be examined on postinjection day 1 and 3. Bilateral injections on the same day should not be done. If both eyes are to be injected, the second eye should be injected after a minimum of 3 days to avoid an increased level of circulating drug in the system. In patients with uncontrolled blood sugar, injections should be avoided to decrease the risk of endophthalmitis.

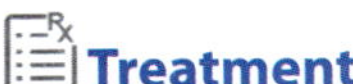

Treatment

Raman R et al. reported that 8/13 of their patients with postinjection endophthalmitis underwent vitrectomy with intravitreal antibiotics and remaining 5/13 managed with intravitreal antibiotics alone.[22]

Another report showed that all but one patient underwent primary vitreous tap with intravitreal injection of antibiotics (vancomycin and ceftazidime). Of those who underwent primary tap/inject, 6 of the 15 total underwent subsequent pars plana vitrectomy, with the decision to proceed to surgery based on persistent vitritis.[28] Treatment of postintravitreal endophthalmitis needs be tailored depending upon individual cases. The treatment in postintravitreal endophthalmitis should be more aggressive as the infection tends to be more aggressive with worse prognosis. While, intravitreal antibiotics seem to be the most common first treatment in postcataract surgery endophthalmitis, early surgical intervention should be preferred in postintravitreal endophthalmitis. With advancement and advent in surgical techniques and equipments, the aim of surgery is to achieve complete vitrectomy with PVD induction, thereby removing the infectious nidus and substantially decreasing toxic and inflammatory load.

POST-TRABECULECTOMY ENDOPHTHALMITIS

Post-trabeculectomy endophthalmitis has been classified as early or late onset with 4 weeks being taken as an arbitrary cut-off point (Table 51.5).

In a study at a single tertiary eye care institute in the period between 1996 and 2001, bleb associated endophthalmitis formed 22% (61/278) of the total cases of endophthalmitis, of which 11 cases were of acute onset and the remaining 50 were of chronic onset.[1]

POST-PPV ENDOPHTHALMITIS

An incidence of 0.046% of culture-proven endophthalmitis following pars plana vitrectomy (PPV) has been reported (Table 51.6).[52] A study reported that out of the 12 patients who developed endophthalmitis post-PPV, those presenting with acute onset were 0.043% (9/20,835) and those with chronic onset were 0.014% (3/20,835).[4] Benz et al.[1] reported a total of 5 cases of post-PPV endophthalmitis which formed 2% of the total 278 cases of endophthalmitis. All the five cases were of acute onset.

Table 51.5: Post-trabeculectomy endophthalmitis.					
Study	*Date of collection*	*Procedure*	*Total no of patients*	*Cases (%)*	*Location*
Levison[18]	Review	Overall		0.2–9.6	Global
Wallin[49]	1990–2012	Trabeculectomy ± MMC	7402	28, 0.38	Sweden
Jambulingam[4]	2000–2007	Overall	7692	2, 0.026	Southern India
Ang[50]	Review till 2010	TRAB Plain		0.2–1.5	Global
Ang[50]	Review till 2010	GDD		0.3–5.0	Global
TVT Study[51]	5 years	TRAB + MMC	105	1.9	USA

(Trab: Trabeculectomy; MMC: Mitomycin C; GDD: Glaucoma drainage device).

Table 51.6: Post-pars plana vitrectomy (PPV) endophthalmitis.

Study	Date of publication	Procedure 20 g (%)	Procedure 23 g (%)	Procedure 25 g (%)	Location
Ho and Tolentino[53]	1984	0.14 (4/2,800)			
Kuminoto and Kaiser[54]	2007	0.018 (1/5,498)		0.23 (1/3,103)	
Scott[55]	2008	0.03 (2/6375)		0.84 (11/1,307)	
Wani[56]	2009		0.12 (3/2,564)		
Oshima[57]	2010	0.034 (10/29,030)	0.054 (8/14,838)		
Jambulingam[4]	2010	Gauge not mentioned 0.057 (12/20,835)			Southern India
Wu[58]	2011	0.021 (4/19,865)	0.029 (3/10,845)	0.022 (1/4717)	
Scott[59]	2011	0.02 (1/4,403)	0.03 (1/3,362)	0.13 (1/789)	
Dave[60]	2016	3 [Total = 0.052 (20/38,591)]	15	2	Southern India

Table 51.7: Postcorneal procedures (except refractive surgeries).

Study	Date of publication	PKP (%)	Keratoprosthesis (%)	Other corneal lamellar surgery (%)	Location
Kunimoto[61]	2004	1.3 (14/1,074)			USA
Jambulingam[4]	2010	0.5 (10/1,949)			Southern India
Levison[18]	2013	0.2–0.4	0–12.5		Review (Global)
New York Eye and Ear Infirmary[62]				DSAEK-0.8% (1/126)	USA
Du[63]	2014	0.11–1.05			USA
Alshihry[64]	2014 (2006–2012)	0.254 (4/1,573)			Saudi Arabia
Behlau[65]	Review 2014 (1990–2012)		Total: 4,729 Boston I/II USA: (1–12.5) Others (upto 17%)		Global
Chen[66]	2015	0.67 (76/11,320)			UK

(PKP: Penetrating keratoplasty; DSAEK: Descemet stripping automated endothelial keratoplasty).

POSTCORNEAL PROCEDURE ENDOPHTHALMITIS

The incidence of endophthalmitis occurring within 6 weeks of surgery was 0.16% (Table 51.7).[66]

ORGANISMS CAUSING ENDOPHTHALMITIS

A series of 278 endophthalmitis from January 1996 to January 2001 isolated 313 microorganisms.[1] The distribution of organisms based on their frequency was: *Staphylococcus epidermidis*—87 (27.8%), *Streptococcus viridans*—40 (12.8%), Coagulase negative staphylococcus (CoNS)—29 (9.3%), *Staphylococcus aureus*—24 (7.7%), propionibacterium acnes—22 (7%), gram negative rods (other)—16 (5.1%) etc. The most frequent organisms that they found were: (1) acute onset postoperative: *S. epidermidis*, 46.9%; (2) delayed onset postoperative: *S. epidermidis*, 22.7%.

Organisms Causing Post-cataract Surgery Endophthalmitis

Organisms causing postcataract endophthalmitis in various studies and their distribution are described here.

Common organisms held responsible for early postoperative endophthalmitis are: CoNS, *Staphylococcus aureus*, beta-hemolytic streptococci, gram negative bacteria including *Pseudomonas aeruginosa* and fungi including Candida spp., Aspergillus spp., Fusarium spp. etc.

Organisms commonly held responsible for chronic or delayed postcataract endophthalmitis are *Propionibacterium acnes*, Corynebacterium spp., *S. epidermidis* and fungi (Tables 51.8 and 51.9).

ESCRS[67] found gram negative microorganisms in up to 35% of positive cultures, significantly higher as compared to

Table 51.8: Organisms causing post-cataract endophthalmitis.

Organisms	EVS[70]	Swedish National Study[71] (using Intracameral Cefuroxime)	China[72]	Netherlands[73]
Gram positive			73.9	
Coagulase negative *Staphylococcus*	70	26	45.5	53.6
S. aureus	10		12.4	12
Streptococcus spp.	9	7	6.2	19
Enterococcus spp.	2	31	7.2	1.8
Other gram-positive	3	6	2.6	5.2
Gram-negative	6	13	13.4	6
Fungal	—		12.7	—

Table 51.9: Organisms causing postcataract endophthalmitis (Indian).

Organisms	Jambulingam (All intraocular surgeries)[4]	Kunimoto[69]	Jindal[74]	R Ramakrishnan (all intraocular surgeries)[3]
Gram-positive		53.1	36.4	74.7
Coagulase negative *Staphylococcus*	18.6	33.3	15.2	36.89
S. aureus	11.4	—	—	3.1
Streptococcus spp.	2.9	10.3	21.2	32
Enterococcus spp.	1.4	—	—	
Other gram-positive	10	—	3	
Gram-negative	42	26.2	21.2	20
Fungal	7.1	16.7	33.3	5.3

the reported 4% in the Endophthalmitis Vitrectomy Study (EVS).[68] The incidence of postprocedure fungus endophthalmitis is variable (8–13%) and depends on the climate.[69] In tropical locations, the fungal isolates can reach upto 20% of positive cultures. The most common organisms isolated are Aspergillus and Candida spp.[55]

Gupta et al.[75] in their study of endophthalmitis cases post-cataract surgery in northern India reported a different microbiology spectrum with equivocal microbiological positivity seen in 22 (18%), bacterial 12 (10%), fungal 27 (21.5%), polymicrobial 8 (6.5%) and negative 55 (44%).

POLYMICROBIAL ENDOPHTHALMITIS

The incidence of polymicrobial infection in the report of the EVS Group was 9.3%. The incidence of polymicrobial endophthalmitis after open-globe injuries has been reported from 5.3% to 47.6%, while it has been reported to be 0.0% to 17% in various postoperative endophthalmitis series.[74]

Jindal[74] reported cases of polymicrobial endophthalmitis in their group of endophthalmitis cases from 2000 to 2010. Polymicrobial endophthalmitis was diagnosed in 43/1107 (3.88%) of the culture proven endophthalmitis cases. 42 patients grew two organisms on culture and one grew three organisms. Overall, the presenting visual acuity was light perception in 38 patients and was greater than or equal to hand motion in 5 patients. In all the patients, the organisms were isolated from the first vitreous biopsy or vitrectomy. The most common isolates were Gram positive organisms (n = 53; 60.9%) followed by Gram-negative organisms (n = 22; 25.3%) and fungi (n = 12; 13.8%). The most common organisms isolated were *Staphylococcus epidermidis* (n = 14; 16.1%) and *Streptococcus pneumoniae* (n = 13; 14.9%) The cause of endophthalmitis was open-globe injury (31/43; 72.1%), postoperative endophthalmitis (9/43; 20.9%), and endogenous endophthalmitis (3/43; 6.9%).

Gram-positive bacteria was most sensitive to vancomycin (100%) and chloramphenicol (96%). Gram-negative bacteria was most sensitive to ciprofloxacin (86.4%) and ofloxacin (81.2%).

A series of endophthalmitis in northern India reported 8 (6.5%) cases of polymicrobial endophthalmitis.[75]

Pathengay et al.[76] in their study from January 2000 to December 2007 reported 807 cases of culture proven endophthalmitis. Out of these 807 patients, 42 patients (5.2%) were found to be multidrug resistant on culture. Multidrug resistance was more common in gram-negative bacteria (33; 78.6%) compared with gram-positive bacteria (9; 21.4%). Pseudomonas spp. (24 isolates) was the most common isolated bacteria. Fifteen (45%) of the 33 gram-negative isolates were resistant to ceftazidime, 18 (54.5%) were resistant to amikacin, and 11 (33.3%) were resistant to both amikacin and ceftazidime. Five (55.56%) of the 9 gram-positive isolates were resistant to vancomycin.

Organisms Causing Post-trabeculectomy Endophthalmitis

A study reported fastidious gram-negative rods (20.4%) as the most frequently isolated microorganisms in delayed onset bleb-associated endophthalmitis. Bleb-associated endophthalmitis in this study confirmed those reports, with 28% of cases caused by streptococcal species and 25% of cases caused by gram-negative organisms.[1]

Wallin O[49] reported that the predominant organisms causing endophthalmitis in their series of patients post-trabeculectomy were staphylococci and streptococci.

In early postoperative endophthalmitis the most common pathogen is CoNS, but in late-onset infection the microorganisms are often more virulent. In 2010, Al-Turki et al. found that 79.2% of organisms were Gram-positive and 20.8% were Gram-negative. Fifty percent of the cases were due to Streptococcus spp.[77]

Other organisms causing endophthalmitis post-PPV are *S. aureus, P. stutzeri, P. aeruginosa,* Klebsiella spp. etc. The organisms causing endophthalmitis in post-PPV are given in Table 51.10.

RISK FACTORS FOR EXOGENOUS ENDOPHTHALMITIS (TABLE 51.11)

Risk Factors for Post-trabeculectomy Endophthalmitis

Anti-mitotic agents, inferior blebs, , exposed glaucoma drainage devices, young age, uncontrolled DM, periocular infections.

Risk Factors for Post-pars Plana Vitrectomy Endophthalmitis

Inadequate wound closure, hypotony, vitreous Wick syndrome, type of intraocular tamponade (like BSS), contamination of vitreous cavity.

Organisms Causing Post-traumatic Endophthalmitis and Associated Risk Factors

A study reported a total of 217 cases of endophthalmitis post-penetrating ocular injuries out of their total of 955 cases.[3] They could isolate organisms in 141 (65%) of those cases. The most commonly isolated organism was filamentous fungi (31/141). Other organisms isolated were CoNS, bacillus cereus, Pseudomonas species, Corynebacterium species, etc. Endophthalmitis can occur in up to 13% of cases of penetrating injury

Table 51.10: Organisms causing endophthalmitis in post-pars plana vitrectomy.

Reference	Year	Culture positivity rate	Culture positive cases	Predominant organism
Cohen[78]	1995	89%	16/18	CoNS
Joondeph[79]	2005	100%	5/5	CoNS
Jambulingam[4]	2010	100%	12/12	CoNS

(CoNS: Coagulase negative staphylococcus).

Table 51.11: Risk factors for exogenous endophthalmitis.

Postoperative endophthalmitis

Preoperative	*Intraoperative*	*Postoperative*
1. Active ocular surface infections	1. Posterior capsular rupture and vitreous loss	1. Wound leak
2. Blepharitis	2. Wound abnormalities	2. Inappropriately buried sutures
3. Poor hygiene	3. Contaminated fluids	3. Delaying postoperative topical antibiotics
4. Lacrimal drainage system infection or obstruction	4. Intraocular lens implantation	4. Poor hygiene
5. DM (uncontrolled)	5. Vital dyes used during surgery	
6. Chronic steroid use	6. Complicated and long duration surgery	
7. Contaminated eye drops	7. Incision size	
	8. Surgeon's experience	

Table 51.12: Organisms causing endogenous endophthalmitis.

Reference	Year	Culture positivity rate	Predominant organism	Other organisms
Benz[1]	1996–2001	22/22 (100%): Only culture proven cases taken	Aspergillus (20.8%)	—
Keswani[80]	2000–2004	8/12 (66%)	Candida (3/8)	*Aspergillus, S. aureus, S. pneumoniae, Pseudomonas, Klebsiella*
Connell[81]	1997–2007	41/64 (64.1)	Fungus (27/41) Mainly *Candida albicans*	*Staphylococcus aureus, Propionibacterium acnes, Klebsiella pneumoniae,* etc.

to the globe. Specifically, those with pure corneal injuries, intraocular foreign bodies, lens rupture, or needle-related injuries have a higher incidence. Most objects that penetrate the eye are contaminated with infectious agents as the trauma usually occurs in a non-sterile environment with the highest risk being in the rural settings.

Traumatic endophthalmitis is usually caused by staphylococcal, streptococcal, and *Bacillus* species. *B cereus* is specifically known to occur with traumatic cases causing a severe infection. A history of penetrating trauma with intraocular foreign body contaminated with organic matter implicates Bacillus species.

Individuals at risk for developing endogenous endophthalmitis usually have comorbidities that predispose them to infection (Table 51.12). These include conditions such as diabetes mellitus, chronic renal failure, cardiac valvular disorders, systemic lupus erythematosus, AIDS, leukemia, gastrointestinal malignancies, neutropenia, lymphoma, alcoholic hepatitis, and bone marrow transplantation.

Invasive procedures, which may result in bacteremia, such as hemodialysis, bladder catheterization, gastrointestinal endoscopy, total parenteral nutrition, chemotherapy, and dental procedures, also can lead to endophthalmitis.

Recent nonocular trauma or surgery, prosthetic heart valves, immunosuppression, and intravenous drug abuse may predispose to endogenous endophthalmitis.

Sources for endophthalmitis include meningitis, endocarditis, urinary tract infection, and wound infection. Additionally, pharyngitis, pulmonary infection, septic arthritis, pyelonephritis, and intra-abdominal abscess also have been implicated as source of infection.

Upto 50% of cases of endogenous endophthalmitis can occur due to fungi.[5] *Candida albicans* is by far the most frequent cause (75–80% of fungal cases). Aspergillosis is the second most common cause of fungal endophthalmitis in west however in Indian subcontinent *Aspergillus* is most common, especially in IV drug users. Less frequent are other candidal species and Torulopsis, Sporotrichum, Cryptococcus, Coccidioides, and Mucor species.

S. aureus is the most common gram-positive organism, usually seen with chronic systemic diseases and skin infections. The other common gram-positive organisms isolated are *Streptococcus pneumoniae, Streptococcus viridans,* and group A streptococci. Other streptococcal species, e.g. group B in newborns with meningitis or group G in elderly patients with wound infections or malignancies, also have been isolated. *Bacillus cereus* has been implicated in intravenous drug abuse and intravenous injections. *Clostridium* species is seen in association with bowel carcinomas.

Among gram negative bacteria, *E coli* is the most common. However, *Haemophilus influenza, N. meningitidis, Klebsiella pneumoniae,* Serratia species, and *Pseudomonas aeruginosa* also can cause endogenous endophthalmitis.

Nocardia asteroides, Actinomyces species, and *Mycobacterium tuberculosis* are acid-fast bacteria that may cause endogenous endophthalmitis.

PATHOGENESIS

Exogenous Endophthalmitis

The pathogenesis of exogenous endophthalmitis is given in Flowchart 51.3.

Endogenous Endophthalmitis

The pathogenesis of endogenous endophthalmitis is given in Flowchart 51.4.

CLINICAL FEATURES

Bacterial endophthalmitis usually presents acutely with decreased visual acuity, pain, redness and lid swelling. Also, some bacteria (e.g. *Propionibacterium acnes*) may present with a more chronic course and milder symptoms. This organism is typical of skin flora and usually is inoculated at the time of intraocular surgery.

Fungal endophthalmitis present with an indolent course over days to weeks. Symptoms are decreased visual acuity and pain. A history of penetrating injury with an organic matter like plant substance or soil-contaminated foreign body may often be elicited. Individuals with candidal infection may present with high fever, followed several days later by ocular symptoms. Persistent fever of unknown origin (FUO) may be associated with an occult retinochoroidal fungal infiltrate.

Flowchart 51.3: Pathogenesis of exogenous endophthalmitis.

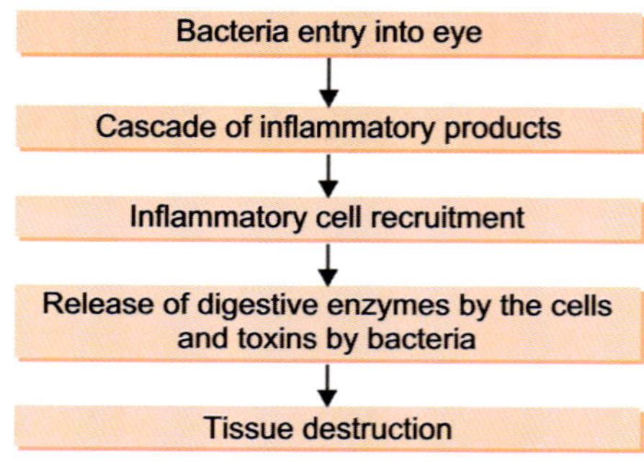

Flowchart 51.4: Pathogenesis of endogenous endophthalmitis.

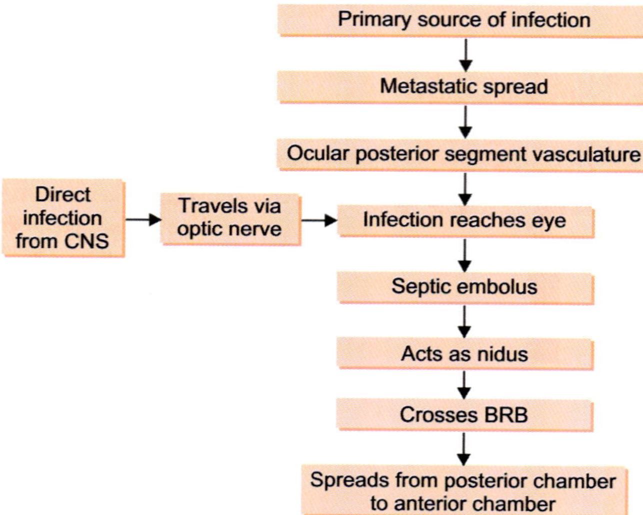

(CNS: Central nervous system; BRB: Blood retinal barrier)

Table 51.13: Timeline of postsurgical endophthalmitis.

No. of days postoperatively	EVS[60]	ESCRS[59]
0–3 days	24%	31%
4–7 days	37%	31%
8–13 days	17%	24%
2–6 weeks	22%	14%

(EVS: Endophthalmitis Vitrectomy Study; ESCRS: European Society of Cataract and Refractive Surgeons).

History of ocular surgery, ocular trauma, and hammering steel, working with baling wire, or working in an industrial setting may be elicited.

In cases of postsurgical endophthalmitis, infection most often occurs approximately 1 week after surgery but may occur months or years later as in the case of *P. acnes* (Table 51.13).

Symptoms

Symptoms may include the following:
- Decrease in vision
- Pain and irritation in the eye
- Headache
- Photophobia
- Ocular discharge
- Redness in the eye
- Visual symptoms in any hospitalized patient or patient taking immunosuppressive therapy.

Signs

Ocular signs correlate with the structures involved and degree of infection or inflammation. A thorough eye examination should be performed which includes visual acuity, external examination, fundoscopic examination, and slit-lamp examination. Urgent referral to an ophthalmologist skilled in handling cases of endophthalmitis should be considered as the patient may be found febrile on systemic examination. The following ocular signs should be looked for:.
- Eyelid swelling and erythema
- Injected conjunctiva and sclera
- Chemosis
- Hypopyon
- Cells and flare in the anterior chamber on slit-lamp examination
- Vitritis
- Reduced or absent red reflex
- Proptosis (a late finding in panophthalmitis)
- Papillitis
- Cotton-wool spots
- Corneal edema and infection
- White lesions in the choroid and retina
- Chronic uveitis
- Vitreal mass and debris
- Purulent discharge

Note: Absence of pain and hypopyon do not rule out endophthalmitis, particularly in the chronic indolent form of *P. acnes* infection.

In cases of endogenous endophthalmitis, the attending ophthalmologist needs to further evaluate the patient for the underlying source of infection.

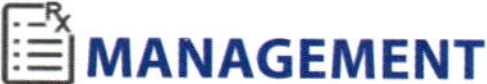 MANAGEMENT

Endophthalmitis Vitrectomy Study[68]

The study was conducted between January 1990 and January 1994. It was a prospective, randomized, multicenter trial on 420 eyes to determine whether it is necessary to use systemic antibiotics in acute postoperative endophthalmitis or to perform immediate vitrectomy. The cases were divided into four categories:

	Vitrectomy	*No vitrectomy*
IV antibiotics	106	100
No IV antibiotics	112	102

Advantages of Doing a Prompt Vitrectomy

- Improves retinal oxygenation
- Diagnostic: provides a large specimen for diagnostic evaluation
- Allows definite treatment at a time when the organism (and its virulence) is still unknown (i.e. antibiotic selection is based on statistical probability, not on case-specific information)
- Decrease the inflammatory load in the vitreous cavity
- Allows direct inspection of the retina by removing the nontransparent medium, thereby permitting timely treatment of coexisting or developing pathologies
- Increases the access to the retina of intravitreally administered pharmacological agents
- Reduces the duration of the disease, thus accelerating visual rehabilitation
- Reduces the incidence and severity of retinal, especially macular complications.

Advantages of Doing a Delayed Vitrectomy

- Easier to operate on a non-inflamed eye
- Less friable tissue
- Better visualization

The EVS evaluated the role of immediate PPV versus intraocular antibiotic injection and systemic antibiotics in the treatment of acute postoperative endophthalmitis. Acute postoperative endophthalmitis (presenting within 6 weeks) and secondary IOL implantation patients who were having an initial visual acuity between 20/50 and light perception, and had a view sufficient to perform a vitrectomy were included in the study. 420 patients were randomized to immediate initial TAP or vitrectomy. There was no difference in final visual outcomes in patients who underwent initial TAP or vitrectomy if presenting visual acuity was better than light perception. However, in patients presenting with light perception vision, those who underwent initial vitrectomy were three times more likely to achieve 20/40 vision or better, twice as likely to maintain 20/100 vision or better, and had a nearly 50% reduction in the risk of severe visual loss (< 5/200), compared to patients who underwent TAP. No long-term difference occurred in media clarity between the treatment groups.

Pitfalls of EVS

Endophthalmitis Vitrectomy Study included postcataract patients when ECCE was performed at much higher rate which is not the case now when ECCE surgeries are more or less obsolete.

Hand movements were checked at a distance of 2 feet with source of light being behind the patient. The patient had to appreciate hand motion at least 4 times out of 5 to be labeled the same or else he was labeled to have a vision of light perception only. This technicality might have caused the patients with vision better than light perception to be included in the early vitrectomy group.

EVS included endophthalmitis cases where the cornea was clear enough to visualize the iris and so the more severe forms of endophthalmitis were not included which could have led to better visual outcomes.

EVS excluded patients with postoperative endophthalmitis who underwent any procedure other than cataract surgery, so the results cannot be generalized to every case of endophthalmitis.

Chronic postoperative endophthalmitis (caused by *P. acnes* or fungus) was also excluded in EVS.

EVS included intravenous amikacin and ceftazidime to check the effect of these drugs on their subset of endophthalmitis and found that they were not effective. Newer generation systemic antibiotics can achieve good concentration inside the eye and helps in reducing the infection with a good outcome.

Technological advancements in vitreoretinal surgery since EVS (MIVS systems etc.) have minimized the risks associated with vitrectomy favoring the initial use of vitrectomy in less severe cases also.

Guidelines from EVS

According to the EVS, vitrectomy was reserved for the most severe cases, and this vitrectomy was limited to core vitrectomy and no attempt should be made to excise the cortical vitreous.[6]

Complete and Early Vitrectomy for Endophthalmitis (CEVE) Study[82]

Argument for complete vitrectomy: In the EVS, no attempt was made to induce a vitreous detachment if there was no vitreous detachment at the time of surgery and the posterior cortical vitreous was not aggressively removed (Fig. 51.6). The goal of surgery was to remove at least 50% of the vitreous gel in eyes with no vitreous separation. The part that is left behind is the posterior half. Detaching the posterior hyaloid allows complete removal of the pus and debris that have accumulated on the macula, what is termed as macular hypopyon, as contrary to popular belief, the posterior vitreous cortex remains attached to the retina in the majority of cases hence there is also a high incidence of vitreoschisis in these cases.

APPROACH AND MANAGEMENT OF A CASE OF INFECTIVE ENDOPHTHALMITIS

1. History of presenting illness
a. *Predisposing event:* Surgery; trauma; endogenous; contiguous spread (corneal ulcer, scleral abscess)
b. *Onset:* Fulminant, acute, sub-acute or chronic
c. *Progression:* Rapid or gradual

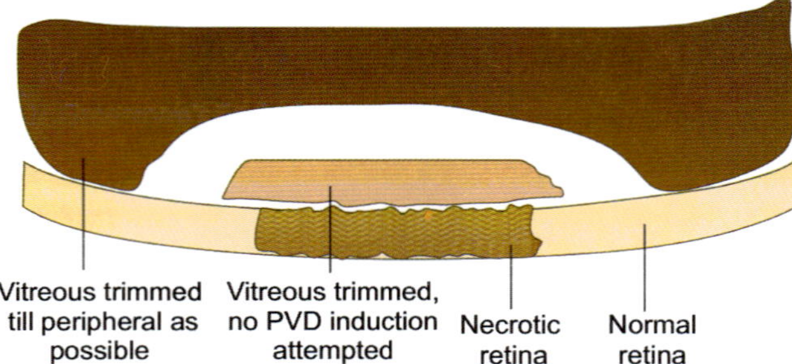

Fig. 51.6: Schematic diagram for vitrectomy in endophthalmitis.

d. *Symptoms*: Pain, redness, diminution of vision, watering
e. *Systemic illness/personal history*: Uncontrolled diabetes, hospitalization, abscesses (most commonly in liver), intravenous drug abuse, chronic debilitating diseases, mode of injury.

2. Workup

a. Ophthalmic evaluation
  i. Best corrected visual acuity
  ii. Examination of the lids and adnexa
  iii. Examination of surgical wounds (clear corneal or scleral tunnel, bleb, side ports, sclerotomies and trauma sites for entry wounds and foreign bodies)
  iv. Anterior segment examination
  v. Intraocular pressure
  vi. Extraocular movements to rule out onset of panophthalmitis
  vii. Dilated fundus evaluation
  viii. Ultrasound B scan in case of hazy media to look for vitritis, retinal detachment, choroidal thickness, T-sign, choroidal detachment, retained lens fragments and or retained intraocular foreign body
  ix. Written informed consent for further management
  x. Anterior chamber tap (for initial microbiological evaluation)
  xii. Initiate empirical therapy (systemic, intravitreal, topical in combination)
  xiii. Admit and close watch
b. Inform the patient and relatives about the seriousness of the condition
c. Inform the concerned medical staff (surgeon, nursing staff, operation theater staff)
d. In case of endophthalmitis post-intravitreal injection, records of the vial used and the patients injected upon on the same day/from the same vial/in the same operation theater should be noted and if need arises other patients who have not presented to the clinic should be called up for evaluation.

3. Perform anterior chamber tap

  i. Explain the procedure to the patient in detail.
  ii. Check the written and informed consent.
  iii. Wash hands thoroughly and air dry (preferred).
  iv. Wear gloves, clean the periocular area with povidone iodine scrubs.
  v. Put proparacaine eye drops (avoid lignocaine, as this is bacteriostatic).
  vi. Apply lid speculum.
  vii. Plan the site of tap based on AC depth, visibility, ease of access and the area of maximum exudation.
  viii. With patient looking in primary gaze, introduce 30G/27G needle through the selected site on the limbus tangentially in a lamellar fashion, keeping direction oblique over the iris surface (avoid direction towards lens).
  ix. With active suction, aspirate as much aqueous and exudates/hypopyon as possible (without collapsing the AC) (approximately 0.1–0.2 mL).
  x. Apply cotton tip applicator and withdraw the needle.
  xi. The syringe can be sent in a sterile transport tube to the microbiology laboratory.
  xii. Administer the intravitreal antibiotics (as per the initial smear report/empirical if a delay is expected in reporting) and patch with topical povidone iodine.
  xiii. The patch should be removed after half an hour and topical medications started.

4. Delivering intravitreal antibiotics

  i. In continuation to the steps mentioned in 3 (i–vi).
  ii. Prepare the intravitreal injections fresh maintaining adequate sterility.
  iii. Mix the drug thoroughly with a small air bubble to dissolve the antibiotic with solvent.
  iv. Remove the air completely and dispose the excess drug to prepare the required amount.
  v. In phakic/pseudophakic eye: With 30G needle directed toward the mid-vitreous cavity, enter through pars plana (pars plicata in children less than 1 year of age) and inject the required amount of drug (loaded in 1 mL tuberculin syringe).
  vi. In aphakic eye: Limbal entry with antibiotic injected into the vitreous cavity through the anterior chamber.
  vii. Apply cotton tip applicator to the injection site, examine the fundus and check the eye pressure digitally.
  viii. AC paracentesis may be needed if the IOP is high and a second injection is needed.
  ix. Label the antibiotic vial and store in refrigerator (do not freeze).
  x. To be used within 3–5 days of preparation (either for topical or repeat intravitreals).
  xi. *In the bag technique*:
    a. In case of subacute endophthalmitis with suspected *Propionibacterium acnes* colonies sequestered in the capsular bag, a 27G needle can be directly introduced from the opposite quadrant at the limbus, the anterior capsule is gently lifted and sequestered organisms are aspirated.
    b. The intravitreal antibiotics can also be directly injected in the capsular bag behind the IOL after gently lifting

Table 51.14: Dosage of intravitreal antibiotics.

S. No.	Antibiotic (available dose)	Intravitreal dose (per 0.1 mL)
1.	Vancomycin (500 mg)	1 mg
2.	Ceftazidime (1,000 mg)	2.25 mg
3.	Amikacin (250 mg/2 mL)	125 µg
4.	Amphotericin B (50 mg)	5 µg
5.	Voriconazole (200 mg)	50–100 µg
6.	Imipenem (250 mg)	50–100 µg
7.	Piperacillin/Tazobactam (2.25 g)	225 µg
8.	Ticarcillin (with clavulanate) (3.1 g)	3,000 µg

the anterior capsule with the needle, taking care to inject small quantities and avoiding sudden injection (to prevent rupture of the capsular bag).

Dose alterations: Vitrectomized eyes (increased frequency/daily injections intravitreally), silicone oil filled eyes (half dose injections intravitreally, due to compartmentalization), pediatric age group (half volumes injected, due to smaller globe volumes) (Table 51.14).

5. Vitreous tap
a. To be avoided (or performed with utmost care) in phakic non-vitrectomized eyes.
b. Indicated in recurrent/nonresolving endophthalmitis in a vitrectomized eye.
c. Use a sterile 27G needle with 2 cc or 5 cc syringe, enter through pars plana, aspirate gently (0.2–0.3 mL approximately), avoiding forceful suction.
d. Keeping the same needle in situ (vitrectomized eye tends to collapse after vitreous tap), the syringe is disconnected and antibiotic loaded tuberculin syringe can be connected and injected to avoid repeat entry sites.

6. Vitreous biopsy
a. Planned along with vitrectomy (20/23/25G).
b. Initial vitreous specimen without turning on the infusion fluid (undiluted sample).
c. Approximately 0.3–0.5 mL of vitreous sample is collected.
d. Techniques:
   i. 5 mL syringe is connected to suction port of vitrectomy cutter, gentle manual aspiration is applied by the assistant along with vitrectomy. The syringe can be sent in a sterile container to the microbiology lab.
   ii. Instructor technique (Insight instruments, Inc., Stuart, FL): one port vitrectomy (23G) technique (portable, battery powered vitrectomy system), using the illumination from the operating microscope or the indirect ophthalmoscope, used for collection of vitreous sample in selective cases.

iii. Microbiological evaluation of the filter (rarely)/cassette used during vitrectomy.

Consent for evisceration to be taken in fulminant cases or cases with no light perception at presentation with detailed explanation to the patient and relatives prior to performing the surgery.

7. Microbiology
a. Samples:
   i. Aqueous: AC tap
   ii. Vitreous: Vitreous tap/Vitreous biopsy.
   iii. Others: IOL (with/without bag contents), IOFB, suture, abscised iris tissue, collection from the vitrectomy cassette.
   iv. After collection of sample, the air in the syringe is expelled and the needle is mounted into a sterile rubber cork placed in a large sterile test tube container, sealed and sent to the laboratory for smear and culture.
   v. In case of other material, the collected specimen is to be sent in a sterile bottle without any solution or preservative.
b. *Culture media*
   i. For isolation of aerobic bacteria and fungi:
      A. Solid media: blood agar, chocolate agar, MacConkey agar, Sabouraud's dextrose agar.
      B. Liquid media: brain heart infusion broth.
   ii. For isolation of anaerobic bacteria:
      A. Solid media: Brucella blood agar.
      B. Liquid media: thioglycollate broth.
c. *Inoculation and sending the samples to microbiology laboratory*
   i. One drop each to be carefully inoculated (not to be spread) in agar media in the center of the plate and into the Brain heart infusion broth and thioglycolate broth.
   ii. It is essential that the inoculation of media is done first (since the number of microorganisms are likely to be low, every chance needs to be given to them to multiply and grow in the culture media)
   iii. Growth for anaerobic microorganisms and fungus is observed for 12 days.
   iv. Samples in odd hours may be inoculated in Brain heart infusion broth and thioglycollate broth and kept at room temperature, 25–30°C (with label). The remaining sample can also be capped onto the needle and kept in the refrigerator at 4°C compartment to be transported at the earliest (for PCR and making smears).

Role of Systemic Antibiotics and Steroids

Systemic antibiotics (antibacterials/antifungals) play a key role in the management of endogenous endophthalmitis. Since the half-life of intravitreal antibiotics is short, the systemically administered antibiotics are given to maintain therapeutic levels for prolonged periods. The investigations including the samples for microbiology tests should ideally be sent before starting systemic antibiotics on empirical basis.

Steroids are important in combating the intraocular inflammation that is particularly severe due to the release of toxins from the infecting organisms. Steroids are to be used judiciously in patients with diabetes and active Koch's infection and are contraindicated in fungal endophthalmitis.

REFERENCES

1. Benz M, Scott I, Flynn H, et al. Endophthalmitis isolates and antibiotic sensitivities: a 6-year review of culture-proven cases. Am J Ophthalmology. 2004;137(1):38-42.
2. Sharma S, Padhi TR, Basu S, et al. Endophthalmitis patients seen in a tertiary eye care centre in Odisha: a clinicomicrobiological analysis. Indian J Med Res. 2014;139(1):91-8.
3. Ramakrishnan R, Bharathi M, Shivkumar C, et al. Microbiological profile of culture-proven cases of exogenous and endogenous endophthalmitis: a 10-year retrospective study. Eye. 2008;23(4):945-56.
4. Madhavan H, Jambulingam M, Parameswaran S, et al. A study on the incidence, microbiological analysis and investigations on the source of infection of postoperative infectious endophthalmitis in a tertiary care ophthalmic hospital: an 8-year study. Indian J Ophthalmology. 2010;58(4):297.
5. Sadiq M, Hassan M, Agarwal A, et al. Endogenous endophthalmitis: diagnosis, management, and prognosis. J Ophthalmic Inflamm Infect. 2015;5:32.
6. Chakrabarti A, Shivaprakash M, Singh R, et al. Fungal endophthalmitis. Retina. 2008;28(10):1400-7.
7. Kim D, Moon H, Joe S, et al. Recent Clinical manifestation and prognosis of fungal endophthalmitis: a 7-year experience at a tertiary referral center in Korea. J Korean Med Sci. 2015;30(7):960.
8. Leopold I. Incidence of endophthalmitis after cataract surgery. Trans Ophthalmology Soc UK.1971;191:575-609.
9. Allen HF, Mangiaracine AB. Bacterial endophthalmitis after cataract extraction: a study of 22 infections in 20,000 operations. Arch Ophthalmology.1964;72:454-62.
10. Aaberg TM Jr, Flynn HW Jr, Schiffman J, et al. Nosocomial acute-onset postoperative endophthalmitis surgery: a ten-year review of incidence and outcomes. Ophthalmology.1998;105:1004-10.
11. West ES, Behrens A, McDonnell PJ, et al. The incidence of endophthalmitis after cataract surgery among U.S. Medicare population increased between 1994 and 2001. Ophthalmology. 2005;112:1388-94.
12. Jensen MK, Fiscella RG, Moshirfar M, et al. Third- and fourth-generation fluoroquinolones: retrospective comparison of endophthalmitis after cataract surgery performed over 10 years. J Cataract Refract Surg. 2008;34:1460-7.
13. Moshirfar M, Feiz V, Vitale AT, et al. Endophthalmitis after uncomplicated cataract surgery with the use of fourth generation fluoroquinolones: a retrospective observational case series. Ophthalmology. 2007;114:686-91.
14. Freeman EE, Roy-Gagnon MH Fortin E, et al. Rate of endophthalmitis after cataract surgery in Quebec, Canada 1996-2005. Arch Ophthalmology. 2010;128:230-4.
15. Ravindran RD, Venkatesh R, Chang DF, et al. Incidence of post-cataract endophthalmitis at Aravind Eye Hospital: outcomes of more than 42,000 consecutive cases using standardized sterilization and prophylaxis protocols. J Cataract Refract Surg. 2009;35(4):629-36.
16. Sheng Y, Sun W, Gu Y, et al. Endophthalmitis after cataract surgery in China, 1995-2009. J Cataract Refract Surg. 2011;37(9):1715-22.
17. Wykoff CC, Parrott MB, Flynn HW J, et al Nosocomial acute-onset postoperative endophthalmitis at a university teaching hospital (2002-2009). Am J Ophthalmology. 2010;150(3):392-8.
18. Levison A, Mendes T, Bhisitkul R. Postprocedural endophthalmitis: a review. Exp Rev Ophthalmology. 2013;8(1):45-62.
19. Tan C, Lim L, Cheong K. Reevaluating intracameral cefuroxime as a prophylaxis against endophthalmitis after cataract surgery. J Cataract Refract Surg. 2015;41(5):1125-6.
20. VanderBeek B, Bonaffini S, Ma L. The Association between Intravitreal Steroids and Post-Injection Endophthalmitis Rates. Ophthalmology. 2015;122(11):2311-2315.e1.
21. Sigford DK, Reddy S, Mollineaux C, et al. Global reported endophthalmitis risk following intravitreal injections of anti-VEGF: a literature review and analysis. Clin Ophthalmology (Auckland, NZ). 2015;9:773-81.
22. Raman R, Singh HS, Appanraj R, et al. Five-year incidence and visual outcomes in postintravitreal injection endophthalmitis. Ophthalmology. 2016;123(5):1162-4.
23. Rosenfeld PJ, Brown DM, Heier JS, et al. MARINA Study Group. Ranibizumab for neovascular age-related macular degeneration. N Engl J Med. 2006;355(14):1419-31.
24. Brown DM, Michels M, Kaiser PK, et al. ANCHOR Study Group. Ranibizumab versus verteporfin photodynamic therapy for neovascular age-related macular degeneration: two-year results of the ANCHOR study. Ophthalmology. 2009;116(1):57-65.e5.
25. Nguyen QD, Brown DM, Marcus DM, et al. RISE and RIDE Research Group. Ranibizumab for diabetic macular edema: results from 2 Phase III randomized trials: RISE and RIDE. Ophthalmology. 2012;119(4):789-801.
26. Bhavsar AR, Ip MS, Glassman AR. DRCRnet and the SCORE Study Groups. The risk of endophthalmitis following intravitreal triamcinolone injection in the DRCRnet and SCORE clinical trials. Am J Ophthalmology. 2007;144(3):454-6.
27. Martin DF, Maguire MG, Fine SL. Ranibizumab and bevacizumab for treatment of neovascular age-related macular degeneration: two-year results. Ophthalmology. 2012;119(7):1388-98.
28. Sachdeva M, Moshiri A, Leder H, et al. Endophthalmitis following intravitreal injection of anti-VEGF agents: long-term outcomes and the identification of unusual micro-organisms. J Ophthalmic Inflamm Infect. 2016;6(1):2.
29. Simunovic MP, Rush RB, Hunyor AP, et al. Endophthalmitis following intravitreal injection versus endophthalmitis following cataract surgery: clinical features, causative organisms and post-treatment outcomes. Br J Ophthalmology. 2012;96:862-6.
30. Chen E, Lin MY, Cox J, et al. Endophthalmitis after intravitreal injection: the importance of viridans streptococci. Retina. 2011;31:1525-33.
31. Kumar A, Ravani R. Using intravitreal bevacizumab (Avastin®)—Indian scenario. Indian J Ophthalmology. 2017;65(7):545-8.
32. Roth DB, Jonna G, Prenner JL, et al. Inferior Intravitreal Injection Site Associated With Higher Incidence of Endophthalmitis. Invest Ophthalmology Vis Sci. 2009;50:35-66.
33. Shah CP, Garg SJ, Vander JF, et al. Post-Injection Endophthalmitis (PIE) Study Team. Outcomes and risk factors associated with endophthalmitis after intravitreal injection of anti-vascular endothelial growth factor agents. Ophthalmology. 2011;118(10):2028-34.
34. McCannel CA. Meta-analysis of endophthalmitis after intravitreal injection of anti-vascular endothelial growth factor agents: causative organisms and possible prevention strategies. Retina. 2011;31:654-61.
35. Wen JC, McCannel CA, Mochon AB, et al. Bacterial dispersal associated with speech in the setting of intravitreous injections. Arch Ophthalmology. 2011;129:1551-4.

36. Sato T, Emi K, Ikeda T, et al. Severe Intraocular inflammation after intravitreal injection of bevacizumab. Ophthalmology. 2010;117:512-6.

37. Yamashiro K, Tsujikawa A, Miyamoto K, et al. Sterile endophthalmitis after intravitreal injection of bevacizumab obtained from a single batch. Retina. 2010;30:485-90.

38. Wickremasinghe SS, Michalova K, Gilhotra J, et al. Acute intraocular inflammation after intravitreous injections of bevacizumab for treatment of neovascular age related macular degeneration. Ophthalmology. 2008;115:1911-5.

39. Sinha S, Vashisht N, Venkatesh P, et al. Managing bevacizumab-induced intraocular inflammation. Indian J Ophthalmology. 2012; 60:311-3.

40. Chen E, Cox J, Brown DM, et al. Endophthalmitis after intravitreal injection: the importance of viridans streptococci. Retina. 2011;31:1525-33.

41. Rishi E, Bhende P. Intravitreal Injection Guidelines. Sci J Med Vis Res Foun. 2015;XXXIII:80-2.

42. Storey P, Dollin M, Pitcher J, et al. The role of topical antibiotic prophylaxis to prevent endophthalmitis after intravitreal injection. Ophthalmology. 2014;121:283-9.

43. Garg SJ, Dollin M, Hsu J, et al. Effect of a strict 'No-Talking' policy during intravitreal injection on post-injection endophthalmitis. Ophthalmic Surg Lasers Imaging Retina. 2015;46:1028-34.

44. Bakri SJ, Synder MR, Pulido JS, et al. Six month stability of Bevacizumab (Avastin) binding to vascular endothelial growth factor after withdrawal into a syringe and refrigeration or freezing. Retina. 2006;26:519-22.

45. Rodrigues EB, Grumann A Jr, Penha FM, et al. Effect of needle type and injection technique on pain level and vitreal reflux in intravitreal injection. J Ocul Pharmacol Ther. 2011;27(2):197-203.

46. Rodrigues EB, Meyer CH, Grumann A Jr, et al. Tunneled scleral incision to prevent vitreal reflux after intravitreal injection. Am J Ophthalmology. 2007;143(6):1035-7.

47. Knecht PB, Michels S, Sturm V, et al. Tunnelled versus straight intravitreal injection: intraocular pressure changes, vitreous reflux, and patient discomfort. Retina. 2009;29(8):1175-81.

48. De Stefano VS, Abechain JJ, de Almeida LF, et al. Experimental investigation of needles, syringes andtechniques for intravitreal injections. Clin Experiment Ophthalmology. 2011;39(3):236-42.

49. Wallin O, Al-ahramy AM, Lundstrom M, et al. Endophthalmitis and severe blebitis following trabeculectomy. Epidemiology and risk factors; a single-centre retrospective study. Acta Ophthalmology. 2014;92(5):426-31.

50. Ang GS, Varga Z, Shaarawy T. Postoperative infection in penetrating versus non-penetrating glaucoma surgery. Br J Ophthalmology. 2010;94(12):1571-6.

51. Gedde SJ, Schiffman JC, Feuer WJ, et al. Tube Versus Trabeculectomy Study Group. Three-year follow-up of the tube versus trabeculectomy study. Am J Ophthalmology. 2009;148(5): 670-84.

52. Aaberg TM Jr, Flynn HW Jr, Schiffman J, et al. Nosocomial acute-onset postoperative endophthalmitis survey. A 10-year review of incidence and outcomes. Ophthalmology. 1998;105(6):1004-10.

53. Ho PC, Tolentino FI. Bacterial endophthalmitis after closed vitrectomy. Arch. Ophthalmology. 1984;102(2):207-10.

54. Kunimoto DY, Kaiser RS. Wills Eye Retina Service. Incidence of endophthalmitis after 20- and 25-gauge vitrectomy. Ophthalmology. 2007;114(12):2133-7.

55. Wykoff CC, Flynn HW Jr, Miller D, et al. Exogenous fungal endophthalmitis: microbiology and clinical outcomes. Ophthalmology. 2008;115(9):1501-7.e1.

56. Wani VB, Al Sabti K, Kumar N, et al. Endophthalmitis after vitrectomy and vitrectomy combined with phacoemulsification: incidence and visual outcomes. Eur. J Ophthalmology. 2009;19(6): 1044-9.

57. Oshima Y, Kadonosono K, Yamaji H, et al. Japan Microincision Vitrectomy Surgery Study Group. Multicenter survey with a systematic overview of acute-onset endophthalmitis after transconjunctival microincision vitrectomy surgery. Am J Ophthalmology. 2010;150(5):716-25.e1.

58. Wu L, Berrocal MH, Arévalo JF, et al. Endophthalmitis after pars planavitrectomy: results of the Pan American Collaborative Retina Study Group. Retina (Philadelphia, PA). 2011;31(4):673-8.

59. Scott IU. Flynn HW Jr, Acar N, et al. Incidence of endophthalmitis after 20-gauge vs 23-gauge vs 25-gauge pars planavitrectomy. Graefes Arch Clin Exp Ophthalmology. 2011;249(3):377-80.

60. Dave VP Pathengay A, Schwartz SG, et al. Endophthalmitis following pars planavitrectomy: a literature review of incidence, causative organisms, and treatment outcomes. Clin Ophthalmology. 2014:8 2133-8.

61. Kunimoto D, Tasman W, Rapuano C, et al. Endophthalmitis after penetrating keratoplasty: microbiologic spectrum and susceptibility of isolates. Am J Ophthalmology. 2004;137(2):343-5.

62. Shih CY, Ritterband DC, Rubino S, et al. Visually significant and nonsignificant complications arising from Descemet stripping automated endothelial keratoplasty. Am J Ophthalmology. 2009;148(6):837-43.

63. Du DT, Wagoner A, Barone SB, et al. Incidence of endophthalmitis after corneal transplant or cataract surgery in a medicare population. Ophthalmology. 2014;121(1):290-8.

64. Alshihry A. Epidemiology of Postoperative Endophthalmitis (POE) in a Specialized Eye Hospital. Epidemiol. 2014;04(01):145.

65. Behlau I, Martin KV. Martin JN, et al. Infectious endophthalmitis in Boston keratoprosthesis: incidence and prevention. Acta Ophthalmology. 2014;92(7):e546-55.

66. Chen J, Jones M, Srinivasan S, et al. Endophthalmitis after penetrating keratoplasty. Ophthalmology. 2015;122(1):25-30.

67. Barry P, Gardner S, Seal D, et al. ESCRS Endophthalmitis Study Group. Clinical observations associated with proven and unproven cases in the ESCRS study of prophylaxis of postoperative endophthalmitis after cataract surgery. J Cataract Refract Surg. 2009;35(9):1523-31.e1.

68. Results of the Endophthalmitis Vitrectomy Study. A randomized trial of immediate vitrectomy and of intravenous antibiotics for the treatment of postoperative bacterial endophthalmitis. Endophthalmitis Vitrectomy Study Group. Arch Ophthalmology. 1995;113(12):1479-96.

69. Kunimoto DY, Das T, Sharma S, et al. Microbiologic spectrum and susceptibility of isolates: part I. Postoperative endophthalmitis. Endophthalmitis Research Group. Am J Ophthalmology. 1999; 128(2):240-2.

70. Han DP, Wisniewski SR, Wilson LA, et al. Spectrum and susceptibilities of microbiologic isolates in the EndophthalmitisVitrectomy Study. Am J Ophthalmology 1996;122:1-17.

71. Friling E, Lundström M, Stenevi U, et al. Six-year incidence of endophthalmitis after cataract surgery: Swedish national study. J Cataract Refract Surg. 2013;39:15-21.

72. Sheng Y, Sun W, Gu Y, et al. Endophthalmitis after cataract surgery in China, 1995-2009. J Cataract Refract Surg. 2011;37:1715-22.

73. Pijl BJ, Theelen T, Tilanus MA, et al. Acute endophthalmitis after cataract surgery: 250 consecutive cases treated at a tertiary referral center in the Netherlands. Am J Ophthalmology. 2010;149:482-7.

74. Jindal A, Moreker M, Pathengay A, et al. Polymicrobial endophthalmitis: prevalence, causative organisms, and visual outcomes. J Ophth Inflamm Infect. 2013;3(1):6.

75. Gupta A, Gupta V, Gupta A, et al. Spectrum and clinical profile of post cataract surgery endophthalmitis in North India. Ind J Ophthalmology. 2013;51(2):139-45.

76. Pathengay A, Moreker M, Puthussery R, et al. Clinical and microbiologic review of culture-proven endophthalmitis caused by multidrug-resistant bacteria in patients seen at a tertiary eye care center in southern India. Retina. 2011;31(9):1806-11.

77. Al-Turki TA, Al-Shahwan S, Al-Mezaine HS, et al. Microbiology and visual outcome of bleb-associated endophthalmitis. Ocul Immunol Inflamm. 2010;18(2):121-6.

78. Cohen SM, Flynn HW Jr, Murray TG, et al. Endophthalmitis after pars plana vitrectomy. The postvitrectomy endophthalmitis study Group. Ophthalmology. 1995;102(5):705-12.

79. Joondeph B, Blanc J, Polkinghorne P. Endophthalmitis after pars planavitrectomy. Retina. 2005;25(5):587-9.

80. Keswani T, Ahuja V, Changulani M. Evaluation of outcome of various treatment methods for endogenous endophthalmitis. Ind J Med Sci. 2006;60(11):454.

81. Connell P, O'Neill E, Fabinyi D, et al. Endogenous endophthalmitis: 10-year experience at a tertiary referral centre. Eye. 2010;25(1): 66-72.

82. Kirchhof B, Wong D. Vitreo-retinal surgery. Berlin: Springer; 2007.

Newer Innovations and Techniques in Vitreoretinal Surgery

Atul Kumar, Rohan Chawla

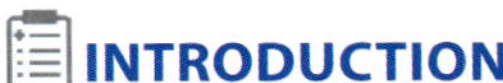

INTRODUCTION

The last decade has seen major advances in the field of vitreoretinal surgery. There have been many technological breakthroughs, which have expanded the indications of vitreoretinal surgery. The efficiency, speed, and safety of posterior segment surgeries have markedly improved. Few recently introduced technologies, like intraoperative optical coherence tomography (iOCT) guided vitreoretinal surgery, have opened new frontiers for us that are yet to be explored. In this chapter, we shall brief through few of the important technological advances which have reduced surgical risks, improved visual outcomes, provided many other potential benefits to the patients and surgeons and most importantly, have paved the way for a future revolution in the surgical management of vitreoretinal conditions.

SMALL GAUGE VITRECTOMY

Vitrectomy was first performed by Robert Machemer[1] in 1970 with a vitreous infusion suction cutter (VISC) which was a 17 gauge instrument (1.5 mm external diameter). We have now come a long way from then, with the availability of instruments as small as 41-gauge (0.1 mm diameter) in the present time. The newer thinner cannulas are used for creating small retinotomies to create perimacular subretinal blebs[2] required for submacular surgeries. These small retinotomies do not require to be laser-delimited at the conclusion of surgery. Such thin cannulas find versatile applications such as to inject subretinal tissue plasminogen activator (tPA) for rapid dissolution of hemorrhage for cases of massive submacular bleeds.[3] One of the authors has reported good functional outcomes with vitrectomy combined with the use of 41G needle for subretinal delivery of air, tPA and anti-VEGFs for faster displacement and dissolution of thick subretinal bleeds.[4]

The vitrectomy cutter size has also considerably reduced. Till about 2002, only the 20G (0.9 mm) vitrectomy cutters developed by O'Malley and Heintz were available.[5] However, cutters of 23G (0.6 mm), 25G (0.5 mm), and even 27G (0.4 mm) are now commercially available. Small gauge single step entry trocar and cannulas have been developed to make ports for insertion of these smaller instruments. These small gauge cannulated ports have several merits. Firstly, beveled incisions made using these instruments can be left sutureless or require only a single 7-0 Polyglactin 910 (Vicryl) (Ethicon, Somerville, NJ) to close them. These incisions can be made transconjunctival, obviating the need to suture the conjunctiva separately. These cannulas prevent herniation of vitreous and retina into the ports in cases of bullous retinal detachments. In our experience, the incidence of port site dialysis and subsequent development of postoperative retinal detachments has also reduced with smaller gauge instrumentation. Le Rouic JF et al. have shown that the risk of development of a retinal detachment as a complication of macular hole surgery is lower with small gauge vitrectomy.[6] These small gauge cannulas can also be valved to reduce turbulence and intraocular pressure variation in the vitreous cavity during insertion and removal of instruments through the ports during surgery. Smaller sutureless incisions enhance postoperative patient comfort and reduce healing time. A comparison of 23G and 25G vitreoretinal surgery by one of the authors revealed less postoperative pain and discomfort with the smaller gauge.[7]

The smaller cutters have an added advantage of the port being closer to the distal tip of the cutter. It is only about 0.23 mm from the tip in 25G cutters as compared to 0.43 mm in 20G cutters (Fig. 52.1). This enhances the ability of the surgeon to go closer to the retina and use the cutter itself in place

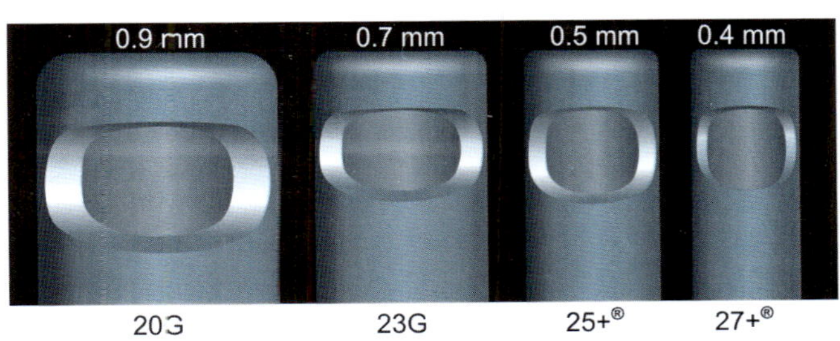

Fig. 52.1: Cutter port is closer to tip in small gauge cutters (23-25-27G), making surface membrane shaving easier.

of a forceps or scissors for membrane dissection and removal. Smaller cutters can also be navigated through smaller gaps between fibrovascular membranes and the retina to create cleavage planes for easier dissection in complicated cases of diabetic tractional detachments. 27G cutters may be even more efficient at this. However in reducing the probe thickness, we also reduce its stiffness. This can sometimes reduce the surgeon's ability to accurately direct the instrument in the required direction. Also, bending these instruments to remove peripheral vitreous may actually alter the shape of the instruments. The malleability of the instruments has been reduced in 25G instrumentation by addition of a stiffening sleeve. 27G and perhaps the future 29G cutters would also need to address this issue.

Another issue with reducing cutter diameter and increasing cut rate is reduction in flow and aspiration rate of the vitreous. This can significantly increase surgical time taken to remove the vitreous. This has been offset by technological advances, which improve the duty cycle and opening time of the cutter port. Alcon has introduced a "dual pneumatic drive design" in which a second pneumatic piston aids in faster opening of the cutter blade.[8] Dutch Ophthalmic Research Center (DORC) has introduced a "twin duty cycle" cutter design which has an additional cutting port drilled into the closed cutter so that the vitreous is again cut while the blade is pushed back to reopen the port. These innovations have enabled the cutting rate to be improved from 750 cpm to 7,500 cpm. Such faster cut rates drastically reduce the vitreous drag during vitrectomy. This reduces traction at the retinal surface, which in turn reduces the incidence of iatrogenic breaks. Less traction significantly enhances the surgeon's ability to go closer to the retina for shaving the vitreous for a much more efficient vitreous removal from areas such as the vitreous base and lattices. With the current technology, the laws of physics prevent improving vitreous flow rates at further small gauges and higher cutting rates. Thus, scientists are looking at other options to improve flow rates in the next generation of smaller and faster cutters. One possible step in this direction is reduction of the viscosity of the vitreous itself. Some strategies, which have been suggested to achieve this, are cutting the vitreous using ultrasound or thinning it using enzymes or electrochemically. A prototype of an ultrasonic vitreous cutter with cutting speeds of 1,000,000 cpm and a 100% duty cycle has been developed by Carl Awh.[9] Another suggested approach is the use of piezoelectrically driven cutters with frequencies lower than that of the phacoemulsification probes and yet good enough to provide a motor speed of around 22,500 cpm.[10]

IMPROVED VIEWING AND ILLUMINATION

Small gauge vitrectomy would not have become popular, had viewing and illumination sources not improved hand in hand (Figs. 52.2A to F).

Both contact and noncontact wide angle viewing systems are extensively used for viewing the retinal periphery and

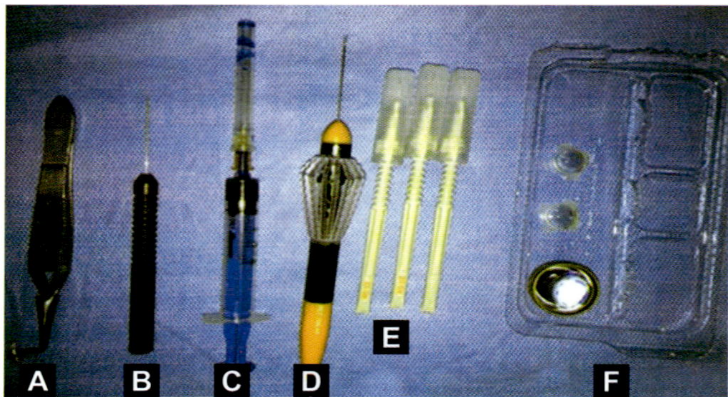

Figs. 52.2A to F: Small gauge surgical accessories. (A) 23G vent used with valved cannulas; (B) 23G diamond dusted membrane scraper; (C) 23G dual-bore cannula attached to a syringe to inject BBG dye; (D) 23G internal limiting membrane forceps; (E) 23G trocar-cannulas (valved); (F) Chalam self-retaining vitrectomy (flat) lenses and SSV MiniQuad wide—field viewing lens.
(BBG: Brilliant blue G; SSV: Self stabilizing vitrectomy).

getting a "panoramic view" of the retina including the periphery (Figs. 52.3A and B).

Illumination sources are varied including halogen, xenon, and light-emitting diode (LED) sources. Reducing the caliber of the fiber optic light pipe does significantly reduce illumination. However, development of brighter sources of illumination such as xenon has enhanced the intensity of light manifold. Though there have been concerns regarding phototoxicity from such sources, animal models have been developed which have demonstrated safety of these light sources.[11] Retinal pigment epithelial cell lines laden with A2E (a lipofuscin component) are used to test phototoxic effects of such light sources.[11] In the future, a new concept of using LEDs to illuminate the retina may come in vogue. Here, the light source itself is placed at the distal end of the probe. This obviates the need of expensive xenon light sources and fiber optic cables. It has been shown to be safe and effective in animal models.[12]

Bimanual vitreoretinal surgery for difficult situations has also become more popular with availability of small gauge chandelier illumination. This can be used as a single chandelier (25G) or a combination of twin chandeliers (29G) placed diametrically opposite to each other. In the author's experience, these provide better illumination and less shadowing than previous attempts at bimanual surgery using illuminated instruments or illuminated infusion cannulas. Bimanual surgeries are extremely helpful in managing complicated diabetic tractional retinal detachments. Placement of a chandelier can also let the surgeon use one of his/her hands for indentation and the other for vitrectomy for peripheral vitreous removal. Phacofragmentation in the vitreous cavity by impaling and stabilizing the dropped lens by one hand and using a phacofragmatome in the other under chandelier illumination has also been described.

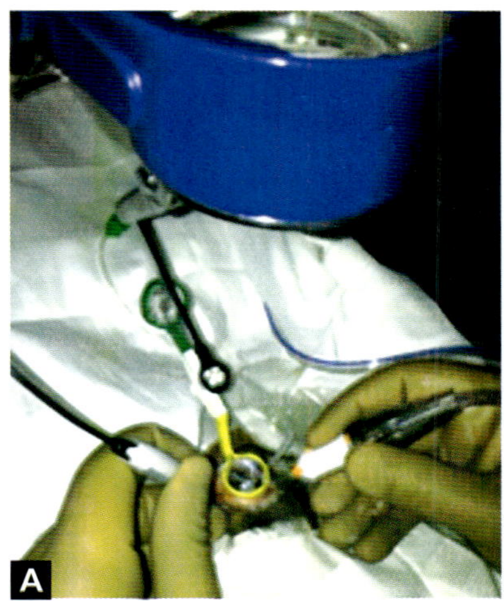 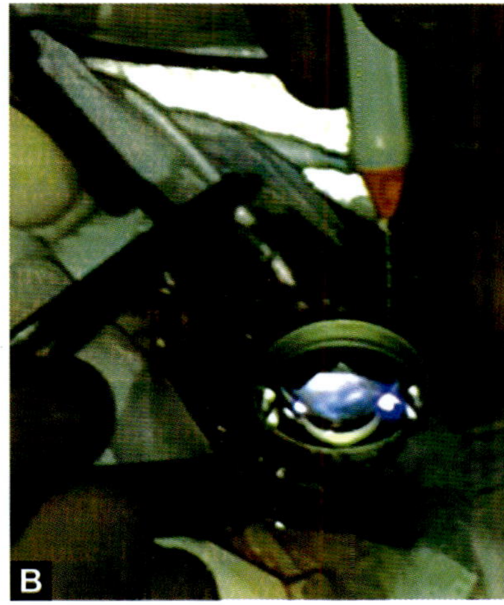

Figs. 52.3A and B: (A) Small gauge surgery being performed using a "RESCAN", a noncontact wide-angle viewing system (WAVS); (B) Flanged self-stabilizing vitrectomy (SSV) lens—"MiniQuad XL" used for wide-angle viewing. This is a contact variety of WAVS that are used in modern vitrectomy.

INTRAOPERATIVE SURGICAL MICROSCOPE WITH INTEGRATED OPTICAL COHERENCE TOMOGRAPHY AND HEADS-UP DISPLAY

Optical coherence tomography is a rapid, noncontact, and noninvasive high-resolution optical biopsy of tissue microstructure, which has revolutionized our understanding of the pathology of various retinal disease and guides therapeutic decision-making. Seamless integration of this technology into ophthalmic surgery has now laid the foundation for a new paradigm in the surgical management of ophthalmic disease.

Spectral domain-OCT (SD-OCT) provides more advantage over conventional time-domain OCT systems in being faster obtaining more images in a shorter period of time (approximately 20,000 A-scans per second compared with 400 A-scans per second on time-domain OCT) with higher resolution and coverage of larger retinal area.

An important limitation of typical OCT setup is that they are nonmobile units and, thus, require a compliant patient who can sit upright. Thus, OCT imaging in uncooperative patients, pediatric patients, and those with musculoskeletal disorders becomes challenging.

To overcome these problems, handheld mobile OCT machines came into use. A portable SD-OCT unit (Bioptigen Inc., Research Triangle Park NC) has made imaging of such patients possible. An additional value of the handheld SD-OCT system is the ability to obtain noncontact, high-resolution, cross-sectional retinal images intraoperatively in the supine position.[13,14] Studies have shown hand held SD-OCT imaging provided an efficient method for visualizing macular pathology. This technology may, in certain cases, help to confirm or identify diseases that may be difficult to visualize during surgery.[15] But the disadvantages include the fact that the surgeon had to halt the surgery to obtain images of the retinal architecture, remove all instruments from the eye, stabilize the eye and move the microscope away from the surgical field in order to position the scanner over the eye. It did not gain popularity because its use was time consuming and tedious.

To ensure maintenance of sterility, improve image quality and reproducibility and reduce image capture time, a mount was built that was attached to the operating microscope used for vitreoretinal surgery at the Emory Eye Center. This allowed the surgeon or assistant to move the device above the patient's eye using the microscope foot pedal. Thus, came the evolution of microscope-mounted OCT. Studies showed that the use of a microscope-mounted SD-OCT unit that is easy to assemble, maintains a sterile surgical field, and produces reproducible and more time efficient images in an intraoperative setting. As with any new technology, it also had a learning curve.[16] It also had disadvantages like a need to bring the OCT unit into alignment with microscope and hence real-time visualization of the surgical steps was not possible. The lack of true coaxiality made it difficult to focus on specific regions of interest.

This gave birth to the technology of microscope-integrated OCT (MIOCT) device, which facilitated simultaneous surgical visualization along with high-resolution SD-OCT imaging. This was made possible by folding the optical OCT path into the full beam path of the operating microscope to aid imaging.[17]

Microscope-integrated Optical Coherence Tomography Design

A high-resolution MIOCT prototype device was developed to interface with an ophthalmic operating microscope (Leica

Microsystems, Heerbrugg, Switzerland).[18] Briefly, a dichroic mirror allows folding of the MIOCT optical path into the surgical microscope above the objective lens to permit simultaneous imaging during surgical manipulations without altering the surgeon's view. This prototype microscope-integrated scanner was coupled with a Bioptigen SD-OCT imaging engine with a center wavelength of 865 nm and a spectrometer equipped to acquire images at a rate of 20,000 A-scans per second. The lateral resolution was 15 µm, and the field of view was 10 × 10 mm. The axial resolution was 5 µm and the depth range was 1.55 mm.

The other MIOCT systems that have been recently developed are the integrated OCT (iOCT) (Haag-Streit, Wedel, Germany) and RESCAN 700 (Carl Zeiss Meditec, Oberkochen, Germany).[19,20] High-definition OCT images appear directly in the LUMERA 700 microscope eyepiece providing the surgeon a clear view below the surface of the surgical field, thus enabling them to alter, refine and improve their surgical decision making.[21] It takes 27,000 A-scans per second to produce real time 2-dimensional images. The RESCAN 700 stabilizes images by using Z-tracking system.

The microscope-integrated system permits stereoscopic heads-up display (HUD) without interfering with the surgical field of view. All the functions of the OCT can be controlled from the microscope's foot pedal and joystick, allowing the surgeon to capture images and record videos without interrupting the surgery. The surgical field can be seen in real time in both cross-sectional and planar-view by the stereoscopic display. Different capture modes like volume cube, raster scan, etc. are available.

Optical coherence tomography scans can also be stored and recalled for later review and "fly through" via CALLISTO

eye from ZEISS. RESIGHT lens systems are used for posterior segment viewing. The Prospective Intraoperative and Perioperative Ophthalmic Imaging with Optical Coherence Tomography (PIONEER) Study: 2-year Results and the recent Discover study revealed that MI-OCT tended to influence the surgical decision-making in retinal surgery.

Clinical Utilizes of Microscope-integrated Optical Coherence Tomography

Macular Hole

Intraoperative SD-OCT imaging of the macula could provide additional information to predict visual outcomes. MIOCT enables a clear visualization and real-time visualization of the internal limiting membrane (ILM) peeling. This helps one to avoid any inadvertent trauma to the underlying nerve fiber layer. It will clearly show the area from where ILM has been peeled. With the latest surgical technique of inverted internal limiting flap, the surgeon can ensure that the ILM flap covers the hole completely (Fig. 52.4).

One can opt out of the usage of vital dyes to visualize the ILM as the MIOCT imaging would guide the procedure. In cases of failed macular hole surgeries, area of peeled ILM can be easily visualized. Intraoperative imaging could identify changes in the macular anatomy that occur during surgery that affect visual recovery.

Epiretinal Membranes and Vitreomacular Traction

Epiretinal membrane (ERM) and vitreomacular traction (VMT) cause definite alterations in the retinal contour and diminution of vision. MIOCT helps the surgeon to assess the area and strength of the vitreomacular adhesion. It enables

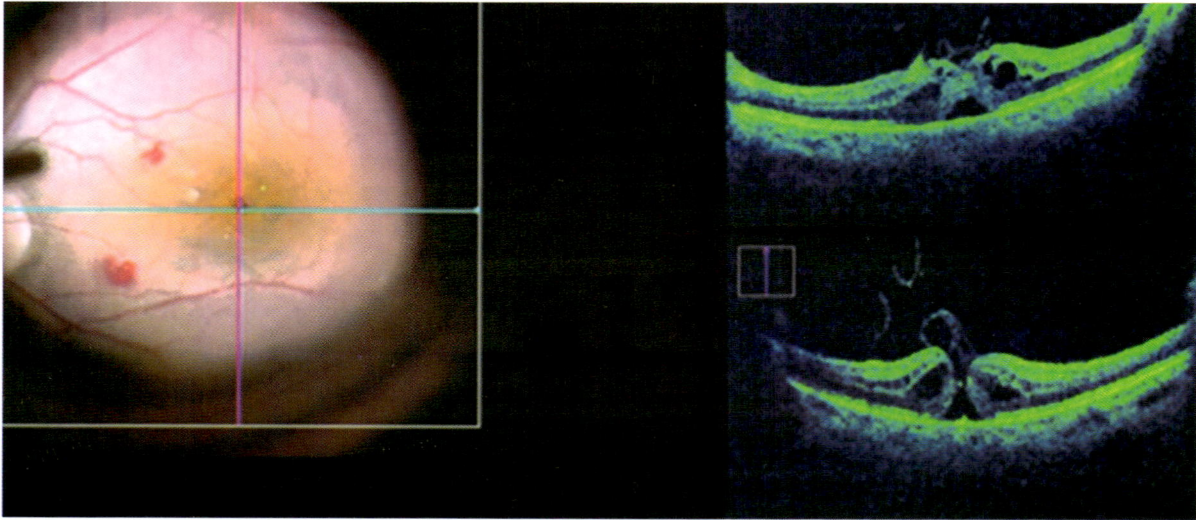

Fig. 52.4: iOCT reveals a macular hole with surgically placed ILM flap lying over the macular hole. (iOCT: Integrated optical coherence tomography; ILM: Internal limiting membrane).

one to identify and carefully peel the membranes without deroofing the foveal cyst. Immediate normalization of the retinal contour can be seen after removal of the membranes (*see* Figs. 52.2A to F).

Retinal Detachment (RD)

In tractional retinal detachment, a safe plane to initiate delamination and segmentation can be obtained with the aid of MIOCT. It helps in determining any residual traction and the adequacy of membrane peeling (*see* Figs. 52.3A and B). In rhegmatogenous retinal detachment, any residual subretinal fluid in the posterior pole can be identified and a complete fluid-air exchange can be achieved (*see* Fig. 52.4). MIOCT helps omit the step of posterior vitreous detachment (PVD) induction while operating RD. Its also useful in removal of any subretinal bubble of perfluorocarbon at the fovea.

Myopic Tractional Maculopathy

In myopic traction maculopathy, along with foveoschisis, there are multiple layers of vitreoschisis (Figs. 52.5A and B). A complete removal of the posterior cortical vitreous with utmost care of not damaging the fovea is required. Multiple stains are used to stain the retained hyaloid and the ILM. With the MIOCT, identification of any remnant of cortical vitreous and peeling of ILM becomes easy and safe, thus averting any iatrogenic breaks. A study by the author (Kumar A et al.) demonstrated outcomes of microscope integrated intraoperative OCT with center-sparing ILM peeling showed good functional and anatomical outcomes with relatively less incidence of intraoperative and postoperative complications.[22] The use of MIOCT allows seamless, high-resolution and real-time imaging of ILM peeling and traction removal. This also allows visualization of ILM, especially in cases of myopic foveoschisis wherein ILM visibility is difficult due to poor contrast. MIOCT also allows visualization of thin cystic areas, where ILM peeling can then be avoided to prevent intraoperative macular hole formation thus improving surgical outcomes.[22]

Disadvantages

The optical properties of surgical instruments affect the visualization of the underlying retina. Metallic instruments (e.g. forceps and needles) showed high reflectivity with total shadowing below the instrument. Polyamide material had a moderate reflectivity with subtotal shadowing. Silicone instruments, such as Tano's diamond dusted membrane scrapper, show partial transmission and, therefore, affect visualization of underlying retinal structures.[23] All the more, faster acquisition speeds have to be developed.

The microscope does not have an inbuilt calibration system to measure the dimensions of the tissue structure visualized. The measurements are taken from the screen and with the aid of a correction factor; the surgeons are able to derive a measurement. An inbuilt calibration system with good agreement with preoperative OCT measurements could be of great help to the surgeons.

However, the microscope along with the Callisto is bulky setup. A sleek, less bulky model is awaited. Though of immense use, the cost of the microscope cannot be ignored.

Clinical Impact

Intraoperative OCT appears to improve surgical decision making. In fact, in 10% or more cases, the OCT data actually causes surgeons to change their mind. For example, if the surgeons think they have completed peeling all of the

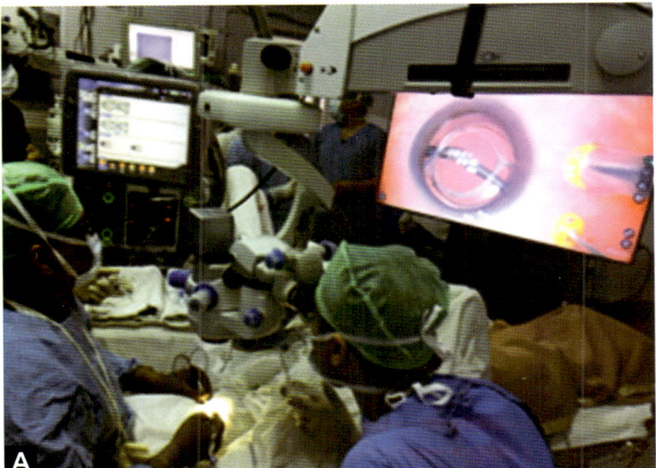
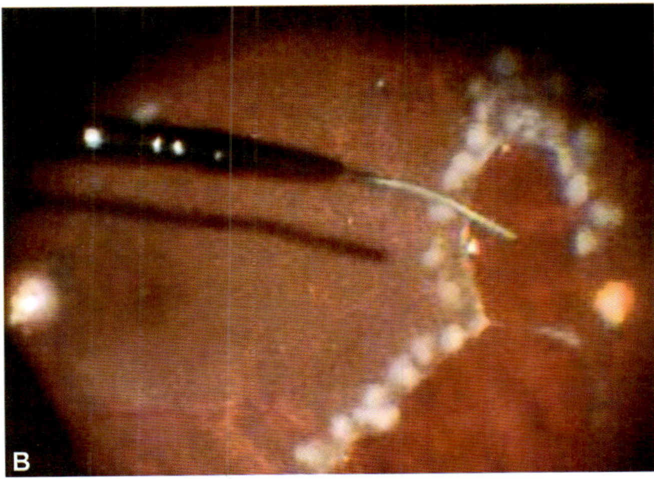

Figs. 52.5A and B: (A) A three-dimensional (3D) high definition (HD) "heads-up" viewing and vitrectomy surgery in progress with the surgeon, assistant, and others in the operation theater viewing an HD 55-inch 4K (8 million pixels) OLED display monitor using polaroid spectacles to achieve an HD 3D image of the surgery. The system works by attaching two HD cameras (one for each eye, attached to the microscope after laser filter) to the microscope and displaying a horizontally disparate stereoscopic image on the HD-screen which is perceived as a 3D image when viewed through the polaroid glasses (B) Complex retinal detachment surgeries with giant retinal tears being done with the help of 3D HD "heads-up" vitrectomy system.

membrane, they may look at the OCT and realize that there is some residual membrane that still requires peeling; while some surgeons, who had decided to continue peeling still more, iOCT enabled them to assess completeness of membrane removal and then change their decision. Also, in ILM peeling with inverted flaps surgery for macular hole, the real time OCT permits visualization of the flaps bridging the hole.

Future Directions

This new visualization technology promised to change ophthalmic surgery especially for retina and cornea surgeons, opening for us a whole new realm of ophthalmic surgeries.

However, the speed of SD-OCT is slow and is probably not real time in the actual sense. Hence, it is not ideal for truly guiding the surgeon during the surgeries. Dr Toth is currently helping to develop a swept source OCT system with an HUD and different display options, including Goggle Glasses at Duke University.[24]

Intratissue targeted delivery of drugs using real-time OCT guided microscope will be a reality in near future.

THREE-DIMENSIONAL VIEWING IN VITREORETINAL SURGERY

Performing long hours of surgery looking down through a microscope has an impact on the health of the cervical spine of vitreoretinal surgeons. To reduce this, three-dimensional (3D) high definition (HD) screen based viewing systems ("heads-up" viewing systems) for performing these long surgeries have been developed (NGENUITY® 3D Visualization System, TrueVision®, Alcon). Using these, the surgeon just looks straight ahead at a screen to get a 3D view of the operative field just as he/she would get looking down through a microscope.[25] NGENUITY® provides an HD digitally processed real-time image to the operating surgeon, also known as, digitally assisted vitreoretinal surgery (DAVS). This technology provides sharper, high contrast, and real-time magnified video display without the loss of stereopsis or field of view. It not only improves surgeon's physical comfort due to its ergonomic design, it also improves peroperative visibility under lower illumination conditions avoiding patient's eyes to inadvertent phototoxicity. Its invaluable role as a teaching tool, since everyone in the operating theater can experience the 3D surgery by wearing polaroid glasses, cannot be overlooked (*see* Figs. 52.5A and B). Integration of intraoperative OCT with screen-based surgery has also been developed.

VITREOUS SUBSTITUTES

Vitreoretinal surgeons have always desired a perfect vitreous substitute, which may be left in the vitreous cavity without worrying about its removal or complications. The present day substances like silicone oil, heavy silicone oil, gases, and perfluorocarbon liquids which may be used to fill the vitreous cavity following vitrectomy are far from an ideal vitreous substitute (Fig. 52.6). It is difficult to develop artificial vitre-

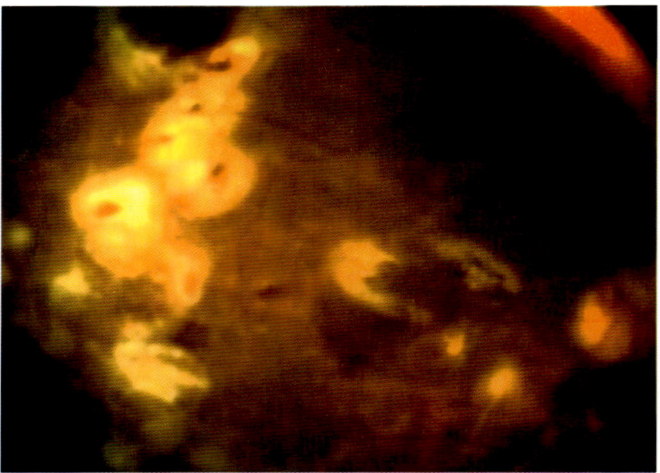

Fig. 52.6: Oil-filled vitreous cavity postoperatively in an eye with pre-existing diabetic tractional retinal detachment (TRD).

ous as vitreous is not just an inert gel but has active cellular components which prevent inflammation and infection, and also play a role in neovascularization.[26]

Hydrogels appear to be promising molecules in this quest for an ideal vitreous substitute. Polyvinyl alcohol gel has been studied in animal models. It has a structure similar to vitreous and has demonstrated good biocompatibility.[27]

Another approach is regeneration of human vitreous itself. There has been some progress towards cloning of human vitreous tissue derived cells.[28]

ROBOTIC EYE SURGERY

Ophthalmic microsurgery especially macular surgery requires considerable expertise. Minimal amount of excess force used during manipulation of a few microns thick tissues such as the ILM can lead to serious complications. Development of tremor with age can also increase possibility of iatrogenic tissue damage. Robotic surgery based on a master and slave concept seems a promising solution to these issues. Further robotic surgery may be able to manipulate retinal tissue in a manner not comprehensible by the human hand. Subretinal surgery and retinal vessel cannulation might become more reproducible using robotic tissue manipulation. The da Vinci robotic surgical system in which the surgeon (master) operates the slave (robot) from a distance looking through a stereoscopic viewfinder has been tested for vitreoretinal surgery in porcine eyes. However, it was not found to be very satisfactory.[29] To overcome the drawbacks of this system a new platform—Intraocular Robotic Interventional Surgical System (IRISS) has been developed by Jules Stein Eye Institute and the UCLA Department of Mechanical and Aerospace Engineering.[30] Though most of these are still investigational techniques being tested on animal eyes, tremendous amount of work has already been done in this field. Sakai T et al. have developed a miniature parallel robot weighing only 770 g

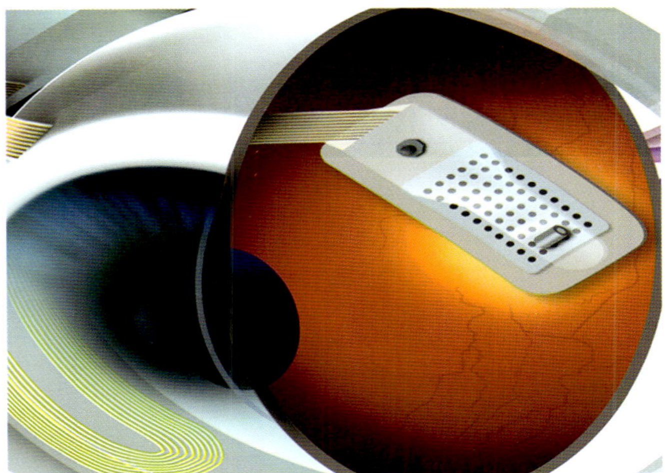

Fig. 52.7: The Argus II implant.

which can remove the ILM with a tracing accuracy of 40 μm.[31] To improve dexterity, a submillimeter intraocular robotic head called Integrated Robotic Intraocular Snake (IRIS) which has a diameter of 0.9 mm and a length of just 3 mm is being tested.[32]

Force sensors are being developed for the tips of such robotic arms which will be able to detect amount of force applied below levels of human perception.[33,34] This could finely regulate the amount of force applied on the retina during procedures like membrane peeling. Telerobotic systems will enhance vitreoretinal surgery by steadying instrument motion[35] and improving accuracy.[36]

RETINAL IMPLANTS

There is a total loss of photoreceptor function in the advanced stages of various degenerative disorders of the retina like retinitis pigmentosa (RP). Despite this, the inner retinal elements might still retain some function. The aim of retinal implant technology is to provide an appropriate stimulus to these inner layers in response to light. This stimulus is further transmitted to the brain and some sort of visual perception is appreciated by the patient. Further training of the patient in analyzing this visual perception enables the patient attain a certain degree of visual acuity which would help the patient in better navigation and comprehension as compared to a similar blind person without the implant. However, the patient who is eligible for an implant needs to have a functioning inner retina and optic nerve.

Currently available retinal implants are Argus II (Fig. 52.7), Boston Retinal Implant, Epi-Ret 3, Intelligent Medical Implants, and Alpha-IMS. Of these, Argus II has got Food and Drug Administration (FDA) approval and CE approval and Alpha-IMS has CE approval and the rest are still under investigational stage.[37-39] Manufactured by Second Sight Medical Products and coinvented by Mark Humayun of the USC Eye Institute, the Argus II Retinal Prosthesis System (bionic eye) was first approved by the US-FDA in 2013 to treat adult patients with advanced RP. The basic design of all these implants consists of a camera, which captures the image. This image is converted into a signal by a processor. This signal is transmitted to an array of electrodes, which can be placed either subretinal or epiretinal fixed to the retina with a tack. These electrodes further send a stimulus to further stimulate the cells of the inner retina. The processor and the electrode array are generally connected by transscleral wires.

The Alpha-IMS implant is a bit different as it does not involve an external camera, but the implant itself has an array of photodetectors, which transmit the signal to associated electrodes. The placement of these implants involves a very tedious surgery. Accurate positioning of the elements of the inner retina[40] implant and its electrodes is of utmost importance for proper stimulation of the functioning.

Risks with such implants include failure of the bionic eye to function, endophthalmitis, retinal detachment, conjunctival erosion, etc.

REFERENCES

1. Machemer R, Buettner H, Norton EW, et al. Vitrectomy: a pars plana approach. Trans Am Acad Ophthalmol Otolaryngol. 1971;75(4):813-20.
2. Zacharias LC, Nóbrega PF, Takahashi WY. Surgical correction of retinal folds involving the fovea. Ophthalmic Surg Lasers Imaging Retina. 2014;45(1):50-3.
3. Haupert CL, McCuen BW 2nd, Jaffe GJ, et al. Pars plana vitrectomy, subretinal injection of tissue plasminogen activator, and fluid-gas exchange for displacement of thick submacular hemorrhage in age-related macular degeneration. Am J Ophthalmol. 2001;131(2):208-15.
4. Kumar A, Roy S, Bansal M, et al. Modified Approach in Management of Submacular Hemorrhage Secondary to Wet Age-related Macular Degeneration. Asia Pac J Ophthalmol (Phila). 2016;5(2):143-6.
5. O'Malley C, Heintz RM Sr. Vitrectomy with an alternative instrument system. Ann Ophthalmol. 1975;7(4):585-8.
6. Le Rouic JF, Becquet F, Ducournau D. Does 23-gauge sutureless vitrectomy modify the risk of postoperative retinal detachment after macular surgery? A comparison with 20-gauge vitrectomy. Retina. 2011;31(5):902-8.
7. Kumar A, Duraipandi K, Gogia V, et al. Comparative evaluation of 23- and 25-gauge microincision vitrectomy surgery in management of diabetic macular traction retinal detachment. Eur J Ophthalmol. 2014;24(1):107-13.
8. Diniz B, Ribeiro RM, Fernandes RB, et al. Fluidics in a dual pneumatic ultra high-speed vitreous cutter system. Ophthalmologica. 2013;229(1):15-20.
9. Awh C. Advances in Vitreoretinal Surgery Instrumentation. Hamburg, Germany: Euretina; 2013.
10. Rizzo S, Faraldi F. The future of small gauge vitrectomy. Retina Today. 2014.
11. Yanagi Y. Retinal phototoxicity from endoilluminators for vitrectomy. Nippon Ganka Gakkai Zasshi. 2008;112(11):975-83.
12. Kölbl PS, Lindner C, Lingenfelder C, et al. Fiberless miniature chandelier LED endoilluminator for pars plana vitrectomy. Ophthalmologe. 2016;113(1):47-51.

13. Scott AW, Farsiu S, Enyedi LB, et al. Imaging the infant retina with a hand-held spectral-domain optical coherence tomography device. Am J Ophthalmol. 2009;147:364.e2-73.e2.

14. Chong G, Farsiu S, Freedman SF, et al. Abnormal foveal morphology in ocular albinism imaged with spectral domain optical coherence tomography. Arch Ophthalmol. 2009;127:37-44.

15. Dayani PN, Maldonado R, Farsiu S, et al. Intraoperative use of handheld spectral domain optical coherence tomography imaging in macular surgery. Retina. 2009;29:1457-68.

16. Ray R, Barañano DE, Fortun JA, et al. Intraoperative microscope-mounted spectral domain optical coherence tomography for evaluation of retinal anatomy during macular surgery. Ophthalmology. 2011;118:2212-7.

17. Ehlers JP, Tao YK, Farsiu S, et al. Integration of a spectral domain optical coherence tomography system into a surgical microscope for intraoperative imaging. Invest Ophthalmol Vis Sci. 2011; 52:3153-9.

18. Tao YK, Ehlers JP, Toth CA, et al. Intraoperative spectral domain optical coherence tomography for vitreoretinal surgery. Opt Lett. 2010;35:3315-17.

19. Binder S, Falkner-Radler CI, Hauger C, et al. Feasibility of intra-surgical spectral-domain optical coherence tomography. Retina. 2011;31:1332-36.

20. Ehlers JP, Kaiser PK, Srivastava SK. Intraoperative optical coherence tomography using the RESCAN 700: preliminary results from the DISCOVER study. Br J Ophthalmol. 2014;98:1329-32.

21. Au J, Goshe J, Dupps WJ Jr, et al. Intraoperative Optical Coherence Tomography for Enhanced Depth Visualization in Deep Anterior Lamellar Keratoplasty from the PIONEER Study. Cornea. 2015;34(9):1039-43.

22. Kumar A, Ravani R, Mehta A, et al. Outcomes of microscope integrated intraoperative optical coherence tomography guided center sparing internal limiting membrane peeling for myopic traction maculopathy: a novel technique. Int Ophthalmol. 2017.

23. Hahn P, Migacz J, O'Connell R, et al. Unprocessed real-time imaging of vitreoretinal surgical maneuvers using a microscope-integrated spectral-domain optical coherence tomography system. Graefes Arch Clin Exp Ophthalmol. 2013;251:213-20.

24. Christopher Kent. Intraoperative OCT Coming into Focus. Review of Ophthalmology. 2014.

25. Eckardt C, Paulo EB. Heads-up surgery for vitreoretinal procedures: an experimental and clinical study. Retina. 2016;36(1):137-47.

26. Kleinberg TT, Tzekov RT, Stein L, et al. Vitreous substitutes: a comprehensive review. Surv Ophthalmol. 2011;56(4):300-23.

27. Maruoka S, Matsuura T, Kawasaki K, et al. Biocompatibility of polyvinylalcohol gel as a vitreous substitute. Curr Eye Res. 2006;31(7-8):599-606.

28. Kashiwagi Y, Nishitsuka K, Takamura H, et al. Cloning and characterization of human vitreous tissue-derived cells. Acta Ophthalmol. 2011;89(6):538-43.

29. Bourla DH, Hubschman JP, Culjat M, et al. Feasibility study of intraocular robotic surgery with the da Vinci surgical system. Retina. 2008;28(1):154-8.

30. Pitcher JD, Wilson JT, Tsao TC, et al. Robotic eye surgery: past, present, and future. J Comput Sci Syst Biol. 2012;S3:001.

31. Sakai T, Harada K, Tanaka S, et al. Design and development of miniature parallel robot for eye surgery. Conf Proc IEEE Eng Med Biol Soc. 2014;2014:371-4.

32. He X, van Geirt V, Gehlbach P, et al. IRIS: Integrated Robotic Intraocular Snake. IEEE Int Conf Robot Autom. 2015;2015:1764-9.

33. He X, Balicki M, Gehlbach P, et al. A Novel dual force sensing instrument with cooperative robotic assistant for vitreoretinal surgery. IEEE Int Conf Robot Autom. 2013;2013:213-8.

34. Gonenc B, Handa J, Gehlbach P, et al. Design of 3-DOF force sensing micro-forceps for robot assisted vitreoretinal surgery. Conf Proc IEEE Eng Med Biol Soc. 2013;2013:5686-9.

35. Ida Y, Sugita N, Ueta T, et al. Microsurgical robotic system for vitreoretinal surgery. Int J Comput Assist Radiol Surg. 2012;7(1): 27-34.

36. Noda Y, Ida Y, Tanaka S, et al. Impact of robotic assistance on precision of vitreoretinal surgical procedures. PLoS One. 2013;8(1):e54116.

37. Rizzo JF III. Update on retinal prosthetic research: the Boston retinal implant project. J Neuroophthalmol. 2011;31:160-8.

38. Fujikado T, Kamei M, Sakaguchi H, et al. Testing of semichronically implanted retinal prosthesis by suprachoroidal-transretinal stimulation in patients with retinitis pigmentosa. Invest Ophthalmol Vis Sci. 2011;52:4726-33.

39. Matthaei M, Zeitz O, Keserü M, et al. Progress in the development of vision prostheses. Ophthalmologica. 2011;225:187-92.

40. Kusnyerik A, Greppmaier U, Wilke R, et al. Positioning of electronic subretinal implants in blind retinitis pigmentosa patients through multimodal assessment of retinal structures. Invest Ophthalmol Vis Sci. 2012;53:3748-55.

Ocular Trauma

Chapter 53

Classification of Ocular Trauma and Evaluation of Patient

Thirumalesh MB, Astha Jain, Sumeet Agarwal

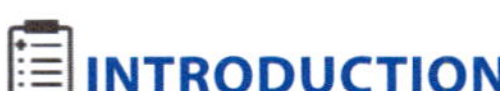 INTRODUCTION

Ocular trauma is a significant disabling public health problem in both developed and developing countries. The 5-year incidence of ocular trauma was 1.6% and cumulative lifetime prevalence was 19.8%, in the Beaver Dam Eye Study.[1]

Negrel and Thylefors reported that around 55 million eye injuries, restricting activities for more than 1 day, occur every year with around 750,000 cases requiring hospitalization. There are approximately 1.6 million blind from injuries, 2.3 million people with bilateral low vision and around 19 million with unilateral blindness or low vision.[2]

Ocular injuries are reported to be more common in males than in females and also are more common in younger population less than 40 years.[3] The most common causes in males were outdoor-related (30.9%), work-related (25.4%) and sports-related (17.5%) injuries; and in females were home-related (52.2%) and outdoor-related injuries (30.4%). Road accidents were more common in urban areas and work-related injuries in rural areas.[4] Intraocular foreign body (IOFB) following work-related injuries were more common in rural than in urban areas. Involvement of posterior segment indicates a poor prognosis with increased risk of blindness.[5] The rate of hospitalization was 8.9 per 100,000 persons aged 20 years or less for pediatric eye injuries in the United States in 2000. The highest percent for hospitalizations among young adults were aged between 18 years and 20 years.[6] The American National Safety Council estimates that $300 million accounts to work-related eye trauma annually.[7]

CLASSIFICATION

Ocular trauma can be classified into nonmechanical and mechanical injuries. The nonmechanical injuries consist of thermal, chemical, radiational, and electrical injury. Mechanical injuries of the eye can further be classified according to various classification systems, namely the Birmingham Eye Trauma Terminology System (BETTS)[8] and the Ocular Trauma Classification system.[9] The BETTS system of classification is shown in Flowchart 53.1.

Flowchart 53.1: Birmingham Eye Trauma Terminology System (BETTS).

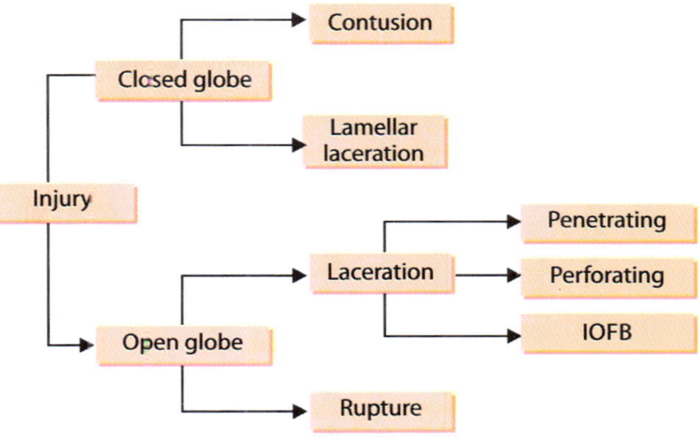

(IOFB: Intraocular foreign body).

The definition of the terms used in ocular trauma is as follows:

- *Eye wall*: Cornea and sclera
- *Closed globe injury*: Injury not causing a full-thickness wound of the eyewall
- *Open globe injury*: Injury causing a full-thickness wound of the eyewall
- Closed globe injury can be further classified as:
  - *Contusion*: Injury is generally by a blunt object. It is caused by energy transferred directly from the object or due to changes in the shape of the globe
  - *Lamellar laceration*: It is a partial-thickness wound of the eyewall usually caused by a sharp object.
- Open globe injury can be further classified as:
  - *Rupture*: It is a full-thickness wound of the eyewall caused due to blunt injury, which causes a momentary rise in IOP leading full-thickness wound at the weakest point (insertion of the recti where sclera is the thinnest or an old cataract surgery wound. The wound is created by an inside out mechanism).

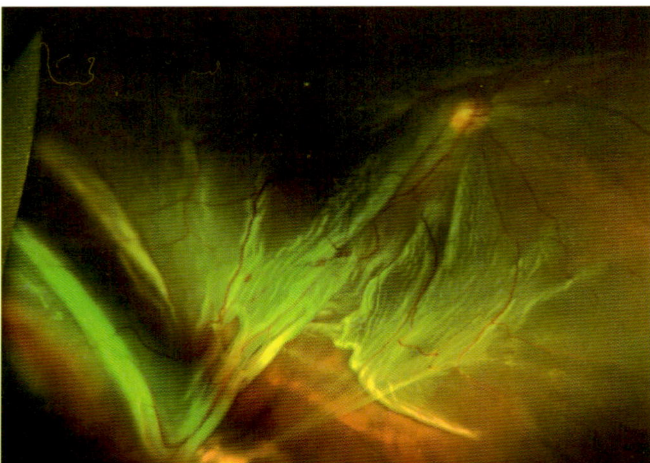

Fig. 53.1: Fundus photograph showing retinal incarceration developing near the exit wound after a perforating injury.

Table 53.1: Ocular trauma classification system.

Type of injury	Open-globe	Closed-globe
A	Rupture	Contusion
B	Penetrating injury	Lamellar laceration
C	Intraocular foreign body	Superficial foreign body
D	Perforating injury	Mixed
E	Mixed	N/A
Visual acuity	*Grade*	
20/40	1	
20/50 to 20/100	2	
19/100 to 5/200	3	
4/200 to light perception	4	
No light perception	5	
Relative afferent pupillary defect	*Response*	
Present	Positive	
Absent	Negative	

- *Laceration*: It is a full-thickness wound of the eyewall caused by a sharp object at the impact site. The lacerating injury can be penetrating or perforating:
  - *Penetrating injury*: Single full-thickness wound
  - *Perforating injury*: Two full-thickness wounds (entrance and exit) of the eyewall (Fig. 53.1).

The Ocular Trauma Classification group classifies both open globe and closed globe injuries according to four parameters: (1) type of injury; (2) grade of injury (visual acuity in the injured eye at first examination); (3) pupil [presence or absence of a relative afferent pupillary defect (RAPD)]; and (4) zone of injury, based on the extent of the injury. The classification is shown in Table 53.1.

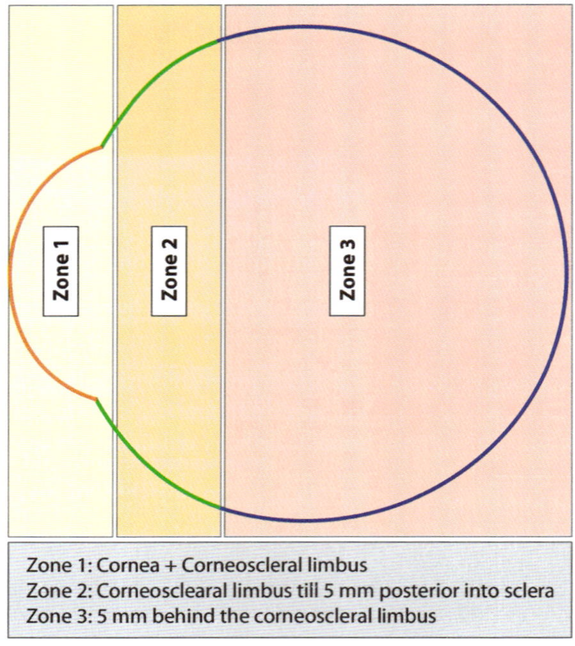

Zone 1: Cornea + Corneoscleral limbus
Zone 2: Corneosclearal limbus till 5 mm posterior into sclera
Zone 3: 5 mm behind the corneoscleral limbus

Fig. 53.2: Zone of injury as defined by the Ocular Trauma Society.

The zone of injury is defined as the posteriormost extent of full-thickness opening of the globe for open globe injuries or the anatomic location of the injury for closed globe injuries (Fig. 53.2).

- *Zone 1*: Within the cornea and corneoscleral limbus.
- *Zone 2*: From the limbus up to 5 mm posterior into the sclera and anterior segment.
- *Zone 3*: Posterior to zone 2 of the sclera and posterior segment.

The ocular trauma score was developed by Kuhn et al. for prognosticating the functional outcome after serious eye injury.[10] It is shown in Tables 53.2 and 53.3.

MECHANISM OF OCULAR INJURY

Blunt trauma causes ocular damage by the coup mechanism, the contrecoup mechanism or equatorial expansion. Coup injury occurs due to direct impact, e.g. subconjunctival hemorrhage, choroidal hemorrhage. Contrecoup mechanism of ocular injury was described by Wolter et al.[11] Contrecoup injury is caused due to transmitted shock waves, e.g. commotio retinae. Equatorial expansion occurs when blunt trauma causes compression along the anteroposterior axis. Eye is a closed space and its volume cannot be changed. Compression of the eye along the anteroposterior axis causes expansion along the equatorial axis as shown in Figure 53.3.

Table 53.2: Ocular trauma score: parameters and raw points.

Variables	Raw points
Initial vision	
No light perception (NPL)/enucleation/evisceration	60
Light perception (LP)/hand motion (HM)	70
1/60–5/60	80
6/60–6/15	90
≥6/12	100
Rupture	−23
Endophthalmitis	−17
Perforating injury	−14
Retinal detachment	−11
Relative afferent pupillary defect (RAPD)	−10

Table 53.3: Calculating the ocular trauma score (OTS): Conversion of raw points into an OTS category and calculating the final visual acuity in five categories.

Sum of raw points	OTS	No light perception	Light perception/Hand movement	1/60–5/60	6/60–6/15	≥6/12
0–44	1	74%	15%	7%	3%	1%
45–65	2	27%	26%	18%	15%	15%
66–80	3	2%	11%	15%	31%	41%
81–91	4	1%	2%	3%	22%	73%
92–100	5	0%	1%	1%	5%	94%

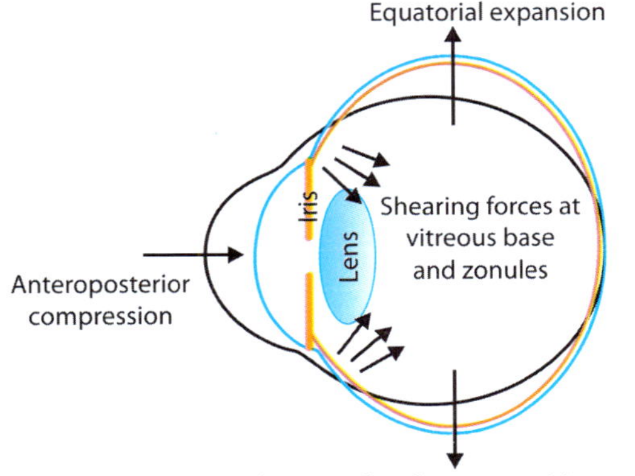

Fig. 53.3: Mechanism of injury due to blunt ocular trauma.

When a blunt object strikes the globe, the kinetic energy of the object is transferred to the globe. This energy alters the shape of the globe by compression and decompression followed by overshoot and oscillations. During the oscillation, each ocular layer moves at a different speed due to different elasticity. Shear forces develop at these interfaces of tissues with different elasticity causing ocular damage.

Size, hardness and velocity of the object contribute to the extent of ocular damage along with the force imparted to the eye. When an object larger than the orbital opening causes injury, there is a rise in the intraorbital pressure leading to fracture of the orbital walls. When the injury is by an object smaller than the orbital opening, the energy is directly absorbed by the eyeball causing a rise in IOP and consequently greater ocular damage.

EVALUATION OF A CASE OF OCULAR TRAUMA

The patient must be seen as a whole and not just as a case of ocular trauma. Before evaluating the ocular injury and the extent of damage, it should be made sure that the patient is systemically stable and any other occult life-threatening injury should be noted.

History

Detailed history regarding the nature and mechanism of injury goes a long way in determining the preferred approach for the patient.

A detailed history should be elicited for both management and for documentation for medicolegal purpose. The history should record the mechanism of injury, type of injury (blunt or penetrating), the time of onset and the possibility of IOFB. History of any previous surgery or a preexisting eye disease should be noted.

After global assessment and history, one should proceed to ocular examination. A thorough examination is done from anterior to posterior segment beginning with gross external inspection and assessment of visual acuity in each eye.

Ocular Examination

Baseline visual acuity should be noted, as it is important to establish the grade of damage and provide a foundation to determine the prognosis. It is also important for medicolegal reasons.[12] Perception of light should be carefully assessed using bright light in a dark room with the other eye properly closed. Projection of rays should also be assessed when light perception is present.

It is then followed by examination of the adnexal structures and gross external examination of the eye. Each globe should be evaluated for protrusion or proptosis and examined for signs of penetration or presence of foreign body. Ocular movements should be noted in the cardinal directions of gaze and any restriction recorded. The orbital rims should be similarly inspected and palpated for any crepitus or obvious bony deformities.

Optic nerve function should be evaluated by looking for RAPD, confrontational visual field testing, color vision and identifying any subjective difference in brightness perception. If possible, the intraocular pressure should be recorded and a detailed slit-lamp examination along with a dilated indirect ophthalmoscopy should be done.

In the presence of hyphema, fundus examination must be done gently to avoid precipitating a secondary hemorrhage. Scleral depression should be deferred for at least 2–3 weeks. All patients must be followed until peripheral retinal examination is complete, to avoid missing any retinal break or impacted foreign body (Fig. 53.4).

Simple penlight examination can often appreciate an obvious open globe injury.

Globe rupture can sometimes be occult and its signs include significantly low IOP, irregular pupil suggesting that the peripheral wound is plugged by iris, shallow or deep anterior chamber compared to the fellow eye and the presence of significant chemosis, usually 360° hemorrhagic, suggesting that there may be bleeding through a scleral rupture. As soon as the diagnosis of ruptured globe is made, the examination should be stopped and the eye should be covered by a protective shield. The complete evaluation and the repair should be done by an eye surgeon in the operating room. Uncooperative patients must be examined under general anesthesia in the operating room.

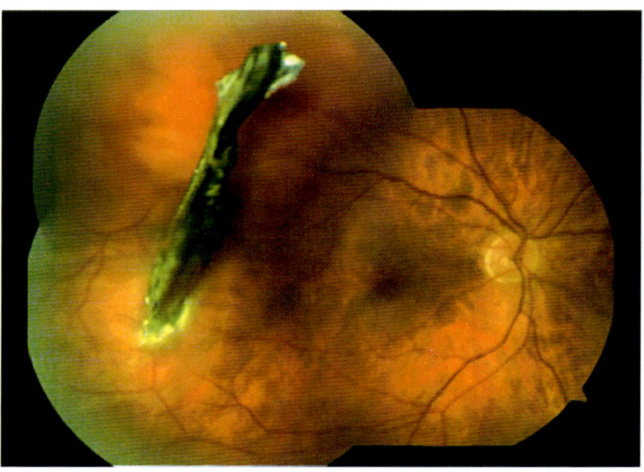

Fig. 53.4: Color fundus image shows intraocular foreign body (IOFB) lying impacted on the retina, temporal to the macula.

Ocular Imaging

Ancillary testing (primarily CT and ultrasonography) can be utilized to obtain additional information. They are very helpful to know the presence and location of any IOFB, to detect any bony damage, if present and to evaluate the posterior segment in cases of hyphema or vitreous hemorrhage.

X-ray

X-ray may be regarded as an archival mode of imaging which has been largely superseded by computed tomography. X-ray is used to detect IOFB and orbital fractures. The detection rate of metallic IOFB by plain X-ray is almost 90%, whereas it is just about 70% for glass and 0–15% for other materials like wood and graphite.[13] The standard views to detect a foreign body includes Water's, Caldwell, and lateral views but, these projections may demonstrate the presence and not the location of the IOFB (Figs. 53.5A and B).

Before the development of computed tomography (CT), plain X-rays with metal locators were used to localize metallic foreign bodies. The limbal ring by Stallard[14] is sutured over the limbus and two views are taken (posteroanterior and lateral). Other locators which were used are Roper-Hall,[15] Berman,[16] and Bronson-Turner.[17] Roper-Hall locator uses electroacoustic waves to detect foreign bodies. Metallic foreign bodies transmit continuous signals whereas nonmetallic foreign bodies transmit interrupted signals.

Bone free method[18] is another technique, which uses rotational movements of the eyes, and the foreign body is located in relation to the films taken at different views. Several radiological techniques[19] have been described of which Sweet method, Comberg method and modified spectacle frame method[20] are of historical importance. Sweet method utilizes metal detectors placed at 10 mm from the vertex cornea and

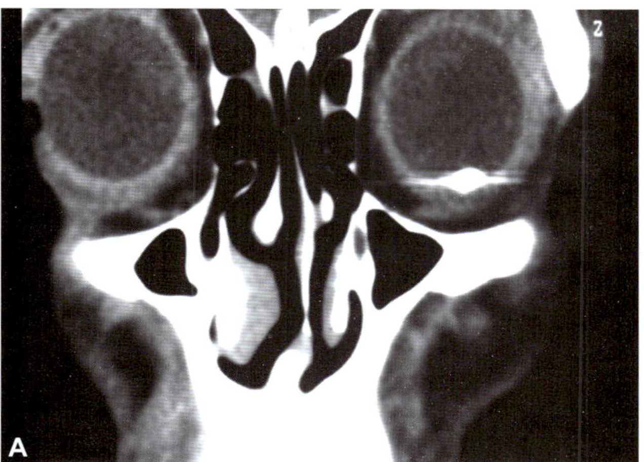
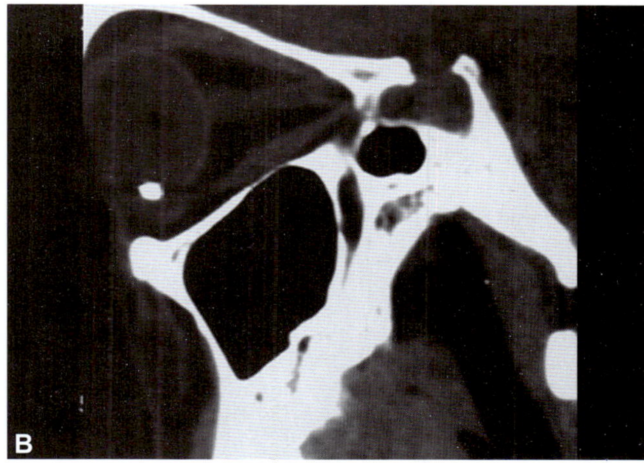

Figs. 53.5A and B: Hyperdense foreign body in the inferior aspect of the left globe with the presence of streak artifact and beam hardening artifact.

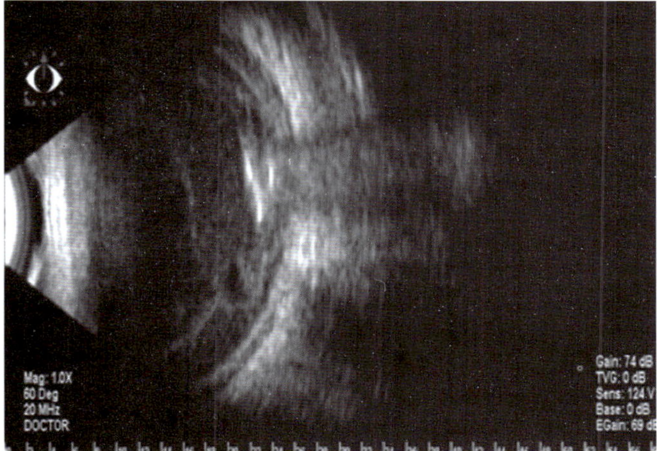

Fig. 53.6: Impacted intraocular foreign body (IOFB) lying on the retina with evidence of shadowing behind it.

films from two views are taken. There have been reports of injecting a radiopaque dye in tenon's space and taking films subsequently but the risk of air embolism and allergic reaction were high. In the present setting, all the above modalities have become obsolete and plain X-ray is being performed as a first-step investigation due to its accessibility, low cost, documentation, and medicolegal purpose.

Ultrasonography

Ultrasonography (USG) allows the ophthalmologist to have an instantaneous look at the posterior segment in presence of opaque ocular media (Fig. 53.6). It is superior to other modalities as it allows real-time imaging and detecting soft tissue abnormalities. It is noninvasive, inexpensive, accessible, and can be easily performed as a routine outpatient procedure or in the emergency room.

It is reliable in detecting retinal detachment, posterior vitreous detachment, vitreous hemorrhage and opacities, choroidal detachment (serous and hemorrhagic), vitreous incarceration, scleral, and choroidal ruptures and IOFBs. The sensitivity and specificity of USG in case of ocular trauma is 91.5% and 93.87%, respectively[21] making it an accurate and indispensable modality of investigation.

B-scan ultrasonic (US) probe of 10 MHz is classically used in case of ocular trauma. In open globe injuries, it is advisable to do a primary repair before subjecting the patient to USG. Anterior segment examination can be done using immersion technique or water-balloon technique.[22]

Integrity of the posterior capsule of lens can be confirmed on USG. Presence of posterior capsule rupture can be confirmed which helps to determine the best approach for cataract extraction. USG also helps in determining the position of a posteriorly dislocated crystalline lens[23] or intraocular lens in patients with opaque media. The mobility of the lens can be confirmed by asking the patient to move his eyes.

Posttraumatic vitreous hemorrhage per se is not an indication for emergency surgery, but presence of retinal detachment and IOFB warrants an early intervention. USG helps in identifying such cases. In mild hemorrhage, dots are seen on B-scan and A-scan shows multiple low amplitude spikes. As the hemorrhage becomes denser, more opacities are displayed on B-scan and they show high reflective spikes on A-scan. Vitreous hemorrhage can accompany with different degrees of PVD. Detached vitreous is smooth on B-scan but may be thick posteriorly when its surface is layered with blood. PVD can be distinguished from retinal detachment as it shows undulating after-movements on kinetic USG. However, they may look similar on USG and the distinction between both may be quite challenging.

Retinal detachment typically appears on USG as a high reflectivity and continuous membrane within the vitreous. A 100% spike is displayed on A-scan when the sound beam is directed perpendicular to the detachment.

Giant retinal tears (GRT)[24] and retinal dialysis may also be identified using B-scan. A characteristic feature of giant retinal tears found on B-scan ultrasonography is the "double linear echo" sign. There are two high-amplitude linear echoes starting from the optic disc and lying parallel and adjacent to each other. The linear echo that is continuous with the globe corresponds to the detached retina, and the adjacent linear echo which is not continuous with the globe is interpreted as the inverted posterior flap of the GRT.

Choroidal detachment can also occur in ocular trauma. It can be seen as a smooth, dome-shaped, thick membrane with little after-movements on B-scan. On A-scan, a thick 100% high spike is produced.

B-scan USG has also been very valuable for detecting and localizing IOFBs.[25] It appears acoustically white in contrast to the acoustically black vitreous and is visible even after the gain is reduced to less than 30 db. It causes strong sound attenuation and causes shadowing of the ocular and orbital tissues behind it[26] (Fig. 53.6). Mobility and location of the IOFB can be determined by taking scans from different probe positions and views. A-scan shows a steeply rising wide spike with a reflectivity of 100% and no spikes between the IOFB and sclera. Other associated intraocular damage like retinal detachment, vitreous hemorrhage, endophthalmitis or vitreous incarceration in scleral wound can be determined with USG scan.

Optic nerve avulsion can also be obscured as it is commonly associated with vitreous hemorrhage. On B-scan, it can be seen as a linear split in the continuity of sclera or a "retinal step sign" in the horizontal B-scan.[27] Color Doppler ultrasonography shows decreased blood flow in the central retinal artery in cases of traumatic optic neuropathy.[28] B-scan USG has recently been used to measure thickness of optic nerve in case of posttraumatic optic neuropathy.

Exploration of globe under general anesthesia in the operating room is recommended when clinical examination and investigations are not definitive for any diagnosis. Photo documentation should be done whenever possible for medicolegal purposes.

REFERENCES

1. Wong TY, Klein BE, Klein R. The prevalence and 5-year incidence of ocular trauma. The Beaver Dam Eye Study. Ophthalmology. 2000;107(12):2196-202.
2. Négrel AD, Thylefors B. The global impact of eye injuries. Ophthalmic Epidemiol. 1998;5(3):143-69.
3. Pandita A, Merriman M. Ocular trauma epidemiology: 10-year retrospective study. N Z Med J. 2012;125(1348):61-9.
4. Cillino S, Casuccio A, Di Pace F, et al. A five-year retrospective study of the epidemiological characteristics and visual outcomes of patients hospitalized for ocular trauma in a Mediterranean area. BMC Ophthalmology. 2008;8:6.
5. Kuhn F, Morris R, Witherspoon CD, et al. Epidemiology of blinding trauma in the United States Eye Injury Registry. Ophthalmic Epidemiol. 2006;13(3):209-16.
6. Brophy M, Sinclair SA, Hostetler SG, et al. Pediatric eye injury-related hospitalizations in the United States. Pediatrics. 2006;117(6):e1263-71.
7. United States Eye Injury Registry. Epidemiology. [online] Available from: https://useir.org/epidemiology/ [Accessed December, 2017].
8. Kuhn F, Morris R, Witherspoon CD, et al. A standardized classification of ocular trauma. Ophthalmology. 1996;103(2):240-3.
9. Pieramici DJ, Sternberg P Jr, Aaberg TM Sr, et al. A system for classifying mechanical injuries of the eye (globe). Am J Ophthalmology. 1997;123(6):820-31.
10. Kuhn F, Maisiak R, Mann L, et al. The ocular trauma score (OTS). Ophthalmology Clin North Am. 2002;15(2):163-5.
11. Wolter JR. Coup-contrecoup mechanism of ocular injuries. Am J Ophthalmology. 1963;56:785-96.
12. Khaw PT, Shah P, Elkington AR. Injury to the eye. BMJ. 2004;328(7430):36-8.
13. Bray LC, Griffiths PG. The value of plain radiography in suspected intraocular foreign body. Eye (Lond). 1991;5(Pt 6):751-4.
14. Poon KY. Use of limbal ring-rod for radiological localisation of ocular foreign body. Br J Ophthalmology. 1989;73(8):645-50.
15. Roper-Hall MJ. An intra-ocular foreign body locator. Trans Opthal Soc U K. 1957;77:239-50.
16. Alvis BY. The use of the Berman locator in removal of intra-ocular foreign bodies. Eye Ear Nose Throat Mon. 1946;25:247-54.
17. Bronson NR 2nd, Turner FT. Practical characteristics of metal locators. Arch Ophthalmology. 1972;88(2):199-203.
18. Lindblom K. Bone-free radiography of the eye. A new projection and a film holder. Acta Radiologica. 1934;15(6):615-19.
19. Ahlbom H. A new method of localizing foreign bodies in the eye. Teleradiography with visualization of the cornea. Acta Radiologica. 1931;12(3):212-35.
20. Little LE, LaPiana FG. Localization of intraorbital foreign bodies. Ann Ophthalmology. 1976;8(5):541-4.
21. Shazlee MK, Ali M, Saad Ahmed M, et al. Diagnostic accuracy of ultrasound B-scan using 10 MHz linear probe in ocular trauma; results from a high burden country. Pak J Med Sci. 2016;32(2):385-8.
22. Chugh JP, Susheel, Verma M. Role of ultrasonography in ocular trauma. Indian J Radiol Imaging. 2001;11:75-9.
23. Ojaghi Haghighi SH, Morteza Begi HR, Sorkhabi R, et al. Diagnostic accuracy of ultrasound in detection of traumatic lens dislocation. Emer (Tehran). 2014;2(3):121-4.
24. Shunmugam M, Ang GS, Lois N. Giant retinal tears. Surv Ophthalmology. 2014;59(2):192-216.
25. McNicholas MM, Brophy DP, Power WJ, et al. Ocular trauma: evaluation with US. Radiol. 1995;195(2):423-7.
26. Wang K, Liu J, Chen M. Role of B-scan ultrasonography in the localization of intraocular foreign bodies in the anterior segment: a report of three cases. BMC Ophthalmology. 2015;15:102.
27. Talwar D, Kumar A, Verma L, et al. Ultrasonography in optic nerve head avulsion. Acta Ophthalmology (Copenh). 1991;69(1):121-3.
28. Mariak Z, Obuchowska I, Ustymowicz A, et al. Color Doppler ultrasonography in diagnosis of post-traumatic optic neuropathy. Klin Oczna. 1999;101(2):105-10.

Chapter 54

Blunt Ocular Trauma

Thirumalesh MB, Astha Jain, Alisha Kishore

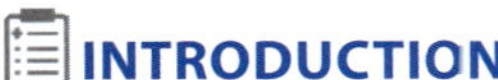 INTRODUCTION

Blunt trauma can cause ocular injury by three mechanisms—coup, contrecoup, or equatorial expansion. Coup injury occurs due to direct impact, for example, subconjunctival, choroidal or vitreous hemorrhage. Contrecoup injury is caused due to transmitted shock waves as in commotio retinae. Equatorial expansion occurs when blunt trauma causes compression along the anteroposterior axis, causing ocular damage (Fig. 54.1).

VITREOUS HEMORRHAGE

Vitreous hemorrhage results from trauma to the retina, choroid, or ciliary body. It may be associated with a retinal tear and hence a detailed fundus evaluation with scleral indentation should be performed when media permits (Fig. 54.2). However, if an occult scleral rupture is suspected, scleral depression should be deferred and globe exploration should be performed along with repair of the perforation, if found. If the fundus is not visible due to vitreous hemorrhage, a thorough ocular ultrasonographic examination of the posterior segment should be done to look for any associated conditions like retinal detachment, choroidal detachment, and optic nerve damage. If vitreous hemorrhage is not associated with evidence of any other intraocular ailment, the patient can be observed and reassured. However, there is always a risk of retinal detachment occurring later and thus the patient should be followed- up every 2–4 weeks for at least 3 months along with ultrasonographic evaluation till complete fundus evaluation is clinically possible.

Surgical indications include vitreous hemorrhage associated with retinal detachment, where immediate surgery is required, or a nonresolving vitreous hemorrhage, which is usually defined as a vitreous hemorrhage that does not clear up in 3 months. The visual prognosis depends on associations such as choroidal rupture, macular hole, retinal detachment, and optic nerve damage.

Poor prognostic factors:

- Visual acuity—light perception or worse
- Presence of hyphema

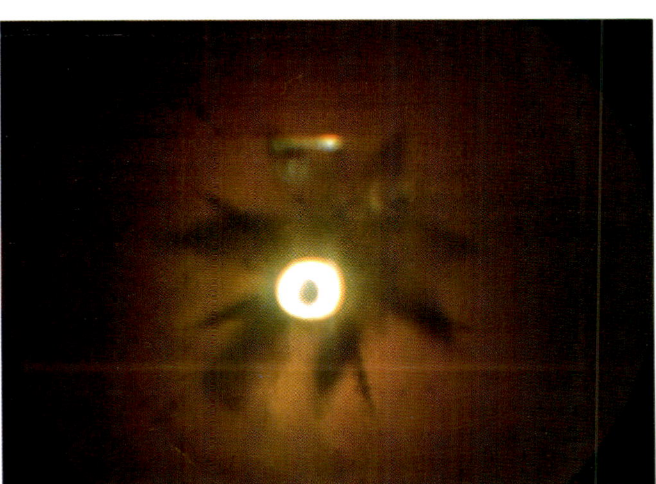

Fig. 54.1: Rosette cataract in an eye with closed globe injury.

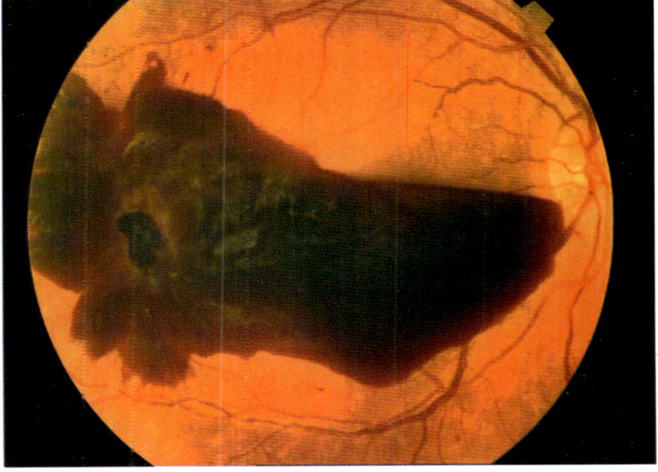

Fig. 54.2: Subhyaloid hemorrhage in a case of blunt trauma.

- Presence of traumatic cataract
- Age less than 55 years.[1]

Macular scar and traumatic optic neuropathy are the most important causes associated with poor visual outcome.

COMMOTIO RETINAE

Berlin first described commotio retinae in 1873 also known as Berlin's edema.[2] It makes up for 9.4% of all the posterior segment manifestations of trauma.[3] It is characterized by transient grayish white discolouration and opacification of neurosensory retina caused by blunt ocular trauma by contrecoup mechanism. It can be classified as concussion or contusion type. Concussion type is mild with visual acuity better than 20/200 or 6/60 and no leakage on fundus fluorescein angiography (FFA), while the latter one is severe with visual acuity worse than 20/200 with leakage on FFA and it may or may not be associated with vitreous hemorrhage. Posterior pole and periphery can be involved. The retina may initially appear normal. Retinal whitening may take hours to develop and becomes normal in a few days[3] (Fig. 54.3).

Fluorescein angiography shows blocked choroidal fluorescence in areas of opaque retina. There is no leakage of dye suggesting that there is no alteration in retinal vascular permeability[4] showing that it is not a true edema. The opacification is due to fragmentation of the photoreceptor outer segment and in more severe cases, retinal pigment epithelium (RPE) damage may also be associated.[5,6]

The major site of injury in commotio retinae is at the level of the photoreceptor outer segment—RPE junction. Experimental injuries in primates have shown photoreceptor degeneration and photoreceptor outer segment disruption.[6] Histopathological findings in a human eye enucleated within 24 hours of clinically observed commotio retinae also revealed photoreceptor outer segment disruption and damage to the RPE.[5] Optical coherence tomography (OCT) reports have further affirmed the damage to be at the photoreceptor RPE interface conforming with the histopathological findings.[7,8]

There is no treatment modality of proven benefit for this condition. Visual acuity can be normal only if the peripheral retina is involved and there is no other ocular damage. Macula involving lesions may lead to loss of central vision. Associated retinal injuries such as macular hole and choroidal rupture can also lead to permanent visual loss. Central and peripheral vision tends to improve as the retinal whitening resolves. However, in some cases (40%), central vision loss may be permanent, associated with RPE changes and pigment migration.[9] The RPE may phagocytose the degenerating photoreceptor cells and may migrate into the inner retinal layers.[6] The peripheral pigmentary changes when present can mimic retinitis pigmentosa.[10]

CHOROIDAL RUPTURE

Choroidal rupture is a break in vascular choroid, Bruch's membrane, and RPE, due to anteroposterior compression and equatorial expansion of the globe due to blunt ocular trauma (Figs. 54.4A and B). Bruch's membrane and RPE

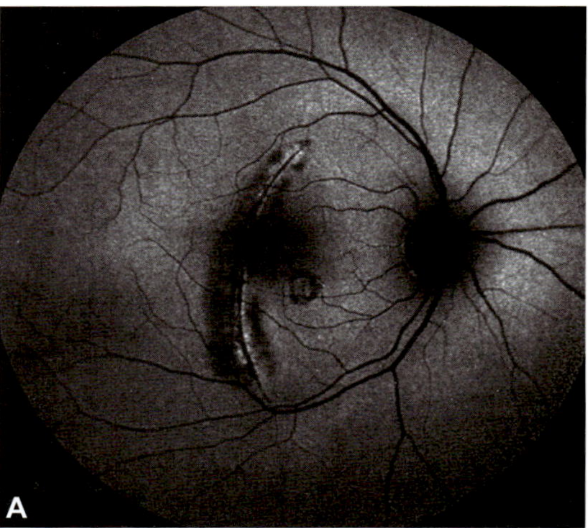

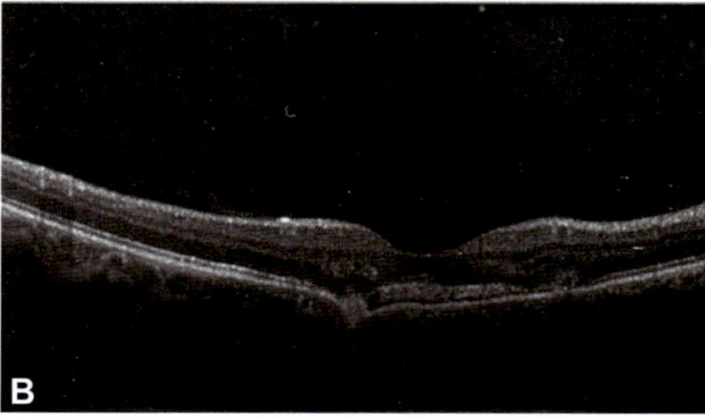

Figs. 54.4A and B: (A) FAF imaging shows a crescentic, linear Bruch's membrane rupture; (B) also visible on OCT scan.
(FAF: Fundus autofluorescence; OCT: Optical coherence tomography).

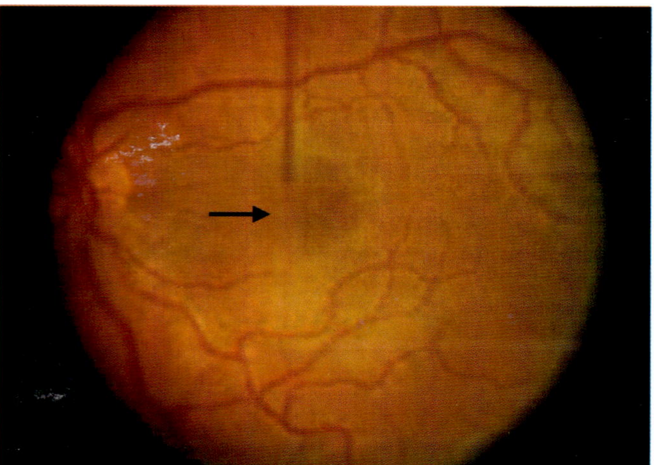

Fig. 54.3: Color fundus image showing commotio retina with loss of foveal reflex (arrow).

are prime targets for rupture as they are the least elastic structures. The deep choroidal vessels remain intact in most cases. Choroidal ruptures are seen in almost 5–10% of closed globe injury cases.[11] The retinal tissue is relatively elastic and flexible and the sclera is relatively tough because of the collagen, thus both these structures are less likely to rupture during blunt ocular trauma.

However, the RPE, Bruch's membrane, and choriocapillaris are relatively inelastic and have a tendency to rupture. The less common direct choroidal ruptures occur directly at the site of impact, found anterior to the equator and are parallel to ora. Indirect choroidal ruptures occur due to contrecoup injury, located at the posterior pole. Indirect choroidal rupture accounts for around 80% of all cases.[12] They occur concentric to the disc due to stabilizing action of optic nerve (as shown in Figs. 54.5A and B). They are mostly temporal to the disc and involve fovea, but can also occur nasally. They are usually single but can be multiple.[12] Patients with increased brittleness of Bruch's membrane such as angioid streaks are prone to choroidal rupture than others.

Choroidal rupture is commonly seen along with intraretinal, subretinal, and intrachoroidal hemorrhage, which may obscure the presence of the rupture. A white continuous streak can be seen as the blood resorbs which is mostly concentric to the disc or elsewhere. Choroidal rupture can be seen on FFA and indocyanine green (ICG) even when not visi-ble clinically. Choroidal rupture appears as hyperfluorescent streaks on FFA and hypofluorescent on ICG angiography (ICGA). ICGA often demonstrates broader area of pathology as compared to FFA and also delineates the choroidal rupture.[13]

Healing of choroidal rupture involves fibrovascular proliferation from the choroid that evolves into a dense fibrous

scar with RPE hyperplasia.[14] Choroidal neovascularization (CNV) can develop in up to 5–10% of choroidal rupture cases,[15] and the chance of CNV development increase with involvement of the macula, older age, and greater extent of the rupture.[5] Management options include photodynamic therapy (PDT) and intravitreal anti vascular endothelial growth factor (VEGF).[16–18] Most of the post-traumatic CNV are subfoveal and hence not amenable to laser treatment[18] (Figs. 54.6A and B).

Visual prognosis depends on the site of rupture and the baseline visual acuity. Rupture involving the fovea and poor initial visual acuity is associated with poor visual outcome.[15] Development of late complication such as CNV can also affect the long- term visual outcome. Fovea sparing lesions usually have a good prognosis as the overlying nerve fiber layer is never injured. Therefore, even if a rupture is located between the disc and the macula, the visual outcome may be good. Multiple choroidal ruptures do not necessarily predict a poor visual outcome.[9]

Secondary CNVMs following a choroidal rupture can lead to a submacular bleed, which can further deteriorate the prognosis. Various treatment options which have been tried for large subretinal bleeds are use of intraocular gas, subretinal and intravitreal tissue plasminogen activator (tPA), and anti-VEGF agents. The authors recommend the use of a combination therapy, which has helped them to achieve excellent results with displacement of the subretinal hemorrhage within first 24 hours of surgery. Following vitrectomy, a small neurosensory detachment is created by injecting subretinal balanced salt solution using a 41G needle. Then tPA (0.4 mL with 50 µg dose) plus 0.4 mL air is injected with a 41 gauge cannula below the retina causing pneumatic displacement of blood. Additionally, bevacizumab can be injected in case a CNV is suspected.

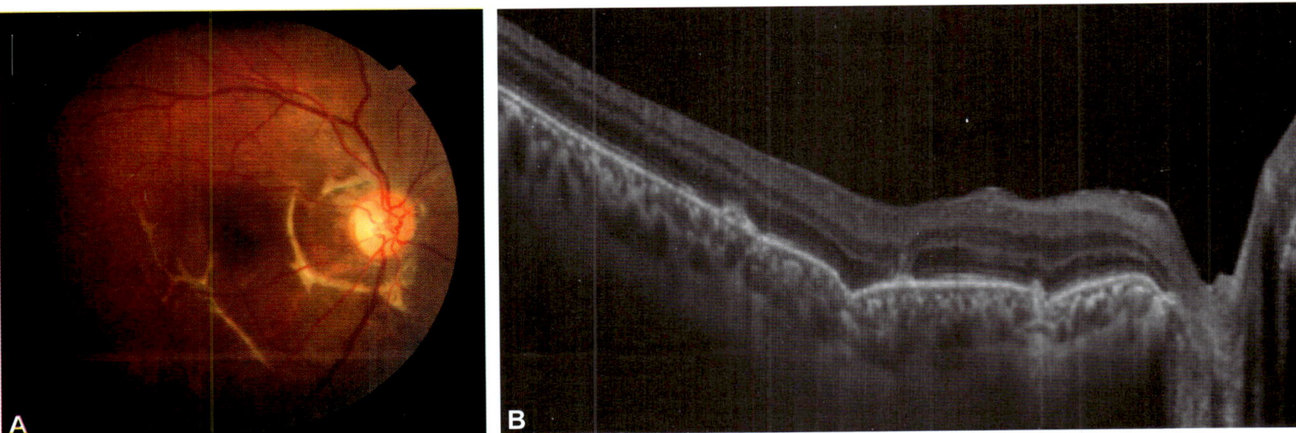

Figs. 54.5A and B: (A) Circumferential multiple choroidal ruptures visible on fundus color picture and (B) breaks in RPE–Bruch's complex is seen on SS-OCT.
(RPE: Retinal pigment epithelium; SS-OCT: Swept source-optical coherence tomography).

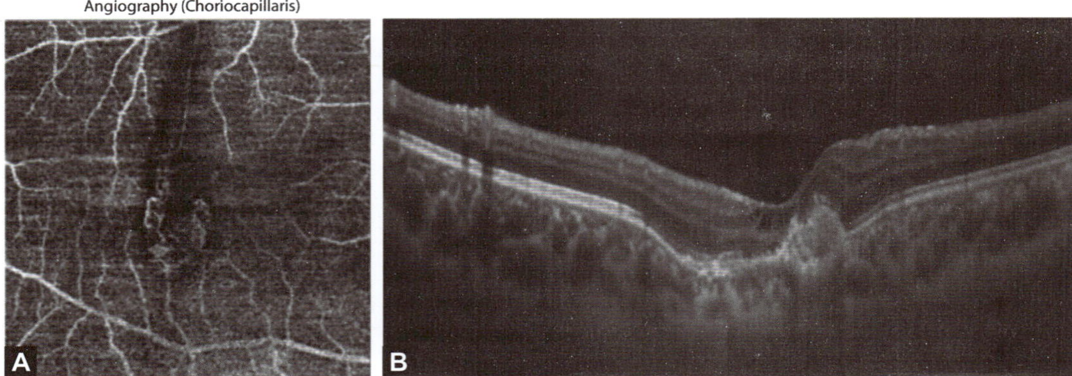

Figs. 54.6A and B: (A) Eye shows choroidal rupture with CNV visible on SS-OCTA and (B) RPE rip with CNV growing through it on SS-OCT. (CNV: Choroidal neovascularization; RPE: Retinal pigment epithelium; SS-OCTA: Swept source- optical coherence tomography angiography).

TRAUMATIC MACULAR HOLE

Traumatic macular hole (Figs. 54.7A and B) was first described by Knapp in 1869.[20] It accounts for 10% of cases.[21,22] The pathophysiological mechanism of traumatic macular hole formation is still unclear. It is likely to be related to increased vitreomacular traction forces occurring during axial compression and equatorial expansion in a contrecoup injury.[23] Other theories described are—cystic degeneration following severe cystoid macular edema, vascular mechanism following subretinal hemorrhage, contusion necrosis, and whiplash separation of vitreous. Macular hole can occur immediately after trauma or several days following it. Huang et al. in a study characterized the difference between traumatic and idiopathic macular hole.[24] They found that traumatic macular hole was more common in younger patients with worse initial presenting vision. OCT comparison by Huang et al. found that traumatic holes had a thinner average retinal thickness with a larger basal diameter and basal area and these holes are not usually associated with posterior vitreous detachment (PVD). Traumatic macular holes tend to possess a more irregular configuration compared to the smooth circular edges of idiopathic macular holes.

Traumatic macular holes may close spontaneously. Young patients with small holes without a fluid cuff and without intraretinal cystic changes[25] tend to close spontaneously. The mechanism of spontaneous closure may be proliferation of RPE and glial cells at the edge of the hole, filling the defect.[26] Yamada et al. proposed to wait for 6 months before surgery to allow spontaneous closure of the hole. Cases which do not close spontaneously can be taken up for pars plana vitrectomy with or without peeling of internal limiting membrane (ILM) with internal tamponade. Johnson et al. described a good success rate with successful closure in 96% of his patients and improvement in visual acuity of two or more lines in 84% patients following vitrectomy and peeling.[27] Platelet concentrate, autologous plasmin or autologous blood, have been used as adjunctive agents in surgical

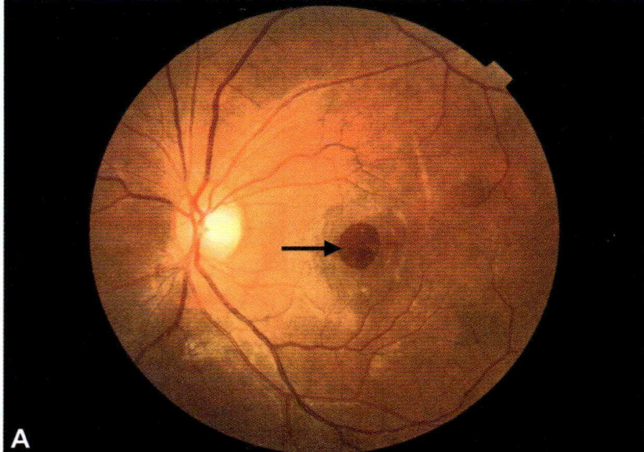

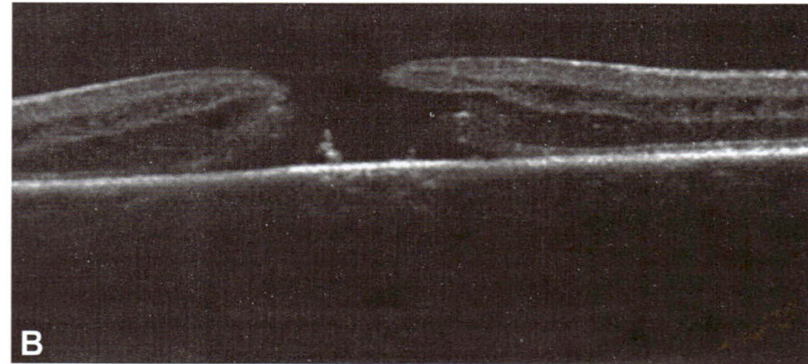

Figs. 54.7A and B: (A) Color fundus pictures showing traumatic macular hole (arrow) with choroidal rupture; (B) OCT picture showing traumatic macular hole with ragged edge. (OCT: Optical coherence tomography).

repair.[28,29] Eyes with associated choroidal or RPE injury have a poorer visual prognosis despite successful surgical closure.

RETINITIS SCLOPETARIA

The term chorioretinitis sclopetaria (Fig. 54.8) was introduced by Goldzieher in 1901.[30] Currently, the term traumatic chorioretinal rupture is more acceptable. It is

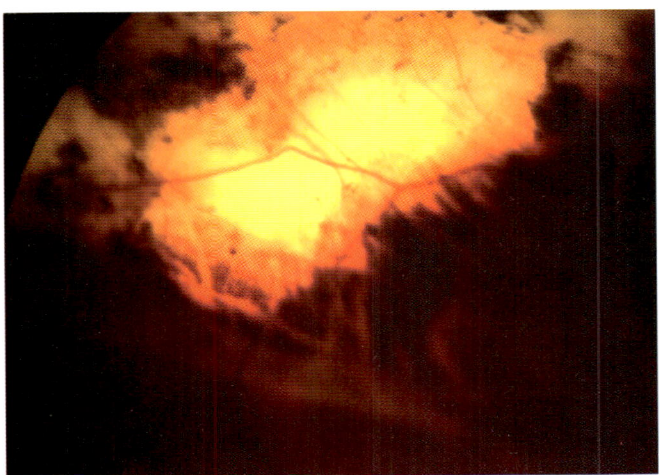

Fig. 54.8: Color fundus picture showing retinal sclopetaria.

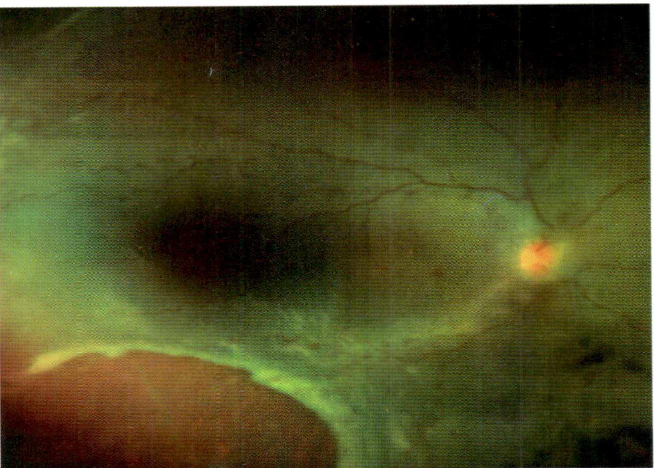

Fig. 54.9: Large posttraumatic retinal dialysis with RD. (RD: Retinal detachment).

characterized by rupture of the retina and choroid caused by a nonpenetrating ocular injury caused by a high-velocity projectile usually a bullet passing close to the globe without causing a scleral rupture. The impact of the injury causes full thickness chorioretinal rupture with associated hemorrhage. Bare sclera is revealed as the choroid and sclera retracts. Direct injury is caused along the direction of the high-velocity object and indirect injury by shock waves that get transmitted to the eye.[31]

Both posterior pole and peripheral retina may be involved. Marked retinal and choroidal hemorrhage is present. Fundus may be initially obscured due to overlying vitreous hemorrhage, intraretinal, and subretinal hemorrhage. With resolution of the hemorrhage, chorioretinal defect with bare sclera, pigment proliferation, marked fibrovascular proliferation, and scar formation may become visible.[32]

Retinal detachment occurs rarely despite severe chorioretinal injury because of the firm adhesion between retina, choroid, and sclera caused by marked proliferation of fibrous tissue.[33] A study by Papakostas et al. showed three cases of sclopetaria who developed retinal detachment within 1 month of injury.[32] In such cases, a break at a different site can cause late detachment.[34]

Management is mainly nonsurgical and continued observation is required for early detection of any late complications.[34] Surgical management may rarely be required in case of a retinal detachment or nonresolving vitreous hemorrhage.[35] Making an accurate diagnosis of sclopetaria is important to avoid unwarranted surgical intervention.[33] A retained intraorbital foreign body following injury is usually well tolerated and can be followed- up without surgical intervention.[33] The visual prognosis is often poor due to initial severity of injury. However, few cases with a good visual gain have been reported.[34,36]

RETINAL DETACHMENT

Blunt trauma is the most common cause of retinal trauma in younger individuals, especially males. Most common break in traumatic retinal detachment is retinal dialysis (Figs. 54.9 and 54.11). The patients with traumatic retinal detachment are younger and hence have formed vitreous which typically have a slow progression, unless a giant retinal tear (Figs. 54.10A and B) is present. The causative break in 87% of all traumatic retinal detachment is found at the vitreous base.

SCLERAL RUPTURE

Scleral rupture occurs when a blunt object strikes the orbit, compressing the globe along the anteroposterior axis with a rise in intraocular pressure to a point that the sclera ruptures. Rupture is most common at the site where sclera is thinnest, that is at the site of muscle insertion (0.3 mm thick) or at the limbus or at the site of previous surgical incision if any. Rupture may be associated with a foreign body retained inside the globe. The diagnosis of globe rupture is obvious when the shape of the globe is altered with uveal tissue seen prolapsing out of the scleral wound (Fig. 54.12). More often than not, on presentation, an occult scleral rupture may be present. Signs suggestive of occult scleral rupture are reduction of visual acuity to light perception, subconjunctival hemorrhage with conjunctival edema, ocular hypotension, pupillary distortion, hyphema, limitation of ocular movements, or vitreous hemorrhage.[37] The size of maximal conjunctival chemosis may indicate the quadrant of globe involved in rupture.[38]

Ultrasonography and computed tomography (CT scan) are adjunctive diagnostic tools in identifying the presence of an associated vitreous hemorrhage, choroidal or retinal detachment, and foreign body. While examining a case of

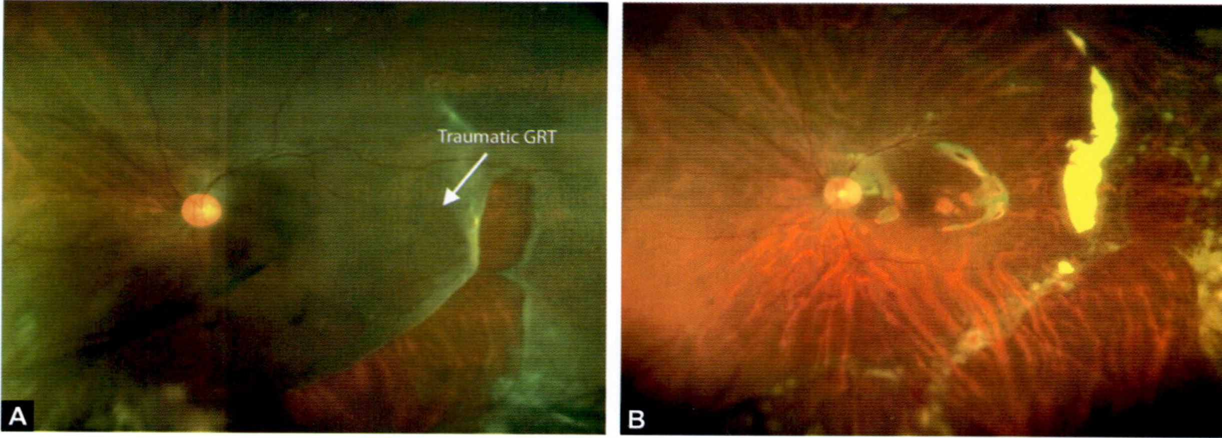

Figs. 54.10A and B: (A) Traumatic GRT showing large break preoperatively (B) attached retina postoperatively at 1 month done using the Ngenuity 3D device for viewing intraoperatively.
(GRT: Giant retinal tear).

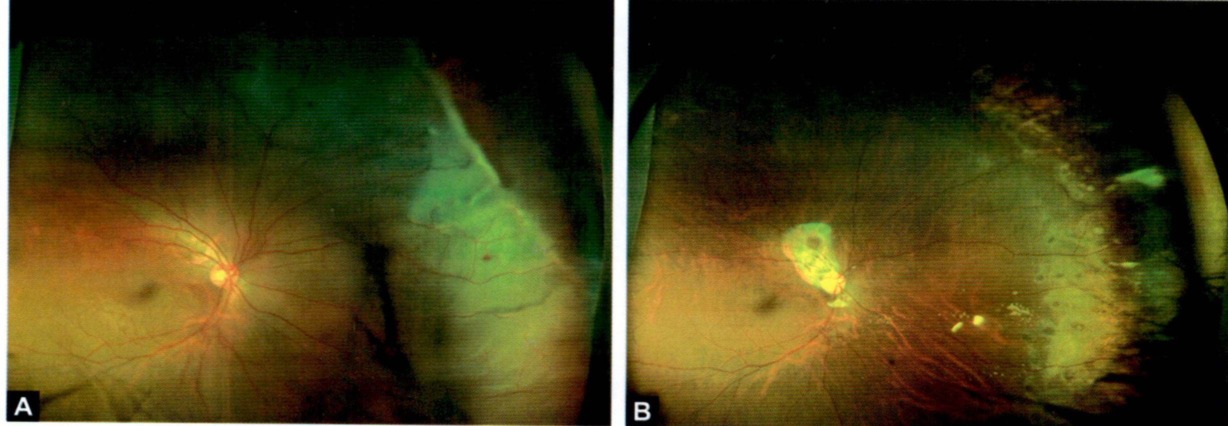

Figs. 54.11A and B: Ulra-widefield optos image showing (A) traumatic superonasal retinal dialysis with RD preoperatively and (B) attached retina under oil postoperatively at 1 month, laser marks are visible.
(RD: Retinal detachment).

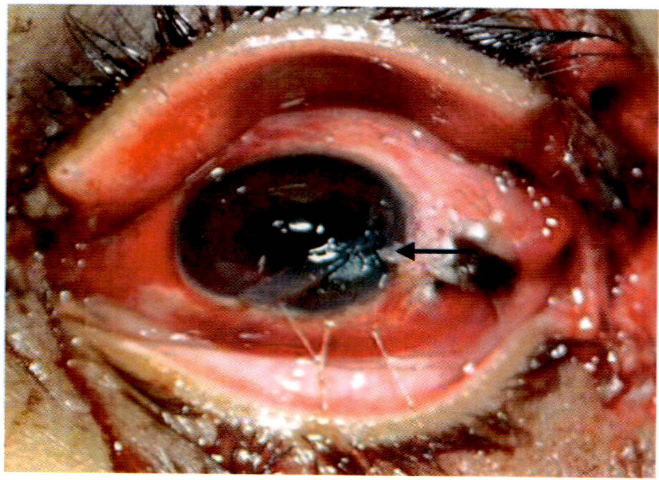

Fig. 54.12: Scleral rupture with uveal prolapse (arrow).

scleral rupture, no undue pressure must be applied on the globe to prevent further prolapse of intraocular contents. In case of younger patients who do not allow examination, globe exploration should be done under general anesthesia.

Management involves urgent wound closure. Associated ocular injuries can be addressed at the time of primary repair or at a later date after the initial inflammation has subsided. Prophylactic intravitreal antibiotics given at the time of primary repair decreases the occurrence of post-traumatic endophthalmitis.[39] Visual prognosis following scleral rupture is usually guarded because of the underlying damage to the choroid, the retina or the optic nerve.

REFERENCES

1. Yeung L, Chen TL, Kuo YH, et al. Severe vitreous hemorrhage associated with closed-globe injury. Graefes Arch Clin Exp Ophthalmology. 2006;244(1):52-7.

2. Berlin R. Zur sogenannten Commotio retinae. Klin Monatsbl Augenheilkd. 1873;1:42-78.

3. Youssri AI, Young LH. Closed-globe contusion injuries of the posterior segment. Int Ophthalmology Clin. 2002;42(3):79-86.

4. Pulido JS, Blair NP. The blood–retinal barrier in Berlin's edema. Retina. 1987;7(4):233-6.

5. Mansour AM, Green WR, Hogge C. Histopathology of commotio retinae. Retina. 1992;12(1):24-48.

6. Sipperley JO, Quigley HA, Gass JD. Traumatic retinopathy in primates: the explanation of commotio retinae. Arch Ophthalmology. 1878;96(12):2267-73

7. Ismail R, Tanner V, Williamson TH. Optical coherence tomography imaging of severe commotio retinae and associated macular hole. Br J Ophthalmology. 2002;86(4):473-4.

8. Bradley JL, Shah SP, Manjunath V, et al. Ultra-high-resolution optical coherence tomographic findings in commotio retinae. Arch Ophthalmology. 2011;129(1):107-8.

9. Duke-Elder S. System of Ophthalmology. St Louis: CV Mosby; 1972. p. 165.

10. Bastek JV, Foos RY, Heckenlively J. Traumatic pigmentary retinopathy. Am J Ophthalmology. 1981;92(5):621-4.

11. Lavinsky D, Martins EN, Cardillo JA, et al. Fundus autofluorescence in patients with blunt ocular trauma. Acta Ophthalmology. 2011;89(1):89-94.

12. Moon K, Kim KS, Kimb YC. A case of expansion of traumatic choroidal rupture with delayed-developed outer retinal changes. Case Rep Ophthalmology. 2013;4(2):70-5.

13. Kohno T, Miki T, Shiraki K, et al. Indocyanine green angiographic features of choroidal rupture and choroidal vascular injury after contusion ocular injury. Am J Ophthalmology. 2000;129(1):38-46.

14. Aguilar JP, Green WR. Choroidal rupture. A histopathologic study of 47 cases. Retina. 1984;4(4):269-75.

15. Ament CS, Zacks DN, Lane AM, et al. Predictors of visual outcome and choroidal neovascular membrane formation after traumatic choroidal rupture. Arch Ophthalmology. 2006;124(7):957-66.

16. Shah N, Shah U. Combination of photodynamic therapy with intravitreal bevacizumab for peribulbar anesthesia (penetrating trauma)-persistent choroidal neovascular membrane. Indian J Ophthalmology. 2008;56(2):163-4.

17. Conrath J, Forzano O, Ridings B. Photodynamic therapy for subfoveal CNV complicating traumatic choroidal rupture. Eye. 2004;18:946-7.

18. Yadav NK, Bharghav M, Vasudha K, et al. Choroidal neovascular membrane complicating traumatic choroidal rupture managed by intravitreal bevacizumab. Eye (lond). 2009;23(9):1872-3.

19. Raman SV, Desai UR, Anderson S, et al. Visual prognosis in patients with traumatic choroidal rupture. Can J Ophthalmology. 2004;39(3):260-6.

20. Knapp H. Ueber Isolirte zerreissungen der aderhaut infolge von traumen auf augapfel. Arch Augenheilkd. 1869;1:6-29.

21. Aaberg TM. Macular holes. Surv Ophthalmology. 1970;15:162.

22. Oehrens AM, Stalmans P. Optical coherence tomographic documentation of the formation of a traumatic macular hole. Am J Ophthalmology. 2006;142(5):866-9.

23. Fernandez MP, Modi YS, John VJ, et al. Accidental Nd:YAG laser-induced macular hole in a pediatric patient. Ophthalmic Surg Lasers Imaging Retina. 2013;44(6):7-10.

24. Huang J, Liu X, Wu Z, et al. Comparison of full-thickness traumatic macular holes and idiopathic macular holes by optical coherence tomography. Graefes Arch Clin Exp Ophthalmology. 2010;248(8):1071-5.

25. Chen H, Chen W, Zheng K, et al. Prediction of spontaneous closure of traumatic macular hole with spectral domain optical coherence tomography. Sci Rep. 2015;5:12343.

26. Yamada H, Sakai A, Yamada E, et al. Spontaneous closure of traumatic macular hole. Am J Ophthalmology. 2002;134(3):340-7.

27. Johnson RN, McDonald HR, Lewis H, et al. Traumatic macular hole: observations, pathogenesis and results of vitrectomy surgery. Ophthalmology. 2001;108(5):853-7.

28. Wachtlin J, Jandeck C, Potthofer S, et al. Long-term results following pars plana vitrectomy with platelet concentrate in pediatric patients with traumatic macular hole. Am J Ophthalmology. 2003;136(1):197-9.

29. Wu W, Drenser K, Trese M, et al. Pediatric traumatic macular hole: results of autologous plasmin enzyme-assisted vitrectomy. Am J Ophthalmology. 2007;144(5):668-72.

30. Goldzieher W. Beitrag zur Pathologie der orbitalen Schussverletzungen. Z Augenheilkd. 1901;6:277-85.

31. Pe'rez-Carro G, Junceda-Moreno C. Dual cause of blindness: chorioretinitis sclopetaria and homonymous hemianopsia. Arch Soc Esp Oftalmol. 2006;81(2):119-22.

32. Papakostas TD, Yonekawa Y, Wu D, et al. Retinal detachment associated with traumatic chorioretinal rupture. Opthhalmic Surg Lasers Imaging Retina. 2014;45(5):451-5.

33. Ahmadabadi MN, Karkhaneh R, Roohipoor R, et al. Clinical presentation and outcome of chorioretinitis sclopetaria: a case series study. Injury. 2010;41(1):82-5.

34. Martin DF, Awh CC, McCuen BW 2nd, et al. Treatment and pathogenesis of traumatic chorioretinal rupture (sclopetaria). Am J Ophthalmology. 1994;117(2):190-200.

35. Williams DF, Mieler WF, Williams GA. Posterior segment manifestations of ocular trauma. Retina. 1990;10(suppl 1):35-44.

36. Carvalho GC, Zacharias LC, Albhy CM, et al. Blindness reversal in corioretinitis sclopetaria. Rev Bras Oftalmol. 2014;73:6.

37. Wang YS, Xu JF, Guo CM. Clinical characteristics of occult scleral rupture Zhonghua Yan Ke Za Zhi. 2008;44(5):431-5.

38. Benjamin L, Wormald R. Diagnosis of scleral rupture. Eye. 1987;1:757-61.

39. Narang S, Gupta V, Gupta A, et al. Role of prophylactic intravitreal antibiotics in open globe injuries. Ind J Ophthalmology. 2003;51(1):39-44.

Chapter 55

Optic Nerve Avulsion

Thirumalesh MB, Vineet Mutha, Abhishek Sheemar, Sagnik Sen

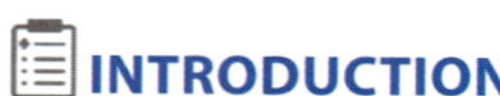 INTRODUCTION

Optic nerve avulsion (Figs. 55.1A and B) is a rare manifestation of ocular trauma. Usually the patient presents with sudden and complete loss of vision following severe blunt trauma due to separation of the optic nerve from the globe. However, it has also been reported with less severe blunt trauma.[1]

MECHANISM

Jameson Evans in his review on optic nerve injuries in 1909 had described slower traumatic avulsion injuries in which the optic nerve had separated from the globe and cases where massive gunshot injuries to the orbit spared the eye but the nerve was completely separated.[2]

Different mechanisms have been described:

1. Rapid extreme rotation of the globe[2]
2. Rapid anterior displacement of the globe
3. Rapid rise in intraocular pressure (IOP) leading to the avulsion of nerve out of scleral canal.[3]

Two trajectory-dependent mechanisms (rotational avulsion and rebound evulsion) have been postulated while studying the impact of paintball on the globe.

1. *Tangential glancing* blows produce strain-rate rotational avulsion, avulsing the optic nerve without major internal globe disruption.
2. *Off-center direct impact* produces slower rotational-rebound evulsion, injuring the globe and breaking through the nerve posteriorly.

The second mechanism is more common and is masked by accompanying intraocular trauma.[4]

Vitreous hemorrhage usually obscures the presence of optic nerve avulsion. Otherwise it is quite apparent on fundus examination. It is seen as a *crescent-shaped excavation and a ring-shaped hemorrhage* in the disc area. Usually the vision is no light perception with a profound depression of the optic nerve head and hemorrhage at the rim.

Electrodiagnostic tests such as visually evoked response (VER) shows an extinguished response. Computed tomo-

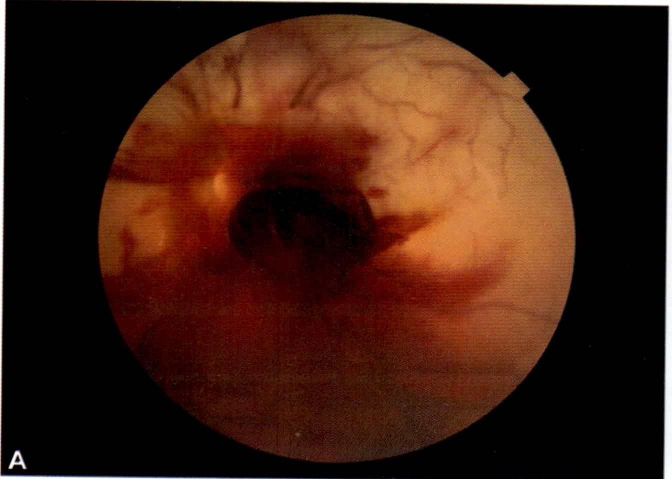
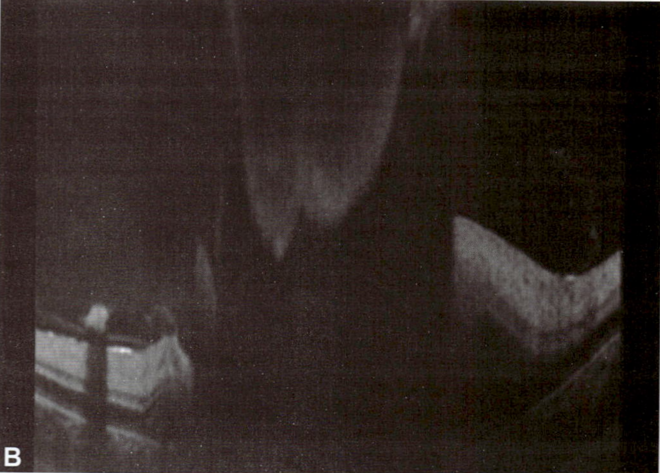

Figs. 55.1A and B: (A) Color fundus image in a case of optic nerve head (ONH) avulsion showing posterior vitreous clot formation just anterior to disc head; (B) Optical coherence tomography (OCT) reveals a clot-induced shadowing and excavation in the region of ONH.

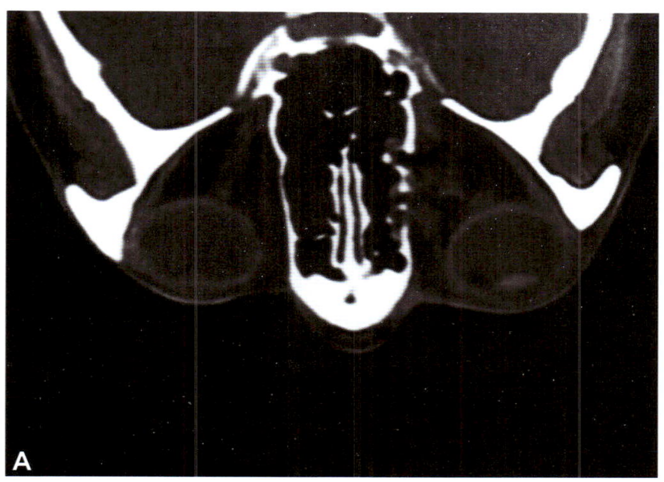 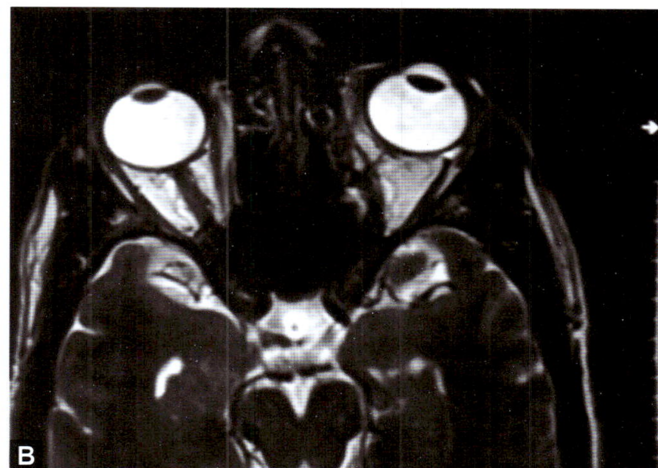

Figs. 55.2A and B: (A) Computed tomography (CT) picture showing left optic nerve avulsion; (B) T2-weighted (T2W) magnetic resonance imaging (MRI) scan showing absent left optic nerve.

graphy (CT) scan can reveal if the avulsion is total or partial or presence of an intact nerve sheath (Figs. 55.2A and B).

Talwar et al.[5] reported hypoechoic defect along the posterior ocular surface at the site of optic nerve on B-scan whereas an A-scan reveals widening of the optic nerve due to edema and bleed within the optic nerve sheath.

TREATMENT

Usually the patients present with no light perception. Intravenous high-dose steroids have been used but are unwarranted and do not have any beneficial effect in the final outcome. Supportive treatment for pain relief should be provided.

REFERENCES

1. Foster BS, March GA, Lucarelli MJ, et al. Optic nerve avulsion. Arch Ophthalmology. 1997;115(5):623-30.
2. Evans JJ. Observations on injuries to the optic nerve. Br Med J. 1909;2(2541):645-6.
3. Hykin PG, Gardner ID, Wheatcroft SM. Optic nerve avulsion due to forced rotation of the globe by a snooker cue. Br J Ophthalmology. 1990;74:499-501.
4. Sponsel WE, Gray W, Scribbick FW, et al. Blunt eye trauma: empirical histopathologic paintball impact thresholds in fresh mounted porcine eyes. Invest Ophthalmology Vis Sci. 2011;52: 5157-66.
5. Talwar D, Kumar A, Verma L, et al. Ultrasonography in optic nerve head avulsion. Acta Ophthalmology (Copenh). 1991;69:121-3.

Chapter 56

Sympathetic Ophthalmia

Aditya Modi, Neha Pareka Sudhakar, Thirumalesh MB, Aswini Behera, Raghav Ravani

DEFINITION

A bilateral granulomatous panuveitis that occurs following surgery or penetrating trauma to the other eye. The injured eye is called the exciting or inciting eye and the noninjured eye is called the sympathizing eye. There is no definite scientific explanation for the term "sympathetic ophthalmia (SO)". It could be due to activation of sympathetic pathways causing uveitis from the inciting eye to the sympathizing eye.[1]

HISTORY

The first conceptual script regarding SO was described in writings of Hippocrates.[2] Complete clinical understanding of the disease was given by Mackenzie of Edinburgh in the third edition of his book on the "Disease of eye" early in 19th century.[1] He postulated that the inflammation is transferred via optic nerve and chiasma from exciting eye to sympathizing eye and coined the term *sympathetic ophthalmia*. First detailed histopathologic study was done by Schirmer followed by Fuchs in 1905 whose histopathological findings formed the counterpart to Mackenzie's clinical description.[3] Dalen-Fuchs nodules were described independently by Fuchs and Dalen as nodular aggregates of inflammatory cells.

EPIDEMIOLOGY

Though not common, it remains the most dreadful disease entity in ophthalmology as both the eyes are involved and the prognosis is poor. Newer observations have helped to put this disorder into perspective. The time of onset of SO can be from 2 weeks to many years from trauma/surgery, with 90% of the cases developing within 1 year.[4-7] Recent studies cited incidence ranging from 0.2% to 0.5% after trauma and 0.01% after surgery[8,9] and prevalence as 0.03 out of 100,000 per year.[10] SO developed in patients with a retained foreign body within 3 months in about 80% and within 1 year in about 90% of cases.[4] SO accounts for approximately 0.3% of all cases of uveitis.[11]

There is no racial, gender, or age predilection, though some case studies suggest that the disease is more common in men as they are more prone to ocular injury[12,13] and in extremes of age, due to the increase in number of ocular surgeries in the aging population[14] and higher incidence of ocular injury in young age.[15]

ETIOLOGY

The etiology of sympathetic ophthalmia is given in Table 56.1.

Table 56.1: Etiology of sympathetic ophthalmia.

Traumatic causes	Surgical causes	Others
Penetrating eye injuries	Couching	Perforated corneal ulcer
Severe blunt trauma	Paracentesis	Radiation for choroidal melanoma
Explosive eye injuries	Cataract extraction	External beam radiation
Projectile foreign body	Evisceration, Enucleation	Helium ion irradiation of a choroidal melanoma
	Vitrectomy	
	Diode cyclophotocoagulation	
	Cyclodialysis	
	Trabeculectomy	
	Transscleral neodymium: yttrium aluminum garnet (YAG) cyclodestruction	
	Keratectomy	

PATHOGENESIS

Over the past 150 years, a vast number of studies have been performed to study the definitive mechanism of SO. Rather than the insight in causation of disease, the state of knowledge developed from these studies is more regarding the mechanism of disease process. The original hypothesis championed by Mackenzie et al. in 19th century was the "nerve theory" where the vague concepts of injury in one eye lead to propagation of inflammation along the nerve and chiasma to the other eye. In the early 20th century, hypersensitivity reaction to melanin was proposed to be responsible for the inflammation. Elschnig postulated that absorption and dissemination of the uveal pigment following injury to the eye produced hypersensitivity reaction.[16]

The current concepts suggest immune dysregulation as a primary etiological mechanism. It is considered within uveomeningeal syndrome spectrum like Vogt-Koyanagi-Harada (VKH) disease. There appears to be a cell-mediated immune response directed against ocular self antigens like retinal soluble antigen (S-antigen),[17] rhodopsin,[18] interphotoreceptor retinoid-binding protein,[19] recoverin[20] found on photoreceptors, retinal pigment epithelium (RPE), and/or choroidal melanocytes. Intraocular antigens do not come in contact with the lymphatics of the eye. Following any breach of the eye wall, these antigens come in contact with the conjunctival lymphatics resulting in a cascade of events of cell-mediated immunity.[21] Rao et al. demonstrated activation of inflammation when retinal antigens were injected subconjunctivally, but not into the eye. The possibility of a concurrent infectious agent with an antigen serving as an adjuvant in this mechanism of sensitization necessary to incite an immune response has also been suggested.[22]

Sympathetic ophthalmia has also been found to be more likely in patients who express HLA-DR4 and closely related HLA-DQw3 and HLA-DRw53 phenotype[23,24] suggesting immune dysregulation to play a role in the pathogenesis of this disease.

Elevated gelatinase B, chemokines like monocyte chemotactic protein-1 (CCL2/MCP-1), and stromal cell-derived factor-1 (CXCL12/SDF-1) present in granulomas of SO may produce epitopes that are present on the surface of antigen-presenting cells which leads to activation of autoimmune T cells contributing to the pathogenesis.[25]

Photoreceptor oxidative stress induced by inducible nitric oxide synthase (iNOS), as well as peroxynitrite (ONOO⁻) and tumor necrosis factor-α (TNF-α) has also been implicated in the pathogenesis of SO.[26]

Oxidative stress following SO also upregulates αA-crystallin (an antiapoptotic protein normally seen in retina).[27]

HISTOPATHOLOGY

Both the exciting and sympathizing eyes exhibit similar inflammatory changes except for the features of trauma in the exciting eye.[28] Histopathological features of SO are diffuse thickening of the uveal tract by infiltration of lymphocytes in which various numbers of nest of epithelioid cells displaying pigment phagocytosis are present. Histopathologically nodular aggregations of lymphocytes, histiocytes, epithelioid cells, and proliferating retinal pigment epithelial cells containing lipofuscin correspond to Dalen-Fuchs nodules.[28] Choroidal infiltrates are predominantly T lymphocytes. CD4⁺ cells are present in the early phase and CD8⁺ cells predominate in late stages (suppressor subset).[29] B lymphocytes comprise less than 5–15% of inflammatory cells[30] suggesting the mechanism of SO to be a type IV hypersensitivity.[31]

The clinical description of the disease gives the impression that SO can be easily diagnosed, however, the suspected diagnosis is confirmed histopathologically in less than one-third of the cases and the diagnosis is not suspected clinically in 15% of the pathologically diagnosed cases. It presents usually as a diffuse nonnecrotizing granulomatous infiltrate relatively sparing choriocapillaris and retina. This preservation could be due to following underlying mechanisms:

- Retinal pigment epithelium cells may liberate factors that downregulate the uveal inflammation.
- Endothelial cells of the choriocapillaris could release anti-inflammatory cytokines.
- The endothelial cells of choriocapillaris may not express adhesion molecules required for attachment and migration of leukocytes.
- Immune complexes may not deposit in the capillaries.

Atypical features due to extension of the granulomatous process into other adjacent structures present as focal, nongranulomatous inflammation of uvea, retinal involvement (retinitis, gliosis, perivasculitis, and detachment),[5,32] focal obliteration of choriocapillaris, choroidal scarring, and optic nerve atrophy.[33]

CLINICAL FEATURES

Symptoms may range from mild visual disturbance to significant visual loss. Other manifestations include pain, photophobia, photopsia, and floaters.[33] The earliest presenting symptom is usually decreased accommodation (difficulty in near vision) while the earliest sign being retrolenticular flare and cells in the fellow eye (Table 56.2).

Patients typically present with bilateral acute anterior uveitis with mutton-fat keratic precipitates.[34] Thickening of iris and synechiae occurs due to lymphocytic infiltration of the iris while intraocular pressure (IOP) may be high or low depending on trabeculitis/trabecular meshwork blockage or ciliary body shutdown, respectively.[35]

Fundus examination shows:

- Acute phase.[4,36–40]
- Chronic phase.[38,39,41]
- Sequelae.

Table 56.2: Clinical presentation in different phases of disease.

Acute phase	Chronic phase	Sequelae
Vitritis	Optic, retinal, and choroidal atrophy	Secondary cataract
Optic nerve edema	Peripheral chorioretinal scars	Glaucoma
Dalen-Fuchs nodules	Sunset glow fundus	Peripheral anterior synechiae
Circumpapillary choroidal lesions	Subretinal fibrosis	Rubeosis iridis
Serous/exudative retinal detachment (RD)	Posterior synechiae	Optic atrophy
Choroidal neovascularization		Exudative RD
Choroiditis		Chorioretinal scarring
Subretinal hemorrhage		Choroidal neovascularization
Vasculitis		Phthisis bulbi
Macular edema		

Table 56.3: Current trends in sympathetic ophthalmia.

Trend	Historical	Current
Cause	Post trauma	Post surgery (especially vitreoretinal)
Patients	Males and children (reflecting trauma peaks)	No gender preference (reflects positive impact of injury prevention program) and increasingly elderly patients (reflects impact of ocular surgery)
Incidence	Considered disappearing 30 years ago	Probably increasing (under diagnosed)
Onset	For 65% within 2–8 weeks, for 90% < 1 year	Many delayed presentations as well
Presentation	Granulomatous panuveitis	Any clinical uveitis
Inciting eye	Enucleation within 2 weeks of trauma for prevention of sympathetic ophthalmia (SO)	Enucleation solely for the prevention of SO is questionable
Visual prognosis	Poor	Reasonable due to modern immunosuppression

White-yellowish lesions are present at RPE which correspond to histopathological Dalen-Fuchs nodules usually seen at equator and beyond but can be located in the posterior fundus.[4] They tend to undergo atrophy with time. These nodules are not pathognomonic of SO as they are seen in other inflammatory diseases as well[35] and they may not be seen in 30–50% of the cases.[42]

SYSTEMIC ASSOCIATIONS

Systemic features more likely seen in VKH syndrome are sometimes seen in SO, such as alopecia, poliosis, vitiligo, and dysacusis (hearing impairment) due to concurrent damage to hair cells of organ of Corti and cells in cerebrospinal fluid.

In humans, the blood supply of uvea is similar to that of kidney, brain, and testes. Hence, it has been speculated that these organs can be susceptible to immune-mediated damage in SO, an entity called serum sickness.

DIAGNOSIS

Good history and clinical examination play a key role in diagnosis of SO. There are no specific laboratory studies to establish the diagnosis, however, focused clinical testing can be used to rule out other disease entities with a similar clinical picture. Changing concepts in presentation are described in Table 56.3.

INVESTIGATIONS

Fundus Photography

Fundus photography aids in:
- Distinguishing acute phase versus chronic phase
- Documentation of sequelae
- Monitoring response to therapy and resolution of clinical findings.

Fundus Fluorescein Angiography

Fundus fluorescein angiography (FFA) helps to confirm and assess the extent of disease (Figs. 56.1A to C).

Acute Phase

Fundus fluorescein angiography shows multiple punctate hyperfluorescent spots at the level of the RPE and choroid in the early venous phase that proceeds to late leakage.[38,39,42] These hyperfluorescent spots can become confluent causing pooling of dye underneath areas of neurosensory detachment in severe cases. Areas of early hypofluorescence are suggestive of Dalen-Fuchs nodules which later on show collection of dye into the nodules exhibiting focal hyperfluorescence. The appearance of these nodules on the angiogram depends on the integrity of RPE and choriocapillaris.[38,39]

Chronic Phase

Dalen-Fuchs nodules undergo atrophy and can be seen as window defects. Disc leak,[40] macular edema, neurosensory detachments and late staining of vessels can also be seen.[4]

Indocyanine Green Angiography

As choroid plays a paramount role, indocyanine green angiography (ICGA) (Fig. 56.2) complements FFA for diagnosing and measuring treatment response. Hypocyanescent areas identified at intermediate phase and not visible in late phase may point out the areas of active choroiditis due to cellular infiltration of the choroid or blockage from subretinal fluid[43] whereas hypocyanescent areas at both phases are suggestive of chorioretinal atrophy.

Optical Coherence Tomography

Spectral domain optical coherence tomography (SD-OCT) (Figs. 56.3A to C) is a useful tool which demonstrates neurosensory detachments, RPE adhesions, RPE tear and intraretinal edema. OCT helps to identify disintegration of RPE and choriocapillaris and disorganization and thinning of the inner retina and disruption of the ellipsoid zone. SD-OCT reveals hyperreflective structures at the region of RPE which corresponds to Dalen-Fuchs nodules.[44]

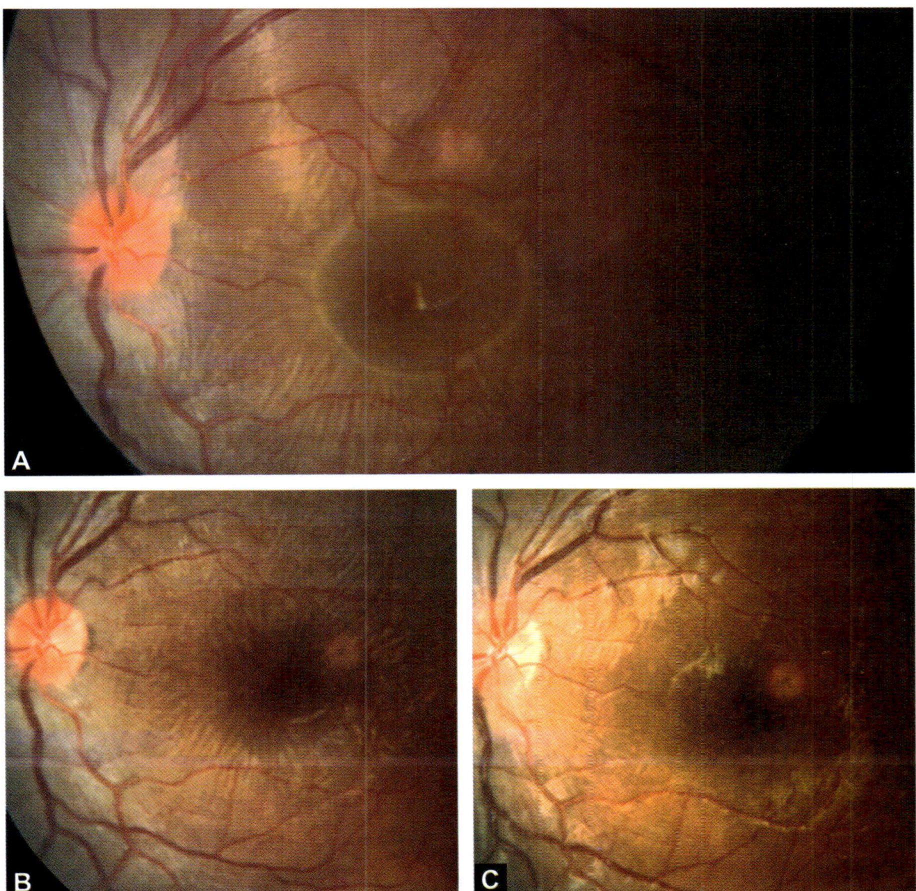

Figs. 56.1A to C: Sympathetic ophthalmia. (A) Treatment naive case of SO showing a large NSD at the fovea; (B) 3rd day on corticosteroids; and (C) 2 weeks on corticosteroids.

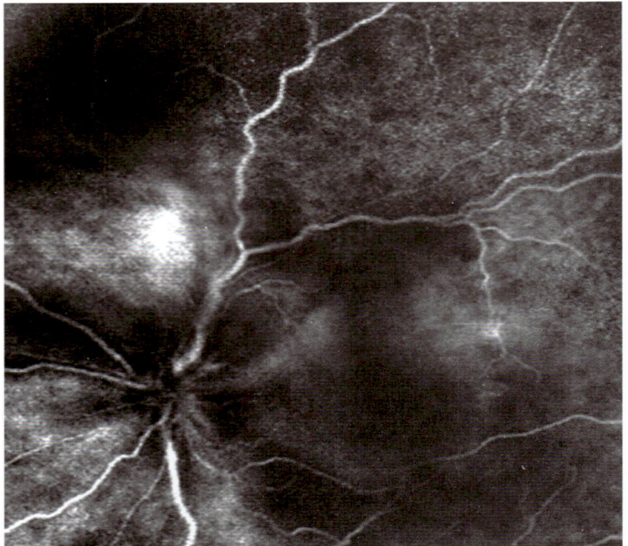

Fig. 56.2: Indocyanine green angiography (ICGA) in sympathetic ophthalmia showing multiple hypocyanescent areas.

Enhanced depth imaging optical coherence tomography (EDI-OCT) can helps us to image beyond the RPE. The choroid can be visualized with much detail and high-definition cross-sectional images can be captured. EDI-OCT of acute VKH shows significant thickening of choroid and RPE undulation which corresponds to the degree of inflammation. This helps in evaluating the degree of SO and response to the medications in a more quantified manner.[45]

Ultrasonography

Diffuse low to medium reflective thickening of choroid is the primary echographic finding. Other findings like vitreous opacities, serous retinal detachment, scleral thickening, and thickening of RPE in the peripapillary region are noted. It also helps in monitoring the response to therapy.[44]

Electrophysiological Tests

Electroretinogram showed diminished photopic and scotopic wave amplitudes. Electroculogram light peak and dark trough are absent and dark adaptation shows elevated cone and rod thresholds.

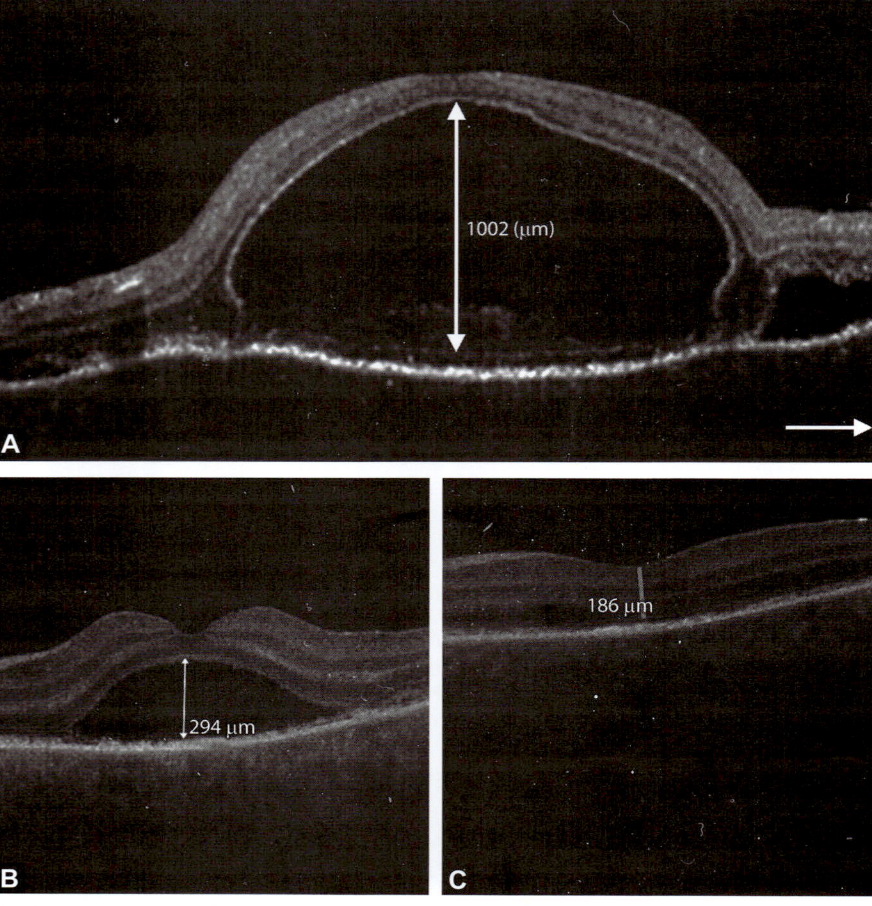

Figs. 56.3A to C: Optical coherence tomography (OCT) image of the same patient showing a large NSD before starting steroids, day 3, and after 2 weeks on steroid.

MANAGEMENT

Medical Management

Corticosteroids

High-dose steroids and immunosuppressives as early as possible play a crucial role in determining the final visual outcome.[6] Steroids such as prednisone should be started at doses ranging from 0.5 mg/kg/day to 2 mg/kg/day.[46]

In severe cases, methylprednisolone pulse therapy (1 g/day) for 3 days has also been recommended. The steroid tapering should be gradual over 2–3 months of period considering the response of the patient.[47] The efficacy of the therapy can be gauged appropriately in 3 months.[4] Even after control of the acute episode of inflammation, maintenance doses of 15–20 mg/day can be given for 3–6 months and alternate day dosing can be done in case of long-term therapy.[4] Cessation of therapy should be done only when the patient has been recorded free of inflammation for at least 6–12 months.[43] Close follow-up of such cases is still required to monitor for flare-ups of inflammation. Side effects of steroid are diabetes mellitus, adrenal insufficiency, hypertension, obesity, decreased immunity to infections, aseptic necrosis of hip and osteoporosis.[48]

Immunosuppressive Therapy

Immunomodulators should be considered in patients in whom steroids are contraindicated, presence of steroid-induced side effects, not responding to steroid therapy, or patients who experience frequent flare-ups of inflammation on decreasing or stopping steroids.[4] Immunosuppressants should be started along with steroids before reducing the dose of steroids. Cyclosporine, cyclophosphamide, azathioprine, and chlorambucil are some of the immunomodulators that have been used and found to be successful. The patient should be followed-up closely as these medications have significant toxicities and a rheumatology consultation is warranted.[35]

Intravitreal Therapy

Intravitreal injections allow targeted delivery at the site of disease. This reduces the use of systemic steroid which can further alleviate the side effects caused by steroids.[49,50] Intravitreal triamcinolone acetonide (IVTA) has been found to be useful in the beginning stages[51] as it has been shown to decrease intraocular inflammation, improve visual acuity, visual field, and decrease the dose of systemic steroids.[52] However, intravitreal steroids can cause cataract, glaucoma, and other complications which may be devastating for patients as they have already lost one eye.[35,49]

Surgical Management

Prophylactic evisceration or enucleation, can be done in eyes that eyes that are badly injured or are blind. However, it is debatable as to which procedure is better and the time of surgery. Chances of SO is very low when a surgery is performed within 10 days of injury, however, when SO sets in, evisceration or enucleation of the traumatized eye does not help and the patient must receive aggressive medical management with steroids and immunosuppressants.[53]

Evisceration has been preferred over enucleation by many surgeons as it is simpler with minimal damage to surrounding soft tissues, better cosmesis, quick recovery, and the movement of the eye is maintained.[51,54] However, the chances of developing SO are still lower (almost negligible) in enucleation compared to evisceration of the inciting eye as there is no residual viable tissue to incite inflammation.[55]

Few studies report that early enucleation does not affect the final outcomes.[55,56]

PROGNOSIS (TABLE 56.4)

It is very important to recognize SO and rule out other differentials (Table 56.5). It is mandatory to follow-up the patient for a long time as the diseases has a tendency to relapse frequently and the treatment options are potentially toxic. It is a dreadful disease as SO eventually leads to loss of vision and phthisis bulbi. The chances of spontaneous recovery are very

Table 56.4: Poor prognostic factors in sympathetic ophthalmia.

Factors	Characteristics
Type of trauma	Penetrating trauma
Surgery	Surgical repair 48 hours after initial injury
Treatment with corticosteroids	Use of local and systemic steroids for more than a week after initial injury
Site of penetrating injury	Ciliary body
Ocular inflammation	Intensity in the inciting eye
Size of wound	Larger than 5 mm
Age of patient	1st decade of life

Table 56.5: Differential diagnosis.

	SO	VKH	Sarcoidosis	Posterior syphilis
Age	All ages	20–50 years	20-40 years	All ages
Racial predisposition	None	Asian and blacks	US: Blacks Europe: Whites	None
Penetrating trauma	Always present	Absent	Absent	Absent
Skin changes	Uncommon	Common	9–37%	Secondary
CNS findings	Uncommon	Common	25–30%	Uncommon
Retinal serous detachment	Rare	Frequently seen	Uncommon	Localized
Choriocapillaris involvement	Usually absent	Frequently seen	Usually absent	Usually absent
CSF findings	Usually normal	Pleocytosis	Usually normal	Abnormal (usually reactive VDRL)

(CNS: Central nervous system; CSF: Cerebrospinal fluid; SO: Sympathetic ophthalmia; VKH; Vogt-Koyanagi-Harada disease).

rare if not treated. The prognosis of SO has improved since the use of corticosteroid and other immunosuppressive agents and with the advancements in microsurgical techniques for wound repair.[57,58] 50% of the patients can achieve a final vision of 6/12 or better in at least one eye. Early diagnosis and treatment can improve the prognosis of this disease and avoid complications like secondary glaucoma, chronic maculopathy, and phthisis bulbi.

REFERENCES

1. Mackenzie W. A Practical Treatise on the Diseases of the Eye, 3rd edition. London: Longmans; 1840. pp. 523-34.
2. Samuels B. Hippocrates. In: Samuels B, Fuchs A (Eds). Clinical Pathology of the Eye: A Practical Treatise of Histopathology. Toronto: Cassell; 1952. pp. 148-64.
3. Fuchs E. User sympathisierende entzündung (nebst bemerkungen überse & etraumatischelritis). Albrecht v Graefes Arch Ophthalmology. 1905;61:365-456.
4. Nussenblatt RB. Sympathetic ophthalmia. In: Nussenblatt RB, Whitcup SM (Eds). Uveitis: Fundamental and Clinical Practice, 3rd edition. Missouri: Mosby; 2004. pp. 311-23.
5. Lubin JR, Albert DM, Weinstein M. Sixty-five years of sympathetic ophthalmia. A clinicopathologic review of 105 cases (1913–1978). Ophthalmology. 1980;87(2):109-21.
6. Chan CC, Roberge RG, Whitcup SM, et al. 32 cases of sympathetic ophthalmia. A retrospective study at the National Eye Institute, Bethesda, Md., from 1982 to 1992. Arch Ophthalmology. 1995;113(5):597-600.
7. Goto H, Rao NA. Sympathetic ophthalmia and Vogt-Koyanagi-Harada syndrome. Int Ophthalmology Clin. 1990;30(4):279-85.
8. Makley TA, Azar A. Sympathetic ophthalmia. A long-term follow-up. Arch Ophthalmology. 1978;96(2):257-62.
9. Marak GE. Recent advances in sympathetic ophthalmia. Surv Ophthalmology. 1979;24(3):141-56.
10. Kilmartin DJ, Dick AD, Forrester JV. Prospective surveillance of sympathetic ophthalmia in the UK and Republic of Ireland. Br J Ophthalmology. 2000;84(3):259-63.
11. Gomi CF, Makdissi FF, Yamamoto JH, et al. An epidemiologic study on uveitis. Rev Med (Sao Paulo). 1997;76:101-8.
12. Liddy L, Stuart J. Sympathetic ophthalmia in Canada. Can J Ophthalmology. 1972;7(2):157-9.
13. Holland G. About indications and time for surgical removal of an injured eye. Klin Monatsbl Augenheilkd. 1964;145:732-40.
14. Kilmartin DJ, Dick AD, Forrester JV. Commentary: sympathetic ophthalmia risk following vitrectomy: should we counsel patients? Br J Ophthalmology. 2000;84:448-9.
15. Albert DM, Diaz-Rohena R. A historical review of sympathetic ophthalmia and its epidemiology. Surv Ophthalmology. 1989;34(1):1-14.
16. Elschnig A. Studies on sympathetic ophthalmia, II: the antigenic effect of eye pigments. Graef Arch Clin Exp. 1910;76(3):365-456.
17. de Kozak Y, Sakai J, Thillaye B, et al. S antigen-induced experimental autoimmune uveo-retinitis in rats. Curr Eye Res. 1981;1(6):327-37.
18. Schalken JJ, Winkens HJ, Van Vugt AH, et al. Rhodopsin-induced experimental autoimmune uveoretinitis in monkeys. Br J Ophthalmology. 1989;73(3):168-72.
19. Gery I, Wiggert B, Redmond TM, et al. Uveoretinitis and pinealitis induced by immunization with interphotoreceptor retinoid-binding protein. Invest Ophthalmology Vis Sci. 1986;27(8):1296-300.
20. Gery I, Chanaud NP, Anglade E. Recoverin is highly uveitogenic in Lewis rats. Invest Ophthalmology Vis Sci. 1994;35(8):3342-5.
21. Chaithanyaa N, Devireddy SK, Kishore Kumar RV, et al. Sympathetic ophthalmia: a review of literature. Oral Surg Oral Med Oral Pathol Oral Radiol. 2012;113(2):172-6.
22. Rao NA, Robin J, Hartmann D, et al. The role of the penetrating wound in the development of sympathetic ophthalmia experimental observations. Arch Ophthalmology. 1983;101(1):102-4.
23. Davis JL, Mittal KK, Freidlin V, et al. HLA associations and ancestry in Vogt-Koyanagi-Harada disease and sympathetic ophthalmia. Ophthalmology. 1990;97(9):1137-42.
24. Shindo Y, Ohno S, Usui M, et al. Immunogenetic study of sympathetic ophthalmia. Tissue Antigens. 1997;49(2):111-5.
25. Abu El-Asrar AM, Struyf S, Van den Broeck C, et al. Expression of chemokines and gelatinase B in sympathetic ophthalmia. Eye (Lond). 2007;21(5):649-57.
26. Parikh JG, Saraswathy S, Rao NA. Photoreceptor oxidative damage in sympathetic ophthalmia. Am J Ophthalmology. 2008;146(6):866-75.

27. Kase S, Meghpara BB, Ishida S, et al. Expression of α-crystallin in the retina of human sympathetic ophthalmia. Mol Med Rep. 2012;5(2):395-9.

28. Easom HA, Zimmerman LE. Sympathetic ophthalmia and bilateral phacoanaphylaxis. A clinicopathologic correlation of the sympathogenic and sympathizing eyes. Arch Ophthalmology. 1964;72:9-15.

29. Chan CC, Benezra D, Rodrigues MM, et al. Immunohistochemistry and electron microscopy of choroidal infiltrates and Dalen-Fuchs nodules in sympathetic ophthalmia. Ophthalmology. 1985;92(4):580-90.

30. Shah DN, Piacentini MA, Burnier MN, et al. Inflammatory cellular kinetics in sympathetic ophthalmia: a study of 29 traumatized (exciting) eyes. Ocul Immunol Inflamm. 1993;1(3):255-62.

31. Müller-Hermelink HK, Kraus-Mackiw E, Daus W. Early stage of human sympathetic ophthalmia. Histologic and immunopathologic findings. Arch Ophthalmology. 1984;102(9):1353-7.

32. Winter FC. Sympathetic uveitis: a clinical and pathologic study of visual field. Am J Ophthalmology. 1955;39:340-7.

33. Croxatto JO, Rao NA, McLean IW, et al. Atypical histopathologic features in sympathetic ophthalmia. A study of a hundred cases. Int Ophthalmology. 1982;4(3):129-35.

34. Ganesh SK, Narayana KM, Biswas J. Peripapillary choroidal atrophy in sympathetic ophthalmia and management with triple-agent immunosuppression. Ocul Immunol Inflamm. 2003;11(1):61-5.

35. Damico F, Kiss S, Young LH. Sympathetic ophthalmia. Semin Ophthalmology. 2005;20(1):191-7.

36. Castiblanco CP, Adelman RA. Sympathetic ophthalmia. Graefes Arch Clin Exp Ophthalmology. 2009;247:289-302.

37. Borkowski LM, Weinberg DV, Delany CM, et al. Laser photocoagulation for choroidal neovascularization associated with sympathetic ophthalmia. Am J Ophthalmology. 2001;132(4):585-7.

38. Power WJ. Sympathetic ophthalmia. In: Foster SC, Vitale AT (Eds). Diagnosis and Treatment of Uveitis. Philadelphia: Saunders; 2002. pp. 742-6.

39. Yanoff M, Duker JS. Ophthalmology. Edinburgh: Mosby/Elsevier; 2009. pp. 861-3.

40. Rao NA. Sympathetic ophthalmia. In: Ryan SJ (Ed). Retina, 3rd edition. New York: Mosby; 2001. pp. 1756-61.

41. Gupta V, Gupta A, Dogra MR. Posterior sympathetic ophthalmia: a single centre long-term study of 40 patients from North India. Eye (Lond). 2008;22(12):1459-64.

42. Chan CC, Wetzig RP, Palestine AG, et al. Immunohistopathology of ocular sarcoidosis. Report of a case and discussion of immunopathogenesis. Arch Ophthalmology. 1987;105(10):1398-402.

43. Bernasconi O, Auer C, Zografos L, et al. Indocyanine green angiographic findings in sympathetic ophthalmia. Graefes Arch Clin Exp Ophthalmology. 1998;236(8):635-8.

44. Castiblanco C, Adelman RA. Imaging for sympathetic ophthalmia: impact on the diagnosis and management. Int Ophthalmology Clin. 2012;52(4):173-81.

45. Behdad B, Rahmani S, Montahaei T, et al. Enhanced depth imaging OCT (EDI-OCT) findings in acute phase of sympathetic ophthalmia. Int Ophthalmology. 2015;35(3):433-9.

46. Gasch AT, Foster CS, Grosskreutz CL, et al. Postoperative sympathetic ophthalmia. Int Ophthalmology Clin. 2000;40(1):69-84.

47. Vote BJ, Hall A, Cairns J, et al. Changing trends in sympathetic ophthalmia. Clin Exp Ophthalmology. 2004;32(5):542-5.

48. Jonas JB, Spandau UH. Repeated intravitreal triamcinolone acetonide for chronic sympathetic ophthalmia. Acta Ophthalmology Scand. 2006;84(3):436.

49. Ozdemir H, Karacorlu M, Karacorlu S. Intravitreal triamcinolone acetonide in sympathetic ophthalmia. Graefes Arch Clin Exp Ophthalmology. 2005;243(7):734-6.

50. Chan RV, Seiff BD, Lincoff HA, et al. Rapid recovery of sympathetic ophthalmia with treatment augmented by intravitreal steroids. Retina. 2006;26(2):243-7.

51. O Donnell BA, Kersten R, McNab A, et al. Enucleation versus evisceration. Clin Exp Ophthalmology. 2005;33:5-9.

52. Jonas JB. Intravitreal triamcinolone acetonide for treatment of sympathetic ophthalmia. Am J Ophthalmology. 2004;137(2):367-8.

53. Gurdal G, Erdener U, Irkec M, et al. Incidence of sympathetic ophthalmia after penetrating eye injury and choice of treatment. Ocul Immunol Inflamm. 2002;10(3):223-7.

54. Timothy NH, Freilich DE, Lindberg JV. Evisceration versus enucleation from the ocularist's perspective. Ophthal Plast Reconstr Surg. 2003;19(6):417-20.

55. Bilyk JR. Enucleation, evisceration, and sympathetic ophthalmia. Curr Opin Ophthalmology. 2000;11(5):372-86.

56. Kumar N, Chang A, Beaumont P. Sympathetic ophthalmia following ciliary body laser cyclophotocoagulation for rubeotic glaucoma. Clin Exp Ophthalmology. 2004;32(2):196-8.

57. Marak GE. Letter to the editor. Ophthalmology. 1982;89:1291.

58. Freidlin J, Pak J, Tessler HH, et al. Sympathetic ophthalmia after injury in the Iraq war. Ophthal Plast Reconstr Surg. 2006;22(2):133-4.

Chapter 57

Post-traumatic Endophthalmitis

Thirumalesh MB, Raghav Ravani, Meghal Gagrani, Alisha Kishore, Prateek Kakkar

INTRODUCTION

Endophthalmitis is a vision-threatening complication of open globe injury and intraocular infections are commonly associated with vitreous exudation after an open globe injury. Post-traumatic endophthalmitis comprises 25–31%[1,2] of all cases of infectious endophthalmitis. The incidence of endophthalmitis after open globe injury (one in 100) is very high compared to endophthalmitis secondary to intraocular surgery (one in 1,000). The incidence of endophthalmitis is reported in up to 12–16% of eyes with open globe injury without intraocular foreign bodies (IOFB).[3] The incidence is found to be higher in penetrating injuries contaminated with organic matter such as soil. Post-traumatic endophthalmitis has a very devastating course compared to postoperative endophthalmitis due to many factors such as associated comorbidities, virulence of microorganisms due to contamination and possible delay in diagnosis and management.

RISK FACTORS

- *Retained intraocular foreign bodies:* The incidence of endophthalmitis is around 6.9–16.5%.[2,4-15] It is especially important if:
  - Low-velocity IOFB
  - Organic nature
- *Delayed wound repair:* Risk of infection increases by four times when primary repair is done after 24 hours of open globe injury.[4]
- *Contamination of wound* with soil, especially more common in rural areas.[5]
- *Vitreous prolapse* through the open wound.
- *Lens rupture:* Gives microbes access to the posterior segment.
- *Large wound size:* Associated larger surface area exposure to contamination.

ETIOLOGY

Many pathogens have been implicated as a cause of post-traumatic endophthalmitis. Most common of these is *Staphy-lococcus epidermidis*, which causes a relatively less virulent form of infective endophthalmitis. It forms a part of normal flora of skin and eyelashes and gets easy access to intraocular structures postinjury.

Bacillus species are also commonly isolated in post-traumatic endophthalmitis cases, particularly in the presence of an IOFB or soil contamination. Such cases are characterized by a fulminant onset (<24 hours), along with severe pain and a rapid decrease in visual acuity. Signs include the presence of chemosis, periorbital edema, proptosis, hypopyon, ring-shaped corneal infiltrates early in the course, followed by rapid progression to panophthalmitis. Its severity is attributed to the presence of enterotoxin, β-lactamase enzyme and a heat-resistant endotoxin-mediated reaction.[16,17]

Polymicrobial infections are more common in open-globe injuries. The most frequently isolated organisms include gram-positive *Staphylococcus epidermidis* and *Streptococcus species*, as they are present in the normal flora and readily contaminate open wounds. *Pseudomonas* and *Clostridium species*[18] can cause fulminant endophthalmitis. Vegetable matter injuries more commonly point the diagnosis toward fungal endophthalmitis. *Candida species* are the most common isolate in fungal endophthalmitis but it may also be caused by molds such as *Aspergillus species*, *Paecilomyces species*, *Fusarium species*, and Dematiaceous fungi (Table 57.1).[19]

CLINICAL FEATURES AND DIAGNOSIS

Penetrating ocular trauma is characterized by a painful diminution of visual acuity.[20] Other symptoms include redness, watering with or without purulent discharge and photophobia (Fig. 57.1). Signs of post-traumatic endophthalmitis are hypopyon, vitritis, corneal ring infiltrates at the site of corneal laceration with or without iris tissue prolapse, intraocular hemorrhage, pupillary peaking, cataract and retinal detachment. Diagnostic imaging must be done in presence of one or more of the above signs.

Ultrasonography is useful in evaluating vitreous cavity for the exudates, the presence of intraocular foreign body, the presence of posterior vitreous detachment, and the

Table 57.1: List of organisms causing post-traumatic endophthalmitis.

Bacterial
- *Gram-positive organisms:*
  - *Staphylococcus epidermidis (Most common)*
  - *Bacillus cereus (Most fulminant)*
  - *Staphylococcus aureus*
  - *Streptococcus sp.*
  - *Clostridium sp.*
  - *Corynebacterium sp.*
  - *Propionibacterium acnes*
- *Gram-negative organisms:*
  - *Pseudomonas sp.*
  - *Proteus sp.*
  - *Moraxella sp.*
  - *Stenotrophomonas maltophila*
  - *Acinetobacter sp.*
  - *Citrobacter sp.*

Fungal
- *Candida albicans (Most common fungal)*
- *Aspergillus sp.*
- *Paecilomyces sp.*
- *Fusarium sp.*
- *Other dematiaceae*

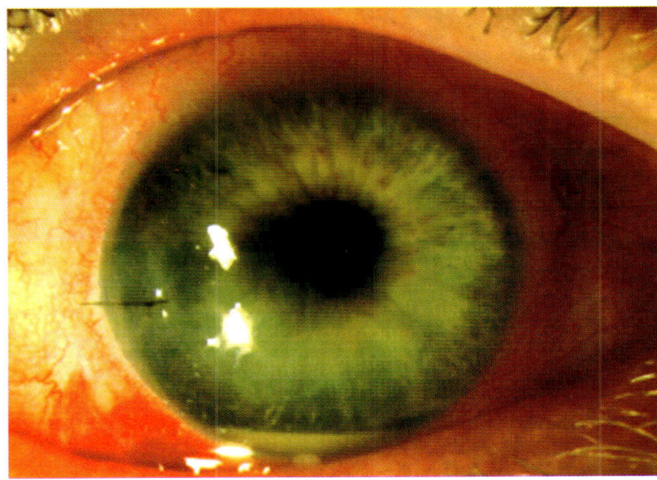

Fig. 57.1: Sutured open globe injury with endophthalmitis.

presence of retinal or choroidal detachment. It is comparatively cheaper than other modalities and allows dynamic assessment of the eye, making it a valuable imaging modality in traumatic cases. It must be done by placing the probe very gently on the eyelid, especially when the wound is open, and not directly over the globe, to avoid inadvertent trauma. It is also useful as a tool to follow-up patients being managed medically or via intravitreal antibiotics only.

A plain orbital radiography must be done to rule out any retained intraocular foreign bodies. Axial computed tomography (CT) scan with 0.5–1 mm cuts with coronal reconstruction images are very useful in detecting and localizing metallic intraocular foreign bodies. It may detect foreign bodies that are as small as 0.5 mm due to its high resolution. Soft tissue windows on CT scan modules can be used to visualize less radiopaque foreign bodies such as wooden or glass foreign bodies. Magnetic resonance imaging (MRI) is another alternative for localizing nonmetallic IOFBs that may be radiolucent on CT scan.

When the diagnosis is made or a patient is suspected to have endophthalmitis, samples of vitreous must be obtained for microbiological evaluation. Cultures can be obtained from the wound, aqueous humor or vitreous humor, though latter has a higher rate of microbiological success. Vitreous samples are obtained either by taking a vitreous biopsy using vitrectomy cutter or a gentle vitreous tap using a large bore needle such as 23G. The former is preferred as it minimizes traction and inadvertent retinal break formation and subsequent retinal detachment. The sample must then be plated on blood and chocolate agar culture plates, and slides prepared for Gram's staining and 10% KOH mount, to help identify the organism early.[21,22] Sabaroud's dextrose agar must be used to rule out fungal etiology.

TREATMENT

Prophylaxis

Tetanus toxoid 0.5 mL should be given intramuscularly in all such cases. The most important prophylaxis for the prevention of post-traumatic endophthalmitis is primary globe repair within 24 hours. It is also recommended to give an intracameral antibiotic wash along with prophylactic intravitreal antibiotic bolus in high-risk open globe injuries.

Systemic antimicrobial prophylaxis is recommended in spite of no level 1 evidence. Levofloxacin 500–750 mg OD is preferred because of its good intraocular penetration. Intravenous, periocular and topical antibiotics should be routinely used in post-traumatic endophthalmitis, unlike postoperative endophthalmitis. The breakdown of the blood-ocular barrier by inflammation following trauma augments the penetration of antibiotics in the ocular tissues. Vancomycin and aminoglycosides are quite useful to cover most of the organisms and are used empirically. Ciprofloxacin may be an alternative in cases of infection by resistant microorganisms.

Intravitreal therapy should be given in the presence of IOFB even in the absence of endophthalmitis as the risk of infection with virulent organisms like gram-negative microbes is higher. A large prospective randomized controlled trial by Soheilian M et al. reported that the risk of developing endophthalmitis decreases in the group receiving prophylactic intracameral and intravitreal antibiotics (0.3%) compared to the control group (2.3%).[23] Only intravitreal injections can achieve high drug concentrations in the vitreous. The commonly used intravitreal antibiotics are vancomycin (1 mg/0.1 mL) and ceftazidime (2.25 mg/0.1 mL) for covering both gram-positive and negative species respectively. Fungal coverage with amphotericin B (5 µg) or voriconazole (100 mg) can be used to cover fungal infections if the patient gives a history of injury with vegetative matter or has a delayed onset of symptoms. Antibiotics can be repeated and changed according to culture and sensitivity report.

Use of steroids by any route is not advised unless fungal involvement is ruled out. Steroids are used after being deferred initially, though its use in post-traumatic endophthalmitis is best described as being controversial. It helps to suppress inflammation due to trauma and infection leading to better overall structural outcome but may lead to increased chances of aggravating fungal infection and delaying wound healing. It is recommended to use steroids cautiously and they must be started only after antibiotic therapy has started.

Vitrectomy and Endophthalmitis

Vitrectomy should be done immediately in cases of endophthalmitis associated with IOFB or retinal detachment.[24] Vitrectomy is done to debulk the vitreous cavity of the toxins, decrease the microorganism load, inflammatory debris and clear the media. Vitreous samples for microbiological evaluation are also obtained.[25,26] A limited vitrectomy is recommended instead of extensive vitreous gel removal. Posterior vitreous detachment must not be attempted to avoid any retinal tear formation in the inflamed and fragile retina. Silicone oil is preferred in most cases because it has shown to prevent the bacterial growth in the vitreous cavity and prevents hypotony, besides providing a long-term tamponade to the globe.[27]

PROGNOSIS

The prognosis of post-traumatic endophthalmitis is usually poor and maybe devastating even after aggressive management. Most important factors contributing to this are the high virulence of organisms, easier access of intraocular tissues to microbes, higher chances of wound contamination, and presence of IOFB acting as a nidus of infection. These are worsened by the presence of associated inflammation due to trauma, the presence of retinal detachment, the use of toxic doses of intravitreal antibiotics and delay in identification or management of such cases. These may be overcome by prophylactic therapy to prevent endophthalmitis in all open-globe injuries along with aggressive management and referral to a higher center.

REFERENCES

1. Brinton GS, Topping TM, Hyndiuk RA, et al. Posttraumatic endophthalmitis. Arch Ophthalmology. 1984;102(4):547-50.
2. Snell Jr AC. Perforating ocular injuries. Am J Ophthalmology. 1945;28:263-81.
3. Cebulla CM, Flynn Jr HW. Endophthalmitis after open globe injuries. Am J Ophthalmology. 2009;147(4):567-8.
4. Thompson JT, Parver LM, Enger CL, et al. Infectious endophthalmitis after penetrating injuries with retained intraocular foreign bodies. Ophthalmology. 1993;100(10):1468-74.
5. Boldt HC, Pulido JS, Blodi CF, et al. Rural endophthalmitis. Ophthalmology. 1989;96(12):1722-6.
6. Edmund J. The prognosis of perforating eye injuries. Acta Ophthalmology. 1968;46:1165-74.
7. Niiranen M. Perforating eye injuries treated at Helsinki University Eye Hospital 1970 to 1977. Ann Ophthalmology. 1981;13:957-61.
8. Barr CC. Prognostic factors in corneoscleral lacerations. Arch Ophthalmology. 1983;101(6):919-24.
9. Affeldt JC, Flynn Jr HW, Forster RK, et al. Microbial endophthalmitis resulting from ocular trauma. Ophthalmology. 1987;94:407-13.
10. Essex RW, Yi Q, Charles PG, et al. Post-traumatic endophthalmitis. Ophthalmology. 2004;111(11):2015-22.
11. Zhang Y, Zhang MN, Jiang CH, et al. Endophthalmitis following open globe injury. Br J Ophthalmology. 2010;94(1):111-4.
12. Colyer MH, Weber ED, Weichel ED, et al. Delayed intraocular foreign body removal without endophthalmitis during Operations Iraqi Freedom and Enduring Freedom. Ophthalmology. 2007;114(8):1439-47.
13. Andreoli CM, Andreoli MT, Kloek CE, et al. Low rate of endophthalmitis in a large series of open globe injuries. Am J Ophthalmology. 2009;147(4):601-8.
14. Yang CS, Lu CK, Lee FL, et al. Treatment and outcome of traumatic endophthalmitis in open globe injury with retained intraocular foreign body. Ophthalmologica. 2010;224(2):79-85.
15. Schrader WF. Epidemiology of open globe eye injuries: analysis of 1026 cases in 18 years. Klin Monatsbl Augenheilkd. 2004;221:629-35.
16. Bhagat N, Nagori S, Zarbin M. Post-traumatic infectious endophthalmitis. Surv Ophthalmology. 2011;56(3):214-51.
17. Thompson JT, Parver LM, Enger CL, et al. Infectious endophthalmitis after penetrating injuries with retained intraocular foreign bodies. Ophthalmology. 1993;100(10):1468-74.
18. Iyer MN, Kranias G, Daun ME. Posttraumatic endophthalmitis involving Clostridium tetani and Bacillus spp. Am J Ophthalmology. 2001;132(1):116-7.
19. Wykoff CC, Flynn Jr HW, Miller D, et al. Exogenous fungal endophthalmitis: microbiology and clinical outcomes. Ophthalmology. 2008;115(9):1501-7.
20. Lieb DF, Scott IU, Flynn Jr HW, et al. Open globe injuries with positive intraocular cultures: factors influencing final visual acuity outcomes. Ophthalmology. 2003;110(8):1560-6.
21. Ariyasu RG, Kumar S, LaBree LD, et al. Microorganisms cultured from the anterior chamber of ruptured globes at the time of repair. Am J Ophthalmology. 1995;119(2):181-8.
22. Axelrod JL, Klein RM, Bergen RL, et al. Human vitreous levels of selected antistaphylococcal antibiotics. Am J Ophthalmology. 1985;100(4):570-5.
23. Soheilian M, Rafati N, Mohebbi MR, et al. Prophylaxis of acute posttraumatic bacterial endophthalmitis: a multicenter, randomized clinical trial of intraocular antibiotic injection, report 2. Arch Ophthalmology. 2007;125(4):460-5.
24. Foster RE, Rubsamen PE, Joondeph BC, et al. Concurrent endophthalmitis and retinal detachment. Ophthalmology. 1994;101(3):490-8.
25. Mittra RA, Mieler WF. Controversies in the management of open-globe injuries involving the posterior segment. Surv Ophthalmology. 1999;44(3):215-25.
26. Mieler WF, Mittra RA. The role and timing of pars plana vitrectomy in penetrating ocular trauma. Arch Ophthalmology. 1997;115(9):1191-2.
27. Azad R, Ravi K, Talwar D, et al. Pars plana vitrectomy with or without silicone oil endotamponade in posttraumatic endophthalmitis. Graefes Arch Clin Exp Ophthalmology. 2003;241(6):478-83.

Chapter 58

Retained Intraocular Foreign Body

Thirumalesh MB, Vineet Mutha, Raghav Ravani, Atul Kumar, Abhidnya Surve

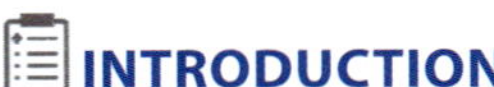

INTRODUCTION

Open-globe injuries with a retained intraocular foreign body (RIOFB) may cause severe vision loss, either due to the trauma or due to secondary events related to IOFB.

HISTORICAL PERSPECTIVE

Historically, IOFBs (magnetic) were removed through the pars plana using an external magnet, after a thorough and meticulous localization with a limbal ring as a reference plane and radiograms taken in anteroposterior and lateral views in various gazes. However, external magnetic extraction of metallic IOFB was associated with a high incidence of intraocular damage. With the development of the pars plana vitrectomy (PPV) and the addition of vitrectomy instrumentation, intraocular magnets (IOMs) and IOFB forceps, both magnetic and nonmagnetic IOFBs could be removed from the vitreous cavity with minimum collateral damage.[1,2]

Intraocular foreign body removal was originally localized using scout films of the orbit. This technique has long been replaced by improvements in ultrasonography and computed tomography (CT) technology.[3] The advances in CT have enabled better preoperative planning by using improved resolution to determine the exact location and size of an IOFB.[4]

Williams et al. published the first large series of visual outcomes using PPV microsurgical techniques, with 60% retaining better than 20/40 best-corrected visual acuity.[5] Chow and colleagues found no difference in visual acuity when comparing an external magnet versus an internal PPV approach for IOFB removal.[6] Over the last 10 years, numerous authors have published their experiences with IOFB removal using a PPV approach.[7-15] Current IOFB removal techniques incorporate the most recent advances in PPV microsurgical instrumentation and technology.[15]

SPECTRUM OF FOREIGN BODIES

A wide spectrum of foreign bodies can affect the eye depending upon the trauma involved. Ninety percent of

Table 58.1: Types of intraocular foreign bodies (IOFBs).	
Inert	*Reactive*
Stone	*Iron*: Siderosis affecting neuroepithelium
Sand	*Copper*: Chalcosis affecting basement membranes
Plastic	*Zinc*: Minimal inflammation
Glass	*Aluminum*: Minimal inflammation
Porcelain	*Nickel*: Purulent inflammation
Plastic	*Mercury*: Rapid phthisis bulbi

the foreign bodies are metallic, out of which 70% are iron and most common mode is chisel-hammer injury. Usually, foreign body enters via the cornea (65%) and mostly the site of lodgement is vitreous cavity (61%).[14] Usually, the size of foreign body is 0.2–2 mm. IOFBs can be differentiated into two types broadly: (1) Inert and (2) Reactive (Table 58.1).

CLINICAL PROFILE

Iron and copper are the most common foreign bodies affecting the eye. Iron is deposited mainly in the neuroepithelial tissues such as retina, ciliary epithelium and iris muscles while copper is philic to basement membranes such as internal limiting membrane (ILM), Descemet's membrane and anterior lens capsule.

Siderosis occurs due to Fenton reaction ($Fe^{3+} + H_2O \rightarrow Fe^{2+} + OH^-$) producing large quantities of hydroxyl ions causing extensive damage. Manifestations of siderosis are brown deposits in corneal stroma, anterior lens capsule and subcapsular area, mydriasis, heterochromia of iris, retinal pigmentation, optic atrophy and secondary glaucoma. Electroretinogram (ERG) may show an extinguished response in extensive siderosis bulbi.

Acute chalcosis is caused by pure copper and is characterized by severe ocular inflammation while chronic disease is caused by copper alloys containing less than 85% copper. In chronic diseases, copper deposits are seen on the Descemet's membrane, anterior lens capsule, on retinal vessels and ILM, and dispersed in aqueous and vitreous. Siderosis and chalcosis can even occur after IOFB removal due to excessive distribution throughout the eye.

STEPWISE APPROACH FOR OPEN-GLOBE INJURY WITH POSSIBLE INTRAOCULAR FOREIGN BODY

The first step in a case of open globe injury with suspected IOFB is preoperative planning and tailored testing. An open-globe injury with a suspected retained IOFB needs a systematic evaluation to rule out any life-threatening emergency if necessary (not needed in a chisel-hammer type of injury but mandatory in blast victims). After ruling out any concomitant injury that may require more urgent attention, an extensive history should be obtained if the patient is conscious and able to communicate. The surgeon should document the etiology of the injury; the type of material that may have entered the eye such as metallic (magnetic/nonmagnetic), nonorganic (stone), organic (plant/wood), or autologous (bone, cilia); time of injury; last meal; and allergy to penicillin.

A complete ophthalmic examination should include an initial visual acuity, pupillary examination to rule out an afferent pupillary defect, slit lamp examination to rule out endophthalmitis, and dilated fundus examination to visualize the IOFB and rule out a retinal detachment. Intraocular pressure and B-scan ultrasonography may be deferred until the primary globe repair is completed. The surgeon should immediately order broad-spectrum antibiotics. Favoured choices for IOFB endophthalmitis prophylaxis include moxifloxacin 400 mg intravenously/orally once per day or levofloxacin 500 mg intravenously/orally once per day. The minimum inhibitory concentration needed to inhibit the growth of 90% of organisms (MIC90) of these two antibiotics penetrating into the vitreous will cover most bacterial causes of posttraumatic endophthalmitis except *Pseudomonas aeruginosa* and *Bacillus cereus*.[16]

The patient should have an urgent helical CT scan of the orbits and the brain. The surgeon should rule out any intracranial foreign bodies or roof fractures that may need neurosurgical consultation. Depending on the etiology of the injury, orbital fractures may need otolaryngology consultation as well. The newer generation helical CT scans can reformat IOFB images in axial, coronal and sagittal views. The high-resolution CT scan generates images as thin as 0.625 mm.[4] The patient with a suspected open-globe injury without a foreign body on the CT scan, can then proceed to the operating room for primary globe repair.

Although CT scan is very sensitive in picking up RIOFB, ultrasonography gives valuable information regarding site of impaction of foreign body, status of posterior vitreous detachment, any associated retinal detachment, and presence of concurrent vitreous hemorrhage or endophthalmitis (Figs. 58.1A and B).

PRIMARY OR STAGED EXTRACTION OF INTRAOCULAR FOREIGN BODY

The timing and type of surgery are the next major decisions in the management of an IOFB. The surgeon can either close the open globe at first stage and secondarily remove the IOFB or combine both surgeries at the same time. An open-globe injury with a retained IOFB must be stable for extended surgery if both a globe repair and IOFB are planned together. An open-globe repair, IOFB removal and intravitreal antibiotics are necessary with posttraumatic endophthalmitis.

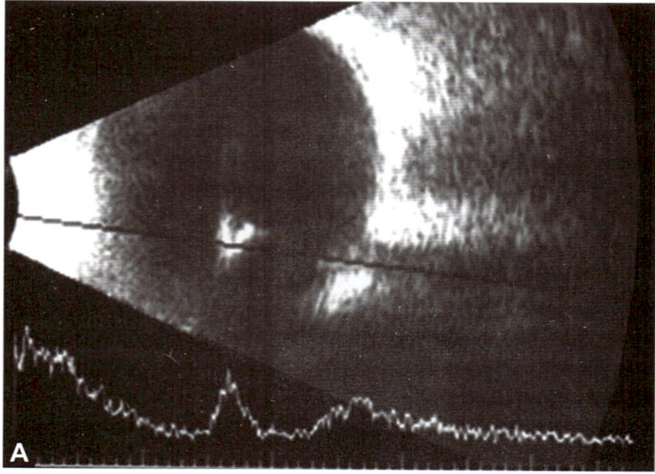
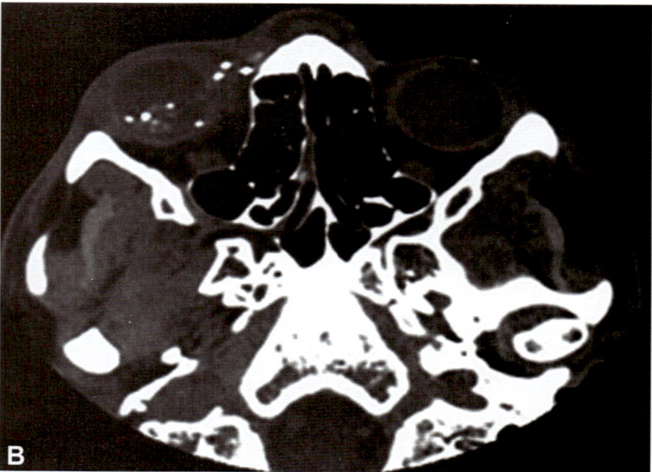

Figs. 58.1A and B: (A) USG B-scan with vector A-scan showing hyperechogenicity in midvitreous cavity with high amplitude spike on A-scan with acoustic shadowing behind the foreign body, suggesting the presence of an IOFB; and (B) Noncontrast orbital CT scan (axial view) showing multiple hyperdense echogenicity in right eye consistent with multiple intraocular foreign bodies. (CT: Computed tomography; USG: Ultrasonography).

A very important factor is the availability of trained operating room personnels who are skilled in assisting during very complicated and lengthy primary open-globe closure and IOFB removal cases. Operating with unskilled personnel after hours may not be the safest setting for an IOFB removal; therefore, primary globe closure with secondary IOFB removal may be a safer option in certain circumstances. Corneal clarity is also a very important consideration when determining primary globe closure with or without IOFB removal. Corneal edema and stromal haze improve dramatically from 7 days to 10 days after primary globe repair.

Once the surgeon decides to remove an IOFB, the operating room planning must include the necessary equipment and supplies needed for the surgical case. The first step is to decide whether the IOFB is isolated in the anterior segment and can be safely removed through a limbal incision and intralenticular IOFBs can be removed after a lens aspiration.

Retained IOFBs in the posterior segment will require a PPV, the vitreoretinal surgeon may choose from a 20-gauge PPV or a small gauge 23/25-gauge PPV. Very small IOFBs less than 0.5 mm can be removed through the cannulas without enlarging the sclerotomy wounds. In case of larger foreign bodies, a hybrid 23 (two ports) and a 20-gauge port at the surgeon's active hand may be used.

CONVENTIONAL 20 GAUGE OR SMALL PORT VITRECTOMY (FIGS. 58.2 TO 58.9)

The 20-gauge PPV uses a micro vitreoretinal blade to create an incision on the sclera and can be enlarged if needed to remove the IOFB. The 20-gauge sutured sclerotomy PPV is better suited for most IOFB injuries, unlike the insertion of a 23/25-gauge trocar, the intraocular pressure does not increase. Trocar insertion in IOFB cases may exacerbate a traumatic optic neuropathy, worsen corneal edema, and cause wound leakage from a recent primary globe closure (all these complication are often preexisting in cases with RIOFB). Suprachoroidal hemorrhage has been documented in 6% of IOFB cases.[15] Visual outcomes after a suprachoroidal hemorrhage are extremely poor, with high rates of no light

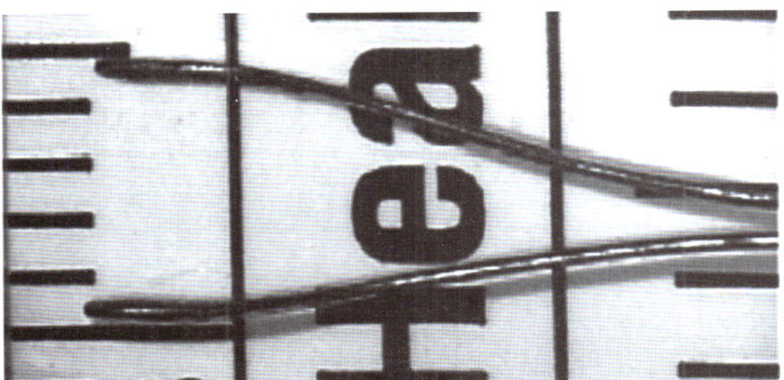

Fig. 58.2: The 20 G diamond dusted Machemer foreign body forceps.

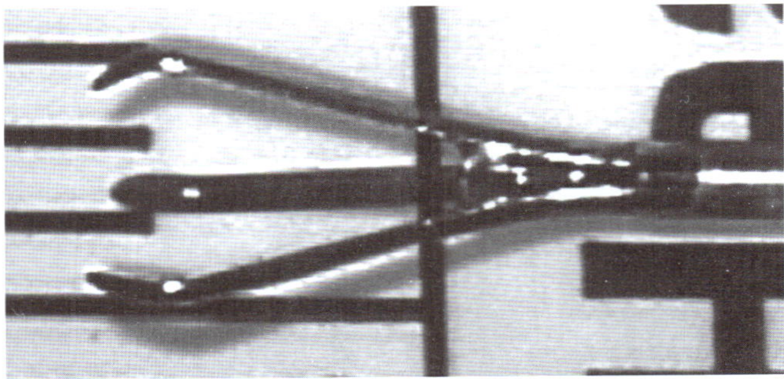

Fig. 58.3: The Pannarale basket foreign body retrieval forceps.

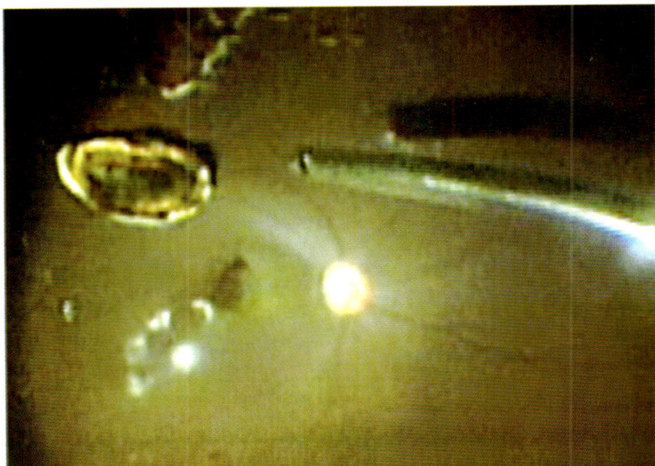

Fig. 58.4: Intraoperative view of retained intraocular foreign body (RIOFB).

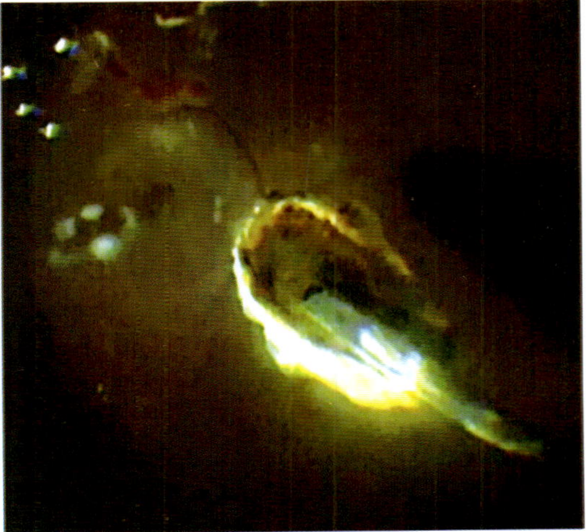

Fig. 58.5: Introperative image of retained intraocular foreign body (RIOFB) picked up using FB forceps.

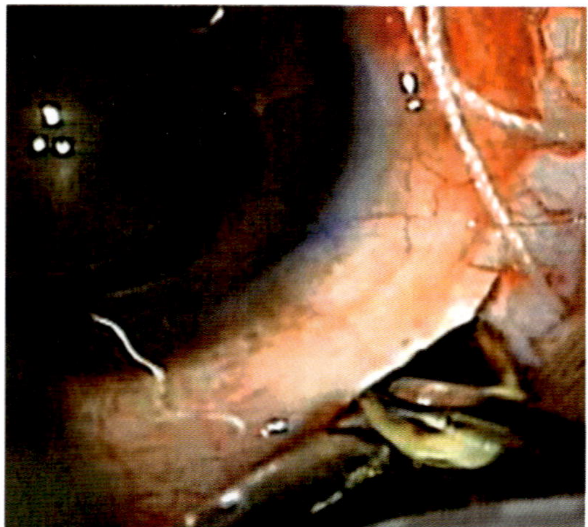

Fig. 58.6: Extraction of the foreign body at the sclerotomy site.

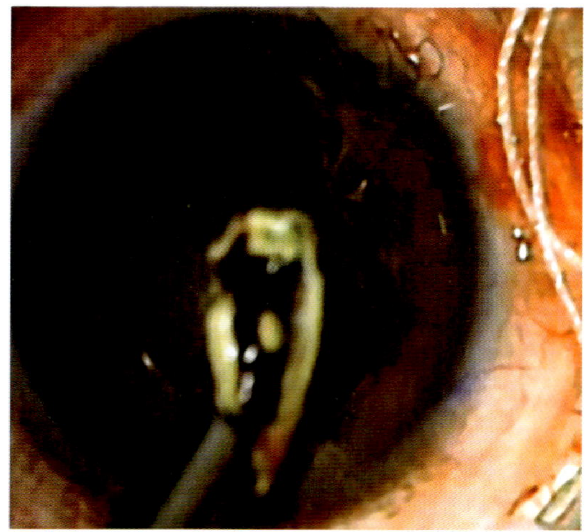

Fig. 58.7: Extracted foreign body.

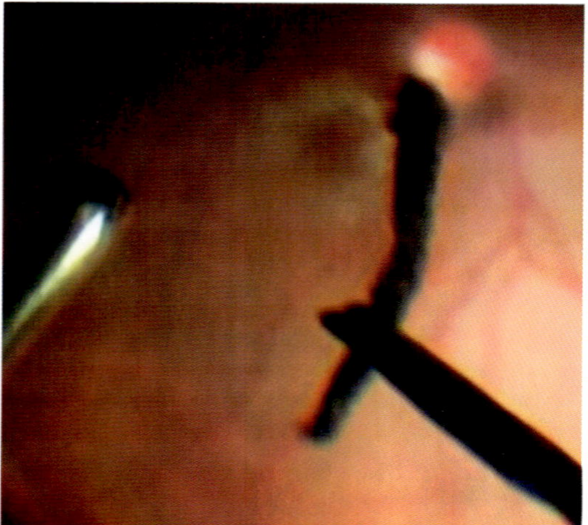

Fig. 58.8: A wooden foreign body held with forceps.

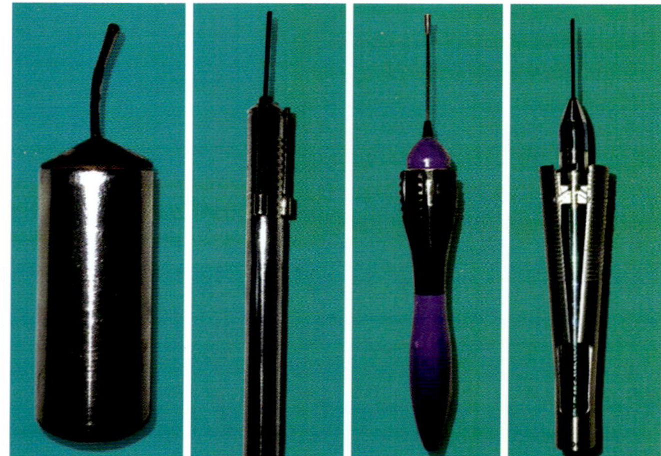

Fig. 58.9: Instruments for foreign body removal—From left to right: Extraocular magnet, intraocular magnet, 20-gauge end grasping forceps and diamond dusted forceps.

perception visual acuity, chronic postoperative hypotony and nonrepairable retinal detachment.[17]

At the beginning of the PPV, a vitreous sample can be obtained and sent for immediate Gram stain and culture. IOFB removal will start with a pars plana lensectomy, if associated with a traumatic cataract. The anterior capsule not damaged by the IOFB should remain intact for possible future intraocular lens (IOL). The most conservative approach is to leave the eye surgically aphakic and return for secondary IOL implantation 3–6 months after IOFB removal. The other option in the case of a retained IOFB with no evidence of endophthalmitis, a preparatory lens aspiration can be done with IOL, if the foreign body is lesser than 5 mm × 5 mm × 5 mm. IOL implantation at the time of IOFB has many pitfalls. The IOL may be decentered postoperative by the gas tamponade used for retinal detachment repair. The IOL may develop synechiae with the iris during the immediate postoperative period, with permanent changes in the pupil.

The artificial IOL implant may lead to a higher risk of delayed endophthalmitis, considering the fact that a contaminated foreign body was removed from the eye at the time of IOL implantation.[18]

Once core vitrectomy is performed, it is important to achieve a complete posterior hyaloid separation from the posterior pole and also from the foreign body site so as to prevent iatrogenic breaks while foreign body retrieval. The size of the IOFB is the most important factor in determining the instrumentation for IOFB removal. A magnetic metallic IOFB less than 1 × 1 × 1 mm in dimension is most easily removed using a positive action by IOFB endomagnet (Grieshaber). This instrument uses the magnet to capture the small IOFB and retracts the IOFB into a sleeve before removal from the sclerotomy site. This prevents the IOFB from catching on the edge of sclerotomy and falling back into the eye. The Grieshaber–

Machemer diamond-coated foreign body forceps are very commonly used in our setup and they are useful for grabbing an IOFB that is 3–5 mm in smallest dimension and are necessary when removing large pieces of glass off the macula. The diamond coating prevents slippage of smooth foreign bodies during retrieval. IOFB ranging in size from 1 mm to 3 mm regardless of composition is best removed with a Grieshaber–Pannarale basket forceps. Sclerotomy incisions larger than 5 mm tend to leak fluid faster than infusion through a 20-gauge infusion line. Globe collapse prevents observation and safe removal of an IOFB. IOFBs requiring larger than 5 mm sclerotomy should be retrieved through a scleral tunnel/limbal incision.

Corneal clarity is the most important aspect of IOFB removal. Injured corneas become more edematous as IOFB cases progress. Particular attention to intraocular pressure is imperative to reduce progression of corneal edema. The illumination of the retina during PPV has significantly improved visualization of IOFBs and retinal tears. The newer generation xenon light sources enable the surgeon to see past an edematous cornea and safely retrieve IOFBs. Xenon-illuminated laser probes enable the management of retinal tears and detachments, especially when used in conjunction with perfluoro-n-octane. Chandelier light sources are also commercially available to perform bimanual removal of large IOFBs. Preservative-free intraoperative triamcinolone is extremely useful in identifying residual cortical vitreous through an edematous cornea.

Without signs of retinal injury, the globe can be left with balanced salt solution, and the sclerotomies closed with 7-0 vicryl (polyglactin). Air may be used as a tamponade after laser retinopexy for retinal tears. After IOFB removal, retinal detachments may be repaired in the standard fashion with or without an encircling band.[19,20] IOFB-related retinal detachments can be repaired with sulfur hexafluoride (SF6), perfluoropropane (C3F8), or silicone oil (1,000 or 5,000 centistoke) depending on the severity of the injury. The most severe IOFB-related retinal detachments and perforating injuries need silicone oil for long-term tamponade to prevent the effects of proliferative vitreoretinopathy (PVR).[21]

PROGNOSIS

Visual outcomes after IOFB injury can vary depending on other concomitant globe injuries. Preoperative visual acuity is usually reduced by traumatic cataract or vitreous hemorrhage. These media opacities are removed during IOFB removal. The major contributing factors for long-term poor visual acuity are traumatic optic neuropathy, corneal scarring, residual effects of posttraumatic endophthalmitis, and suprachoroidal hemorrhage as well as PVR causing irreparable chronic retinal detachment. The most common type of IOFB injury involves a small corneal laceration with traumatic cataract and vitreous hemorrhage in more than 50% of these cases. These IOFB injuries have excellent visual recovery; with most obtaining best-corrected visual acuity 20/40.[22] Corneal scarring and astigmatism are significant factors for vision loss

after an IOFB injury. Anterior segment reconstruction for a traumatic iridodialysis is commonly repaired using a double-armed McCannell suture to repair a sectoral iris defect.[23] Aniridia IOL can be used to manage traumatic aniridia with symptomatic photophobia.[24] Traumatic optic neuropathy can be followed using visual field or multifocal visual evoked potential testing.[25]

The rate of preoperative retinal detachment associated with an IOFB has been reported at 31%.[26] IOFB removal associated with a retinal detachment can be extremely complicated, especially with subretinal IOFBs located away from the entry site of the IOFB. It has been found that an IOFB left in the subretinal space after PPV is a nidus for PVR formation regardless of IOFB composition and recommend removing a subretinal IOFB through the existing retinal hole or another retinotomy site. Postoperative IOFB-related retinal detachment can also contribute to poor visual outcome, with large IOFB and endophthalmitis as the strongest predictive factors. Late rhegmatogenous retinal detachments have been documented after posterior segment IOFB removal.[27] PVR is another major risk factor for vision loss after an IOFB injury. Cardillo and colleagues reported an 11% rate of PVR after IOFB, with vitreous hemorrhage as a major risk factor.[28] PVR can lead to chronic nonrepairable total retinal detachment, with resulting phthisis bulbi and enucleation. Increased depth of IOFB penetration and more extensive intraocular injuries are associated with higher rates of PVR.[28] IOFB injuries, which penetrate through the retina, develop PVR in up to 75% of the cases. On the contrary, an IOFB that penetrates into the vitreous cavity or ricochets off the retina surface, only carries roughly a 5% rate of PVR formation.[28] Posttraumatic endophthalmitis has historically averaged 4–8% of all IOFB injuries, with up to 30% in rural settings.[29] Bacteria such *as Bacillus cereus, Staphylococcus aureus, Streptococcus pneumoniae* and *Pseudomonas aeruginosa* can lead to extremely poor visual results.[30,31] Reported risks factors for posttraumatic endophthalmitis include delay in primary closure, delay in IOFB removal, disruption of the crystalline lens and sustaining ocular trauma in a rural setting.[29,32] Clinical features associated with favorable visual acuity outcomes in posttraumatic endophthalmitis include better presenting visual acuity, culture of a nonvirulent organism, lack of a retinal detachment, absence of clinical endophthalmitis and shorter wound length.[33] Broad-spectrum systemic antibiotics with third- or fourth-generation fluoroquinolones have been increasingly used by ophthalmologists after open-globe injuries. The levels of orally administered fluoroquinolones in the aqueous and vitreous have been shown to exceed the MIC90 of the major organisms causing posttraumatic endophthalmitis.[34] A meta-analysis of all published posttraumatic endophthalmitis cases reported an average rate of 8.7% in open-globe injuries. Recently published studies have suggested a reduction in this rate of posttraumatic endophthalmitis of 1–2% over the last 10 years.[33]

NONREACTIVE OR ENCAPSULATED AND FIXED INTRAOCULAR FOREIGN BODIES

Occasionally there might be some delayed presentation of RIOFB in which the foreign body is although metallic, but with a well-formed encapsulation; or totally inert foreign bodies like large graphite foreign bodies (pencil leads), rubber pellets which are fixed in the vitreous or a few foreign bodies which have pierced in the optic nerve head which carry a huge risk of torrential hemorrhage with attempted removal, these kind of foreign bodies can be safely left alone and the patient can be monitored with clinical examination and electrophysiological test like ERG and visually evoked response (VER). Intervention can be planned if there is a risk of retinal detachment/endophthalmitis.

CONCLUSION

Current IOFB removal techniques have advanced with improving imaging using ultrasound and helical CT scan for localization and preoperative planning and improved technology and instrumentation combined with newer broad-spectrum antibiotics have improved visual outcomes and mitigated complications from IOFB injuries.

REFERENCES

1. Irvine AR. Old and new techniques combined in the management of intraocular foreign bodies. Ann Ophthalmology. 1981;13(1):41-7.
2. Coleman DJ, Lucas BC, Rondeau MJ, et al. Management of intraocular foreign bodies. Ophthalmology. 1987;94(12):1647-53.
3. Kwong JS, Munk PL, Lin DT, et al. Real-time sonography in ocular trauma. AJR Am J Roentgenol. 1992;158(1):179-82.
4. Lakits A, Prokesch R, Scholda C, et al. Multiplanar imaging in the preoperative assessment of metallic intraocular foreign bodies. Helical computed tomography versus conventional computed tomography. Ophthalmology. 1998;105(9):1679-85.
5. Williams DF, Mieler WF, Abrams GW, et al. Results and prognostic factors in penetrating ocular injuries with retained intraocular foreign bodies. Ophthalmology.1988;95(7):911-6.
6. Chow DR, Garretson BR, Kuczynski B, et al. External versus internal approach to the removal of metallic intraocular foreign bodies. Retina. 2000;20(4):364-9.
7. Greven CM, Engelbrecht NE, Slusher MM, et al. Intraocular foreign bodies: management, prognostic factors, and visual outcomes. Ophthalmology. 2000;107(3):608-12.
8. De Souza S, Howcroft MJ. Management of posterior segment intraocular foreign bodies: 14 years' experience. Can J Ophthalmology. 1999;34(1):23-9.
9. El-Asrar AM, Al-Amro SA, Khan NM, et al. Visual outcome and prognostic factors after vitrectomy for posterior segment foreign bodies. Eur J Ophthalmology. 2000;10(4):304-11.
10. Jonas JB, Knorr HL, Budde WM. Prognostic factors in ocular injuries caused by intraocular or retrobulbar foreign bodies. Ophthalmology. 2000;107(5):823-8.
11. Soheilian M, Abolhasani A, Ahmadieh H, et al. Management of magnetic intravitreal foreign bodies in 71 eyes. Ophthalmic Surg Lasers Imaging. 2004;35(5):372-8.
12. Soheilian M, Feghi M, Yazdani S, et al. Surgical management of non-metallic and non-magnetic metallic intraocular foreign bodies. Ophthalmic Surg Lasers Imaging. 2005;36(3):189-96.
13. Wani VB, Al-Ajmi M, Thalib L, et al. Vitrectomy for posterior segment intraocular foreign bodies: visual results and prognostic factors. Retina. 2003;23(5):654-60.
14. Kuhn F, Morris R. Posterior segment intraocular foreign bodies: management in the vitrectomy era. Ophthalmology. 2000;107(5):821-2.
15. Colyer MH, Weber ED, Weichel ED, et al. Delayed intraocular foreign body removal without endophthalmitis during Operations Iraqi Freedom and Enduring Freedom. Ophthalmology. 2007;114(8):1439-47.
16. Hariprasad SM, Shah GK, Mieler WF, et al. Vitreous and aqueous penetration of orally administered moxifloxacin in humans. Arch Ophthalmology. 2006;124(2):178-82.
17. Wirostko WJ, Han DP, Mieler WF, et al. Suprachoroidal hemorrhage: outcome of surgical management according to hemorrhage severity. Ophthalmology. 1998;105(12):2271-5.
18. Pavlovic S. Primary intraocular lens implantation during pars plana vitrectomy and intraretinal foreign body removal. Retina. 1999;19(5):430-6.
19. Ersanli D, Sonmez M, Unal M, et al. Management of retinal detachment due to closed globe injury by pars plana vitrectomy with and without scleral buckling. Retina. 2006;26(1):32-6.
20. Warrasak S, Euswas A, Hongsakorn S. Posterior segment trauma: types of injuries, result of vitreo-retinal surgery and prophylactic broad encircling scleral buckle. J Med Assoc Thai. 2005;88(12):1916-30.
21. Szurman P, Roters S, Grisanti S, et al. Primary silicone oil tamponade in the management of severe intraocular foreign body injuries: an 8-year follow-up. Retina. 2007;27(3):304-11.
22. Woodcock MG, Scott RA, Huntbach J, et al. Mass and shape as factors in intraocular foreign body injuries. Ophthalmology. 2006;113(12):2262-9.
23. Wachler BB, Krueger RR. Double-armed McCannell suture for repair of traumatic iridodialysis. Am J Ophthalmology. 1996;122(1):109-10.
24. Tanzer DJ, Smith RE. Black iris-diaphragm intraocular lens for aniridia and aphakia. J Cataract Refract Surg. 1999;25(11):1548-51.
25. Klistorner A, Fraser C, Garrick R, et al. Correlation between full-field and multifocal VEPs in optic neuritis. Doc Ophthalmology. 2008;116(1):19-27.
26. El-Asrar AM, Al-Amro SA, Khan NM, et al. Retinal detachment after posterior segment intraocular foreign body injuries. Int Ophthalmology. 1998;22(6):369-75.
27. Weissgold DJ, Kaushal P. Late onset of rhegmatogenous retinal detachments after successful posterior segment intraocular foreign body removal. Br J Ophthalmology. 2005;89(3):327-31.
28. Cardillo JA, Stout JT, LaBree L, et al. Post-traumatic proliferative vitreoretinopathy. The epidemiologic profile, onset, risk factors, and visual outcome. Ophthalmology. 1997;104(7):1166-73.
29. Boldt HC, Pulido JS, Blodi CF, et al. Rural endophthalmitis. Ophthalmology. 1989;96(12):1722-6.
30. Lieb DF, Scott IU, Flynn HW, et al. Open globe injuries with positive intraocular cultures: factors influencing final visual acuity outcomes. Ophthalmology. 2003;110(8):1560-6.
31. Al-Omran AM, Abboud EB, Abu El-Asrar AM. Microbiologic spectrum and visual outcome of posttraumatic endophthalmitis. Retina. 2007;27(2):236-42.
32. Thompson JT, Parver LM, Enger CL, et al. Infectious endophthalmitis after penetrating injuries with retained intraocular foreign bodies. National Eye Trauma System. Ophthalmology. 1993;100(10):1468-74.
33. Chhabra S, Kunimoto DY, Kazi L, et al. Endophthalmitis after open globe injury: microbiologic spectrum and susceptibilities of isolates. Am J Ophthalmology. 2006;142(5):852-4.
34. Sakamoto H, Sakamoto M, Hata Y, et al. Aqueous and vitreous penetration of levofloxacin after topical and or oral administration. Eur J Ophthalmology. 2007;17(3):372-6.

Chapter 59

Shaken Baby Syndrome

Pooja Shah, Raghav Ravani, Amit Gadkar

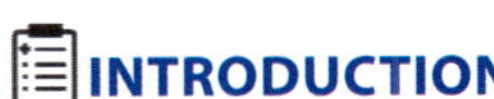
INTRODUCTION

Child abuse is a broad terminology encompassing physical abuse, sexual abuse, emotional abuse, neglect and it remains a compelling cause of morbidity and mortality in children. Shaken baby syndrome (SBS) is a form of physical abuse described by Henry Kempe[1] and Guthkelch,[2] before John Caffey's[3] sentinel work titled "whiplash shaken infant syndrome" based on description of 27 infant injury cases with subdural hematoma, intraocular bleeding and metaphyseal fractures in the absence of external trauma to the head, in the year 1974. Several terms have been used in literature to describe SBS, viz. abusive head trauma, shaken impact syndrome, shaken brain trauma, pediatric traumatic brain injury, however as per recommendation of the Committee on Child Abuse and Neglect of the American Association of Pediatrics (AAP) in 2009, the term "abusive trauma" (AT) should replace the terminology "shaken baby syndrome"; to encompass mechanisms other than shaking resulting in similar outcomes.[4]

INCIDENCE

Nearly 700,000 cases of child abuse and neglect are reported annually in the United States, with figures varying annually.[5] Reported incidence of abusive head trauma (AHT) is estimated at 20–30 cases per 100,000 infants infants are younger than one year age.[6] Fatal cases may be grouped under multiple traumatic injuries while minor injury may be unrecognized.

CLINICAL FEATURES

Violent shaking of infant head with or without impact results in tearing of veins running from cerebral cortex to dural sinuses resulting in subdural hemorrhage. Discrepancy of movement of unmyelinated infant brain versus firm skull with large fontanels induces shear stress producing cerebral contusion. Poor head holding and large head to body ratio amplifies the shear stress.[7,8] Occurrence of retinal hemorrhages has

been explained by several theories including transmission of shear stress via soft tissue connection between brain and eye resulting in traction over retinal vessels, shear forces at vitreoretinal interface, raised intracranial tension and obstruction of retinal vasculature.[9] Skeletal fractures are a result of pressure exerted while holding infant during shaking.[7,8]

Usual victim is less than 5 years of age, particularly children younger than 1 year of age. Increase in prolonged crying episodes start at 2–3 weeks of age, peaks at 6–8 weeks, and declines in majority by 4 months of age.[10] Offender is usually a parent or caregiver who shook an inconsolable crying baby out of frustration; followed by lethargy, drowsiness, poor feeding, seizures, apnea or breathing difficulty. Often a misleading history of antecedent trivial trauma may be present. A reliable medical history may not be always available; however, diagnosis of AHT can be made based on characteristic clinical findings.

Intracranial injury may manifest as subdural hematoma over cerebral convexities or interhemispheric fissure, subarachnoid bleed, cerebral contusion and cerebral edema. Later, cerebral atrophy may be the only evidence of intracranial injury. Neuroimaging shows cerebral edema, ischemia or contusion in acute phase while cerebral atrophy ensues later.

Lack of external signs of trauma except for bruises over trunk or extremities, rib fracture, metaphyseal fractures is a characteristic feature of AHT. It may present with nonspecific signs like bradycardia, apnea, hypothermia, lethargy, irritability, seizures, hypotony, lag in growth and development, bulging fontanels, scalp swelling and injuries in various stages of healing, hence a high index of suspicion must be maintained.

OCULAR MANIFESTATIONS

Ophthalmologist plays a crucial role in identifying AHT since 85% cases show evidence of retinal hemorrhage and 5% cases present with an ocular problem and retinal hemorrhages may be the only evidence of AHT. Retinal hemorrhages are common in nonaccidental head injury (NAHI) while they are infrequently encountered after cardiopulmonary resuscitation and rarely encountered in accidental trauma, e.g. motor vehicle accident, fall from height.[11] Classic ophthalmic findings in AHT include retinal hemorrhages, vitreous hemorrhage, and macular folds. Retinal hemorrhages can be unilateral or typically bilateral, preretinal, flame shaped, deep retinal, or subretinal. Hemorrhages show predilection for the posterior pole, ora serrata and perivascular areas, sites of strong vitreoretinal attachment; rarely involve entire fundus. Preretinal hemorrhage may migrate into vitreous body resulting in vitreous hemorrhage. Extensive retinal hemorrhages frequently accompany intracranial injury. Retinal hemorrhages resolve at variable pace over months to year, usually 4 weeks, posing a difficulty in precisely identifying timing of assault.

Retinal hemorrhages may occur in variety of conditions, however, those secondary to birth trauma seldom persist beyond 1 month of age. Terson syndrome, i.e. vitreous hemorrhage with subarachnoid hemorrhage is uncommon in this age group, so is central retinal vein occlusion which may result in extensive retinal hemorrhages. Other possibilities resulting in retinal hemorrhages in children include coagulopathy, anemia, hypertension, leukemia, raised intracranial pressure, meningitis, retinopathy of prematurity and aminoaciduria.

Other findings which may be encountered include retinal tissue disturbance causing a full thickness retinal fold at the macula with a crater like appearance, traumatic retinoschisis either at the level of nerve fiber layer or deep retina following resolution of retinal hemorrhage. Full thickness retinal break and detachment while common in accidental head trauma are uncommon in AHT. Similarly, choroidal rupture and retinal dialysis are suggestive of closed globe injury rather than AHT. Retinal fold flattens over weeks after injury while schisis cavities which may be of enormous size and partly filled with blood, may persist indefinitely or resolve spontaneously or very rarely progress. Ocular adnexa and anterior segment of the eye are usually uninjured. Optic nerve injury has prognostic significance and should be documented. Traumatic contusion of optic nerve, hemorrhage within the nerve sheath or descending optic atrophy secondary to trauma to geniculate ganglion or chiasma may be the cause, however, signs are apparent late in the course and not helpful in initial diagnosis.[8]

MANAGEMENT

Hospital admission is recommended and any life-threatening injury should be managed on priority basis. Management of SBS warrants integrated efforts from emergency care physician, ophthalmologist, pediatrician, pediatric surgeon, social support and judicial system. Careful history taking, analysis of circumstances of alleged injury, identifying risk factors like step father, absence of mother, single mother, broken family, etc. are important as perpetrator may not confess about the assault.[8,12] Complete physical examination of fully unclothed child in collaboration with a pediatrician is of paramount importance. Baseline visual acuity and pupillary reaction should be documented. Complete blood count, serum biochemistry, CT/MRI brain and abdomen, skeletal survey should be obtained.[13] Fundus photograph to document retinal hemorrhages. Notification of child protection services as per law of state should be done. Pars plana vitrectomy may be indicated for dense vitreous hemorrhage to prevent amblyopia; however, loss of b-wave amplitude on flash electroretinogram (ERG) is suggestive of extensive retinal disruption and confers poor prognosis. Retinal detachment, if present, should be treated with scleral buckling or vitrectomy.

At the time of diagnosis, 40–45% of children have clinical or radiologic evidence of prior brain injury.[14] Most children (68%) who survive AHT will have diagnosed neurologic, visual, cognitive, behavioral, sleep abnormalities, motor disturbances and learning disabilities by 2–5 years of age.[15] Mortality ranges from 6% to 36%.[15-17] Vision loss occurs due to cortical injury or optic neuropathy. Dense vitreous hemorrhage and extensive hemorrhagic retinopathy confer poor prognosis for vision as well as life.[8]

REFERENCES

1. Kempe CH, Silverman FN, Steele BF, et al. The battered-child syndrome. JAMA. 1962;181(1):17-24.
2. Guthkelch AN. Infantile Subdural Haematoma and its Relationship to Whiplash Injuries. Br Med J. 1971;2(5759):430-1.
3. Caffey J. The whiplash shaken infant syndrome: manual shaking by the extremities with whiplash-induced intracranial and intraocular bleedings, linked with residual permanent brain damage and mental retardation. Pediatrics. 1974;54(4):396-403.
4. Christian CW, Block R, The Committee on Child Abuse and Neglect. Abusive head trauma in infants and children. Pediatrics. 2009;123(5):1409-11.
5. Administration for Children and Families, Administration on Children, Youth and Families, Children's Bureau, Washington, DC: Department of Health and Human Services. (2017). Child maltreatment 2015—data tables [online]. Available from: http://www.acf.hhs.gov/programs/cb/research-data-technology/statistics-research/child-maltreatment. [Accessed December, 2017].
6. Using hospital discharge data to track inflicted traumatic brain injury [online]. PubMed Journals. Available from: https://ncbi.nlm.nih.gov/labs/articles/18374268/ [Accessed December, 2017].
7. Caffey J. On the theory and practice of shaking infants. Its potential residual effects of permanent brain damage and mental retardation. Am J Dis Child. 1972;124(2):161-9.
8. Duhaime AC, Gennarelli TA, Thibault LE, et al. The shaken baby syndrome. A clinical, pathological, and biomechanical study. J Neurosurg. 1987;66(3):409-15.
9. Binenbaum G, Forbes BJ. The eye in child abuse: key points on retinal hemorrhages and abusive head trauma. Pediatr Radiol. 2014;44(Suppl 4):S571-7.

10. Barr RG. Crying as a trigger for abusive head trauma: a key to prevention. Pediatr Radiol. 2014;44(Suppl 4):S559-64.

11. Togioka BM, Arnold MA, Bathurst MA, et al. Retinal hemorrhages and shaken baby syndrome: an evidence-based review. J Emerg Med. 2009;37(1):98-106.

12. Hinds T, Shalaby-Rana E, Jackson AM, et al. Aspects of Abuse: Abusive Head Trauma. Curr Probl Pediatr Adolesc Health Care. 2015;45(3):71-9.

13. Berkowitz CD. Physical abuse of children. N Engl J Med. 2017;376(17):1659-66.

14. Ewing-Cobbs L, Kramer L, Prasad M, et al. Neuroimaging, physical, and developmental findings after inflicted and noninflicted traumatic brain injury in young children. Pediatrics. 1998;102(2 Pt 1):300-7.

15. Barlow KM, Thomson E, Johnson D, et al. Late neurologic and cognitive sequelae of inflicted traumatic brain injury in infancy. Pediatrics. 2005;116(2):e174-85.

16. Niederkrotenthaler T, Xu L, Parks SE, et al. Descriptive factors of abusive head trauma in young children—United States, 2000-2009. Child Abuse Negl. 2013;37(7):446-55.

17. Outcome following subdural haemorrhages in infancy [online]. Available from: https://www.ncbi.nlm.nih.gov/pmc/articles/PMC2083697/ [Accessed December, 2017].

Miscellaneous Retinal Conditions

Chapter 60

Cancer Associated and Related Autoimmune Retinopathies

Ruchir Tewari, Rohan Chawla, Atul Kumar

INTRODUCTION

Autoimmune retinopathies are a group of acquired retinal inflammatory degenerative disorders presenting with generalized retinal photoreceptor dysfunction, rapidly progressive bilateral and otherwise, unexplained vision loss and field defects along with circulating antiretinal antibodies. Paraneoplastic retinopathies (PR) display antibodies directed to various retinal proteins with an underlying malignancy whereas, autoimmune retinopathies (AIR) are characterized by autoantibodies directed against retinal proteins without a known malignancy. The onset of visual symptoms and detection of antibodies may precede the diagnosis of malignancy by months to years.

Specific paraneoplastic and autoimmune retinopathies that have been identified include cancer-associated retinopathy (CAR),[1-3] melanoma-associated retinopathy (MAR),[4,5] antienolase retinopathy,[6] anticarbonic anhydrase II retinopathy,[7] and cancer-associated cone dysfunction. The clinical features of paraneoplastic retinopathy and autoimmune retinopathy are similar. Patients typically present with rapid, painless vision loss associated with flashing lights (photopsias) and photosensitivity.[8] The disease is bilateral, occasionally sequential and evolves over weeks to months. In patients with antienolase retinal antibodies, presentation is less acute with a slow progression.[6]

Retinal examination is within normal limits in early stages causing a diagnostic dilemma in some cases. Markedly abnormal electroretinographic (ERG) findings are associated with a definitive diagnosis which can usually be confirmed with immunofluorescence methods for detection of circulating retinal antibodies. Occasionally, a pseudoretinitis pigmentosa like appearance with arteriolar attenuation, waxy disc pallor, pigmentary changes and diffuse retinal atrophy may be seen. Inflammation signs are usually not present.[9,10] The current chapter intends to highlight both our understanding and shortcomings of this rare and ever elusive disease.

EPIDEMIOLOGY

The PR and AIR are rare disorders and the exact prevalence and incidence are unknown. Older adults are affected usually with youngest recorded presentation at 3 years,[8] with no sex predilection. CAR is thought to be the most common form of PR. Malignancy most commonly associated with CAR is small-cell lung cancer, followed by gynecologic (uterine and cervical) and breast cancers.[3] MAR now appears to be increasing in frequency relative to CAR perhaps, because of a decrease in incidence of lung cancer.[4]

No standard set of guidelines for the diagnosis of these conditions exist.[11] Recently, the American Uvea Society has given a set of updates regarding the diagnosis and management of AR although they have not been standardized.[12] A large review of MAR and CAR patients have reported a female predominance (2:1 ratio) with average age of onset around 65 years.[8] Major systemic malignancies associated with CAR included lung (16%), breast (16%), melanoma (16%), hematological (15%, including lymphomas, leukemias and myelomas), gynecological (9%), prostate (7%) and colon (6%).[8] Only 4% patients developed retinopathy prior to development of cancer. Lung cancer and lymphoma associated retinopathy may appear early (weeks to months) while breast and prostate cancer patients may develop the same after years. A shorter latency has been seen to be associated with a rapid visual decline.

A case series of MAR reported a mean age at onset around 57.5 years after a diagnosis of melanoma with a mean latency of 3.6 years (range of 2 months to 19 years).[13] Metastatic disease had shorter latency of around 1.9 years (range 1 month to 15 years). Retinopathy preceding development of melanoma was however, infrequently seen with average latency of 2 years.[13]

PATHOLOGY

Although presence of antiretinal antibodies is a common occurrence in all forms of disease, the exact mechanism of retinal antigen destruction is not fully known.[9,14] A multitude of retinal and nonretinal antigens are associated with retinal dysfunction and the list keeps on growing. The major antigens include—recoverin (23 kDa), carbonic anhydrase II, α-enolase, arrestin, transducin-β, glyceraldehyde-3-phosphate dehydrogenase, Tubby- like protein 1 (TULP1), neurofilament protein, heat shock protein-70 (hsp70), photoreceptor cell-specific nuclear receptor (PNR), bestrophin, antialdolase A and C, Müller cell-specific antigen (35 kDa), transient receptor potential cation channel, subfamily M, member 1 (TRPM1), inter-photoreceptor retinoid binding protein and many other undefined minor antigens.[15-17] While some antigens are specific to the retina (recoverin and inter-photoreceptor retinoid binding protein), others are present elsewhere as well (enolase, carbonic anhydrase II, glyceraldehyde-3-phosphate dehydrogenase and aldolase).

Of all the antigens, recoverin, a 23 kDa calcium channel binding protein present in photoreceptors and enolase, a 48 kDa glycolytic enzyme, have been most exhaustively studied. Enolase has three isoforms: α, β and γ of which, γ isoform is neuronal tissue specific.[18] Anti-enolase is probably the most preva-lent antiretinal antibody, being present in 30% of patients with antiretinal antibodies, many autoimmune disorders and even healthy subjects indicating multifactorial nature of the antigen.[19-22] Recoverin, on the other hand is highly specific for cases with CAR, although association with small cell lung cancer without retinopathy and other nonparaneoplastic retinopathies has been reported.[23-26] Both enolase and recove-rin are highly expressed by tumor cells that makes molecular mimicry between tumor cells and retinal antigens very likely.[6] Similar response may also explain nonparaneoplastic AIR where mimicry between presumed viral, bacterial and retinal antigens may lead to formation of autoantibodies.[6,27,28]

Experimental animal models and in vitro cell cultures have shone some light over the possible pathogenic mechanisms related with autoantibodies. In vitro studies of AIR have demonstrated virulence of autoantibodies that leads to apoptosis of retinal cells after cellular internalization by endocytosis. Caspase pathway and intracellular calcium buildup rather than complement activation have been proposed as possible mediators of cell death. A specific example is extensive rhodopsin phosphorylation by antirecoverin antibodies leading to apoptosis of photoreceptors.

Recoverin mediated cell damage has been extensively studied. The recoverin gene has been mapped to chromosome 17, very close to p53 tumor suppressor gene in patient with recoverin mediated CAR.[29] The initial step in etiopathogenesis of CAR is believed to be a novel germline mutation leading to aberrant systemic expression of recoverin gene by tumor infected cells that causes an immune response in the body. This is followed by buildup of antirecoverin antibodies (thought to be protective from the primary tumor)[30] that in a handful of individuals, cross -react with retinal photorecep-

tors leading to widespread retinal dysfunction and a clinical picture of CAR.[23,27,31] In vivo studies with intravitreal antirecoverin antibody injection have shown retinal cell death and ERG changes.[32-34] A similar response was seen with intravitreal injection of recoverin that incited a uveitogenic response in both Lewis rat and mouse models leading to creation of antibodies and changes in ERG responses.[35,36] Immunization of rabbits and Lewis rats has been shown to cause development of uveitis and retinal dysfunction as well.[37,38] In both in vivo and in vitro studies, cells undergoing apoptosis were recoverin positive which leads credence to a direct pathogenic mechanism of antirecoverin antibodies.[39] Recoverin is usually expressed by photoreceptors that explains the severe scotopic and photopic ERG depression associated with introduction of antirecoverin antibodies.

Other autoantibodies have similar effects on retinal cells. Antienolase antibodies usually target ganglion cells whereas antibodies associated with systemic melanoma [melanoma associated retinopathy (MAR)] are associated with bipolar cell death. The signs and symptoms in most of the cases thus, correlate with the type of retinal autoantibody involved.

CLINICAL FINDINGS

Symptoms and signs are variable. CAR affects both rods and cones whereas, MAR affects bipolar cells that interfere with rod function. Patients with cone-associated retinopathy have dysfunction limited to only cones.

Individuals with cone dysfunction experience photosensitivity, prolonged glare after light exposure (hemeralopia), reduced visual acuity and central vision and loss of color vision. Individuals with rod dysfunction have difficulty seeing in dim illumination (nyctalopia), prolonged dark adaptation and peripheral field loss. In either case, positive visual phenomena are prominent, including flashing lights (photopsia), flickering, smoky or swirling vision and other entoptic symptoms. Some patients report transient dimming of vision, which may be mistaken for retinovascular disease. Occasional cases with overlap features occur.

On examination, patients with CAR usually have prominent involvement of central vision, resulting in markedly decreased visual acuity, loss of color vision and central scotomas. In some cases, visual field testing shows paracentral scotomas that progress to classic ring scotomas. Photo-stress recovery times are typically prolonged. In contrast, patients with MAR often have near-normal visual acuity, color vision and central visual fields early in their course.[12] For example, in the series by Keltner et al. visual acuity was 20/60 or better in 82% at presentation but in only 30% at last follow-up.[12] However, most patients with MAR experience progressive visual loss especially, in the peripheral visual field.

Funduscopic findings at presentation are often normal in all forms of PR and AIR. However, characteristic changes occur over time including attenuation of retinal arterioles with thinning and mottling of the retinal pigment epithelium (RPE) and occasional optic disc pallor. In rare cases of CAR or MAR, vitreous cells, arteriolar sheathing and periphlebitis may be present, particularly late in the course of disease. As reported by Keltner et al., funduscopic findings in 43 patients with MAR were as follows: 19 (44%) patients had normal fundus findings at presentation, 13 (30%) had vascular attenuation and 12 (28%) had RPE changes. Vitreous cells were present in 13 (30%) patients and 10 (23%) had optic disc pallor.[12]

Fluorescein angiography is often performed to exclude other entities as potential causes of vision loss. Findings are usually normal but in occasional cases, there is mild peripheral vascular leakage consistent with vasculitis. Thinning of the inner retinal layers has been demonstrated with optical coherence tomography (OCT) in CAR and in AR.[40]

The findings from full-field (Ganzfeld) ERG are almost always abnormal. Specific findings depend on the predominance of cone versus rod dysfunction. Patients with CAR usually have absent cone responses with reduced a- and b-waves in both photopic and scotopic conditions. Findings in MAR include a markedly reduced or absent dark adapted b wave (electronegative waveform), which indicates bipolar and Müller cell dysfunction with preserved photoreceptor function.[6] Multifocal ERG (MERG) is useful for evaluating selective cases in which visual field loss is localized for monitoring disease progression and for correlating with visual field loss.

WORKUP AND INVESTIGATIONS

It is important to maintain a high index of suspicion for PR or AR in patients who present with newly onset progressive vision loss in the setting of a normal appearing fundus on examination.

The initial workup should include a full assessment of the patient's visual function including color vision and visual field testing. Goldmann perimetry readily tests the peripheral field and because kinetic perimetry may be more sensitive than static for detecting changes in this disorder, Goldmann is preferred. If automated perimetry is performed, the test should be adapted to include the peripheral field. Full-field ERG helps to globally define the retinal involvement and also for localizing the layer of retina involved. In selective cases, MERG may be helpful.

A definitive diagnosis of PR or AR requires the demonstration of antiretinal antibodies. Tests for these antibodies are now available commercially. On occasion, individuals without clinical evidence of retinopathy have these antibodies and in some cases of presumed PR or AR, the antibodies cannot be identified with current techniques. In one report, it is estimated that up to 35% of retinal antibodies are not detected in patients with presumed CAR.[9]

Diagnosing AR becomes all the more difficult as patients do not present with a clinical diagnosis of systemic malignancy. Although history of systemic autoimmune disorders might be present, clinical examination can be normal in the beginning.

Therefore, minor and subtle changes in the fundus such as mild pigmentary mottling or mild arteriolar attenuation should not be overlooked. In any patient with suspected CAR and without a known malignancy, a chest radiograph should be obtained. If the result is normal and the index of suspicion of CAR remains high, a chest CT scanning is appropriate. Additional imaging studies to consider include CT of the abdomen and pelvis, mammography (in women) and total-body positron emission tomography (PET) or CT/PET. Complete physical examination including pelvic and breast examinations for women is also recommended.

Electrophysiological testing plays an important part in evaluating a patient of suspected AIR as it might provide the only clue in otherwise unexplained vision loss.[6] An ERG should be ordered in any young individual with symptoms such as "shimmering", photopsia, photo-aversion, nyctalopia or color disturbances and otherwise normal fundus examination. Specific patterns of ERG response may be seen depending on the type of cell involved. Severe photoreceptor dysfunction (rods more than cones) may lead to severe depression of a- and b-waves on ERG in cases with PR/AIR whereas a negative waveform in scotopic response indicating bipolar cell dysfunction is typically seen in MAR. Impaired dark adaptation may again indicate toward rod photoreceptor dysfunction. A patient with ERG responses suggestive of CAR should undergo an X-ray evaluation as bronchogenic carcinoma is most commonly associated. Similarly, history of cutaneous melanoma should be proactively elicited when MAR is suspected. It often becomes imperative to seek help of an internist for ruling out systemic malignancy. Other imaging tests such as MRI, CT scan and PET scan may be required for detecting an occult malignancy and should be considered after due consultation with a specialist.

Visual field constriction as well development of central and isolated scotomas may be a presenting sign in some cases with AIR. Visual field testing for constriction of visual fields is best done by kinetic perimetry, though it still remains a subjective technique and is marred by issues such as examiner dependence, intertest variability, patient cooperation and lack of standardization. Static perimetry on the other hand, is an objective modality utilized mainly for detection of central and paracentral scotomas. Apart from initial assessment, visual field testing also plays a part in assessing disease progression.

Fundus fluorescein angiography (FFA), optical coherence tomography (OCT) and fundus autofluorescence (FAF) are additional modalities that may help in evaluating a patient with subtle fundus changes. OCT may pick up mild cystic changes in the macula as well as disruption of outer layers especially, the ellipsoid zone that has a bearing on the visual acuity.[41] Cystic changes seen on OCT may not usually leak on FFA and point toward AIR. Typical FAF findings described previously for AIR help in differentiating it from other possible diagnosis that may pose a challenge (Figs. 60.1A to F).[41]

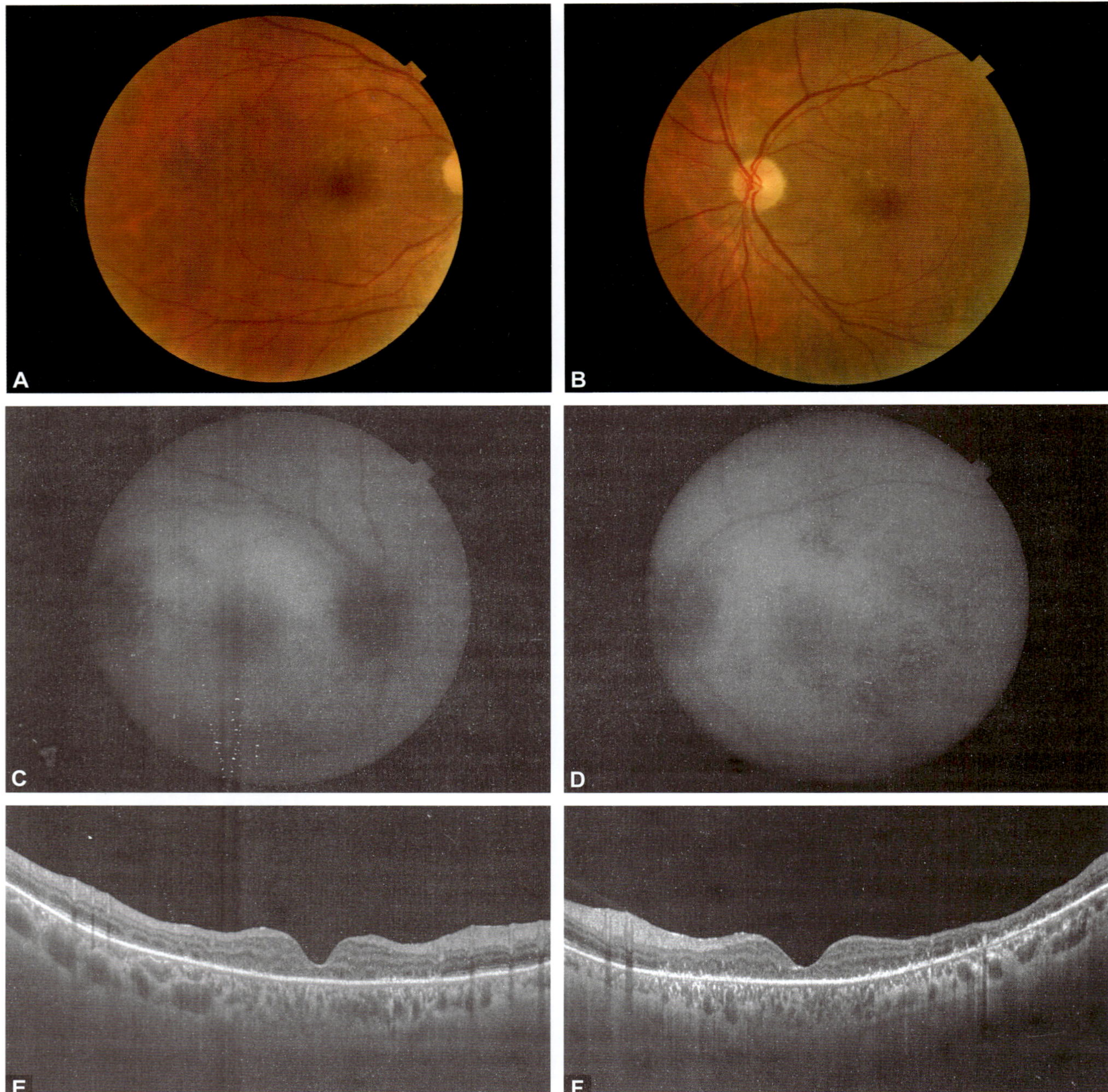

Figs. 60.1A to F: (A and B) Fundus photographs of a 55-year-old male patient with inflammatory bowel disease and autoimmune retinopathy. Both eyes show mild pigmentary mottling at the posterior pole, mild disc pallor and slight attenuation of vessels. (C and D) Fundus autofluorescence images of both eyes show a ring of hyperautofluorescence in the parafoveal region and small punctate hyperautofluorescent lesions temporal to the macula that are surrounded by a hypoautofluorescent halo. (E and F) Swept- source optical coherence tomography (SS-OCT) of both eyes shows foveal atrophy with disorganization of retinal layers and disruption of outer retinal layers extending well into the parafoveal region.

Enzyme-linked immunosorbent assay (ELISA) involves the use of specific proteins loaded in wells that are allowed to bind with different dilutions of patient's serum. A secondary anti-IgG (human immunoglobulin) is then, added to this that detects the antigen-antibody complex using spectrophotometer to detect the concentration. Both antirecoverin and antienolase antibodies have been detected using this technique and it is believed to be quite sensitive.

While interpreting the result, it should be kept in mind that like Western blot, various reports using ELISA fall short on reporting standard curves, positive controls, use of replicates or samples from healthy individuals.[15] This leads to difficulty in achieving acceptable sensitivity, specificity and both positive and negative predictive values.

Immunohistochemistry and western blot are the more widely used tests. As already emphasized, all these techniques lack standardization,[15] it is therefore, best to employ a two-step approach in confirming the presence of antibodies rather than relying on a single test.

DIFFERENTIAL DIAGNOSIS

Acute or subacute unilateral or bilateral vision loss with a normal appearing fundus suggests the possibility of retrobulbar optic neuropathy. Other disorders also to be considered include compressive orbital and intracranial lesions, demyelinating disease, ischemia, toxicity and hereditary disorders.

Inflammatory conditions especially white-dot syndromes such as acute zonal occult outer retinopathy (AZOOR) and multiple evanescent white-dot syndrome (MEWDS) have reportedly been associated with antiretinal antibodies and may be confused with AR.[11,42] AZOOR may present with similar signs, symptoms as well as ERG and visual field changes. It is usually bilateral but asymmetric. Although there have been isolated case reports in AZOOR, antibodies are not thought to play a pathologic role and it is believed to be an epiphenomenon. Also prognosis in such cases is fairly good with stabilization of vision and partial recovery even without treatment. Moreover, FAF in AZOOR shows characteristic hypoautofluorescent lesions that are not visualized in AR.[43] MEWDS is invariably unilateral, presents with afferent pupillary defect, optic nerve swelling and tends to recover spontaneously. It is therefore, easy to differentiate from AR. Inflammatory conditions such as idiopathic retinal vasculitis and uveitic conditions such as VKH, Behcet's disease and sympathetic ophthalmia have also been reported to present with antiretinal antibodies. Infectious pathologies such as viral retinitis, onchocerciasis and toxoplasma retinochoroiditis may also be rarely associated with retinal antibodies. All these disorders have typical history and clinical presentation that sets them apart from PR/AR.

Retinitis pigmentosa (RP) may also present with autoantibodies. Although family history is an important feature of RP, more than half of cases do not present with a positive family history. The clinical picture in most cases of RP is similar to PR/AR. Advanced stages of RP are easy to distinguish from paraneoplastic AIR as by then, a definitive diagnosis of systemic malignancy has already been made. OCT also can be confusing as both may present with macular cysts. Around 90% of patients with RP and macular cysts have circulating antiretinal antibodies as opposed to 13% in RP without macular cyst and 6% healthy subjects.[44] Moreover, RP patients with antibodies may show a progressive downhill course with rapid loss of vision and macular changes. It is still unclear whether antibodies play any role in the pathology or are just an incidental finding.

PROGNOSIS

Data regarding visual prognosis from various reports of antiretinal antibody syndromes is not very encouraging and spontaneous recovery is seldom seen. It is also suggested that the type of antiretinal antibody present may have a bearing on final visual outcome. In cases with CAR and npAIR, antirecoverin antibodies are associated with severe vision loss and final visual outcome as poor as perception of light. This is quite ironical as many reports suggest a rather protective effect of these antibodies with decreased mortality. On the other hand, antienolase antibody associated retinopathy is usually not associated with blindness and reported visual acuity is seldom below 20/300.[6]

In cases with neoplastic AIR it is believed that tumor antigens lead to formation of autoantibodies. A logical extrapolation therefore, would merit the notion that treating the primary malignancy should in fact lead to resolution of visual disturbance. Alas, data on visual improvement with treatment of primary malignancy remains inconclusive. *Idiopathic acute exudative polymorphous vitelliform maculopathy (AEVPM)* is a rare retinal disorder, reported in middle-age to old age patients presenting as visual loss along with yellow material deposited in submacular space. The disease begins with a localized serous detachment in macular area that over few days develops deposits of yellowish-white lipofuscin material mimicking vitelliform material.[45] Smaller lesions regress, though larger lesions later separate into a heavier layer gravitating inferiorly with the hyperautofluorescent material which takes up a curvilinear shape. Fluorescein angiography shows no leakage in initial stages, though later stages may be associated with secondary choroidal neovascularization. OCT shows intraretinal cystic changes without fluorescein leakage and increased choroidal thickness. The pathogenesis is not yet clear, though it is considered to be due to a paraneoplastic etiology most commonly reported with metastatic melanoma of skin or eye.[46] Other etiologies suggested include an auto-immune mechanism or an inflammatory pathology due to occasional reports of favourable response to steroids.[47] The disease closely mimics autosomal recessive bestrophinopathy and paraneoplastic retinopathy.

TREATMENT

The overall prognosis of patients with PR is poor. Treatment of the primary tumor with surgery, chemotherapy and radiation therapy does not appear to alter the visual prognosis. Various immunotherapies may result in modest visual recovery in some cases, but mostly a disease stabilization is achieved.[48] Corticosteroids have been shown to decrease antibody titers in patients with CAR and may stabilize their vision without a reversal of vision loss. Anecdotal reports describe improvement in both CAR and MAR with high-dose intravenous (IV) methylprednisolone, plasmapheresis combined with steroids or IV immunoglobulin (IVIG), however, the treatment results are largely disappointing.[49-51]

A study of 30 patients of PR/AR found positive response with immunosuppressive agents, with the best response seen in CAR (100%).[48] Agents used were corticosteroids (periocular and systemic), azathioprine, IVIG, mycophenolate mofetil, cyclosporine, infliximab and various combinations of these immunomodulatory medications.

CONCLUSION

The AIR is a rare entity that presents as a diagnostic dilemma. With no set of diagnostic guidelines and lack of specificity with current diagnostic tools, it largely remains a clinical diagnosis with supportive laboratory evidence; lack of evidence based treatment protocols compound the difficulties in management. Thus, further research and large scale clinical trials are the need of the hour and essential in prevention and better management of the autoimmune diseases.

REFERENCES

1. Saito W, Kase S, Ohguro H, et al. Slowly progressive cancer-associated retinopathy. Arch Ophthalmology. 2007;125(10):1431-3.
2. Sawyer RA, Selhorst JB, Zimmerman LE, et al. Blindness caused by photoreceptor degeneration as a remote effect of cancer. Am J Ophthalmology. 1976 ;81(5):606-13.
3. Thirkill CE, Roth AM, Keltner JL. Cancer-associated retinopathy. Arch Ophthalmology. 1987;105(3):372-5.
4. Berson EL, Lessell S. Paraneoplastic night blindness with malignant melanoma. Am J Ophthalmology. 1988;106(3):307-11.
5. Weinstein JM, Kelman SE, Bresnick GH, et al. Paraneoplastic retinopathy associated with antiretinal bipolar cell antibodies in cutaneous malignant melanoma. Ophthalmology. 1994;101(7):1236-43.
6. Weleber RG, Watzke RC, Shults WT, et al. Clinical and electrophysiologic characterization of paraneoplastic and auto-immune retinopathies associated with antienolase antibodies. Am J Ophthalmology. 2005;139(5):780-94.
7. Adamus G, Karren L. Autoimmunity against carbonic anhydrase II affects retinal cell functions in autoimmune retinopathy. J Autoimmun. 2009;32(2):133-9.
8. Adamus G. Autoantibody targets and their cancer relationship in the pathogenicity of paraneoplastic retinopathy. Autoimmun Rev. 2009;8(5):410-4.
9. Adamus G, Ren G, Weleber RG. Autoantibodies against retinal proteins in paraneoplastic and autoimmune retinopathy. BMC Ophthalmology. 2004;4:5.
10. Mizener JB, Kimura AE, Adamus G, et al. Autoimmune retinopathy in the absence of cancer. Am J Ophthalmology. 1997;123(5):607-18.
11. Heckenlively JR, Ferreyra HA. Autoimmune retinopathy: a review and summary. Semin Immunopathol. 2008;30(2):127-34.
12. Fox AR, Gordon LK, Heckenlively JR, et al. Consensus on the diagnosis and management of nonparaneoplastic autoimmune retinopathy using a modified delphi approach. Am J Ophthalmology. 2016;168:183-90.
13. Keltner JL, Thirkill CE, Yip PT. Clinical and immunologic characteristics of melanoma-associated retinopathy syndrome: eleven new cases and a review of 51 previously published cases. J Neuroophthalmol. 2001;21(3):173-87.
14. Adamus G. Autoantibody-induced apoptosis as a possible mechanism of autoimmune retinopathy. Autoimmun Rev. 2003;2(2):63-8.
15. Forooghian F, Macdonald IM, Heckenlively JR, et al. The need for standardization of antiretinal antibody detection and measurement. Am J Ophthalmology. 2008;146(4):489-95.
16. Kondo M, Sanuki R, Ueno S, et al. Identification of autoantibodies against TRPM1 in patients with paraneoplastic retinopathy associated with ON bipolar cell dysfunction. PloS One. 2011;6(5):e19911.
17. Adamus G, Brown L, Schiffman J, et al. Diversity in autoimmunity against retinal, neuronal, and axonal antigens in acquired neuro-retinopathy. J Ophthalmic Inflamm Infect. 2011;1(3):111-21.
18. McAleese SM, Dunbar B, Fothergill JE, et al. Complete amino acid sequence of the neurone-specific gamma isozyme of enolase (NSE) from human brain and comparison with the non-neuronal alpha form (NNE). Eur J Biochem. 1988;178(2):413-7.
19. Pancholi V. Multifunctional alpha-enolase: its role in diseases. Cell Mol Life Sci. 2001;58(7):902-20.
20. Forooghian F, Adamus G, Sproule M, et al. Enolase autoantibodies and retinal function in multiple sclerosis patients. Graefes Arch Clin Exp Ophthalmology. 2007;245(8):1077-84.
21. Vermeulen N, Arijs I, Joossens S, et al. Anti-alpha-enolase antibodies in patients with inflammatory bowel disease. Clin Chem. 2008;54(3):534-41.
22. Shin SJ, Kim BC, Kim TI, et al. Anti-alpha-enolase antibody as a serologic marker and its correlation with disease severity in intestinal Behçet's disease. Dig Dis Sci. 201;56(3):812-8.
23. Thirkill CE, Tait RC, Tyler NK, et al. Intraperitoneal cultivation of small-cell carcinoma induces expression of the retinal cancer-associated retinopathy antigen. Arch Ophthalmology. 1993;111(7):974-8.
24. Bazhin AV, Shifrina ON, Savchenko MS, et al. Low titre autoantibodies against recoverin in sera of patients with small cell lung cancer but without a loss of vision. Lung Cancer. 2001;34(1):99-104.
25. Whitcup SM, Vistica BP, Milam AH, et al. Recoverin-associated retinopathy: a clinically and immunologically distinctive disease. Am J Ophthalmology. 1998;126(2):230-7.
26. Heckenlively JR, Fawzi AA, Oversier J, et al. Autoimmune retinopathy: patients with antirecoverin immunoreactivity and panretinal degeneration. Arch Ophthalmology. 2000;118(11):1525-33.
27. Polans AS, Witkowska D, Haley TL, et al. Recoverin, a photoreceptor-specific calcium-binding protein, is expressed by the tumor of a patient with cancer-associated retinopathy. Proc Natl Acad Sci USA. 1995;92(20):9176-80.
28. Matsubara S, Yamaji Y, Sato M, et al. Expression of a photoreceptor protein, recoverin, as a cancer-associated retinopathy autoantigen in human lung cancer cell lines. Br J Cancer. 1996;74(9):1419-22.
29. Kobayashi M, Ikezoe T, Uemura Y, et al. Establishment of a novel small cell lung carcinoma cell line with specific recoverin expression from a patient with cancer-associated retinopathy. Lung Cancer. 2007;56(3):319-26.
30. Matsuo S, Ohguro H, Ohguro I, et al. Clinicopathological roles of aberrantly expressed recoverin in malignant tumor cells. Ophthalmic Res. 2010;43(3):139-44.
31. Ohguro H, Yokoi Y, Ohguro I, et al. Clinical and immunologic aspects of cancer-associated retinopathy. Am J Ophthalmology. 2004;137(6):1117-9.
32. Ohguro H, Ogawa K, Maeda T, et al. Cancer-associated retinopathy induced by both anti-recoverin and anti-hsc70 antibodies in vivo. Invest Ophthalmology Vis Sci. 1999;40(13):3160-7.

33. Adamus G, Machnicki M, Elerding H, et al. Antibodies to recoverin induce apoptosis of photoreceptor and bipolar cells in vivo. J Autoimmun. 1998;11(5):523-33.

34. Adamus G, Machnicki M, Seigel GM. Apoptotic retinal cell death induced by antirecoverin autoantibodies of cancer-associated retinopathy. Invest Ophthalmology Vis Sci. 1997;38(2):283-91.

35. Gery I, Chanaud NP, Anglade E. Recoverin is highly uveitogenic in Lewis rats. Invest Ophthalmology Vis Sci. 1994;35(8):3342-5.

36. Lu Y, He S, Jia L, et al. Two mouse models for recoverin-associated autoimmune retinopathy. Mol Vis. 2010;16:1936-48.

37. Bazhin AV, Slepova OS, Tikhomirova NK. Retinal degeneration under the effect of antibodies to recoverin. Bull Exp Biol Med. 2001;131(4):350-2.

38. Adamus G, Ortega H, Witkowska D, et al. Recoverin: a potent uveitogen for the induction of photoreceptor degeneration in Lewis rats. Exp Eye Res. 1994;59(4):447-55.

39. Williams RC Jr, Peen E. Apoptosis and cell penetration by autoantibody may represent linked processes. Clin Exp Rheumatol. 1999;17(6):643-7.

40. Abazari A, Allam SS, Adamus G, et al. Optical coherence tomography findings in autoimmune retinopathy. Am J Ophthalmology. 2012;153(4):750-6.e1.

41. Pepple KL, Cusick M, Jaffe GJ, et al. SD-OCT and autofluorescence characteristics of autoimmune retinopathy. Br J Ophthalmology. 2013;97(2):139-44.

42. Brown J Jr, Folk JC. Current controversies in the white dot syndromes. Multifocal choroiditis, punctate inner choroidopathy, and the diffuse subretinal fibrosis syndrome. Ocul Immunol Inflamm. 1998;6(2):125-7.

43. Fujiwara T, Imamura Y, Giovinazzo VJ, et al. Fundus auto-fluorescence and optical coherence tomographic findings in acute zonal occult outer retinopathy. Retina. 2010;30(8):1206-16.

44. Heckenlively JR, Jordan BL, Aptsiauri N. Association of antiretinal antibodies and cystoid macular edema in patients with retinitis pigmentosa. Am J Ophthalmology. 1999;127(5):565-73.

45. Gass JD, Chuang EL, Granek H. Acute exudative polymorphous vitelliform maculopathy. Trans Am Ophthalmology Soc. 1988;86354-366.

46. Modi KK, Roth DB, Green SN. Acute exudative polymorphous vitelliform maculopathy in young man: a case report. Retinal Cases Brief Rep. 2014;8(3):200-4.

47. Barbazetto I, Dansingani KK, Dolz-Marco R, et al. Idiopathic acute exudative polymorphous vitelliform maculopathy: clinical spectrum and multimodal imaging characteristics. Ophthalmology. 2018;125(1):75-88.

48. Ferreyra HA, Jayasundera T, Khan NW, et al. Management of autoimmune retinopathies with immunosuppression. Arch Ophthalmology. 2009;127(4):390-7.

49. Guy J, Aptsiauri N. Treatment of paraneoplastic visual loss with intravenous immunoglobulin: report of 3 cases. Arch Ophthalmology. 1999;117(4):471-7.

50. Powell SF, Dudek AZ. Treatment of melanoma-associated retinopathy. Curr Treat Options Neurol. 2010;12(1):54-63.

51. Keltner JL, Thirkill CE, Tyler NK, et al. Management and monitoring of cancer-associated retinopathy. Arch Ophthalmology. 1992;110(1):48-53.

Chapter 61

Toxic Retinopathies

Vinod Kumar, Pradeep Kumar, Akshay Tayade, Ajay Panwar

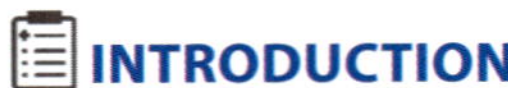 INTRODUCTION

Macular toxicity has been reported with multiple medications and other exogenous substances. Some of these are:

- Antimalarial drugs
- Phenothiazines
- Tamoxifen
- Canthaxanthin
- Talc.

ANTIMALARIALS

Chloroquine (Nivaquine, Avloclor) and hydroxychloroquine (Plaquenil) are used for treatment of malaria and rheumatological disorders (i.e. rheumatoid arthritis, lupus). More than 300 g cumulative oral dose (250 mg/day for 3 years) significantly increases the risk of maculopathy (Figs. 61.1A and B). Maculopathy risk is less with hydroxychloroquine as compared to chloroquine, and as such is typically the preferred medication. Chloroquine-associated ocular side effects can be divided into three categories: (1) accommodation abnormality, which is the most common; (2) corneal deposition; and (3) pre- and true retinopathy. These side effects are in general, completely reversible with drug discontinuation. On the other hand, "bull's eye retinopathy" once developed, is irreversible.[1,2]

The severity of maculopathy is directly related to duration and dose as described here:

1. *Premaculopathy*: Scotoma to a red target between 4° and 9°.
2. *Established maculopathy*: 20/30–20/40 best-corrected visual acuity (BCVA), faint halo of retinal pigment epithelium (RPE) pallor.
3. *Bull's eye maculopathy*: 20/60–20/80 BCVA, dark ring surrounds halo (Figs. 61.1A and B).
4. *Severe maculopathy*: 20/120–20/200 BCVA, pseudohole and atrophy.
5. *End-stage maculopathy*: Legally blind, large RPE atrophy, pigment clumps.

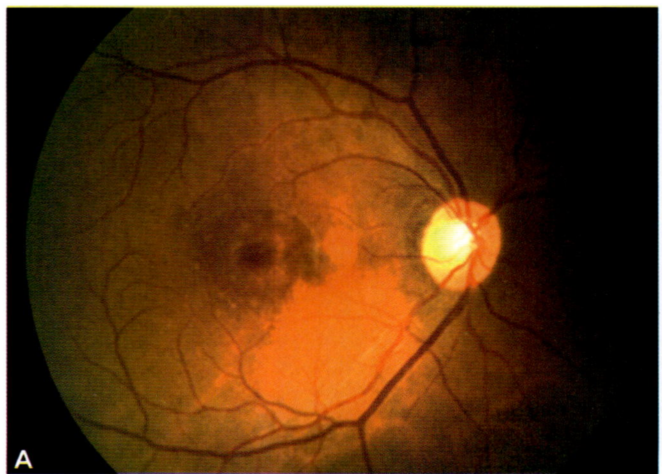
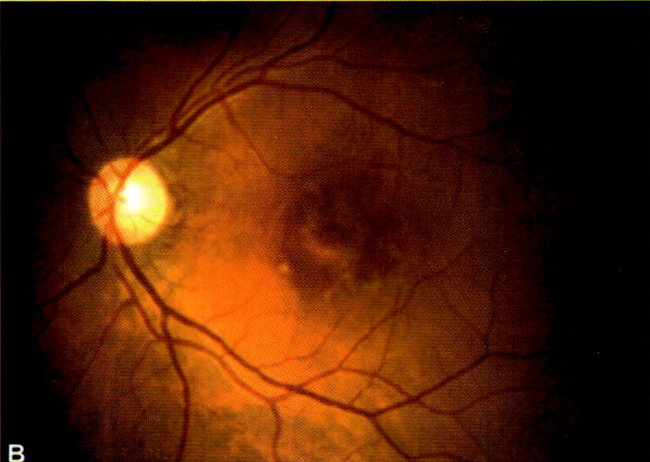

Figs. 61.1A and B: Clinical fundus image showing Bull's eye maculopathy.

Concentration of antimalarials occurs in melanin-containing structures, such as the RPE and choroid. Benign corneal deposits can also occur.

A pretreatment baseline retinal evaluation prior to initiation of therapy is recommended and should include:

- Visual acuity
- Amsler grid
- Color vision
- Visual fields (10–2, macular threshold)
- Dilated retinal examination
- Fundus imaging
- Electroretinography (ERG).

On optical coherence tomography (OCT), chloroquine maculopathy is seen as a disruption of the photoreceptor layer and loss of ellipsoid zone at the fovea (Fig. 61.2A). A foveolar pigmented zone surrounded by a depigmented zone is visible on fundus imaging. Fluorescein angiography and indocyanine green (ICG) imaging highlight these pigmentary abnormalities seen in bull's eye maculopathy (Figs. 61.2B and C).

Multifocal ERG shows depressed amplitudes in the macula in an eye with bull's eye maculopathy (Figs. 61.3A and B).

Differential diagnosis includes cone dystrophy which has a similar presentation on autofluorescence imaging (Figs. 61.4A and B).

Annual post-treatment retinal evaluation with the above tests should be performed, if no signs or symptoms are noted.

Amsler grid charts for daily monitoring of central vision in both eyes should be advised.

Quinine is an alkaloid compound that also reduces nocturnal muscle cramps. An overdose of quinine may cause cinchonism, an ocular complex which has the following findings:

- Visual acuity loss (can also occur with normal dose)
- Fixed and dilated pupils
- Retinal edema (unknown mechanism)
- Attenuated arterioles
- Constricted visual fields
- Optic atrophy (Fig. 61.5).

PHENOTHIAZINE MACULOPATHY

Thioridazine (Mellaril) and chlorpromazine (Largactil) are used in treating schizophrenia and related psychoses. Chlorpromazine is also used as a sedative. The usual dose of thioridazine is 150–600 mg/day, while chlorpromazine is 75–300 mg/day. More than 800 mg/day of thioridazine for a few weeks can cause retinal toxicity, while greater than 2,400 mg/day of chlorpromazine over many weeks is required to cause retinal toxicity. This retinopathy presents as pigment changes that give a "salt and pepper" appearance to the macula (Fig. 61.6). Macular toxicity usually causes decreased visual acuity and poor dark adaptation. Coarse granular-macular pigmentation usually appears first, which may not progress, if the

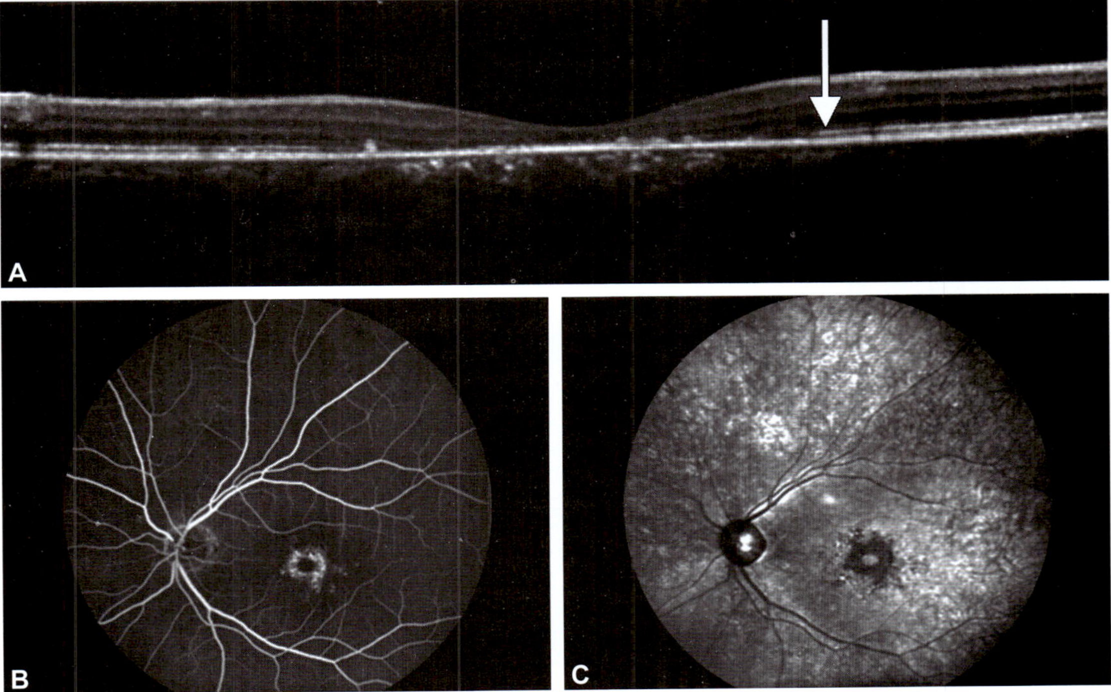

Figs. 61.2A to C: Bull's eye maculopathy. (A) Optical coherence tomography (OCT) showing disruption of ellipsoid zone (arrow); (B) Fundus fluorescein angiography (FFA); (C) Indocyanine green (ICG) showing perifoveal pigmentary changes.

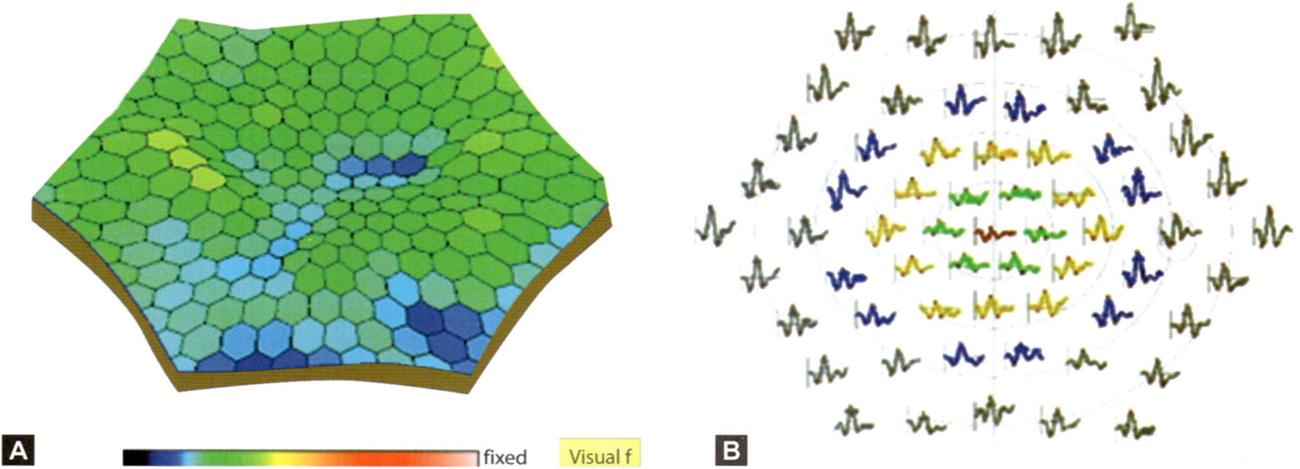

Figs. 61.3A and B: Multifocal electroretinography (ERG) showing depressed amplitudes in bull's eye maculopathy.

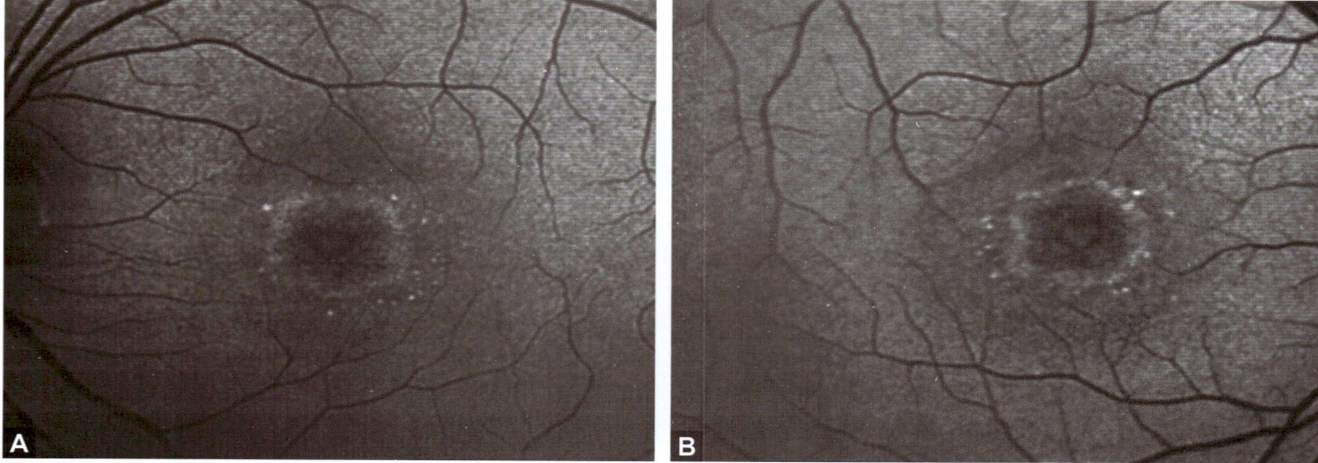

Figs. 61.4A and B: Autofluorescence imaging of cone dystrophy.

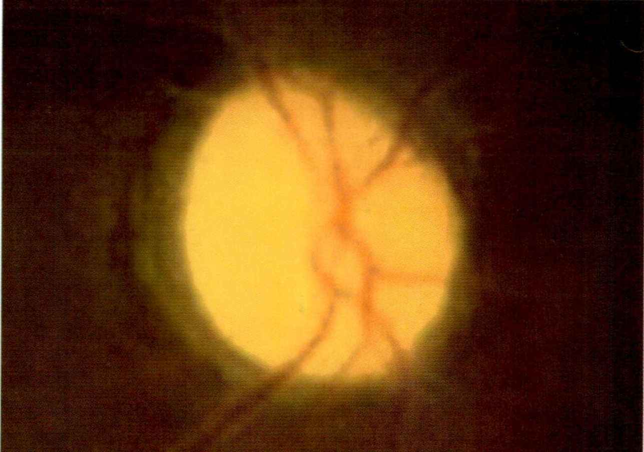

Fig. 61.5: Quinine toxicity showing disc pallor with arteriolar attenuation.

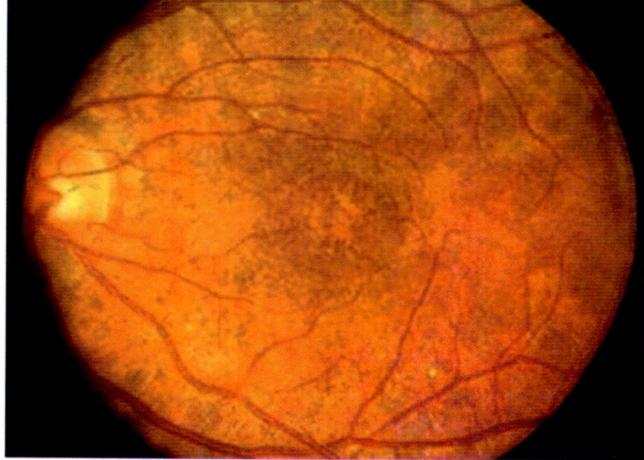

Fig. 61.6: Salt and pepper maculopathy in phenothiazine toxicity.

drug is stopped. With continued use of the drug, geographic RPE/choriocapillaris atrophy with hyperpigmented clumps and plaques may occur.

TAMOXIFEN MACULOPATHY

Tamoxifen (Nolvadex, Emblon, Noltam, Tamofen) is an anti-estrogen used to treat breast carcinoma. It has few systemic side effects at a traditional dose of 20–40 mg/day. Current dosages prescribed today may be even less, reducing the prevalence of side effects. Vortex keratopathy and optic neuritis can rarely occur, which is usually reversible on stopping the therapy.[3] Retinotoxicity presents as multiple superficial yellow crystalline ring-like deposits at the macula that can cause visual acuity loss. Crystalline retinopathy involving the perifoveal region in tamoxifen toxicity, taken for over 2 years, is shown in Figures 61.7A to D.

Crystals may reduce in size and number over 6 months with preservation of 6/6 visual acuity (Fig. 61.8A); However, an active smokestack leak (Fig. 61.8B) may develop at this stage with serous neurosensory detachment on swept-source OCT (Fig. 61.8C).

CANTHAXANTHIN MACULOPATHY

Canthaxanthin is an oral agent that enhances sun tanning. Prolonged used over time can cause maculopathy. It appears as tiny glistening yellow dots arranged in a doughnut-shaped ring around both maculae.[4] These benign deposits appear in the inner retina (ganglion cell layer) (Fig. 61.9).

TALC MACULOPATHY

Talc maculopathy presents as multiple tiny, yellow-white, glistening particles scattered throughout the posterior pole in both eyes (Fig. 61.10). The talc is more numerous in the capillary bed and small arterioles of the perimacular area. Some patients can get macular edema, venous engorgement, punctate and flame-shaped hemorrhages, and arterial occlusion associated with the talc emboli. Talc retinal granulomas and neovascularization can also rarely occur.[5]

Cases of associated paramacular scarring in certain patients who have injected cocaine or methylphenidate (Ritalin) over several years have been noted. Drug abusers typically crush tablets of cocaine, Ritalin or other narcotics

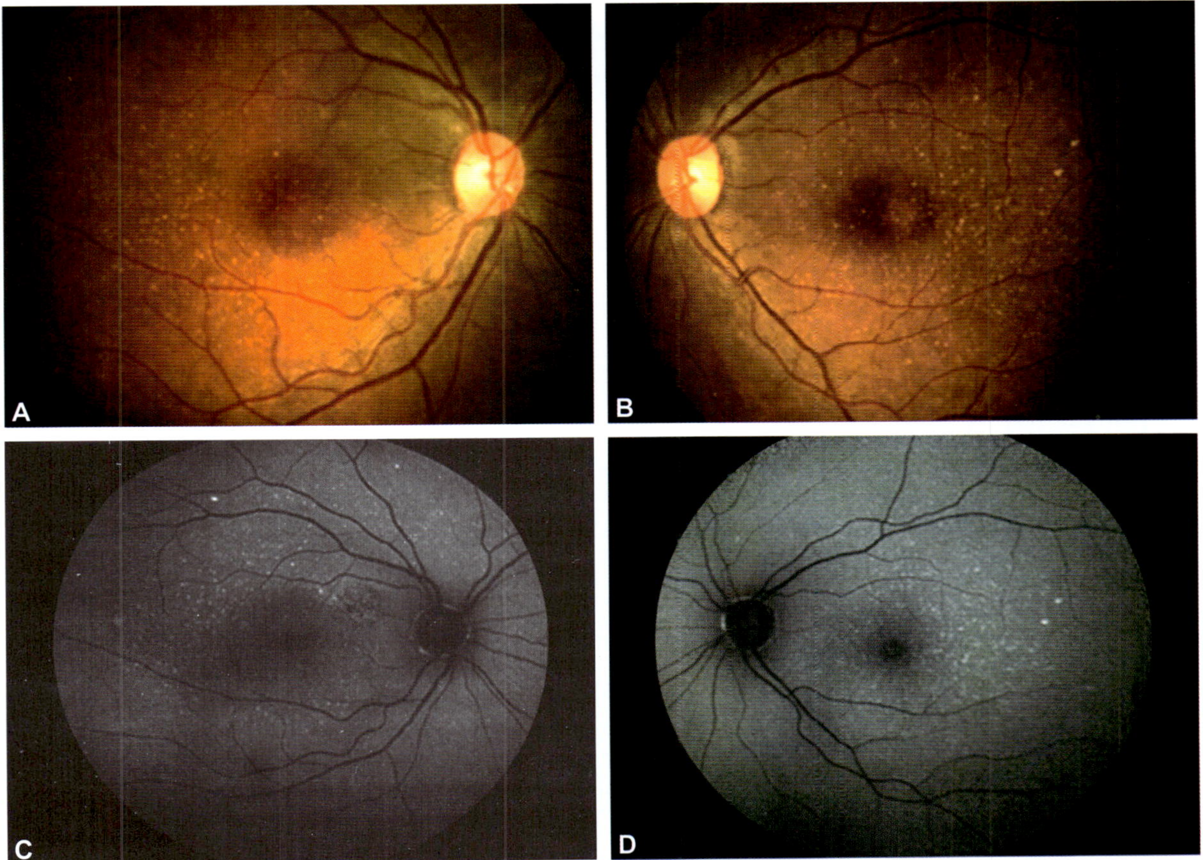

Figs. 61.7A to D: (A and B) Color fundus image of a patient with tamoxifen retinopathy; (C and D) Autofluorescence imaging showing autofluorescent drug deposits.

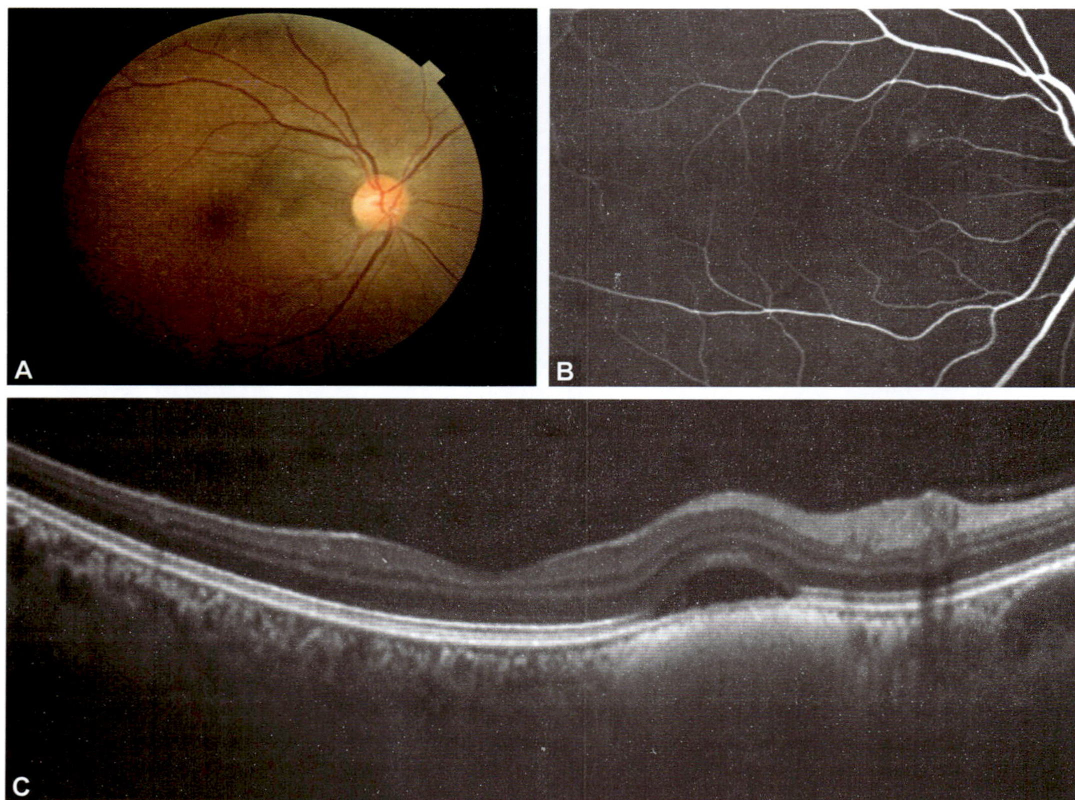

Figs. 61.8A to C: (A) Color fundus photograph showing decreased crystalline deposits; (B) Smokestack leak on fundus fluorescein angiography (FFA); (C) Neurosensory detachment on OCT in advanced retinopathy.
(OCT: Optical coherence tomography).

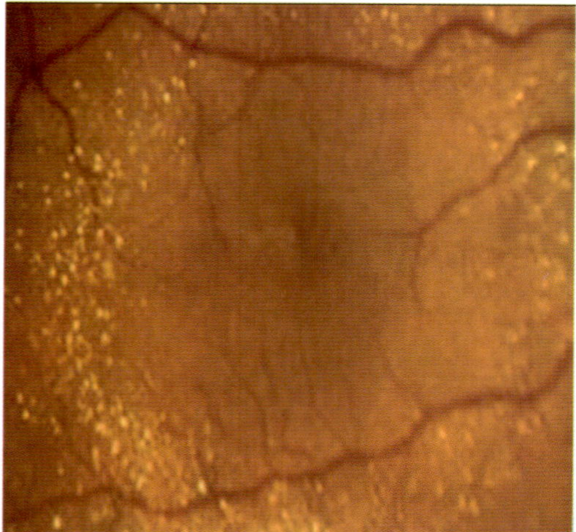

Fig. 61.9: Clinical picture showing crystalline deposits in canthaxanthin maculopathy.

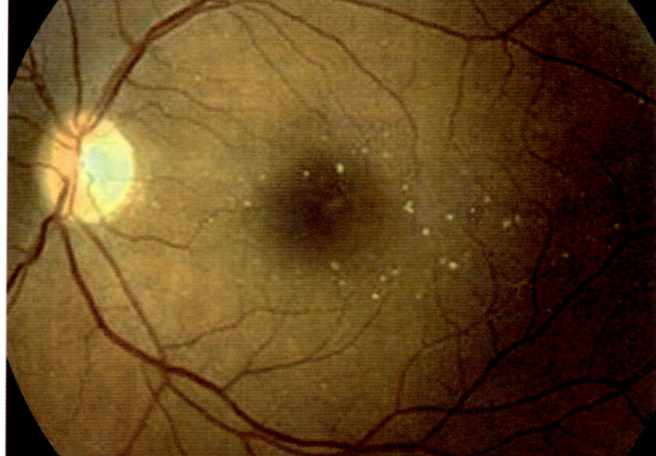

Fig. 61.10: Clinical picture showing talc maculopathy secondary to cocaine abuse.

in water, boil the suspension, and filter it before injecting it. Consumption is typically by intravenous, subcutaneous, and/or intramuscular routes. Talc is used as a filler in many of these tablets. Talc particles enter the circulation and embolize in various tissues. Most parts of bloodstream including the retina

develop talc deposits over a long period of time of injections. A recent study using adaptive optics imaging revealed the talc particles within the retinal microvasculature.

The extent of talc corresponds with amount and duration of drug abuse. It is routinely found, if the person has injected the equivalent of over 12,000 tablets. Most patients have no visual symptoms, and the visual acuity is usually normal. However, blur and/or blind spots in visual field can occur. "Microtalc retinopathy" is a variant of talc retinopathy, involving finer deposits. This type of retinopathy may be associated with nerve fiber layer (NFL) defects and "glaucoma-like" visual field loss.

Patient should be carefully questioned regarding his medicinal and social drug history. Ocular talc indicates excess lung involvement, whereby lung function may be compromised. Drug abuse counseling and possibly a pulmonary consultation may be needed. Annual retinal evaluation with fundus photography and threshold visual field testing are recommended. If there are risk factors of glaucoma along with visual field loss, ocular hypotensive medications may be indicated. High-resolution adaptive optics is used to evaluate the appearance, distribution/extent and location of talc crystals in a case of talc retinopathy. Adaptive optics may be considered as a valuable tool for screening of drug abuse prior to the development of retinopathy/appearance of talc crystals.[6]

FLUPENTIXOL MACULOPATHY

Flupentixol is an antipsychotic neuroleptic drug of thioxanthene class used for treatment of schizophrenia. It is a D1 and D2 receptor antagonist. A cumulative dose of 4,380 mg taken over 2 years has been associated with crystalline retinopathy with mild visual loss.[7] Fundus shows multiple, discrete, yellowish-white refractile intraretinal deposits located over the macula and peripapillary region in a distinct annular fashion (Figs. 61.11A and B), which are hyperautofluorescent (Figs. 61.11C and D). On OCT, the deposits are hyper-reflective

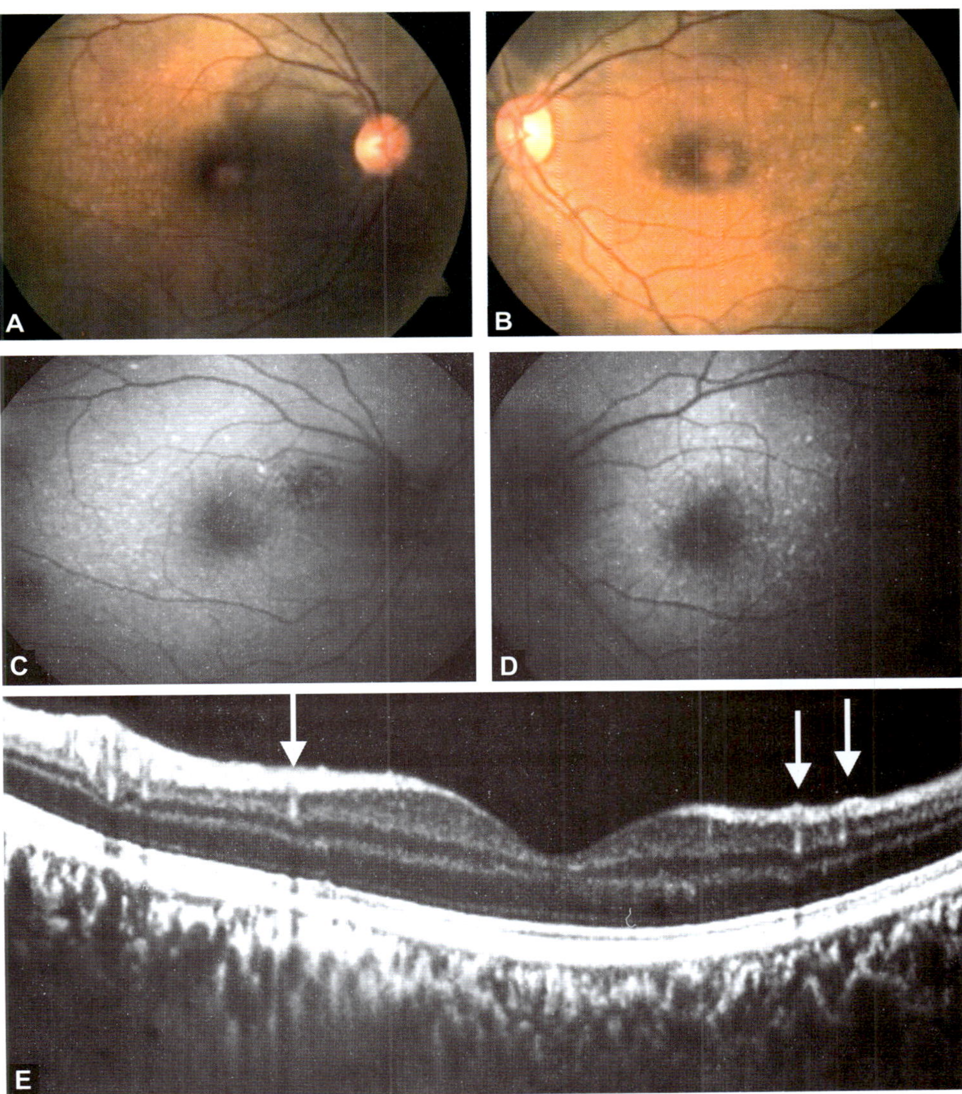

Figs. 61.11A to E: (A and B) Clinical fundus photograph showing multiple yellowish-white crystals over the entire macula in a 36-year-old patient with chronic flupentixol intake; (C and D) Autofluorescence imaging shows hyperautofluorescent crystalline lesions; (E) Swept-source optical coherence tomography (SS-OCT) confirms the inner retinal location of discrete hyper-reflective crystals (arrows).

and located in the inner retina (Fig. 61.11E). Multifocal ERG objectively quantifies the visual dysfunction and adaptive optics examination reveals decrease in cone density at the fovea. Cessation of flupentixol halts the progression of disease but recovery of visual function is partial and the crystalline lesions of retina persist. Regular retinal evaluation is recommended in patients with chronic flupentixol intake.

TOXIC AMBLYOPIA

Toxic amblyopia or toxic optic neuropathy (TON) is a disease entity which often gets misdiagnosed and presents to the ophthalmologist at a stage when the disease is irreversible. The common causes of toxic amblyopia are ethambutol toxicity, isoniazid toxicity, methanol poisoning and tobacco-alcohol abuse. Other drugs causing this disease are linezolid, chloramphenicol, cimetidine, cyclosporine, amiodarone, disulfiram and halogenated hydroquinolones (amebicidal drugs).[8] There is no gender predilection and all ages and races are equally susceptible.

The pathophysiology behind TON is the accumulation of toxins which has been hypothesized to impair the tissue's vascular supply and metabolism. It also impairs mitochondrial oxidative phosphorylation resulting in disruption of ATP production and ultimately impairing the ATP-dependent axonal transport system of the optic nerve. Tobacco and alcohol abuse increase the risk of nutritional optic neuropathy by causing multivitamin deficiency, primarily thiamine (vitamin B_1) and cyanocobalamin (vitamin B_{12}).

A case of toxic amblyopia usually presents with painless, progressive and bilateral visual decline. Dyschromatopsia or color defect is usually the first symptom and red-green is the first color to be affected as in all optic neuropathies. Diminution of vision can range from a relative scotoma to profound generalized visual decline. Patients of methanol poisoning can present with acute loss of vision.

The diagnosis can be established with a detailed medical history and meticulous eye examination. The patient should also undergo physical examination and toxic urinalysis, if needed, to establish a diagnosis in which the specific toxin cannot be identified. Serum B_{12} and red cell folate levels should be obtained in patients with bilateral central scotomas. The pupillary reflex is usually normal unless the patient has gross loss of vision. Optic disc appears normal or shows signs of swelling or hyperemia at early stages. Prolonged exposure to the toxin results in the development of optic atrophy which can be seen as temporal pallor of the optic disc (Figs. 61.12A to E).

A complete examination includes color vision, contrast sensitivity, visual fields and electrophysiological tests, primarily visually evoked response (VER). Color vision tests can show depression of certain colors, especially red-green or a generalized decrease in color perception. Contrast sensitivity can help in early detection of subclinical cases. Visual fields show the classical central or centrocecal scotoma as the papillomacular bundle is primarily affected. VER P100 wave amplitude is markedly reduced with normal or near normal latency in tobacco-alcohol amblyopia.[9]

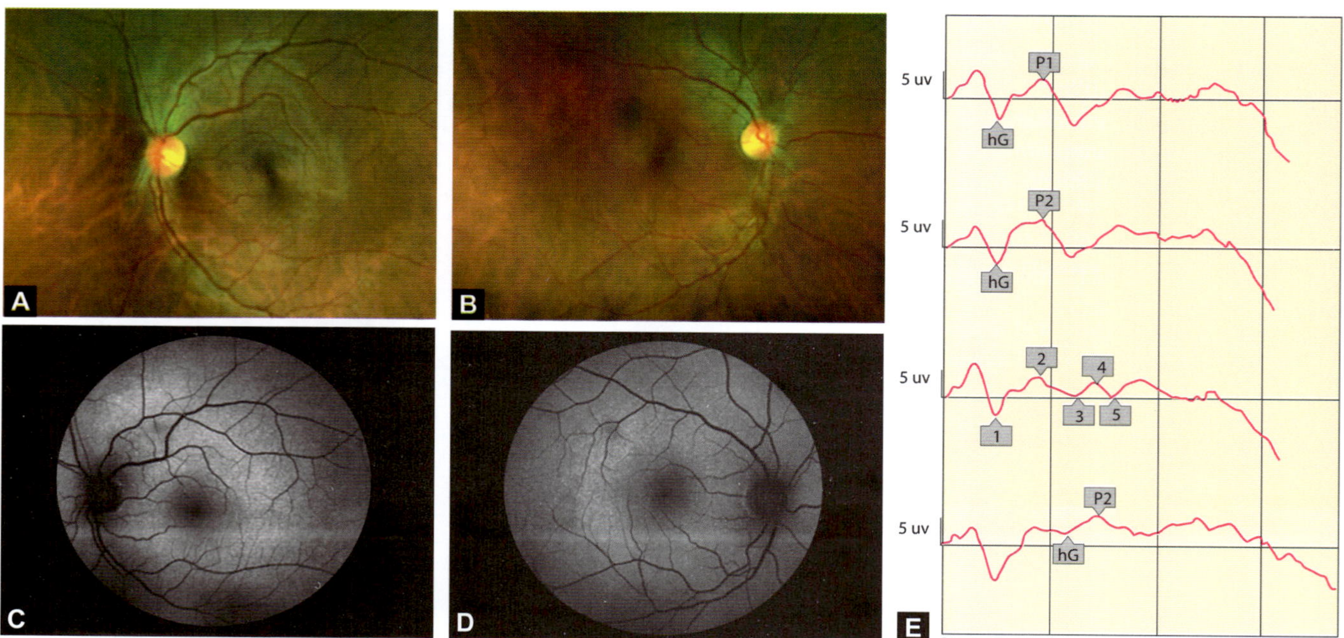

Figs. 61.12A to E: (A to D) Fundus color image and autofluorescence image of a patient with toxic amblyopia showing mild temporal disc pallor. History revealed 7 years of intake of tobacco and alcohol combined and diminution of vision for 3 months. Ishihara plates showed total color vision defect; (E) Subnormal visual evoked response (VER).

The primary management is to remove the offending agent. This may lead to recovery in a few early cases. Vitamin supplementation is the mainstay of treatment and it is most effective in tobacco-alcohol amblyopia.

Ethambutol toxicity usually manifests at 2–8 months. There is no specific treatment other than stopping the drug. OCT can be used to quantify the loss of retinal nerve fiber layer which is a sign of early toxicity. Isoniazid toxicity may be associated with bilateral optic disc swelling or bitemporal hemianopic scotomas. Pyridoxine may help in stabilizing vision, though overall visual outcomes are poor. In a study from our center, of a series of seven consecutive patients with severe visual deficit due to ethambutol toxicity, only 42.2% (3 of the 7 patients) achieved a visual recovery of better than 20/200 after an average follow-up of 8.3 ± 2.1 months after stoppage of the drug. On fluorescein angiography, three cases (42.2%) progressed to optic atrophy during the follow-up with permanent visual damage. There were no predisposing risk factors to contribute toward the poor visual gain. In this background, we recommended discontinuation of ethambutol from the anti-tubercular regimen. As an additional sidelight, the value of visually evoked potential in the monitoring of patients on ethambutol, especially in cases with early periaxial neuritis, had been emphasised.[12]

Methanol is oxidized to formaldehyde and later to formic acid by alcohol dehydrogenase (ADH) in the liver. Accumulation of formic acid within the optic nerve causes classic symptoms of flashes and scintillating scotomas. Treatment of methanol poisoning begins with supportive therapy and correcting electrolyte disturbances. Specific treatment is administration of fomepizole (antidote of methanol) and ethanol which competitively inhibits the action of ADH on methanol. Intravenous pulse steroids have also been tried to salvage vision and the results have been encouraging.[10] But despite all these measures, the prognosis stays grave.

Tobacco-alcohol amblyopia is worsened due to malnutrition. Treatment includes cessation of adverse habits combined with an improved diet and vitamin supplementation (thiamine 100 mg orally twice daily, folate 1 mg once a day, and a multivitamin tablet daily).[11] Injection of hydroxocobalamin has also been effective in treating tobacco-alcohol amblyopia.

REFERENCES

1. Rynes RI, Bernstein HN. Ophthalmologic safety profile of antimalarial drugs. Lupus. 1993;2(Suppl 1):S17-9.
2. Yam JC, Kwok AK. Ocular toxicity of hydroxychloroquine. Hong Kong Med J. 2006;12:294-304.
3. Rolf MM. Clinical implications of tamoxifen ocular toxicity. Clinical Eye and Vision Care. 1998;10(3):135-40. [online] Available from https://www.sciencedirect.com/journal/clinical-eye-and-vision-care/vol/10/issue/3 [Accessed December, 2017].
4. Fraunfelder FW. Corneal toxicity from ocular and systemic medications. Cornea. 2006;25:1133-8.
5. Fraser-Bell S, Capon M. Talc retinopathy. Clin Exp Ophthalmology. 2002;30:432-3.
6. Soliman MK, Sarwar S, Hanout M, et al. High-resolution adaptive optics findings in talc retinopathy. Int J Retina Vitreous. 2015;1:10.
7. Kumar P, Ravani R, Kakkar P, et al. Crystalline retinopathy association with flupentixol intake. Int Ophthalmology. 2017. doi: 10.1007/s10792-017-0624-1 [Epub ahead of print].
8. Sharma P, Sharma R. Toxic optic neuropathy. Indian J Ophthalmology. 2011;59:137-41.
9. Kupersmith MJ, Weiss PA, Carr RE. The visual-evoked potential in tobacco-alcohol and nutritional amblyopia. Am J Ophthalmology. 1983;95:307-14.
10. Sodhi PK, Goyal JL, Mehta DK. Methanol-induced optic neuropathy: treatment with intravenous high dose steroids. Int J Clin Pract. 2001;55:599-602.
11. Kee C, Hwang JM. Optical coherence tomography in a patient with tobacco-alcohol amblyopia. Eye (Lond). 2008;22:469-70.
12. Kumar A, Sandramouli S, Verma L, et al. Ocular ethambutol toxicity, is it irreversible? J Clin Neuro-ophthalmology. 1993;13(1):15-7.

Photic Retinopathy

Aditya Modi, Neha Pareka Sudhakar

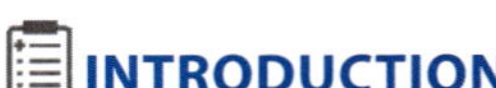 INTRODUCTION

The development and the degree of photic damage to the retina depends primarily on two factors:

- Pre-existing ocular anatomy
- Parameters of the light source (including wavelength, duration and power).[1]

Breakdown of the intrinsic ocular protective mechanisms or exposure to external high-risk conditions can produce light or photic damage to the retina.[1]

SOURCES

- Sun
- Artificial lighting
- Ophthalmic instruments
- Lasers[2]

MECHANISM OF DAMAGE

1. Mechanical
2. Thermal
3. Photochemical[3]

These effects are determined by the:

- Irradiance (W/cm^2) from the light source.
- The wavelength of incident light.
- The duration of exposure.
- The absorption of target tissue.[4]

Mechanical Effects

Mechanical injury results from high irradiance and short-duration exposures (nanosecond to picosecond range). Photic energy produced from the light source strips the electrons from molecules and disintegrates the target tissue into a collection of ions and electrons known as plasma.[5]

Thermal Effects

At moderate irradiance and duration of exposure greater than 1microsecond, the critical temperature rises int he target tissue resuting in deleterious themal effects. An elevation of retinal temperature by 10–20°C produces protein denaturation and enzyme inactivation which results in photocoagulation and associated cellular necrosis and hemostasis.[5] Long visible wavelengths and infrared radiation (IR) produce thermal injury to the retina and choroid during retinal laser photocoagulation.

Photochemical Effects

Photochemical or phototoxic effects occur with low to moderate irradiances below coagulation thresholds and with short wavelengths, particularly UV and visible blue wavelength.[3,6] Damage to cellular components occurs at temperatures too low to cause thermal destruction, which may account for a delay of 24–48 hours before appearance of the lesion. Absorption of a photon by the outer electron produces an excited molecular state, which can drive a chemical reaction. Because the energy per photon is inversely proportional to its wavelength, short-wavelength photons have more energy to induce a photochemical reaction. Long-wavelength visible light can also induce photochemical changes when tissues are sensitized by an exogenous photosensitizer.[7]

OCULAR PROTECTIVE MECHANISMS AGAINST PHOTIC DAMAGE

- The cornea absorbs most UV-B (280–315 nm) and UV-C (less than 280 nm), as well as some IR radiation and reflects up to 60% of incident light that is not perpendicular to its surface.[5]
- The lens absorbs most UV-A (315–400 nm) and visible blue wavelengths.
- Xanthophyll in the retina absorbs shorter wavelengths.
- Choroidal circulation regulates temperature.
- Intracellular eradication of free radicals and toxic molecules.
- Retinal pigment epithelium (RPE) cell recycling of photoreceptors.[5]
- Structural adaptations for protection like the eyebrow ridge, squint and blink reflexes, the aversion response and pupillary miosis.
- With surgical alterations to the eye or with deliberate gazing at a light source, the eye may be prone to damage.

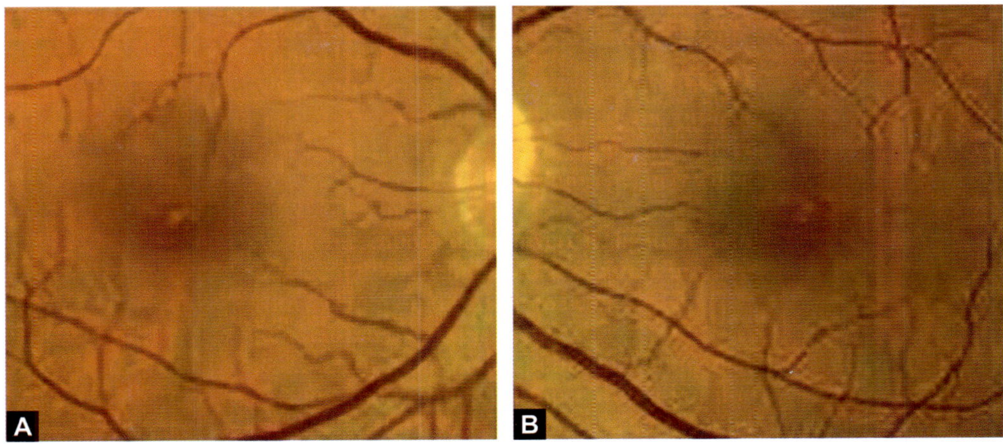

Figs. 62.1A and B: Solar retinopathy: Yellow-white spots and dots in both foveae.
Source: John A Dunbar.

Younger people are at more risk due to more efficient transmission of light through the ocular media.[1,2,5]

SOLAR RETINOPATHY

- Solar retinopathy is an injury to the retina caused by directly or indirectly looking at the sun.[8] Other names for this entity include foveomacular retinitis, photoretinitis and photo maculopathy.
- The extent of retinal injury and the visual prognosis depend on factors like[9]:
  - Interval and spectrum of solar exposure
  - Reduction in the ozone layer
  - Atmospheric conditions
  - The distance from the sun
  - Telescopic viewing
  - Pupil dilatation
  - Elevated body temperature
  - Increased chorioretinal pigmentation
  - Clarity of the ocular media
  - Pre-existing retinal disease
- Emmetropes and hyperopes may be at increased risk due to effective focusing of light on the retina.
- Systemic photosensitizing agents such as tetracycline, hematoporphyrin and psoralen may predispose to photochemical damage.
- Solar retinopathy has also been associated with religious sun gazing, solar eclipse viewing, telescopic solar viewing, sunbathing, psychiatric disorders and the use of psychotropic drugs.[8] More than 90 seconds of looking at the sun through a constricted pupil exceeds the threshold for photochemical retinal damage, while a dilated 7 mm pupil produces a 22°C increase in retinal temperature which crosses photocoagulation limits.

Symptoms

Symptoms appear 1–4 hours after exposure including:
- Unilateral or bilateral loss of vision.
- Metamorphopsia

- Central or paracentral scotoma
- Color vision alteration
- Photophobia
- After image
- Periorbital ache[2]

Signs

- Visual acuity between 20/40 and 20/200.
- A small yellow spot surrounded by a gray margin in the foveolar or parafoveal area (Figs. 62.1A and B).[10]
- The lesion measures up to 200 μm in diameter corresponding to the retinal image of the sun.

Investigations

1. *Fluorescein angiography*: May be normal or reveal transmission defects due to RPE irregularities (Fig. 62.2). Leakage of fluorescein is rarely noted during the acute stage.
2. *Optical coherence tomography*: Abnormal reflectivity in the outer foveal retina, fragmentation, or interruption of

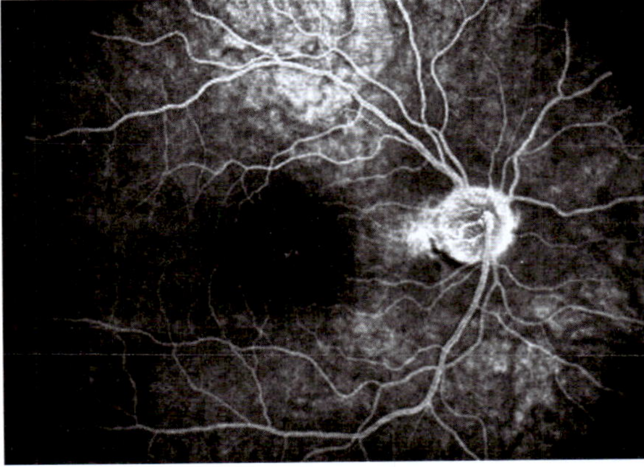

Fig. 62.2: Fundus fluorescein angiography in solar retinopathy: Window defect is evident at the fovea due to retinal pigment epithelial damage.

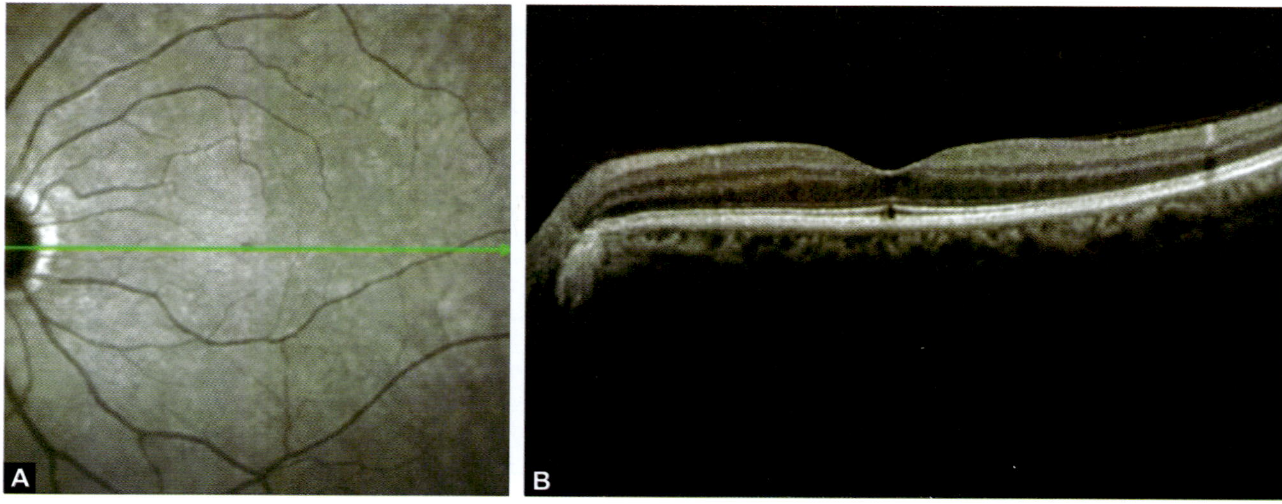

Figs. 62.3A and B: Optical coherence tomography in solar retinopathy: Subtle fragmentation of ellipsoid and interdigitation zone at the fovea.

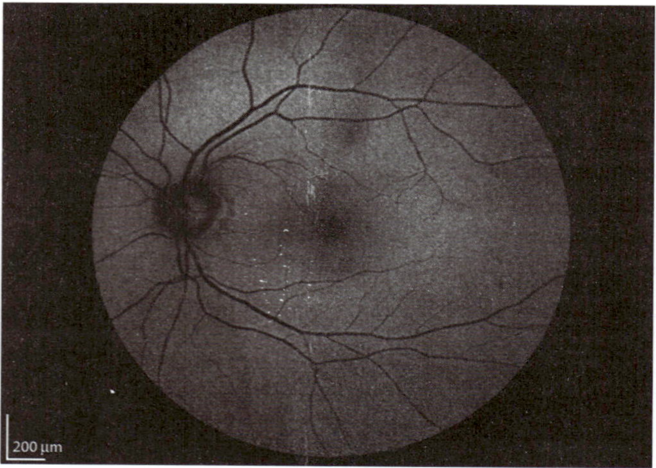

Fig. 62.4: Fundus autofluorescence in solar retinopathy: Central area of hypoautofluorescence surrounded by a ring of hyperautofluorescence.

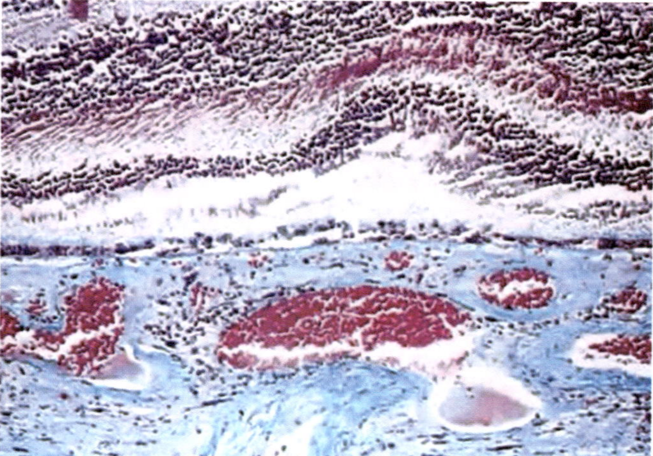

Fig. 62.5: Light-microscopic appearance of photic retinopathy with edematous outer retina and the edematous irregularly thickened retinal pigment epithelium.
Source: Schwartz SG, Gombos SD, Schneider S. Light Toxicity in the Posterior Segment. Duane's Ophthalmology. Philadelphia: Lippincott; 2011.

the inner high reflective layer corresponding to the junction between the photoreceptor inner and outer segments (Figs. 62.3A and B).[11]

3. *Fundus autofluorescence (FAF)*: It shows a well-demarcated hypoautofluorescence that corresponded to the outer retina/RPE defect surrounded by a slightly hyperautofluorescent ring (Fig. 62.4).

4. *Multifocal electroretinogram*:[12] Decrease in P1 and N1 amplitudes of central macular region can be detected by mfERG in eyes with solar retinopathy.

Histopathology/Ultrastructural Changes

Occurs mainly in RPE and photoreceptors:

- RPE necrosis, irregular pigmentation and scattered retinal pigment epithelial cell degeneration (Fig. 62.5).

- Outer segment changes of rod and cones, of foveal or parafoveal region, includes vesiculation and fragmentation of photoreceptor lamellae and the presence of discrete 100–120 nm whorls within disc membranes. Mitochondrial swelling and nuclear pyknosis in photoreceptors.[2]

Prognosis

The yellow lesion is replaced by a permanent focal depression with RPE mottling or a lamellar hole over the weeks following injury. Vision usually improves to 20/20 to 20/40 within 6 months, although scotomata and metamorphopsia can persist.[13] Overall prognosis in solar retinopathy is good and has been attributed to the resistance of foveal cone cells to photochemical damage.

ECLIPSE RETINOPATHY

Eclipse retinopathy is the macular damage resulting from directly viewing a solar eclipse.[14]

The visual morbidity associated with full solar eclipse on August 11, 1999 was evaluated in detail and majority of patients sought treatment within 2 days of viewing the eclipse. 84% people had an abnormal macula. The condition is usually temporary with no cases of continued visual loss after 6 months. Few patients had persistent symptoms till 7 months after.

Albino rat models of retinal damage due to sun showed irreversible neuronal death in retina which was irreversible causing permanent visual impairment. Non-neuronal glial and endothelial cell changes may be responsible for more transient clinical symptoms.[2]

Therapy

- No specific treatment exists for solar or eclipse retinopathy.
- Repetition should be discouraged without adequate use of proper protection.

A beneficial effect of oral steroids in acute phase has not been demonstrated conclusively and vision often improves spontaneously.

WELDING ARC RETINOPATHY

Welding arcs emit radiation. Keratitis due to UV absorption by the cornea is the most common injury in welders.

The temperature of the retina increases not more than photocoagulation thresholds and thus all injury is produced by photochemical effects from UV and short blue wavelength exposure.

Symptoms include unilateral or bilateral decreased vision, scotomata and metamorphopsia.

Retinal manifestations are similar to those of solar retinopathy. A yellow edematous lesion is seen acutely in the fovea which recovers as RPE irregularity or a pseudo -macular hole.

No effective therapy exists but vision generally improves with time, although permanent loss of vision may occur.[2]

LIGHTNING RETINOPATHY

Lightning maculopathy involves acute visual loss and macular changes after injury by lightning. Patients may have macular edema, macular hole, cyst or a solar retinopathy like picture, cataract, retinal detachment, retinal artery occlusions and relative afferent pupillary defect. Severe visual loss may occur with recovery overtime even with severe disease. High-dose intravenous methylprednisolone treatment may play a role in recovery of vision.

RETINAL PHOTOTOXICITY FROM OPHTHALMIC INSTRUMENTS

Operating microscope and fiberoptic endoillumination may act as sources of retinal damage and has been reported after cataract extraction, epikeratophakia, combined anterior segment procedures, and vitreous surgery of which the most frequently cited cause is the operating microscope. The associated injury was described initially after an uncomplicated extracapsular cataract extraction.

This injury occurs via photochemical methods but may be thermally enhanced. Because operating microscopes generates little UV radiation, photochemical damage probably is caused by short-wavelength visible blue and green light. The incorporation of UV and IR filters in the intraocular lens (IOL) and microscope may reduce the risk of photic and thermal effects, respectively.[2]

Immediately after exposure, macula seems normal. A yellow lesion measuring 0.5–2.0 disc diameters at the level of the RPE is observed after 24–48 hours with associated retinal edema (Figs. 62.6A to C). Retinal damage often is inferior

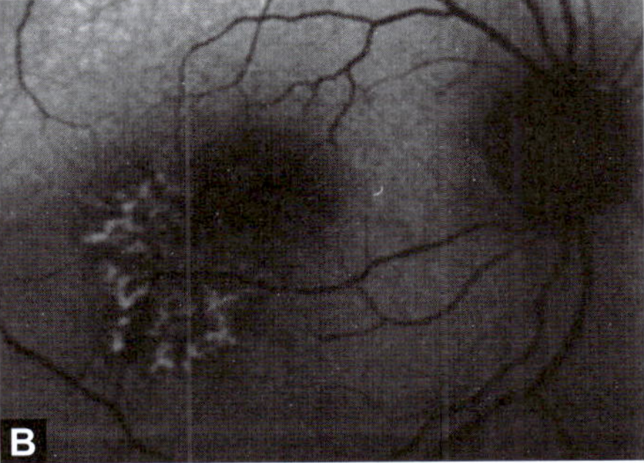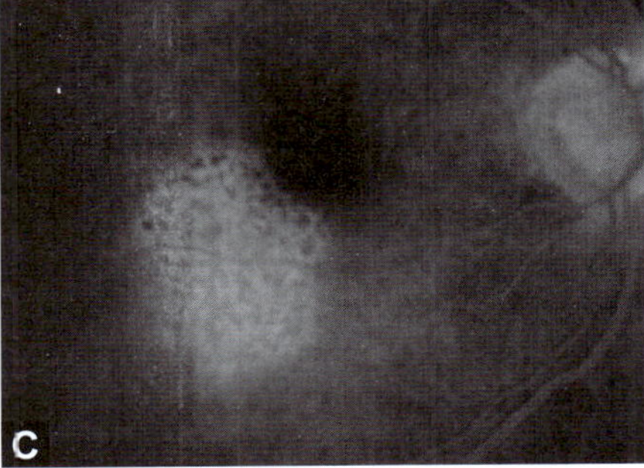

Figs. 62.6A to C: Photic retinopathy in an eye which underwent complicated cataract surgery. (A) The fundus photograph shows a well-demarcated, elliptical, yellowish, mottled retinal pigment epithelium alteration approximately twice the size of the optic disc, and encroaching on the fovea. (B) Autofluorescence image of the posterior pole of the right eye shows a dendritiform pattern of autofluorescence at the inferotemporal macula (BluePeak Blue Laser Autofluorescence, Heidelberg Engineering GmbH, Heidelberg, Germany). (C) Fluorescein angiography shows an irregular fluorescein transmission pattern without leakage.
Source: Mansour MA, Yunis MH, Medawar WA. Ocular coherence tomography of symptomatic phototoxic retinopathy after cataract surgery: a case report. J Med Case Rep. 2011;5:133.

to the fovea due to rotation of the globe by a superior rectus bridle suture, microscope tilt and displacement of the microscope field over the superior limbus. Injury may occur at or superior to the fovea during vitreous surgery or when a superior rectus bridle suture is not used. [15]

The shape of the lesion matches that of the surgical illuminating source. A tungsten filament in the operating microscope produces a horizontal, oval lesion, while the fiberoptic illuminator produces a round lesion.

Fluorescein angiography of the acute lesion may show leak at the level of RPE simulating a choroidal neovascularization. This yellow lesion fades over months and is permanently replaced by areas of RPE clumping and atrophy which correspond angiographically to blocking and transmission defects respectively.[16]Changes also observed are postoperative erythropsia and retinal surface wrinkling.

Histopathological studies have shown that after 60 minutes of operating microscope exposure in primates, photoreceptor damage and disruption of RPE tight junction occur. Their regeneration was noted in 3–5 months after injury. This may account for the recovery of vision after phototoxic injury noted in some human eyes.[16]

Retinal phototoxic lesions after short-duration cataract surgery (defined as surgery for less than 30 minutes) were associated with a refraction within 1.0 D of emmetropia and with diabetic retinopathy.[17] The risk of photic damage may increase after IOL insertion which can focus the incoming light on the retina.

Factors which make a patient more susceptible are increased body temperature, blood oxygenation, chorioretinal pigmentation, pre-existing maculopathy, pupillary dilatation, diabetes mellitus, retinal vascular disease, deficiencies of either ascorbic acid or vitamin A and hydrochlorothiazide or photosensitizer use.

No specific treatment is available for the condition.[4]Prognosis for early visual recovery appears to be good, even with macular lesions. Recommendations for the reduction of risk of phototoxicity include reduction of microscope coaxial illumination and operative time, use of IR and UV filters in the microscope and IOL, placement of an air bubble in the anterior chamber to defocus the light, and use of an eclipse filter or corneal cover to block light from entering the pupil when the incision is sutured.

Light from indirect ophthalmoscope and fundus camera[18]cannot reach beyond experimentally determined retinal injury thresholds. The total energy delivered to the eye is less under nonoperative than operative conditions. Acute retinal injury has not been reported in humans with these everyday instruments, however some retinal lesions have been seen in primates.

LIGHT EXPOSURE AND AGE-RELATED MACULAR DEGENERATION

Histopathological studies of acute photic injury in animals occur at the RPE and photoreceptor level in the macular region and is similar to that observed in age-related macular degeneration (AMD).[19]

The RPE pigmentary irregularities occur which are similar to those in AMD, although unlike in AMD, diffuse thickening of Bruch's membrane is not noted.

In a population-based study of Chesapeake Bay watermen, an association was noted between blue or visible light exposure over the preceding 20 years and the risk of developing advanced AMD (defined as exudative neovascular disease or geographical atrophy).

Although in the Beaver Dam Eye Study, no association was found between the estimated ambient UV-B exposure and AMD. The amount of outdoor leisure time in summer was associated with an increased retinal pigmentation in men and late AMD in both men and women. The use of hats and sunglasses was inversely associated with the prevalence of soft, indistinct drusen.

LASER HAZARD

American National Standards Institute (ANSI) standards define four laser classes:

1. *Class 1*: Maximum power output in the visible spectrum ranges from 0.0004 MW or less for blue or green light to 0.024 MW or less for red light.
2. *Class 2:* Produce laser power that is less than 1 MW.
3. *Class 3a:* Between 1 MW and 5 MW.
4. *Class 3b:* Between 5 MW and 500 MW.
5. *Class 4*: Lasers include potentially hazardous industrial, military, or medical lasers that generate more than 500 MW of laser power.

Laser-induced phototoxicity can occur by thermal, mechanical or photochemical mechanism and can cause small, subtle lesions to extensive hemorrhage and disruption of the retina and choroid. Accidental foveal photocoagulation can produce immediate loss of vision up to 20/200, with a foveal cyst or yellow discoloration of the RPE.

Long-term RPE irregularities, epiretinal membrane, macular hole and gliosis may occur. Recovery of vision is variable and is related to the extent and location of the initial injury. Corticosteroids have been used to treat laser-induced retinal injuries, although their benefit is unproven.

In laser photocoagulation, light scattered from optical interfaces such as contact lenses and mirrors can produce inadvertent harmful effects. Even though lasers for photocoagulation contain filters to protect the operator, protective goggles should be worn by all as there is a chance of the light to reach the eyes of the observers too.

Decreased color discrimination in a tritan color-confusion axis has been noted in ophthalmologists who use the argon blue-green probably due to long-term exposure to reflections from the argon blue aiming beam. Many photocoagulators now employ either a red or green aiming beam to minimize operator risk.

Slit-lamp photocoagulators: Subtle defects in blue-color contrast sensitivity have been documented in long-term operators of argon blue-green laser photocoagulators. The color contrast defects were believed to be due to the cumulative effect of viewing argon blue (488 nm) aiming beam reflections. Modern red aiming beams pose no significant risk for retinal phototoxicity.

Laser pointers: Laser pointers are low-energy lasers with output powers either less than 1 milliwatt (MW) (class 2 devices) or between 1 MW and 5 MW (class 3A devices). Most of the common class 3A laser pointers have power outputs that are 2 MW or less. In contrast, class 3B lasers used by ophthalmologists for retinal therapy have output powers up to or greater than 100 MW. There are very few reports of presumed retinal damage caused by laser pointers. The mechanism of injury is not clear, but it appears due to thermal chorioretinal damage, because the longer red 650 nm- or 635 nm-wavelength light emitted from a laser pointer do not produce significant retinal phototoxicity. Damage manifests as transient visual abnormalities and macular RPE disturbances that correspond to window defect.

NEONATAL INTENSIVE CARE UNIT (NICU) EXPOSURE

Neonatal retinal irradiance depends on many factors, including:

- The geometry and reflectance of NICU walls
- The location and spectral output of room and accessory lighting
- The duration of eyelid closure
- Pupillary size and reactivity
- Neonatal eyelid
- Ocular media transmittance.

Infants have very clear ocular media which transmit short-wavelength blue light and UV radiation more effectively than adult ocular media.

COMMERCIAL TANNING BOOTH EXPOSURE

Modern commercial tanning booths produce high-intensity UV-A and some UV-B radiation. Tanning booth exposure can cause photokeratitis similar to welding. The crystalline lens and cornea protect the retina from most UV tanning booth radiation, but tanning booth users should always wear proper eye protection to reduce the risk of photokeratitis, cataractogenesis and retinal phototoxicity.

REFERENCES

1. Heilig P, Rozanova E, Godnic-Cvar J. Retinal light damage. Spektrum der Augenheilkd. 2009;23(4):240-8.
2. Schwartz SG, Gombos SD, Schneider S. Light Toxicity in the Posterior Segment. Duane's Ophthalmology. Philadelphia: Lippincott; 2011.
3. Reme C, Reinboth J, Clausen M, et al. Light damage revisited: converging evidence, diverging views? GraefesArch Clin Exp Ophthalmology. 1996;234(1):2-11.
4. FN Youssef, N Sheibani , DM Albert. Retinal light toxicity. Eye (Lond). 2011; 25(1):1-14.
5. Organisciak DT, Vaughan DK. Retinal light damage: Mechanisms and Protection. Prog Retin Eye Res. 2010;29(2):113-34.
6. Mainster MA, Turner PL. Ultraviolet-B phototoxicity and hypothetical photomelanomagenesis: intraocular and crystallin lens photoprotection. Am J Ophthalmology. 2010;149(4):543-9.
7. Wu J, Seregard S, Algvere PV. Photochemical Damage of the Retina. Surv Ophthalmology. 2006; 51(5):461-81.
8. Rai N, Thuladar L, Brandt F, et al. Solar retinopathy. A study from Nepal and from Germany. Doc Ophthalmology. 1998;95(2):99-108.
9. Yannuzzi LA, Fisher YL, Slakter JS, et al. Solar retinopathy: A photobiologic and geophysical analysis. Retina.1989;9(1):28-43.
10. Harada T, Koizumi E, Saito A, et al. Three cases with light-induced retinopathy. Doc Ophthalmology. 1988;69(1):11-8.
11. Comander J, Gardiner M, Loewenstein J. High-resolution optical coherence tomography findings in solar maculopathy and the differential diagnosis of outer retinal holes. Am J Ophthalmology. 2011;152(3):413-9.
12. Arda H, Oner A, Multu S, et al. Multifocal electroretinography in solar maculopathy. Doc Ophthalmology. 2007;114(3):159-62.
13. Atmaca LS, Idil A, Can D. Early and late visual prognosis in solar retinopathy. Graefes Arch Clin Exp Ophthalmology. 1995; 233(12): 801-4.
14. Thanos S, Heiduschka P, Romann I. Exposure to a solar eclipse causes neuronal death in the retina. Graefes Arch Clin Exp Ophthalmology. 2001;239(10):794-800.
15. Azzolini C, Brancato R, Venturi G, et al. Updating on intraoperative light-induced retinal injury. Int Ophthalmology. 1995;18(5):269-76.
16. Michels M, Sternberg P Jr. Operating microscope-induced retinal phototoxicity: pathophysiology, clinical manifestations and prevention. Surv Ophthalmology. 1990;34(4):237-52.
17. Cetinkaya A, Yilmaz G, Akova YA. Photic retinopathy after cataract surgery in diabetic patients. Retina. 2006;26(9):1021-8.
18. Kohenan S. Light-induced damage of the retina through slit-lamp photography. Graefes Arch Clin Exp Ophthalmology. 2000;238(12): 956-9.
19. Arnault E, Barrau C, Nanteau C, et al. Phototoxic action spectrum on a retinal pigment epithelium model of age-related macular degeneration exposed to sunlight normalized conditions. PLoS One. 2013;8(8):e71398.

Chapter 63

Phakomatoses

Karthikeya R, Shashwat Behera, Alisha Kishore, Atul Kumar

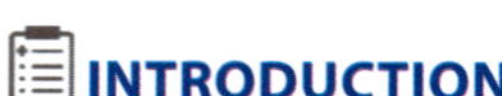 **INTRODUCTION**

Phakomatoses, also known as systemic hamartomatous lesions, are a heterogenous group of conditions manifesting with abnormalities in the eye, skin, central nervous system (CNS), peripheral nervous system and the viscera.[1] Although distinct genetically and etiologically, they all present early in life, are progressive, mostly inherited as an autosomal dominant condition and have predilection for neoplastic proliferation in the nervous system and the viscera. Pathologically, they classically comprise of *hamartomas* (abnormal masses of histologically normal tissue in an expected location) which are usually benign and slow-growing. But malignant neoplastic growths may also occur and can predispose to reduced vision while also shortening patient's life span.[2] Many of the described conditions frequently present to an ophthalmic practitioner first before an internist and, therefore, the importance of prompt recognition of the cutaneous and ocular features aiding in an accurate diagnosis of the systemic condition and subsequent comprehensive care of the patient cannot be overemphasized.

The term *phakomatoses* (from the Greek word *phakomata* or birthmark) was coined by Van der Hoeve in his research paper published in year 1932 in which he described the similarities between tuberous sclerosis (TS) and neurofibromatosis (NF), both of which present with characteristic skin findings.[3] Later, conditions such as Von Hippel–Lindau (VHL) disease, Sturge–Weber syndrome (SWS), ataxia-telangiectasia (AT), Wyburn–Mason syndrome (WMS) and retinal cavernous hemangioma were added to the list. Often the terms 'neurocutaneous syndrome' and 'neurooculocutaneous syndrome' are used synonymously with phakomatosis. But many authors believe that neurocutaneous and neurooculocutaneous are descriptive terms for component lesions and the presence of hamartomas in multiple organ systems is essential to classify a condition under phakomatosis.[4-6] Currently, there are over 50 conditions classified as neurocutaneous syndromes[6] and new conditions continue to be added,[7] even though the definitions of each of these terms still remain ill-defined.[8]

Van der Hoeve was also the first to hypothesize that a defect in the ectodermal germ layer, of which are brain, skin, and eye derivatives which lead to the manifestations of phakomatoses.[9] But the prominent blood vessel and adipose tissue involvement seen in many conditions was not explained by this and led to the hypothesis that a primary defect lies in the neural crest cells and its migration.[10] In the present era of modern genetics, causative gene mutations are identified for NF, TS and VHL diseases, all of which are mutations in tumor suppressor genes, but the role of neural crest cells, especially in complex diseases like TS is still speculated.[11]

The biology of the genes involved in NF, TS and VHL are similar to the *Rb1* gene of the retinoblastoma which is also a tumor suppressor gene. They are all inherited in an autosomal recessive manner at the cellular level and only a homozygous mutation in the alleles can cause tumors, but heterozygous mutation is transmitted as a dominant trait from generation to generation. Mutations may also arise sporadically. Once one of the pair is mutated, the mutation of the wild-type of the pair is a chance phenomenon (Knudson's two hit hypothesis) and when it occurs, it leads to the formation of a tumor such as a neurofibroma or schwannoma.[12] This also explains the 'patchy' nature of the hamartomas found in these conditions. Phakomatoses display high penetrance and variable expressivity i.e. each individual with a mutation will show some signs of the disease, but the severity of presentation varies.

For the purpose of this chapter we will be emphasizing on the three classic hamartomatous conditions[4,12]—NF, TS and VHL disease along with other conditions with prominent ocular manifestations such as SWS, WMS, retinal cavernous hemangiomatosis with particular reference to the retina and choroid.

VON RECKLINGHAUSEN'S NEUROFIBROMATOSIS (TYPE 1)

Neurofibromatosis consists of two genetically and clinically distinct conditions, neurofibromatosis type 1 (NF1) and neurofibromatosis type 2 (NF2), with tumor predilection perhaps being the only one similarity between the two entities. They have an autosomal dominant inheritance with high penetrance and variable expressivity but about one-half of patients with both conditions have a sporadic mutation with a negative family history. NF1 predisposes to tumors along peripheral nerves and NF2 predisposes to tumors in the CNS.

Neurofibromatosis Type 1 is characterized by benign, and occasionally malignant tumors of the Schwann cells and astrocytes. As discussed earlier, they have high penetrance, implying every individual with the mutation manifests at least some features, but variable expressivity, implying, for example, the number of neurofibromas on individuals greatly vary from only a few to thousands. It is a common disorder with a prevalence of 1 in 3,500 people worldwide,[13] affecting males and females equally and occuring among all ethnic groups.[14] It is caused by a mutation in the tumor suppressor gene neurofibromin-1 (*NF1*) located on chromosome 17q11.2. *NF1* gene is expressed in the astrocytes of CNS and Schwann cells of the peripheral nervous system. There are over a 1,000 mutations in this gene that are known to cause NF1.[15] The product of *NF1* gene is neurofibromin protein which acts by inhibiting the activity of an important cell signaling molecule known as *RAS*.[16] *RAS* is a proto-oncogene which when activated leads to a downstream cascade resulting in the transcription of multiple genes ultimately resulting in cell division. Neurofibromin helps in terminating the *RAS* signal and mutations in *NF1* gene lead to uninhibited *RAS* activity, finally leading to neoplasia.

Von Recklinghausen first described the condition in 1882,[17] when it came to known with his name till the current diagnostic criterion was proposed in 1987 by the National Institute of Health Consensus Development Conference which also suggested it to be called NF1.[18] According to this diagnostic criterion, NF1 is clinically diagnosed if at least two of the following seven clinical findings are seen:

1. Six or more café au lait spots, each larger than 5 mm in prepubertal children and each larger than 15 mm in adults
2. Intertriginous freckling
3. Two or more typical cutaneous nodular neurofibromas or one or more plexiform neurofibroma
4. Optic pathway glioma
5. Two or more iris lisch nodules
6. Bony dysplasias in the form of sphenoid dysplasia or congenital tibial dysplasia
7. A first-degree relative with NF1

Systemic Features

The hallmark feature of NF1 is the occurrence of neurofibromas (Figs. 63.1A to C) on skin or subcutaneously along nerves. They are benign neoplastic proliferation of Schwann cells, fibroblasts, perineurial cells and mast cells.[19] There are two important kinds of neurofibromas occurring in NF1.

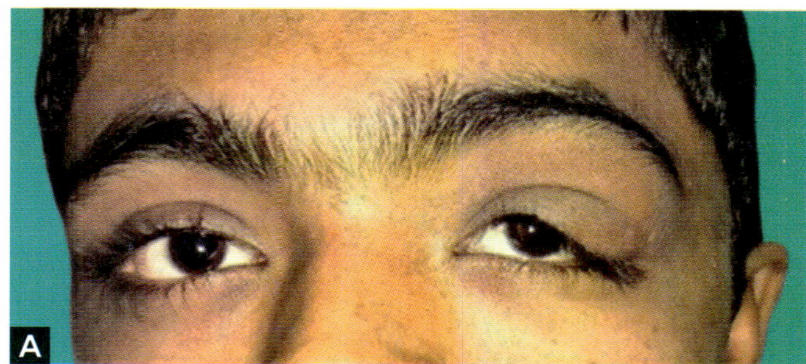
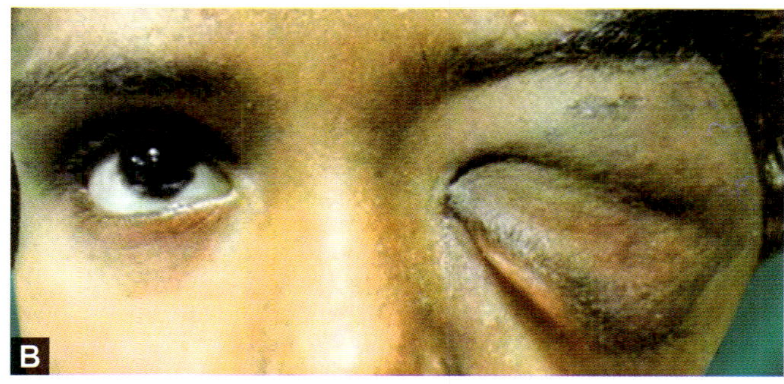
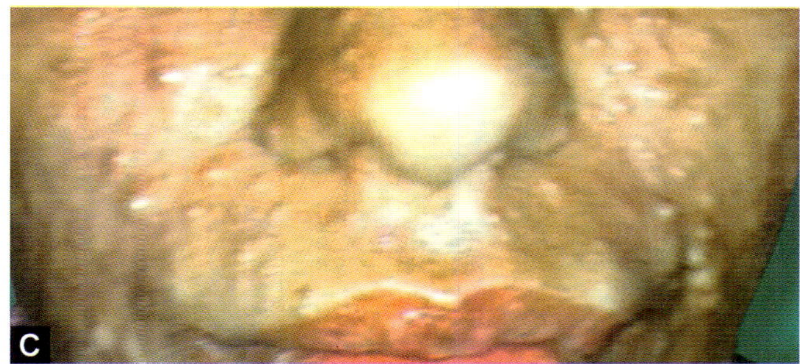

Figs. 63.1A to C: Neurofibromatosis type 1. (A) Plexiform neurofibroma in the left upper eyelid with ptotic lid showing partial encroachment of pupillary axis. Note the characteristic 'S'-shape of the upper lid margin. (B) Severe forms of eyelid neurofibromas can cause skin and conjunctival hypertrophy, complete ptosis and disfiguration. (C) The other form of neurofibromas is dermal nodular.

The dermal neurofibroma (Fig. 63.1C) which is a solitary well-defined firm nodule on the skin or subcutaneous tissue and the plexiform neurofibroma (Figs. 63.1A and B) which is a diffuse form of neurofibroma due to longitudinal involvement of fascicles of a major nerve. The latter is often associated with infiltration of surrounding tissue, hypertrophy of overlying skin and deformity. The plexiform neurofibromas have a predilection for malignant transformation into malignant peripheral nerve sheath tumors and the risk is estimated to be at around 10%.[20] Both forms of neurofibromas can cause disfiguration.

Central nervous system tumors include gliomas in the optic pathway (most common and discussed later), cerebellum and brainstem.[21] Most gliomas are pilocytic astrocytomas but tumors appearing later in life and at sites other than the optic nerve can be higher WHO (World Health Organization) grade tumors. Cognitive impairment is the most common neurological abnormality found in NF1. Specific learning difficulty, behavioral problems, spinal nerve root neurofibromas, Arnold Chiari type 1 malformation and aqueductal stenosis due to subependymal glial cell proliferation are also known. Café-au-lait (Latin; coffee with milk) spots are the most important, earliest and most frequent nontumorous manifestation of NF1. They are hyperpigmented skin macules with smooth margins typically of the 'coffee with milk' color present in 99% of the patients by the age of 5 years and maybe the only cutaneous sign in young children.[22] It must be remembered, though, that about 10% of the normal population have one or two café au lait spots and in patients with NF1 they may fade by adulthood or be hidden by a neurofibroma. Axillary freckling (Crowe's sign) and groin freckling are more common but freckling in the neck, trunk and breast area in females are also known to occur in NF1. It is important to recognize the cutaneous manifestations early since these may be the only manifestations at birth and early childhood and the tumorous features appear gradually with increasing age.[23]

Skeletal dysplasias like scoliosis, tibial bowing and pseudarthrosis, sphenoidal dysplasia, orbital dysplasia are also known with NF1.[24] About one-third of patients with NF1 have short stature because of affection of limb bones. Cardiovascular problems are also well described in NF1.[25] Segmental NF is caused by somatic mutations or mosaicism. Heterozygosity in NF1 mutations is known to cause learning difficulties in children. Other neurocognitive abnormalities in NF1 are also known.

Ocular Features

The eye may be affected in NF1 with multiple possible manifestations (Table 63.1). Even though ocular manifestations are nearly universal in patients with NF1, complications leading to vision loss occurs in about 5% of the patients.[26] They are often multifactorial and profound.[27] Important causes of vision loss include amblyopia, optic pathway gliomas, plexiform neurofibroma, congenital glaucoma and sphenoid dysplasia.[26,27-29]

Lisch nodules are the most common ocular manifestation of NF1. They were first described by Waardenburg in 1918 but were correlated to NF1 by Lisch in 1937, after whom they were named.[24,25] These were thought to be iris melanocytic hamartomas arising from the anterior limiting layer, but recent histopathological studies have revealed that they are composed of pigmented cells, fibroblast-like cells and mast cells, a pattern similar to neurofibroma.[30,31] They start appearing at an early age and may be the only sign of NF1 in young children along with café-au-lait spots. By adulthood, they are present in 100% of patients in NF1 and are unique to NF1.[15,17,26] They are bilateral, clear to yellow-brown in color, dome-shaped elevations projecting from the surface of iris often seen without magnification, prominently distributed in the inferior half of the iris. In young patients they are found more frequently than neurofibromas and

Table 63.1: Ocular manifestations of neurofibromatosis Type 1.	
Region	*Manifestation*

Orbit, periorbital, facial skin and adnexa	• Periorbital nodular neurofibroma
	• Plexiform neurofibroma of the eyelids
	  – Brow ptosis
	  – Upper eyelid infiltration with ptosis
	  – Lower eyelid infiltration
	  – Lateral canthal disinsertion
	  – Conjunctival and lacrimal gland infiltration
	• Functional nasolacrimal duct obstruction
	• Proptosis and subsequent complications
	  – Neurofibromas
	  – Optic pathway gliomas
	  – Schwannomas
	  – Sphenoid dysplasia
	• Pulsatile exophthalmos due to sphenoid dysplasia
	• Enophthalmos due to sphenoid dysplasia
	• Strabismus

Anterior segment	• Congenital glaucoma: Open angle, closed angle and neovascular • Prominent corneal nerves • Conjunctival and scleral neurofibroma • Congenital ectropion uveae • Conjunctival choristoma • Heterochromia • Posterior embryotoxon
Posterior segment	• Choroidal neurofibroma/nodule • Retinal/optic nerve head astrocytoma remove • Choroidal hamartoma/nevi/pigmented lesions • Choroidal neurilemmoma/schwannoma • Uveal melanoma • Increased axial length • Retinoschisis • Congenital hypertrophy of retinal pigment epithelium • Combined hamartoma of the retina and retinal pigment epithelium • Retinal vasoproliferative tumors • Retinal capillary hemangiomas • Retinal microangiopathy • Choroidal ganglioneuroma • Retinal ganglioneuroma • Combined hamartoma of the retina and retinal pigment epithelium
Neuro-ophthalmological	• Optic pathway gliomas • Optic nerve drusen • Cranial nerve palsies • Nystagmus

may aid in the diagnosis.[28] Lisch nodules are differentiated from the more common iris nevi by their elevation from the surface, distinct margins and lighter pigmentation. They are often asymptomatic and are not associated with any complications.

Periorbital, orbital and adnexal involvement of NF1 can lead to significant disfigurement and are challenging cases to manage.[32] Nodular NF is easy to diagnose and can cause complications like mechanical ectropion or ptosis. Plexiform NF of the orbitotemporal region can cause brow ptosis, upper eyelid infiltration with ptosis, lower lid infiltration, lateral canthal disinsertion and conjunctival, lacrimal gland infiltration.[33] The blepharoptosis associated with plexiform neurofibroma has a classical S-shaped deformity because of the temporal part of the eyelid being more infiltrated. Plexiform neurofibroma of the orbit can also cause proptosis, orbital expansion, bone erosion, zygomatic hypoplasia, orbital floor depression, extraocular muscle infiltration and strabismus.[34,35] Sphenoid dysplasia is due to maldevelopment of the sphenoid bone with absence of the greater wing of the sphenoid causing the middle cranial fossa to be connected with the orbit via the superior orbital fissure. This can lead to herniation of the temporal lobe of the brain into the orbit causing pulsatile proptosis or occasionally herniation of orbital contents into the middle cranial fossa causing enophthalmos.[34] Treatment depends on the extent of involvement, tissues involved, visual potential and age. Debulking is often done to reduce the tumor mass but invariably leads to recurrence. Ptosis needs to be corrected with an additional levator resection. Lateral canthal surgery or lateral canthal strip can be used in addition in required cases. Severe involvement of soft tissue and bone may be best managed by exenteration.[32]

Congenital/developmental glaucoma is a rare manifestation of NF1.[36] It usually affects the side of the face affected with orbitotemporal NF and is associated with buphthalmos. Many mechanisms have been hypothesized for the development of glaucoma like angle maldevelopment, infiltration of the angle with a neurofibroma, synechial angle closure due to infiltration of the ciliary body and neovascularization due to retinal ischemia.[37] Visual prognosis is generally poor in these children.

Decreased visual acuity, a large and displaced globe, skull and orbital deformity, and tumor within the orbit and cavernous sinus are potential causes of strabismus in NF1.[38] In a study by Oystreck et al.,[38] 28% patients with orbitofacial NF has no strabismus, 55% had incomitant strabismus, inferiorly displaced globe and limited ductions and 16% had comitant strabismus with poor vision and no abnormality of eye ductions.

An important pathological involvement in NF1 is of the optic nerve (and optic pathway) where it manifests as glioma. Optic nerve glioma or optic pathway gliomas are histologically low-grade pilocytic astrocytomas (WHO grade I astrocytomas) and usually affect the nerve at the chiasma. About one-third of patients with optic pathway glioma have NF1 and among children with NF1 about 15–20% have optic pathway gliomas

out of which a significant one-half to two-third remain clinically indolent[39] which is why they are picked up on routine screening neuroimaging as often as they are picked up due to symptoms.[40] They usually present in children younger than 6 years with impaired visual acuity, strabismus, color vision abnormality, proptosis or optic atrophy. Precocious puberty may also be seen in gliomas impinging on the hypothalamus.[39] Natural course of the tumor is highly variable—they may remain stable, slowly progress or even spontaneously regress. Only progressive tumors, which is about 30% of cases require treatment.[40] Given the severity of visual outcomes in the cases of progressive optic nerve gliomas and to avoid the unnecessary imaging and anxiety the child and the parents go through screening guidelines have been laid down.[41] A newly diagnosed NF1 patient without known, Optic Pathway Glioma (OPG) should undergo a complete ophthalmological examination at diagnosis followed by annual examinations until the age of 7 years and longer intervals thereafter till the age of 18 years.[39,42] Measurement of visual acuity, color vision, squint, visual field charting, visual evoked response and retinal nerve fiber layer thickness with optical coherence tomography have all been used for the assessment of presence and progression of the tumor. Routine MRI screening is not advised.[39] Once diagnosed with an optic pathway glioma, surveillance and treatment need to be tailored depending on the location, evidence of progression, visual impairment and other factors. Chemotherapy with carboplatin and vincristine is the current first-line treatment. Drugs that block RAS pathway could be of benefit and clinical trials to test the same are underway. Surgery is usually undertaken for large orbital tumors with exposure keratopathy and tumors close to hypothalamus. Radiotherapy is contraindicated given the tumor predisposition among the affected individuals. Recently, bevacizumab has also been tried for optic pathway gliomas with good response.[43] Optic pathway gliomas can also appear sporadically and unrelated to NF1 in which case the tumors are more posterior in the optic pathway and are generally more aggressive.

Choroidal neurofibroma often also referred to as choroidal nodule or choroidal abnormality is a common yet subtle finding of neurofibroma often missed on routine fundoscopy.[44,45] There are suggestions that they may be seen as frequently as lisch nodules.[44] They are best appreciated by infrared autofluorescence or near infrared reflectance as bright patchy lesions in the posterior pole and on indocyanine green angiography as hyperfluorescent patches in early and late phase.[46,47] Clinically when apparent, they may appear as a nodule or a yellowish area of retinal pigment epithelial abnormality overlying an area of diffuse choroidal thickening. Pigmented choroidal lesions/hamartomas were the second most common ophthalmic manifestation in a few series.[26,31] They clinically and angiographically resemble choroidal nevi and are usually multiple and bilateral. Both of the above conditions do not require specific therapy. Choroidal schwannomas and melanoma are also known to occur in NF1 and must be treated like any other melanoma in the same location. Astrocytomas are characteristics of TS (discussed later) but can occur in NF1 and do not require treatment. Ganglioneuroma listed in Table 63.1 are primarily a histopathological diagnosis made mostly on enucleated eyes. However, many other entities reported in literature like combined hamartoma of the retina and retinal pigment epithelium, cavernous hemangioma are without histopathological confirmation. Ischemic retinopathy[48] with subsequent neovascular glaucoma,[49,50] vasoproliferative retinal tumors with significant exudation requiring cryotherapy and/or laser are also reported. Author would like to re-emphasize the common undercurrent in the seemingly diverse manifestations of NF1 is the hamartomatous proliferation of cells.

NEUROFIBROMATOSIS TYPE 2

Neurofibromatosis 2 (NF2) was first described by Wishart in 1822 and is characterized by bilateral vestibular schwannomas.[51,52] Other tumors that frequently occur in NF2 are meningiomas, schwannomas of other cranial, spinal and peripheral nerves and ependymomas. It is a less common disease when compared to NF1 with a prevalence of 1 in 60,000.[13] It is inherited in an autosomal dominant fashion with complete penetrance but about 50–60% of the affected individuals show sporadic mutations, 30% of whom are somatic mosaics.[53] Cutaneous signs are not conspicuous in NF2[22] making diagnosis more difficult. Cafe´-au-lait spots are not seen regularly and neurofibromas are infrequent. But this occasional occurrence of skin features similar to NF1 was what had caused this condition to be historically classified under von Recklinghausen disease and only when genes responsible for both the conditions were identified on chromosome 17 and 22 that it was understood that the two diseases were distinct entities. The NIH consensus conference in 1987 called this entity with CNS tumors as NF2.[18]

The causative gene, neurofibromin 2, lies in the locus 22q12 and encodes a protein called as merlin or schwannomin.[54,55] Merlin is a protein localized to the plasma membrane cytoskeleton interface and links cytoskeletal proteins like actin and spectrin to the plasma membrane proteins.[55] It has functions in cell-to-cell adhesion. It is supposed that this protein functions as a tumor suppressor protein by the mechanism of 'contact inhibition of cell division'.[56,57-59]

Multiple sets of diagnostic criteria have been proposed and tested for the diagnosis of NF2 but the Manchester criterion is the most accepted criterion which improves on the NIH criteria of 1991.[51,53,60,61] According to this criteria, NF2 is diagnosed when a patient has:

- Bilateral vestibular schwannomas, or
- When there is a family history of NF2 with:
  - Unilateral vestibular schwannoma, or
  - Any two of the following additional features—meningioma, glioma, neurofibroma, schwannoma, posterior subcapsular cataracts, or

- Unilateral vestibular schwannoma with any two of—meningioma, glioma, neurofibroma, schwannoma and posterior subcapsular cataracts, or
- Two or more meningiomas with unilateral vestibular schwannoma or any two of—glioma, neurofibroma, schwannoma, posterior subcapsular cataract.

Systemic Features

NF2 mostly presents in young adulthood with symptoms related to vestibular schwannoma—unilateral or bilateral progressive sensorineural hearing loss, tinnitus and vertigo. But they can appear at any time in life from early childhood to old age. 95% of NF2 patients manifest a vestibular schwannoma. Unlike NF1, there is only a little malignant potential in these tumors and complications arise from progressive enlargement of these tumors and compression of vital structures and nerves. Sometimes meningiomas (including optic nerve sheath meningiomas) and schwannomas present long before vestibular schwannomas and make diagnosis difficult. The second most common type of tumor in NF2 is meningioma. They can occur intracranially along optic nerve or along the spine. 45% patients develop intracranial meningiomas and are usually multiple. Spinal tumors are also very common in NF2. Up to 90% of the patients have a spinal tumor—schwannomas, meningiomas or ependymomas, but only about one-third of them cause symptoms.[53] Mononeuropathy (most commonly facial nerve), polyneuropathy, focal amyotrophy, polio-like illness, epilepsy are also known in NF2.[22,52,53]

Skin manifestations are not as prominent as seen in NF1. About 70% of NF2 patients have skin tumors, but only 10% have more than 10 skin tumors. Neurofibromas are rare but plaque-like, elevated hyperpigmented, hypertrichotic, skin lesions are common. A lesser common skin manifestation is schwannoma along a superficial nerve which can be felt as a nodule in the subcutaneous tissue. Café-au-lait spots are seen in 40% of the patients.[22]

Ocular Features

Ocular involvement is noted in 86–94% of affected individuals especially prominent in early onset NF2 (Table 63.2).[61] Patients with ophthalmic manifestations present with vision loss earlier than hearing loss. Younger onset disease has a higher chance of ocular involvement and a higher risk of losing vision.[61-63]

Juvenile posterior subcapsular cataracts are the most common ocular finding in NF2 noted in 60–81%.[61] The merlin protein is expressed in the lens and its mutation explains the proliferation of lens epithelial cells which gives rise to the subcapsular opacities noted in these patients. They rarely are symptomatic or cause vision loss and do not generally require surgery. Since cataracts are present from a very early age and tumors associated with NF2 appear only after adolescence, children of patients with NF2, less than 10 years of age are screened for these subcapsular opacities for early diagnosis of NF2.[52] Cortical spokes are also noted in NF2.

Table 63.2: Ocular manifestations of neurofibromatosis type 2.

Region	Manifestation
Anterior segment	• Posterior subcapsular cataracts • Cortical wedge cataracts • Lagophthalmos and exposure keratopathy • Corneal hypoaesthesia and neurotrophic ulcer
Posterior segment	• Combined hamartoma of the retina and retinal pigment epithelium • Epiretinal membranes • Optic disc glioma • Retinal glial hamartoma/astrocytoma • Vitreoretinal degeneration • Astrocytic hamartoma of retina and optic disc
Orbit	• Optic nerve sheath meningiomas • Optic nerve glioma
Neuro-ophthalmic	• Papilledema • Optic atrophy • Cranial nerve palsies • Strabismus • Nystagmus

Lagophthalmos and corneal hypoesthesia are related to vestibular schwannoma per se or its treatment. Involvement of multiple other cranial nerves and subsequent ocular motility disturbance and diplopia are also known.[64] Strabismus due to nerve palsies, sensory deprivation amblyopia and supranuclear palsies are common. Nystagmus can occur due to vestibular nerve compression.[64] Papilledema and optic atrophy can occur due to intracranial tumors or optic nerve sheath meningioma. Optic nerve sheath meningioma occurs in 4th or 5th decade and presents with a classic triad of gradual painless loss of vision, proptosis and optociliary shunt vessels. One-half will present with disc edema and the other half with optic atrophy. Sphenoid wing meningiomas often cause more proptosis and are the ones often associated with NF2. Surgical resection of progressive tumors and observation of the nonprogressive tumors appears prudent.

Epiretinal membranes in NF2 are a common finding in patients with NF2[65] and are closely associated with combined hamartoma of the retina and retinal pigment epithelium.[66] Histopathologic studies have shown that epiretinal membranes are composed of intraretinal and epiretinal proliferation of astrocytes and could be an earlier stage of a retinal or combined retinal and retinal pigment epithelium hamartoma.[65,67,68] Presence of epiretinal membrane indicates a severe phenotype of NF2 with multiple intracranial and spinal tumors.[66] A few NF2 specific features have been observed in these epiretinal membranes like absence of PVD, curled edges, speculated appearance, loss of foveal depression with inner retinal elements overlying the fovea, preservation of the IS-OS junction, absence of cystoid spaces and projection toward vitreous.[68]

Combined hamartoma of the retina and the retinal pigment epithelium are benign tumors composed of pigment epithelial cells, vessels and glial cells noted in the posterior pole and around the optic disc. They present as elevated masses with tortuous vessels and varying degree of pigmentation and gliosis. About 22% of the patients with NF2 have combined hamartomas.[62] Epiretinal membranes are also associated with 78% cases of combined hamartoma of the retina and retinal pigment epithelium and sometimes considered an early manifestation of the hamartoma.[63,68] Visual acuity less than 6/60 ensues in about 50% of the untreated patients.[69] Vitrectomy and epiretinal membrane peeling appears to be an effective treatment in a subgroup of patients with predominantly glial hamartomas.[70,71]

TUBEROUS SCLEROSIS

Tuberous sclerosis is a complex, autosomal dominant, multisystem disorder with hamartomas predominantly involving the CNS, skin, eye, kidney, lung, heart and other viscera.[72-74] It was first described in 1880 by Bourneville in a postmortem clinicopathological study of sclerotic tubers found in the brain of patients with mental retardation and epilepsy and for many years after that was called 'Bourneville's disease'.[74] The clinical manifestations of TS fall on a wide spectrum with some patients showing minimal signs and symptoms with no neurological disability, while others show severe early disease with significant disability and loss of quality of life. The classic triad (Vogt triad) of intractable seizures, cutaneous angiofibromas and mental retardation occurs only in about 25% of the patients.

Tuberous sclerosis is inherited as an autosomal dominant condition with almost complete penetrance and variable expressivity. About 70% of the patients have sporadic mutations.[74] Mosaicism is also common. The genetics of TS is complex and is only beginning to be understood. It is caused by mutations in two tumor suppressor genes, *TSC1*, located on chromosome 9q34, encoding hamartin and *TSC2*, located on 16p13, encoding tuberin. *TSC2* mutations cause TS more frequently and these are also more severe than *TSC1* mutations causing TS. The product of *TSC1* and *TSC2* work in conjunction as a heterodimer and act as a tumor suppressor by inhibiting the activation of mammalian target of rapamycin, mTOR. mTOR has a pivotal role in the control of cell growth and proliferation through its regulation of ribosomal biosynthesis and protein translation.[75,76]

Systemic Features

Tuberous sclerosis affects multiple organ systems and often presents with a constellation of signs and symptoms. No feature, however, is pathognomonic and each feature develops at a distinct developmental stage. For example, cardiac rhabdomyomas and cortical tubers develop during embryogenesis and are therefore typical findings at birth. Adenoma sebaceum develop during late childhood or adolescence and lymphangioleiomyomatosis is found mostly in adolescent girls or women.[72]

Ash leaf spots are hypomelanotic spots founds on the skin of about 90% of patients with TS. They are rounded at one end, pointed at the opposite end; more pronounced on Wood's lamp examination and are found at birth. Adenoma sebaceum (Fig. 63.2A) are pathologically angiofibromas present on the face especially on the nasolabial folds and malar area. They often appear during childhood and adolescence. The Shagreen patch is another important dermatological manifestation produced due to collagen accumulation in the skin to form an irregular-shaped thickened plaque in the lumbosacral region. Stippled hypopigmented lesions (confetti lesions), forehead plaques (Fig. 63.2B), periungual fibromas are other important dermatologic features. Café-au-lait spots are also seen in about 30% of patients with TS. Dental pitting and gingival fibromas also occur in TS.

Neurological manifestations are the most common and the most disabling manifestations of TS. They fall on a spectrum ranging from patients with normal intelligence and no seizures to patients with severe mental retardation and intractable seizures. Seizures are the most common manifestation and the most common cause of morbidity in patients with TS. Seizures occur in about 75–90% of patients. Infantile spasms are the commonest seizure type in infants.[77] As children grow partial motor seizures and generalized tonic-clonic seizures are also found. Mental retardation, behavioral abnormalities, cognitive impairment, autism, attention deficit hyperactive disorder and sleep problems are prominent manifestations of TS. Intracranial tumors include glioneuronal hamartomas—earlier called as cortical tubers, subependymal nodules and subependymal giant cell astrocytoma. Subependymal nodules (<10 mm) are also histologically hamartomas and indistinguishable on histology from giant cell astrocytomas (>10 mm).[76] These can cause seizures, cognitive dysfunction,

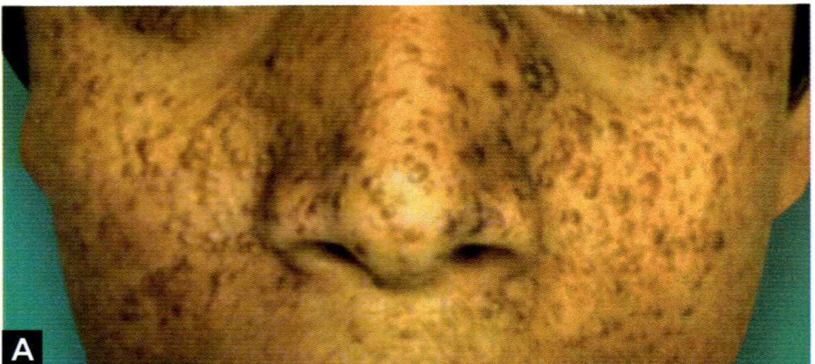

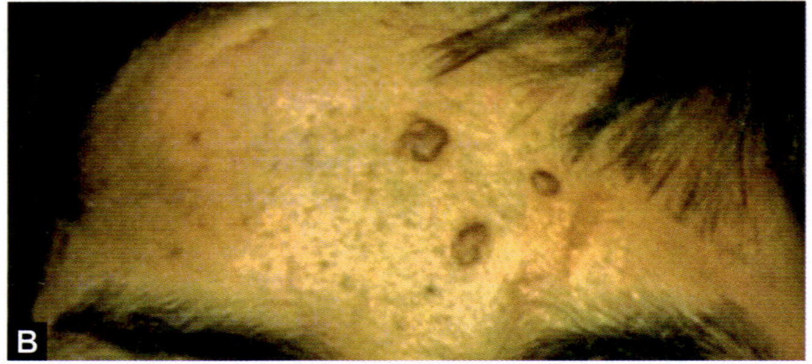

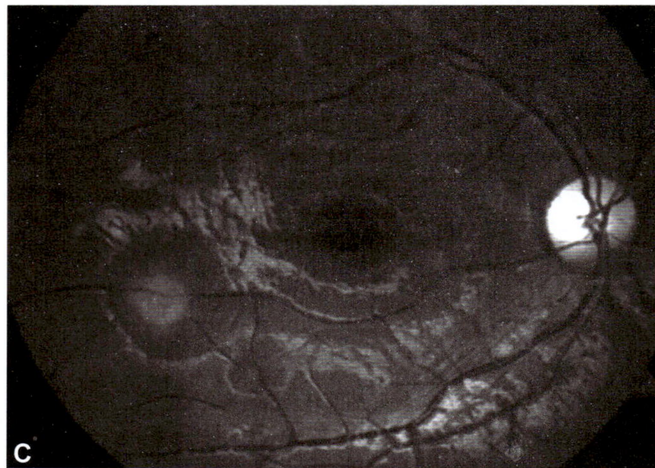

Figs. 63.2A to C: Tuberous sclerosis. (A) Cutaneous manifestations include adenoma sebaceum, and (B) Forehead plaques. They are hamartomatous proliferation in the skin. Ophthalmic manifestation includes retinal astrocytic hamartomas. (C) Red-free fundus photography demonstrates multiple retinal astrocytic hamartomas.

obstructive hydrocephalus and raised intracranial tension. Cortical migration defects also occur in the white matter.

Renal lesions includes multiple bilateral angiomyolipomas, renal cortical cysts and autosomal dominant polycystic kidney disease. Rarely early onset renal cell carcinoma can also occur. In the lungs, TS can cause a chronic progressive cystic lung disease known as lymphangioleiomyomatosis which ultimately leads to a restrictive lung disease. While all manifestations of TS are seen equally in both sexes, renal and pulmonary manifestations are seen more frequently in females. Cardiac rhabdomyomas are also present in about two-third of newborns with TS and can cause heart failure in intrauterine life or immediate neonatal period. They regress later in life but can lead to other problems like valvular disease and arrhythmias. Arterial aneurysms, cysts of the phalangeal bones and hamartomas in the gastrointestinal tract also occur in TS.

The diagnostic criterion for TS was updated in 2012[78] and includes major and minor clinical criteria or a genetic criteria. According to this criterion:

- Identification of a known pathogenic mutation in *TSC1* or *TSC2* from a normal (nonlesional) tissue is sufficient to make a definite diagnosis of TS. But since 10–25% of the patients may not have a mutation identified by a conventional genetic testing, negative result does not exclude the diagnosis of TS.
- Clinical diagnostic criterion is an ordinal criterion which makes a definitive diagnosis of TS if two major features are present or one major with two or more minor features are present. A possible diagnosis of TS is made if either one major feature or two or more minor features are present.
  - Major features are:
    - Three or more hypomelanotic macules (ash leaf spots), each at least 5 mm in diameter
    - Three or more angiofibroma or fibrous cephalic plaque
    - Two or more ungual fibroma
    - Shagreen patch
    - Multiple retinal hamartomas
    - Cortical dysplasia (including tubers and white matter radial migration lines)
    - Subependymal nodules
    - Subependymal giant cell astrocytoma
    - Cardiac rhabdomyoma
    - Lymphangioleiomyomatosis (LAM)
    - Two or more angiomyolipomas
  - Minor features are:
    - 'Confetti' skin lesions
    - Dental enamel pits (>3)
    - Intraoral fibromas (two or more)
    - Retinal achromic patch
    - Multiple renal cyst
    - Nonrenal hamartomas.

Ocular Features

Like elsewhere in the body, TS causes hamartomas in the retina. Retinal hamartomas (Fig. 63.2C) arise from the astrocytes (retinal astrocytic hamartomas, RAH) of the nerve fiber layer and are composed of elongated fibrous astrocytes with predilection for calcification.

They are seen in about 50% of patients with TS in at least one eye and bilaterally in about 25%.[79,80] They are usually located over or around the optic disc but can be found anywhere in the posterior pole of the fundus. RAH can also be seen in association with NF but is more frequently and more

characteristically associated with TS. Occasionally they occur in the absence of any stigmata of phakomatoses in which cases they are usually solitary and have a different clinical course (acquired retinal astrocytoma, discussed below).

Retinal astrocytic hamartomas are mostly endophytic tumors, i.e. tumors growing toward the center of the eye into the vitreous cavity but are occasionally known to be exophytic, i.e. growing away from the center of the eye into the subretinal space. They are usually small, about one-half to two disc diameters in size. There are three morphologic types of RAH described[79]: (1) Type 1 is a flat to slightly elevated, circular or oval, translucent, grayish yellow mass with indistinct borders arising from inner retina, often subtle and only recognized by the altered light reflex around it. This type is not associated with calcification and is the most common variety observed.[79,80] (2) Type 2 lesions are yellow white multi-nodular lesions with areas of chalky white calcification, having irregular surface and margins (mulberry tumors), frequently have calcium and hyaline deposits and are easily recognizable clinically. (3) Type 3 lesions have features of both, type 2 area centrally and type 1 area surrounding it. These tumors are usually nongrowing, requiring decades of follow-up to document progression, if any. Type 1 tumors can change into type 2 or 3 tumors on follow-up. Only very rarely can these tumors show progressive growth to cause confusion with retinoblastoma. They are usually asymptomatic and become symptomatic only when complications occur.

Retinal achromic patches are punched out depigmented fundal lesions found in up to 40% of patients with TS.[80] Their appearance is similar to paving stone degeneration but these occur mid-peripherally as opposed to the peripheral location of paving stone degeneration. Also, some of these lesions do not show large choroidal vessels seen through their base; instead have gray-white plaque like centers. Hyperpigmented lesions similar to those of congenital hypertrophy of retinal pigment epithelium are also known to occur in TS.

On fluorescein angiography, type 1 RAH lesions showed early hypofluorescence due to blockage and late leakage from the tumor. Type 2 and 3 RAH lesions also show late leakage but to a lesser extent as compared to type 1 lesions.[81] Sometime vessels within the tumor can also be imaged on FA. ICG angiography shows blocked fluorescence. On fundus autofluorescence type 2 and type 3 RAH show hyperautofluorescence[81] owing to their calcium and hyaline content while type 1 RAH lesions block the normal background autofluorescence.

Other ocular findings in TS include papilledema, secondary optic atrophy and paralytic squints—all secondary to intracranial hamartomas. Eyelid angiofibromas (Salmon lid), lens and irido-fundal coloboma, strabismus (nonparalytic), poliosis of eyelashes, cataracts, retinal angiomas, persistent pupillary membrane, band shaped keratopathy and sectoral iris depigmentation are also known.[80] Children with TS also have a higher incidence of hypermetropia and amblyopia.

Complications

Retinal astrocytic hamartomas are usually stationary and asymptomatic tumors or grow very slowly with growth documented only with decades of follow-up.[82] Occasionally, however, they do display aggressive behavior and may lead to a diagnostic dilemma. Of the tumors that do behave aggressively, most are located in the peripapillary location. Leakage and macular edema, lipid exudation, serous detachment, vitreous hemorrhage, vitreous seeding, neovascularization over the surface of the tumor are all reported complications of retinal astrocytic hamartomas associated with TS.[83]

In this context, acquired retinal astrocytoma requires a special mention. Unlike the congenital varieties discussed so far, these acquired tumors, although histologically benign, show a locally invasive clinical course. Whereas the congenital variety associated with TS only rarely cause the above-mentioned complications, the acquired variety often results in exudative retinal detachment, massive lipid exudation, vitreous seeding and hemorrhage, retinal vein occlusion, neovascular glaucoma and painful blind eye. Clinically, they are large gelatinous yellow-white tumors, prominently vascular and are not associated with TS. Their growth and aggressive behavior might often lead to misdiagnosis of a retinoblastoma or a tumor of choroidal origin leading to enucleation.[84,85]

Differential Diagnosis

In the setting of inner retinal tumefaction, astrocytic hamartoma is a straightforward diagnosis to make if TS in the patient is already well-established or if there are frank stigmata of the condition. But in the absence of the diagnosis of TS, differential diagnoses like retinoblastoma, medullated nerve fibers, Coat's disease, toxocariasis, toxoplasmosis, choroiditis, choroidal mass lesions, optic disc drusen, optic nerve glioma, etc. need to be considered.

Retinoblastoma is a progressive disease, can be bilateral and is associated with calcification. But Shields et al have stressed on the fact that mulberry like calcification is pathognomonic of TS and that it is only rarely that hamartomas are confused with retinoblastoma. Fine-needle aspiration and cytology may help differentiate between the two. Optic disc drusens are buried in the disc while hamartomas of the optic disc protrude above it and obscure the vessels. Optic nerve gliomas arising from the disc can also be confused with optic disc hamartomas. Cavitation within the hamartoma is reported and might lead to a misdiagnosis.

Treatment

Retinal astrocytic hamartomas are usually benign and asymptomatic tumors often requiring no treatment for the retinal hamartomas per se. But when they are progressive and associated with complications, treatment is indicated. Macular edema associated with hamartomas can be treated with bevacizumab injections.[86] Additional laser photocoagulation of the tumor can be considered if bevacizumab treatment fails or if edema recurs after stopping antivascular endothelial growth factor (VEGF) injections.[87]

The management of acquired astrocytoma remains controversial.[88] Enucleation, laser photocoagulation, cryotherapy, brachytherapy, pars plana vitrectomy and endoresection have been reported as treatment options. Recently photodynamic therapy with verteporfin has been found to be effective in the treatment of acquired retinal astrocytomas.

VON HIPPEL-LINDAU SYNDROME

Von Hippel-Lindau (VHL) syndrome also known as retinocerebellar angiomatosis is an autosomal dominant precancerous condition resulting from mutations in the tumor suppressor VHL gene and causing cystic or highly vascular tumors in multiple organ systems. Affected individuals may show hemangioblastomas of the retina and CNS, renal cysts and clear cell carcinoma of the kidney, pheochromocytoma, pancreatic cysts and neuroendocrine tumors, endolymphatic sac tumor and broad ligament and epididymal cystadenomas.[89] The disease is named after the German ophthalmologist Eugen von Hippel who first described familial retinal angiomas (*angiomatosis retinae*) and the Swedish pathologist Arvid Lindau who discovered the association between retinal, CNS and visceral lesions.

Von Hippel-Lindau syndrome is caused by a germline mutation of the *VHL* gene located on 3p25-26. About 20% have sporadic mutations and do not have a family history.[90] Genotype-phenotype correlation is complex and patients are classified as having VHL type-1 if they have deletions in the gene and as type-2 if they have missense mutations. Type-1 patients infrequently develop pheochromocytoma while in type-2 patients pheochromocytoma is common. Penetrance is age-dependent reaching about 90% by the age of 65.[90-94] It is estimated to have an incidence of 1 in 36,000 to 1 in 53,000.

Elaboration of *VHL* gene and understanding the function of its protein has helped in not only understanding of the VHL syndrome but also of tumor genesis, tumor angiogenesis and cancer biology in general.[95] The product of *VHL* gene, a 213-amino acid protein, pVHL, has pivotal role in many cellular processes and is abundantly expressed in many tissues in both fetal and adult life. Among the many functions, pVHL seems to be pivotal in the processes of regulating the proteolytic degradation of the α-subunits of the hypoxia inducible factors 1 and 2 (HIF-1 and HIF-2 transcription factors) by targeting them for ubiquitination and proteasomal degradation. Under conditions of normal tissue oxygen tension and when *VHL* gene is not mutated and the pVHL is functional, the HIF-α-subunits are rapidly degraded. In conditions of tissue hypoxia or absent/inactive pVHL, HIF-1 and HIF-2 are stabilized and activate the hypoxic gene response that consists of a large repertoire of target genes implicated in diverse processes such as angiogenesis, proliferation, apoptosis and metabolism (e.g. VEGF, PDGFb, TGFa, cyclin D1, etc.).

Systemic Features

Central nervous system hemangioblastomas are the most common tumors seen in patients with VHL syndrome affecting 60–80% of all patients. They present in about three-fourth of the patients at an average age of 33 years.[96] They are usually present infratentorial in cerebellum, spinal cord or brainstem and present with mass effect (truncal or limb ataxia being most common) or with raised intracranial pressure. They are benign tumors with variable growth rate and removal is warranted only in symptomatic and progressive tumors. Surgical removal and stereotactic radiotherapy are the available options for treatment and prognosis has improved over recent years and is generally favorable.

Clear cell renal cell carcinoma is the leading cause of mortality in patients with VHL syndrome. They are usually multiple and bilateral and can lead to distant metastases and death. Renal cysts are also common in VHL and they do not usually cause loss of renal function and have very low malignant potential. RCC is treated with nephrectomy (partial or total) and renal replacement therapy whenever necessary. Radiofrequency ablation is also an option.

Pheochromocytoma in patients with VHL may be adrenal or extraadrenal. Pancreatic cysts and neuroendocrine (nonsecreting islet cell) tumors also occur in VHL syndrome. Endolymphatic sac tumors in VHL present with tinnitus and hearing loss. Bilateral endolymphatic sac tumors are considered pathognomonic for VHL. Among the reproductive adnexal organs, epididymal cystadenoma is more common than broad ligament cystadenoma. Unlike other phakomatoses, VHL syndrome only rarely manifests cutaneous cafe-au-lait spots.

Ocular Features

The primary manifestation of VHL syndrome in the eye is in the posterior segment in the form of retinal capillary hemangioma (RCH) or retinal hemangioblastoma (Figs. 63.3 and 63.4). Anterior segment manifestations are secondary to the RCH in the retina or the optic nerve and there could also be neuro-ophthalmic manifestations like optic nerve and chiasmal compression secondary to mass effect of the tumors in the cranial cavity. About one-half of all patients with VHL have ophthalmic manifestations.[97]

Retinal capillary hemangioma is the most common manifestation of VHL and is seen in 85% of patients with VHL and is often the lesion with which patients with VHL present first to any physician.[97,98] RCH is traditionally referred in ophthalmologic literature as retinal angioma and the former is only a histopathologically more accurate description of the same

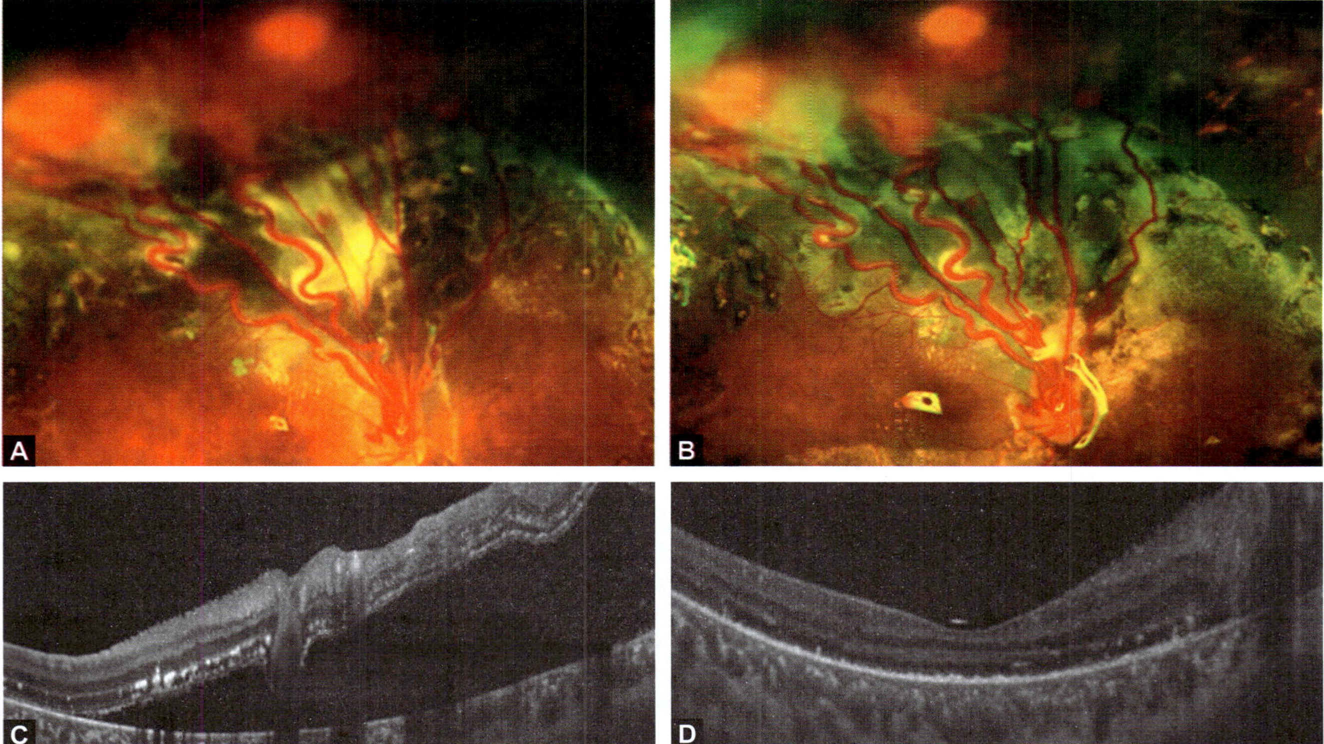

Figs. 63.3A to D: (A and C) Von Hippel angiomatosis with detached macula, dilated feeder vessels and extensive subretinal exudation on color picture and OCT (with presenting visual acuity as only hand motions close to face); (B and D) Postoperatively, at 6 weeks postvitrectomy the exudation has markedly reduced and macula is attached (visual acuity improved to 6/60).
(OCT: Optical Coherence Tomography).

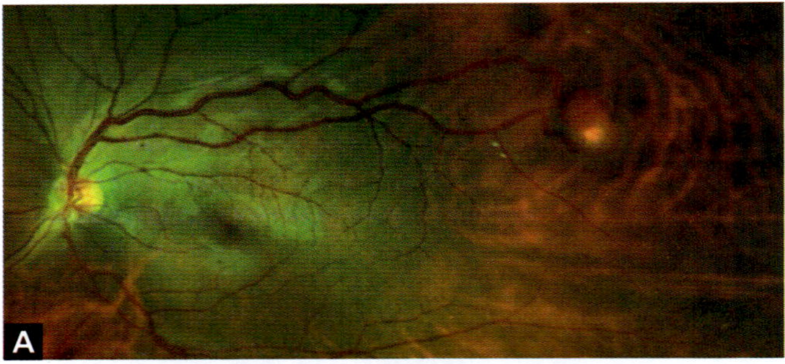

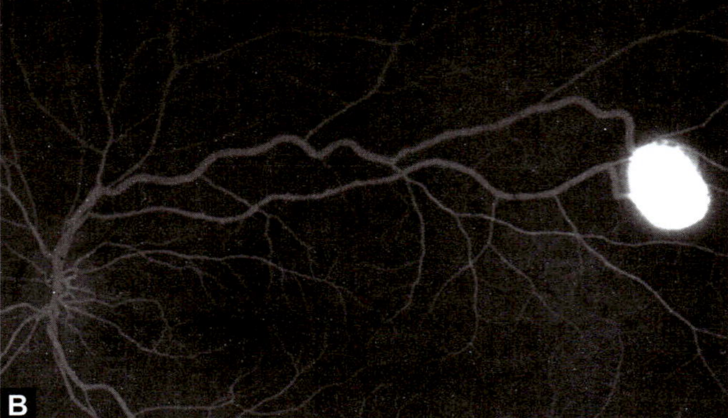

Figs. 63.4A and B: (A) Widefield imaging (Optos P200MA, Optos PLC) of the fundus showing a retinal capillary hemangioma along with dilated tortuous vessels feeding and draining the lesion. (B) Corresponding fundus fluorescein angiography shows a solitary hyperintense lesion with leakage into surrounding tissue. The lesion was asymptomatic and was detected on routine examination.

lesion. They are usually solitary tumors being bilateral in about half of the patients and multiple in about a third. They usually present in the 3rd decade of life but can be noted in adolescence and childhood in some.

Clinically, they are orange-red well-circumscribed nodular retinal lesions with dilated tortuous vessels feeding and draining them (Fig. 63.4A and B). They are mostly located in the periphery (superotemporal and inferotemporal quadrants being the most frequently involved) but peripapillary location is also well known. Distinguishing a vein from an arteriole around these lesions is often difficult. Even RCH as small as 1.5 mm in diameter located in the periphery are associated with prominent retinal vessels emerging from the optic disc and this can be used as a hint to identify the peripherally located tumor.

Morphologically there are three types of RCH noted— exophytic, endophytic and sessile. A peripapillary exophytic RCH may be difficult to distinguish from chronic papilledema and a sessile variant may be often too subtle and missed. Based on their secondary effect on the retina they could be classified as exudative or tractional. The exudative variety leaks fluid and lipids into the retina and subretinal space (Figs. 63.4A and B). The tractional variety can cause epiretinal glial proliferation and lead to tractional retinal detachments

or macular pucker. In late stages, total retinal detachment, peripheral retinal ischemia, neovascularization of retina and iris, vitreous hemorrhage, cataract and painful blind eye can occur. Other reported manifestations of VHL in the eye are vascular hamartomas of the retina and retinal 'twin vessels.' The twin vessels are defined as a paired retinal arteriole and venule that are separated by less than the diameter of one venule. Twin vessels are of normal caliber and look like normal retinal vessels except for their course. Retinal neovascularization mimicking proliferative diabetic retinopathy has also been described.[97]

Von Hippel-Lindau syndrome accounts for over 50% of RCH. The rest of them are not associated with VHL (a germline mutation) but are associated with acquired VHL gene mutation and usually present later in life than the VHL associated hemangiomas. Multiple tumors are likely to be associated with VHL syndrome and may be an indication for genetic testing in patients who do not show any other signs of VHL syndrome on workup.

Most RCH are progressive but a minority can remain stable for many years or even spontaneously regress with gliosis. A progressive RCH has been classified into four stages by Vail.[98,99]

- *Stage I*: Stage of dilation of feeding and draining vessels and RCH formation.
- *Stage II*: Stage of development of hemorrhages and exudation.
- *Stage III*: Stage of exudation and retinal detachment.
- *Stage IV*: Stage of uveitis, absolute glaucoma, and loss of the eye.

A reddish nodular retinal lesion with associated exudation and dilated vessels do not lead to any diagnostic differentials but differentials (Figs. 63.5A and B) may need to be considered when the RCH is small or when the hemangioma is obscured by vitreous hemorrhage or exudative detachment.

Coats' disease, racemose hemangioma, retinal cavernous hemangioma and retinal artery microaneurysms are the usual differentials that may mimic clinical findings of RCH. Coats' disease is a unilateral disease in young male patients with telangiectatic vessels and no localized nodular proliferation. The family history and the other clinical findings of VHL are lacking in Coats. In racemose hemangioma, the abnormal vessels do not lead to an angioma and there is no exudation. Cavernous hemangioma lacks feeder vessels and exudation and retinal microaneurysms are usually present in the posterior pole and present with subretinal or intraretinal hemorrhage more frequently than exudation. Rarely retinal vasoproliferative tumor, retinal pigment epithelial adenoma and uveal melanoma with retinal invasion may mimic a RCH.

On fluorescein angiography, the RCH has fine capillary filling which rapidly becomes homogenous. There is progressive hyperfluorescence (Figs. 63.6 and 63.7) with late leakage of dye into the surrounding structures. Fluorescein angiography is especially helpful in establishing the diagnosis of juxtapapillary RCH by revealing the fine vascular pattern on the

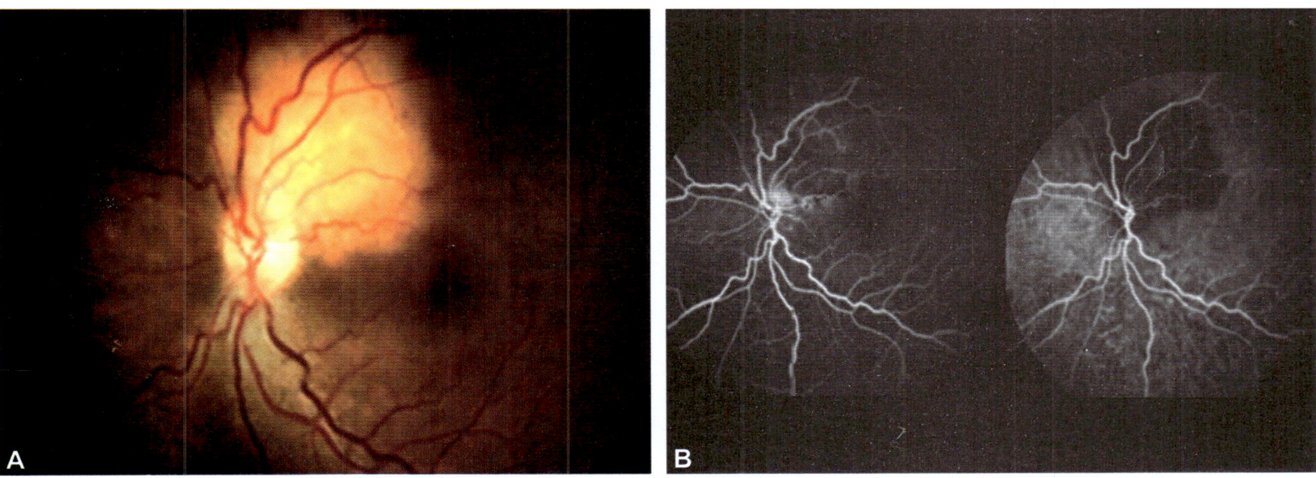

Figs. 63.5A and B: (A) Choroidal osteoma; (B) Choroidal osteoma revealing hypofluorescence on FA and ICG, a differential diagnosis of hemangioma.
(FA: Fluorescein angiography; ICG: Indocyanine green).

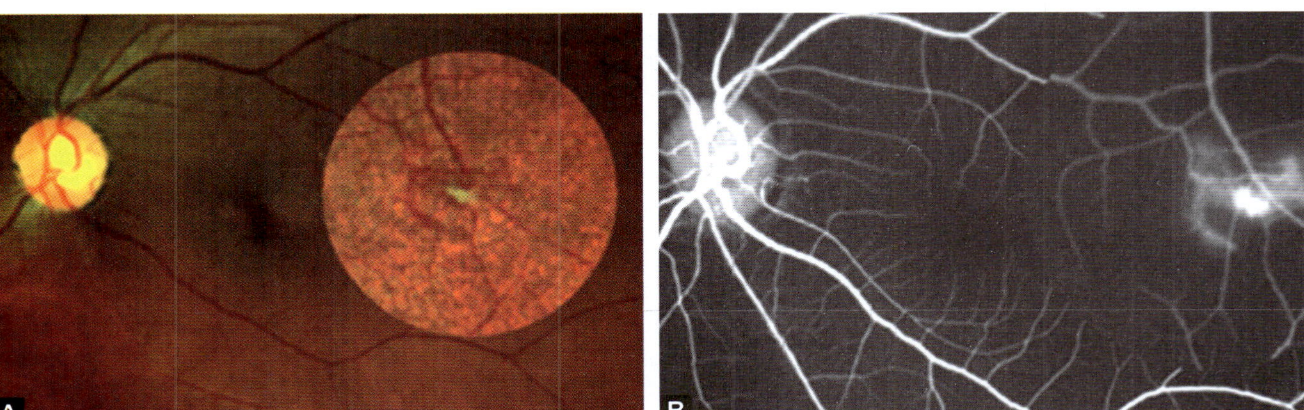

Figs. 63.6A and B: (A) Retinal capillary angioma in a patient with VHL (using enhancement on the UWF device); (B) Fluorescein angiogram of the angioma showing late leakage into surrounding structures.

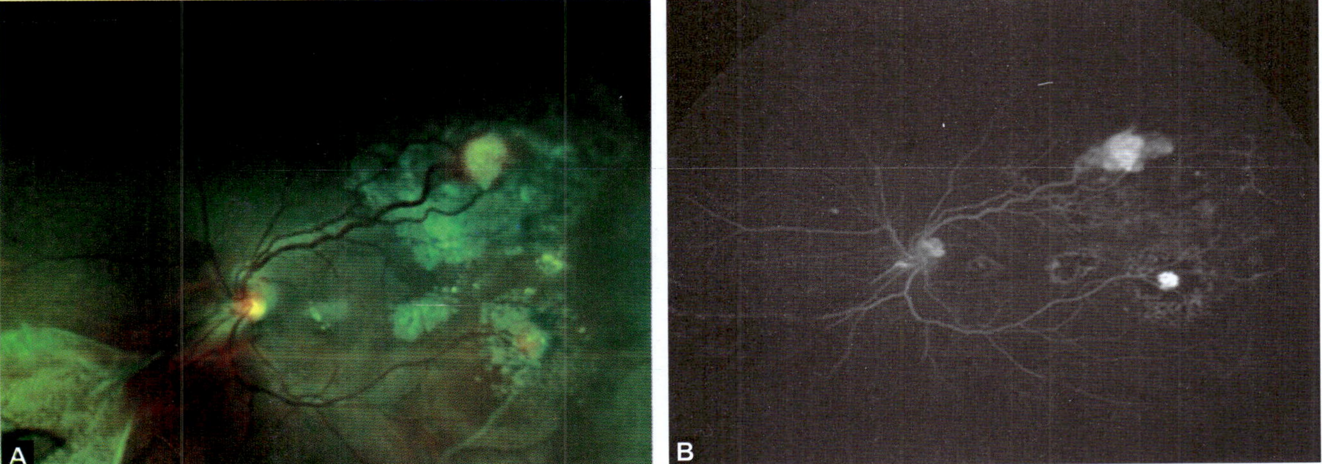

Figs. 63.7A and B: (A) Ultra-widefield imaging and (B) fluorescein angiography (Optos P200MA, Optos PLC, Dunfermline, Scotland, UK) in a patient of VHL with multiple lasered retinal capillary hemangiomas. Note the quiescent untreated superonasal angiomas. Note the exudative superotemporal lesions and the tractional inferonasal lesions.

angiogram. On A-scan ultrasonography the tumor shows high internal reflectivity.

Histopathologically these tumors are composed of thin vascular capillary-like channels lined by endothelial cells and pericytes and separated by foamy stromal cells, which is identical to the histopathological features of CNS hemangioblastomas. It is believed that the true neoplastic components are the stromal cells which harbor the VHL mutation.

Diagnostic Criterion

When a patient comes to the ophthalmologist with a RCH it is important to rule in or rule out VHL in a patient for subsequent management and screening of the patient and at risk family. If there is a confirmed family history of VHL disease, a diagnosis of VHL disease can be made by finding a single VHL tumor (e.g. RCH or central nervous system hemangioblastoma, clear cell RCC, pheochromocytoma, pancreatic endocrine tumor or endolymphatic sac tumor) in an at-risk relative. All of the tumors typically found in VHL disease can occur as a sporadic (nonfamilial) event and so a clinical diagnosis of VHL disease in a patient without a positive family history requires the presence of two tumors (e.g. two hemangioblastomas or a hemangioblastoma and a visceral tumor).

Treatment

The decision to treat retinal capillary hemangioma and the method of management is determined by various factors like the size, location and number of the lesions; associated findings such as extent of subretinal fluid, evidence of retinal traction, and overall effect or threat of the clinical findings on the visual potential of the eye. The available treatment options are observation, laser photocoagulation, cryotherapy, photodynamic therapy, plaque radiotherapy, vitreoretinal surgery, anti-VEGF agents. Electrolysis and diathermy are only of historical interest and are not discussed.[99]

1. *Observation:*[100] Small RCHs (<500 μm) without associated exudation or vessel tortuosity especially the ones on the nasal side with less risk of visual deterioration can be observed. Peripapillary RCHs also are candidates for observation in view of their different biologic behavior and since treating them entails significant risk of visual loss due to damage to the optic disc. But more and more authorities prefer to treat all RCHs irrespective of size and progression.
2. *Laser photocoagulation:*[101] Lasers can be used to treat small posterior RCHs. Lasers are preferred modality due to their precision, repeatability, smaller spot size and the ability to use different wavelengths.[102] Two strategies are generally used during photocoagulation—application directly to the tumor or to the feeder artery. Direct treatment of the angioma has a potential risk of causing hemorrhage and exudative detachment; therefore, some prefer treatment of the feeding arteriole. Laser treatment causes transient increase in exudation which is termed as 'ablatio fugax'. Pre- and postoperative steroids may be

tried to reduce this phenomenon. Multiple sittings may be necessary to achieve complete regression of the RCH. Argon, krypton, diode, and yellow dye laser have been used and currently frequency doubled Nd:YAG is also used.

3. *Photodynamic therapy (PDT):* Concentrating the verteporfin dye into the angiomatous tumor and applying 689 nm wavelength diode laser causes release of singlet oxygen and oxidative damage to the angioma with variable results. At our centre, when laser photocoagulation shows minimal effect in large angiomas, we have occasionally tried full fluence PDT to such lesions.
4. *Cryotherapy:* Cryotherapy is another mainstay ablative procedure for the treatment of RCHs. It is usually used in tumors larger than 3 mm in size, peripheral and in RCHs associated with significant subretinal fluid in which case laser reaction might be weak. At least two cycles of freeze-thaw are recommended. The entire angioma needs to be frozen before thawing is begun. Cryotherapy may be associated with lesser increase in posttreatment exudation.
5. *Anti-VEGF:* As has been discussed earlier, the molecular mechanism of tumorigenesis in VHL involves VEGF and many angiogenic factors. This knowledge was tried in the treatment of RCH in the form of systemic and intravitreal anti-VEGF therapy. Systemic anti-VEGF therapy with SU5416, a VEGFR2 inhibitor did not show promising results. Intravitreal bevacizumab and ranibizumab also do not cause any change in the tumor size but have been used to treat the macular edema and reduce the exudation associated with the condition. They may have a special role in optic disc and macular hemangiomas.[103,104]
6. *Surgery:* Pars plana vitrectomy is usually necessary in cases of tractional retinal detachment and in cases with vitreous hemorrhage. Advanced VHL disease with exudative detachment and treatment resistant RCH has also been subjected to PPV with poor late postoperative results in view of progressive disease.[105]
7. *Others:* Other modalities are generally reserved for large RCHs (more than 4.5 mm in diameter). Photodynamic therapy with verteporfin and doubled light exposure with/without simultaneous anti-VEGF agent has been reported. Transpupillary thermotherapy[106] uses diode laser to increase the temperature within the tumor and cause tumor destruction. This modality has been used in peripapillary RCH but can cause optic atrophy. Plaque brachytherapy, external beam radiotherapy, and proton beam radiotherapy all have been used with plaque brachytherapy showing favorable results in large RCHs. Anecdotal reports of response to oral propranolol, acetazolamide and oral prednisone are also present.

Screening

Screening of patients and at risk relatives is important to prevent avoidable morbidity and mortality and increase life expectancy. Early diagnosis of most VHL complications improves prognosis and all VHL patients and at risk relatives should be enrolled into a comprehensive screening program in childhood. Since retinal hemangioblastomas are one of the earliest lesions noted, screening for them should begin in infancy or early childhood and a comprehensive ophthalmic examination including direct and indirect ophthalmoscopy should be done. Screening for CNS hemangioblastoma starts in adolescence with MRI scans of the head every 12–36 months. Annual screening for renal cell carcinoma and pancreatic tumors is done with MRI scans or ultrasound, although CT is more sensitive in picking up renal tumors, to avoid cumulative radiation dose. Pheochromocytoma screening strategy varies based on the risk of this tumor in the kindred (See genotypic types discussed earlier) and can vary from annual blood pressure monitoring and urinary metanephrines to annual adrenal imaging beginning from the age of 8 years.

Sturge-Weber Syndrome

Sturge-Weber syndrome is a neurocutaneous disorder characterized by avascular malformation involving the skin, eye, and brain. It consists of facial port-wine stain (PWS) involving the ophthalmic division of the trigeminal nerve, ipsilateral buphthalmos and vascular abnormalities of the eye along with ipsilateral leptomeningeal angioma affecting primarily the occipital cortex.[107-109] It is also called as encephalofacial angiomatosis. Unlike other phakomatoses, SWS is a sporadic condition with no inheritance pattern or family history, although genes responsible for the condition, such as *RASA1* and *GNAQ* genes have recently been identified.[110,111] It is a heterogenous condition with a spectrum of clinical manifestations which can range from isolated brain involvement, isolated eye involvement, eye and skin or eye and brain involvement, to PWS associated with both brain and skin involvement.[112] The incidence varies from 1 in 20,000 to 1 in 50,000. What we today know as SWS was first described in 1860 by Schirmer as an association between facial angioma and ipsilateral buphthalmos.[109] William Alan Sturge in 1879 described the association of this condition with the neurological manifestations and in 1922 Parkes Weber provided the radiological details to prove that ipsilateral leptomeningeal vascular abnormality was the cause of the contralateral neurological features.

Embryologically, the ectoderm forming the upper facial skin is in close proximity with the neuroectoderm which later forms the parieto-occipital lobes. It is hypothesized that an acquired somatic mutation in the precursor of the primitive venous plexus in this region leads to faulty regression/maturation of the plexus in the first trimester and leads to the vascular lesion of the SWS.[108,109,113]

Systemic Features

Facial PWS (i.e. nevus flammeus) is a characteristic manifestation of SWS but is also commonly present in many infants without SWS. PWS occurs in about 0.3% of all live births and the overall risk of SWS associated with *any kind* of facial cutaneous vascular malformation is approximately 8%. The risk varies with the extent of the cutaneous malformation with the ones affecting the entire V1 dermatome having a risk of SWS of up to 78% and minor/partial involvement of V1 segment having a risk of about 26%.[114] SWS is also reported with PWS in sites apart from the usual cephalofacial location. Bilateral PWS increases the risk of associated SWS. PWS is a venous-capillary vascular malformation and can cause maxillary hypertrophy, facial asymmetry, lid hypertrophy and conjunctival hyperplasia, amblyopia, sinus and ENT problems and dental problems.

Leptomeningeal angiomatosis is another important feature of SWS. They are usually unilateral, located over the occipital cortex, associated with calcification and lead to neurological signs and symptoms based on the location. About 15% of patients have bilateral leptomeningeal angiomas. Pathologically they consist of abnormally dilated and tortuous pial vessels with thickened leptomeninges and abnormality in underlying cortical venous drainage leading to venous ischemia of the brain and long-term atrophy of the brain. Neurological features include intractable seizures, hemiparesis and stroke-like episodes, migraine-like headache, behavioral problems, cognitive impairment, mental retardation, and visual field defects. About 75–100% of patients have seizures and are usually partial motor.[115]

Classic neuroimaging sign described in older children with SWS on X-ray skull is the 'tram-track calcification'. Currently the modality of choice for imaging is contrast-enhanced MRI imaging which shows leptomeningeal changes with enlargement of transmedullary and periventricular veins, associated dilation and enhancement of the choroid plexus on the involved side, dilated deep draining venous vessels underlying the affected cortical region. In advanced cases, atrophy and calcification are evident.

Ocular Features

Sturge-Weber syndrome affects the eye in about 50% of the cases and leads to vascular malformation in the periorbital skin and in conjunctiva, episclera, retina and choroid. Eyelid hemangioma, episcleral hemangioma, dilated conjunctival and episcleral vessels, heterochromia iridis are known manifestations of SWS in the eye. The circulation of the eye is usually affected if the ipsilateral upper eyelid skin is involved in the PWS (Anderson's rule).

Glaucoma is the most important ocular feature of SWS. 30–70% of patients with SWS will develop glaucoma.[116] Glaucoma is almost always unilateral and ipsilateral to the PWS, although contralateral or bilateral glaucoma with unilateral cutaneous lesions have been reported. The risk is higher when the PWS involves both the upper and the lower eyelids or when it involves more than one segment of the trigeminal nerve or if there are bilateral PWS. Presentation is trimodal, with the first peak being the largest within 1 year of birth, second peak between 5-8 years and the third peak after 20 years.[117] The early form of the disease is caused by maldevelopment of the angle much like primary congenital glaucoma with similar gonioscopic findings.[118,119] The late onset glaucomas are usually a result of elevated episcleral venous pressure or angle closure due to forward displacement of ciliary body because of choroidal hemangioma. Neovascular glaucoma in cases of chronic exudative detachment is also known. Hypersecretion of aqueous is another hypothesis for the glaucoma caused by SWS. Whatever be the mechanism, uncontrolled pressures lead to optic neuropathy and field loss. Management is challenging, often requiring surgical intervention. Goniotomy and trabeculotomy are first-line surgical treatment in infants but results are often poor requiring filtering procedures. But filtering procedures have high-risk of choroidal hemorrhage owing to the presence of a hemangioma in the choroid. Preprocedural management of the choroidal hemangioma may reduce the risk of expulsive hemorrhage.

Choroidal hemangiomas are of two types—diffuse and focal or circumscribed. SWS is associated with the diffuse variety of choroidal hemangioma and is present in as many as 40–50% of the patients.[116] They are usually present at birth, ipsilateral to the side of the PWS and are associated with an orange-colored diffuse choroidal elevation and a bright red pupillary reflex in the involved eye called the 'tomato ketchup' fundus. Normal choroidal markings are obscured and this may be the only sign seen in early cases. There may be associated retinal vein tortuosity and varying degree of pigmentary changes. Focal hemangiomas can occasionally be seen along with a diffuse hemangioma. There may also be focal areas of nodularity in a diffuse hemangioma mimicking a solitary focal hemangioma. Hyperopia, exudative detachment, overlying choriocapillary and RPE atrophy are the usual causes of vision loss in SWS. On ultrasound B scan they show diffuse choroidal thickening with overlying retinal detachment and A scan shows high internal reflectivity. On fluorescein angiography (Figs. 63.8A to C) they show early hypofluorescence

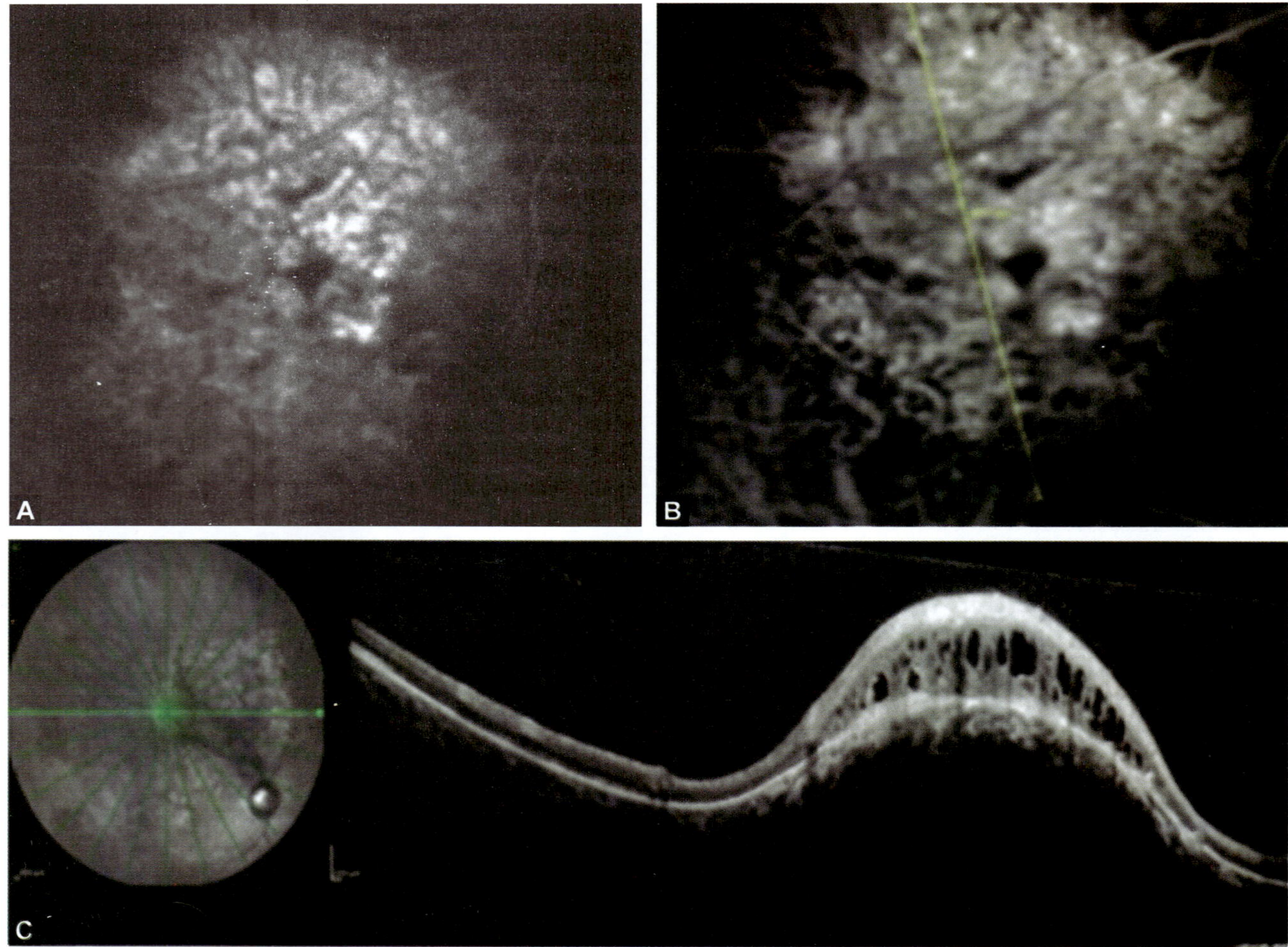

Figs. 63.8A to C: Solitary hemangioma showing hyperfluorescence on (A) FFA and (B) ICG. (C) OCT reveals a choroidal mound with internal reflectivity and overlying cystic retina in a patient with SWS.
(FFA: Fundus fluorescein angiography; ICG: Indocyanine green angiography; OCT: Optical coherence tomography; SWS: Sturge–Weber syndrome).

and late dye leakage. The choroidal angiomatosis grows slowly and usually remains asymptomatic in childhood. During adolescence or adulthood, marked thickening of the choroid sometimes becomes evident with secondary changes in the overlying ocular structures.

Treatment options for symptomatic diffuse choroidal hemangioma includes external beam radiation therapy, proton beam therapy, brachytherapy, photodynamic therapy and possibly anti-VEGF therapy.[120]

- Low-dose lens sparing external beam radiation therapy can help in the resolution of subretinal fluid with minimal effects on tumor size. But late complications like subretinal fibrosis due to RPE metaplasia can lead to dramatic loss of visual acuity.[121]
- Plaque brachytherapy using ruthenium-106 plaques and cobalt-60 applicators have been reported to be of benefit in cases of diffuse choroidal hemangioma with total resorption of fluid, flattening of the tumor, no recurrence of exudation and no radiation-related adverse effects.[122-124]
- Proton beam radiotherapy delivers a homogenous dose of radiation avoiding neighboring structures and provides an advantage over external beam radiotherapy and plaque brachytherapy. Favorable results have been found even in children with diffuse choroidal hemangioma.[125-127]
- Anti-VEGF agents (bevacizumab and pegaptanib) have been used singly or in combination with PDT for exudation associated with SWS. Favorable results have been reported.[128-130]
- Photodynamic therapy (PDT) has multiple reports for circumscribed choroidal hemangioma but has also been tried for the diffuse variety with good success. Multiple spots need to be given to cover the entire area of hemangioma which covers more than half of the fundus.[120,131-133]
- Oral propranolol is a newer modality of treatment reported for diffuse choroidal hemangioma. Propranolol use in infantile capillary hemangioma is well-established although the mechanism of action is not completely elucidated. Similar effect is also reported in choroidal diffuse hemangioma associated with SWS.[134,135]

As soon as SWS is first suspected or documented, a complete ophthalmological evaluation is essential to rule out glaucoma. Infants need to be on a frequent screening program, the frequency of which can be tapered as the child grows old but needs to be continued well into adulthood when annual comprehensive examination may suffice.

OTHER PHAKOMATOSES

Racemose Hemangiomatosis

Like SWS, Racemose hemangiomatosis is a sporadic condition. Cutaneous manifestations are very few. This condition leads to abnormal arteriovenous communications in the retina, midbrain, maxilla, mandible and the calvarial bones. When retinal lesion is associated with ipsilateral midbrain racemose hemangiomas, it is known as Wyburn-Mason syndrome. About 30% of patients with retinal findings have a brain finding while only about 8% of the patients with brain lesions have a corresponding retinal lesion. The brain lesion usually presents with hemorrhage causing stroke or a focal neurological deficit in a young adult. The retinal lesion is classified by Archer into three groups. In Group 1, there is an abnormal capillary bed between the dilated arteriole and venule and there are usually no symptoms and CNS manifestations are rare. In Group 2 lesions, there is direct communication between artery and vein but usually asymptomatic and can be associated with CNS lesions. In Group 3, there are extensive arteriovenous communications often associated with vision loss. There are dilated arteries and veins arising from the disc in this group. These lesions do not leak on fluorescein angiography and there is no exudation clinically. There is a risk of vitreous hemorrhage and BRVO in Group 3 lesions. They are treated with vitrectomy and anti-VEGFs respectively.

Klippel-Trenaunay Syndrome

The Klippel-Trenaunay syndrome (KTS) is a rare sporadic multisystem disorder with a characteristic triad of PWS, varicose veins, and bony and soft-tissue hypertrophy. When this clinical picture is associated with arteriovenous shunting the condition has also been called the Parkes Weber syndrome.[136] The PWS in KTS is distributed in the limbs and trunk and rarely on the face. Many authors consider KTS and SWS to be similar diseases on the same spectrum. The most common ophthalmic abnormality seen associated with KTS is choroidal hemangioma and glaucoma, like is seen in SWS. Other ocular abnormalities reported include conjunctival telangiectasia, orbital varix, strabismus, oculosympathetic palsy, Marcus-Gunn pupil, iris coloboma and heterocromia, cataracts, persistent fetal vasculature, chiasmal and bilateral optic nerve gliomas, drusen of the optic disc, acquired myelination of the retinal nerve fiber layer, and retinal dysplasia with astrocytic proliferation of the nerve. Treatment of the condition is similar to SWS.

Phakomatosis Pigmentovascularis

Phakomatosis pigmentovascularis (PPV) was first described by Ota et al. in 1947. It is a condition associated with port-wine stain (PWS) and pigmentary nevi involving the eye (ocular melanocytosis) or the face and body (oculodermal melanocytosis).[136] The pigmentary nevus can be a Mongolian spot or a nevus of Ota. Nevus of Ota (i.e. ocular melanocytosis) is when the skin along the ophthalmic, maxillary, and rarely the mandibular branch of the trigeminal nerve is involved and if the hyperpigmentation only involves the eye it is termed melanosis oculi. It is often found in association with SWS or KTS. The pathophysiology is thought to be defective migration of neural crest cells.

Ophthalmic manifestations in PPV include hyperpigmentation of the ocular structures that contain melanin like the conjunctiva, sclera, episclera, iris, choroid and the trabecular meshwork. Iris mammillations are also found in association with melanosis oculi which can be confused with Lisch nodules typical of NF type 1. 10% of patients with oculodermal melanocytosis present with glaucoma and the mechanism can be due to angle hyperpigmentation or the increase in aqueous outflow resistance due to melanocytes or due to abnormal neural crest development which leads to anomalous anterior chamber angle. Patients with oculodermal melanocytosis especially with melanocytosis of the fundus have a greater risk to develop melanoma of the uvea and conjunctiva, 1 in 400 white patients with oculodermal melanocytosis with respect to 6 per million for the general population.

Organoid Nevus Syndrome

Organoid nevus syndrome is an atypical phakomatoses because it is a condition that gives rise to complex choristomas (abnormal mass of histologically normal tissue in an unexpected location) as opposed to hamartomas seen in all other phakomatoses. The genetics is also not well understood and therefore it is more appropriately only classified as a neurocutaneous syndrome and not a phakomatoses. The features in this condition include the sebaceous nevus of Jadassohn, cerebral atrophy, arachnoidal cyst, epibulbar complex choristoma, eyelid coloboma, posterior calcified scleral cartilage, cardiac and renal abnormalities including patent ductus arteriosus, ventricular septal defect, coarctation of the aorta, nephroblastomatosis, horseshoe kidney, vitamin D-resistant rickets and liver cysts.

The significant ocular manifestations apart from epibulbar choristomas include a posterior scleral cartilage. This lesion is present in infancy and produces a peculiar yellow-white discoloration of the fundus in the area of involvement and needs to be differentiated from other conditions such as retinoblastoma and choroidal osteoma. CT scan shows a bone density plaque at the level of the choroid and sclera that corresponds to cartilage in the posterior sclera and not bone as seen with an osteoma.

REFERENCES

1. Shields JA, Shields CL. Systemic hamartomatoses ("Phakomatoses"). In: Shields JA, Shields CL (Eds). Intraocular tumors. A Text and Atlas. WB Saunders; 1992. pp. 513-39.
2. Traboulsi EI, Singh AD. The Phakomatoses. In: Albert DM, Miller JW, Azar DT, Blodi BA, Cohan JE, Perkins T (Eds). Albert and Jakobiec's Principles and Practice of Ophthalmology. New York: Saunders Elsevier; 2008. pp. 5009-24.
3. Hoeve V der. The Doyne memorial lecture. Eye symptoms in phakomatoses. Trans Ophthalmology Soc U K. 1932;52:380-401.
4. Palena PV, Augsburger JJ. Phakomatoses. In: Tasman W, Jaeger EA (Eds). Duane's Clinical Ophthalmology on CD-ROM. Philadelphia, US: Lippincott Williams & Wilkins; 2005.
5. Developmental diseases of the nervous system. In: Ropper A, Samuels M, Klein J (Eds). Adams and Victor's Principles of Neurology, 10th Edition. New York: McGraw Hill Professional; 2014. pp. 1012-3.
6. L. Flores-Sarnat, HB Sarnat. Embryology of neurocutaneous syndromes. In: Ruggieri M, Castroviejo IP, Rocco CD (Eds). Neurocutaneous Disorders: Phakomatoses & Hamartoneoplastic Syndromes. Berlin: Springer Science & Business Media; 2009. pp. 1-17.
7. Tucker M, Goldstein A, Dean M, et al. National Cancer Institute Workshop Report: The Phakomatoses Revisited. J Natl Cancer Inst. 2000;92(7):530-3.
8. Augsburger JJ, Bolliing JP. Phakomatoses. In: Yanoff M, Duker JS (Eds). Ophthalmology. New York: Elsevier Health Sciences; 2009. pp. 937-42.
9. Hoeve V der. Eye symptoms in tuberous sclerosis of the brain. Trans Ophthalmology Soc UK. 1920;20:329-34.
10. Sarnat HB, Flores-Sarnat L. Embryology of the neural crest: its inductive role in the neurocutaneous syndromes. J Child Neurol. 2005;20(8):637-43.
11. Delaney SP, Julian LM, Stanford WL. The neural crest lineage as a driver of disease heterogeneity in Tuberous Sclerosis Complex and Lymphangioleiomyomatosis. Front Cell Dev Biol. 2014;2:69.
12. Korf BR. The phakomatoses. Clin Dermatol. 2005;23(1):78-84.
13. Evans DG, Howard E, Giblin C, et al. Birth incidence and prevalence of tumor-prone syndromes: estimates from a UK family genetic register service. Am J Med Genet A. 2010;152A(2):327-32.
14. Huson SM, Harper PS, Compston DA. Von Recklinghausen neurofibromatosis.A clinical and population study in south-east Wales. Brain J Neurol. 1988;111(Pt 6):1355-81.
15. Friedman JM. Neurofibromatosis 1. In: Pagon RA, Adam MP, Ardinger HH, Wallace SE, Amemiya A, Bean LJ (Eds). GeneReviews(®) [Internet]. Seattle (WA): University of Washington, Seattle; 1993. [online] Available from: http://www.ncbi.nlm.nih.gov/books/NBK1109/ [Accessed December, 2017].
16. Lau N, Feldkamp MM, Roncari L, et al. Loss of neurofibromin is associated with activation of RAS/MAPK and PI3-K/AKT signaling in a neurofibromatosis 1 astrocytoma. J Neuropathol Exp Neurol. 2000;59(9):759-67.
17. Recklinghausen F von. Ueber die multiplen Fibrome der Haut und ihre Beziehung zu den multiplen Neuromen: Festschrift zur Feier des fünfundzwanzigjährigen Bestehens des pathologischen Instituts zu Berlin Herrn Rudolf Virchow [Internet]. Berlin : A. Hirschwald; 1882. p. 170. [online] Available from: http://archive.org/details/ueberdiemultiple00reck [Accessed December, 2017].
18. Neurofibromatosis. Conference statement. National Institutes of Health Consensus Development Conference. Arch Neurol. 1988;45(5):575-8.
19. Rubinstein LJ. The malformative central nervous system lesions in the central and peripheral forms of neurofibromatosis.A neuropathological study of 22 cases. Ann NY Acad Sci. 1986;486:14-29.
20. Evans DGR, Baser ME, McGaughran J, et al. Malignant peripheral nerve sheath tumours in neurofibromatosis 1. J Med Genet. 2002;39(5):311-4.
21. Ferner RE, Huson SM, Thomas N, et al. Guidelines for the diagnosis and management of individuals with neurofibromatosis 1. J Med Genet. 2007;44(2):81-8.
22. Ferner RE. The neurofibromatoses. Pract Neurol. 2010;10(2):82-93.
23. Korf BR. Diagnostic outcome in children with multiple café au lait spots. Pediatrics. 1992;90(6):924-7.
24. Crawford AH, Schorry EK. Neurofibromatosis in children: the role of the orthopaedist. J Am Acad Orthop Surg. 1999;7(4):217-30.
25. Friedman JM, Arbiser J, Epstein JA, et al. Cardiovascular disease in neurofibromatosis 1: Report of the NF1 Cardiovascular Task Force. Genet Med. 2002;4(3):105-11.
26. Huson S, Jones D, Beck L. Ophthalmic manifestations of neurofibromatosis. Br J Ophthalmology. 1987;71(3):235-8.

27. Oystreck DT, Morales J, Chaudhry I, et al. Visual loss in orbitofacial neurofibromatosis type 1. Ophthalmology. 2012;119(10):2168-73.

28. Lubs ML, Bauer MS, Formas ME, et al. Lisch nodules in neurofibromatosis type 1. N Engl J Med. 1991;324(18):1264-6.

29. Lisch K. Ueber Beteiligung der Augen, insbesondere das Vorkommen von Irisknötchen bei der Neurofibromatose (Recklinghausen). Ophthalmologica. 1937;93(3):137-43.

30. A Richetta SG. Lisch nodules of the iris in neurofibromatosis type 1. J Eur Acad Dermatol Venereol JEADV. 2004;18(3):342-4.

31. Lewis RA, Riccardi VM. Von Recklinghausen neurofibromatosis. Incidence of iris hamartomata. Ophthalmology. 1981;88(4):348-54.

32. Erb MH, Uzcategui N, See RF, et al. Orbitotemporal neurofibromatosis: classification and treatment. Orbit Amst Neth. 2007;26(4):223-8.

33. Lee V, Ragge NK, Collin JRO. Orbitotemporal neurofibromatosis. Clinical features and surgical management. Ophthalmology. 2004;111(2):382-8.

34. Jackson IT, Carbonnel A, Potparic Z, et al. Orbitotemporal neurofibromatosis: classification and treatment. Plast Reconstr Surg. 1993;92(1):1-11.

35. Altan-Yaycioglu R, Hintschich C. Clinical features and surgical management of orbitotemporal neurofibromatosis: a retrospective interventional case series. Orbit Amst Neth. 2010;29(5):232-8.

36. Morales J, Chaudhry IA, Bosley TM. Glaucoma and globe enlargement associated with neurofibromatosis type 1. Ophthalmology. 2009;116(9):1725-30.

37. Edward DP, Morales J, Bouhenni RA, et al. Congenital ectropion uvea and mechanisms of glaucoma in neurofibromatosis type 1: new insights. Ophthalmology. 2012;119(7):1485-94.

38. Oystreck DT, Alorainy IA, Morales J, et al. Ocular motility abnormalities in orbitofacial neurofibromatosis type 1. J AAPOS Off Publ Am Assoc Pediatr Ophthalmology Strabismus Am Assoc Pediatr Ophthalmology Strabismus. 2014;18(4):338-43.

39. Listernick R, Ferner RE, Liu GT, et al. Optic pathway gliomas in neurofibromatosis-1: controversies and recommendations. Ann Neurol. 2007;61(3):189-98.

40. King A, Listernick R, Charrow J, et al. Optic pathway gliomas in neurofibromatosis type 1: the effect of presenting symptoms on outcome. Am J Med Genet A. 2003;122A(2):95-9.

41. Listernick R, Louis DN, Packer RJ, et al. Optic pathway gliomas in children with neurofibromatosis 1: consensus statement from the NF1 Optic Pathway Glioma Task Force. Ann Neurol. 1997;41(2):143-9.

42. Cassiman C, Legius E, Spileers W, et al. Ophthalmological assessment of children with neurofibromatosis type 1. Eur J Pediatr. 2013;172(10):1327-33.

43. Avery RA, Hwang EI, Jakacki RI, et al. Marked recovery of vision in children with optic pathway gliomas treated with bevacizumab. JAMA Ophthalmology. 2014;132(1):111-4.

44. Yasunari T, Shiraki K, Hattori H, et al. Frequency of choroidal abnormalities in neurofibromatosis type 1. Lancet Lond Engl. 2000;356(9234):988-92.

45. Klein RM, Glassman L. Neurofibromatosis of the choroid. Am J Ophthalmology. 1985;99(3):367-8.

46. Byun YS, Park YH. Indocyanine green angiographic findings of obscure choroidal abnormalities in neurofibromatosis. Korean J Ophthalmology KJO. 2012;26(3):230-4.

47. Makino S, Tampo H. Choroidal abnormalities in a patient with neurofibromatosis type 1. Intern Med Tokyo Jpn. 2013;52(12):1445-6.

48. Dansingani KK, Jung JJ, Belinsky I, et al. Ischemic retinopathy in neurofibromatosis type 1. Retin Cases Brief Rep. 2015;9(4):290-4.

49. Al Freihi SH, Edward DP, Nowilaty SR, et al. Iris neovascularization and neovascular glaucoma in neurofibromatosis type 1: report of 3 cases in children. J Glaucoma. 2013;22(4):336-41.

50. Fichi F, Morara M, Lembo A, et al. Neovascular Glaucoma Induced by Peripheral Retinal Ischemia in Neurofibromatosis Type 1: Management and Imaging Features. Case Rep Ophthalmology. 2013;4(1):69-73.

51. Baser ME, Friedman JM, Wallace AJ, et al. Evaluation of clinical diagnostic criteria for neurofibromatosis 2. Neurology. 2002;59(11):1759-65.

52. Evans DGR. Neurofibromatosis type 2 (NF2): a clinical and molecular review. Orphanet J Rare Dis. 2009;4:16.

53. Lloyd SKW, Evans DGR. Neurofibromatosis type 2 (NF2): diagnosis and management. Handb Clin Neurol. 2013;115:957-67.

54. Trofatter JA, MacCollin MM, Rutter JL, et al. A novel moesin-, ezrin-, radixin-like gene is a candidate for the neurofibromatosis 2 tumor suppressor. Cell. 1993;72(5):791-800.

55. Rouleau GA, Merel P, Lutchman M, et al. Alteration in a new gene encoding a putative membrane-organizing protein causes neurofibromatosis type 2. Nature. 1993;363(6429):515-21.

56. Asthagiri AR, Parry DM, Butman JA, et al. Neurofibromatosis type 2. The Lancet. 2009;373(9679):1974-86.

57. Korf BR. Neurofibromatosis. Handb Clin Neurol. 2013;111:333-40.

58. Evans DGR, Baser ME, O'Reilly B, et al. Management of the patient and family with neurofibromatosis 2: a consensus conference statement. Br J Neurosurg. 2005;19(1):5-12.

59. Acoustic neuroma. Consens Statement NIH Consens Dev Conf Natl Inst Health Consens Dev Conf. 1991;9(4):1-24.

60. Baser ME, Friedman JM, Joe H, et al. Empirical development of improved diagnostic criteria for neurofibromatosis 2. Genet Med. 2011;13(6):576-81.

61. Bosch MM, Boltshauser E, Harpes P, et al. Ophthalmologic findings and long-term course in patients with neurofibromatosis type 2. Am J Ophthalmology. 2006;141(6):1068-77.

62. Ragge NK, Baser ME, Klein J, et al. Ocular abnormalities in neurofibromatosis 2. Am J Ophthalmology. 1995;120(5):634-41.

63. Sachdeva R, Rothner DA, Traboulsi EI, et al. Astrocytic hamartoma of the optic disc and multiple café-au-lait macules in a child with neurofibromatosis type 2. Ophthalmic Genet. 2010;31(4):209-14.

64. Feucht M, Griffiths B, Niemüller I, et al. Neurofibromatosis 2 leads to higher incidence of strabismological and neuro-ophthalmological disorders. Acta Ophthalmology (Copenh). 2008;86(8):882-6.

65. Kaye LD, Rothner AD, Beauchamp GR, et al. Ocular findings associated with neurofibromatosis type II. Ophthalmology. 1992;99(9):1424-9.

66. Meyers SM, Gutman FA, Kaye LD, et al. Retinal changes associated with neurofibromatosis 2. Trans Am Ophthalmology Soc. 1995;93:245-57.

67. McLaughlin ME, Pepin SM, Maccollin M, et al. Ocular pathologic findings of neurofibromatosis type 2. Arch Ophthalmology Chic Ill 1960. 2007;125(3):389-94.

68. Sisk RA, Berrocal AM, Schefler AC, et al. Epiretinal membranes indicate a severe phenotype of neurofibromatosis type 2. Retina Phila Pa. 2010;30(4 Suppl):S51-8.

69. Schachat AP, Shields JA, Fine SL, et al. Combined hamartomas of the retina and retinal pigment epithelium. Ophthalmology. 1984;91(12):1609-15.

70. Zhang X, Dong F, Dai R, Yu W. Surgical management of epiretinal membrane in combined hamartomas of the retina and retinal pigment epithelium. Retina Phila Pa. 2010;30(2):305-9.

71. Vinekar A, Quiram P, Sund N, et al. Plasmin-assisted vitrectomy for bilateral combined hamartoma of the retina and retinal pigment epithelium: histopathology, immunohistochemistry, and optical coherence tomography. Retin Cases Brief Rep. 2009;3(2):186-9.

72. Crino PB, Nathanson KL, Henske EP. The tuberous sclerosis complex. N Engl J Med. 2006;355(13):1345-56.

73. Rosser T, Panigrahy A, McClintock W. The diverse clinical manifestations of tuberous sclerosis complex: a review. Semin Pediatr Neurol. 2006;13(1):27-36.

74. Leung AKC, Robson WLM. Tuberous sclerosis complex: a review. J Pediatr Health Care Off Publ Natl Assoc Pediatr Nurse Assoc Pract. 2007;21(2):108-14.

75. DiMario FJ, Sahin M, Ebrahimi-Fakhari D. Tuberous sclerosis complex. Pediatr Clin North Am. 2015;62(3):633-48.

76. Crino PB. Evolving neurobiology of tuberous sclerosis complex. Acta Neuropathol (Berl). 2013;125(3):317-32.

77. Riikonen R, Simell O. Tuberous sclerosis and infantile spasms. Dev Med Child Neurol. 1990;32(3):203-9.

78. Northrup H, Krueger DA, International Tuberous Sclerosis Complex Consensus Group. Tuberous sclerosis complex diagnostic criteria update: recommendations of the 2012 International Tuberous Sclerosis Complex Consensus Conference. Pediatr Neurol. 2013;49(4):243-54.

79. Nyboer JH, Robertson DM, Gomez MR. Retinal lesions in tuberous sclerosis. Arch Ophthalmology Chic Ill 1960. 1976;94(8):1277-80.

80. Rowley SA, O'Callaghan FJ, Osborne JP. Ophthalmic manifestations of tuberous sclerosis: a population based study. Br J Ophthalmology. 2001;85(4):420-3.

81. Mennel S, Meyer CH, Eggarter F, et al. Autofluorescence and angiographic findings of retinal astrocytic hamartomas in tuberous sclerosis. Ophthalmologica. 2005;219(6):350-6.

82. Zimmer-Galler IE, Robertson DM. Long-term observation of retinal lesions in tuberous sclerosis. Am J Ophthalmology. 1995;119(3):318-24.

83. Arora S, Bhushan G, Thirumalai S, et al. Exudative retinal detachment as the presenting feature of tuberous sclerosis complex. Retin Cases Brief Rep. 2016;10(2):121-6

84. Shields CL, Shields JA, Eagle RC, et al. Progressive enlargement of acquired retinal astrocytoma in 2 cases. Ophthalmology. 2004;111(2):363-8.

85. Tuncer S, Cebeci Z. Dramatic Regression of Presumed Acquired Retinal Astrocytoma with Photodynamic Therapy. Middle East Afr J Ophthalmology. 2014;21(3):283-6.

86. Tomida M, Mitamura Y, Katome T, et al. Aggressive retinal astrocytoma associated with tuberous sclerosis. Clin Ophthalmology Auckl NZ. 2012;6:715-20.

87. Saito W, Kase S, Ohgami K, et al. Intravitreal anti-vascular endothelial growth factor therapy with bevacizumab for tuberous sclerosis with macular oedema. Acta Ophthalmology (Copenh). 2010;88(3):377-80.

88. House RJ, Mashayekhi A, Shields JA, et al. Total regression of acquired retinal astrocytoma using photodynamic therapy: Retin Cases Brief Rep. 2016;10(1):41-3.

89. Richard S, Graff J, Lindau J, et al. Von Hippel-Lindau disease. Lancet Lond Engl. 2004;363(9416):1231-4.

90. Maher ER, Neumann HP, Richard S. von Hippel-Lindau disease: a clinical and scientific review. Eur J Hum Genet. 2011;19(6):617-23.

91. Chittiboina P, Lonser RR. Von Hippel-Lindau disease. Handb Clin Neurol. 2015;132:139-56.

92. Haddad NMN, Cavallerano JD, Silva PS. Von hippel-lindau disease: a genetic and clinical review. Semin Ophthalmology. 2013;28(5–6):377-86.

93. Schmid S, Gillessen S, Binet I, et al. Management of von hippel-lindau disease: an interdisciplinary review. Oncol Res Treat. 2014;37(12):761-71.

94. Lonser RR, Glenn GM, Walther M, et al. von Hippel-Lindau disease. Lancet Lond Engl. 2003;361(9374):2059-67.

95. Richard S, Gardie B, Couvé S, et al. Von Hippel-Lindau: how a rare disease illuminates cancer biology. Semin Cancer Biol. 2013;23(1):26-37.

96. Slater A, Moore NR, Huson SM. The natural history of cerebellar hemangioblastomas in von Hippel-Lindau disease. AJNR Am J Neuroradiol. 2003;24(8):1570-4.

97. Chew EY. Ocular manifestations of von hippel–lindau disease: clinical and genetic investigations. Trans Am Ophthalmology Soc. 2005;103:495-511.

98. Singh AD, Shields CL, Shields JA. von Hippel–Lindau disease. Surv Ophthalmology. 2001;46(2):117-42.

99. Vail D. Angiomatosis retinae, eleven years after diathermy coagulation. Am J Ophthalmology. 1958;46(4):525-34.

100. Singh AD, Nouri M, Shields CL, et al. Treatment of retinal capillary hemangioma. Ophthalmology. 2002;109(10):1799-806.

101. Lane CM, Turner G, Gregor ZJ, et al. Laser treatment of retinal angiomatosis. Eye. 1989;3(1):33-8.

102. Annesley WH, Leonard BC, Shields JA, et al. Fifteen year review of treated cases of retinal angiomatosis. Trans Sect Ophthalmology Am Acad Ophthalmology Otolaryngol. 1977;83(3 Pt 1):OP446-453.

103. Hrisomalos FN, Maturi RK, Pata V. Long-term use of intravitreal bevacizumab (avastin) for the treatment of von hippel-lindau associated retinal hemangioblastomas. Open Ophthalmology J. 2010;4:66-9.

104. Slim E, Antoun J, Kourie HR, et al. Intravitreal bevacizumab for retinal capillary hemangioblastoma: a case series and literature review. Can J Ophthalmology. 2014;49(5):450-7.

105. Krzystolik K, Stopa M, Kuprjanowicz L, et al. Pars plana vitrectomy in advanced cases of von hippel-lindau eye disease. Retina Phila Pa. 2016;36(2):325-34.

106. Kim H, Yi JH, Kwon HJ, et al. Therapeutic outcomes of retinal hemangioblastomas. Retina Phila Pa. 2014;34(12):2479-86.

107. Comi AM. Update on Sturge–Weber syndrome: diagnosis, treatment, quantitative measures, and controversies. Lymphat Res Biol. 2007;5(4):257-64.

108. Nabbout R, Juhász C. Sturge-Weber syndrome. Handb Clin Neurol. 2013;111:315-21.

109. Sudarsanam A, Ardern-Holmes SL. Sturge-Weber syndrome: from the past to the present. Eur J Paediatr Neurol. 2014;18(3):257-66.

110. Revencu N, Boon LM, Mendola A, et al. RASA1 mutations and associated phenotypes in 68 families with capillary malformation-arteriovenous malformation. Hum Mutat. 2013;34(12):1632-41.

111. Shirley MD, Tang H, Gallione CJ, et al. Sturge-Weber syndrome and port-wine stains caused by somatic mutation in GNAQ. N Engl J Med. 2013;368(21):1971-9.

112. Comi A. Current therapeutic options in Sturge-Weber syndrome. Semin Pediatr Neurol. 2015;22(4):295-301.

113. Maiuri F, Gangemi M, Iaconetta G, et al. Sturge-Weber disease without facial nevus. J Neurosurg Sci. 1989;33(2):215-8.

114. Ch'ng S, Tan ST. Facial port-wine stains—clinical stratification and risks of neuro-ocular involvement. J Plast Reconstr Aesthetic Surg. 2008;61(8):889-93.

115. Jagtap S, Srinivas G, Harsha KJ, et al. Sturge-Weber syndrome: clinical spectrum, disease course, and outcome of 30 patients. J Child Neurol. 2013;28(6):725-31.

116. Maslin JS, Dorairaj SK, Ritch R. Sturge-Weber syndrome (encephalotrigeminal angiomatosis): recent advances and future Challenges. Asia-Pac J Ophthalmology Phila Pa. 2014;3(6):361-7.

117. Cibis GW, Tripathi RC, Tripathi BJ. Glaucoma in Sturge-Weber syndrome. Ophthalmology. 1984;91(9):1061-71.

118. Tripathi BJ, Tripathi RC. Neural crest origin of human trabecular meshwork and its implications for the pathogenesis of glaucoma. Am J Ophthalmology. 1989;107(6):583-90.

119. Tanwar M, Sihota R, Dada T, et al. Sturge-Weber syndrome with congenital glaucoma and cytochrome P450 (CYP1B1) gene mutations. J Glaucoma. 2010;19(6):398-404.

120. Tsipursky MS, Golchet PR, Jampol LM. Photodynamic therapy of choroidal hemangioma in sturge-weber syndrome, with a

review of treatments for diffuse and circumscribed choroidal hemangiomas. Surv Ophthalmology. 2011;56(1):68-85.

121. Schilling H, Sauerwein W, Lommatzsch A, et al. Long-term results after low dose ocular irradiation for choroidal haemangiomas. Br J Ophthalmology. 1997;81(4):267-73.

122. Murthy R, Hanovaz SG, Naik M, et al. Ruthenium-106 plaque brachytherapy for the treatment of diffuse choroidal haemangioma in Sturge-Weber syndrome. Indian J Ophthalmology. 2005;53(4): 274-5.

123. Kubicka-Trząska A, Karska-Basta I, Oleksy P, et al. Management of diffuse choroidal hemangioma in Sturge-Weber syndrome with Ruthenium-106 plaque radiotherapy. Graefes Arch Clin Exp Ophthalmology Albrecht Von Graefes Arch Für Klin Exp Ophthalmology. 2015;253(11):2015-9.

124. Zografos L, Bercher L, Chamot L, et al. Cobalt-60 treatment of choroidal hemangiomas. Am J Ophthalmology. 1996;121(2):190-9.

125. Chan RVP, Yonekawa Y, Lane AM, et al. Proton beam irradiation using a light-field technique for the treatment of choroidal hemangiomas. Ophthalmology J Int Ophtalmol Int J Ophthalmology Z Für Augenheilkd. 2010;224(4):209-16.

126. Zografos L, Egger E, Bercher L, et al. Proton beam irradiation of choroidal hemangiomas. Am J Ophthalmology. 1998;126(2):261-8.

127. Yonekawa Y, MacDonald SM, Shildkrot Y, et al. Standard fractionation low-dose proton radiotherapy for diffuse choroidal hemangiomas in pediatric Sturge-Weber syndrome. J AAPOS Off Publ Am Assoc Pediatr Ophthalmology Strabismus Am Assoc Pediatr Ophthalmology Strabismus. 2013;17(3):318-22.

128. Anaya-Pava EJ, Saenz-Bocanegra CH, Flores-Trejo A, et al. Diffuse choroidal hemangioma associated with exudative retinal detachment in a Sturge-Weber syndrome case: photodynamic therapy and intravitreous bevacizumab. Photodiagnosis Photodyn Ther. 2015;12(1):136-9.

129. Paulus YM, Jain A, Moshfeghi DM. Resolution of persistent exudative retinal detachment in a case of Sturge-Weber syndrome with anti-VEGF administration. Ocul Immunol Inflamm. 2009;17(4):292-4.

130. Shoeibi N, Ahmadieh H, Abrishami M, et al. Rapid and sustained resolution of serous retinal detachment in Sturge-Weber syndrome after single injection of intravitreal bevacizumab. Ocul Immunol Inflamm. 2011;19(5):358-60.

131. Ang M, Lee SY. Multifocal photodynamic therapy for diffuse choroidal hemangioma. Clin Ophthalmology Auckl NZ. 2012;6:1467-9.

132. Monteiro S, Casal I, Santos M, et al. Photodynamic therapy for diffuse choroidal hemangioma in sturge-weber syndrome. Case Rep Med. 2014;2014:452372.

133. Nugent R, Lee L, Kwan A. Photodynamic therapy for diffuse choroidal hemangioma in a child with Sturge-Weber syndrome. J AAPOS Off Publ Am Assoc Pediatr Ophthalmology Strabismus Am Assoc Pediatr Ophthalmology Strabismus. 2015;19(2):181-3.

134. Thapa R, Shields CL. Oral propranolol therapy for management of exudative retinal detachment from diffuse choroidal hemangioma in Sturge-Weber syndrome. Eur J Ophthalmology. 2013;23(6): 922-4.

135. Dave T, Dave VP, Shah G, et al. Diffuse choroidal hemangioma masquerading as central serous chorioretinopathy treated with oral propranolol. Retin Cases Brief Rep. 2016;10(1):11-4.

136. Abdolrahimzadeh S, Scavella V, Felli L, et al. Ophthalmic alterations in the Sturge-Weber syndrome, Klippel-Trenaunay syndrome, and the phakomatosis pigmentovascularis: an independent group of conditions? Bio Med Res Int. 2015;2015:786519.

Index

Page numbers followed by *b* refer to box, *f* refer to figure, *fc* refer to flowchart, and *t* refer to table.